FOR REFERENCE

Do Not Take From This Room

Mollison's
Blood Transfusion in
Clinical Medicine

Mollison's Blood Transfusion in Clinical Medicine

11TH EDITION

Harvey G. Klein MD

President of the American Association of Blood Banks;
Chief, Department of Transfusion Medicine
Warren G Magnuson Clinical Center
National Institutes of Health
Bethesda
Maryland, USA;
Adjunct Professor of Medicine and Pathology,
The Johns Hopkins School of Medicine

and

David J. Anstee PhD FRCPath FMedSci

Director, Bristol Institute for Transfusion Science
National Blood Service
Bristol, UK;
Honorary Professor of Transfusion Science, University of Bristol

**A revision of the 10th edition written by
P.L. Mollison, C.P. Engelfriet and Marcela Contreras**

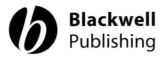

Blackwell Publishing

First published 1951	Fifth edition 1972	Ninth edition 1993
Second edition 1956	Reprinted 1974	Reprinted 1994 (twice)
Third edition 1961	Sixth edition 1979	Tenth edition 1997
Reprinted 1963, 1964	Seventh edition 1983	Eleventh edition 2005
Fourth edition 1967	Eighth edition 1987	
Reprinted 1967	Reprinted 1988	

Library of Congress Cataloging-in-Publication Data

Klein, Harvey G.
    Mollison's blood transfusion in clinical medicine. – 11th ed. /
Harvey Klein and David Anstee.
        p. ; cm.
    Rev. ed. of: Blood transfusion in clinical medicine / P.L. Mollison,
C.P. Engelfriet, Marcela Contreras. 10th ed. c1997.
    Includes bibliographical references and index.
    ISBN-13: 978-0-632-06454-0
    ISBN-10: 0-632-06454-4
    1. Blood--Transfusion.   2. Blood groups.   I. Mollison, P. L.
(Patrick Loudon)   II. Anstee, David J.   III. Mollison, P. L.
(Patrick Loudon). Blood transfusion in clinical medicine.   IV. Title.
V. Title:
    Blood transfusion in clinical medicine.
    [DNLM: 1. Blood Transfusion.   WB 356 K64m 2005]
    RM171.M6 2005
    615′.39–dc22

                                    2005012644

A catalogue record for this title is available from the British Library

Set in 9/11.5pt Sabon by Graphicraft Limited, Hong Kong
Printed and bound in the United Kingdom by TJ International Ltd, Padstow, Cornwall

Development Editor: Rebecca Huxley
Commissioning Editor: Maria Khan
Production Controller: Kate Charman

For further information on Blackwell Publishing, visit our website:
http://www.blackwellpublishing.com

The publisher's policy is to use permanent paper from mills that operate a
sustainable forestry policy, and which has been manufactured from pulp
processed using acid-free and elementary chlorine-free practices. Furthermore,
the publisher ensures that the text paper and cover board used have met
acceptable environmental accreditation standards.

Contents

Foreword

The first edition of *Blood Transfusion in Clinical Medicine* was published in 1951, at a time when the subject was, if not in its infancy, certainly in its very early childhood. Transfusions were given for the treatment of acute blood loss or for the relief of chronic anaemia. Platelet and leucocyte transfusions were not attempted and plasma fractions were not available. Only a few red cell antigen systems were recognized and leucocyte or platelet antigens were unknown. It was understood that syphilis and malaria could be transmitted by transfusion, and it had recently been discovered that hepatitis could also be transmitted although no test for the virus was available. Evidently, attempting to summarize knowledge of the whole subject in 1951 was not a very daunting task.

My own position in the years that followed made it possible for me to devote a great deal of time to trying to keep the book up to date in successive editions as the subject expanded in all directions. However, by the time that the eighth edition was being planned I recognized that, even with a great deal of help from others, I could not give an adequate account of leucocyte and platelet antigens or of diseases transmitted by transfusion. Professors Paul Engelfriet and Marcela Contreras, who had immense experience of these and many other aspects of the subject, became joint authors, greatly strengthening the scientific background of the book.

After the tenth edition was published in 1997, the three of us decided not to continue, but Blackwell Publishing felt that as the book was an established text in the field of transfusion they would like to commission a new edition. I must point out that, although we are clearly responsible for such parts of the text of the tenth edition as have been retained, credit for the revision is due entirely to the new authors, who have had no help of any kind from us. It is fortunate that two people so highly qualified as Harvey Klein and David Anstee have been willing to undertake this task.

Harvey Klein is one of the very ablest practitioners of transfusion medicine in existence and has a wide understanding of all the clinical aspects of the subject. David Anstee's research has vastly increased knowledge of the molecular structure of red cell antigens; the chapters he has revised – particularly the chapter on the Rh blood group system – now provide what must be the best available source of information on this subject. Both authors have dealt in an authoritative way with the still rapidly expanding specialty, and the eleventh edition of the book will be of the greatest value to all who are interested in the scientific and practical aspects of blood transfusion in clinical medicine.

Professor P.L. Mollison
2005

Preface to eleventh edition

The huge challenge of revising this seminal work has been both daunting and immensely rewarding. Mollison's textbook is an icon. *Blood Transfusion in Clinical Medicine* arose from the concept of the transfusionist as both scientist and expert consultant. For many years, this text provided the primary, and often the sole, reference for detailed information and practical experience in blood transfusion. A generation of scientists and clinicians sought and found in its pages those fine points of immunohaematology that helped them manage their patients and satisfy their intellectual curiosity. The last two decades have witnessed an explosion of scientific knowledge, the proliferation of textbooks, handbooks, systematic reviews and specialty journals, not to mention immediate access to manuscripts not yet in print via the Internet. The current authors determined to distil from this mass of information the relevant biology and technology for a timely, comprehensive and clinically useful textbook – without altering the spirit and character that has made Mollison's textbook a cherished companion.

Mollison's textbook has recorded the development of blood transfusion practice and its scientific basis for more than half a century. The first edition focused mainly on the recognized blood groups and their clinical implications. Immunohaematology was confined largely to the red cell. The marvellous complexity of blood was defined by agglutination, and subsequently by the mixed lymphocyte reaction, lymphocytotoxicity and serum protein electrophoresis. Red cell survival, a tool both for investigating clinical problems and for exploring fundamental information regarding haemolytic processes and red cell pathology, was estimated 'with the comparative precision of differential agglutination'. Whole blood was still transfused by the bottle. Today, tens of millions of units of blood components are transfused annually. The immune response is analysed by a wide array of sophisticated techniques and the diversity of human blood is routinely examined at the molecular level. Circulating cells and their survival still teach us about immunology and cellular biology, but we can now track the persistence of transfused lymphocyte subpopulations with molecular assays of microchimerism. This text endeavours to continue the tradition of integrated biology, technology and clinical practice that characterized the original book and all subsequent editions.

Since the last edition, major changes in practice and advances in our understanding have occurred in some aspects of the field, but not in others. The human genome has been sequenced. Informatics and computational biology have revolutionized the approach to biodiversity. Advances in DNA-based technology, from microarrays to recombinant proteins, have had a major impact on many aspects of blood transfusion practice. Transfusion medicine now involves mobilization and selection of haematopoietic progenitor cells for transplantation, storage of umbilical cord blood, and manipulation of mononuclear cells by culture and gene insertion to offer potential therapies for a wide range of diseases. This edition has been revised to reflect this remarkable progress. Enormous advances in protein structure determination have occurred since the last edition and these too are reflected in the revised edition. It is particularly satisfying to record the three-dimensional structure of the glycosyltransferase responsible for the ABO blood groups just over a century after Landsteiner's discovery made safe blood transfusion a possibility. In contrast, Mollison's text has traditionally been used as a source of 'classic' studies and information not available elsewhere, and we have been careful to retain that information in this edition.

We have not attempted to remake this edition into an exhaustive textbook. By intent, we have eschewed separate chapters on medicolegal issues, detailed methods of blood collection, administrative practices, quality systems, facilities management and cost–benefit analysis. Instead, we have integrated elements of these important topics into discussions of clinical problems.

In summary, we have endeavoured to provide the reader with a comprehensive and authoritative clinical text on the broad subject of transfusion medicine. We anticipate that this volume will be used most frequently by the physician specialist practising in transfusion medicine. However, we hope that the book will have equal appeal to the non-specialist (and non-physician) and would be particularly gratified if it finds favour among those doctoral and postdoctoral students with a burgeoning interest in the past, present and future of blood transfusion in clinical medicine.

We are indebted to many people for advice, support and assistance. DJA owes particular thanks to Sherrie Ayles, Nick Burton, Geoff Daniels, Kirstin Finning, Gary Mallinson, Tosti Mankelow, Peter Martin, Clare Milkins, Robin Knight and Steve Parsons. HGK thanks the many physicians and scientists who provided critique, helpful comments and invaluable expert advice, particularly Drs James Aubuchon, Mark Brecher, George Garratty, Dennis Goldfinger, Brenda Grossman, David Stroncek, Franco Marincola, Maria Bettinotti, Paul Holland, Paul Schmidt, Jay Menitove, Paul Mintz, Gary Moroff, Peter Page, Edward Snyder, Richard Weiskopf and Charles Bolan, and to Mr Boyd Conley and Ms Patricia Brooks for technical assistance. HGK is especially grateful to John I. Gallin and David K. Henderson, who provided him the time and opportunity to work on this edition, and to Sigrid Klein, without whose support it would not have been completed.

We owe a special debt of gratitude to Professors Patrick Mollison, C. Paul Engelfriet and Marcela Contreras, upon whose solid foundation this edition was built, and to Maria Khan of Blackwell Publishing, who kept the book on track.

Harvey G. Klein
David J. Anstee
2005

x

Preface to first edition

Blood was once regarded as a fluid of infinite complexity, the very essence of life. The blood of each person seemed to carry in it the secrets of individuality. As recently as 1666 it was natural for Mr Boyle, in writing to Dr Lower, to speculate in the following terms about the possible effect of cross-transfusion: '. . . as whether the blood of a mastiff, being frequently transfused into a bloodhound, or a spaniel, will not prejudice them in point of scent'.

If each person's blood were as individual as this, transfusion would indeed be complex and would deserve to rank as the most refined branch of medicine. However, this early view of the subtlety of transfusion was eclipsed at the beginning of the century by the discovery that the blood of all human beings could be divided into four groups. It seemed that, provided blood of the same group was transfused, one person's blood was indistinguishable from another's. Indeed, it came to be believed that people who belonged to the common group O could give their blood to anyone whatsoever. This point of view reached its widest acceptance in the early 1940s, when hundreds of thousands of bottles of group O blood were given as a general panacea for the injuries of war, with remarkably satisfactory effects. As a result of this experience, a generation of medical men has grown up believing that blood transfusion is one of the simplest forms of therapy.

And yet, this view of the interchangeability of blood has to be reconciled with the growing knowledge of its immense complexity. There are so many possible combinations of blood group antigens that the commonest of them all occurs in only 2% of the English population. Indeed, such is the individuality of the blood that, in Race's striking phrase, certain combinations 'may never have formed the blood of an Englishman'.

The explanation of this apparent paradox – the potential complexity of transfusion and its actual simplicity – lies in the fact that many blood group factors are so weakly antigenic in man that they are not recognized as foreign by the recipient. However, it can no longer be maintained that a knowledge of the ABO system constitutes an adequate equipment for the transfusionist, for the role of some of the other systems is by no means negligible. Thus, a book on blood transfusion requires a special account of blood groups, in which the emphasis laid on any one of the antigens depends upon the part that it plays in incompatibility.

A good understanding of the effects of transfusion requires two further accounts: one of the regulation of blood volume and of the effects of transfusion on the circulation, and one of the survival of the various elements of blood after transfusion. The survival of transfused red cells has become a matter of special interest. Red cells survive for a longer period than any of the other components of blood, and their survival can be estimated with comparative precision by the method of differential agglutination. A study of the survival of transfused red cells has proved to be of great value in investigating haemolytic transfusion reactions. In addition, it has contributed strikingly to fundamental knowledge in haematology by demonstrating the diminished survival of pathological red cells and the existence of extrinsic haemolytic mechanisms in disease. Transfusions are now not uncommonly given for the purpose of investigation as well as of therapy.

This book is thus composed mainly of an account of blood groups from a clinical point of view and of descriptions of the effects of transfusion on the circulation and of the survival of transfused red cells; it also contains chapters designed to fill in the remaining background of knowledge about the results of transfusion in man. Finally, it contains a rather detailed account of haemolytic disease of the newborn. It is addressed to all those who possess an elementary knowledge of blood transfusion and are interested in acquiring a fuller understanding of its effects.

In preparing this book I have had the help and advice of many friends. Dr J.V. Dacie read through almost all the typescript and made innumerable suggestions for improvements. Dr A.C. Dornhorst gave me the most extensive help in writing about the interpretation of red cell survival cures, and he is responsible for the simple rules for estimating mean cell life, which I hope that many besides myself will find useful; he has also read through the book during its preparation and given me the benefit of his very wide general

knowledge. Dr J.F. Loutit, Dr I.D.P. Wootton and Dr L.E. Young are amongst those who have read certain sections and helped me with their expert advice.

I am even more indebted to Miss Marie Cutbush, who has given an immense amount of time to helping to prepare this book for the press and has, on every page, suggested changes to clarify the meaning of some sentence. In addition, she has most generously encouraged me to quote many joint observations which are not yet published.

Miss Sylvia Mossom was responsible for typing the whole book, often from almost illegible manuscript. I am indebted to her for her skill and patience.

The *British Medical Journal, Clinical Science* and *The Lancet* have been so good as to allow the reproduction of certain figures originally published by them.

Professor P.L. Mollison
1951

Abbreviations

not including abbreviated names of blood group systems or
of any antigens or antibodies

aa	amino acid		CAT	column agglutination technique
ACD	acid citrate dextrose		CAVG	coronary artery vein graft
AChE	acetylcholinesterase		CBPC	cord blood progenitor cells
ADCC(L)	antibody-dependent cell-mediated cytotoxicity test, using lymphocytes		CD	cluster differentiation (designation)
ADCC(M)	antibody-dependent cell-mediated cytotoxicity test, using monocytes		CDC	Centers for Disease Control and Prevention
ADP	adenosine diphosphate		cDNA	complementary DNA
Adsol	(an) adenine–dextrose solution		CDR	Communicable Disease Report
AET	2-amino-ethyl-isothiouronium		CFU	colony-forming units
AHG	anti-human globulin		CGD	chronic granulomatous disease
AIDS	acquired immune deficiency syndrome		CHAD	cold haemagglutinin disease
AIHA	autoimmune haemolytic anaemia		CL	chemiluminescence
AITP	autoimmune thrombocytopenic purpura		CMV	cytomegalovirus
			COMPRIA	competitive radioimmunoassay
ALT	alanine aminotransferase		CPD	citrate phosphate dextrose
AML	acute myeloid leukaemia		CR	complement receptor
AMP	adenosine monophosphate		CREGS	crossreactive groups
AMT	aminomethyl-trimethyl (psoralen)		CSF	colony-stimulating factor
APC	antigen-presenting cells		CTL	cytotoxic T lymphocytes
ARC	AIDS-related complex		CVP	central venous pressure
ARDS	adult respiratory distress syndrome		DAF	decay accelerating factor
ASO	allele-specific oligonucleotides		DAT	direct antiglobulin test
ASP	allele-specific primers		DDAVP	desmopressin (1-deamino-8-D-arginine vasopressin)
ATLS	acute trauma life support (system)			
ATP	adenosine triphosphate		DEAE	diethylaminoethyl
BC	buffy coat(s)		DEHP	di (2-ethylhexyl) phthalate
BHTC	butyryl-*n*-trihexyl citrate		DHTR	delayed haemolytic transfusion reaction
BP	blood pressure		DIC	disseminated intravascular coagulation
BSA	bovine serum albumin		DL	Donath–Landsteiner
BSS	buffered saline solution		DMSO	dimethyl sulphoxide
C8bp	C8 binding protein		DNA	deoxyribonucleic acid
CABG	coronary artery bypass graft		DPG	2,3-diphosphoglycerate
CAH	chronic active hepatitis		DR	(HLA) D-related
			DSTR	delayed serological transfusion reaction

xiii

DTT	dithiothreitol	HTR	haemolytic transfusion reaction
EBV	Epstein–Barr virus	IAT	indirect antiglobulin test
ECP	extracorporeal photopheresis	IHTR	immediate haemolytic transfusion reaction
EDTA	ethylene diamine tetra-acetic acid		
EIOP	endoimmuno-osmopheresis	IL	interleukin
ELAT	enzyme-linked antiglobulin test	ICSH	International Committee for Standarization in Haematology
ELISA	enzyme-linked immunosorbent assay		
EPO	erythropoietin	i.m.	intramuscular
ESR	erythrocyte sedimentation rate	ISBT	International Blood Transfusion Society
EVS	extravascular space	iu	international units
Fab	fragment, antigen-binding	i.v.	intravenous
FBS	fetal blood sampling	IVIG	intravenously administered IgG
Fc	fragment, crystallizable	LAIR	Letterman Army Institute of Research
FCIT	flow cytometric immunofluorescence test	LAK	lymphokine-activated killer (cells)
FcγR	Fcγ receptor	LAV	lymphocyte-associated virus
FFP	fresh-frozen plasma	LCT	lymphocytotoxicity test
FUT	fucosyl transferase	LDL	low-density lipoprotein
FVIIIC	factor VIII coagulant activity	LIP	low-ionic-strength polybrene
GAC	G antibody capture	LIS	low ionic strength
G-CSF	granulocyte colony-stimulating factor	LISS	low-ionic-strength solution
GIFT	granulocyte immunofluorescence technique	MAC	membrane attack complex
		MAIEA	monoclonal antibody-specific immobilization of erythrocyte antigens
GM-CSF	granulocyte–macrophage colony-stimulating factor		
		MAIGA	monoclonal antibody-specific granulocyte assay
GP	glycophorin		
CPI	glycosyl-phosphatidylinositol	MAIPA	monoclonal antibody-specific immobilization of platelet antigens
GvHD	graft-versus-host disease		
HAM	HTLV-associated myelopathy	MARIA	monoclonal anti-Ig radioimmunoassay
HAV	hepatitis A virus	MHC	major histocompatibility complex
HBLV	human B lymphotropic virus	MIRL	membrane inhibitor of reactive lysis
HBV	hepatitis B virus	MMA	monocyte monolayer assay
HCC	hepatocellular carcinoma	MPS	mononuclear phagocyte system
HCV	hepatitis C virus	MPT	manual polybrene test
HDN	haemolytic disease of the (fetus and) newborn	MRC	Medical Research Council (UK)
		MSBOS	maximum surgical blood order schedule
HDV	hepatitis delta virus		
HEMPAS	hereditary erythroblastic multinuclearity with a positive acidified serum test	NANA	N-acetyl neuraminic acid
		NANB	non-A non-B hepatitis
		NASBA	nucleic acid sequence-based amplification
HES	hydroxyethyl starch		
HGV	hepatitis G virus	NATP	neonatal alloimmune thrombocytopenia (fetus and newborn)
HHV-6	human herpes virus-6		
HIV	human immunodeficiency virus		
HLA	human leucocyte antigen	NIH	National Institutes of Health (USA)
HPA	human platelet antigen	NHS	National Health Service (UK)
HPV B19	human parvovirus	NPBI	Nederlands Productie Laboratorium von Bloedtransfusie Apparatur en Infusievloeistoffer
HRF	homologous restriction factor		
HTC	homozygous typing cells		
HTLV	human lymphotropic virus		

PBPC	peripheral blood progenitor cells		S-D	solvent–detergent (treatment)
PC	progenitor cells *or* platelet concentrate		SDS-PAGE	sodium dodecyl sulphate-polyacrylamide gel electrophoresis
PCC	prothrombin complex concentrate		Se	secretor of ABH substances
PCH	paroxysmal cold haemoglobinuria		SGP	sialoglycoprotein
PCR	polymerase chain reaction		sHLA	soluble HLA class I antigen
PCS	plasma collection system		SLE	systemic lupus erythematosus
PCWP	pulmonary capillary wedge pressure		SIRS	system inflammatory response syndrome
PEG-IAT	polyethylene glycol indirect antiglobulin test		SRBC	sheep red blood cells
PKA	prekallikrein activator		SSO	sequence-specific oligonucleotides
PLAP	placental alkaline phosphatase		SSP	sequence-specific primers
PNH	paroxysmal nocturnal haemoglobinuria		STS	serological test for syphilis
PPF	plasma protein fraction		TAA	transfusion-associated AIDS
PPP	platelet-poor plasma		TA-GvHD	transfusion-associated GvHD
PRP	platelet-rich plasma		tPA	tissue plasminogen activator
PTH	post-transfusion hepatitis		TOTM	tri-(2-ethylhexyl) trimellate
PTP	post-transfusion purpura		TPE	therapeutic plasma exchange
PUBS	percutaneous umbilical blood sampling		TPH	transplacental haemorrhage
PVP	polyvinyl pyrrolidone		TPHA	*Treponema pallidum* haemagglutination assay
RAS	red cell additive solution			
RFLP	restriction fragment length polymorphism		TPO	thrombopoietin
			TRALI	transfusion-related acute lung injury
rgp	recombinant glycoprotein		TSP	tropical spastic paraparesis
rHuEPO	recombinant human erythropoietin		TTP	thrombotic thrombocytopenic purpura
RIA	radioimmunoassay		u	unit(s)
RIBA	recombinant immunoblot assay		VDRL	Venereal Disease Research Laboratory serological test for syphilis
RIPA	radioimmunoprecipitation assay			
RNA	ribose nucleic acid		VWF	von Willebrand factor
SAG-M	saline–adenine–glucose–mannitol		WAIHA	warm antibody type of AIHA
SCF	stem cell factor		WB	Western blot
SD	standard deviation		ZZAP	reagent containing papain and DTT

Amino acids and their symbols

One-letter code	Abbreviation	Amino acid	One-letter code	Abbreviation	Amino acid
A	Ala	Alanine	M	Met	Methionine
C	Cys	Cysteine	N	Asn	Asparagine
D	Asp	Aspartic acid	P	Pro	Proline
E	Glu	Glutamic acid	Q	Gln	Glutamine
F	Phe	Phenylalanine	R	Arg	Arginine
G	Gly	Glycine	S	Ser	Serine
H	His	Histidine	T	Thr	Threonine
I	Ile	Isoleucine	V	Val	Valine
K	Lys	Lysine	W	Trp	Tryptophan
L	Leu	Leucine	Y	Tyr	Tyrosine

1 Blood donors and the withdrawal of blood

Bloodletting was once the treatment for almost all maladies and, when carried out in moderation, caused little harm. This chapter includes a discussion of therapeutic phlebotomy but is mainly concerned with the withdrawal of blood or its constituent parts from healthy donors for transfusion to patients. The chapter addresses qualification of the donor, statistics regarding collection and use, blood shortages and conditions that disqualify donors. Complications of blood donation including iron loss, syncope and needle injuries, and other less common adverse events are discussed. Some applications of therapeutic phlebotomy and blood withdrawal during neonatal exchange transfusion are outlined.

Blood donation

The blood donor

General qualifications

Qualification of blood donors has become a lengthy and detailed process, a 'donor inquisition' some would say. Yet blood collection depends on this system of safeguards to protect the donor from injury and the recipient from the risks of allogeneic blood (see Chapters 15 and 16). Sensitive screening tests have been considered the cornerstone of blood safety for more than three decades. However, testing represents only one component of this system. Additional 'layers of safety' include detailed donor education programmes prior to recruitment, pre-donation informational literature, stringent donor screening selection and deferral procedures, post-donation product quarantine, and donor tracing and notification when instances of disease transmission are detected. Each element plays a role in preventing 'tainted' units from entering the blood inventory. Most transfusion services have developed evidence-based standards and regulations for the selection of donors (UKBTS/NIBSC Liaison Group 2001; American Association of Blood Banks 2004) and quality systems to assure excellence in all phases of their application (Brecher 2003). Other standards derive from 'expert opinion' and 'common sense', and these policies need to be revisited as scientific information becomes available.

Blood donors should have the following general qualifications: they should have reached the age of consent, most often 18 years, but 17 in some countries such as the USA and the UK; they should be in good health, have no history of serious illness, weigh enough to allow safe donation of a 'unit' and not recognize themselves as being at risk of transmitting infection (see below). Ideally, donation should be strictly voluntary and without financial incentive (see Chapter 16). Some blood services impose an arbitrary upper limit on age, commonly 65 years, or up to age 70 in Denmark and the UK; however, it seems curiously subjective to exclude donors on the basis of age alone if they are otherwise in good health (Schmidt 1991; Simon et al. 1991). The Blood Collection Service should provide informational literature for prospective blood donors. After information and counselling about criteria for donor selection, donors should consent in writing to the terms of donation, including the use of the donated blood, the extent of testing, the use of testing results (including donor notification of positive results) and the future use of any stored specimens. Donors should be told about the possibility of delayed fainting and about other significant risks of the donation procedure.

Blood donation has potential medicolegal consequences. If a donor becomes ill shortly after giving blood, the illness may be attributed to blood donation. For this reason, among others, it is important to ensure that donors have no history of medical conditions such as brittle diabetes, hypertension, poorly controlled epilepsy and unstable cardiopulmonary disease that might be associated with an adverse event following phlebotomy. Pregnancy might be adversely affected by the donation process and ordinarily excludes a donor. Donors who become ill within 2 weeks of donation should be encouraged to inform the transfusion service, which may wish to discard the donated blood, recall any plasma sent for fractionation or follow up recipients of the blood components as appropriate. Donors who develop hepatitis or HIV infection within 3–6 months of donation should also inform the Blood Collection Service.

Donor interview

The donor interview should be conducted by staff trained and qualified to administer questions and evaluate responses. The donor interview should be conducted in a setting sufficiently unhurried and private as to permit discussion of confidential information. With current practices in the USA, approximately 2% of volunteer donors still disclose risks that would have led to deferral at the time of donation (Sanchez et al. 2001). Introduction of standardized and validated questionnaires and the application of interactive computer-assisted audiovisual health history may reduce errors and misinterpretations during conduct of the donor interview (Zuck et al. 2001).

Physical examination

Blood collectors perform a limited physical examination designed to protect donor and recipient. Screeners routinely assess the donor's general appearance and defer those who do not appear well or are under the influence of alcohol. A normal range of pulse and blood pressure is defined, although variances may be granted for healthy athletes. Body weight and temperature are measured by some collection services. Both

arms are examined for evidence of illicit drug use and for lesions at the venepuncture site.

Volume of donation

The volume of anticoagulant solutions in collection bags is calculated to allow for collection of a particular volume of blood, which, in the UK, is 450 ± 45 ml. In the USA often 500 ml, but in no case more than 10.5 ml/kg including the additional volume of 20–30 ml of blood collected into pilot tubes. From donors weighing 41–50 kg, only 250 ml of blood is collected into bags in which the volume of anticoagulant solution has been appropriately reduced. In some countries, the volume collected routinely is less than 450 ml, for example 350–400 ml in Turkey, Greece and Italy, and 250 ml in some Asian countries such as Japan, where donors tend to be smaller.

Record-keeping

It should be possible to trace the origin of every blood donation and records should be kept for several years, depending on the guidelines for each country. In many countries, a system employing unique bar-coded eye-readable donation numbers is now in use. This system makes it possible to link each donation to its integral containers and sample tubes and to the particular donor session record. Information concerning previous donations, such as records of blood groups and microbiology screening tests, antibodies detected, donor deferrals and adverse reactions are important for subsequent attendances. Electronic storage of donor information greatly facilitates accurate identification, release, distribution and traceability of units of blood and blood products. An international code, ISBT 128, is intended to be used by all countries for the accurate identification of donors and donations (Doughty and Flanagan 1996). These records must be protected from accidental destruction, modification or unauthorized access.

Frequency of donors in the population

Although in many Western countries, some 60% of the population are healthy adults aged 18–65 years and thus qualified to be blood donors, the highest annual frequency of donation in the world corresponds to about 10% of the population eligible to give blood donating once per year, as in Switzerland (Linden *et al.* 1988; Hassig 1991). The frequency in most developing countries is less than 1% (Leikola 1990).

The number of units collected per 1000 US inhabitants of usual donor age (18–65) was 88.0 in 2001, up from 80.8 in 1999. Although this number compares favourably with the rate of 72.2 per 1000 in 1997, it pales in comparison with the 100 units per 1000 population collected in Switzerland. As treacherous as it may be to interpret these figures, the numbers suggest that US collecting facilities are progressively improving efficiency. Data from the American National Red Cross indicate that the average volunteer donates about 1.7 times a year. Losses from outdated red cells accounted for 5.3% of the supply but, given the fact that red cells can be transfused only to compatible recipients, the number of usable units outdated appears to be extremely small. More than 99% of group O units and 97% of group A units were transfused (National Blood Data Resource Center 2001).

Blood utilization and shortages

Despite the constant rise in collections, blood collectors report frequent shortages and emergency appeals for blood are disturbingly common. Some 14 million units of red cells and 12 million units of platelets are collected annually in the USA. With the current shelf life, the blood supply more closely resembles a pipeline than a bank or reservoir. A few days of under collection can have a devastating effect on supply. Although most national supermarket chains have developed efficient bar code-based information systems to monitor perishable inventory on a daily basis, few national blood services have as accurate an accounting of blood component location and availability by group and type. Furthermore, there is little general agreement about what constitutes a shortage. Measures of postponed surgery and transfusion, as well as increased rates of RhoD-positive transfusions to RhoD-negative recipients provide some indication of shortage at the treatment level. In a national survey in the USA in 2001, 138 out of 1086 hospitals (12.6%) reportedly delayed elective surgery for 1 day or more, and 18.9% experienced at least 1 day in which transfusion was postponed because blood needs could not be met (National Blood Data Resource Center 2002). A separate government-sponsored study revealed seasonal

fluctuations of blood appeals and cancellations of surgery for lack of platelet transfusion support (Nightingale *et al.* 2003). In the former survey, blood utilization approached 50 units per 1000 of the population, an increase of 10% over the previous survey 2 years earlier and the average age of a transfusion recipient was 69 years. The USA decennial census 2000 projects that, by the year 2030, the population of Americans over the age of 65 will increase from 12% to 20%; this figure will be even higher in most countries in western Europe (Kinsella and Velkoff 2001). Given these projections, developed countries may expect blood shortages to become a way of life unless substantial resources are invested in donor recruitment and retention. In developing countries, this is already the case.

The shrinking donor pool: the safety vs. availability conundrum

Donor deferrals and miscollected units have an increasing role in blood shortages. In a 1-year study at a regional blood centre, nearly 14% of prospective donors were ineligible on the day of presentation and more than 3.8% of donations did not result in the collection of an acceptable quantity of blood (Custer *et al.* 2004). Short-term deferral for low haemoglobin (Hb) was the overwhelming reason for the deferral of female donors in all age groups, representing more than 50% of all short-term deferrals. In first-time female donors, low Hb accounted for 53–67% of deferrals within different age groups, and for repeat female donors 75–80% of deferrals. In both first-time and repeat male donors aged 40 years and older, the most common reason for short-term deferral was blood pressure or pulse outside allowed limits. For persons aged 16–24 years, regardless of sex and donation status, the most common reason for lengthy deferral was tattoo, piercing or other non-intravenous drug use needle exposure. For 25- to 39-year-old female donors, needle exposure was also the most common reason, whereas for male donors, travel to a malarial area was more common. For all ages over 40, the most common reason for long-term deferral was travel to a malarial area.

Measures introduced to increase blood safety may have the unintended consequence of decreasing blood availability. Results from demographic studies indicate that certain donor groups or donor sites present an unacceptable risk of disease transmission. For example, blood collectors no longer schedule mobile drives at prisons or institutions for the disabled because of the recognized high prevalence of transfusion-transmissible viruses. Few would argue the risk–benefit analysis of these exclusions. More questionable were the temporary exclusions of US soldiers exposed to multiple tick bites at Fort Chaffee, Arkansas, and the lengthy deferrals of veterans who served in Iraq and Kuwait because of the fear that they might harbour *Leishmania donovani*, an agent infrequently associated with transfusion risk. Donors who have received human growth hormone injections have been indefinitely deferred because of the possible risk of transmitting Creutzfeldt–Jakob disease (CJD); however, relatives of patients with 'sporadic' CJD are still deferred in the US (except for preparation of plasma fractions) despite evidence of their safety. There have now been five case–control studies of more than 600 CJD cases, two look-back studies of recipients of CJD products, two autopsy studies of patients with haemophilia and mortality surveillance of 4468 CJD deaths over 16 years without any link to transmission by transfusion (Centers for Biologic Evaluation and Research, US Food and Drug Administration 2002). Although the impact of this deferral on the US blood supply has been negligible, the recent indefinite deferral of donors who resided in the UK for a total of 3 months or longer between 1980 and 1996, and the complicated deferral policy for residents and visitors to the European continent, designed to reduce a calculated risk of transmission of the human variant of 'mad cow disease' (variant Creutzfeldt–Jakob disease, vCJD), has had a substantial impact, a loss of as much as 10% by some estimates, particularly on apheresis donors (Custer *et al.* 2004). Additional donor exclusions appear to be on the horizon.

Donor medications constitute another significant area of deferral losses. Certain medications, for example etretinate (Tegison), isotretinoin (Accutane), acitretin (Soriatane), dutasteride (Avodart) and finasteride (Proscar), have been identified as posing potential risk to transfusion recipients because of their teratogenic potential at low plasma concentrations. Such exclusions have little impact on blood safety but each shrinks the potentially eligible volunteer donor pool.

More troublesome, although not as numerous, are donor deferrals resulting from false-positive infectious disease screening tests. This problem has been recog-

nized since the introduction of serological tests for syphilis. However, during the past 15 years, the introduction of new screening tests and testing technologies has resulted in numerous deferrals for 'questionable' test results and either complex re-entry algorithms or no approved method to requalify such donors. Surrogate tests used for screening have proved particularly troublesome (Linden *et al.* 1988). However, even specific tests result in inappropriate deferrals. Of initial disease marker-reactive donations, 44% proved to be indeterminate or false positive (Custer *et al.* 2004). Each year an estimated 14000 donors are deferred from donating blood for an indefinite period because of repeatedly reactive enzyme immunoassay (EIA) screening tests for human immunodeficiency virus (HIV) and hepatitis C virus (HCV), and several hundred donors are deferred for apparently false-positive nucleic acid testing (NAT) results (L Katz MD, personal communication).

Registry of bone marrow donors

Voluntary blood donors are highly suitable to become bone marrow or peripheral blood stem cell donors for unrelated recipients, and many transfusion services now recruit them for this purpose. From its founding in 1986 until August 2003, the National Marrow Donor Program in the USA had registered more than 5 million bone marrow and blood stem cell donors, and Bone Marrow Donors Worldwide in the Netherlands records more than 8 million donors from 51 registries in 38 countries. Standards for acceptance of stem cell donors are based on blood donor eligibility. A uniform donor history is being developed.

Conditions that may disqualify a donor

Carriage of transmissible diseases

The most important infectious agents transmissible by transfusion are the hepatitis viruses B and C, HIV, human T-lymphotropic viruses (HTLVs), bacteria and the agents causing malaria and Chagas' disease. Increasing attention is being paid to the risks of 'emerging' agents and newly recognized infectious risks of transfusion such as West Nile virus, babesiosis and vCJD. Steps that should be taken to minimize the risk of infecting recipients with the agents of these and other diseases involve exclusion based on geographical residence, signs and symptoms of disease, high-risk activity and demographics associated with risk transmission (American Association of Blood Banks 2003); see also Chapter 16. Donors who have been exposed to an infectious disease and are at risk of developing it should be deferred for at least the length of the incubation period.

Recent inoculations, vaccinations, etc.

To avoid the possibility of transmitting live viruses (e.g. those of measles, mumps, rubella, Sabin oral polio vaccine, yellow fever, smallpox), donors should not give blood during the 3 weeks following vaccination. In subjects immunized with killed microbes or with antigens (cholera, influenza, typhoid, hepatitis A and B, Salk polio, rabies, anthrax, tick-borne and Japanese encephalitis) or toxoids (tetanus, diphtheria, pertussis), the interval is normally only 48 h. These recommendations apply if the donor is well following vaccination. Plasma from recently immunized donors may be useful for the manufacture of specific immunoglobulin preparations. Donors who have received immunoglobulins after exposure to infectious agents should not give blood for a period slightly longer than the incubation period of the disease in question. If hepatitis B immunoglobulin has been given after exposure to the virus, donation should be deferred for 9 months to 1 year; similarly, if tetanus immunoglobulin has been given, donation should be deferred for 4 weeks. When rabies vaccination follows a bite by a rabid animal, blood donations should be suspended for 1 year. In developed countries, tetanus and diphtheria immunoglobulin is derived from human sources. However, horse serum is still used in some parts of the world. Donors who have received an injection of horse serum within the previous 3 weeks should not donate blood because traces of horse serum in their blood might harm an allergic recipient. The administration of normal human immunoglobulin before travelling to countries where hepatitis A is endemic is not a cause for deferral.

Group O subjects may develop very potent haemolytic anti-A following an injection of tetanus toxoid, typhoid-paratyphoid (TAB), vaccine or pepsin-digested horse serum, which may contain traces of hog pepsin. In the past, the use of such subjects as 'universal donors' sometimes led to severe haemolytic transfusion reactions in group A subjects. Platelet concentrates collected by apheresis from subjects with hyperimmune anti-A should not be used for transfusion to group A or AB patients in view of the large volume of plasma needed to suspend the platelet concentrate.

Ear-piercing, electrolysis, tattooing, acupuncture

All of these procedures carry a risk of transmission of hepatitis or HIV infection when the equipment used is not disposable or sterilized, and blood donation should then be deferred for 12 months. In the UK, donors are accepted if the acupuncture is performed by a registered medical practitioner or in a hospital. Although the association between tattooing and exposure to hepatitis C is generally acknowledged (Haley and Fischer 2003), less clear is whether a tattoo performed by licensed and inspected facilities carries more risk than a trip to the dentist's surgery.

'Allergic' subjects

Subjects who suffer from very severe allergy are unacceptable as donors because their hypersensitivity may be passively transferred to the recipient for a short period (see Chapter 15). Subjects with seasonal allergy (e.g. hay fever) may donate when not in an active phase of their hypersensitivity. A screening test for immunoglobulin E (IgE) antibodies would not help to identify those allergic individuals with an increased chance of passively transferring their hypersensitivity (Stern et al. 1995).

Blood transfusions and tissue grafts

Donations should not be accepted for at least 12 months after the subject has received blood, blood components or grafts. Increasingly, donors who have received transfusion in the UK are being deferred indefinitely as a precaution against transmission of vCJD.

Surgery and dental treatment

When surgery has been carried out without blood transfusion, donation may be considered when the subject has fully recovered. Uncomplicated dental treatments and extractions should not be a cause for prolonged deferral, as utensils are sterilized and the risk of bacteraemia persisting for more than 1 h is negligible (Nouri et al. 1989).

Medication

Many subjects taking medication are not suitable as donors because of their underlying medical condition. Others are unsuitable as donors because the drugs they are taking, for example anticoagulants or cytotoxic agents, may harm the recipients (Mahnovski *et al.* 1987). Subjects who have taken aspirin within the previous week are unsuitable when theirs are the only platelets to be given to a particular recipient. Ingestion of oral contraceptives or replacement hormones such as thyroxine is not a disqualification for blood donation. On the other hand, recipients of human growth hormone (non-recombinant) should be permanently deferred from blood donation as should subjects who have used illicit injected drugs. Deferral for specific medication use is usually an issue of medical discretion; the US Armed Services Blood Program has made its drug deferral list available online (http://military-blood.dod. mil/library/policies/downloads/medication_list.doc).

Donors with relatively minor red cell abnormalities

In some populations, a considerable number of donors have an inherited red cell abnormality. The three conditions most likely to be encountered are: glucose-6-phosphate dehydrogenase (G-6-PD) deficiency, sickle trait (HbAS) and thalassaemia trait.

G-6-PD deficiency. This is the most common red cell enzyme defect; hundreds of molecular variants have been catalogued. Although most G-6-PD-deficient red cells have only slightly subnormal survival and lose viability on storage with adenine at only a slightly increased rate (Orlina *et al.* 1970), some enzyme variants render the cells unsuitable for transfusion. With the African variant Gd^{A-} present in 10% of African Americans, a relatively small number of red cells are severely affected. However, the Mediterranean variant $Gd^{Mediterranean}$ and others render the red cell particularly sensitive to oxidative stress. If the recipient of one of these units develops an infectious illness or ingests fava beans or one of any number of drugs (phenacetin, sulfonamides, vitamin K, primaquine, etc.), rapid destruction of the donor's G-6-PD-deficient cells may result. Neonatologists avoid using G-6-PD-deficient blood for exchange transfusion, and subjects who have evidenced G-6-PD-related haemolysis should be permanently deferred from donation (Beutler 1994).

Sickle trait (HbAS). Sickle trait red cells survive normally in healthy subjects, even after storage. However, in patients subject to various types of hypoxic stress, these cells survive poorly. HbS polymerizes at low oxygen tension and the cells are trapped in the spleen (Krevans 1959). Blood from donors with sickle cell trait should not be used for infants or for patients with sickle cell disease who undergo exchange transfusion. Patients, other than those with sickle Hb, who require general anaesthesia should have no problems if transfused with HbAS red cells provided that adequate oxygenation is maintained. Red cells from subjects with HbAS are usually unaffected by collection via apheresis, but those with sickling haemoglobinopathies should not donate by apheresis and are not suitable for intraoperative salvage. If blood from donors with sickle cell trait is glycerolized for storage in the frozen state, extra wash solution must be used during the deglycerolization procedure (Castro *et al.* 1981). Sickle trait prevents effective WBC reduction by filtration (Stroncek *et al.* 2004).

Thalassaemia trait. This is associated with little or no reduction in red cell lifespan in most subjects with a normal Hb concentration and these subjects may be accepted as donors.

Special conditions in which normally disqualified donors may donate

In some circumstances, a donor may give blood or components to be used for a special purpose, even although the requirements for normal donation are not met. For example, a donor who is mildly anaemic or who has recently given birth may give plasma or platelets by apheresis; the plasma may be needed for reagent preparation, for example HLA antibodies, or the platelets may be needed for transfusion to the newborn infant. Donors at risk for carrying malaria may give plasma for fractionation. The usual interval between donations may be waived for important medical indications. The donor age limitation and a number of other screening criteria may be modified for components directed to the recipient of the donor's bone marrow. In every case, medical evaluation should ensure that there is no increased risk to the donor's health and that the value of the component outweighs any perceived increase in risk. Under these circumstances, informed consent regarding the variance and documentation of the circumstances is mandatory.

Donation of whole blood

Frequency of donation

The volume lost from a single unit donation is replaced within 48–72 h. Red cell mass recovers more slowly, requiring 3–6 weeks. Some collection services bleed donors no more than two or three times a year; most do not bleed women who are pregnant or those who have been pregnant within the previous 6 weeks. The primary objective of this policy is to protect the donor from iron deficiency.

There is a wide variation in the recommended minimum interval between donations. For example in the US, in line with World Health Organization (WHO) recommendations, the interval can be as short as 8 weeks and a maximum of 3 l of blood per year may be collected (American Association of Blood Banks 2003). Premenopausal women should not donate as frequently as men (see below). In the Netherlands, men are bled every 3 months and women every 6 months.

Because few red cells are lost during platelet and plasmapheresis, these procedures may be performed more often and at shorter intervals. Standards vary by country; in the USA plateletpheresis donors may be drawn every 48 h up to twice per week and 24 times per year. Commercial plasmapheresis donors are bled even more frequently; however, physical examination is more rigorous and laboratory testing more extensive for these donors. As combinations of components, such as two-unit red cells, are drawn by apheresis, volumes and intervals become individualized, but generally limited by the loss of red cells.

Effect of blood donation on iron balance

Failure to meet the Hb standard is the most common reason for donor disqualification and iron deficiency, as a result of frequent donation, most often causes rejection.

Kinetics of iron loss

More than one-half of the total iron in the body is in the form of Hb. Adult males have approximately 1000 mg of storage iron, whereas adult females typically have only 250–500 mg. A twice-per-year blood donor loses more blood than does the average menstruating woman, whose annual loss does not normally exceed 650 ml. In men, iron lost from a 450-ml donation (242 ± 17 mg) is made up in about 3 months by enhanced absorption of dietary iron. For women (217 ± 11 mg), almost 1.5 years would be required to replace iron lost at donation. Based on these data, the interval between donations would appear to be no less than 3 months for men and 6 months or more for women (Finch 1972). However, even when these intervals are observed, blood donation seems to cause iron deficiency. Generally, iron stores are adequate between the first and second donations. Thereafter, an increase in iron absorption is necessary to sustain the increased plasma iron turnover and maintain iron balance (Garry *et al.* 1995). In total, 8% of males who donate four or five times per year and 19% of those who donate every 8 weeks will become iron deficient. If these male donors continue to donate, some may still meet the Hb and/or Hct standard for donation, but develop red cell indices consistent with iron deficiency. Some men will qualify to donate even although their Hb is substantially below their baseline value; others will be deferred as their Hb level drops below the 12.5-g requirement (Simon *et al.* 1981). In a group of healthy young men who gave blood every 2 months and received no iron therapy, one-third had no stainable iron in the marrow after four donations (Lieden 1975). In another study of donors deferred because of low Hb concentration, more than 70% had evidence of iron deficiency (Finch *et al.* 1977). Similarly, even male donors who gave blood only twice per year had a significant fall in mean ferritin levels accompanied by a lower Hb, red cell count and mean corpuscular Hb concentration (MCHC) if they had donated more than 10 times (Green 1988). Iron stores are exhausted in virtually all female donors regardless of the frequency of blood donations (Conrad 1981).

Oral iron supplementation

The suggestion that repeat blood donors receive iron supplementation raises a number of scientific, medical and ethical questions of which the scientific ones are most easily answered. Oral iron supplementation, if prescribed in sufficient doses and if taken by the donor, can increase annual donation frequency without the risk of iron deficiency (Bianco *et al.* 2002). The sub-optimal doses found in daily multivitamins will not. In a study of donors who had given blood either 15 times or 50 times at the rate of five donations per year and had received a supplement of 600 mg of Fe^{2+} after each donation, about 75% had no stainable iron in the marrow (Lieden 1973). These subjects were not anaemic and had normal serum iron levels. In a further study in which blood was donated every 2 months, resulting in an average daily loss of 3.5 mg of iron, iron stores were not maintained at the initial level, even when the subjects received 100 mg of iron per day (Lieden 1975). On the other hand, in 12 regular blood donors with subnormal serum ferritin levels who gave blood every 8 weeks, the ingestion of 5600 mg of iron between phlebotomies was sufficient to restore serum ferritin levels to normal and to provide a small store of iron in the bone marrow (Birgegard *et al.* 1980). Despite this finding, some experts believe that frequent bleeding even with iron supplementation is not justified and that the maximum annual rate of donation should be twice for men and once for women (Jacobs 1981).

When the interval between donations is 3 months or less, iron supplementation in the form of ferrous iron may be given to try to prevent iron deficiency. In the past, ferrous sulphate and ferrous gluconate have been prescribed but some preparations are not well absorbed, cause gastrointestinal disturbances in many donors and are potentially fatal if ingested in large doses by children. For all of these reasons, carbonyl iron, a small particle preparation of highly purified metallic iron with high bioavailability and almost no risk of accidental poisoning in children, seems better suited for this purpose. A series of studies by Gordeuk and co-workers (1990) showed that, with a regimen of 100 mg of carbonyl iron taken daily at bedtime for 56 days, the minimum interval between donations in the USA is well tolerated and provides enough absorbable iron to replace whatever is lost at donation in 85% of donors. A higher dose of carbonyl iron given for a shorter period of time (600 mg of iron three times daily for 1 week) caused gastrointestinal side-effects similar to those seen with ferrous sulphate (Gordeuk *et al.* 1987). In a controlled trial designed to prevent iron deficiency in qualifying female blood donors, women who received carbonyl iron (100 mg at bedtime for 56 days) increased their mean number of donations per year from 2.4 to 3.6 while increasing their iron stores (Bianco *et al.* 2002).

Iron supplementation programmes are difficult to implement and maintain (Skikne 1984). Even ongoing programmes may have limited effectiveness if the iron preparation is unpalatable or poorly absorbed (Monsen *et al.* 1983). Many blood collectors remain reluctant to become 'community clinics', whereas others raise concerns about prescribing medication for normal volunteers in order to extract additional donations. Finally, some physicians are concerned about overlooking occult gastrointestinal malignancy as the stool turns dark with the iron preparation and occult blood may be lost without the resulting anaemia.

Laboratory monitoring of iron status

Laboratory monitoring can help manage the repeat blood donor. In normal, well-nourished subjects, serum ferritin concentration is a good indicator of iron stores (Worwood 1980), although red cell ferritin may be a better indicator of body iron status (Cazzola and Ascari 1986). Red cell ferritin is affected only slightly by factors other than tissue iron stores (e.g. inflammation, increased red cell turnover), whereas these factors may cause a rise in serum ferritin. Several studies of ferritin estimations in large series have confirmed that iron stores may be seriously depleted in blood donors (Finch *et al.* 1977; Bodemann *et al.* 1984; Skikne 1984). For serial blood donors who have complete blood counts performed, a progressive drop in the red cell indices [mean cell volume (MCV), MCHC] provides an even easier and less expensive method of following functional iron status (Leitman *et al.* 2003).

Screening test to detect anaemia

Subjects should be tested before donation to make sure that they are not anaemic. A convenient test is to allow a drop of blood to fall from a height of 1 cm into a selected solution of copper sulphate and thus to determine its Hb concentration from the specific gravity. A more accurate, portable photometric method avoids some of the environmental hazards of the copper sulphate technique at a higher cost (James *et al.* 2003). In some countries, such as France, the Hb level is no longer determined before donation. Instead, the Hb level and the packed cell volume (PCV) of blood donations are estimated. Donors found to be anaemic are recalled for investigation.

The lowest acceptable Hb levels for male and female blood donors, defined by the specific gravity of whole blood, correspond reasonably well with limits defined by conventional spectrophotometric analysis of venous samples. In a series of 200 healthy subjects, the range (mean ± 2 SD) was 121–165 g/l for males and 120–147 g/l for females (Bain and England 1975). Similar values were reported in a review of normal Hb concentrations based on published data (Garby 1970). Haematologic differences have been found between African–Americans and white people; reference standards for Hb, PCV and MCV differ among ethnic groups (Beutler 2005).

In the UK, the National Blood Transfusion Service accepts male donors whose blood contains at least 135 g Hb/l as judged by the observation that a blood drop sinks in a copper sulphate solution of specific gravity 1.055, and female donors whose Hb concentration is not less than 125 g/l as measured by a copper sulphate solution of specific gravity 1.053. If a donor fails the copper sulphate test, rapid microhaematocrit or Hb determinations can be done at the donor station from skin-prick blood, using accurate portable photometry instruments (Cable 1995). In London, these supplementary determinations reveal that in approximately 50% of cases a donation can be taken, thus saving the donor from unnecessary anxiety (James *et al.* 2003). When donors are found to be anaemic (2–3% of London donors, mostly women), venous samples should be taken and retested by conventional haemoglobinometry. Donors who are confirmed as anaemic should be referred to their general practitioner. In the US, the minimum acceptable level of Hb for donors is 125 g Hb/l (American Association of Blood Banks 2003).

Errors in technique in using the copper sulphate method, for example incorporation of air bubbles or the use of an inadequate height for dropping the blood, tend to result in underestimating the Hb concentration so that donors may be rejected unnecessarily. On the other hand, in rare cases in which the plasma protein concentration is greatly raised, anaemic donors may be accepted as normal, each extra g/dl of plasma protein being equivalent to 0.7 g/dl Hb (Mannarino and MacPherson 1963). Falsely high positive results in the copper sulphate method may also be due to a high white cell count associated with granulocyte mobilization or leukaemia.

The source of the blood sample may determine acceptance or rejection of a donor in borderline cases.

Based on microhaematocrit methods, blood obtained by ear lobe puncture was found to give values about 6% higher than those obtained simultaneously by fingerprick puncture (Avoy *et al.* 1977), and blood from fingerprick was found to have an Hb value 2% lower than that of venous blood obtained simultaneously (Moe 1970). Ear lobe sampling is unreliable and is now considered obsolete in the US.

Hb regeneration after normal blood donation

In 14 normal healthy subjects bled of about 400 ml of blood (8% of their blood volume), circulating reticulocytes increased minimally but significantly, and peaked on the ninth day after bleeding. The Hb level was lowest 1 or 2 weeks after bleeding, and increased rapidly thereafter, reaching predonation levels at 3–4 weeks (Fig. 1.1). In a study in which total red cell volumes were measured in subjects who had donated about 190 ml of red cells, about 50 ml of red cells were restored after 1 week and restoration was almost complete at 6 weeks (Heaton and Holme 1994).

Untoward effects during or shortly after venesection

When light-headedness and bruising at the venepuncture site are included, some 11–36% of blood donors will suffer a phlebotomy-related reaction (Newman 1997; Trouern-Trend *et al.* 1999; Newman 2003). The majority of these reactions are mild. However, a small number, some of which are avoidable, result in donor injury and disability. Reaction rates are higher in autologous donors, some of whom have significant degrees of medical debility (see Chapter 17).

Fainting or the vasovagal attack

The mere sight of blood being taken from another person can precipitate a 'vasovagal attack' in certain subjects. Withdrawing a sufficient quantity of blood will provoke syncope in everyone. After the loss of as little as 400 ml of blood, some subjects remain liable to faint even several hours later if they rise suddenly from a sitting or lying position or if they remain standing for prolonged periods. In view of this risk, all donors should be observed for at least 15 min after donation and should be questioned about their occupation. Donors in whom fainting would be especially hazardous

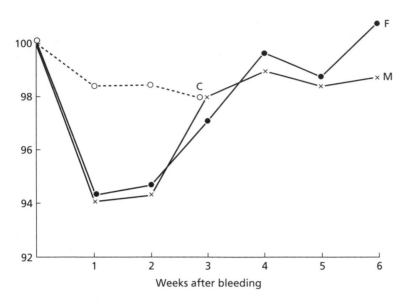

Figure 1.1 Mean Hb concentration in seven women (F) and seven men (M) at weekly intervals after being bled about 8% of blood volume. The dotted line indicates the change in mean Hb concentration for four men and four women who were not bled (C) (Wadsworth 1955).

to themselves or to others (e.g. pilots, surgeons and bus drivers) should probably refrain from work or potentially dangerous hobbies for up to 12 h after giving blood. Donors who experience a delayed faint should be indefinitely deferred from blood donation, regardless of their occupation.

Pathophysiology. The vasovagal attack appears to be a hypothalamic response mediated by either a central neural pathway or a peripheral pathway associated with the baroreceptors. While blood is being drawn, warning of oncoming fainting may be presaged by a fall in flow rate, as already noted in the seventeenth century (Harvey 1628). Vasovagal reactions are typically biphasic, originating with a stress-induced elevation in pulse and blood pressure, and rapidly followed by the commonly recognized signs and symptoms of fainting. As the syndrome develops, the donor feels weak and dizzy. Clinical characteristics include sweating and pallor, cool extremities, strikingly slow and faint pulse, low or undetectable blood pressure, vomiting and, less commonly, tetany and urinary and faecal incontinence. Loss of consciousness may follow and convulsions are seen occasionally. These effects result primarily from the action of the autonomic system, causing slowing of the heart, vomiting and sweating and, perhaps most important, dilatation of the arterioles, leading to a sudden fall in blood pressure (Barcroft *et al.* 1944). The slow pulse rate (30–60 per min) in the vasovagal attack is the most useful single sign in differential diagnosis.

Donor characteristics and frequency. Estimates of the frequency with which fainting occurs in blood donors vary according to the definition of the term 'faint'. In the Medical Research Council's inquiry (1944), 'fainting' was defined as the manifestation of any of a series of signs or symptoms such as pallor, sweating, dimness or nausea (MRC 1944). By this definition, some 5–6% of donors fainted. A similar frequency of vasovagal symptoms (5.3%) was noted by interviewers who solicited this information from 1000 donors 3 weeks after blood donation (Newman 2003). In a series of 10 000 cases, only 2.8% of donors fainted, but the term 'fainting' was applied only to those who lost consciousness or could not stand or sit without doing so (Poles and Boycott 1942). Moderate to severe reactions are reported in 0.08–0.34% of donations (Newman 1997).

Vasovagal reactions occur more commonly on the first occasion of giving blood. Among 1000 donors studied over a period of several years, more than one-half experienced their only symptoms at the time of their first donation; the incidence of reactions fell progressively over a period of 6 years (Beal 1972). In 40 437 donations studied, fainting was found to be more common in female donors; 4.9% of first-time female donors suffered vasovagal reactions compared with 3.8% of first-time male donors. The figures were less than half in repeat donors of both sexes, 1.9% and 1.1% respectively (Tomasulo *et al.* 1980). However, gender may be a surrogate measure for body weight. In a case–control study, age, weight and first-time donor status were significant predictors of syncope (Trouern-Trend *et al.* 1999).

One early study noted a relation between the incidence of fainting and the amount of blood donated. The incidence was 3.8% in those giving 440 ml, but 8.5% in those giving 540 ml (Poles and Boycott 1942). In normal males from whom 800–1000 ml of blood was taken, the incidence was 11 out of 28, and in those from another series, loss of consciousness was observed in 5 out of 6 (Ebert *et al.* 1941). In experiments in which up to 1500 ml of blood was withdrawn from normal volunteers, fainting could be produced in all subjects if enough blood was withdrawn within a limited time (Howarth and Sharpey-Schafer 1947).

Management of vasovagal reactions: science, custom and myth

Subjects who display these signs but who have not lost blood recover rapidly when they are placed supine and positioned so that the head is lower than the rest of the body (Trendelenburg position). Time-honoured measures include applying an ice pack or cold towel to the (donor's) forehead or back of the neck or using a paper bag rebreathing technique to elevate CO_2 and cerebral blood flow. The effectiveness of such techniques is unknown. Inhalation of ammonia salts adds very little other than irritating the respiratory membranes and the donor. Intravenous infusion, inotropic agents and cholinergic blockade are rarely necessary. Donor room personnel should be cautioned against the precipitous use of external defibrillation and cardiopulmonary resuscitation, as these techniques will invariably cause more harm than good to a donor suffering from a vasovagal attack.

Some consequences of syncope. Syncope can have serious consequences. Skull and facial bone fractures, scalp lacerations, chipped teeth and extremity fractures have all been reported (Boynton and Taylor 1945). A retrospective analysis of 178 vasovagal reactions from 194 000 donations found that 10% of these donors sustained a head injury and 6% required additional medical care in an emergency room. One injured donor developed post-concussion syndrome and suffered headaches and other symptoms for more than 1 year (Newman and Graves 2001). Although 12% of the reactions occurred off site, the majority within 1 h of donation, more than 60% occurred at the refreshment table, an observation that should stimulate serious thought about the design and oversight of the donor recovery area.

Some other untoward effects

Bruising. Bruising is one of the commonest complications of blood donation, and is reported in 9–16% of donations (Boynton and Taylor 1945; Newman 1997). In the majority of cases, the haematoma is restricted to a small area in the antecubital fossa. However, very large, incapacitating and painful haematomas develop occasionally following blood donation. Inattention to an enlarging haematoma can result in a forearm compartment syndrome with consequent neural and vascular compromise and massive tissue necrosis. Instruction regarding pressure dressing, cold compresses and medical follow-up can prevent a large bruise from turning into a medical emergency.

Phlebitis and cellulitis. Mild phlebitis at the venepuncture site in the antecubital fossa is common, self-limited and usually of little consequence. Mild discomfort, warmth and local linear or surrounding erythema may be difficult to distinguish from mild cellulitis or reaction to the topical antiseptic, particularly if the latter contains iodine. Despite their benign appearance, local reactions merit close medical follow-up to prevent extension of these lesions to abscess formation or septic phlebitis. Early application of warm compresses, oral anti-inflammatory agents and administration of antibiotics when indicated are prudent. Newman reports an incidence of local reactions of 1 in 50 000 to 1 in 100 000 (Newman 1997).

Nerve injury. The proximity of cutaneous branches of the medial and ulnar nerves to the large-bore needle access to the antecubital vein makes occasional injury to these structures inevitable. The injuries are generally transient and rarely a source of donor distress. In most instances the donor reports a localized area of numbness or tingling (paraesthesia). In 419 000 donations over a 2-year period, Newman and Waxman (1996) reported an incidence of peripheral nerve injury of 1 in 6300, with 78% of donors reporting their injury on the day of donation. Symptoms were almost evenly divided between paraesthesias and radiating pain, although eight donors reported loss of arm strength. Almost one-quarter of these reports were associated with haematoma formation at the venepuncture site. In total, 70% of donors recovered completely within 1 month; 52 out of 56 recovered completely and four donors reported a small area of persistent numbness.

Puncture of an artery. This leads to an unusually rapid flow of bright red blood; when the needle is withdrawn, there may be severe leakage of blood, followed by extensive bruising. If an arterial puncture is suspected, the needle should be withdrawn immediately and firm pressure applied for at least 10 min, followed by a pressure dressing. If the radial pulse is not palpable, the donor should be referred to a vascular specialist. Rare complications of arterial injury include pseudoaneurysm formation and development of an arteriovenous fistula (Lung and Wilson 1971; Popovsky *et al.* 1994).

Tetany. Tetany is occasionally observed in blood donors (incidence 1 in 1000), characteristically in nervous subjects, and is thought to be due to hyperventilation. Manifestations may include carpopedal spasm, laryngismus, stridulus and a positive Chvostek's sign. Rapid relief can be obtained by rebreathing from a paper bag or inhaling 5% CO_2 from a cylinder, an unlikely method of management in the modern blood centre (Frazer and Fowweather 1942).

Convulsions. These are rare. If seizures occur, the donor should be immobilized on the bed or on the floor to prevent injury, and an open airway ensured.

Air embolism during blood donation. When blood is taken into plastic bags that contain no air, there is no possibility of air embolism. On the other hand when blood is drawn into glass bottles (as is still the practice in some countries), air embolism may occur. The prime cause of air embolism in this circumstance is obstruction to the air vent of the bottle (for details and further references, see seventh edition, p. 6). Apheresis devices include inline filters and air detector alarm systems to prevent air from a defective seal from being pumped into a donor.

Fatalities attributed to blood donation. In 1975, the Food and Drug Administration of the USA published regulations requiring the reporting of deaths associated with blood collection, plasmapheresis and transfusion. In the 10 years from 1976 to 1985, three deaths attributed to blood donation were reported out of 100 million units of donated blood. Two deaths were due to myocardial infarction and one was in a patient with phaeochromocytoma (Sazama 1990). In 1999, of 48 deaths reported to the FDA in some 20 million donations, four fatalities occurred in donors. Two of these were donors of autologous units and all deaths were attributed to underlying disease.

Potential health benefits of blood donation

For the volunteer donor, the chief benefit lies in the satisfaction of selfless concern for the welfare of others. However, two studies suggest that there may be more tangible health benefits, particularly for middle-aged men, such as lowering the risk of cardiovascular disease (Meyers *et al.* 1997; Salonen *et al.* 1998). The proffered explanation derives from the so-called 'iron hypothesis': menstrual iron loss protects women against cardiovascular disease; iron stores correlate with cardiovascular disease across European populations and heart failure is a hallmark of disorders of iron surplus (Sullivan 1981). One proposed mechanism for this association is generation of oxygen free radicals that induce oxidation of lipids (McCord 1991). However the Johns Hopkins Hospital autopsy registry found less coronary artery disease in hearts from patients with haemochromatosis and haemosiderosis than in hearts of age- and sex-matched controls (Miller and Hutchins 1994).

Salonen and co-workers (1998) conducted a prospective 9-year follow-up study of 2862 men aged 42–60 from eastern Finland, who had participated in the Kuopio Ischemic Heart Disease Risk Factor Study (Salonen *et al.* 1998). Only one man out of 153 who had donated blood in the 24 months prior to baseline examination suffered a myocardial infarction, compared with 316 (12.5%) of the 2529 non-donors. Meyers and co-workers (1997) compared the rate of cardiovascular events of 665 blood donors with that of 3200 non-donors in a telephone survey of a cohort selected from the Nebraska Diet Heart Survey. By multivariate analysis, non-smoking men who had donated at least once in the previous 3 years had a significantly lowered risk of cardiovascular events; no additional benefit was derived from longer or more frequent donation. Numerous cofactors confound these studies, and the validity of this statistical association has been questioned (Ford 1997).

Although the hypothesis remains intriguing, it is premature to suggest that health benefits, other than those attributable to altruism, will derive from blood donors – even for non-smoking middle-aged men.

Directed donations

Directed donations are those given exclusively for named patients, usually by relatives or friends. The use of directed donations contravenes the normal principles of voluntary blood donation, fails to increase safety (Cordell et al. 1986; Strauss 1989) and finds medical justification in vanishingly few circumstances: (1) in patients with rare blood groups when the only available compatible donors may be close relatives; (2) in occasional patients awaiting renal transplants, for whom donor-specific transfusions may still play a role (Salvatierra et al. 1981; Anderson et al. 1985; see also Chapter 14); (3) in infants with neonatal alloimmune thrombocytopenia or haemolytic disease of the newborn, for whom maternal platelets or red cells are occasionally invaluable; (4) in children requiring open-heart or extensive orthopaedic surgery, for whom the total requirements for blood and components can be collected preoperatively, as for autologous transfusion but from designated relatives or parents, thus minimizing the number of donor units to which the children are exposed (Brecher et al. 1988); and (5) in patients with leukaemia in relapse after bone marrow transplantation, for whom donor leucocytes are used as adoptive immunotherapy to induce graft-versus-leukaemia (GvL) effect (Sullivan et al. 1989; Kolb et al. 1990).

The practice of transfusing parental blood to premature newborn infants is not without risks. Mothers may have antibodies against antigens (inherited from the father) on the infant's red cells, platelets or white cells and maternal plasma should not be used. Fathers should not serve as cell donors because they may have antigens present on their red cells, which are incompatible with maternally derived antibodies present in the fetus. Moreover, in view of partial histocompatibility, transfusion of cells from parents and close relatives may result in graft-versus-host disease (GvHD) in the infants, or older children, especially if the infants are immunodeficient (Bastian et al. 1984; Strauss 1989). Circumstances such as these, in which blood or platelet

suspensions should be irradiated, are described in Chapter 15.

The practice of transfusing parents with blood from their offspring can also be dangerous. Fatal GvHD occurred in two immunocompetent adult patients who were transfused with fresh whole non-irradiated blood from their children during cardiac surgery. In both cases, one of the donors was homozygous for one of the recipient's HLA haplotypes (Thaler et al. 1989). When such transfusions are indicated, and except for instances in which adoptive immunotherapy is intended, the components should be treated with 25 Gy gamma irradiation (see Chapter 15).

People who donate for friends and family lose their anonymity and may be subject to influences not placed upon community donors. Such donors may provide less than candid answers to sensitive donor questions, either because they believe that unsafe blood will inevitably be detected by testing procedures or because they wish to conceal information from the recipient or the blood collector. Two examples follow:

1 A 28-year-old male first-time donor qualified to give a unit of blood for his mother's scheduled heart surgery. The unit tested positive for anti-HIV. During a subsequent confidential interview, the donor acknowledged untruthful answers to the high-risk activity questions on the donor interview form. When asked why he would donate for his mother when he was aware of the increased risk of his blood, he responded that any exposure to a transfusion-transmitted disease would surely be detected by testing. He indicated that refusal to donate for his mother would have signalled either lack of filial devotion or a lifestyle unacceptable to his mother. Furthermore, he interpreted the fact that he had been detected by testing as validation of his approach.

2 A child with a 19-year history of aplastic anaemia was found to harbour a chronic parvovirus B19 infection (Kurtzman et al. 1987). Treatment with immune plasma was planned on an investigational protocol. Among numerous donors tested for antibody to this virus, the child's parents were found to have the highest titred plasma by several factors. Each had an unremarkable medical history and physical examination. Because both parents qualified to donate blood and insisted that they were the safest donors for their child, units of plasma were drawn and prepared for immunotherapy. Neither parent had donated blood previously. During routine sample testing, extremely high alanine aminotransferase (ALT) levels were detected in specimens from both parents, and subsequent medical evaluation revealed that both parents had chronic hepatitis. After persistent questioning

about this finding, the parents recalled several episodes of intravenous drug use some 16 years earlier.

A variant of directed donation is the compulsory 'replacement donation' extracted from relatives and friends of patients admitted to hospital in many countries in the developing world. Such donations are often purchased and are generally less safe than true voluntary donations (Sarkodie *et al.* 2001).

Use of cadaver blood

Administration of cadaver blood seems to be of prime interest to journalists and reporters. The collection of blood from cadavers (for further details see seventh edition, p. 9) has been practised in only a few centres in Russia (Agranenko and Maltseva 1990). Reports of widespread use and benefits have attained mythical proportions.

Therapeutic phlebotomy

Blood centres and transfusion services, with their expertise in safe blood withdrawal and donor management, present a logical setting for performing therapeutic phlebotomy. Even although many subjects referred for therapeutic phlebotomy are as healthy as volunteer donors, and in the case of hereditary haemochromatosis have been volunteer donors, others are true patients who deserve close medical supervision. Blood collected from these procedures may be unsuitable for transfusion because of the patient/donor's underlying medical condition or because the subject fails to qualify as a donor for other reasons. By tradition, therapeutic phlebotomy services have been located in an area separate from volunteer blood donation and have required a medical prescription from an attending physician. However, as otherwise healthy subjects with hereditary haemochromatosis are being identified by screening programmes, the distinction between patient and donor has blurred. Some countries require that blood drawn from such donors (see below) be so labelled, and that the recipient be informed of the source of the transfusion.

Polycythaemia vera. Phlebotomy remains the overwhelming choice for the initial therapy of polycythaemia vera (Streiff *et al.* 2002). Although red cells from such patients survive normally, polycythaemia vera is a clonal, progressive, myeloproliferative dis-

order and patients are at increased risk for developing leukaemia. As a rule, this blood is not used for transfusion, although the risk of acquiring a graft of malignant cells from the donor seems to be negligible, even in recipients whose immune mechanisms are suppressed by disease or drugs. Although the target level for phlebotomy remains controversial, studies of blood viscosity and thromboembolic disease suggest that patients be maintained at a PCV < 44%, a level usually reached by weekly to monthly phlebotomy until iron stores are depleted (Streiff *et al.* 2002).

Other conditions associated with polycythaemia. Erythrocytosis may occur in a variety of congenital states, such as mutations in the erythropoietin receptor gene and in the Hb molecule, in residents of high-altitude locations and in patients with respiratory insufficiency, cyanotic congenital heart disease and a variety of neoplasms. It may be useful to measure oxygen consumption and exercise tolerance to help determine whether therapeutic phlebotomy is helpful in these disorders and, if so, what the target level for phlebotomy should be (Winslow *et al.* 1983; 1985).

Hereditary haemochromatosis

Hereditary haemochromatosis is one of the most common inherited disorders of white people, occurring in 1 in 250 individuals of northern European descent (Olynyk 1999). It is uncommon in other racial groups, although sporadic cases occur. A point mutation in the HFE gene, Cys282Tyr, is found in 85–100% of white people (Gilbert *et al.* 1989). Failure of the HFE gene product to bind to the transferrin receptor on gut mucosal cells leads to inappropriately high gastrointestinal absorption of iron, with progressive iron deposition in the skin, liver, heart and other tissues. Hepatic fibrosis, cirrhosis, endocrine insufficiency, heart failure and arthritis may ensue. However, the clinical penetrance of the disorder is variable and a substantial number of subjects with the mutation remain unaffected or asymptomatic for years.

Management of phlebotomy. Phlebotomy remains the most effective therapy for haemochromatosis. If phlebotomy is initiated before the onset of cirrhosis, patients can lead a normal life (Barton *et al.* 1998). Phlebotomy is generally initiated on a weekly basis, with removal of approximately one unit of blood (500 ml)

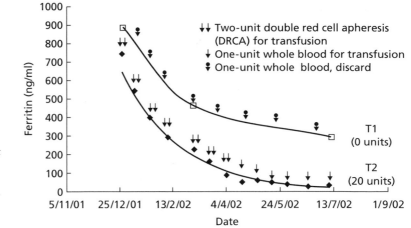

Figure 1.2 Twin brothers with hereditary haemochromatosis undergoing therapeutic phlebotomy. Twin 2 (T2) was treated with two-unit apheresis phlebotomy that resulted in more rapid iron depletion than his twin (T1) who received manual single-unit bleeding. Subject A required fewer treatment visits.

per session. Clinical and laboratory endpoints of induction (weekly) therapy differ widely from centre to centre (Bolan *et al.* 2001). Recent guidelines target a transferrin saturation ranging from less than 20–30% as a guide to the pace of maintenance phlebotomy. However, the transferrin saturation may rebound rapidly after initial iron depletion owing to the dysregulation of iron cycling associated with hereditary haemochromatosis, and may not accurately reflect the true total body iron burden. Monitoring the Hb and MCV in combination provides a reliable, accurate and inexpensive method for indicating the onset of iron-limited erythropoiesis and guiding the endpoints of therapy (Bolan *et al.* 2001; Leitman *et al.* 2003). Furthermore, sustained maintenance of the MCV at exactly this level (5–10% below baseline) was found to keep subjects with hereditary haemochromatosis just on the verge of iron-limited erythropoiesis and could be used to define a phlebotomy interval that prevented iron reaccumulation during maintenance therapy, while allowing Hb levels to rise well into the normal range (above 14 g/dl). Two-unit apheresis affords a rapid method for removing iron on a schedule convenient for most subjects. The efficiency can be seen by comparing twins with haemochromatosis, one of whom was treated with manual single-unit phlebotomy, whereas the other underwent the apheresis procedure (Fig. 1.2).

Use of blood for transfusion. Several countries use blood withdrawn from subjects with haemochromatosis for allogeneic transfusion. However in the US, federal regulations require disease labelling of blood

derived from therapeutic phlebotomy and additional donation conditions must be met before labelling for hereditary haemochromatosis is waived by the FDA (Guidance for Industry. Variances for Blood Collection from Individuals with Hereditary Hemochromatosis. Rockville MD: Center for Biologics Evaluation and Research. August 2001. Accessed August 13, 2002, at http://www.fda.gov/cber/gdlns/hemchrom.htm). One oft-voiced concern has been that the cost to the patient of therapeutic phlebotomy provides sufficient financial incentive that patients might withhold risk activity information from the donor service ('paid donors'). A confidential survey conducted by the REDS group determined that the prevalence of deferrable risks concealed at the time of donation was similar in patients with haemochromatosis (2.0%) and non-health-related volunteer donors (3.1%) as was the overall prevalence of positive screening test results (1.3% of patients with haemochromatosis vs. 1.6% of non-health-related donors). The authors conclude that significant numbers of patients with haemochromatosis already donate blood for therapeutic reasons and do not present a greater risk to blood safety than do other donors (Sanchez *et al.* 2001).

During the first 27 months of a hospital-based study, donors with haemochromatosis were contributing 14% of all units entering the hospital inventory (Leitman *et al.* 2003); 75% of subjects referred for therapeutic phlebotomy were found to meet donor suitability criteria. A pre-phlebotomy Hb of 12.5 g/dl, the normal threshold for all allogeneic donations, also proved to be an excellent indicator of readiness for phlebotomy, ensuring both the potency of the component and the avoidance of unnecessary anaemia in the subject. An MCV decline of 3% was similarly a reproducible indicator of total body iron depletion, as confirmed by ferritin and transferrin saturation assays during induction and maintenance phases of therapy. The number of allogeneic red cell units that could potentially be made available for transfusion in the US if haemochromatosis donor programmes were widely implemented, perhaps as part of a national programme, could make an impact on blood availability. Even if a conservative model is used, and only donors in the maintenance phase of therapy undergoing a mean of five donations per year are incorporated into the equation, a net increase of 16% (2.27 million units) in the US red cell supply could be realized (Conry-Cantilena 2001).

References

Agranenko VA, Maltseva IY (1990) Cadaver blood transfusion. Transfusion Today 5: 11

American Association of Blood Banks (2004) Standards for Blood Banks and Transfusion Services. Bethesda, MD: AABB Press

Anderson CB, Tyler JD, Sicard GA (1985) Renal allograft recipient pretreatment with immunosuppression and donor-specific blood. Transplant Proc 17: 1047–1050

Avoy DR, Canuel ML, Otton BM (1977) Haemoglobin screening in prospective blood donors: a comparison of methods. Transfusion 17: 261

Bain BJ, England JM (1975) Normal haematological values: sex difference in neutrophil count. Br Med J i: 306

Barcroft H, Edholm OG, McMichael J (1944) Post-haemorrhagic fainting: study by cardiac output and forearm flow. Lancet i: 489

Barton JC, McDonnell SM, Adams PC et al. (1998) Management of hemochromatosis. Hemochromatosis Management Working Group. Ann Intern Med 129: 932–939

Bastian JF, Williams RA, Ornelas W (1984) Maternal isoimmunisation resulting in combined immunodeficiency and fatal graft-versus-host disease in an infant. Lancet i: 1435–1437

Beal RW (1972) Vaso-vagal reactions in blood donors. Med J Aust 2: 757

Beutler E (1994) G6PD deficiency. Blood 84: 3613–3636

Beutler E, West C (2005) Hematologic differences between African-Americans and whites: the roles of iron deficiency and alpha-thalassemia on hemoglobin levels and mean corpuscular volume. Blood 106: 740–745

Bianco C, Brittenham G, Gilcher RO et al. (2002) Maintaining iron balance in women blood donors of childbearing age: summary of a workshop. Transfusion 42: 798–805

Birgegard G, Hogman C, Johansson A (1980) Serum ferritin in the regulation of iron therapy in blood donors. Vox Sang 38: 29–35

Bodemann HH, Rieger A, Bross KJ (1984) Erythrocyte and plasma ferritin in normal subjects, blood donors and iron deficiency anaemia patients. Blut 48: 131–137

Bolan CD, Conry-Cantilena C, Mason G et al. (2001) MCV as a guide to phlebotomy therapy for hemochromatosis. Transfusion 41: 819–827

Boynton MH, Taylor ES (1945) Complications arising in donors in a mass blood procurement project. Am J Med Sci 209: 421–436

Brecher ME (ed) (2003) Technical Manual. Bethesda, MD: AABB Press

Brecher ME, Moore SB, Taswell HF (1988) Minimal exposure transfusion: a new approach to homologous blood transfusion. Mayo Clin Proc 63: 903–905

Cable RG (1995) Hemoglobin determination in blood donors. Transfusion Med Rev 9: 131–144

Castro O, Hardy KP, Winter WP et al. (1981) Freeze preservation of sickle erythrocytes. Am J Hematol 10: 297–304

Cazzola M, Ascari E (1986) Red cell ferritin as a diagnostic tool. Br J Haematol 62: 209–213

Centers for Biologic Evaluation and Research. US Food and Drug Administration (2002) Guidance for Industry. Revised Preventive Measures to Reduce the Possible Risk of Transmission of Creutzfeldt-Jakob Disease (CJD) and Variant Creutzfeldt-Jakob Disease (vCJD) by Blood and Blood Products. 1. 2002. US Food and Drug Administration

Conrad ME, Crosby WH, Jacobs A et al. (1981) In International Forum: The Hippocratian principle of 'primum nil nocere' demands that the metabolic state of a donor should be normalized prior to a subsequent donation of blood or plasma. How much blood, relative to his body weight, can a donor give over a certain period, without a continuous deviation of iron metabolism in the direction of iron deficiency? Vox Sang 41: 336–343

Conry-Cantilena C (2001) Phlebotomy, blood donation, and hereditary hemochromatosis. Transfusion Med Rev 15: 136–143

Cordell RA, Yalon VA, Cigahn H (1986) Experience with 11,916 designated donations. Transfusion 26: 485–486

Custer B, Johnson ES, Sullivan SD et al. (2004) Quantifying losses to the donated blood supply due to donor deferral and miscollection. Transfusion 44: 1417–1426

Doughty R, Flanagan P (1996) ISBT Code 128 and code changes as part of the implementation of a national IT system for the English National Blood Service. Transfusion Med 6: 299–301

Ebert RV, Stead EA, Gibson JG (1941) Response of normal subjects to acute blood loss, with special reference to the mechanism of restoration of blood volume. Arch Intern Med 68: 578

Finch CA (1972) In International Forum. Which measures should be taken in order to prevent iron deficiency in blood donors? Vox Sang 23: 238

Finch CA, Cook JD, Labbe RF *et al.* (1977) Effect of blood donation on iron stores as evaluated by serum ferritin. Blood 50: 441–447

Ford I (1997) Is blood donation good for the donor? Heart 78: 107

Frazer WF, Fowweather FS (1942) Tetany in blood donors. Br Med J i: 759

Garby L (1970) Annotation: the normal haemoglobin level. Br J Haematol 19: 429

Garry PJ, Koehler KM, Simon TL (1995) Iron stores and iron absorption: effects of repeated blood donations. Am J Clin Nutr 62: 611–620

Gilbert GL, Hayes K, Hudson IL *et al.* (1989) Prevention of transfusion-acquired cytomegalovirus infection in infants by blood filtration to remove leucocytes. Neonatal Cytomegalovirus Infection Study Group. Lancet 1: 1228–1231

Gordeuk VR, Brittenham GM, Hughes MA *et al.* (1987) Carbonyl iron for short-term supplementation in female blood donors. Transfusion 27: 80–85

Gordeuk VR, Brittenham GM, Bravo J *et al.* (1990) Prevention of iron deficiency with carbonyl iron in female blood donors. Transfusion 30: 239–245

Green ES, Hewitt PE, England JM (1988) Iron depletion in male donors bled at three monthly intervals is not accompanied by changes in haematological parameters. Proceedings of the 20th Congress of the International Society of Blood Transfusion (London), p. 124.

Haley RW, Fischer RP (2003) The tattooing paradox: are studies of acute hepatitis adequate to identify routes of transmission of subclinical hepatitis C infection? Arch Intern Med 163: 1095–1098

Harvey W (1628) De Motu Cordis, Frankfurt. Oxford: Blackwell Scientific Publications

Hassig A (1991) [50 years of blood transfusion services of the Swiss Red Cross]. Schweiz Med Wochenschr 121: 156–159

Heaton A, Holme S (1994) Blood donation and red cell volume (RCV) regeneration in donors of different weights (Abstract). Vox Sang 67 (Suppl.) 2: 3

Howarth S, Sharpey-Schafer EP (1947) Low blood pressure phases following haemorrhage. Lancet i: 19

Jacobs A (1981) In International Forum: The Hippocratic principle of 'primum nil nocere' demands that the metabolic state of a donor should be normalized prior to a subsequent donation of blood or plasma. How much blood, relative to his body weight, can a donor give over a certain period, without a continuous deviation of iron metabolism in the direction of iron deficiency? Vox Sang 41: 336–343

James V, Jones KF, Turner EM *et al.* (2003) Statistical analysis of inappropriate results from current Hb screening methods for blood donors. Transfusion 43: 400–404

Kinsella K, Velkoff VA (2001) An Aging World: 2001. Washington DC: US Government Printing Office

Kolb HJ, Mittermuller J, Clemm C *et al.* (1990) Donor leukocyte transfusions for treatment of recurrent chronic myelogenous leukemia in marrow transplant patients. Blood 76: 2462–2465

Krevans JR (1959) *In vivo* behaviour of sickle-trait erythrocytes when exposed to continuous hypoxia. Clin Res 7: 203

Kurtzman GJ, Ozawa K, Cohen B *et al.* (1987) Chronic bone marrow failure due to persistent B19 parvovirus infection. N Engl J Med 317: 287–294

Leikola J (1990) Formulation of a national blood programme. In: Management of Blood Transfusion. SR Hollan, W Wagstaff, J Leikola, and F Lothe (eds). Geneva: World Health Organization

Leitman SF, Browning JN, Yau YY *et al.* (2003) Hemochromatosis subjects as allogeneic blood donors: a prospective study. Transfusion 43: 1538–1544

Lieden G (1973) Iron state in regular blood donors. Scand J Haematol 11: 342–349

Lieden G (1975) Iron supplement to blood donors. I. Trials with intermittent iron supply. Acta Med Scand 197: 31–36

Linden JV, Gregorio DI, Kalish RI (1988) An estimate of blood donor eligibility in the general population. Vox Sang 54: 96–100

Lung JA, Wilson SD (1971) Development of arteriovenous fistula following blood donation. Transfusion 11: 145

Mahnovski V, Cheung MH, Lipsey AI (1987) Drugs in blood donors. Clin Chem 33: 189

Mannarino AD, MacPherson CR (1963) Copper sulfate screening of blood donors: report of a donor passing the test with less than eight grams of hemoglobin. Transfusion 3: 398

McCord JM (1991) Is iron sufficiency a risk factor in ischemic heart disease? Circulation 83: 1112–1114

Meyers DG, Strickland D, Maloley PA *et al.* (1997) Possible association of a reduction in cardiovascular events with blood donation. Heart 78: 188–193

Miller M, Hutchins GM (1994) Hemochromatosis, multiorgan hemosiderosis, and coronary artery disease. JAMA 272: 231–233

Moe PJ (1970) Hemoglobin, hematocrit and red blood cell count in 'capillary' (skin-prick) blood compared to venous blood in children. Acta Paediatr Scand 59: 49

Mollison PL (1983) Blood Transfusion in Clinical Medicine. Oxford: Blackwell Scientific Publications

Monsen ER, Critchlow CW, Finch CA (1983) Iron balance in superdonors. Transfusion 23: 221–225

MRC (1944) Report prepared by a Sub-committee of the Blood Transfusion Research Committee. Fainting in blood donors. Br Med J i: 279

National Blood Data Resource Center (2001) Comprehensive report on blood collection and transfusion in the United

States in 1999. National Blood Data Resource Center, Bethesda, MD: AABB Press

National Blood Data Resource Center (2002) Comprehensive report on blood collection and transfusion in the United States in 2001. National Blood Data Resource Center, Bethesda, MD: AABB Press

Newman BH (1997) Donor reactions and injuries from whole blood donation. Transfusion Med Rev 11: 64–75

Newman BH (2003) Vasovagal reaction rates and body weight: findings in high- and low-risk populations. Transfusion 43: 1084–1088

Newman BH, Waxman DA (1996) Blood donation-related neurologic needle injury: evaluation of 2 years' worth of data from a large blood center. Transfusion 36: 213–215

Newman BH, Graves S (2001) A study of 178 consecutive vasovagal syncopal reactions from the perspective of safety. Transfusion 41: 1475–1479

Nightingale S, Wanamaker V, Silverman B et al. (2003) Use of sentinel sites for daily monitoring of the US blood supply. Transfusion 43: 364–372

Nouri A, Macfarlane TW, Mackenzie D (1989) Should recent dental treatment exclude potential blood donors? Br Med J 298: 295

Olynyk JK (1999) Hereditary haemochromatosis: diagnosis and management in the gene era. Liver 19: 73–80

Orlina AR, Josephson AM, McDonald BJ (1970) The post-storage viability of glucose-6-phosphate dehydrogenase-deficient erthrocytes. J Lab Clin Med 75: 930

Poles FC, Boycott M (1942) Syncope in blood donors. Lancet ii: 531

Popovsky MA, McCarthy S, Hawkins RE (1994) Pseudoaneurysm of the brachial artery: a rare complication of blood donation. Transfusion 34: 253–254

Salonen JT, Tuomainen TP, Salonen R et al. (1998) Donation of blood is associated with reduced risk of myocardial infarction. The Kuopio Ischaemic Heart Disease Risk Factor Study. Am J Epidemiol 148: 445–451

Salvatierra O Jr, Amend W, Vincenti F (1981) Pretreatment with donor-specific blood transfusion in related recipients with high MLC. Transplant Proc 13: 142–149

Sanchez AM, Schreiber GB, Bethel J et al. (2001) Prevalence, donation practices, and risk assessment of blood donors with hemochromatosis. JAMA 286: 1475–1481

Sarkodie F, Adarkwa M, Adu-Sarkodie Y et al. (2001) Screening for viral markers in volunteer and replacement blood donors in West Africa. Vox Sang 80: 142–147

Sazama K (1990) Reports of 355 transfusion-associated deaths: 1976 through 1985. Transfusion 30: 583–590

Schmidt PJ (1991) Blood donation by the healthy elderly. Transfusion 31: 681–683

Simon TL, Garry PJ, Hooper EM (1981) Iron stores in blood donors. JAMA 245: 2038–2043

Simon TL, Rhyne RL, Wayne SJ et al. (1991) Characteristics of elderly blood donors. Transfusion 31: 693–697

Skikne B (1984) Iron and blood donation. In: Blood Transfusion and Blood Banking. WL Bayer (ed.). London: WB Saunders

Stern A, Hage-Hamsten M, Sondell K (1995) Is allergy screening of blood donors necessary? Vox Sang 69: 114–119

Strauss RG (1989) Directed and limited-exposure donor programmes for children. In: Contemporary Issues in Pediatric Transfusion Medicine. RA Sacher and R Strauss (eds). Arlington, VA: Am Assoc Blood Banks, pp. 1–11

Streiff MB, Smith B, Spivak JL (2002) The diagnosis and management of polycythemia vera in the era since the Polycythemia Vera Study Group: a survey of American Society of Hematology members' practice patterns. Blood 99: 1144–1149

Stroncek DF, Rainer T, Sharon V et al. (2002) Sickle Hb polymerization in RBC components from donors with sickle trait prevents effective WBC reduction by filtration. Transfusion 42: 1466–1742

Sullivan JL (1981) Iron and the sex difference in heart disease risk. Lancet 1: 1293–1294

Sullivan KM, Storb R, Bucker CD (1989) Graft versus host disease as adoptive immunotherapy in patients with advanced hematologic neoplasms. N Engl J Med 320: 828–834

Thaler M, Shamis A, Orgad S (1989) The role of blood from HLA-homozygous donors in fatal transfusion-associated graft-versus-host disease after open-heart surgery. N Engl J Med 321: 25–28

Tomasulo PA, Anderson AJ, Paluso MB (1980) A study of criteria for blood donor deferral. Transfusion 20: 511–518

Trouern-Trend JJ, Cable RG, Badon SJ et al. (1999) A case-controlled multicenter study of vasovagal reactions in blood donors: influence of sex, age, donation status, weight, blood pressure, and pulse. Transfusion 39: 316–320

UKBTS/NIBSC Liaison Group (2001) Guidelines for the Blood Transfusion Services. London: HMSO

Wadsworth GR (1955) Recovery from acute haemorrhage in normal men and women. J Physiol (Lond) 129: 583

Winslow RM, Butler WM, Kark JA et al. (1983) The effect of bloodletting on exercise performance in a subject with a high-affinity hemoglobin variant. Blood 62: 1159–1164

Winslow RM, Monge CC, Brown EG et al. (1985) Effects of hemodilution on O_2 transport in high-altitude polycythemia. J Appl Physiol 59: 1495–1502

Worwood M (1980) Serum ferritin. In: Iron. Biochemistry and Medicine. A Jacobs (ed.). New York: Academic Press

Zuck TF, Cumming PD, Wallace EL (2001) Computer-assisted audiovisual health history self-interviewing. Results of the pilot study of the Hoxworth Quality Donor System. Transfusion 41: 1469–1474

2 Transfusion of blood, blood components and plasma alternatives in oligaemia

This chapter follows the development of transfusion as treatment in oligaemia from its early underpinnings through the Blundell's proof of principle using clinical trial methods to the current understanding of the physiology and pathology of blood loss. The modern approach to monitoring and managing blood loss with blood and components as well as with non-blood volume expanders is reviewed. Transfusion approaches for some special clinical settings such as in patients who refuse transfusion, burns, elective non-cardiac surgery, cardiac surgery and acute respiratory distress syndrome (ARDS) are discussed. Red cell substitutes (oxygen therapeutics) are discussed in Chapter 18.

History

Notes on the early history of transfusion

Intravenous injection. The work of William Harvey on the circulation of the blood provided the necessary climate for the trial of blood transfusion (Harvey 1628). In 1656, Christopher Wren, who at the age of 16 was assisted in dissections by Harvey's pupil Charles Scarburgh, infused morphia suspended in sack into the veins of a dog procured for him by the soon-to-be legendary physicist, Robert Boyle. Whether it was the narcotic or the Oxonian sherry suspension, the dog rapidly became lethargic. Following discussions with his Oxford colleagues, Wren subsequently tested the effects of several other intravenous substances. When Sprat (1667) wrote the early history of the Royal Society (of which Wren was one of the small group of founders) he wrote presciently of Wren and his work:

He was the first author of the Noble Anatomical experiment of injecting liquors into the veins of animals, an experiment now vulgarly known but long since exhibited by the meetings at Oxford. By this operation, divers creatures were immediately purged, vomited, intoxicated, killed or revived. Hence arose many new experiments and chiefly that of transfusing blood, which the Society has prosecuted in sundry instances that will probably end in extraordinary success.

Sprat (1667)

Extraordinary success did not come quickly. Blood transfusions to humans – although not from human donors – were first carried out later in the seventeenth century. These experiments are known more for the boldness of concept and the great skill with which they were carried out than for evidence of efficacy.

The first transfusion to a human. The first transfusion from an animal to a human was performed by Professor J. Denis with the help of a surgeon, Mr C. Emmerez, in France in June 1667 (see Chapter 10), and the first transfusion of this kind was performed in England in November of the same year by Lower and King (*Philosophical Transactions* 1667, p. 557).

Beginnings of modern transfusion

By the nineteenth century, physicians realized that the most dramatic effects that could be achieved with blood transfusion would likely be in the treatment of acute blood loss. Dr James Blundell, an obstetrician on the staff of the United Hospitals of St Thomas and Guy, is generally credited with performing the first human-to-human blood transfusion. Before he administered his first transfusion to a human, he had established two central principles: the first was that a dog that had been bled an otherwise lethal volume could be revived by a transfusion of dog's blood, and the second was that transfusion to a dog of even a small amount (114 ml) of the blood of another species (human) could be fatal (Blundell 1824).

Convinced that only human blood was suitable for transfusion to humans, Blundell began cautious experiments in humans, attempting transfusion only when the patient seemed beyond hope (Blundell 1818, 1824). Finally, he recorded a successful case in which a patient who had suffered a postpartum haemorrhage was transfused by means of a special syringe with some 8 oz (227 ml) of blood. The patient reported that 'she felt as if *life* were infused into her body' (Blundell 1829). One interesting footnote is Blundell's observation that the risk of transfusion approximated the risk of amputation of an extremity, a procedure with a significant mortality in the nineteenth century. The same comparison might be made today.

Blundell may not, in fact, have been the first physician to carry out a transfusion from one human to another. Schmidt recounts that Dr Philip Syng Physic almost certainly carried out such a transfusion in Philadelphia in 1795 (Schmidt 1968). No more than a reference in a footnote is known about the circumstances. In any case, Blundell deserves the main credit for initiating human transfusion because, through a remarkably modern approach, he performed careful preliminary experimental studies, established proof of principle, proceeded in humans only when risk seemed low and potential benefit high, and published full details of his work.

For those who desire a more thorough treatment of the subject, Starr (1998) has written a detailed and eloquent history of blood transfusion.

The response to blood loss

The response to acute blood loss results in very reproducible changes in numerous parameters including mean arterial pressure (MAP), central venous pressure (CVP), acute base deficit (ABD) and peripheral pulse and blood pressure. However, absolute values provide little help because of patient variability. The resting pulse and blood pressure of a well-conditioned athlete

may be well below the established 'norms', whereas an obese male with chronic obstructive pulmonary disease may have misleading 'elevation' of packed cell volume (PCV), CVP and blood pressure in the face of haemorrhage. In the clinical setting, the effects of acute haemorrhage may be confused with signs and symptoms connected with the cause of the haemorrhage – head trauma, crush injury or pain, for example. Moreover, it is seldom possible to estimate with precision the amount of blood that has been lost. However, the changes in the pulse, PCV, MAP and CVP can be extraordinarily informative. Studies of the effect of sudden loss of blood, produced by the venesection of volunteers, have provided valuable information about the effects produced by haemorrhage alone.

Circulatory effects of blood loss

In healthy adults, the loss of 430 ml of blood in 4 min produces only trivial effects on the circulation. As a rule no change in blood pressure or pulse rate takes place, although venous pressure may fall slightly and take more than 30 min to regain its initial level (Loutit et al. 1942).

In normal subjects the rapid withdrawal of about 1 l of blood often produces no fall in blood pressure as long as the subject remains supine, but if the subject sits up blood pressure may fall and even lead to loss of consciousness (Ebert et al. 1941; Wallace and Sharpey-Schafer 1941). The loss of 1500–2000 ml leads to a fall in right atrial pressure and a diminished cardiac output; the subject becomes cold, clammy and slightly cyanotic and may display air hunger (Howarth and Sharpey-Schafer 1947).

Changes in CVP reflecting right atrial pressure mirror changes in blood volume. A fall in CVP leads to a fall in cardiac output, which in turn leads to a fall in arterial pressure. These changes produce adrenergic stimulation, an increase in heart rate and force of contraction, constriction of the veins and venules, and regional increases in peripheral resistance, chiefly in the skin, muscles, kidney and gut (Skillman et al. 1967a). The increase in resistance is mainly precapillary, so that capillary pressure is reduced and plasma volume is restored at the expense of extracellular and intracellular fluid. If the inadequate peripheral flow continues, precapillary resistance ceases to respond to adrenergic stimulation, while the veins still respond so that irreversible shock with still further loss of fluid from the circulation ensues (Mellander and Lewis 1963; Skillman *et al.* 1967b).

Spontaneous restoration of blood volume

When healthy normal males sustain a sudden loss of about 1 l of blood, restoration of blood volume may take more than 3 days (Skillman *et al.* 1967c; Adamson and Hillman 1968). The rate at which PCV falls depends to some extent on the activity of the subject. In the experiments just referred to, subjects were encouraged to walk immediately after venesection and PCV had not fallen significantly at 10 h in four out of six subjects. The average plasma volume replacement at about 3 days was only 76%. On the other hand, in a series in which subjects rested in bed for 24 h after venesection, blood volume was usually restored at 36 h (Ebert *et al.* 1941). Even after the loss of as little as 0.5 l, only about one-half of the decrease in blood volume has been replaced at the end of 24 h (Pruitt *et al.* 1965). In summary, for at least 48 h after haemorrhage, the PCV alone is misleading as an index of the extent of acute blood loss in normal subjects.

Following acute haemorrhage, plasma protein concentration barely changes because protein transfers readily from the extravascular space to the plasma (Adamson and Hillman 1968).

Oligaemic shock

When the amount of blood lost rapidly is equivalent to 30% of the blood volume, a subject may develop oligaemic shock. The shock syndrome was defined graphically by the nineteenth century physician Samuel V. Gross (1872) as 'the rude unhinging of the machinery of life'. A more physiological if less elegant definition describes shock as 'loss of effective circulating blood volume which produces abnormal micro-circulatory perfusion and attendant cellular metabolic derangements' (Schumer 1974) or more simply as 'inadequate capillary perfusion' (Hardaway 1974). Shock may be classified further by aetiology as hypovolaemic, traumatic, cardiogenic, septic or anaphylactic.

Investigations carried out during the First World War showed that in 'wound (hypovolaemic) shock' blood volume was reduced and the severity of the clinical picture roughly paralleled the degree of reduction in blood volume (Keith 1919; Robertson and Bock 1919). In a landmark treatise in 1923, Walter B. Cannon concluded that shock on the battlefield most often resulted from intravascular volume deficits and should be treated by restoration of blood volume (Cannon 1923).

Assessment of the degree of haemorrhage

Except in the operating room, the amount of blood lost immediately is rarely obvious to the observer. Usually, the extent of bleeding has to be deduced from the nature of the injury that caused the haemorrhage, from the physical signs in the patient's cardiovascular system, from any evidence of impaired organ perfusion and from the patient's response to treatment of the oligaemia.

Estimates of blood loss

Assessment of haemorrhage around the site of injury. Swelling surrounding the area of the wound is due to loss of blood into the tissues and thus often indicates a gross reduction in circulating blood volume. In severe injuries without external blood loss there is a tendency to underestimate the amount of blood that has been lost into the tissues (Noble and Gregersen 1946).

Patients with wounds involving large muscles of the extremities frequently need transfusion of an amount of fluid equal to their initial blood volume. Continued loss of blood into the tissues appears to be important in bringing about the extensive loss of circulatory volume (Prentice *et al.* 1954). A single injury to the thigh may be associated with a blood loss of 2.5 l or more (Clarke *et al.* 1955). Perforating wounds of the chest or abdomen are frequently associated with considerable haemorrhage into the pleural or peritoneal cavities, and pelvic fractures often cause massive haemorrhage into retroperitoneal tissues.

In battle casualties in whom gross tissue disruption occurs, the size of the wound itself correlates fairly well with the degree of blood loss. Thus, Grant (1951) and Reeve found that for each area of tissue damage corresponding to the size of the patient's hand, a loss of 10% of the patient's blood volume should be assumed. Patients with extensive soft tissue injuries have a high death rate, often from pulmonary insufficiency. Good correlation exists between the general severity of the clinical picture and signs of disseminated intravascular coagulation (DIC), another marker of compromised tissue perfusion (String *et al.* 1971).

Oligaemia in 'accidental' haemorrhage. From 29 cases of 'accidental' (placental) haemorrhage in which plasma volume was estimated, Tovey and Lennon (1962) conclude that when the blood pressure has fallen by 20 mmHg or more and the pulse rate has risen to 100 or above, chances are at least 6:1 that the patient has suffered a loss of 30% or more of blood volume.

Blood loss at operation. Even operations associated with very little apparent blood loss may be accompanied by a decrease in circulating red cell volume. In a series of nine patients undergoing meniscectomy, red cell volume decreased on average by 7% from the day before operation until 3 days after operation. In the following week, a further fall of 2% occurred (Davies and Fisher 1958).

Measurement of blood volume changes after operative procedures has confirmed that volume decreases more than 'estimated blood loss'. For example, the average total blood loss associated with partial gastrectomy has been estimated at 1400 ml (Wiklander 1956). Of this volume, about 650 ml was lost at operation; an additional 300 ml was lost from the circulation in the next 24 h, and a further 450 ml in the following week. The loss determined by weighing swabs at operation was only about 70% of that determined from estimates of blood volume (Wiklander 1956). This observation agrees well with the finding that weighing of sponges at operation underestimates blood loss by 25%, partly as a result of evaporation of fluid from the sponges before weighing and partly due to bleeding into tissues that was not taken into account (Caćeres and Whittembury 1975).

Circulatory signs

The cardinal signs of oligaemia in non-medicated subjects are tachycardia, peripheral cooling and colour change (vasoconstriction), hypotension and a reduced jugular venous pressure. Medications such as beta-adrenergic antagonists (beta-blockers) or calcium channel blockers may interfere with interpretation of the compensatory mechanisms or response to therapeutic volume challenge. As acidosis develops and organ systems are compromised, respirations increase, urinary output falls and mental status deteriorates. Based on these signs, the American College of Surgeons has defined four classes of shock and provided fluid resuscitation guidelines for each (American College of Surgeons Committee on Trauma 1997).

Peripheral vasoconstriction. In subjects who have lost large amounts of blood, the skin remains cool, even after the subject has been lying for some time in reasonably warm surroundings. In subjects suffering from shock of diverse aetiology, toe temperature correlates with cardiac index (Joly and Weil 1969). Toe

temperature has been superseded by more sophisticated measures of peripheral vasoconstriction.

Hypotension does not occur if mild oligaemia is adequately compensated by tachycardia and vasoconstriction. Blood pressure is a reliable guide to the degree of hypovolaemia only if the patient's pressure before haemorrhage is known. A young woman with a systolic pressure of 90 mmHg may be perfectly well; in an elderly patient with arterial disease such a figure may represent severe circulatory decompensation.

Central venous pressure. Empty peripheral veins and low jugular venous pressure are features of poor circulatory filling. The right atrial pressure (central venous pressure, CVP) may be measured directly by cannulating the superior vena cava through a peripheral vein. The normal range of values is wide and the zero level (that of the right atrium) difficult to estimate consistently. It is usually taken at the angle of Louis in a patient propped up at an angle of 45°, and at the mid-axillary line in one lying flat, so that the level has to be moved as the patient's position changes. A single measurement of the CVP, therefore, has little value in assessing the degree of haemorrhage. Changes in CVP in response to circulatory refilling are, however, a valuable guide to the adequacy of therapy (Sykes 1963).

Confirmation of CVP line location is essential. Without radiological confirmation, only 64% of lines were found to be correctly positioned (Johnston and Clark 1972). Use of a pressure transducer can also establish catheter position without the need for a radiograph.

Left atrial pressure. The use of CVP measurements as a guide to cardiac performance or to circulatory filling rests on the assumption that the right and left ventricles function similarly. The right and left atrial pressures would thus be similar; at the very least, they could be expected to move in the same direction at the same time. In a number of circumstances, this underlying assumption may be false. Many cardiac disorders affect one side of the heart more than the other. In oligaemia, especially in the elderly, hypotension and tachycardia impair coronary perfusion, affecting mainly the performance of the left ventricle. Continued filling of the normally functioning right ventricle will thus overfill the left atrium and pulmonary oedema will result. There is a place, therefore, for measuring left atrial pressure itself. The least invasive method of doing so is to float a catheter through the superior vena cava, right atrium and right ventricle into the pulmonary artery as far as possible. The inflation of a balloon at the end of the catheter wedges it into a pulmonary capillary and the pressure is then recorded. Pulmonary capillary wedge pressure (PCWP) is a good indication of left atrial pressure (Swan *et al.* 1970). Although often helpful, PCWP need not be measured in every bleeding patient and unnecessary use is not without hazard. Placement of the Swan–Ganz catheter is associated with an increased risk of pulmonary embolism and retrospective studies suggest a negative impact on long-term survival. Its value is questionable in patients who are being ventilated with positive end-expiratory pressure (Lozman *et al.* 1974; Leading 1980).

Further uses of pulmonary artery catheters. Catheterization of the pulmonary artery is an essential step towards measuring cardiac output. If the catheter is fitted with a thermistor, the method of thermodilution may be used. Cardiac output computers, if primed with appropriate data, will derive other variables. For example, the systemic vascular resistance can be calculated if the cardiac output and blood pressure are known, and O_2 delivery if the arterial O_2 content is measured as well as cardiac output. Fibre optic oximeters have been incorporated into pulmonary artery catheters and can provide a continuous estimate of mixed venous O_2 saturation, a useful guide to the adequacy of tissue oxygenation (Armstrong *et al.* 1978).

Organ damage resulting from oligaemia

The combination of hypotension and arterial vasoconstriction causes a reduction of blood flow in most organs. The blood supply to some vital organs, notably heart, brain and kidneys, is protected to some extent by local vasodilatation ('autoregulation'), but severe oligaemia invariably leads to underperfusion. Impaired renal perfusion is associated with a low output of concentrated urine and renal failure may ensue if oligaemia is not corrected. Restoration of urine output to at least 0.5 ml/kg of body weight/min is one of the aims of resuscitation and one of the measures of success.

Cerebral and myocardial damage may also follow oligaemia, especially in elderly patients whose arteries are sclerotic (Weisel *et al.* 1978). Hepatic hypoperfusion

associated with severe hypovolaemia may determine the onset of jaundice in patients transfused with non-viable red cells in stored blood (see Chapter 11). Such patients may develop ischaemic hepatitis with striking elevation of ALT and lactate dehydrogenase (LDH), as well as glucose intolerance (Gitlin and Serio 1992).

Splanchnic vasoconstriction may, if prolonged, cause ischaemic damage to the intestinal mucosa, and toxic substances may be absorbed from the lumen of the bowel (Silverman 1991). Hypovolaemia may thus be complicated by endotoxaemia and systemic sepsis, now more commonly referred to as the systemic inflammatory response syndrome (SIRS); macrophages release cytokines, causing fever, generalized vasodilatation, hypotension and capillary leakage (ACCP-SCCM Consensus Conference 1992). Multiple organ failure, including the adult respiratory distress syndrome, may develop. Low pH within the gastric and colonic mucosal cells (pHi) has been used as a measure of the inadequacy of splanchnic perfusion (Silverman 1991) and gastric pHi can be measured by sampling saline from a balloon tonometer placed in the lumen of the stomach (Fiddian-Green 1991). Critically ill patients in whom gastric pHi was monitored and corrected at levels of pHi below 7.32 were more likely to survive than those who were resuscitated on the strength of cardiovascular monitoring alone (Gutierrez *et al.* 1992). On the other hand, the validity of this measurement as a true measure of intracellular pH has been questioned, and a small prospective study suggests that measurements of metabolic acidosis obtained from routine blood gas analysis yield the same information far more simply (Boyd *et al.* 1993).

Restoration of intravascular volume by blood, blood components and plasma alternatives

The goal of early volume replacement is to delay or prevent the chain of events that leads to irreversible shock. Early restoration of blood volume, reversal of acidosis and management of metabolic derangements can restore blood pressure and cardiac output temporarily, even in prolonged shock. Delay in treatment is usually fatal (Guyton and Hall 2005). In haemorrhagic shock, the main management strategies are the arrest of bleeding and the replacement of circulating volume. During much of the second half of the twentieth century, aggressive fluid administration was encouraged

(Shires *et al.* 1964; American College of Surgeons Committee on Trauma 1997). Over the last decade, however, this approach has been re-examined, at least in the pre-hospital setting when haemostasis has not been achieved. Intravenous fluids appear to improve haemodynamic indices in the short term, but most regimens also have adverse consequences on haemostatic mechanisms that may result in exacerbation of blood loss (Dries 1996). Bleeding may be worsened by injudicious fluid administration as a consequence of a dilutional coagulopathy and of clot disruption from increased blood flow, increased perfusion pressure and decreased blood viscosity. The clinical setting, for example uncontrolled haemorrhage or the presence of head trauma, may dictate the nature of the resuscitation solution(s), the volume that is administered and its timing in relation to definitive haemostasis.

Physiological considerations in fluid replacement

The aim of fluid replacement in the oligaemic patient is to provide an adequate supply of O_2 to the tissues. Oxygen delivery is calculated from the equations (Nunn and Freeman 1964a):

arterial delivery (ml/min)
= cardiac output (ml/min) × arterial O_2 content

$$(2.1)$$

arterial O_2 content (ml/dl)
= Hb concentration (g/dl) × ml O_2 carried/g Hb

$$(2.2)$$

If normal values are substituted in the equations above, a healthy adult male of 70 kg body weight will have an O_2 delivery of about 1000 ml/min. His basal O_2 consumption at rest, which is given by the equation:

O_2 consumption
= cardiac output × arteriovenous O_2 content difference

$$(2.3)$$

and will be about 250 ml/min. Fortunately evolution has blessed the O_2 delivery system with substantial reserve capacity. Provided that the cardiac output and arterial O_2 saturation are maintained within the normal range, a fair degree of anaemia can be tolerated.

There is some evidence that O_2 delivery may be enhanced by a moderate degree of acute normovolaemic anaemia. In dogs rendered acutely anaemic by the withdrawal of blood, and kept normovolaemic by the simultaneous infusion of dextran, calculated O_2 delivery peaked at an Hb level of 100 g/l, and fell below the pre-phlebotomy level at an Hb level of about 85 g/l. The apparent improvement in O_2 delivery was attributed to a fall in blood viscosity and a doubling of the cardiac output (Messmer *et al.* 1972). Subsequent human studies appeared to confirm these findings (Messmer 1987). However, Weiskopf and co-workers (1998), in a careful study of non-medicated volunteers, measured no rise and peak in O_2 delivery as the Hb declines and found that O_2 delivery begins to fall at a lower Hb value that is age and sex dependent (males = 70 g/l; females = 60 g/l). At lower Hb levels, when O_2 content is reduced, demand for O_2 is met by increased extraction of O_2. The mixed venous O_2 content then falls (Wilkerson *et al.* 1987). In chronic normovolaemic anaemia, the low arterial O_2 content is further compensated by a shift of the O_2 dissociation curve to the right.

Some organs normally extract more O_2 from the blood that perfuses them than do others. Thus, although the whole body arteriovenous O_2 content difference is normally 5 ml/dl at rest, corresponding to an extraction ratio of 25%, the heart normally extracts 55% of the O_2 from the blood it receives and the brain 35–40%. Substantial increases in coronary and cerebral blood flow will therefore be required to maintain O_2 delivery to the heart and brain in the presence of normovolaemic anaemia. In normovolaemic humans, cerebral blood flow rises when the PCV is reduced to 0.28 (Paulson *et al.* 1973). The reduction in blood viscosity that results from haemodilution of this order appears to be beneficial in patients with focal cerebral ischaemia (Kee and Wood 1984). Animal studies suggest that coronary blood flow increases out of proportion to the rise in cardiac output in normovolaemic anaemia (von Restorff *et al.* 1975; Biro 1982), but that the combination of severe acute anaemia with coronary stenosis results in myocardial ischaemia (Most *et al.* 1986; Biro *et al.* 1987; Levy *et al.* 1993). Studies of acute isovolaemic haemodilution confirm that reduction of circulating haemoglobin (Hb) concentration to 50 g/l in conscious healthy resting volunteers does not produce inadequate systemic O_2 delivery as measured by decreased O_2 consumption, increased lactate production or electrocardiographic changes (Leung *et al.* 2000); however, acute isovolemic anaemia slows human reaction time, degrades memory, increases heart rate and decreases energy level to a significant if subtle degree (Weiskopf *et al.* 2002).

The implications for the restoration of blood volume in oligaemic patients are that: first, it is crucial to maintain the cardiac output by prompt restoration of the circulating blood volume; second, a moderate degree of anaemia should be well tolerated at least in previously healthy subjects provided that normovolaemia is maintained; and third, in patients whose coronary or cerebral arteries are diseased, or whose cardiac reserves are already depleted, any diminution in the O_2 delivery may be damaging.

The rate of transfusion

As emphasized above, the primary aim in treating oligaemia is to maintain an adequate supply of O_2 to vital organs. Provided that the cardiac output is maintained, some degree of anaemia can be tolerated. Although cardiac output can be maintained and even increased with anaemia, it is not maintained with oligaemia. If haemorrhage is moderate or severe, restoring the circulating volume immediately with a rapid infusion of crystalloid or colloid is preferable to delaying resuscitation until blood has been crossmatched. The added risks of uncrossmatched blood (universal donor) are discussed elsewhere (see Chapters 10 and 11).

When it is necessary to transfuse a unit of blood in a few minutes or less, rapid transfusion is safe as long as the patient is carefully monitored. Very fast rates of transfusion cannot be attained by gravity infusion through a small cannula inserted in a peripheral vein. Methods of increasing the rate of flow are discussed below.

Technique of rapid transfusion

The internal bore of the cannula. This is an important factor in limiting the rate of flow. Kestin (1987) measured the flow rates generated through all the intravenous cannulae available in the UK using a test prescribed by the British Standards Institution (BSI 1972). Distilled or deionized water was run under a pressure of 10 kPa (76 mmHg) from a constant level tank at 22°C via 110-cm tubing with an internal bore of 4 mm. The mean flow obtained through 14-SWG cannulae of all brands was 286 ± 35 ml/min, whereas through 16-, 18- and 20-SWG cannulae it was 162 ± 35, 91 ± 17 and 54 ± 14 ml/min respectively. However, the internal bore of the cannula and not necessarily the gauge (outside diameter) is the critical factor.

The viscosity of the blood. Blood is more viscous than water. Under test conditions at room temperature, the flow of blood (PCV = 0.45) through cannulae is only 50–60% of the flow of water (Farman and Powell 1969). When blood was infused at constant pressure through needles of various bore sizes, raising the Hb concentration from 12.6 to 14.3 g/dl slowed the flow rate by about 10% (Chaplin and Chang 1955). As blood temperature drops, blood viscosity increases. Warming blood with a PCV of 0.42 from 10°C to 36°C doubles the rate of flow (Knight 1968).

Venous spasm. Infusing cold blood may cause local discomfort and venospasm, which will slow transfusion. The transfusion of warm blood or plasma may also induce venous spasm due to vasoconstrictor substances in plasma [see Mollison (1983), pp. 746–747]. In patients with peripheral circulatory failure due to oligaemia, the veins are constricted, so that the rate of flow of transfusion may be slower than is required. Local warming of the arm helps to relieve venous spasm, as does transdermal nitroglycerine applied as a patch distal to the infusion site (Wright *et al.* 1985). Despite the potential disadvantages, rapid transfusion of 1–2 units of blood taken straight from the refrigerator seems to be safe. Transfusion of large amounts of very cold blood is undesirable (see Chapter 15).

Positive pressure. Quadrupling the pressure gradient from a litre bag of 0.9% saline down an infusion set and cannula by enclosing the bag in a pressure cuff at 300 mmHg only doubles the flow rate through the cannula (Chen *et al.* 2002). The rather small increment in flow rate may be due both to the physics of flow through a tube and to the development of turbulence. When rapid transfusion is required, insertion of a large cannula is more efficacious than reliance on pressurizing the infusate through a smaller one. In practice, both pressurized infusion and large bore cannulae are used. Central venous cannulation with catheters of wide bore (for example, a pulmonary artery catheter of 8.5 gauge) is frequently performed in the management of severe haemorrhage, but a shorter 14-G peripheral catheter is usually more efficient. Pumps may be employed to transfuse or re-infuse blood at operations in which blood loss is massive, for example liver transplantation. Multiple infusion sites are commonly used as well.

How long to continue transfusion in oligaemia

Transfusion with appropriate fluids should be continued until haemostasis has been achieved and clinical evidence of hypovolaemia has resolved.

A rise in systolic pressure to 100 mmHg is not an indication for stopping the transfusion. A relatively small transfusion given to an injured person may produce considerable clinical improvement without fully restoring blood volume. Evans and co-workers (1944) made serial estimations of plasma volume in injured subjects with peripheral signs of circulatory failure. They noted that after a small transfusion, for example 500 ml of blood, blood pressure might rise and the patient might appear much improved. Nevertheless, blood volume remained low for as long as 4 days. During the intervening period, the patient might easily pass into shock again. Grant (1951) and Reeve suggested that the patient's blood volume should be raised to at least 80% of normal before taking a patient to operation. Most practitioners aim to return circulating volume to normal values if possible and if bleeding can be controlled. However, operation may be required at low circulatory volume if bleeding cannot be otherwise controlled. Global measures of organ perfusion such as base deficit and serum lactate may help guide fluid management during the first 24 h (Ivatury *et al.* 1996).

Failure to respond to transfusion

When an injured person's blood pressure fails to respond to transfusion, two situations should be considered immediately. First, the patient may still be losing blood, so that transfusion is not succeeding in restoring blood volume to an adequate level. Much later, infection may develop, so that the patient develops sepsis in addition to hypovolaemia. Operation should not be further delayed if the patient's condition does not improve after transfusion of a reasonable volume, as surgery may help to deal with both underlying causes. A third concern when patients fail to respond to volume challenge is a cardiogenic cause; in this situation, if acute pericardial tamponade is not the issue, non-operative management may be the most prudent course.

Overloading of the circulation

Although blood loss is commonly underestimated and circulatory overload of a patient who has lost blood through injury is unusual, volume overloading, characterized by engorgement of the neck veins and moist sounds on auscultation, does occur. Overloading is best prevented by close attention to the state of the patient's circulation. Frequent or continuous monitoring of central venous pressure provides the most reliable guide. The heart rate, arterial pressure, and core and peripheral temperatures can add helpful supplementary information about the degree of filling.

Choice of intravenous fluid in oligaemia: use of whole blood

A long-sanctified fallacy maintained that no other fluid is superior to whole blood in the treatment of haemorrhage, even with the proviso that blood, after storage in the cold for several weeks, contains membrane-modified, relatively inflexible, 2,3-DPG-depleted red cells that may be temporarily less effective than fresher red cells in delivering and releasing O_2 to the tissues (Klein 2003). No evidence supports this contention and its proponents appear to be dwindling. In any case, whole blood is not often available and rarely ordered even when it is.

Several factors oppose the routine use of whole blood. From a public health perspective, blood is a scarce resource and should not be used when the major requirement is volume replacement and when an adequate substitute is available. From a patient care perspective, blood transfusion involves many hazards, of which the transmission of human immunodeficiency virus (HIV) is but one (Chapters 11, 15 and 16). Because a degree of anaemia can be tolerated by most patients, moderate haemorrhage can usually be managed effectively by the infusion of a crystalloid or colloid solution. If haemorrhage is severe enough to require the transfusion of red cells, red cell concentrates combined with crystalloid or artificial colloid solutions may be more appropriate than transfusion of whole blood. Infusion of red cell concentrates in combination with albumin fractions, a rich man's reconstituted blood, has not been found superior to less expensive approaches to volume expansion (see below).

Whole blood still has its place in the treatment of massive haemorrhage. Many clinicians who treat rapidly bleeding patients agree with Schmidt (1978) that in hospital practice, a small but real need for whole blood exists. On the other hand, Lundsgaard-Hansen and co-workers (1978) issued 80% of units as packed cells and supplemented these units with modified fluid gelatin when treating large haemorrhages.

The need for plasma fractionation: the use of albumin

At present, plasma fractionation is driven by demand for two protein concentrates: albumin and immunoglobulin. Specific indications for the latter are well documented, whereas the need for albumin is a more controversial matter. Albumin is an effective plasma expander. An estimated 90–95% of infused albumin solution remains in the intravascular space (Payen *et al.* 1997). Normal colloid osmotic pressure is 28 mmHg and albumin accounts for 21.8 mmHg. Each gram of albumin attaches 18 g of water. However, fractionated human albumin is easily the most expensive volume expander available and several non-human-derived alternatives exist. Furthermore, the effect of albumin infusion varies significantly among patients and over time for any given patient (Schwartzkopff *et al.* 1980). Theoretical volume expansion of a 500-ml infusion of 4% albumin is approximately 400 ml. However, the effect is influenced by hydration status, endogenous albumin stores and accelerated albumin leakage into the extravascular space as a result of an underlying disease. In a prospective, randomized study of 475 patients admitted to an intensive care unit, albumin was found to offer no advantage over gelatin in terms of mortality, length of stay or incidence of pulmonary oedema or renal failure. Not surprisingly serum albumin levels were lower in the patients who received gelatin, although no clinical importance attaches to this observation (Stockwell *et al.* 1992a,b). A flawed meta-analysis has concluded that albumin administration may increase mortality in critically ill patients (Cochrane Injuries Group Albumin Reviewers 1998). However, this analysis included studies of albumin used for what might charitably be called uncommon indications as well as studies with small numbers of patients, so that the warning of possible increased risk when albumin is used as a volume expander may not be warranted. A more recent analysis of the Cochrane database that reviewed 57 trials and 3659 participants concluded that no single colloid solution is more effective or safe than any other (Bunn *et al.* 2003). A large randomized controlled trial in critically ill patients has confirmed the apparent equivalence of albumin and saline as resuscitation fluids (The SAFE Study Investigators 2004).

Infusions of saline: crystalloid or colloid?

Because delay is associated with the emergency provision of blood components, resuscitation guidelines generally recommend early infusion of universally available crystalloid or colloid solutions. Debate rages as to whether crystalloid or colloid is preferable in the initial management of haemorrhagic shock. The proponents of both views base their case on Starling's equation, which states that the flow of fluid outwards through the walls of the capillaries (J_v) is proportional to the hydrostatic pressure (P) gradient between the capillaries and the interstitial space and inversely proportional to the protein oncotic pressure (π) gradient, namely:

$$J_v = Kf(P_c - P_t) - \sigma(\pi_c - \pi_t) \qquad (2.3)$$

where P_c is capillary hydrostatic pressure; P_t is interstitial fluid hydrostatic pressure; π_c is plasma protein oncotic pressure; π_t is interstitial fluid oncotic pressure; Kf is the filtration coefficient representing the permeability of the capillary membrane to fluids; and σ is the reflection coefficient representing the permeability of the capillary membrane to proteins.

The protein concentration of plasma is normally considerably higher than that of interstitial fluid. It seems logical to suppose that infusions of albumin or of other substances of equal or greater molecular weight would, given normal capillary permeability, remain in the intravascular space longer than would saline, which diffuses throughout the extracellular compartment. Based on an understanding of Starling's law, colloid solutions have been developed and used for more than 70 years as volume expanders. Increasing osmotic pressure with colloidal products has remained an attractive theoretical premise for volume resuscitation. Colloids do increase osmotic pressure in clinical practice, but the effects are short-lived. Lower molecular weight colloids exert a large, if transient, initial osmotic effect, as the small molecules are rapidly cleared from the circulation. Larger molecules exert a smaller osmotic pressure, but one that is sustained longer. The main drawback to colloid therapy lies in pathological states with endothelial injury and capillary leak, precisely the clinical scenario in which colloids might be needed and are commonly given. The colloid solution may leak into the interstitium and exert an osmotic gradient, pulling additional water into the interstitium.

Four general types of colloid are available for clinical use. Albumin, the predominant plasma protein exerting some 80% of normal colloid osmotic pressure, remains the standard against which other colloids are compared (see Chapter 14). Dextrans of various molecular weights have been used to restore plasma volume and to prevent deep venous thrombosis in postoperative settings. Hydroxyethyl starch (HES), widely used as a plasma volume expander, provides equivalent plasma volume expansion to albumin, but has been shown to affect haemostasis and clotting assays. Although severe coagulopathies have been reported in sporadic cases, the newer HES formulations have not been shown to increase postoperative bleeding compared with albumin therapy, even in large doses (3 l per day). Gelatins have been used extensively in some European countries, but have never been licensed in the USA and have now been largely replaced by HES in other countries.

Measurements in rabbits have suggested that colloid solutions are more effective and persistent expanders of the plasma volume than is isotonic saline (Farrow 1967, 1977). In sheep that had about one-half of their blood volume removed, restoration of the left atrial pressure and cardiac output to baseline values with Ringer's lactate required the infusion of two and a half times the volume of the blood withdrawn, whereas a second similarly bled group needed only to have the shed blood returned to achieve the same result. The authors could find no evidence of pulmonary capillary damage after this degree of haemorrhage (Demling et al. 1980). In a study of elderly patients resuscitated with either HES or Ringer's lactate, together with packed red cells, much smaller volumes were required and a lower incidence of pulmonary oedema was observed in the group receiving colloid (Rackow et al. 1983). Despite the theoretical advantages compared with crystalloid therapy, these colloids have not been shown to decrease the risk of acute lung injury or to improve survival. The case for colloids has been summarized by Rady (1994).

An opposing case has also been presented. Several estimates of the protein concentration of pulmonary interstitial fluid have suggested that it is higher than in interstitial fluid elsewhere in the body (Staub 1974). In baboons that were subjected to haemorrhage and treated with either albumin or Ringer's lactate plus their own shed blood, pulmonary oedema was more frequent when albumin was used, and albumin appeared to be extravasated into the pulmonary tissue (Holcroft and Trunkey 1974; Lewis et al. 1979).

Numerous clinical studies support these animal findings. Virgilio and co-workers (1979) compared the results of infusing albumin and Ringer's lactate, both with packed red cells, in two groups of patients undergoing major vascular surgery. To achieve a pre-determined circulatory state and urine output, the patients who were given albumin required the infusion of smaller volumes than did those who were given crystalloid, but showed a higher incidence of pulmonary oedema. Moss and co-workers (1981) studied a series of young injured patients who were given washed red cells and Ringer's lactate, supplemented in one-half of the cases with albumin. No patient developed pulmonary oedema and the total volume of Ringer's lactate required to correct hypovolaemia was not reduced by the addition of protein (Pearl et al. 1988).

Clinical and experimental studies support the concept that haemorrhagic shock leads to a cellular insult that promotes interstitial fluid expansion at the expense of the plasma volume after successful control of haemorrhage. This expansion of interstitial fluid is associated with plasma protein reduction; the degree of hypoproteinaemia is directly related to the shock insult as measured by a systolic pressure below 80 mmHg and by the number of transfusions required during phase I. During the interstitial fluid expansion period, the percentage of protein exiting the plasma volume is below normal so that the interstitia fluid protein accumulates because even less protein returns to the plasma space. During the subsequent mobilization phase, the plasma proteins increase progressively as the interstitial fluid space contracts. This increase in the plasma proteins occurs when the percentage of extravascular albumin flux is actually increased so that the mechanism for increased plasma proteins must reflect an even greater increase in the protein flux out of the interstitial fluid space into the plasma. The supplementation of the resuscitation regimen with any colloid forces an even greater amount of colloid flux from the plasma into the interstitial fluid during the fluid sequestration phase and prolongs the re-entry of proteins from the interstitial fluid space into the plasma during the subsequent mobilization phase. This phenomenon is associated with multiple adverse effects on organ function and coagulation and an increase in the mortality rate (Lucas and Ledgerwood 2003).

In the face of such conflicting evidence, conclusions are difficult to draw. The human studies were conducted on widely differing groups of patients, often involved different measurements, and all had different endpoints. In a few instances, they seem designed to reinforce the preconceived ideas of the workers concerned. The results of animal studies are also at variance, and, illuminating though such studies may be, are not necessarily applicable to human subjects. A landmark randomized study of resuscitation involving nearly 7000 critically ill patients found that 4% albumin and normal saline were associated with equivalent overall mortality in a heterogeneous population of patients in the intensive care unit (The SAFE Study Investigators 2004). Subgroup analyses revealed no significant differences between patients who received saline and those who received albumin, but in the 1126 trauma patients, albumin was associated with a trend towards increased mortality, and among the 1218 patients with severe sepsis, albumin was associated with a trend towards reduced mortality. Both findings merit further study.

It seems reasonable to conclude that in previously fit young patients, timely restoration of the blood volume is more important than how the restoration is accomplished, whether with a colloid or a crystalloid solution. Clinical judgement, convenience and cost should dictate the choice of solution infused. Despite the theoretical advantages compared with crystalloid therapy, colloid solutions have not been shown to decrease the risk of acute lung injury or to improve survival. Most experts agree that when crystalloid solutions are used, the volume infused should equal at least three times the estimated volume of shed blood, although dilution kinetics depend on the specific solutions used (Drobin and Hahn 2002). In the SAFE study, the ratio of the volume of albumin to the volume of saline administered over the first 4 days was only 1:1.4 (The SAFE Study Investigators 2004). In the elderly or in patients with poor renal or cardiac function, it may be prudent to avoid massive infusions of saline as well as rapid infusions of a highly concentrated (25%; 12.5 g of albumin in 50 ml of buffered saline with an oncotic pressure of 100 mmHg) albumin solution that might lead to cardiac decompensation (Roberts and Bratton 1998). Characteristics of commonly used crystalloid and colloid solutions are found in Table 2.1.

The Advanced Trauma Life Support (ATLS) Programme for Physicians, initiated in the USA and adopted by at least 15 other countries, directs attention to the management of patients in the first 'golden' hour after injury when a high proportion of deaths occurs and when proper care might be expected to improve outcome. The ATLS protocols on hypovolaemia include guidelines on the clinical assessment of the degree of haemorrhage and advocate aggressive fluid replacement with crystalloid (2000 ml for an adult, 20 ml/kg for children), supplemented by red cells, if necessary, infused through two large-bore (14-G) cannulae placed peripherally (American College of Surgeons Committee on Trauma 1997).

Infusions of hypertonic saline

Infusions of small volumes (about 4 ml/kg body weight) of hypertonic solutions (7.2–7.5% sodium chloride) over a short period (2 min) have been used in the initial resuscitation of both patients and experimental animals with hypovolaemic shock since 1980 (Kramer et al. 1986; Holcroft et al. 1987). Dramatic instantaneous improvements in cardiac output, arterial pressure, acid–base balance and urine flow, persisting for a few hours, have been observed. Hypertonic solutions produce their beneficial effects by expanding the circulating volume at the expense of the intracellular volume. Several studies have shown that the efficiency of hypertonic saline may be enhanced by the addition of dextran (Wade et al. 2003). Hypertonic saline solutions, with or without supplementary colloid, appear to have a place in the immediate management of an injured patient; an infusion may be started at the site of the accident before the patient is removed to hospital (see Messmer 1988). An early study found a survival advantage for patients who required surgery, and the hypertonic saline dextran group appeared to have fewer complications (Mattox et al. 1991). Multicentre trials, however, comparing lactated Ringer's solution and hypertonic saline with dextran, fail to show convincing overall differences in survival. The advantages of hypertonic saline resuscitation include its haemodynamic effects and its effects on lowering intracranial pressure in brain-injured patients. Recently, multiple studies have suggested further benefits in modulating the inflammatory response that occurs during shock. Unfortunately, analyses of controlled trials do not provide guidance. A meta-analysis in the Cochrane database concludes from an analysis of 12 studies of patients with trauma burns

Table 2.1 Characteristics of selected resuscitation fluid.

Fluid	Fluid compartment	Osmolarity (mOsM/l)	pH	Na⁺ (meq/l)	Cl⁻ (meq/l)	K⁺ (meq/l)	Mg²⁺ (meq/l)	Ca²⁺ (meq/l)	Dextrose (g/l)	Buffer
Blood										
Plasma	Intravascular	308	7.4	140	100	4	0	0	0–4	Protein; bicarbonate
Crystalloid										
0.9% saline	Extracellular	308	5	154	0	0	0	0	None	None
Lactated Ringer's solution	Extracellular	275	6.5	130	109	4	0	3	0	Lactate
Plasmalyte-A	Extracellular	294	7.4	140	98	5	3	0	0	Acetate; gluconate
Normosol-r	Extracellular	295	5.5–7.0	140	98	5	3	0	0	Acetate; gluconate
7.0% saline	Extracellular	2396	5	1197	1197	5	3	0	0	None
5% dextrose in water	Extracellular	252	4	0	0	0	0	0	50	None
Colloid										
5% albumin	Intravascular	309	6.4–7.4	130–160	130–160	<1	0	0	0	Sodium bicarbonate, sodium hydroxide. Or acetic acid
25% albumin	Intravascular	312	6.4–7.4	130–160	130–160	<1	0	0	0	Sodium bicarbonate, sodium hydroxide. Or acetic acid
Frozen plasma	Intravascular	300	Variable	140	110	4	0	0	0–4	Protein; bicarbonate
6% hetastarch	Intravascular	310	5.5	154	154	0	0	0	0	None
10% pentastarch	Intravascular	326	5	154	154	0	0	0	0	None
Dextran 40	Intravascular	311	3.5–7.0	154	154	0	0	0	0	None
Dextran 70	Intravascular	310	3.0–7.0	154	154	0	0	0	0	None
Oxypolygelatin	Intravascular	200	7.4	155	100	0	0	1	0	None

Adapted from Committee on Fluid Resuscitation for Combat Casualties (1999).

or surgery that insufficient data exist to recommend between hypertonic and isotonic saline (Bunn *et al.* 2002; Kwan *et al.* 2003).

Hypertonic saline resuscitation may be most useful in the pre-hospital setting. A report from the US Institute of Medicine analysed issues with crystalloid resuscitation using lactated Ringer's solution and concerns regarding colloid resuscitation. The report recommended a single bolus (4 ml/kg) of hypertonic saline as the initial resuscitation measure for military casualties (Committee on Fluid Resuscitation for Combat Casualties 2003). Hypertonic saline is currently not approved by the US Food and Drug Administration.

Plasma alternatives (substitutes)

The immediate effect of blood transfusion in haemorrhage derives mainly from the sustained increase in blood volume that it produces. Bayliss (1919) showed that a fluid that contained colloids with an osmotic pressure similar to that of plasma proteins could be used as a substitute for blood. Plasma is a complex solution containing numerous lipids, proteins, hormones, electrolytes and functions; solutions designed to restore or sustain blood volume should probably be referred to as 'plasma alternatives,' but as the name 'plasma substitute' has gained widespread acceptance, the terms will be used interchangeably.

Many substances have been tried as plasma substitutes but not one of these has entirely fulfilled the theoretical requirements. For example, gum arabic, introduced by Bayliss, fell into disrepute because it was found to be stored in the tissues. Human serum albumin has been widely used as a plasma substitute since the Second World War. Characteristics of albumin plasma protein fractions are discussed in Chapter 14.

The main qualities required of a plasma substitute are: (1) retention in the circulation for relatively long periods after infusion; (2) minimal risk of allergic reactions; (3) freedom from unwanted side-effects, including coagulopathy and transmission of infection; (4) complete metabolism after clearance from the circulation; (5) immunological compatibility; (6) long shelf-life under practical storage conditions; and (7) reasonable cost. No product providing all of these features is available.

A problem that arises with all artificial colloids is that, unlike albumin, they are polydisperse, composed of mixtures of molecules of widely varying size and molecular weight. Ideally, a preparation should contain no molecules of molecular weight below 70 kDa, as these will be rapidly excreted by the kidney. On the other hand, to ensure that only a small proportion of such molecules are present, it may be necessary to accept some molecules with a molecular weight greater than 250 kDa.

Size counts. In describing the average molecular weight of preparations that contain molecules of widely varying size, it makes a substantial difference whether one gives the number average ($\overline{M}_n$) or weight average ($\overline{M}_w$).

($\overline{M}_n$) is obtained by dividing the total weight of all molecules present by the total number of molecules. ($\overline{M}_w$) is obtained by summing the products of the weights of all molecules of a particular size multiplied by their molecular weight and dividing the sum by the total weight of all the molecules. For mixtures of different molecular weight, ($\overline{M}_w$) is always greater than ($\overline{M}_n$) and the ratio ($\overline{M}_w$)/($\overline{M}_n$) gives a good measure of the degree of scatter of molecular weights in the mixture. Values of $\overline{M}_w$ and ($\overline{M}_n$) for dextran and gelatin preparations provided in this chapter are either taken from the monograph by Gruber (1969) or have been obtained from manufacturers.

Clinical dextran

Dextrans are polydisperse glucose polymers produced by bacteria grown on sucrose-containing media. Commercial dextran preparations can be stored at room temperature. Dextrans are not used widely in the USA where they have been generally supplanted by HES and albumin solutions.

Two preparations of clinical dextran are commonly used, namely dextran 70 ($\overline{M}_w$ 70 kDa, $\overline{M}_n$ 39 kDa) and dextran 40 ($\overline{M}_w$ 40 kDa, $\overline{M}_n$ 25 kDa). The effects on the plasma volume of rabbits of these two dextrans, and also of dextran 110, modified fluid gelatin and a 'plasma protein (albumin) preparation', were compared by Farrow (1967, 1977). The main conclusions were as follows: the expansion of plasma volume depends mainly upon the weight of dextran in the circulation and is not directly related to the molecular weight of the preparation. However, in terms of maintenance of expanded plasma volume, the average molecular weight of the infused dextran is very important because of the rapid excretion of small molecules. Dextran 40 is supplied as a 10% solution, whereas other dextran preparations are supplied as 6% solutions, so that for equivalent volumes the immediate effect of dextran 40 is considerably greater; the infusion of a volume equivalent to 22% of the rabbit's plasma volume produces an immediate increase of about 35%. Nevertheless, the effect is maintained for only a few hours. Higher molecular weight dextrans tend to aggregate red cells *in vitro*, which can cause some confusion during compatibility testing (see below). Compared with dextran 110, dextran 70 has the advantage of producing negligible red cell rouleaux formation, but the duration of plasma volume expansion is sacrificed and the material remains effective for only about 24 h, whereas at the end of this period dextran 110 continues to produce some increase in plasma volume. Plasma protein fraction produces a much smaller increase in plasma volume than an equivalent volume of 6% dextran, but the effect is well maintained. Physiogel has a very short survival in the circulation, similar to that of dextran 40 and is therefore not particularly effective as a plasma volume expander.

Dextran 40 as a plasma volume expander is contraindicated in the treatment of shock, because it may obstruct the renal tubules (Rush 1974). Similarly, the infusion of large amounts of dextran 40 in patients who already have slight impairment of renal function may precipitate acute renal failure; six cases were reported by Feest (1976), who advised that not more than 1 l per day should be given and that if urinary output falls, the infusions should be stopped and the patient given diuretics and a high fluid intake.

More recently, a 3% solution of dextran 60 (molecular weight 60 kDa) has been introduced in Europe. Despite its low concentration of dextran, dextran 60 seems to be an effective plasma substitute. For example, in a small, randomized study of patients undergoing aortic surgery, and receiving fluid replacement of red cells with either Ringer's lactate or 3% dextran 60, almost three times the volume of crystalloid was needed to achieve adequate circulatory filling with Ringer's lactate in comparison with the dextran solution (Dawidson *et al.* 1991).

Allergic reactions to dextran

Many types of clinical dextran are capable of acting as antigens in humans. Moreover, anti-dextrans may be found in the serum of individuals who have never received dextran infusions (Kabat and Berg 1953).

The sera of elderly people and of patients with inflammatory disease of the intestinal tract may contain large quantities of dextran and reactive antibodies of the immunoglobulin G (IgG) class, suggesting that dextran may be ingested in food or produced by microorganisms in the gut (Palosuo and Milgrom 1980).

Severe reactions to dextran infusions are confined to individuals who have high titres of IgG anti-dextran before they receive any dextran parenterally (Hedin and Richter 1982). The clinical manifestations result from the formation of immune complexes between the dextran infused and the antibodies already present (Hedin *et al.* 1979). The inhibition of immune complex formation by a hapten (dextran 1) prevents severe dextran-induced anaphylactic reactions (Messmer *et al.* 1980). The routine use of dextran 1 immediately before the infusion of dextran 70 or dextran 40 has been associated with a reduction in the reported incidence of severe reactions in Sweden (from 22 per 100 000 units between 1975 and 1979 to 1.2 per 100 000 units between 1983 and 1985) (Ljungstrom *et al.* 1988), although cases continue to be reported (Berg *et al.* 1991).

Unwanted side-effects of dextrans

Abnormal bleeding. Dextran may interfere with haemostasis, apparently by affecting platelet function. A fall in factor VIII levels was observed when as little as 500 ml of 6% dextran was given to 16 volunteers; no such change occurred in three others who were given normal saline (Aberg *et al.* 1979). These observations have led many authorities to advise that the total dosage of dextran administered should not exceed 1.5 g/kg, i.e. about 1.5 l of 6% solution for a 70-kg patient. However, some clinicians have given twice this amount to patients who are undergoing elective orthopaedic surgery, with no apparent ill effects. The platelet counts were lowered in these patients but factor VIII levels were unchanged (Bergmann *et al.* 1990). Dextran has been reported to have fibrinolytic properties that may contribute to its anticoagulant effects (Eriksson and Saldren 1995).

Interference with crossmatching. The tendency of dextran to cause rouleaux formation increases with molecular weight; with a molecular weight of 60 kDa, a concentration of 2% is needed, but with a molecular weight of 270 kDa, only 0.4% (Thorsen and Hint

1950). Despite the wide range of molecular weights in dextran preparations, the infusion of presently available preparations does not lead to rouleaux formation in tests with untreated red cells. On the other hand, if enzyme-treated cells are used, even infusions of dextran 40 can lead to intense aggregation. When the possibility exists that large amounts of dextran will be administered, blood should be taken for cross-matching before the infusion is begun.

Gelatin

Gelatins are prepared from bovine collagen treated with alkali and suspended in aqueous solution. Preparations of a molecular size large enough to be well retained in the circulation do not remain fluid at low temperatures, a serious disadvantage in a preparation that is essentially needed for emergency conditions. The $T_{1/2}$ of injected modified fluid gelatin, such as that of dextran 40, was found to be 2–3 h compared with 6 h for dextran 60 and HES (Ring *et al.* 1980).

Two types of gelatins that remain fluid under normal ambient temperatures are available (Saddler and Horsey 1987). In all gelatin preparations, the range of molecular weights is wide; about 70% of molecules are below the renal threshold.
1 *Succinylated gelatin (modified fluid gelatin)*, for example Physiogel, Plasmagel, Gelofusine (4% in electrolyte solution), $(\overline{M}_w)$ 35 kDa, $(\overline{M}_n)$ 22.6 kDa;
2 *Urea-linked gelatin*, supplied as Haemaccel (3.5% in electrolyte solution), $(\overline{M}_w)$ 35 kDa, $(\overline{M}_n)$ 24 kDa.

Gelatin-induced volume expansion lasts about 3 h in healthy subjects but may be reduced in patients with sepsis (Salmon and Mythen 1993). The urea-linked gelatins contain high concentrations of calcium, so they must be used cautiously when infused with citrated blood components or clotting may occur. As mentioned below, allergic reactions seem to be somewhat more common after gelatin than after other plasma substitutes.

Perhaps the greatest advantage of modified fluid gelatin over other plasma substitutes is its apparent lesser tendency to contribute to bleeding. Compared with dextran and HES, gelatins have only a slight effect on platelets; whereas both dextran and HES lengthen the partial thromboplastin time, gelatin has no effect (Harke *et al.* 1976). In experiments on irradiated thrombocytopenic dogs that were subjected to rapid haemorrhage of 25 ml of blood per kilogram,

replaced either by oncotically equivalent volumes of 15 ml/kg of 6% dextran or 4% modified fluid gelatin, the output of red cells into the thoracic duct lymph was three times greater in three out of six dogs treated with dextran, but was no greater than before bleeding in the dogs treated with gelatin (Lundsgaard-Hansen 1978). Furthermore, in a controlled prospective study of patients undergoing elective surgery, in those patients receiving 1000 ml of 6% dextran 70, bleeding times postoperatively were 50 s greater than preoperatively, whereas in patients receiving 1500 ml of 4% modified fluid gelatin, the increase was insignificant (3.8 s). Three patients survived after receiving more than 10 l of modified fluid gelatin within 24 h (Tschirren *et al.* 1973).

Hydroxyethyl starch

Hydroxyethyl starch (HES) is a modified natural polymer that has been used frequently for plasma volume expansion in trauma and surgery. Because native starches are rapidly hydrolysed by [α-]amylase, commercially available HES preparations are extremely polydisperse polymers of natural amylopectin, chemically modified by hydroxyethylation at the glucose subunit carbon atoms (C2, C3 or C6). The molar substitution (moles of hydroxyethyl residues per mole of glucose subunits), the pattern of hydroxyethylation (C2/C6 ratio) and the *in vivo* mean molecular weight $(\overline{M}_w)$ are important characteristics that affect the *in vivo* function of different preparations. The higher the molar substitution and C2/C6 ratio, the slower the starch is metabolized. $\overline{M}_w$ is less important. The physicochemical characteristics of HES solutions are related to different safety profiles of various HES types with respect to coagulation and renal function. In particular, after the repeated administration of certain HES solutions with high MS and, to a lesser extent, a higher mean $\overline{M}_w$, large molecules may accumulate in plasma because of decelerated enzymatic degradation. Macromolecules that accumulate in plasma are known to decrease plasma concentrations of coagulation factor VIII, von Willebrand factor (VWF) and ristocetin cofactor, although the pathogenetic mechanism responsible for the adverse effect on factor VIII/VWF complex is not fully understood (Treib *et al.* 1999). Some of the older, less readily metabolized HES products reportedly lead to deterioration of renal function.

In the US, HES is supplied as a 6% solution in 0.9% saline ($\overline{M}_w$ 450 kDa, $\overline{M}_n$ 65 kDa), a 5% solution, and 6% HES in balanced electrolyte solution. A variety of other formulations are available in Europe and other countries (Dieterich 2003). As far as initial retention in the circulation is concerned, HES appears to be similar to dextran 70 [Gruber (1969), p. 140], although small amounts of HES tend to persist in the circulation for long periods (see below).

HES has a relatively low tendency to cause allergic reactions. In one study, only eight untoward reactions were observed in just over 10 000 recipients; only one of the reactions was of a severe anaphylactic type (see below).

Like dextran, HES interferes with blood coagulation, although to a lesser extent (Karlson *et al.* 1967). Coagulopathy resulting from HES administration is well documented for high-molecular-weight, highly substituted HES solutions (Treib *et al.* 1996). Particular concern has been expressed about reports of increased bleeding in patients who undergo open-heart surgery, especially as cardiopulmonary bypass independently induces a decline in platelet von Willebrand receptor glycoprotein IB. Some centres add 6% HES to the pump prime solution. In a review of 444 patients with coronary artery bypass graft (CABG), blood loss at 4 and 24 h was significantly increased in the 234 patients who received intraoperative HES (Knutson *et al.* 2000). A meta-analysis that included 653 patients arrived at the same conclusion (Wilkes *et al.* 2001).

A variety of other HES solutions that differ greatly in their pharmacological properties exist worldwide. Slowly degradable high-molecular-weight HES 450/0.7 and medium-molecular-weight HES 200/0.62 have a high *in vivo* molecular weight and are eliminated slowly via the kidneys. As a result, these starches have a relatively long-lasting volume effect. When higher volumes (> 1500 ml) are infused, large molecules accumulate in the plasma. This can result in bleeding complications due to decreased factor VIII/von Willebrand factor, platelet function defects, incorporation into fibrin clots and an unfavourable effect on rheological parameters. Rapidly degradable medium-molecular-weight HES 200/0.5 or low-molecular-weight HES 70/0.5 is quickly split *in vivo* into smaller, more favourable molecule sizes, resulting in faster renal elimination, shorter volume effect and fewer adverse effects on coagulation and rheological parameters. For historical and marketing reasons, only slowly

degradable, high-molecular-weight HES (480/0.7) is available in the US. In Europe, a large variety of HES solutions are available, dominated by medium-molecular-weight, easily degradable HES (200/0.5). HES 130/0.4, a recently developed solution, was especially designed to minimize influence on coagulation (Franz *et al.* 2001). Because of the availability of newly developed starches, it is important to be aware of the pharmacological properties of HES and the advantages/disadvantages of the individual preparations (see Treib *et al.* 1999).

HES is commonly used to increase the yield of granulocytes from donors giving blood via cell separators (see Chapter 17).

Comparisons between plasma substitutes

Comparisons may be made on the grounds of retention in the circulation, incidence of allergic reactions, unwanted side-effects, such as interference with platelet function, catabolism and excretion from the body, and cost.

1 Dextran 70 and HES appear to be retained about equally well, but gelatin preparations, with smaller molecular weights, are excreted more rapidly.

2 All plasma substitutes have been associated with allergic reactions. In a prospective survey, reported in 1977, the incidence of reactions of all kinds, from skin symptoms alone at one extreme to cardiac arrest at the other, was 0.69% for dextran 60/75; 0.007% for dextran 40; 0.085% for HES; 0.115% for gelatin; and 0.014% for plasma protein solutions (either whole serum or albumin). About one-quarter of the reactions were life threatening; the highest incidence was found with gelatin solutions (0.039%), the next with dextran 60/75 (0.017%), then HES (0.006%) followed by plasma protein solutions (0.004%), with dextran 40 last with 0.002% (Ring and Messmer 1977).

3 Gelatin is less likely than the other two plasma substitutes to interfere with platelet function (as is HES molecular weight 130 000) and thus less likely to provoke bleeding.

4 Gelatin is rapidly catabolized, and dextran is also completely broken down, but some doubts remain about HES, which, in any case, tends to persist for long periods in the circulation. In volunteers infused with 7 ml/kg of HES or dextran 60, after 17 weeks the plasma HES concentration was still 1% of the post-

infusion level, whereas after 4 weeks, dextran was undetectable (Boon *et al.* 1977).

Red cell substitutes

Synthetic and Hb-based O_2 carriers (blood substitutes, red cell substitutes, O_2 therapeutic) are discussed in Chapter 18.

Transfusion in special clinical settings

Massive transfusion

A transfusion is conventionally regarded as massive when a volume equivalent to the patient's normal blood volume is given within 24 h. This definition is clearly arbitrary. The complications of this syndrome, bleeding, hypothermia, acidosis and a variety of electrolyte derangements, may occur when one-half of this volume is given over a few hours or when several blood volumes are replaced over a period of days (Rutledge *et al.* 1986).

The clinical problems that arise in massively transfused patients are due first to the condition that caused the haemorrhage, and second to the effect of replacing normal whole blood with stored citrated blood, possibly supplemented by plasma substitutes. Although a detailed consideration of clinical conditions associated with haemorrhage is beyond the scope of this book, some of these conditions, for example disseminated intravascular coagulation and sepsis, produce effects that may be attributed to the massive transfusion.

Some of the consequences of replacing large volumes of the patient's blood with similar volumes of stored citrated blood are as follows:

1 There is a shift to the left in the O_2 dissociation curve, because stored red cells have a diminished 2,3 DPG content (see Chapter 9). This may be one of the few situations in which the other compensatory mechanisms in the O_2 transport system have been maximized and red cell O_2 affinity becomes clinically important.

2 There may be direct toxic effects from citrate as well as dangerous changes in electrolytes and in plasma pH if infusion of plasma-containing components approaches 1 unit every 5 min (see Chapter 15).

3 There may be a precipitous fall in the recipient's body temperature, which may reach dangerous levels if blood is transfused straight from the refrigerator.

Furthermore, viscosity increases as blood cools, so that warming blood will facilitate the flow of the transfusion. The current standard of care is to warm blood components during massive transfusion.

4 Microaggregates from stored blood may be transfused into the recipient (see Chapter 15).

5 Dilutional thrombocytopenia occurs as platelets do not survive in stored blood. Moreover, the residual population of the patient's own platelets may be damaged. Clinically important dilution of labile clotting factors such as factors V and VIII occurs much less frequently (Counts *et al.* 1979; Ciavarella *et al.* 1987).

A haemorrhagic state following massive transfusion

Adults transfused with large amounts of stored blood are at risk for excessive bleeding. Abnormal bleeding associated with thrombocytopenia has been observed after transfusions of volumes of stored blood as small as 5 l (Stefanini *et al.* 1954; Krevans and Jackson 1955). In a later series of 27 patients with major trauma, massive gastrointestinal haemorrhage or ruptured aortic aneurysm, who received an average of 33 units of blood, eight developed a haemostatic abnormality within 48 h of admission. Thrombocytopenia, most frequently due to the loss of large numbers of the patient's own platelets from the circulation and replacement with platelet-poor stored blood, was the most important factor in causing the haemostatic abnormality seen in massively transfused patients (Counts *et al.* 1979).

If dilution of platelets alone was responsible for abnormal bleeding in massively transfused patients, one might expect that, first, every patient given a transfusion of predictable volume would bleed, and that second, bleeding could be suppressed by the prophylactic administration of platelets. However, even although thrombocytopenia and prolongation of the prothrombin time occur regularly in massively transfused patients (Leslie and Toy 1991), abnormal bleeding does not. In a prospective study of 33 patients, who were transfused with approximately 20 units of modified whole blood (range 12–41 units), only six developed abnormal bleeding (Reed *et al.* 1986); 17 of the 33 patients were given 6 units of prophylactic platelets, while a control group of 16 received 2 units of fresh-frozen plasma (FFP) for every 12 units of blood transfused. Although all of the patients developed thrombocytopenia, the platelet count in the two groups did not differ; the frequency of abnormal bleeding was identical (three patients per group). Only one out of the six patients who bled responded promptly to further platelet transfusion. The authors concluded that platelet consumption as a result of the injuries necessitating massive transfusion accounted for the abnormal bleeding seen in the other five.

Inadequate and delayed transfusion, not massive transfusion itself, may be responsible in part for the development of a haemorrhagic diathesis (Collins 1987). This view is supported by a study of 36 patients, which found no correlation between the degree of coagulopathy and the volume of blood transfused, but demonstrated that the longer the patients remain hypotensive after severe haemorrhage, the more severe the ensuing coagulopathy (Harke and Rahman 1980).

In addition, the hypothermia that results from massive transfusion, and from the injury or surgery that necessitated it, may induce coagulopathy (Iserson and Huestis 1991). Platelet dysfunction, reversible on rewarming, has been demonstrated in hypothermic, massively transfused baboons and in normal subjects (Valeri et al. 1987; Michelson et al. 1994). In a retrospective study of 45 injured patients who required massive transfusion, those who were hypothermic and acidotic developed abnormal bleeding despite adequate blood, plasma and platelet replacement (Ferrara et al. 1990).

To best guard against a haemorrhagic state caused by massive transfusion, therefore, transfusion should be prompt and of adequate volume, and both the blood and the patient should be warmed. Coagulation should be monitored and deficiencies corrected. A Consensus Development Conference recommended that platelets should be transfused only when the platelet count is 50×10^9 or less (NIH 1987). The use of a thrombo-elastograph (TEG) to detect abnormalities of coagulation in massively transfused patients has been reported to reduce the demands for blood products by 30% (Spiess 1994); however, use of TEG is operator dependent and its use has not been validated.

Indications for fresh-frozen plasma

A definition of FFP and a discussion of the indications for giving FFP to normovolaemic patients can be found in Chapter 14. In the present chapter, only the indications for giving FFP to oligaemic patients are discussed.

A conference at the National Institutes of Health (NIH 1985) found no justification for the use of FFP as a volume expander or nutrition source, although reportedly 50% of FFP was given solely for such reasons (Silbert et al. 1981). The NIH conference also advised that in treating abnormal bleeding after massive transfusion FFP should be used only after demonstrating an abnormality of blood coagulation.

There is no evidence that the prophylactic administration of FFP benefits management of massive transfusion. A comparative study demonstrated that the transfusion of 1 unit of FFP for every 3 units of whole blood or packed red cells was associated with neither a reduction in the amount of blood transfused nor with any improvement in the results of tests of coagulation (Mannucci et al. 1982). Similarly, in a controlled experiment in which dogs were resuscitated by massive transfusion after severe haemorrhage, prophylactic administration of FFP was no better than electrolyte solution in restoring coagulation activity (Martin et al. 1985).

Transfusion in elective surgery

Preoperative Hb levels in the surgical patient

Friedman and co-workers (1980) introduced the term 'transfusion trigger' to describe the constellation of factors that precipitate blood transfusion. In their study of 535 031 male and female surgical patients, they confirmed both the importance of the PCV as a component of this transfusion trigger in clinical practice and the arbitrary nature of its use.

Anaesthesia practice long maintained that a preoperative Hb concentration of 100 g/l was the lowest value acceptable for safe elective surgery. If the three major determinants of O_2 availability – cardiac output, arterial O_2 saturation and Hb concentration – are all reduced by one-third, O_2 availability will be only 300 ml/min (Nunn and Freeman 1964b). The work of Messmer and co-workers (1972) provided some scientific support for a value of 100 g/l. Considerable variation in red blood cell transfusion practices still exists in the surgical specialties, in large part related to difficulties in defining specific transfusion threshold criteria (Khanna et al. 2003). Some clinicians, mindful that anaesthesia may be associated with a fall in cardiac output and that surgery often results in sudden haemorrhage, continue to insist on preoperative transfusion to attain 100 g Hb/l. Nunn and Freeman (1964b) pointed out that a great deal of surgery throughout the world is performed on patients with Hb concentrations of less than 80 g/l, and most patients survive. More recent experimental evidence suggests that a level lower than 70 g/l may be acceptable (Weiskopf et al. 1998) and the American Society of Anesthesiologists (1996) suggest that levels of 60 g/l are appropriate in some situations. Increased awareness on the part of the medical profession and its patients that transfusion carries risks has led to a more conservative approach to preoperative transfusion (Stehling 1990). A Consensus Conference (1988) emphasized the folly of relying on a single Hb value as an indication for transfusion but suggested acceptance in certain circumstances of Hb levels as low as 70 g/l. There is, however, no better justification for a value of 70 g/l, and even less theoretical support, than there is for a value of 100 g/l.

In practice, each case must be considered on its merits, and clinicians must satisfy themselves that they are bringing patients to surgery in the best possible condition that the circumstances permit, and are not accepting unnecessary risks because they will probably 'get away with it'. For example, an Hb concentration of 70 g/l might be perfectly acceptable as part of the normocytic normochromic anaemia in a patient with chronic renal failure. If a patient scheduled for elective surgery unexpectedly turns out to have a preoperative Hb level of 70 g/l, it is more important to discover the cause of the anaemia and treat it than it is to ligate the patient's varicocele. If an Hb concentration of 70 g/l is due to recent bleeding which surgery is expected to stop and the patient is known to have coronary artery disease, transfusion may be indicated.

Haemodilution

The term acute normovolaemic haemodilution (ANH) has been used to describe the deliberate production of a low Hb level immediately before surgery, by taking blood from the patient, with the objects of (1) improving the microcirculatory flow owing to a reduction in the viscosity of the blood and (2) obtaining autologous blood and so reducing the amount of allogeneic blood required for transfusion. The blood lost after ANH will have a lower concentration of red cells and the withdrawn blood can be returned to the patient as needed. In this form of autologous transfusion, blood is taken before surgery. However, because phlebotomy

is carried out in the operating suite, this practice is widely, although inaccurately, referred to as 'intraoperative haemodilution'. ANH can produce large amounts of autologous blood (see below), is much more convenient for the patient than preoperative deposit and yields fresh blood with viable platelets if kept at room temperature. ANH is a procedure that lends itself to ready mathematical modelling. Analyses have shown that effective haemodilution requires high initial PCV, low PCV after ANH ('target') and a surgical blood loss that exceeds a specific minimum value (Weiskopf 2001).

Messmer and co-workers (1972) described one way in which haemodilution could be used in patients immediately before surgery: 1800–2000 ml of blood are withdrawn with simultaneous infusion of a colloid solution, producing a fall in the PCV to about 0.25. Cardiac output increases, but CVP and mean arterial pressure remain essentially unchanged. Although heart rate increases linearly in proportion to the degree of anaemia in non-medicated conscious subjects (Weiskopf et al. 2003), heart rate changes are anaesthetic dependent in the surgical patient. As blood is lost during operation, the decision to initiate retransfusion of autologous blood will depend on the Hb nadir achieved after haemodilution and the transfusion trigger. A mathematical model predicts that surgical blood loss should exceed 50% of the patient's blood volume (fractional surgical blood loss = blood volume loss/blood volume) for ANH to begin to 'save' erythrocytes and 70% of the patient's blood volume for ANH to save 1 unit of erythrocytes for the usual surgical patient with an initial PCV of 0.32–0.36 and a transfusion 'trigger' PCV of 0.18–0.21 (Weiskopf 2001). Matot and co-workers (2002) have confirmed this prediction. This study removed approximately 2 l of blood during ANH, reducing the patients' haematocrit from 41% to 24%, and found that the technique significantly decreased the fraction of patients requiring allogeneic transfusion (from 36% to 10%). Furthermore, there was a range of blood loss, above and below which ANH did not result in avoidance of allogeneic transfusion. When blood loss was within the range of potential efficacy (70–90% of the estimated blood volume), none of nine patients in whom ANH was performed required allogeneic blood, whereas all 10 patients in the control group did. The study was not adequately powered to address the safety of ANH.

Messmer and co-workers (1972) emphasized that: (1) an increase in cardiac output must be regarded as an indispensable compensatory mechanism; (2) the tolerance and safe limits of clinical haemodilution are dependent on the contractile state of the myocardium; and (3) the following are to be regarded as contraindications: myocardial failure, coronary artery disease, obstructive lung disease and pre-existing anaemia. Thus ANH efficacy is limited and restricted to specific clinical circumstances. ANH safety has not been demonstrated by a prospective randomized trial of adequate size.

Preoperative ('pre-deposit') autologous collection and autologous blood collected from the operative field (cell salvage) and from surgical drainage sites are discussed in Chapter 18.

Cardiopulmonary bypass

Since the introduction of coronary artery bypass grafting, the number of operations involving cardiopulmonary bypass (CBP) increased enormously. The annual requirement for CABG in the UK has been estimated as 400–450 per million of the population (Joint Cardiology Committee of the Royal College of Physicians of London and the Royal College of Surgeons of England 1985). The number of such operations performed in the USA far exceeds this figure, although aggressive percutaneous placement of stents and 'beating heart' surgery may reduce these numbers. As the number of operations has risen, the number of units of blood used at each operation has fallen. In 1971, a survey of 88% of hospitals performing cardiopulmonary bypass in the USA revealed an average use of almost 8 units per operation (Roche and Stengle 1973). In 1974, however, Sandiford and co-workers (1974) referred to a previously published series of 100 consecutive patients who underwent open-heart surgery at the Texas Heart Institute with an average transfusion requirement of 1.4 units of blood per patient; 35 out of the 100 patients required no blood whatever and a further 31 received only a single unit. In a more recent study of 1235 consecutive patients undergoing primary CABG over a period of 2 years (1999 and 2000), 681 patients underwent coronary surgery with use of CPB and 554 patients underwent off-pump surgery using a median sternotomy incision. The 881 males and 354 females averaged 3.4 red blood cell transfusions for patients on

CPB with 1.6 units for the off-pump group. Patients on CPB received more frequent red cell transfusion (72.5%) compared with 45.7% of off-pump patients. The average number for males was 2.2 units compared with 3.6 units for females (Scott et al. 2003). Finally, they reported a series of aortocoronary bypass operations on 36 Jehovah's Witnesses in whom no blood was used. The estimated blood loss during operation was 530 ml (range 200–1200 ml) and the mean blood loss from chest tubes during the first two postoperative days was 250 ml in all but one patient. Only two patients died and in neither case was the death related to the lack of transfusion. The average Hb concentration fell from 149 g/l before operation to 112 g/l in the immediate postoperative period, and was at its lowest about 6 days after operation, with an average of 92 g/l.

Numerous additional reports have confirmed an average use of 3 units or fewer per patient, and verified that a significant proportion of patients require no allogeneic blood at all (Cosgrove et al. 1981; McCarthy et al. 1988; Ramnath et al. 2003). Several factors (see below) have helped to reduce the need for blood.

Priming of pump-oxygenators with electrolyte solution

Pump-oxygenators are normally primed with electrolyte solution but in exceptional circumstances, for example for children or for patients with severe renal failure, it may be necessary to use blood.

Use of autologous transfusion

Haemodilution, together with the use of electrolyte priming solution, can produce PCVs as low as 0.20 during bypass (Cosgrove et al. 1981). The safety of such low PCV levels is disputed (Messmer 1987).

Postoperative defibrinated blood shed through mediastinal drains can be collected and transfused (Thurer et al. 1979). Because the blood loss after cardiac surgery is usually small, the adoption of this manoeuvre is unlikely to bring about a great saving in transfusion requirements. The return of unwashed red cells is also subject to criticism (Griffith et al. 1989) and has the potential for inducing hypotension, possibly caused by the infusion of cytokines.

Haemostasis after cardiopulmonary bypass

Haemorrhage does not occur through the walls of intact blood vessels, and it is reasonable to suppose that improved surgical technique and devices have contributed to the diminished need for allogeneic blood transfusion that has been observed in cardiac surgical patients over the past 20 years. In 1964, the commonest cause of serious bleeding after cardiopulmonary bypass was found to be failure to ligate blood vessels (Bentall *et al.* 1964). Apart from better surgical haemostasis, the routine use of vasodilators to prevent hypertension after cardiac surgery may help to reduce blood loss. There has been a suggestion, not entirely convincing, that application of positive end-expiratory pressure may reduce severe bleeding in cardiac surgical patients (Ilabaca *et al.* 1980).

Defective haemostasis may be due to reduction in numbers of platelets and to an impairment of platelet function (Moriau *et al.* 1977; Mammen *et al.* 1985; Musial *et al.* 1985). Platelets may be damaged in the oxygenator and preoperative factors such as the administration of aspirin or calcium channel blockers may contribute to a prolonged bleeding time. Bleeding after cardiopulmonary bypass may also be due to inadequate neutralization of heparin or excess administration of protamine sulphate. Dilution of clotting factors occurs in oxygenators primed only with electrolytes but seldom affects tests of coagulation.

Desmopressin acetate (DDAVP), which increases the plasma concentration of VWF and has a direct effect on platelet function, has been shown to reduce bleeding in patients who have undergone cardiac surgery (Czer and Czer 1985; Salzman *et al.* 1986). However, a double-blind, randomized trial involving 150 patients undergoing cardiac surgery failed to demonstrate any favourable effect when DDAVP was administered after bypass in place of a placebo (Hackmann *et al.* 1989) (see Chapter 18).

Aprotinin, a serine proteinase inhibitor, when administered in very large doses, has brought about significant reductions in blood loss and transfusion requirements in both complicated cardiac surgery (Royston *et al.* 1987; Bidstrup *et al.* 1988) and routine CABG (Dietrich *et al.* 1990). Aprotinin is believed to inactivate kallikrein (Emerson 1989) and to preserve platelet function (van Oeveren *et al.* 1987). Aprotinin is also a plasmin inhibitor, and the level of circulating tissue plasminogen activator (tPA) during cardiopulmonary bypass is lower in patients who have been given aprotinin than in those who have not (van Oeveren *et al.* 1987; Marx *et al.* 1991). Concern has been expressed that the use of aprotinin may cause premature graft occlusion (Cosgrove *et al.* 1992) but, in a prospective series of 96 patients, each with three or four coronary grafts, no difference in the rate of graft occlusion in the early postoperative period was found between those patients who had been given aprotinin during surgery and those who had not (Bidstrup *et al.* 1993). Aprotinin is a bovine protein, and presents a risk of antibody formation, with anaphylactic reactions on second exposure, i.e. at re-operation. The incidence of severe reactions has been estimated to be less than 1% (Freeman *et al.* 1983). Because regrafting may be required after 10 years, and blood loss is greater at re-operation, some surgeons prefer to reserve aprotinin for second operations (Hardy and Desroches 1992) (see Chapter 18).

Fibrinolysis is commonly associated with cardiopulmonary bypass, and fibrinolytic inhibitors might be expected to reduce blood loss. Small, but significant, reductions have been demonstrated in randomized, double-blind studies using E-aminocaproic acid (van der Salm *et al.* 1988) and tranexamic acid (Horrow *et al.* 1990) but these substances are not used routinely (see Chapter 18).

Complement activation during cardiopulmonary bypass

During cardiopulmonary bypass, plasma levels of C3a increase steadily; although plasma levels of C5a do not increase, granulocytopenia follows the re-establishment of cardiopulmonary circulation, suggesting that C5a-activated granulocytes are trapped in pulmonary vessels. Complement activation is promoted by contact of blood with plastic surfaces (e.g. nylon mesh liner and bubble oxygenator) as well as by vigorous oxygenation of the whole blood. The production of C3a and C5a during extracorporeal circulation may contribute to the pathogenesis of the so-called post-pump syndrome (Chenoweth *et al.* 1981). The interaction of heparin and protamine is another potential source of complement activation (Rent *et al.* 1975; Chenoweth *et al.* 1981; White 1981).

Selected patients have coronary surgery performed on the beating heart without extracorporeal circulation. This procedure appears to require less allogeneic blood than does the on-pump procedure (Aldea *et al.* 2003; Ramnath *et al.* 2003). However, the apparent blood savings may depend less on the procedure than on the selection of a relatively low-risk cohort of CABG patients.

Transfusion for Jehovah's Witnesses. Some patients decline transfusion for religious reasons. Jehovah's Witnesses will not accept blood and most blood products for themselves or their children. In the setting of acute, life-threatening haemorrhage, this refusal poses both ethical and medicolegal problems. For an unconscious adult in urgent need of a transfusion, many clinicians feel duty bound to administer transfusions even although relatives oppose it. They do so at some risk. However, physicians should provide the best medical practice (including transfusion) unless there are clear legal grounds to do otherwise. The expressed wishes of a conscious patient must be respected. For children below the age of consent, clinicians should seek a court order for doing what is needed for the child's welfare, irrespective of the wishes of the parents. However, even without blood components, such patients tolerate surgical bleeding well when blood volume is maintained (see also Chapter 9). In a retrospective cohort study of 1958 patients of 18 years and older who underwent surgery and declined blood transfusion for religious reasons, the 30-day mortality was 1.3% for patients with preoperative Hb of 120 g/l or greater, and 33.3% in patients with preoperative Hb less than 60 g/l. The increase in risk of death associated with low preoperative Hb was more pronounced in patients with cardiovascular disease than in patients without (Carson *et al.* 1996). The effect of blood loss on mortality was greater for patients with low preoperative Hb than for those with higher preoperative Hb. A full discussion of the problems raised when transfusion is clinically indicated for Jehovah's Witnesses, and evidence that the decisions of courts in different countries may well differ, can be found in a series of articles in *Transfusion Medicine Reviews* (1991, vol. 5, no. 4).

Transfusion in burns

After thermal injury, considerable and continual leakage of salt- and protein-containing fluid from the damaged tissue occurs with consequent falls in circulating blood volume and cardiac output. The volume of fluid lost depends on the size and thickness of the burn.

Arturson (1961) showed that in dogs, extensive third-degree (full thickness) burns were associated with an increase in capillary permeability in unburned areas. He emphasized, however, that the capillary membrane in such areas remained impermeable to protein molecules, although there was a leakage of dextran of molecular weight 40 000.

It is generally agreed that the patient's circulating volume should be restored with intravenous fluids containing salt and water. However, the number of different infusion formulae is limited only by the number of burn units. Most protocols agree that the volume of fluid infused should be related to the surface area of the burn and that most of this large volume (2–4 ml/kg) must be given in the first 24 h after injury. One-half of the total requirements of the first 24 h should be administered during the initial 8 h and the balance over the next 16 h. The patient's circulatory state, PCV and urine output must be carefully monitored.

In calculating the area of the burn, the figures shown in Table 2.2 for the relative areas of the different parts of the body are helpful (Berkow 1931).

Experts disagree about the desirability of giving colloid solutions such as albumin to burned patients. The formulations of Bull (1954) and Evans and co-workers (1952) recommended that one-half of the fluid infused should contain protein, or some form of colloidal plasma substitute. This plan is still followed in the UK (Settle 1982). A mixture of a gelatin solution and Ringer's lactate was used successfully in the Falkland Islands campaign (Williams *et al.* 1983). In the USA, as a result of the finding that infusion of plasma into burned patients is not followed by a significant and persistent rise in blood volume until 24 h after injury (Baxter 1974), there has been widespread acceptance of the case for giving no colloid until the protein

Table 2.2 Estimate of percentage body burn.

Head	6%	6%
Trunk and neck (back and front together)	38%	38%
Upper limb: hand alone, 2.5%	9% × 2	18%
Lower limb: thigh alone, 9.5%	19% × 2	38%
Lower limb: leg alone, 6.5%		
Lower limb: foot alone, 3.0%		
Total		100%

leak has ceased (Pruitt 1978); only saline solutions are used for fluid replacement during the first 24 h. A number of centres in the USA now follow the practice of administering larger volumes of crystalloid if albumin is used as well as electrolyte solution (Goodwin *et al.* 1983).

In order to keep the volume of fluid infused to a minimum, Monafo and colleagues (1973) suggested that hypertonic saline solutions might be infused. The extracellular fluid volume would then be maintained at the expense of some intracellular dehydration. As yet this regimen has shown no advantage over standard crystalloid resuscitation (Bunn *et al.* 2002).

Red cells are destroyed in burned tissue (Shen *et al.* 1943). Anaemia of unclear cause may persist in burned patients despite their elevated erythropoietin levels and reticulocytosis (Deitch and Sittig 1993). These patients tolerate moderate anaemia and a PCV of 15–20% is now common practice for patients without cardiovascular disease. In patients with large burns, transfusions of red cells may be needed, although retrospective studies suggest that the need is most pressing when multiple operative procedures are anticipated (Topley *et al.* 1962).

The adult respiratory distress syndrome ('shock lung'; traumatic wet lung)

Adult respiratory distress syndrome (ARDS) is a diffuse pulmonary parenchymal injury in which microvascular endothelial damage develops and leads to increased capillary permeability and oedema. The clinical features include progressive hypoxaemia, with widespread radiological shadowing and reduced compliance (Murray *et al.* 1988). Some purists insist that the left atrial pressure must be established as being within normal limits, to exclude pulmonary oedema due to left ventricular failure.

It has been proposed that the diagnosis of ARDS in any patient should be accompanied by reference to its underlying cause and that possible underlying causes fall into two general categories. In the first are specific agents such as toxic gases, fat emboli, gastric contents and infectious microorganisms that damage the lungs directly, the resultant injury being confined to the lungs. The second category comprises generalized disorders, involving many organs as well as the lungs, with a high mortality rate due to multiple organ failure. For example, systemic sepsis, acute pancreatitis

and multiple injuries are frequent precursors of ARDS, DIC and hepatic and renal dysfunction (American-European Consensus Conference on ARDS 1994). The relatively high mortality rates of acute lung injury/ acute respiratory distress syndrome are primarily related to the underlying disease, the severity of the acute illness and the degree of organ dysfunction (Vincent *et al.* 2003).

Repeated large volume transfusions have been associated with the development of ARDS, suggesting the possibility that blood loss is an important factor. However, in experimental animals oligaemia alone does not seem to produce the syndrome (Tobey *et al.* 1974). Possibly the translocation of bacteria and endotoxin from the bowel into the circulation, during an episode of hypovolaemia severe enough to warrant transfusion is responsible for the relationship between transfusion and ARDS (Parsons *et al.* 1989).

A serious pulmonary injury known as transfusion-related acute lung injury (TRALI) that is most often caused by passively transfused antibodies to leucocytes is characterized by fever, dyspnoea, hypotension and radiographic changes in the lungs (Chapter 15). Radiographic interpretation has not readily distinguished these differing pulmonary syndromes (Silliman *et al.* 2004).

Evidence that microaggregates infused with stored blood cause pulmonary damage is at best inconclusive (Chapter 15).

References

Aberg M, Hedner U, Bergenz S-E (1979) Effect of dextran on Factor VIII and platelet function. Ann Surg 189: 243–247

ACCP-SCCM Consensus Conference (1992) Definitions for sepsis and organ failure and guidelines for the use of innovative therapies in sepsis. Chest 101: 1644–1655

Adamson J, Hillman RS (1968) Blood volume and plasma protein replacement following acute blood loss in normal man. JAMA 205; 609

Aldea GS, Goss JR, Boyle EM, Jr *et al.* (2003) Use of off-pump and on-pump CABG strategies in current clinical practice: the Clinical Outcomes Assessment Program of the state of Washington. J Card Surg 18: 206–215

American College of Surgeons Committee on Trauma (1997) ACS Advanced Trauma Life Support for Doctors. Chicago: American College of Surgeons

American Society of Anesthesiologists Task Force on Blood Component Therapy (1996) Practice Guidelines for blood component therapy: A report by the American Society of Anesthesiologists Task Force on Blood Component Therapy. Anesthesiology 84: 732–747

American–European Consensus Conference on ARDS (1994) Definitions, mechanisms, relevant outcomes and clinical trial co-ordination. Am J Respir Crit Care Med 149: 818–824

Armstrong RF, Secker WJ, St Andrew D (1978) Continuous monitoring of mixed venous oxygen tension in cardio-respiratory disorders. Lancet ii: 632–634

Arturson G (1961) Capillary permeability in burned and non-burned areas in dogs. Acta Chir Scand 274 (Suppl.): 55

Baxter CR (1974) Fluid volume and electrolyte changes of the early postburn period. Clin Plastic Surg 1: 4–709

Bayliss WM (1919) Intravenous injection to replace blood. Spec Rep Ser Med Res Cttee (Lond) No. 25

Bentall HH, Smith B, Omeri MA (1964) Blood loss after cardiopulmonary bypass. Lancet ii: 277

Berg EM, Fasting S, Sellevold OFM (1991) Serious complications with dextran-70 despite hapten prophylaxis. Anaesthesia 46: 1033–1035

Bergman A, Andreen M, Blomback M (1990) Plasma substitution with 3% dextran-60 in orthopaedic surgery: influence on plasma colloid osmotic pressure, coagulation parameters, immunoglobulins and other plasma constituents. Acta Anaesthes Scand 34: 21–29

Berkow SG (1931) Value of surface-area proportions in the prognosis of cutaneous burns and scalds. Am J Surg 11: 315

Bidstrup BP, Royston D, Taylor KM (1988) Effect of aprotinin on need for blood transfusion in patients with septic endocarditis having open-heart surgery (Letter). Lancet i: 366–367

Bidstrup BP, Harrison J, Royston D et al. (1993) Aprotinin therapy in cardiac operations: a report on use in 41 cardiac centers in the United Kingdom. Ann Thorac Surg 55: 971–976

Biro GP (1982) Comparison of acute cardiovascular effects and oxygen-supply following haemodilution with dextran, stroma-free haemoglobin solution and fluorocarbon suspension. Cardiovasc Res 16: 194–204

Biro CP, White FC, Guth BD (1987) The effect of hemodilution with fluorocarbon or dextran on regional myocardial flow and function during acute coronary stenosis in the pig. Am J Cardiovasc Path 1: 99–114

Blundell J (1818) Experiments on the transfusion of blood by the syringe. Med-Chir Trans 9: 56

Blundell J (1824) Researches Physiological and Pathological. London: E Cox and Son

Blundell J (1829) A successful case of transfusion. Lancet i: 431

Boon JC, Jesch F, Messmer K (1977) Intravascular persistence of hydroxyethyl starch in man. Eur Surg Res 8: 497

Boyd O, Mackay CJ, Lamb G (1993) Comparison of clinical information gained from routine blood-gas analysis and from gastric tonometry for intramural pH. Lancet 341: 142–146

BSI (1972) BS4843, Sterile Intravenous Cannulae for Single Use. London: British Standards Institution

Bull JP (1954) Shock caused by burns and its treatment. Br Med Bull 10: 9

Bunn F, Roberts I, Tasker R et al. (2002) Hypertonic versus isotonic crystalloid for fluid resuscitation in critically ill patients. Cochrane Database Syst Rev CD002045

Bunn F, Alderson P, Hawkins V (2003) Colloid solutions for fluid resuscitation. Cochrane Database Syst Rev CD001319

Cáceres E, Whittembury G (1975) Behavior of human haematopoietic stem cells in cord blood and neonatal blood (Letter). Haematologica 60: 492

Cannon WB (1923) Traumatic Shock. New York: D. Appleton

Carson JL, Duff A, Poses RM et al. (1996) Effect of anaemia and cardiovascular disease on surgical mortality and morbidity. Lancet 19: 348, 1055–1060

Chaplin HJ, Chang E (1955) In vitro comparison of the effects of four different preservative solutions on single donor blood with special emphasis on rate of flow. J Lab Clin Med 46: 234

Chen IY, Huang YC, Lin WH (2002) Flow-rate measurements and models for colloid and crystalloid flows in central and peripheral venous line infusion systems. IEEE Trans Biomed Eng 49: 1632–1638

Chenoweth DE, Cooper SW, Hugh TE (1981) Complement activation during cardiopulmonary bypass: evidence for generation of C3a and C5a anaphylatoxins. N Engl J Med 304: 497–503

Ciavarella D, Reed RL, Counts RB et al. (1987) Clotting factor levels and the risk of diffuse microvascular bleeding in the massively transfused patient. Br J Haematol 67: 365–368

Clarke R, Topley E, Flear CTG (1955) Assessment of blood loss in civilian trauma. Lancet i: 629

Cochrane Injuries Group Albumin Reviewers (1998) Human albumin administration in critically ill patients: systematic review of randomised controlled trials. BMJ 317: 235–240

Collins JA (1987) Recent developments in the area of massive transfusion. World J Surg 11: 75–81

Committee on Fluid Resuscitation for Combat Casualties (2003) In: Fluid Resuscitation. A Pope, G French, D Longnecker (eds). Washington, DC: National Academy Press, pp. 1–195

Consensus Conference (1988) Perioperative red blood cell transfusion. JAMA 260: 2700–2703

Cosgrove DM, Loop FD, Lytle BW (1981) Blood conservation in cardiac surgery. Cardiovasc Clin 12: 165–175

Cosgrove DM, Heric B, Lyde BW (1992) Aprotinin therapy for preoperative myocardial revascularization: a placebo-controlled study. Ann Thorac Surg 54: 1031–1038

Counts RB, Haisch C, Simmon TL (1979) Hemostasis in massively transfused trauma patients. Ann Surg 190: 91–99

Czer L, Czer L. (1985) Prospective trial of DDAVP in treatment of severe platelet dysfunction and hemorrhage after cardiopulmonary bypass. Circulation 72 (Suppl. 3): section III, 130.

Davies JWL, Fisher MR (1958) Red cell and total blood volume changes following a minor operation. Clin Sci 17: 537

Dawidson IJ, Willms CD, Sandor ZF et al. (1991) Ringer's lactate with or without 3% dextran-60 as volume expanders during abdominal aortic surgery. Crit Care Med 19: 36–42

Deitch EA, Sittig KM (1993) A serial study of the erythropoietic response to thermal injury. Ann Surg 217: 293–299

Demling RH, Manohar M, Will JA (1980) Response of the pulmonary microcirculation to fluid loading after hemorrhagic shock and resuscitation. Surgery 87: 552–559

Dieterich HJ (2003) Recent developments in European colloid solutions. J Trauma 54: S26–S30

Dietrich W, Spannagl M, Jochum M (1990) Influence of high-dose aprotinin treatment on blood loss and coagulation patterns in patients undergoing myocardial revascularisation. Anesthesiology 73: 1119–1126

Dries DJ (1996) Hypotensive resuscitation. Shock 6: 311–316

Drobin D, Hahn RG (2002) Kinetics of isotonic and hypertonic plasma volume expanders. Anesthesiology 96: 1371–1380

Ebert RV, Stead EA, Gibson JG (1941) Response of normal subjects to acute blood loss, with special reference to the mechanism of restoration of blood volume. Arch Intern Med 68: 578

Emerson TE (1989) Pharmacology of aprotinin and efficacy during cardiopulmonary bypass. Cardiovasc Drug Rev 7: 127–140

Eriksson M, Saldren T (1995) Effect of dextran on plasma tissue plasminogen activator (t-PA) and plasminogen activator inhibitor-1 (PAI-I) during surgery. Acta Anaesthes Scand 39: 163–166

Evans EI, James GW, Hoover MJ (1944) Studies in traumatic shock. II. The restoration of blood volume in traumatic shock. Surgery 15: 420

Evans EI, Purnell OJ, Robinett RW (1952) Fluid and electrolyte requirements in severe burns. Ann Surg 135: 804–807

Farman JV, Powell D (1969) The performance of disposable venous catheters, needles and cannulae. Br J Hosp Med Equipment (Suppl.) 37–45

Farrow SP (1967) Effects of infusion of various colloid solutions upon the circulatory volumes of rabbits. Thesis, University of Birmingham, UK

Farrow SP (1977) Comparative effects of dextran and plasma protein solutions. Burns 3: 202

Feest TG (1976) Low molecular weight dextran: a continuing cause of acute renal failure. BMJ ii: 1275

Ferrara A, Macarthur JD, Wright HK (1990) Hypothermia and acidosis worsen coagulopathy in the patient requiring massive transfusion. Am J Surg 160: 575–578

Fiddian-Green RG (1991) Should measurements of tissue pH and PCO2 be included in the routine monitoring of intensive care patients? Crit Care Med 19: 141–143

Franz A, Braunlich P, Gamsjager T et al. (2001) The effects of hydroxyethyl starches of varying molecular weights on platelet function. Anesth Analg 92: 1402–1407

Freeman JG, Turner GA, Venables CW et al. (1983) Serial use of aprotinin and incidence of allergic reactions. Curr Med Res Opin 8: 559–561

Friedman BA, Burns TL, Schork MA (1980) An analysis of blood transfusion of surgical patients by sex: a question for the transfusion trigger. Transfusion 20: 179–188

Gitlin N, Serio KM (1992) Ischemic hepatitis: widening horizons. Am J Gastroenterol 87: 831–836

Goodwin CW, Dorethy J, Lam V (1983) Randomised trial of efficacy of crystalloid and colloid resuscitation on hemodynamic response and lung water following thermal injury. Ann Surg 197: 520–529

Grant RT, Reeve EB (1951) Observations on the general effects of injury in man, with special reference to wound shock. Spec Rep Ser Med Res Coun (Lond) p. 277

Griffith LD, Billman GF, Daily PO (1989) Apparent coagulopathy caused by infusion of shed mediastinal blood and its prevention by washing of the infusate. Ann Thorac Surg 47: 400–406

Gruber UF (1969) Blood Replacement. New York: Springer-Verlag

Gutierrez G, Bismar H, Dantzker DR (1992) Comparison of gastric mucosal pH with measures of oxygen transport and consumption in critically ill patients. Crit Care Med 20: 451–457

Guyton A, Hall JE (2005) Circulatory shock and physiology of its treatment. In: Textbook of Medical Physiology, 11th edn. Philadelphia, PA: WB Saunders

Hackmann T, Gascoyne RD, Naiman SC (1989) A trial of desmopressin (1-desamino-8-d-arginine vasopressin) to reduce blood loss in uncomplicated cardiac surgery. N Engl J Med 321: 1437–1443

Hardaway RM, III (1974) Vasoconstrictors vs. vasodilators. In: Treatment of Shock: Principles and Practice. WSAL Nyhus (ed.). Philadelphia, PA: Lea & Febiger

Hardy JF, Desroches J (1992) Natural and synthetic antifibrinolytics in cardiac surgery. Can J Anaesth 39: 353–365

Harke H, Rahman S (1980) Hemostatic disorders in massive transfusion. Bibl Haematol 46: 179–188

Harke H, Thoenies R, Margraf et al. (1976) Der Einfluss verschiedener Plasmaersatzmittel auf Gerinnungssystem

</br>

und Thrombocytenfunktion während und nach operativen Eingriffen. Vorläufige Ergebnisse einer klinischen Studie. Anaesthetist 25: 366–373

Harvey W (1628) De Motu Cordis, Frankfurt. Oxford: Blackwell Scientific Publications

Hedin H, Richter W (1982) Pathomechanisms of dextran-induced anaphylactoid/anaphylactic reactions in man. Int Arch Allergy Appl Immunol 68: 122–126

Hedin H, Kraft D, Richter W (1979) Dextran reactive antibodies in patients with anaphylactoid reactions to dextran. Immunology 156: 289–290

Holcroft JW, Trunkey DD (1974) Extravascular lung water following hemorrhagic shock in the baboon: comparison between resuscitation with Ringer's lactate and Plasmanate. Ann Surg 180: 408–417

Holcroft JW, Vassar MJ, Turner JE et al. (1987) 3% NaCl and 7.5% NaCl/dextran 70 in the resuscitation of severely injured patients. Ann Surg 206: 279–288

Horrow JC, Hlavacek J, Strong MD (1990) Prophylactic tranexamic acid decreases bleeding after cardiac operations. J Thorac Cardiovasc Surg 99: 70–74

Howarth S, Sharpey-Schafer EP (1947) Low blood pressure phases following haemorrhage. Lancet i: 19

Ilabaca PA, Ochsner JL, Mills NL (1980) Positive end-expiratory pressure in the management of the patient with a postoperative bleeding heart. Ann Thorac Surg 30: 281–284

Iserson KV, Huestis DW (1991) Blood warming: current applications and techniques. Transfusion 31: 558–571

Ivatury RR, Simon RJ, Islam S et al. (1996) A prospective randomized study of end points of resuscitation after major trauma: global oxygen transport indices versus organ-specific gastric mucosal pH. J Am Coll Surg 183: 145–154

Johnston AOB, Clark RG (1972) Malpositioning of central venous catheters. Lancet ii: 1395

Joint Cardiology Committee of the Royal College of Physicians of London and the Royal College of Surgeons of England (1985) Provision of services for the diagnosis and treatment of heart disease in England and Wales. Br Heart J 53: 477–482

Joly HR, Weil MH (1969) Temperature of the great toe as an indication of the severity of shock. Circulation 39: 131

Kabat EA, Berg D (1953) Dextran – an antigen in man. J Immunol 70: 514

Karlson KE, Gaczon AA, Shaftan GW (1967) Increased blood loss associated with administration of certain plasma expanders: Dextran 75, Dextran 40 and hydroxyethyl starch. Surgery 62: 670

Kee DB Jr, Wood JH (1984) Rheology of the cerebral circulation. Neurosurgery 15: 125–131

Keith NM (1919) Blood volume in wound shock. Spec Rep Ser Med Res Cttee (Lond) No. 27

Kestin IG (1987) Flow through intravenous cannulae. Anaesthesia 42: 67–70

Khanna MP, Hebert PC, Fergusson DA (2003) Review of the clinical practice literature on patient characteristics associated with perioperative allogeneic red blood cell transfusion. Transfusion Med Rev 17: 110–119

Klein HG (2003) Getting older is not necessarily getting better. Anesthesiology 98: 807–808

Knight RJ (1968) Flow rates through disposable intravenous cannulae. Lancet ii: 665–667

Knutson JE, Deering JA, Hall FW et al. (2000) Does intra-operative hetastarch administration increase blood loss and transfusion requirements after cardiac surgery? Anesth Analg 90: 801–807

Kramer GC, Perron PR, Lindsey DC et al. (1986) Small-volume resuscitation with hypertonic saline dextran solution. Surgery 100: 239–247

Krevans JR, Jackson DP (1955) Hemorrhagic disorder following massive whole blood transfusions. JAMA 159: 171

Kwan I, Bunn F, Roberts I (2003) Timing and volume of fluid administration for patients with bleeding. Cochrane Database Syst Rev CD002245

Leading A (1980) Haemodynamic monitoring in the intensive care unit. BMJ 280: 1035–1036

Leslie SD, Toy PTCY (1991) Laboratory hemostatic abnormalities in massively transfused patients given red blood cells and crystalloid. Am J Clin Path 96: 770–773

Leung JM, Weiskopf RB, Feiner J et al. (2000) Electrocardiographic ST-segment changes during acute, severe isovolemic hemodilution in humans. Anesthesiology 93: 1004–1010

Levy PS, Kim SJ, Eckel PK et al. (1993) Limit to cardiac compensation during acute isovolemic hemodilution: influence of coronary stenosis. Am J Physiol 265: H340–H349

Lewis FR, Elings VB, Sturm JA (1979) Bedside measurement of lung water. J Surg Res 27: 250–261

Ljungstrom K-G, Renck H, Hedin H (1988) Hapten inhibition and dextran anaphylaxis. Anaesthesia 43: 729–732

Loutit JF, Mollison MD, van der Walt ED (1942) Venous pressure during venesection and blood transfusion. BMJ ii: 658

Lozman J, Powers SP Jr, Older T (1974) Correlation of pulmonary wedge and left atrial pressures. Arch Surg 109: 270

Lucas CE, Ledgerwood AM (2003) Physiology of colloid-supplemented resuscitation from shock. J Trauma 54: S75–S81

Lundsgaard-Hansen P (1978) Modified fluid gelatin as a plasma substitut. In: Blood Substitutes and Plasma Expanders. GA Jamieson, TJ Greenwalt (eds). New York: Alan R Liss

McCarthy PM, Popovsky MA, Schaff HV (1988) Effect of blood conservation efforts in cardiac operations at the Mayo Clinic. Mayo Clin Proc 63: 225–229

Mammen EF, Koets MN, Washington BC (1985) Hemostasis during cardiopulmonary bypass surgery. Semin Thromb Hemost 11: 281–292

Mannucci PM, Federici AB, Sirchia G (1982) Hemostasis testing during massive blood replacement. Vox Sang 42: 113–123

Martin DJ, Lucas CE, Ledgerwood AM (1985) Fresh frozen plasma supplement to massive red blood cell transfusion. Ann Surg 202: 505–511

Marx G, Pokar H, Reuter H (1991) The effects of aprotinin on hemostatic function during cardiac surgery. J Cardiothorac Vasc Anesthes 5: 467–474

Matot I, Scheinin O, Jurim O et al. (2002) Effectiveness of acute normovolemic hemodilution to minimize allogeneic blood transfusion in major liver resections. Anesthesiology 97: 794–800

Mattox KL, Maningas PA, Moore EE et al. (1991) Prehospital hypertonic saline/dextran infusion for posttraumatic hypotension. The USA Multicenter Trial. Ann Surg 213: 482–491

Mellander S, Lewis DH (1963) Effect of hemorrhagic shock on the reactivity of resistance and capacitance vessels and on capillary filtration transfer in cat skeletal muscle. Circ Res 11: 105

Messmer KF (1987) Acceptable haematocrit levels in surgical patients. World J Surg 11: 41–46

Messmer K (1988) Characteristics, effects and side-effects of plasma substitutes. In: Blood Substitutes. Preparation, Physiology and Medical Applications. KC Wwe (ed.). Chichester: Ellis Horwood, pp. 51–70

Messmer K, Lewis DH, Sunder-Plassman L (1972) Acute normovolemic hemodilution. Eur Surg Res 4: 55

Messmer K, Ljungstrom K-G, Gruber U-F (1980) Prevention of dextran-induced anaphylactoid reactions by hapten inhibition (Letter). Lancet i: 975

Michelson AD, MacGregor H, Barnard MR et al. (1994) Reversible inhibition of human platelet activation by hypothermia in vivo and in vitro. Thromb Haemost 71: 633–640

Mollison PL (1983) Blood Transfusion in Clinical Medicine. Oxford: Blackwell Scientific Publications

Monafo WW, Chuntrasakul C, Ayvazian VH (1973) Hypertonic sodium solutions in the treatment of burn shock. Am J Surg 126: 778–783

Moriau M, Masure R, Hurler A (1977) Haemostasis disorders in open heart surgery with extracorporeal circulation. Importance of the platelet function and the heparin neutralization. Vox Sang 32: 41

Moss GS, Lowe RJ, Jilek J (1981) Colloid or crystalloid in the resuscitation of hemorrhagic shock; a controlled clinical trial. Surgery 89: 434–438

Most AS, Ruocco NA, Gewirtz H (1986) Effect of a reduction in blood viscosity on maximal oxygen delivery distal to a moderate coronary stenosis. Circulation 74: 1085–1092

Murray JF, Matthay MA, Luce JM et al. (1988) An expanded definition of the adult respiratory distress syndrome. Am Rev Resp Dis 136: 720–723

Musial J, Niewiarowski S, Hershock D (1985) Loss of fibrinogen receptors from the platelet surface during simulated extracorporeal circulation. J Lab Clin Med 105: 514–522

National Institutes of Health (NIH) (1985) Fresh frozen plasma. Indications and risks. JAMA 253: 551–553

National Institutes of Health (1987) Consensus Development Conference. Platelet transfusion. JAMA 257: 1777–1780

Noble RP, Gregersen MI (1946) Blood volume in clinical shock. II. The extent and cause of blood volume reduction in traumatic, hemorrhagic, and burn shock. J Clin Invest 25: 172

Nunn JF, Freeman J (1964a) Problems of oxygenation and oxygen transport during haemorrhage. Anaesthesia 19: 120

Nunn JF, Freeman J (1964b) Problems of oxygenation and oxygen transport during anaesthesia. Anaesthesia 19: 206

van Oeveren W, Nansen J, Bidstrup (1987) Effects of aprotinin on hemostatic mechanisms during cardiopulmonary bypass. Ann Thorac Surg 44: 640–645

Palosuo T, Milgrom F (1980) Appearance of dextrans and anti-dextran antibodies in human sera. Int Arch Allergy Appl Immunol 57: 153–161

Parsons PE, Worthen GS, Moore ER (1989) The association of circulating endotoxin with the development of the adult respiratory distress syndrome. Am Rev Resp Dis 240: 249–310

Paulson OB, Parring H-H, Olsen J (1973) Influence of carbon monoxide and of hemodilution on cerebral blood flow and blood gases in man. J Appl Physiol 35: 111

Payen JF, Vuillez JP, Geoffray B et al. (1997) Effects of preoperative intentional hemodilution on the extravasation rate of albumin and fluid. Crit Care Med 25: 243–248

Pearl RG, Halperin BD, Mihm FG (1988) Pulmonary effects of crystalloid and colloid resuscitation from hemorrhagic shock in the presence of oleic acid-induced pulmonary capillary injury in the dog. Anesthesiology 68: 12–20

Prentice TC, Olney JM Jr, Artz CP (1954) Studies of blood volume and transfusion therapy in the Korean battle casualty. Surg Gynecol Obstet 99: 542

Pruitt BA, Moncrief JA, Mason AD (1965) Effect of Buffered Saline Solution upon the Blood Volume of Man after Acute Measured Hemorrhage. Texas: Annual Research Progress Report, US Army Surgical Research Unit

Pruitt BJ (1978) Advances in fluid therapy and the early care of the burn patient. World J Surg 2: 139–150

Rackow EC, Falk JL, Fein A (1983) Fluid resuscitation in circulatory shock: a comparison of the cardiorespiratory effects of albumin, hetastarch and saline solutions in patients with hypovolemic and septic shock. Crit Care Med 11: 839–850

Rady M (1994) An argument for colloid resuscitation for shock. Acad Emerg Med 1: 572–579

Ramnath AN, Naber HR, de Boer A *et al.* (2003) No benefit of intraoperative whole blood sequestration and auto-transfusion during coronary artery bypass grafting: results of a randomized clinical trial. J Thorac Cardiovasc Surg 125: 1432–1437

Reed RL, Heimbach DM Counts RB (1986). Prophylactic platelet administration during massive transfusion. Ann Surg 203: 40–48

von Restorff W, Höfling B, Holtz J (1975) Effect of increased blood fluidity through hemodilution on coronary circulation at rest and during exercise in dogs. Pflügers Arch 357: 15–34

Rent R, Ertel N, Eisenstein R (1975) Complement activation by interaction of polyanions and polycations. I. Heparin-protamine induced consumption of complement. J Immunol 114: 120

Ring J, Messmer K (1977) Incidence and severity of anaphylactoid reactions to colloid volume substitutes. Lancet i: 466

Ring J, Sharkofl D, Richter W (1980) Using HES in man. Vox Sang 39: 181–185

Roberts JS, Bratton SL (1998) Colloid volume expanders. Problems, pitfalls and possibilities. Drugs 55: 621–630

Robertson OH, Bock AV (1919) Memorandum on blood volume after haemorrhage. Spec Rep Ser Med Res Cttee (Lond) No. 25

Roche JK, Stengle JM (1973) Open-heart surgery and the demand for blood. JAMA 225: 1516–1521

Royston D, Bidstrup BP, Taylor KM (1987) Effect of aprotinin on need for blood transfusion after repeat open heart surgery. Lancet ii: 1289–1290

Rush BF (1974) Volume replacement: when, what and how much? In: Treatment of Shock: Principles and Practice. W Schume, LM Nyhus (eds) Philadelphia, PA: Lea & Febiger

Rutledge R, Sheldon GF, Collins ML (1986) Massive transfusion. Crit Care Clin 2: 791–805

Saddler JM, Horsey PJ (1987) The new generation gelatins. Anaesthesia 42: 998–1004

van der Salm TJ, Ansell JE, Okike ON (1988) The role of epsilon-aminocaproic acid in reducing bleeding after cardiac operation; a double-blind randomised study. J Thorac Cardiovasc Surg 95: 538–540

Salmon JB, Mythen MG (1993) Pharmacology and physiology of colloids. Blood Rev 7: 114–120

Salzman EW, Weinstein MJ, Weintraub RM (1986) Treatment with desmopressin acetate to reduce blood loss after cardiac surgery. N Engl J Med 314: 1402–1406

Sandiford FM, Chiariello L, Hallman GL (1974) Aorto-coronary bypass in Jehovah's witnesses. Report of 36 patients. J Thorac Cardiovasc Surg 68: 1

Schmidt PJ (1968) Transfusion in America in the eighteenth and nineteenth centuries. N Engl J Med 279: 1319

Schmidt PJ (1978) Red cells for transfusion. N Engl J Med 299: 1411

Schumer W (1974) Preface to treatment of shock. In: Principles and Practice. W Schumer (ed.). Philadelphia, PA: Lea & Febiger

Schwartzkopff W, Schwartzkopff B, Wurm W *et al.* (1980) Physiological aspects of the role of human albumin in the treatment of chronic and acute blood loss. Dev Biol Stand 48:7–30: 7–30

Scott BH, Seifert FC, Glass PS *et al.* (2003) Blood use in patients undergoing coronary artery bypass surgery: impact of cardiopulmonary bypass pump, hematocrit, gender, age, and body weight. Anesth Analg 97: 958–963

Settle JAD (1982) Fluid therapy in burns. J R Soc Med 75 (Suppl.) 1: 6–11

Shen SC, Ham TH, Fleming EM (1943) Studies in destruction of red blood cells. III. Mechanism and complications of hemoglobinuria in patients with thermal burns: spherocytosis and increased osmotic fragility of red blood cells. N Engl J Med 229: 701

Shires T, Coln D, Carrico J *et al.* (1964) Fluid therapy in hemorrhagic shock. Arch Surg 88: 688–693

Silbert JA, Bove JR, Dubin S (1981) Patterns of fresh frozen plasma use. Connecticut Med 45: 507–511

Silliman CC, Ambruso DR, Boshkov LK (2005) Transfusion-related acute lung injury (TRALI). Blood 105: 2266–2273

Silverman HJ (1991) Gastric tonometry: an index of splanchnic tissue oxygenation? Crit Care Med 19: 1223–1224

Skillman JJ, Lauler DP, Hickler RB *et al.* (1967a) Hemorrhage in normal man: effect on renin, cortisol, aldosterone, and urine composition. Ann Surg 166: 865–885

Skillman JJ, Awwad HK, Moore FD (1967b) Plasma protein kinetics of the early transcapillary refill after hemorrhage in man. Surg Gynecol Obstet 125: 983–996

Skillman JJ, Olson JE, Lyons JH *et al.* (1967c) The hemodynamic effect of acute blood loss in normal man, with observations on the effect of the Valsalva maneuver and breath holding. Ann Surg 166: 713–738

Spiess BD (1994) Cardiac anesthesia risk management. Hemorrhage, coagulation and transfusion: a risk-benefit analysis. J Cardiothorac Vasc Anesthes 8 (Suppl. 1): 19–22

Sprat T (1667) The History of the Royal Society of London, for the Improving of Natural Knowledge. Printed by TR for J Martyn at the Bell without Temple-bar and J Allestry at the Rose and Crown in Duck-lane, Printers to the Royal Society

Starr D (1998) Blood: An epic History of Medicine and Commerce. New York: Alfred A Knopf, pp. 1–441

Staub NC (1974) Pulmonary edema. Physiol Rev 54: 678–811

Stefanini M, Mednicoff IB, Salomon L (1954) Thrombocytopenia of replacement transfusion: a cause of surgical bleeding. Clin Res Proc 2: 61

Stehling L (1990) Trends in transfusion therapy. Anesthesiol Clin N Am 8: 519–531

Stockwell MA, Scott A, Day A (1992a) Colloid solutions in the critically ill. A randomised comparison of albumin and polygeline. Serum albumin concentration and incidences of pulmonary oedema and renal failure. Anaesthesia 47: 7–9

Stockwell MA, Soni N, Riley B (1992b) Colloid solutions in the critically ill. A randomised comparison of albumin and polygeline. 1. Outcome and duration of stay in the intensive care unit. Anaesthesia 47: 3–6

String T, Robinson AJ, Blaisdell FW et al. (1971) Massive trauma. Effect of intravascular coagulation on prognosis. Arch Surg 102: 406

Swan HJC, Ganz W, Forester J (1970) Catheterisation of the heart in man with use of a flow-directed balloon-tipped catheter. N Engl J Med 283: 447

Sykes MK (1963) Venous pressure as a clinical indication of adequacy of transfusion. Ann R Coll Surg 33: 185

The SAFE Study Investigators (2004) A comparison of albumin and saline for fluid resuscitation in the intensive care unit. N Engl J Med 350: 2247–2256

Thorsen G, Hint H (1950) Aggregation, sedimentation and intravascular sludging of erythrocytes. Acta Chir Scand (Suppl.): 154

Thurer RL, Lytle BW, Cosgrove DM (1979) Autotransfusion following cardiac operations: a randomized prospective study. Ann Thorac Surg 27: 500–507

Tobey RE, Kopriva CJ, Homer LD (1974) Pulmonary gas exchange following hemorrhagic shock and massive transfusion in the baboon. Ann Surg 179: 316

Topley E, Jackson DM, Cason JS (1962) Assessment of red cell loss in the first two days after severe burns. Ann Surg 155: 581

Tovey GH, Lennon GG (1962) Blood volume studies in accidental haemorrhage. J Obstet Gynaecol Br Cwlth 5: 749

Treib J, Haass A, Pindur G et al. (1996) All medium starches are not the same: influence of the degree of hydroxyethyl substitution of hydroxyethyl starch on plasma volume, hemorrheologic conditions, coagulation. Transfusion 36: 450–455

Treib J, Baron JF, Grauer MT et al. (1999) An international view of hydroxyethyl starches. Intens Care Med 25: 258–268

Tschirren B, Affolter U, Elstisser R (1973) Der klinische Plasmaersatz mit Gelatine: zwölf Jahre Erfahrungen mit 39320 Einheiten Physiogel. Infusionstherapie 1: 651–662

Valeri CR, Feingold H, Cassidy G (1987) Hypothermia-induced reversible platelet dysfunction. Ann Surg 205: 175–181

Vincent JL, Sakr Y, Ranieri VM (2003) Epidemiology and outcome of acute respiratory failure in intensive care unit patients. Crit Care Med 31: S296–S299

Virgilio RW, Rice CL, Smith DE (1979) Crystalloid vs. colloid resuscitation: is one better? Surgery 85: 129–139

Wade CE, Grady JJ, Kramer GC (2003) Efficacy of hypertonic saline dextran fluid resuscitation for patients with hypotension from penetrating trauma. J Trauma 54: S144–S148

Wallace J, Sharpey-Schafer EP (1941) Blood changes following controlled haemorrhage in man. Lancet ii: 393

Weisel RD, Dennis RC, Manny J (1978) Adverse effects of transfusion therapy during abdominal aortic aneurysmectomy. Surgery 83: 682

Weiskopf RB (2001) Efficacy of acute normovolemic hemodilution assessed as a function of fraction of blood volume lost. Anesthesiology 94: 439–446

Weiskopf RB, Viele MK, Feiner J et al. (1998) Human cardiovascular and metabolic response to acute, severe isovolemic anemia. JAMA 279: 217–221

Weiskopf RB, Feiner J, Hopf HW et al. (2002) Oxygen reverses deficits of cognitive function and memory and increased heart rate induced by acute severe isovolemic anemia. Anesthesiology 96: 871–877

Weiskopf RB, Feiner J, Hopf H et al. (2003) Heart rate increases linearly in response to acute isovolemic anemia. Transfusion 43: 235–240

Weiskopf RB, Toy P, Hopf HW et al. (2005) Acute isovolemic anemia impairs central processing as determined by P300 latency. Clin Neurophysiol 116: 1028–1032

White JV (1981) Complement activation during cardiopulmonary bypass (Letter). N Engl J Med 305: 51

Wiklander O (1956) Blood volume determinations in surgical practice. A comparative analysis of the Evans blue dye method, the radioactive phosphorus method and the alveolar CO method, with special reference to determinations under pre- and post-operative conditions. Acta Chir Scand (Suppl.): 208

Wilkerson DK, Rosen AL, Gould SA (1987) Oxygen extraction ratio: a valid indicator of myocardial metabolism in anemia. J Surg Res 42: 629–634

Wilkes MM, Navickis RJ, Sibbald WJ (2001) Albumin versus hydroxyethyl starch in cardiopulmonary bypass surgery: a meta-analysis of postoperative bleeding. Ann Thorac Surg 72: 527–533

Williams JG, Riley TRD, Moody RA (1983) Resuscitation experience in the Falkland Islands campaign. BMJ 286: 775–777

Wright A, Hecke IF, Lewis GBH (1985) Use of transdermal glyceryl trinitrate to reduce failure of intravenous infusion due to phlebitis and extravasation. Lancet ii: 1148–1150

Immunology of red cells

In this chapter, blood groups as a whole are discussed with special emphasis on immunological aspects; in subsequent chapters, some of the blood group systems are considered in more detail.

Although all inherited differences in the blood may fall within the widest meaning of the term *blood groups*, in this book the term is usually used simply for red cell antigens. When the inheritance of one series of antigens is independent of another series the antigens are said to belong to different blood group systems.

Discovery of the blood group systems

The ABO system

Antigenic differences between different species were recognized before differences within a species. Landois (1875, p. 185) discovered that when the red cells of an animal, for example a lamb, were mixed with the serum of another animal (a dog) and incubated at 37°C they might be lysed within 2 min.

Landsteiner (1900, 1901) was prompted by the work of Landois to see whether it was possible to demonstrate differences, although presumably slighter ones, between individuals of the same species. As he later explained (Landsteiner 1931), he chose the simplest plan of investigation and simply allowed serum and red cells from different human individuals to interact. For his resulting discovery of the ABO blood group system, which proved to be of vast importance for blood transfusion, he received the Nobel Prize, although it is said that he would much rather that it had been awarded to him for his work on the chemical basis of the specificity of serological reactions.

The Hh and Le systems were much later discovered to be biochemically related to the ABO system.

MN and P systems

After the discovery of the ABO system, no new blood group systems were found for 25 years. Landsteiner and Witt (1926) examined human sera for antibodies other than anti-A and anti-B but could find only weak agglutinins active at low temperatures. It occurred to Landsteiner and Levine (1927) that they might be able to reveal other antigens by injecting different samples of human red cells into rabbits. Antibodies identifying three new human antigens were obtained; to the first of these the letter M was given to indicate that the antigen had been identified with immune serum ('I' was avoided because of confusion with the numeral 1; Levine 1944).

The Rh system

Antibodies demonstrating Rh polymorphism in humans were found in two different ways. Landsteiner and Wiener (1940, 1941) injected the red cells of rhesus monkeys into rabbits and guinea pigs and tested the resulting serum against human red cells. Meanwhile, Levine and Stetson (1939) found an antibody (which subsequently proved to be anti-Rh D) in the serum of a recently delivered woman whose fetus had died *in utero*. Although the dates quoted here seem to establish priorities clearly, it is in fact very difficult to give a short answer to the question 'who discovered the Rh blood group system?'

According to RE Rosenfield (1977, supplemented by personal communication), L Buchbinder, a PhD student of Karl Landsteiner, had discovered Rh polymorphism at some time in the 1930s, but Landsteiner had refused to permit further studies or publication (Buchbinder's studies on the antigenic structure of erythrocytes of humans and *Macacus* rhesus were published in 1933).

A Wiener, who worked with Landsteiner in the late 1930s, stated, in the preface to his book *Rh-Hr Blood Types* published in 1954, that he had known about Rh polymorphism in 1937. In 1940, he described the results of tests on three patients who had had severe transfusion reactions; with the rabbit anti-rhesus serum available in Landsteiner's laboratory, the patients typed as Rh negative and the donors as Rh positive; moreover, haemagglutinins of the same specificity as the rabbit anti-rhesus serum were present in the patients' plasma (Wiener and Peters 1940). Landsteiner (Landsteiner and Wiener 1940) now agreed to publish the results of human blood typing with the animal anti-rhesus sera. Rosenfield (1977) pointed out that in this latter paper no data were published on adsorption and elution experiments; Rosenfield added, 'if Landsteiner remembered that this had been done by Buchbinder he forgot that it had not been published by Buchbinder [in 1933]'. Rosenfield concluded that if only Landsteiner and Wiener had published their findings in 1937, the question of priorities would not have arisen. As it was, Levine and Stetson's (1939) case (see Chapter 12) was the first published evidence of polymorphism related to Rh and thus could be claimed to take priority over the rabbit anti-rhesus data not published by Landsteiner and Wiener before 1940, even although Levine and Stetson failed to give a name to the specificity they had discovered. For further details of the Levine–Wiener argument, see Rosenfield (1989).

Other blood group systems

As Table 3.1 shows, the Lutheran (Lu), Kell (K), Duffy (Fy) and Kidd (Jk) systems were discovered by finding alloantibodies in the serum of transfused patients or of mothers of infants with haemolytic disease of the newborn (HDN). Other systems since discovered in the same way are Diego (Di), Cartwright (Yt), Xg, Scianna (Sc), Dombrock (Do), Colton (Co), Chido/Rodgers (Ch/Rg), Kx, Gerbich (Ge), Cromer (Cr), Knops (Kn) and Indian (In).

Terminology of blood groups

Blood group terminology is inconsistent. In some systems, for example ABO, antigens are given capital

Table 3.1 The first 10 blood group systems to be discovered.

Blood group system	Year of discovery	Antibody defining the system first found in
ABO	1901	Normal subjects
Le	1946	
MN*	1927	Rabbits injected with human red cells
P	1927	
LW	1930s	Rabbits injected with *rhesus* monkey red cells
Rh	1939	Mother of stillborn infant
	1940	Transfused patients
Lu	1945	Transfused patients or mothers of infants with HDN
K	1946	
Fy	1950	
Jk	1951	

* The S and s antigens were later discovered to be part of the same (MNSs) systems.

HDN = haemolytic disease of the newborn.

letters (e.g. B) or capital letters with subscripts (e.g. A_2); the corresponding alleles are denoted by italics, with superscripts when relevant (e.g. A^2). Although the alleles of the ABO system are all thought to be alternative forms at a single locus, this is not indicated by the nomenclature (e.g. one allele of A^2 is O). In other systems (e.g. Kell) the main alleles are denoted by large and small letters, thus *K* and *k*; here the terminology indicates that the alleles are alternative forms. The MNS system follows a blend of these two systems of nomenclature, the first antigens to be described being called M and N, and the next pair S and s.

The Le, Lu, Fy, Jk, Di, Yt, Do, Co, Kn and In systems follow a uniform pattern; the first alleles to be recognized are denoted thus Lu^a, Lu^b; phenotypes are written, for example, Lu(a+b–) and the corresponding antibody, anti-Lu^a. However, in almost all the systems, more than two alleles have been discovered and these additional alleles have usually been given numbers, for example, Fy^3. In the Xg, P_1, Hh and Kx systems only one antigen has been demonstrated so far, i.e. Xga, P_1, H and Kx respectively. The silent allele of Xg^a is termed *Xg* and that of H is *h*; those of P^1 and

Kx have no names. In the Sc system, the antigens are termed Sc1 and Sc2. In most cases the full name of the system is that of the subject in whom the antibody that led to the recognition of the system was first found. For the Rh system there were for a long time two nomenclatures, although now the CDE nomenclature is almost always used in preference to Wiener's. In several systems (Rh, K) a numerical system has for long been preferred by some for the identification of antigens and antibodies.

A standard numerical nomenclature, consisting of six numbers was devised by a Working Party of the International Society of Blood Transfusion (Lewis *et al.* 1985) and is regularly revised (Daniels *et al.* 2003). The first three numbers represent the blood group system, for example 001, ABO; 002, MNSs; 003, P; 004, Rh, and the second three numbers represent a particular antigenic specificity within that system, for example 001001, A; 004001, D.

In total, 29 blood group systems have been given numbers so far. In numerical order, systems 001–029 are: ABO, MNSs, P, Rh, Lu, K, Le, Fy, Jk, Di, Yt, Xg, Sc, Do, Co, LW, Ch/Rg, Hh, Kx, Ge, Cr, Kn, In, Ok, Raph, JMH, I, Globoside and GIL (Daniels *et al.* 2003). In the standard nomenclature, designed to be suitable for computers, the initials of the system are given in capitals, for example RH, but we have preferred to keep to the old style (Rh) in this book.

Further series of numbers have been established to encompass related families of antigens ('collections') as well as those high-frequency antigens ('public' antigens, the 901 series) and those low-frequency antigens ('private' antigens, the 700 series), which are not currently known to be genetically linked to any of the established 29 systems. At present, the collections comprise Cost (205), antigens Cs^a and Cs^b, i (207), Er (208), antigens Er^a and Er^b, Glob (209), antigens P^k and LKE and 210, antigens Le^c and Le^d, and the Vel (211) antigens, Vel and ABTI.

The relative clinical importance of different blood group systems

The clinical importance of a blood group system depends mainly on (1) the frequency with which alloantibodies of the system occur and (2) the characteristics of the alloantibodies, namely, Ig class and, if IgG, subclass, thermal range and ability to fix complement. These characteristics in turn determine the capacity of the antibody to cause red cell destruction and to be transferred across the placenta and cause HDN.

In the ABO and Lewis systems, the presence of soluble blood group antigens in the plasma is sometimes of clinical significance. In the fetus and newborn infant, A and B in the plasma may be partially protective against maternal anti-A and -B; and in transfusion recipients with potent anti-Le^a, who are transfused with Le(a+) blood, the presence of Le^a in the donor's plasma neutralizes the antibody and protects against red cell destruction.

ABO is easily the most important blood group system because anti-A and -B are found as naturally occurring antibodies in virtually all subjects who lack the corresponding antigens and these antibodies often cause intravascular haemolysis when incompatible red cells are transfused. The Rh system is next in importance because Rh D-negative subjects readily form anti-D and this antibody is capable of causing haemolytic transfusion reactions and HDN.

There are some systems in addition to ABO in which naturally occurring antibodies are sometimes found but these antibodies are usually inactive at body temperature and are then incapable of causing red cell destruction. Naturally occurring antibodies active at 37°C are often found in the Lewis system but, for reasons described later, very seldom cause haemolytic transfusion reactions.

There are other systems that have some similarities to Rh in that naturally occurring antibodies are rare and immune antibodies relatively frequent, particularly in patients who have been transfused many times. The most important of these systems, Kell, is very much less important than Rh, and the importance of the many other blood group systems, also described in Chapter 6, becomes progressively less until one reaches a system such as Colton in which very few antibodies have ever been encountered.

Red cell antigens

The red cell membrane

Like other cell membranes, the red cell membrane (see Plate 3.1 shown in colour between pages 528 and 529) is an assembly of lipid and protein molecules. The lipids, which together make up almost one-half of the mass of the membrane, are phospholipids (60%), cholesterol (30%) and glycolipids (10%). The lipid molecules are arranged as a continuous double layer, 4–5 nm thick.

The properties of mechanical strength and deformability that the red cell exhibits allow it to undergo the extensive deformation in the microvasculature necessary for O_2 delivery to the tissues over its 120-day lifespan. These properties are imparted by the skeleton, a network of proteins lying just beneath the red cell membrane, and tethered to the lipid bilayer primarily through interactions with the transmembrane proteins band 3 and glycophorin C. The major component of the skeleton, spectrin, consists of two subunits α (240 kDa) and β (220 kDa), which associate to form heterodimers. The heterodimers associate head to head to form tetramers. The tails of the tetramers interact at junctional complexes with a variety of proteins, including actin, protein 4.1, dematin (protein 4.9), tropomyosin and adducin (Gilligan and Bennett 1993; Peters and Lux 1993).

The spectrin lattice is linked to the plasma membrane mainly by ankyrin (protein 2.1) and actin. Ankyrin, in association with protein 4.2 (pallidin) attaches spectrin tetramers to the amino terminal cytoplasmic domain of the transmembrane protein band 3. Protein 4.1, in addition to its role in junction complexes, interacts with the cytoplasmic domain of protein glycophorin C.

The term 'Band' and the numbers given above, for example 4.1, refer to results obtained by the technique known as SDS-PAGE. In this technique, washed red cell ghosts are mixed with the ionic detergent sodium dodecyl sulphate (SDS), which solubilizes membrane proteins by displacing lipids from transmembrane regions. The solubilized proteins can be separated according to size by electrophoresis through a polyacrylamide gel, which acts as a molecular sieve: large glycoproteins tend to move more slowly than small ones (PAGE = polyacrylamide gel electrophoresis). When the separated proteins were visualized by staining with a protein stain (Coomassie blue) a number of bands were seen and these were numbered according to their apparent molecular size so the band of highest apparent molecular weight became band 1, the next largest band 2 and so on (Steck, 1974). In the intervening years some of the bands numbered in this way have acquired other names, the two subunits of spectrin were originally bands 1 and 2, while others, band 3, band 4.1 and band 4.2, have remained in common usage.

Surface proteins of the red cell

The blood group antigens of 22 blood group systems (MNS, Rh, Lu, K, Fy, Jk, Di, Yt, Xg, Sc, Do, Co, LW, Kx, Ge, Cr, Kn, In, Ok, Raph, JMH and GIL) are found on red cell surface proteins. The primary sequences of all these proteins are known and in most cases the molecular bases of the antigens in the systems are also known (see Chapters 5 and 6). These blood group active proteins constitute a diverse array of structures and functions. A minority of proteins at the red cell surface are not known to express blood group antigens defined by their protein sequence at the time of writing. These include the glucose transporter (GLUT1), the Rh-associated glycoprotein (RhAG), CD47 (IAP), CD58, CD59(MIRL), lactate transporter (MCT-1), prion protein (PRP) and a nucleoside transporter. The major surface proteins (defined as those with an abundance of 200 000 copies/red cell or more), and most of the minor surface proteins (50 000 copies/red cell or less), are listed in Table 3.2, and models of the structures of some of the blood group active proteins are shown in Plate 3.2 (shown in colour between pages 528 and 529). Some of the minor proteins (LW, CD47) associate with the major protein band 3 complex depicted in Plate 3.1 while others, particularly the GPI-anchored proteins, are located in microdomains known as 'lipid rafts' in areas of the red cell membrane remote from the major skeletal linked protein complexes (Brown and London 2000). The antigens of the Ch/Rg system are defined by the protein sequence of the fourth component of complement (see Chapter 6, page 209). The antigens of the remaining six systems (ABO, P, Le, H, I and Globoside) are formed by the action of glycosyltransferases and these are discussed in detail in Chapter 4. Carbohydrate structures at the red cell surface occur on both proteins and lipids and so antigens defined by carbohydrate structure alone are on several different molecules. There are two major oligosaccharide stuctures found on proteins, N-glycans and O-glycans. N-glycans are formed by the attachment of sugars to asparagine (N) in the polypeptide chain when it is part of a signal sequence N-X-S/T, where X is any other amino acid except proline and S/T is serine or threonine. N-glycans can be very large branched structures (Kameh et al. 1998). O-glycans are heavily sialylated and generally smaller than N-glycans. They are found mainly on the glycophorins but other proteins may also carry

Table 3.2 Surface proteins of the red cell (based on Anstee 1990, 1993).

	Synonym	Copies per cell $\times 10^5$	Antigens carried
Major proteins			
Anion transporter	band 3	10	ABH, Ii
Glycophorin A	SGP α	10	M, N
Glucose transporter	band 4.5	5	ABH, Ii
Glycophorin B	SGP δ	2.5	Ss, 'N'
Aquaporin1	CHIP	2	Co^a, Co^G
Rh polypeptides (D; CE)		1–2	Rh
RhAG	Rh glycoprotein	1–2	
Glycophorin C	SGP β	0.6–1.2	Ge
Glycophorin D	SGP γ	0.15–0.2	

	Synonym	Copies per cell $\times 10^3$	Antigens carried
Minor proteins			
Acetylcholinesterase (AChE)		3–10	Yt^a, Yt^b
Dombrock	–	?	Do^a, Do^b, Gy^a, Hy, Jo^a
Duffy	DARC	10–12	Fy^a, Fy^b
Kell		4–18	K
Kx		?	Kx
Kidd	RUT-B1	14	Jk^a, Jk^b, Jk^3
Lutheran		1–4	Lu antigens
LW	ICAM-4	3–5	LW^a, LW^b, LW^{a+b}
Xg^a		?	Xg^a
JMH	CDW108, semaphorin 7A	?	JMH
Ok^a	EMMPRIN, CD147	?	Ok^a
Scianna	ERMAP	?	Sc1, Sc2, Rd
CD35	CR1 (C3 receptor)	<1	Kn^a, McC^a, Sl^a, Yk^a
CD44		5–10	In^a/In^b
CD47		10–50	
CD55	Decay-accelerating factor	10–20	Cromer antigens
CD59	Membrane inhibitor of reactive lysis	20–40	
CD151	RAPH	<1	MER2

them (CD55 syn DAF for example, Lukacik *et al.* 2004).

The A, B, H, I and i antigens are carbohydrate structures (N-glycans) carried mainly on Band 3 and the glucose transporter (GLUT1). These proteins together account for about 2 million potential N-glycans/red cell but other glycoproteins, for example RhAG and aquaporin 1, and glycolipids also carry these antigens; see the section on the chemistry of ABH and other carbohydrate antigens in Chapter 4.

Transmembrane proteins contain stretches of around 20 hydrophobic amino acids (transmembrane domains), which lock them into the double layer of phospholipids in the cell membrane. There are three structural types of transmembrane protein in the red cell membrane. Many are type I membrane proteins, having a single membrane traverse with the amino terminus on the outside of the cell and the carboxyl terminus on the inside (glycophorins A, B and C, Lutheran, Xg, Sc, LW, Kn, In, Ok, CD47). The Kell protein is a type II membrane protein. It has a single transmembrane domain but its amino terminus is on the inside of the red cell and its carboxyl terminus on the outside. Several transmembrane proteins have more than one transmembrane domain and so are predicted to pass through the lipid bilayer several times, band 3 (14 times), glucose transporter (10 times), aquaporin 1 (six times), Rh polypeptides and Rh glycoprotein (RhAG, 12 times each), Jk protein (urea transporter, 10 times), Kx protein (10 times), Fy protein (DARC, seven times), Raph glycoprotein (CD151, four times), nucleoside transporter (12 times) and GIL protein (aquaporin 3, six times). Other proteins are attached to the membrane through a glycosylphosphatidyl inositol (GPI) anchor and do not have transmembrane domains (Yt (AchE), Cr(CD55,DAF), CD58,Do, JMH(CDw108), CD59(MIRL) and PRP (see Plate 3.2). Notable in this latter group are the complement-inhibiting proteins DAF (decay-accelerating factor, CD55), MIRL (membrane inhibitor of reactive lysis, CD59) and C8bp (C8 binding protein), also known as HRF (homologous restriction factor). Patients with paroxysmal nocturnal haemoglobinuria have deficiencies in the enzymes that assemble the GPI anchor and so lack all GPI-linked proteins from their red cells. Their red cells are highly sensitive to lysis by complement primarily because of the lack of CD59 (Inoue *et al.* 2003). Further information about red cell antigens carried on proteins is given in Chapters 5 and 6.

The antigenic determinant

The antibody-binding portion of an antigenic determinant, the 'epitope', which is the region of the antigen that is complementary to the combining site of the antibody, has an area of between one and seven sugar residues (0.5–3.5 nm) for the carbohydrate moiety of glycoproteins or glycolipids, and of four or five amino acids for protein. That part of the antigenic determinant that is bound most strongly is called the immunodominant group and is often the terminal non-reducing sugar residue. Antigenic determinants may be sequential, as in linear polysaccharides or polypeptides, or may be conformational and involve structures brought into proximity by folding, as in proteins.

Inheritance of red cell antigens

Two similar sets of chromosomes – one set inherited from each parent – are present in all cells of the body except the germ cells; each set is composed of 22 autosomes and one sex chromosome so that the total number of chromosomes is 46. In the female, the sex chromosomes are equal in size and are termed X chromosomes but in the male there is one X chromosome and one much smaller chromosome, termed Y.

A simple but incomplete definition of a gene is that segment of chromosomal DNA which determines a particular polypeptide. Alternative forms of genes at a particular locus are termed alleles, for example *A*, *B* and *O*. With one exception (see below), for all genes carried on autosomes an individual may be homozygous (both alleles the same, e.g. *AA*) or heterozygous (alleles dissimilar, e.g. *AO*). Whereas the term *genotype* is used for the sum of inherited alleles of a particular gene, for example *AA*, *AO*, *phenotype* refers only to the recognizable product of the alleles. As *O* has no serologically recognizable product, the genotypes *AO* and *AA* both have the phenotype *A*. The only X-borne blood group genes are *Xgª* and *Xᵏ*, the gene which determines Kx. Females may be homozygous or heterozygous for *Xgª* (*XgªXgª* or *XgªXg*) but males can only be *Xgª* or *Xg* and are said to be hemizygous.

Although *O* has no recognizable product, the DNA structure of this silent allele differs only slightly from that of the *A* and *B* alleles. However, in the Rh system, the gene *D* has no allele. At the corresponding position on the homologous chromosome, there is either another *D* gene or a *D* gene altered in such a way that *D* polypeptide cannot be made. Subjects who have *D* on either or both of the pair of chromosomes concerned are *D* positive and those in whom *D* is lacking from both chromosomes are *D* negative.

A distinction between the red cells of some homozygotes and heterozygotes (e.g. *DD* and *D*, *AA* and *AO*) cannot be made reliably with serological methods but can be achieved using molecular methods (see Chapter 12, page 510).

Genes that are far apart on the same chromosome, for example *Rh* and *Fy*, or genes that are carried on different chromosomes are inherited independently and the antigens they determine are said to belong to different blood group systems; see Table 3.1 for an example and see the following section for the chromosomal location of the different blood group genes.

In bacteria, genes consist of a single stretch of DNA, which directly encodes its protein product but in man (and in all eukaryotes) the coding region is almost always interrupted by at least one stretch of DNA, known as an intron, which does not code for a protein. The introns are spliced out of the RNA prior to its translation into the protein. The coding sections are referred to as exons.

In some cases, more than one protein is produced from a single gene and thus one allele determines more than one polypeptide (see Ge in Chapter 6).

Red cell antigens that are proteins (e.g. Rh) are direct products of genes, but those that are carbohydrate (e.g. *A*) are determined indirectly by enzymes (glycosyltransferases) that are the gene products; these enzymes transfer the appropriate sugar, determining specificity, on to a structure whose synthesis may be determined by one or more unrelated genes.

In most cases there appears to be a simple correspondence between genes and antigens, so that if a person inherits a given gene the antigen can be detected on the red cells. It is not uncommon for one gene to interfere with the expression of another, carried on a different chromosome. For example, the expression of *Le* is modified by *A* and *B* (see Chapter 4) and that of *Lu* may be modified by inhibitor genes (see Chapter 6).

Gene (allele) frequencies

Gene frequency means simply the frequency of the allele in the population as a whole; the term *allele frequency* would be more precise but it is not generally used. From a knowledge of the frequencies of the gene (allele) in a blood group system, phenotype frequencies are readily derived. For example, based on testing almost 200 000 white British subjects, the frequencies of the three main alleles in the ABO system were calculated to be: *A*, 0.2573; *B*, 0.0600; and *O*, 0.6827 (Dobson and Ikin 1946). (Note that in calculating the frequency of the *O* allele one must count not only people of group O with a double dose of the allele but also those people whose genotype is *AO* or *BO*.) From the above gene frequencies, the frequency of group O is 0.6827×0.6827, or 0.47 (47%); that of group AB is $(0.2573 \times 0.0600) \times 2$, or 0.03 (3%). The '× 2' is accounted for by the fact that *A* can combine with *B*, as well as *B* with *A*. In this book, unless otherwise stated, frequencies of alleles and phenotypes refer to a mainly white population in the UK. Frequencies for other populations are given by Mourant and co-workers (1976).

In different races the proportion of individuals belonging to a particular blood group varies widely; some examples of differences between Chinese, Europeans and West Africans are given in Table 3.3.

Table 3.3 Appoximate frequencies (as percentages) of some blood group antigens in Chinese, Europeans and West Africans.

	Chinese	Europeans	W. Africans
B	35	9	20
P_1	31	80	95
Rh D	100	84	95
V(ce^s)	?0	<1	40
K	0	9	<1
Js^a	0	0	20
Fy^a	99	65	20
Di^a	5	0	0

Several techniques are now available for determining the genotype of a polymorphic gene directly at the DNA level. These techniques are described in Chapter 8. The performance of these techniques is dependent on amplification of the relevant stretches of DNA, using the polymerase chain reaction (PCR) with appropriate primers. For a description of the PCR, see Chapter 16 and Plate 16.1.

Chromosomal location of different blood group genes

The locations are: on chromosome 1, *Rh*, *Fy*, *Sc*, *Cr* and *Kn*; on 2, *Ge*; on 4, *MNSs*; on 6, *HLA*, genes for several complement components including C2 and the C4A and C4B markers Ch and Rg; on 7, *Co*, *K*, and *Yt*; on 9, *ABO* and *GIL*; on 11, *In* and *Raph*; on 12, *Do*; on 15, *JMH*; on 17, *Di*; on 18, *Jk*; on 19, *H*, *Le*, *Lu*, *LW* and *Ok*; on 22, *P*; and on the X chromosome, *Xg*, together with *Xk* and the X-linked suppressor of *Lu*.

Inherited markers on blood cells and predisposition to disease

The relation between a genetic marker and disease may be expressed as linkage, i.e. the marker and disease susceptibility are inherited together, or as association, i.e. the particular marker is more frequent in subjects with the disease than in normal subjects.

The majority of HLA-associated diseases display a higher frequency of a particular HLA-DR antigen, for example in immunoglobulin A (IgA) deficiency and in several autoimmune diseases, the frequency of HLA-DR3 is increased (see Lechler 1994).

The associations between red cell groups and disease are not as strong as those between HLA groups and disease and the risk, for individuals carrying the associated red cell antigen, of acquiring a particular disease is, as a rule, only slightly larger than for those subjects negative for the red cell antigen. The first of such associations to be established was that between group A and carcinoma of the stomach (Aird and Bentall 1953), the risk of group A subjects being 1.2 times that of group O or B subjects (see review by Roberts 1957).

There is an association between group O and peptic ulcer (Aird et al. 1954), the risk for group O being 30–40% (1.3 times) higher than non-O (Mourant et al. 1978). There is also an association between non-secretors (of ABH) and peptic ulcer; non-secretors are almost 50% (1.5 times) more likely than secretors to have a duodenal ulcer (Clarke et al. 1956). The increased risk for group O and non-secretors is multiplicative, being about 2.5 times that of non-group O secretors (Doll et al. 1961). A partial explanation for these associations is that the Le[b] antigen (present only in secretors) is an epithelial receptor for *Helicobacter pylori*, a bacterium associated with gastritis, gastric ulcer and adenocarcinoma. The bacterium will not bind to Le[b] molecules to which A or B determinants have been added and the binding is inhibited by Le[b] substance and by anti-Le[b] (Borén et al. 1993, discussed further in Chapter 4).

An association of interest to haematologists is that between the levels of factor VIII, von Willebrand factor (vWF) and ABO group. Blood group O individuals have approximately 25% lower plasma levels of both factor VIII and vWF than individuals of group A,B or AB (Gill et al. 1987; O'Donnell and Laffan 2001). This variance may have an influence on the diagnosis of von Willebrand disease (vWd). Gill et al. found that 88 of 114 patients with type I vWd were group O and suggested that some individuals of group AB with a genetic defect of vWF may have their diagnosis overlooked because of the elevated levels of vWF in their blood group. Conversely, high levels of FVIII-vWF found in A,B and AB individuals may confer an increased risk of thrombosis and myocardial infarction (von Beckerath et al. 2004; Schleef et al. 2005).

Red cell markers on functionally important membrane structures

Some red cell antigens are situated on important structures on the cell membrane so that absence or presence of the antigen is associated with some structural abnormality of the cell, associated with functional change. Examples of such associations are as follows: (1) between Rh_{null} or Rh_{mod} and haemolytic anaemia (see Chapter 5); (2) between the rare McLeod phenotype (see Kell blood group system, Chapter 6) and acanthocytosis; (3) between absence or depression of certain red cell antigens and elliptocytosis (see Chapter 6); (4) between Fy-related antigens and susceptibility to malaria (see Chapter 6); (5) between Cr-null (Inab phenotype) red cells and absence of decay-accelerating factor (see Chapter 6); and (6) between expression of the normally hidden antigen Tn and deficiency of sialic acid (see Chapter 7).

Effect of neoplastic change and dyserythropoiesis on blood group antigens

Cell surface antigens and neoplastic change

Neoplastic change in cells may be accompanied by changes in cell surface antigens. Some of these changes are due to incomplete synthesis of antigens normally present; others are due to abnormal synthesis, giving rise to neoantigens. As an example of the first kind of change, in some subjects with acute leukaemia, A, B and I antigens may be depressed (see Chapter 4); similarly, in some subjects with carcinoma, ABH determinants are lost due to incomplete synthesis, and precursor substances accumulate (Hakomori 1984a). Loss of A,B and H antigens is frequently found in myeloid malignancies (Bianco et al. 2001). T and Tn antigens, which are normally covered by attached sialic acid, are commonly exposed on the surface of malignant cells (see Chapter 7).

The first recorded example of the production of a neoantigen by malignant tissue was that of Levine et al. (1951a). The patient was a woman with a gastric adenocarcinoma, whose serum contained the rare antibody anti-Tj[a] (later renamed anti-PP[1]P[k]). As expected, the patient's red cells were Tj (a−) but a dried extract of the tumour specifically inhibited the antibody in her serum, suggesting that Tj[a] antigen had been formed by the malignant tissue and might have

55

evoked production of the anti-Tj^a. Thirty years later, biochemical analysis of lyophilized tumour tissue showed that glycolipids with P and P$_1$ activity were present (Hakomori 1984a). Similarly, some tumours derived from gastrointestinal tissue of group O or B individuals contain an A-like antigen, different from Forsmann antigen, and some tumours from Forsmann-negative tissue contain Forsmann antigen, which is similar to blood group A (Hakomori 1984a). The overlapping functions of A and B transferases provide an explanation for the apparent expression of blood group antigens in certain tumours; changes in biochemical pathways in tumour tissue may provide appropriate substrates for the transfer of the 'wrong' sugars, giving rise, in subjects with exceptionally potent transferases, to A or B antigens not expected from the ABO genotype of the individual (Yates *et al.* 1983).

Various types of human adenocarcinoma accumulate a large quantity of fucolipids and their sialated derivatives as well as fucosylated glycoproteins with type II chains (see Chapter 4). Monoclonal antibodies directed against some of these structures have been produced and may prove to be useful diagnostic and therapeutic tools.

Dyserythropoiesis

In acquired dyserythropoiesis associated with a variety of haematological disorders (e.g. megaloblastic anaemia, sideroblastic anaemia) there is an increase in i and, in tests with some antisera, of I. In inherited (congenital) dyserythropoietic anaemia of type I and type II (HEMPAS), i is increased but I is probably not increased; see review by Worlledge (1977). Congenital dyserythropoietic anaemias (CDAs) are a rare group of inherited diseases in which erythropoeisis is altered quantitatively and qualitatively. Seven types of CDA are recognized by Wickramasinghe (1998). The clinical features of all types are reviewed by Delauney and Iolascon (1999). CDA II (HEMPAS) is the most common and best characterized. Examination of bone marrow under the light microscope shows that about 10–40% of more mature erythroblasts are multinucleated. Under the electron microscope a double membrane is seen. This double membrane comprises the plasma membrane and elongated vesicles that run parallel and beneath the plasma membrane derived from endoplasmic reticulum (Alloisio *et al.* 1996). Hypoglycosylation of the major red cell anion transport protein is a characteristic but not exclusive feature of CDA II. Zdebska and colleagues (2001) report that glycosylation abnormalities of band 3, glycophorin A and glycolipids can be found in CDA I, II and III. These glycosylation abnormalities presumably account for the altered expression of I and i antigens reported in such cases. Paw and co-workers (2003) describe a zebrafish band 3 mutation with an erythroid phenotype very similar to that of CDA II. However, mutation in band 3 cannot be the explanation for most cases of CDA II in man, where the disease maps to chromosome 20q11.2 rather than 17q21-q22, the locus of band 3 (Perrotta *et al.* 2003).

CDA VII is associated with severe transfusion-dependent anaemia and was described in a Danish patient who had persistence of embryonic and fetal haemoglobins. The blood group phenotype of this patient [In(a–b–), AnWj–,Co(a–b–)] was remarkable and further investigation showed the red cells lacked CD44 and that aquaporin-1 was expressed at only 10% of normal levels (Agre *et al.* 1994; Parsons *et al.* 1994).

Myeloproliferative disease

Myeloproliferative disease is thought to be due to a mutation of haemopoietic stem cells, giving rise to an abnormal clone of cells. In several cases, Rh mosaicism has been observed; for example, in a patient whose probable genotype was originally *DCe/dce*, a proportion of the red cells typed as D negative (Mannoni *et al.* 1970). In another case, a man who had originally been D positive was found to have become D negative. An anomaly was found involving chromosome 1, on which the *Rh* genes are known to be located. The patient developed anti-D (and -C) following transfusion, demonstrating loss of immunological tolerance to self-antigens following the loss of ability to express these antigens (Copper *et al.* 1979).

Tn polyagglutination (Chapter 7), which is a form of mosaicism affecting red cells (and other blood cells), has also been observed in myelofibrosis (Bird *et al.* 1985).

Development of red cell antigens

Red cell antigens in embryos and newborn infants

During ontogeny, ABH and Lewis activity is at its highest from the fifth week after fertilization. ABH

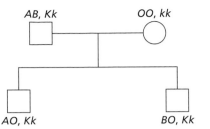

Fig 3.1 Independent inheritance of the ABO and Kell genes. In this example, the father passes on *A* to one son and *B* to the other, but passes on *K* to both.

antigens are found in large amounts on endothelial cells, on most epithelial primordia and in practically all early organs, for example in the blood islands of the yolk sac, on digestive tube epithelia, etc. The central nervous system, liver, adrenal glands and secretory tubules show no activity at this stage. From the end of the 12th–14th weeks of gestation, there is regression of ABH expression from epithelial cell walls and from thyroid and other glands and organs (Szulman 1980). Similarly, although P_1 is only weakly expressed on the red cells of newborn infants, on the red cells of embryos with a crown–rump length of less than 10 cm it is expressed almost as strongly as in the adult (Ikin *et al.* 1961). The reason for the regression of expression of these various antigens is unknown.

I, Le^a, Le^b and Sd^a are very weakly expressed on the red cells of newborn infants, and A, B, P_1, Lu^a, Lu^b, Yt^a, Xg, Vel and Ch/Rg and antigens of the Cost collection are more weakly expressed on infants' red cells than on adults' red cells. The antigens of the Rh, K, Fy, Jk, MNSs, Di, Sc, Do, Co and Ge systems, as well as Au^a of the Lu system, appear to be fully developed at birth.

Red cell antigens on red cell precursors

Reticulocytes are as strongly agglutinated as mature red cells by anti-A and anti-B (Maizels and Patterson 1940; Winkelstein and Mollison 1965). Although A can be demonstrated even on early erythroblasts (Reyes *et al.* 1974; Gourdin *et al.* 1976), anti-A and anti-B do not inhibit the growth of colony-forming units (CFUs) or erythrocyte burst-forming units (BFU-Es) *in vitro* (Hershko *et al.* 1980) nor do they delay the engraftment of ABO-incompatible bone marrow *in vivo* (Dinsmore *et al.* 1983). The following red cell

antigens have also been demonstrated on erythroblasts: A_1, B and H (Yunis and Yunis 1963), I and those of the Rh, MNSs, P, Lu, K, Le, Fy and Jk systems (Yunis and Yunis 1964). The amount of D antigen on pronormoblasts is about one-quarter as great as that on mature red cells (Rearden and Masouredis 1977).

It seems that the onset of Hb synthesis and expression of glycophorins at the cell surface occur at the same stage of differentiation (Gahmberg *et al.* 1978). The temporal appearance of blood group antigens during erythropoiesis has been studied using *in vitro* culture of CD34^+ cells derived from cord blood or adult peripheral blood in the presence of SCF, IL3 and EPO (Bony *et al.* 1999; Southcott *et al.* 1999). The earliest blood group markers expressed are ABO, Kell and the Rh-related glycoprotein RhAG followed by glycophorin A, band 3 and the Rh polypeptides. Lutheran appears late in the cultures.

Red cell antibodies

Antibodies are immunoglobulins (Igs), a family of proteins that are structurally related and all of which have two functions: to combine with antigen; and then to mediate various biological effects. Thus, all antibody molecules have antigen-combining sites and various effector function sites.

The common structural feature of all Ig molecules is an arrangement of a pair of identical, relatively large, 'heavy' (H) polypeptide chains joined, by covalent (disulphide) and non-covalent bonds, to each other and to a pair of identical 'light' (L) chains (Fig. 3.2). The covalent bonds are mainly in the hinge region (see below). Five different classes of Ig are recognized, IgG, IgM, IgA, IgD and IgE, and these have different H chains, termed γ, μ, α, δ and ϵ. Igs of all five classes have the same L chains, although these may be either kappa (κ) or lambda (λ). In each IgG molecule, the two L chains are the same, e.g. a molecule may be $\gamma\gamma\kappa\kappa$ or $\gamma\gamma\lambda\lambda$. IgG molecules occur as monomers, IgM molecules as pentamers, e.g. $(\mu_2\lambda_2)_5$ (see below), and IgA molecules as monomers or dimers. All Ig molecules have carbohydrate (CHO) attached to their H chains. For example, in IgG there is a short-branched CHO chain (approximately nine residues) attached to each H chain in the $C\gamma2$ domain (see Fig. 3.2). The CHO chains lie in the space between the two $C\gamma2$ domains and may help to keep them apart. IgM has short CHO chains attached to each of the

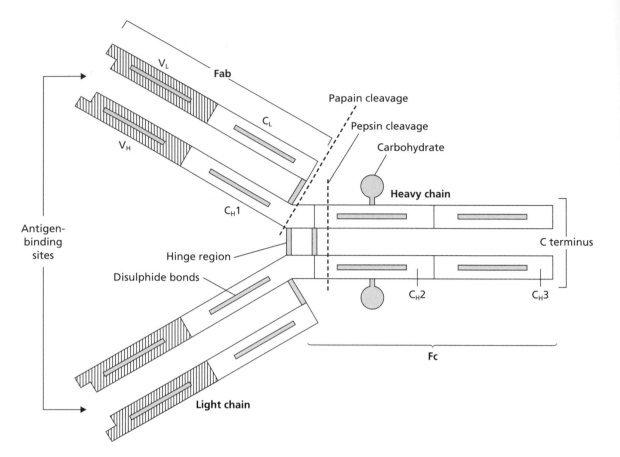

Fig 3.2 The IgG molecule. The constant (C) and variable (V) domains of the heavy (H) and light (L) chains are shown, together with the intra- and interchain disulphide bonds (▨) that hold them together. The antigen-binding site is situated in the groove between the terminal parts of the V_H and V_L regions. The sites of attachment of carbohydrate chains indicated in the figure are, in fact, internal. After treatment with papain, the IgG molecule is cleaved into two Fab fragments and one Fc fragment; after treatment with pepsin, the two Fab fragments remain joined by disulphide bonds as an $(Fab')_2$ fragment and the Fc fragment disintegrates. Slightly modified from Roitt *et al.* (1989).

constant domains. The function of these CHO chains is not definitely known, although there is often loss of functional activity when the CHO is absent.

H and L chains are made up of regions ('domains'), each of about 110 amino acids with the same basic structure. Both H and L chains take part in combining with antigen. The first 110–120 amino acids at the amino terminal end of each chain form the variable (V) domains, each of which contains hypervariable regions (four for V_H and three for V_L). The hypervariable regions on a pair of H and L chains, each consisting of fewer than 10 amino acids, come together in the folded molecule to form the antigen-binding site. The peptide sequences joining the hypervariable regions do not take part in binding to antigen but form an essential framework. The rest of the H and L chains are constant regions (C_H and C_L) with characteristic amino acid sequences. IgG and IgA have three constant regions per H chain but IgM and IgE have four. L chains each have only one C region. The different biological activities of each class of Ig molecule are affected by the amino acid sequences of the C regions. Flexibility is conferred on Ig molecules by a hinge region which, in IgG, is situated between the Cγ1 and Cγ2 domains (see Figs 3.2 and 3.3) and in IgM in the Cγ2 domain (Fig. 3.4). Flexibility is believed to be very

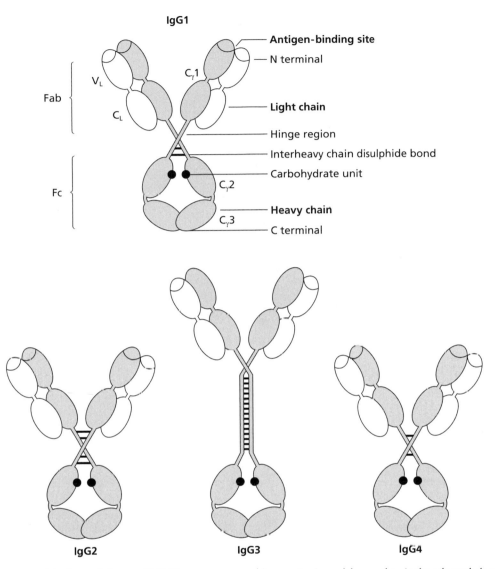

IgG1

Antigen-binding site

N terminal

V_L

$C_\gamma 1$

Fab

C_L

Light chain

Hinge region

Interheavy chain disulphide bond

Carbohydrate unit

Fc

$C_\gamma 2$

Heavy chain

$C_\gamma 3$

C terminal

IgG2　　　　IgG3　　　　IgG4

Fig 3.3 Structure of the four subclasses of IgG. The arrangement and number of the interheavy chain disulphide bonds are different in each of the subclasses. In IgG3 the hinge region is much longer than in the other subclasses. From Roitt *et al.* (1989).

important in enabling the molecule to fulfil its effector functions.

In IgG1 and IgG3, the site for binding C1q, and thus for activating the complement pathway (see later), is found on $C_\gamma 2$, as is the site for binding to Fc receptors on mononuclear phagocytic cells. Sites on both the $C_\gamma 2$ and $C_\gamma 3$ domains are involved in binding IgG to Fc receptors on placental tissue. In IgM, the site for binding C1q is on the $C_H 3$ domains (see Fig. 3.4).

By treatment with papain, the IgG molecule can be split, between the $C_\gamma 1$ and $C_\gamma 2$ domains (see Fig. 3.2), into two Fab (fragment antigen-binding) fragments, each of which carries a single antigen-combining site, and one Fc (fragment crystallizable) fragment that carries sites for various effector functions (see above). As Fig. 3.2 implies, the Fab fragment consists of the whole of the L chain and part of the H chain; in both chains, regions (V_L and V_H) at the amino terminal end

(a)

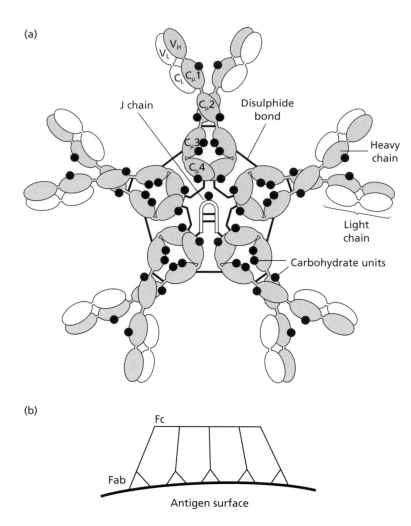

Fig 3.4 (a) The IgM molecule, showing the way in which the five subunits are held together by disulphide bonds and joined by joining, J, chain. As in Fig. 3.1, the position of attachment of carbohydrate chains is shown, but their size and structure are not indicated. Slightly modified from Roitt *et al.* (1989). (b) Staple form (as opposed to star form shown in (a) of IgM molecule). This configuration is observed when the molecule binds to a surface on which antigen sites are sufficiently close together to permit two or more antigen-combining sites of the same IgM molecule to bind (Feinstein *et al.* 1971).

of the fragment are joined to the single C region of the L chain and the Cγ1 region of the H chain. IgG can also be split into fragments by pepsin but in this case the molecule is cleaved nearer the carboxy terminal end (Fig. 3.2) and the two Fab fragments are left joined together to form an F(ab')$_2$ fragment, the rest of the molecule being broken up (Porter 1967).

Characteristics of different immunoglobulins

The main immunoglobulins in serum are shown in Table 3.4.

IgG

IgG is the most abundant Ig in plasma, having a mean concentration of about 12 g/l (range 8–16 g/l), so that the total plasma content, taking the plasma volume to be 40 ml/kg, is about 0.5 g/kg or, in a subject weighing 70 kg, 35 g; there is an approximately equal amount of IgG in the extravascular space, so that, in the example taken, total body IgG would be about 70 g, or 1 g/kg. The rate of transfer of IgG between the extra- and intravascular compartments is described briefly in Chapter 14.

Four subclasses of IgG are recognized and their mean concentrations in normal adult serum (in g/l) are as follows: IgG1, 6.63; IgG2, 3.22; IgG3, 0.58; IgG4, 0.46 (Morell *et al.* 1971). The subclasses differ in structure and function; thus, the number of inter-H-chain disulphide bonds varies in the different subclasses and, for example, IgG3 differs from the other

Table 3.4 The main immunoglobulins in serum.

	IgG	IgM	IgA
Heavy chains	γ	μ	α
Light chains	κ and λ	κ and λ	κ and λ
Molecular forms	$\gamma_2\kappa_2$	$(\mu_2\kappa_2)_5 J$	$(\alpha_2\kappa_2)_1$ or $_2$
	$\gamma_2\lambda_2$	$(\mu_2\lambda_2)_5 J$	$(\alpha_2\kappa_2)_1$ or $_2$
Molecular weight	150 000	970 000	160 000
Sedimentation coefficient	7S	19S	7S, 9S and 11S
Concentration in plasma (g/l)			
Adult*	8–16	0.5–2.0	1.4–4.0
Newborn	Similar	Approx. 0.1	Undetectable
Catabolic rate, $t_{1/2}$ (d)[†]	21	5	6
Percentage of total which is intravascular[†]	52	74	40
Transferred across placenta?	Yes	No	No
Binds to Fc receptors?	Yes	No	Yes
Usual serological behaviour as red cell antibody	Incomplete antibody	Agglutinin	Agglutinin (dimers only)
Serological activity after heating to 56°C for 3 h	Unaffected	Reduced	Unaffected
Effect of reducing agents on serological activity	May develop agglutinating activity	No longer agglutinates	Partially inactivated

* Roitt (1988).
[†] Wells (1980).
J = J chain.

subclasses in having a much longer hinge region (see Fig. 3.3).

Several membrane-bound receptors recognize the Fc region of antibodies. FcRI, FcRII and FcRIII recognize sites on the lower hinge region (CH2) of IgG (Sondermann and Oosthuizen 2001) (Plate 3.3). Monomeric IgG1 and IgG3 bind to FcRI; polymeric IgG1 and IgG3 bind, in addition, to FcRII and FcRIII. Three closely linked genes encode three different types of FcRII: FcRIIa, FcRIIb and FcRIIc. FcRIIa has two variants, one binds only weakly to IgG2 but the other, present in 30% of white people, binds strongly (Warmerdam et al. 1991). IgG4 binds weakly to both forms of FcRIIa. Glycosylation is essential for some functions of IgG, including adherence to Fc receptors.

IgG is the only Ig to be transferred across the placenta from mother to fetus, a fact that explains the role of IgG antibodies in the aetiology of alloimmune cytopenias of the fetus and newborn. The transfer of IgG across the placenta from mother to fetus is mediated by the neonatal Fc receptor (FcRn) (see Chapter 12 and Plate 12.1). FcRn has a different structure from the other Fc receptors and consists of a heavy chain complexed with beta2 microglobulin (Burmeister et al. 1994).

IgG1 and IgG3 activate complement strongly but IgG2 activates only weakly and IgG4 not at all. IgG1, IgG2 and IgG4 myeloma proteins have catabolic rates that are similar to those of total IgG, i.e. they have a $t_{1/2}$ of about 21 days but the $t_{1/2}$ of IgG3 is about 7 days (Morell et al. 1970). The foregoing estimates were derived from measurements on myeloma proteins. Similar half-lives have been found for monoclonal Rh D antibodies, namely for IgG1, 21–22 days (Callaghan et al. 1993; Goodrick et al. 1994) and for IgG3, 10 days (Goodrick et al. 1994).

IgM

The plasma concentration of IgM is 0.5–2.0 g/l; about 74% of total body IgM is intravascular; the plasma

$t_{1/2}$ is 5 days. IgM molecules are held together by a J (joining) chain (see Fig. 3.3).

IgM is more effective than IgG in activating complement. The difference is due to the fact that C1 is activated only when it is attached by two of its C1q heads to the activating molecule. Thus, whereas a single bound IgM molecule can activate C1, at least two IgG molecules bound at closely adjacent sites are needed. Several of the antigen-binding sites on a single IgM molecule may bind to antigen sites on the cell surface, giving the molecule the appearance of a staple (see Fig. 3.4b), in contrast to the normal star form shown in Fig. 3.4a.

IgA

The plasma concentration of IgA is 1.4–4.0 g/l; about 40% of total body IgA is intravascular; the plasma $t_{1/2}$ is 6 days.

IgA is the only Ig present in epithelial secretions. Whereas, in plasma, IgA is predominantly monomeric, in secretions it occurs mainly as dimers, which are held together by a J chain. In secretions, IgA has a 'secretory piece' that prevents the molecule from being digested. The presence of IgA in secretions is believed to be due almost entirely to local production rather than to transport from plasma. The function of IgA is evidently to neutralize antigens that might otherwise enter the body via mucosal routes.

There are two subclasses of IgA, a major component, IgA1, and a minor component, IgA2, which has two serologically distinguishable variants, A2m(1) and A2m(2). Both IgA1 and IgA2 bind to an Fc receptor for IgA (CD89) on monocytes and macrophages. Inhibition of IgA binding to CD89 by staphylococcal superantigen-like proteins leads to increased survival of staphylococcal bacteria in blood (Langley *et al.* 2005).

IgD and IgE

Both of these Igs act mainly as cell receptors. No free antibodies made of IgD have been described, although IgD is synthesized by, and demonstrable on, the surface of B lymphocytes and is probably involved in the activation of these cells by antigen.

IgE is synthesized by plasma cells and is present in the plasma in very low concentrations. It has a very high affinity for Fc receptors (FcεRI) on basophils and mast cells. The binding of antigen to IgE antibody on the surface of these cells leads to crosslinking of receptors and produces degranulation with release of vasocative amines, such as histamine, and of cytokines as well as synthesis of inflammatory mediators of arachidonic acid (e.g. leukotrienes). These mediators are responsible for producing such atopic phenomena as asthma and hay fever. The role of IgE antibodies in reactions to atopens is discussed in Chapter 15.

Markers on immunoglobulin molecules

Idiotypic markers. Idiotypic determinants arise from the unique configuration of the antigen-combining site of an antibody molecule, which gives the molecule its specificity.

The idio*type* of a particular antibody specificity is composed of several individual determinants called idio*topes*, in much the same way that the Rh polypeptides expressed by the R^1 haplotype encompass several Rh determinants (i.e. D, C, G, e, Rh17, Rh18, Rh29, Rh34, Rh44, Rh46, Rh47, etc.). Some of the individual idiotopes arise from the unique amino acid sequences in the hypervariable region that come into contact with the antigen in the antibody-binding site; others arise from framework amino acid sequences. Antisera can be raised to both sets of idiotopes.

Some idiotypes (public idiotypes) are common to all antibodies of a single specificity; each individual can make 10^6–10^7 different antibody specificities. Other idiotypes (private idiotypes) are restricted to only a few clones producing antibodies of similar specificity but each differing slightly (by one or two amino acids) in their hypervariable region; a typical polyclonal immune response can be composed of 10^4 different species of antibody molecules of similar specificity, each species being the product of a separate B cell clone. Sometimes, antibodies of quite distinct specificities, for example anti-albumin and anti-influenza virus can exhibit common idiotypes; these are called the major crossreactive idiotypes and represent common amino acid sequences in the framework regions of their binding sites.

Every antibody is capable of inducing the formation of auto- or allo-anti-idiotypes. The formation of auto-anti-idiotypes is believed to be important in regulating the immune response.

Allotypic markers. These are antigens, found on γ, α and κ chains, the inheritance of which is controlled by alleles of the gene coding for a particular Ig chain. For example, H chains of IgG subclass 1 can carry either G1m(z) or G1m(f), the difference being determined by a single amino acid substitution. Further details are given in Chapter 13.

Isotypic markers. These are antigenic determinants on H chains and on certain L chains, which define and characterize the class or subclass of Ig molecules and which are sequences on the C region of γ and μ chains or on the C region of κ and λ chains. Isoallotypic markers (formerly called non-markers) are those which are isotypic markers for one subclass but are allotypic markers in another subclass. For example, G4m(a) is an allotype in subclass IgG4 but is an isotype in IgG2.

Immunoglobulins in fluids other than plasma

Immunoglobulins are found in the following fluids.

Colostrum and saliva. In colostrum, the IgA concentration is about 90% and in saliva is about 20% of that in normal serum (Chodirker and Tomasi 1963). By contrast, concentrations of IgG and IgM in colostrum are respectively 1% and 5–10% of the amounts in normal serum, and in saliva only faint traces of IgG and IgM are present (Adinolfi *et al.* 1966). The titre of IgA antibody tends to be higher in colostrum than in serum (Tomasi *et al.* 1965; Adinolfi *et al.* 1966). Colostrum frequently contains potent IgA anti-A and anti-B, but in saliva these antibodies are usually present only in low concentration (see Chapter 4).

Ascitic fluid. Several alloantibodies have been harvested from ascitic fluid; anti-Yt^a (Eaton *et al.* 1956); anti-c and -Le^a (MM Pickles, quoted by Race and Sanger 1968, p. 255); and anti-E (Zeitlin *et al.* 1958) and anti-K (Longster and Major 1975). In the last mentioned case the titre of the antibody was about the same in serum as in ascitic fluid and the antibody was probably IgG; in contrast to that of anti-K, the titres of anti-A and anti-B were slightly lower in ascitic fluid than in serum.

Amniotic fluid. The IgG concentration at or near term is about 0.1–0.2 g/l, i.e. 1/50–1/100 of that in normal adult serum.

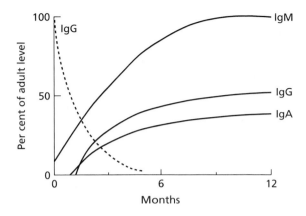

Fig 3.5 Concentration of IgG, IgM and IgA in the first year of life, as percentages of the normal adult levels (based on the data of West *et al.* 1962). The dotted line indicates IgG derived from the mother by placental transfer.

Production of immunoglobulin in the fetus and infant

Changes in Ig levels in the first year of life are summarized in Fig. 3.5.

IgG. Although most of the IgG in the serum of newborn infants is derived from the mother by placental transfer, a small amount is of fetal origin as shown by the fact that it has the father's Gm allotype (Mårtensson and Fudenberg 1965).

The time at which the synthesis of substantial amounts of IgG begins after birth was studied by Zak and Good (1959) in two normal infants born to mothers with severe hypogammaglobulinaemia. The IgG level, which was negligible at birth, started to increase between 3 and 6 weeks; antibodies were first demonstrable at about 2 months, by which time the IgG level had reached 2 g/l. At 10–18 months, IgG levels are about 60% of adult values (Buckley *et al.* 1968).

IgM. IgM is not transferred across the placenta. The concentration in cord serum is between 5% and 10% of that found in adult serum. IgM antibodies of various specificities can be found in cord serum: anti-I in most infants (see Chapter 7); anti-A and anti-B in occasional infants (see Chapter 4); anti-Gm in most infants (see Chapter 13) and anti-A chain in about 10% of infants (Epstein 1965). Within 2 or 3 days of birth the concentration of IgM starts to rise and reaches 50% of

63

the adult level at 2–3 months and 100% at about 9 months; between the ages of 9 months and 3 years values remain at the adult level, although between 5 and 9 years they are at the lower end of the adult range (West *et al.* 1962).

IgA. This protein cannot be detected in cord serum. By the age of 2 months, the amount in the serum has reached about 20% of the adult level (West *et al.* 1962) and by the age of 5 years about 50% (Buckley *et al.* 1968).

Immunoglobulin class and subclass of red cell alloantibodies

Red cell alloantibodies may be naturally occurring or immune. When naturally occurring they are most often IgM but may be partly IgG or, occasionally, predominantly IgG (see also p. 80); when immune they are most often IgG, but may be IgM or a mixture of IgM and IgG; they are sometimes partly IgA. Cells derived from a single clone make antibodies of the same specificity but any given cell can make only one class of antibody.

Determination of the subclass of antibodies is difficult. There is more than 95% sequence homology between most of the C regions of human IgG subclasses. There are therefore few subclass-specific epitopes and it is difficult to raise antibodies against them (Michaelsen and Kornstad 1987). If insufficiently absorbed sera are used, false-positive results are obtained. If well-absorbed sera are used, some antibodies fail to react with all subclass sera.

Investigations of the subclass composition of different blood group antibodies are referred to in the three following chapters.

Immunoglobulins on B lymphocytes

The Ig on the surface of lymphocytes gives them the capacity to react with an antigen of corresponding specificity and to develop into active antibody-secreting cells. The two major classes of Ig demonstrable on the surface of immature B lymphocytes are IgM and IgD; the latter appears to have a role in triggering the cell's response to antigen.

In subjects immunized to Rh D, anti-D-bearing lymphocytes can be demonstrated by incubating D-positive red cells with the blood of the immunized

subjects and observing 'rosettes', i.e. single lymphocytes surrounded by many adherent erythrocytes. Rosetting could be demonstrated in two out of eight women immunized by pregnancy and in five out of five hyperimmunized volunteers following a booster injection of red cells; in these latter subjects the number of rosettes increased to a maximum on about the 10th day after re-stimulation (Elson and Bradley 1970).

The Ig superfamily

The name Ig superfamily is given to all those molecules that contain domains within their structures that are related to either the variable or constant domains of immunoglobulins. Most of the molecules concerned play an important role in antigen recognition at the cell surface in cell–cell adhesive interactions or in cell–extracellular matrix interactions. The Ig superfamily includes the antigen receptors, i.e. immunoglobulins and T-cell receptors, Fc receptors, as well as several other lymphocyte cell surface molecules, such as CD4 and CD8 and MHC class I and II molecules. It also includes several blood group active molecules on red cells (Lutheran, LW, Ok[a], see Chapter 6).

Methods of separating and identifying immunoglobulins

IgG can be affinity purified with particle-bound bacterial proteins A and G. Protein A and Protein G although structurally distinct both bind to the Fc portion of antibody molecules at the interface of the CH2 and CH3 domains (Sauer-Eriksson *et al.* 1995). Protein A binds human IgG1, IgG2 and IgG4 but not IgG3.

Immunoglobulins may be separated according to their different charges, for example by ion-exchange chromatography or by their different sizes, i.e. by passage through a 'molecular sieve' as in gel filtration.

The greater positive charge on IgG compared with other plasma proteins is exploited in one method of preparing anti-D IgG for immunoprophylaxis, IgG being separated from plasma on a diethylaminoethyl (DEAE)-cellulose column (Hoppe *et al.* 1973). This method of separating IgG from plasma has a much higher yield than that of cold-ethanol precipitation.

Some IgG antibodies can be separated from one another by fractionation on carboxymethyl (CM) cellulose or hydroxyapatite columns, and results with

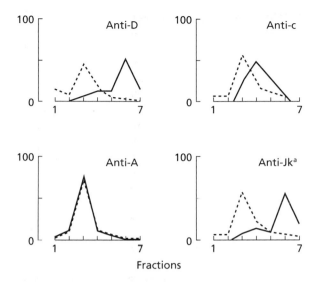

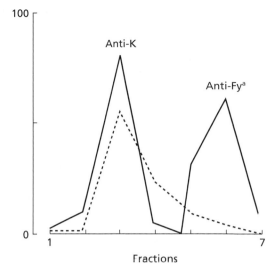

Fig 3.6 Distribution of the total IgG (– – – –) and of particular antibodies (——) in fractions eluted from carboxymethyl-cellulose (using buffers or increasing molarity), expressed as percentages of the total amount recovered from the columns. The four small figures show the distribution of single antibodies in four sera; the larger right-hand figure shows the elution of two antibodies from one serum. From Frame and Mollison (1969).

these methods will be briefly described, as the methods do not seem to have been fully exploited so far.

Anti-D, and some other red cell alloantibodies, are more positively charged than the bulk of IgG in the serum and can thus be partially separated from it. Similarly, the charge on different alloantibodies varies. Examples of separation of anti-D from the bulk of IgG and of other alloantibodies from one another, on carboxymethyl-cellulose columns, are shown in Fig. 3.6.

Identification of immunoglobulins using the antiglobulin test

Determination of the Ig class of red cell antibodies is most conveniently performed using Ig class-specific antiglobulin reagents (Polley *et al.* 1962; Adinolfi *et al.* 1966).

Effect of reduction on different immunoglobulins

Effect on IgM. Mild reduction of human IgM with sulphydryl compounds cleaves intersubunit (IgMs–IgMs), intersubunit-J chain and intrasubunit (H–H, H–L) disulphide bonds. Intersubunit bonds are more sensitive than intrasubunit bonds to reduction. Mild reduction releases J chain from the IgM molecule.

Treatment of serum with a reducing agent abolishes the agglutinating activity of most IgM antibodies. IgM subunits of anti-D, anti-A and anti-B retain their ability to combine with red cell antigens, but subunits of IgM anti-Lea have no serological activity, indicating that their binding affinity is very low (Holburn 1973).

If a monoclonal IgM is mildly reduced and then dialysed against saline to remove the reducing agent, the subunits may slowly reassemble, if the suspending medium does not contain non-specific IgM. It would therefore be expected that if a purified IgM antibody, or for example an eluate, were treated in the same way, the serological activity of the antibody would be partially restored. On the other hand, when an IgM antibody in whole serum is mildly reduced and the serum is then dialysed, restoration of serological activity is not expected, because the subunits of IgM reassemble at random and most of the IgM molecules in the serum are of different antibody specificities.

The reassembly of IgM subunits to form 19S IgM can be prevented by treatment with alkylating agents, such as iodoacetamide (IAA). Such agents irreversibly block the SH groups which have been liberated by

65

reduction of the protein, as well as any free SH groups originally present.

Effect on IgG. After mild reduction, some IgG incomplete antibodies such as anti-D become weakly agglutinating (Chan and Deutsch 1960; Romans *et al.* 1977). The changes in the properties of the IgG molecule are brought about by the breaking of the disulphide bonds in the hinge region of the molecule, permitting the two antigen-binding sites to move further apart and thus bridge the distance between red cells. The two halves of the molecule remain held together by strong non-covalent bonds between the C_H3 domains (see Fig. 3.2). Reduced IgG3 anti-D monoclonals are more potent direct agglutinators than reduced IgG1 anti-D monoclonals (Scott *et al.* 1989).

The modification of the properties of the IgG molecule produced by mild reduction are stabilized by treatment with alkylating reagents (e.g. IAA).

Practical applications. Treatment of serum with the reducing agents 2-mercaptoethanol (2-ME), dithiothreitol (DTT) or its isomer dithioerythritol (DTE), is commonly used in blood group serology to distinguish between IgG and IgM antibodies as, if the agglutinating activity is abolished, it is virtually certain that the antibody in question is IgM.

DTT is preferred to 2-ME for the following reasons: first, it is more efficient in maintaining reduction; second, it is more resistant to oxidation in air; and third, it lacks an offensive odour.

Serum that has been treated with 2-ME may be tested for agglutination without preliminary dialysis (Reesink *et al.* 1972), although if the mixture of undiluted serum and 2-ME is tested by the indirect antiglobulin test, false-positive reactions occur (Freedman *et al.* 1976). False-positive reactions also occur occasionally if DTT-treated undiluted serum is left with red cells for more than 2 h. False-positive reactions are not observed when dilutions of 2-ME-treated or DTT-treated serum are tested.

Heat lability of different immunoglobulins

Heating at 56°C for 3 h has little effect on anti-D (IgG) but produces a just detectable fall in anti-P titre (IgM). Heating at 63°C for 3 h decreases the IgG anti-D titre by about one-third, whereas heating at 63°C for only 1 h almost completely inactivates anti-P_1 (Adinolfi

1965). IgA antibodies, like IgG antibodies, are unaffected by heating at 56°C for 3 h (Adinolfi *et al.* 1966).

Naturally occurring antibodies

In blood group serology, the term naturally occurring is used for antibodies (Table 3.5) found in the serum of a subject who has never been transfused or injected with red cells containing the relevant antigen or been pregnant with a fetus carrying the relevant antigen.

Landsteiner (1945) concluded that natural antibodies had a dual origin, antigen induced and spontaneous. As examples of the first kind, anti-A and -B may be cited. These antibodies are believed to be heteroagglutinins produced as a response to substances in the environment, which are antigenically similar to red cell alloantigens (Wiener 1951b).

In 'germ-free' chicks, no heteroagglutinins against group B human red cells developed in the first 60 days of life, whereas in ordinary chicks such agglutinins usually develop within the first 30 days. In germ-free chicks, anti-B developed promptly after the administration by mouth of *Escherichia coli* O_{86}; the antibodies had serological characteristics similar to the 'naturally occurring' agglutinins; that is, they reacted slightly more strongly at 0°C than at 37°C. In germ-free chicks, very weak agglutinins developed 2–3 months after hatching but this was attributed to traces of non-living antigenic contaminants.

Although the stimulus to the formation of these naturally occurring agglutinins was traced to the environment, the authors pointed out that there was evidence that the time of onset and extent of the response depended upon genetic factors (Springer *et al.* 1959).

A direct demonstration that anti-B titres can be increased in humans by the ingestion or inhalation of suitable bacteria was provided by Springer and Horton (1969). In both infants and adults, the oral administration of killed *E. coli* O_{86}, with blood group B specificity, produced rises in anti-B titre in a proportion of subjects; responses were commoner in subjects with an intestinal disorder, suggesting that antigen was absorbed more readily when the mucosal surface was damaged. Four out of 12 adults showed an increase in anti-B titre after receiving a nasal spray of *E. coli* O_{86}. Similar observations have been reported for anti-T and anti-Tn (Springer and Tegtmeyer 1981).

Other antibodies which may be heteroagglutinins include anti-H, -PP_1^{pk} and -P^k, found in virtually all

Table 3.5 Naturally occurring alloantibodies to red cell antigens.

System (or antigen)	Specificity of antibodies	Subjects in whom antibodies occur
ABO/Hh	A, B, H	All without corresponding antigen
	A_1	1–8% of A_2
		22–35% of A_2B
	HI	Occasional A_1 and A_1B
Lewis	Le^a	20% of Le (a–b–), ABH secretors
	Le^b	Often accompanies anti-Le^a; rare on its own
P/P_1	P^k, PP_1P^k	All without corresponding antigen
	P_1	Common in P_2
I	I	Most i
MNSs	M	0.02% of M–N+
	N	0.002% of M+N–
	S	Very rare in S–
	V^w, M^g	1–2% of population
Rh	E	0.1% of D positives
	C, C^w, C^x	Very rare
	D (cold)	0.15–0.3% of D negatives
Sd	Sd^a	1–2% of population
Di	Wr^a	1% of population
Ge		Rare
Kk	K	Rare
Lu	Lu^a	0.02% of population

The list is incomplete: specificities that have been found occasionally include anti-In^a, -Lu^b, -LW and -Yt^a amongst others; naturally occurring antibodies to several low-frequency antigens other than V^w, M^g and Wr^a are common; the figures given for frequencies are only approximate; further details are given in the relevant chapters on blood groups.

subjects who lack the corresponding antigen, and anti-A_1, -HI, -Le^a and -P_1, found in only some subjects who lack the corresponding antigen. In some cases, the formation of anti-K has evidently been due to infection with a microorganism producing a K-like substance.

There is abundant evidence that some natural antibodies are spontaneous, i.e. generated without the intervention of antigens: natural antibodies are present in newborn nude, germ- and antigen-free mice, sometimes in higher proportions than in normal mice (Avreamas 1992).

Examples of red cell antibodies that are probably spontaneous in origin are anti-E and various others in the Rh system (see Chapter 5), antibodies to low-incidence antigens, and anti-Lu^a, -Di^a and -Xg^a (see Chapter 6) and anti-HLA, found in about 1% of normal donors (see Chapter 13). In autoimmune

haemolytic anaemia, it is common to find several antibodies to low-incidence antigens, for example to Wr^a, Sw^a, C^x, Mi^a and V^w, to which the patient has clearly not been exposed (Cleghorn 1960).

Further evidence that antibodies are produced in the absence of antigenic stimulation is supplied by work referred to on p. 74: antibodies such as anti-D, -E and -Kp^b were grown from heavy and light chains of serum from normal subjects.

Naturally occurring antibodies and class of immunoglobulin

Most, but by no means all, naturally occurring antibodies are cold agglutinins (IgM) and immune antibodies of the same specificity are either warm IgM or IgG antibodies.

Anti-A and anti-B are always partly IgM and may be wholly IgM; in group O subjects anti-A and -B are always partly IgG and may be partly IgA. Anti-A_1 in A_2 and A_2B subjects seems always to be wholly IgM, but anti-A1 separated from group O serum may be only IgG (see Chapter 4). Examples of anti-HI and -H have been solely IgM (Adinolfi et al. 1962; Chattoraj et al. 1968).

Although most examples of anti-Le[a] behave on ordinary serological testing as if they were solely IgM, an IgG component can often be demonstrated by appropriate methods. Rare examples of anti-Le[a] and -Le[b] are solely IgG. Naturally occurring antibodies of the MNSs system may be IgM or IgG.

In the past, many examples of naturally occurring anti-E were considered to be solely IgM because they gave a negative indirect antiglobulin test but, with the introduction of more sensitive methods, an IgG component is usually detectable and some examples may be solely IgG. Rather surprisingly, cold-reacting anti-D, demonstrable in the AutoAnalyzer, has been found to be IgG. References supporting the foregoing statements and further details will be found in Chapters 4–6.

Naturally occurring antibodies to low-frequency antigens (e.g. anti-Wr[a]) are mainly IgM but a large proportion of them have an IgG component and some are solely IgG (Lubenko and Contreras 1989).

Immune responses to red cell antigens

Immune responses to foreign antigens are mediated by lymphocytes. There are two types of immune response, humoral and cellular, but only humoral responses are relevant to blood transfusion. In the humoral response, antigen is recognized by receptors on T cells, which subsequently stimulate B lymphocytes. The T-cell receptors are extremely diverse and are capable of recognizing all of the foreign molecules that may be encountered. A few antigens can stimulate B cells directly. Stimulation of B lymphocytes results in their proliferation and, eventually, in the production of plasma cells. Some of the primed B cells do not differentiate and remain, in the absence of further antigenic stimulation, as memory cells. On re-stimulation, memory cells mount a secondary (anamnestic) response; this response is characterized by the rapid production of antibody that is more potent and specific than that produced in the primary response.

Antigen recognition

Before a humoral response can be mounted, antigen must be brought into contact with antibody-forming cells, i.e. B lymphocytes. The way in which this is done and the role of HLA antigens in the process are described in Chapter 13.

Primary and secondary responses to red cell antigens

Primary responses to any particular antigen can, by definition, be studied only in subjects who have not previously encountered the antigen. In the case of some antigens, for example A and B, it can be presumed that there has been previous exposure, as antigens identical with or similar to the human ones are found in a wide variety of organisms, and in the case of others, for example Le[a], P_1, previous exposure to the antigen is possible. Although it is difficult or impossible to study primary responses to these antigens, such responses can be studied in many other systems, for example Rh, K, Fy and Jk, in which naturally occurring antibodies are rare. As Rh D is the most immunogenic of the latter antigens, it has been used in most of the systematic work that has been done. As described in Chapter 5, after a first injection of 1 ml of D-positive red cells to D-negative subjects who have not previously been exposed to the antigen and who have no trace of anti-D in their serum, antibody can first be detected in some subjects after about 4 weeks; in these subjects, the concentration of antibody increases slowly and after 6–10 weeks reaches peak values not exceeding about 4 μg/ml (Samson and Mollison 1975; Contreras and Mollison 1981). In other subjects, antibody can first be detected only after two injections, given at an interval of 3 months or more; less commonly, antibody is first detected only after three or more injections. There is evidence that in all subjects in whom antibody is ultimately detected, primary immunization is induced by the first injection of red cells because in such subjects red cells injected on the second occasion invariably have a shortened survival (see Chapter 10). There are some subjects in whom no antibody is formed even after many injections given over a period of 2–3 years, and these subjects are classified as non-responders. In these subjects, D-positive red cells have a strictly normal survival even after many injections of D-positive red cells have been given.

The production of anti-D after a first injection of D-positive red cells cannot be hastened by injecting a much larger amount of red cells, although the number of responders increases, as does the amount of antibody produced in the primary response (see Chapter 5).

It is known that in animals, after a first injection of antigen has been given, there is a certain period during which the animal will not respond well to a second injection. For example, in horses injected with tetanus toxoid, the period was at least 3 months, although less than a year (Barr and Glenny 1945). In humans, the number of D-negative subjects forming anti-D within 6 months did not appear to be greater when injections were given every 6 weeks than when only a single injection was given (Archer et al. 1969).

In subjects already immunized to Rh D, following a (further) transfusion of D-positive red cells, the concentration of anti-D in the serum starts to increase about 3 days after transfusion and then rises logarithmically to reach a peak value, which may be as high as about 1000µg/ml (i.e. 10% of the total IgG), some 10–20 days later (see Chapters 5 and 11). The response to a first injection of group A or B red cells in a group O subject is similar in that antibody concentration rises rapidly and reaches a peak within about 12 days (see Figs 4.1 and 4.2), indicating that these responses should be regarded as secondary.

The differences between primary and secondary responses to the D red cell antigen in humans are very similar to those between primary and secondary responses to bacterial toxins in animals (Burnet and Fenner 1949).

There have been few systematic studies of immune responses to alloantigens other than D; the production of serologically detectable anti-K, -E and -C within 4 weeks of a first transfusion has been reported in children with burns (Bacon et al. 1991). The production of anti-Jk^a and anti-P$_1$ within 2 weeks of a first transfusion has been reported in a 7-year-old child (Cox et al. 1992).

Class of immunoglobulin produced in red cell alloimmunization

In the primary response it is usual for IgM antibody to be formed initially and for production then to be switched to IgG antibody, but it has proved difficult to confirm that this generalization applies to the production of red cell alloantibodies in humans. For example,

in investigating responses to the Rh D antigen, using manual tests, anti-D can often first be detected by the agglutination of enzyme-treated red cells at a time when the indirect antiglobulin test is negative. As it is known that both IgM and IgG anti-D in low concentrations will agglutinate enzyme-treated cells, and as all serological reactivity is usually lost if attempts are made to fractionate serum containing such antibodies, it is usually impossible to decide the Ig class of the antibody present.

Although it is not known with certainty whether IgM antibody is the first to be made in subjects responding to the Rh D antigen, it is quite clear that in the majority of subjects IgG antibody soon predominates and is often the only type that can be identified at any time. In a minority of subjects IgM antibody is also produced in substantial amounts. In hyperimmunized donors anti-D is also quite often partly IgA (see Chapter 5).

Responses to several other red cell antigens, for example K, Fy^a and Jk^a, appear to be similar to responses to D; that is to say, most antibodies are predominantly IgG, although in some subjects a mixture of IgM and IgG antibodies is found. Lutheran antibodies may sometimes be partly IgA (see Chapter 6).

Blood group systems in which naturally occurring antibodies are found demand separate consideration. In the ABO system perhaps all subjects should be regarded as immunized. Moreover, ABO-incompatible pregnancies and injections of various animal products cause both quantitative and qualitative changes in anti-A and anti-B (see Chapter 4). Perhaps the most interesting fact about the production of ABO antibodies is that immune anti-A and anti-B are predominantly IgM in A or B subjects but may be largely IgG (and partly IgA) in group O subjects.

Alterations in binding constant. IgG antibody formed late in the immune response tends to have a higher binding constant than antibody formed early in the response; for example, an increase in the binding constant of anti-D during the secondary Rh D immunization was demonstrated by Holburn et al. (1970).

Increased heterogeneity of antibody in hyperimmunized subjects

There is evidence that as immunization progresses the antibody tends to be more diverse with regard to Ig class and subclass. Data with regard to anti-D are given in Chapter 5.

Persistence of IgM and IgG antibodies

IgM antibodies tend to decline rapidly in concentration after the last stimulus and usually become undetectable after 1–2 years. Some IgG antibodies (e.g. anti-Rh D) decline far more slowly and may be readily detectable 30 years after the last stimulus (see Chapter 5); others (e.g. anti-Jk^a) may become undetectable a few months after the last stimulus. In a follow-up with a median period of 10 months, of 160 patients in whom 209 antibodies had been detected, some of the findings were as follows: of 39 antibodies belonging to the Lewis, MN or P$_1$ systems (presumably IgM), 28 became undetectable, whereas of 170 belonging mainly to the Rh, K, Fy and Jk systems, which were presumably IgG, only 49 became undetectable. Antibodies of the Kidd system became undetectable more frequently than those of the Rh system, in 11 out of 21 compared with 27 out of 98, although this difference may have been partly due to the relative potency of the antibodies concerned; of antibodies (of all specificities) with initially weak reactions, 41 out of 84 became undetectable whereas of those with initially very strong reactions, only 1 out of 18 became undetectable (Ramsey and Larson 1988). In a retrospective study, 5–10 years after first being identified, 14 out of 36 alloantibodies could no longer be detected on at least one occasion. Of a further 22 antibodies looked for after more than 10 years, only 10 could still be detected (Ramsey and Smietana 1994).

Relation between immunoglobulin class of antibody and serological behaviour

IgM antibodies. Most IgM antibodies will agglutinate red cells suspended in saline. Agglutination by some IgM antibodies, for example anti-A (Polley *et al.* 1963) is not enhanced in a medium of serum whereas that of some other antibodies is. Using purified IgM anti-D, it was found that the agglutinin titre was greater by four or five doubling dilutions when using serum rather than saline as a diluent; the effect was observed with serum diluted up to 1 in 32 (Holburn *et al.* 1971a). The enhancing effect of serum is, therefore, important only when comparing sera with titres of more than 32 or when determining the titre of purified antibodies.

The titre of IgM antibodies is about four times higher with enzyme-treated red cells than with untreated cells (Aho and Christian 1966; Holburn *et al.* 1971a). Evidently, very weak IgM antibodies may be detectable only with enzyme-treated red cells.

Naturally occurring IgM antibodies of the ABO, Lewis and P systems agglutinate red cells more strongly at 0°C than at higher temperatures. For example, the titre of anti-A and anti-B is about eight times higher at 0°C than at 37°C (Kettel, cited by Wiener 1943, p. 19). Although anti-A and -B almost invariably agglutinate appropriate red cells at 37°C, other antibodies of the aforenamed systems, for example anti-A$_1$, -HI, -Le^a -Le^b and -P$_1$, do not usually agglutinate red cells above 20–25°C; occasional examples of these antibodies will agglutinate up to about 30°C and even give trace reactions at 37°C; examples with such a wide thermal range as this will invariably bind complement. The behaviour of anti-Le^a is slightly different in that although it will usually not agglutinate cells above a temperature of about 20–25°C, it will usually bind to red cells and fix complement at 37°C and thus give a strongly positive indirect antiglobulin test.

Anti-D agglutinins produced in an immune response are 'warm', i.e. they are as active at 37°C as at lower temperatures (Levine *et al.* 1941). A few IgM antibodies are 'incomplete', for example occasional examples of anti-Jk^a (Adinolfi *et al.* 1962; Polley 1964).

IgG antibodies. In most blood group systems IgG antibodies will not agglutinate untreated red cells suspended in saline; such non-agglutinating antibodies used to be described as 'incomplete'.

The term 'incomplete' was introduced by Pappenheimer (1940) for horse antibodies against ovalbumin that produced no visible precipitation but inhibited the reaction of precipitating antisera. The term was subsequently introduced into blood group serology by Race (1944) to describe the behaviour of Rh D antibodies that failed to agglutinate D-positive red cells suspended in saline but blocked the subsequent agglutination of the red cells by an agglutinating anti-D serum; such antibodies were described as 'blocking' by Wiener (1944).

Potent examples of IgG anti-D either in undiluted serum, or in some cases in serum diluted 1:2 in saline, will agglutinate saline-suspended red cells (Hopkins 1969, 1970). In fact, it has subsequently become clear that really potent IgG anti-D, even at a dilution of 1 in 10 or more, will agglutinate saline-suspended cells (unpublished observations, M. Contreras). Potent IgG anti-K and anti-M may also agglutinate saline-suspended red cells.

IgA antibodies. IgA fractions containing anti-A and anti-B will agglutinate red cells suspended in saline; the titre is increased about four-fold by using the indirect antiglobulin test with an anti-IgA serum (Adinolfi *et al.* 1966). Sera containing IgA anti-D as well as IgG anti-D do not as a rule agglutinate red cells suspended in saline although they sensitize red cells to agglutination by anti-IgA. A serum containing potent IgA anti-D, such as a purified IgA fraction from the same serum, which did agglutinate saline-suspended red cells, is mentioned in Chapter 5. In tests on five murine IgA monoclonals, three anti-A and two anti-A,B, agglutinating activity was associated only with tetramers or higher polymers (Guest *et al.* 1992).

Individual differences in response

Individuals vary widely in their response to different antigens. The recognition of nearly all antigens depends on their presentation, bound to HLA class II molecules by antigen-presenting cells, i.e. dendritic cells. Evidently then, specific immune responsiveness is influenced by the products of the HLA-DR alleles (see review by Benacerraf 1981; see also Chapter 13). Control of antibody responses is also influenced by genes outside the HLA system and segregating independently from it, which control the quantitative production of antibody.

Alterations in antibody response in disease

Subjects with autoimmune disease appear to have an increased risk of forming red cell alloantibodies. One early example was a patient with systemic lupus erythematosus, who formed five different immune alloantibodies (Race and Sanger 1950, p. 240). There have been several reports of a high incidence of alloantibodies in patients with the warm-antibody type of autoimmune haemolytic anaemia (WAIHA) who have been transfused. In three series, the frequency was 32–38% and was as high as 75% in patients who had received more than five transfusions (Branch and Petz 1982; James *et al.* 1988; reviewed by Garratty and Petz 1994). In these three series, the patient's serum was absorbed with autologous red cells before being

tested for alloantibodies. In another series it was found that 44% of alloantibodies could not be detected before autoabsorption (Wallhermfechtel *et al.* 1984). There has been one report indicating that red cell allo-immunization is rare in WAIHA (Salama *et al.* 1992) but the patients' sera were not absorbed with autologous red cells before being tested and alloantibodies may have been overlooked.

Subjects with hypogammaglobulinaemia have a greatly diminished capacity to form alloantibodies. As described in Chapter 4, their serum may lack anti-A and anti-B. In one case a patient of group A whose serum lacked anti-B was given a series of injections of B substance of animal origin but failed to form anti-B (Barandun *et al.* 1956).

Among patients with various diseases, receiving regular transfusion over a period of a year or so, only those with chronic lymphocytic leukaemia failed to produce any new red cell alloantibodies; in contrast, patients with acute myeloid leukaemia on intensive chemotherapy produced alloantibodies as frequently as those with aplastic anaemia or gastrointestinal bleeding (Blumberg *et al.* 1983).

In another study of patients receiving regular transfusions, the frequency of formation of red cell alloantibodies was significantly lower in patients with chronic lymphocytic leukaemia than in those with other diagnoses (Blumberg *et al.* 1984). Patients on haemodialysis may have a reduced tendency to form red cell alloantibodies; of 405 patients who had received a total of almost 7000 red cell transfusions, only seven developed alloantibodies attributable to the transfusion (Habibi and Lecolier 1983).

Formation of immune red cell alloantibodies in infants

The immune response in newborn infants appears to be similar to that of newborn mice; the response is typically limited to the production of low-titre IgM antibodies, with reduced switching to IgG production and the repertoire of available antibody specificities is highly restricted. In the mouse, the repertoire is 100 times smaller in the newborn than in the adult. In newborn human infants, class II HLA molecules are weakly expressed (Riley 1992) although the response to foreign antigens is normal (Roncarolo *et al.* 1994). It is uncommon for red cell alloantibodies other than anti-A and -B to be produced in the first few months of life. Some examples are: (1) anti-c in a 7-week-old child of phenotype CCDee, who had been transfused during surgery 6 weeks previously (S Kevy, unpublished observations, reported by Konugres 1978); (2) anti-Lu^b in a 2-month-old infant who had been transfused 1 month previously (unpublished observations, M. Contreras); (3) IgG anti-E in an infant aged 11 weeks who had received 31 transfusions in the previous 6 weeks, all from donors whose plasma had been screened for alloantibodies (DePalma *et al.* 1991); and (4) anti-K in a premature infant born at 30 weeks and given 28 red cell transfusions in the first 2 months, anti-K was found for the first time 18 days after the last transfusion; the antibody was still present 1 year later (Maniatis *et al.* 1993).

In two series of newborn infants transfused with blood from an average of nine donors during the first few months of life no unexpected red cell antibodies were detected. The first series consisted of 53 premature infants, about one-half of whom were tested at least 5 months after birth (Floss *et al.* 1986) and the second of 90 full-term infants tested not less than 3 weeks after their last transfusion (Ludvigsen *et al.* 1987). In contrast, in a series of adults, primary immunization to red cell antigens was observed in some 6% of subjects (see below).

Role of the spleen

In splenectomized subjects, the response to sheep red blood cells (SRBC) is much lower than in control subjects (Rowley 1950; McFadzean and Tsang 1956). However, the spleen is not essential in the formation of antibodies against red cell antigens. For example, the patient described by Collins and colleagues (1950), who formed so many blood group antibodies, had had her spleen removed before receiving the series of blood transfusions that immunized her. Moreover, in subjects with sickle cell disease, whose spleens are usually infarcted and functionless, alloimmunization is no less frequent than in other patients (see later in text).

Association between weakening of red cell antigens and the appearance of allo- or autoantibodies in the serum

There are many examples of this phenomenon.
1 In pregnant women, the agglutinability of red cells with Lewis antibodies tends to diminish (see

Chapter 4), a change that appears to be correlated with an increase in the frequency with which Lewis antibodies are detected in the serum.
2 Transient weakening of Rh D antigens has been observed in an infant with autoimmune haemolytic anaemia (AIHA) (see Chapter 5).
3 Temporary weakening of LW may be associated with the appearance of anti-LW in the serum (see Chapter 5).
4 The appearance of Kell antibodies in the serum may be associated with weakening of Kell antigens; in one case there was a second episode in which a Lutheran antibody appeared concomitantly with weakening of Lu antigens (see Chapter 6).
5 In a patient whose red cell phenotype changed from Jk(a+ b−) to Jk(a− b−), loss of Jk^a was associated with the appearance in the serum of anti-Jk3 (see Chapter 6).
6 In a patient in whose serum anti-Glycophorin C appeared, Glycophorin C was temporarily absent from the red cell membrane; when Glycophorin C reappeared, the antibody disappeared; the cells now reacted with serum taken earlier (Daniels *et al.* 1988).
7 Temporary depression of AnWj has been associated with the presence of auto-anti-AnWj (see Chapter 6).

Monoclonal antibodies

Each kind of antibody molecule is made by a line of plasma cells derived from a single lymphocyte. The progeny of a single cell is called a clone and a monoclonal antibody population consists of the identical molecules produced by such a clone. When an antigen is injected into an animal, numerous different lymphocytes, each producing antibodies with the capacity to react to some extent with the antigen, are stimulated. Polyclonal antibodies consist of such collections of molecules.

In 1975, Köhler and Milstein described a method of obtaining monoclonal antibodies, which depended on fusing mouse lymphocytes with mouse myeloma cells. The lymphocytes were obtained from the spleen of mice immunized with a particular antigen. Unfused splenic lymphocytes die in laboratory culture within 48 h and unfused myeloma cells in the culture die because the composition of growth medium is selected so that it does not support DNA synthesis in these cells. As a result, the fused 'hybridoma' cells flourish and cell lines secreting specific antibody that grow indefinitely in culture can be obtained by cloning.

Cloning is achieved by culturing the hybrid cells at low cell concentrations in microplates, recovering cells from the well containing the antibody of interest, and then repeating the process two or three times to obtain a stable clone of cells. When stable clones secreting antibody of interest at high concentrations (50–100 µg/ml) are obtained it is possible to culture the cells in large fermenters to obtain grams of antibody for diagnostic or therapeutic use.

The ability to make monoclonal antibodies has proved to be of vast importance, on both a theoretical and a practical level.

Mouse monoclonal antibodies

Some monoclonal antibodies produced from lymphocytes from mice injected with human red cells have specificities corresponding to those of human alloantibodies, for example anti-A, -B, -A,B, -H Type 1, -H Type 2, -P, -P_1, -P^k, -I, -Y (as in Le^y), -Le^a, -Le^b, -M, -N, -T, -Tn, -k, -Lu^b (First and Second International Workshop on Monoclonal Antibodies 1987, 1990) and -Ge3 (Loirat et al. 1992). Others react with structures carrying the antigenic determinants rather than the antigens themselves. For example, they may react with glycophorin A, rather than with M or N; or they may react with Rh-related glycoprotein and thus with all human red cells except those that are Rh_{null}; or they may react with Kell glycoprotein and thus with all except K_O cells (see Chapter 6). Murine monoclonal antibodies against A and B and against complement components have largely replaced polyclonal reagents in diagnostic blood typing procedures.

Human monoclonal antibodies

The first human monoclonal antibodies with blood group specificity were produced by transformation of human B lymphocytes with Epstein–Barr virus (EBV). The lymphoblastoid cells that result have the property of growing in tissue culture and of secreting antibody. By taking lymphocytes from Rh D-immunized donors, both IgG (Koskimies 1980) and IgM (Boylston et al. 1980) anti-D have been obtained. EBV-transformed cell lines are unstable, often ceasing to produce antibody after a few months (Melamed et al. 1985), although many stable EBV-transformed cell lines have been described (Goosens et al. 1987; Kumpel et al. 1989a). Another way of obtaining stable cell lines is to fuse human lymphocytes with murine myelomas to form heteromyelomas (see review by Thompson and Hughes-Jones 1990).

Examples of monoclonal anti-D have been used in analysing the different D epitopes (see Chapter 5) and in the experimental clearance of D-positive red cells from the circulation of volunteers (see Chapter 10); they are used routinely in blood grouping (see Chapter 8). Other human monoclonal antibodies available as diagnostic reagents include anti-C, -c, -E, -e, -G, -K, -Jk^a, -Jk^b, -H, -Le^a, -Le^b, -IgG and –C3d.

Some disadvantages of monoclonal antibodies

As mentioned elsewhere in this chapter, changes in pH alter the binding affinity of antibodies. The effect is particularly striking with monoclonal antibodies and may have a profound effect on apparent specificity in tests in a system such as HLA, which involves many similar but non-identical antigens. Monoclonal antibodies which give non-specific reactions at normal pH can be made monospecific by lowering pH to 6.0 (Mosmann et al. 1980).

A problem associated with some high-affinity monoclonal antibodies is crossreactivity. It may seem paradoxical that an antibody apparently specific for a single antigenic determinant should crossreact at all. Nevertheless, single antibody molecules are not specific for one particular epitope. The combining site on the end of the Fab arm is capable of binding closely with a number of different epitopic configurations (Talmage 1959). The higher the affinity of an antibody, the more it tends to crossreact (Steiner and Eisen 1967). Presumably, the more strongly an antibody combines with any particular determinant, the more certain it is to bind to some extent to related antigenic determinants. By no means all monoclonal antibodies have a high affinity. On the contrary, the affinities of monoclonal antibodies produced by different clones are similar to those of polyclonal antibodies, although all antibodies of a single clone have the same affinity, whereas the antibodies in a polyclonal population have a range of affinities. Monoclonal antibodies even of average affinity are more likely than polyclonal antibodies to crossreact. This is because all the molecules of a monoclonal antibody population have the same paratope and will therefore all recognize the same crossreacting antigen. In contrast, in a population of polyclonal antibodies, the paratopes will differ and only a proportion of the molecules will recognize any particular crossreacting antigen.

Crossreactivity explains the demonstration that certain examples of monoclonal anti-D react with the cytoplasmic component vimentin (Thorpe 1989, 1990), giving rise to the false conclusion that D is present on tissue cells. On the other hand, the reaction of certain monoclonal anti-A with B cells and of certain monoclonal anti-B with A cells is due to the potency of the antibodies concerned which enables them to detect the small amounts of B and A, respectively produced by A and B subjects (see Chapter 4).

A different problem is provided by monoclonal antibodies with 'pseudo-specificity', for example: (1) an anti-glycophorin B, which, in agglutination tests, behaved as anti-S but in other tests reacted with both s+ and S+ red cells (Green *et al.* 1990a) and (2) an anti-J chain that reacted more strongly with Gm(a+) than with Gm(a–) molecules but could be shown to be reacting with the same determinant on the γ chain in both cases (De Lange 1988).

Copying variable regions and constructing new antibodies

For the construction of new antibodies, the genes encoding the V regions can be amplified using the PCR and can then be cloned into expression vectors (e.g. bacteriophage). Complete antibody V domains with specificity identical to the parent antibody can then be displayed on the surface of the bacteriophage. Completely new antibodies can be constructed (McCafferty *et al.* 1990). Another approach has been to link V_H and V_L gene repertoires together at random to encode a repertoire of single-chain F_V (scF_V) antibody fragments, which are then displayed on the surface of bacteriophage. Phage are selected by binding to the surface of mobilized antigen (red cells) and then used to infect *E. coli*. Antibodies produced include anti-B, -D, -HI, -E and -Kp[b] (Marks *et al.* 1993) and -HPA-1a (Griffin and Ouwehand 1995).

Frequency of immune red cell alloantibodies

By definition, an immune red cell alloantibody is one that develops in a subject who has been exposed to a red cell alloantigen. Evidently then, the frequency of immune red cell antibodies will be zero in subjects who have never been transfused or been pregnant, and will

be greatest in subjects who have received many transfusions. For two reasons, pregnancies constitute a smaller stimulus than transfusions: first, the number of foreign antigens is limited to those possessed by the father of the fetus (although, of course, some women have infants by more than one man), and, second, in many pregnancies the amount of red cells transferred from fetus to mother is too small to stimulate a primary response.

The frequency of alloantibodies is expected to be relatively low in blood donors compared with patients in hospital requiring blood transfusion; blood donors have a lower average age and are far less likely to have received blood transfusions in the past. The frequency with which particular antibodies are found depends on the sensitivity of testing (usually relatively low in screening healthy donors) and on the ethnic group being tested (e.g. anti-D is rare in Chinese people).

D is the most immunogenic red cell antigen (excepting A and B), but the frequency of immunization to D has been reduced to a low level, first, by using only D-negative donors for transfusion to D-negative subjects and, second, by administering anti-D Ig to D-negative women who would otherwise become immunized as a result of a pregnancy with a D-positive infant. As a result of these measures, the frequency with which anti-D is encountered has fallen greatly in the last few decades.

In contrast with the diminishing frequency of anti-D, that of anti-K, -Fy[a], etc. has increased, evidently due to the increased number of multitransfused patients and the absence of measures for preventing immunization to antigens other than D.

Frequency of immune anti-D (including anti-DC and anti-DE)

In healthy blood donors. In more than 200 000 donors screened between 1971 and 1975 in Seattle, the frequency was 0.22% (Giblett 1977). In 36 000 donors screened in London in 1988, the frequency (0.25%) was almost identical although in 35 000 screened in 1990 the frequency was 0.16% (R Knight, personal communication).

In pregnant women. Before the introduction of immunoprophylaxis, anti-D was found in approximately 1 in 170 pregnant white women, both in England (Walker 1958) and in North America (Walker 1984). Following the introduction of immunoprophylaxis with anti-D in the late 1960s, the frequency with which anti-D is found has fallen progressively and was, for example, 1 in 963 in 1988 in one North American survey (RH Walker, personal communication 1991) and 1 in 1600 in another (Heddle *et al.* 1993). The frequency in one English region for 1988 had fallen to a lesser extent, being 1 in 497 (GJ Dovey, personal communication), although a slightly greater fall, namely to one in 584, was found in another English region for 1993–95 (A Rankin, personal communication). Figures for the changing incidence of HDN are given in Chapter 12.

In pre-transfusion tests on potential recipients. Although there appears to have been a fall between the mid-1950s and mid-1970s in the frequency with which anti-D (and -DC) was found in transfusion recipients, there has been no obvious fall since then. Some figures are as follows: in 1956–57, 0.77%; in 1974–75, 0.52%, based on testing 60 000 patients in Seattle (Giblett 1977); in 1970–75, 0.55%, in 1976–81, 0.29% and in 1982–87, 0.27%, based on screening about 100 000 patients in each 5-year period in Michigan (Walker *et al.* 1989). In a smaller series (more than 12 000 patients) tested in England in 1990, 0.56% (J Sangster, personal communication).

In recipients following solid organ transplants. The frequency with which anti-D develops in D-negative recipients of D-positive grafts and the apparent influence of cytotoxic drugs is mentioned in Chapter 5.

Frequency of immune red cell antibodies other than anti-D

In healthy blood donors. In the two series referred to above, the frequencies were 0.10% in Seattle in 1975 (Giblett 1977) and in London 0.19% in 1988 and 0.18% in 1990 (unpublished observations, M. Contreras). In the London series, about 30% of the antibodies were anti-E and 20% were anti-K.

In pregnant women. In approximately 175 000 women (about 85% of whom were D positive), antibodies other than anti-D were found in 0.14%; rather more than one-half of these were within the Rh system and, of these, one-half were anti-E; the next commonest antibody, found in 0.025% of the women, was anti-K (Kornstad 1983). In a more recent survey,

clinically significant antibodies other than anti-D were found in 100 out of 17 568 women, but in 58 instances the antibody was present in the first trimester and it was concluded that the frequency of antibodies stimulated by the current pregnancy was 42 out 17 568 or approximately 0.24% (Heddle *et al.* 1993).

In pre-transfusion tests on potential recipients. Frequencies were: in 1974–75, 1.12% (Giblett 1977); in 1970–75, 0.39%; in 1976–81, 0.45% and in 1982–87, 0.6% (Walker *et al.* 1989).

In random recipients following transfusion. The figures in the preceding paragraph are for patients, only some of whom had been transfused or been pregnant previously. In a prospective study of 452 patients, all of whom had been transfused in relation to elective surgery, pre-transfusion samples and 10 serial, 2-weekly, post-transfusion samples were taken. Additional red cell alloantibodies developed in 38 out of 452 (8.2%) patients between 2 and 18 weeks after transfusion, but 10 of these had been transfused before and one had been pregnant, leaving an apparent frequency of primary immunization of about 27 out of 441 (6.1%); 13 out of the 27 antibodies were anti-E and if these are excluded (because their immune nature is in some doubt) the frequency falls to 14 out of 428 (3.3%). Of all the newly found antibodies, 50% were initially detectable only by a two-stage papain technique or by the manual polybrene test, and not by the indirect antiglobulin test (IAT) (Redman *et al.* 1996).

Relative frequencies of antibodies other than anti-D

Combined figures from 20 different blood grouping laboratories were reported by Grove-Rasmussen (1964); these figures and those from a much smaller series reported by Tovey (1974) are shown in Table 3.6. No information was given as to the relative numbers of parous women and transfusion recipients in the two series. As will be seen, Rh antibodies (other than anti-D) constituted about 54% of the total and anti-K and -Fy^a about 40%, leaving only 5% for all other specificities. In the series of Walker and colleagues (1989), if the figures for the three 5-year periods (in each of which approximately 100 000 patients were screened) are pooled, the absolute frequencies for antibodies of various specificities were as follows: Rh

Table 3.6 Relative frequency of immune red cell antibodies* (excluding anti-D, -CD and -DE): (a) and (b) in transfusion recipients (and some pregnant women), (c) associated with immediate haemolytic transfusion reactions and (d) associated with delayed haemolytic transfusion reactions.

	No. of cases	Blood group systems within which the various alloantibodies occurred (%)				
		Rh (excluding -D)[†]	K	Fy	Jk	Others
(a)	4523	51.8	28.6	10.2	4.2	5.2
(b)	705	61.4	24.7	10.2	2.4	1.3
(c)	142	42.2	30.3	18.3	8.5	0.7
(d)	82	34.2	14.6	15.9	32.9	2.4

(a) Grove-Rasmussen, 1964; (b) Tovey, 1974; (c) Grove-Rasmussen and Huggins, 1973; (d) data from the Mayo Clinic and Toronto General Hospital; for further details see Chapter 11.

* That is, excluding antibodies of the ABO, Lewis and P systems and anti-M and anti-N.

[†] Almost all anti-E or -c.

antibodies other than anti-D, 0.22%; anti-K, 0.19%; anti-Fy^a, 0.05%; and anti-Jk^a, 0.035%.

Patients with thalassaemia are usually transfused about once per month, starting in the first few years of life. In some series in which patients have been transfused with blood selected only for ABO and D compatibility, antibodies, mainly of Rh or K specificities, have been found in more than 20% of patients. For example, out of 973 thalassaemics transfused with an average of 18 units per year from about the age of 3 years, 21.1% had formed clinically significant antibodies after about 6 years; 84% of the antibodies were within the Rh or K systems; about half the immunized patients made antibodies of more than one specificity. Of 162 patients transfused from the outset with red cells matched for Rh and K antigens, only 3.7% formed alloantibodies compared with 15.7% of 83 patients of similar age, transfused with blood matched only for D (Spanos *et al.* 1990).

The incidence of antibody formation is less when transfusion is started in the first year of life (Economidou *et al.* 1971). The induction of immunological tolerance by starting repeated transfusions at this time was believed to account for the low rate of alloimmunization, namely 5.2%, observed in a series of 1435 patients (Sirchia *et al.* 1985).

Alloimmunization in sickle cell disease

In a survey of 1814 patients from many centres, the overall rate of alloimmunization was 18.6%. The rate increased with the number of transfusions and, although alloimmunization usually occurred with less than 15 transfusions, the rate continued to increase as more transfusions were given. The commonest specificities were anti-C, -E and -K; 55% of immunized subjects made antibodies with more than one specificity (Rosse *et al.* 1990). In another series, the incidence of alloimmunization was somewhat higher; out of 107 patients who received a total of 2100 units, 32 (30%) became immunized and 17 of these formed multiple antibodies; 82% of the specificities were anti-K, -E, -C or -Jk^b. Those patients who formed antibodies had had an average of 23 transfusions; those who did not had had an average of 13; 75% of antibodies had developed by the time of the 21st transfusion (Vichinsky *et al.* 1990).

The finding that the percentage of patients forming antibodies increases with the number of transfusions has been documented in previous series (Orlina *et al.* 1978; Reisner *et al.* 1987). In the latter series, 50% of patients who had received 100 or more transfusions had formed antibodies.

It has been suggested that in sickle cell disease the rate of alloimmunization is due partly to racial differences between donors (predominantly white people) and patients (black people). The antibodies formed most commonly are anti-K, -C, -E and -Jk^b, and the frequencies of each of the corresponding antigens are significantly higher in white people than in black people (Vichinsky *et al.* 1990). It has been pointed out that when one considers the probability of giving at least one incompatible unit when 10 units are transfused, the differences for C, E and Jk[b] between white and black donors become very small, only that for K remaining substantial, namely 0.178 with black donors and 0.597 with white (Pereira *et al.* 1990), so that the use of white donors for black donors may not play a large role in inducing the formation of red cell alloantibodies. In any case, the conclusion is that for patients with sickle cell disease, as for those with thalassaemia, it is worth giving blood matched for Rh antigens and for K. This conclusion is implied by the findings of Rosse and co-workers (1990) and was reached earlier by Davies co-workers (1986). These latter authors found that two of their patients, both of the phenotype Dccee, which is much commoner in black people than in white people, had developed anti-C and anti-E, and they recommended that Dccee patients with sickle cell disease should be given C-negative, E-negative blood.

Alloimmunization following solid organ transplants. Out of 704 recipients of transplants of heart, lung or both, who were followed up, new alloantibodies appeared, usually only transiently in 2.1%. The frequency with which anti-D was formed is mentioned in Chapter 5; the commonest other specificities were anti-E and anti-K. The low incidence was attributed to immunosuppressive therapy (Cummins *et al.* 1995).

Relative importance of different alloantibodies in transfusion

As discussed in Chapter 11, anti-A and anti-B must be regarded as overwhelmingly the most important red cell alloantibodies in blood transfusion because they are most commonly implicated in fatal haemolytic transfusion reactions. Rh antibodies are the next most important mainly because they are commoner than other immune red cell alloantibodies. For example, in the series of Grove-Rasmussen and Huggins (1973), out of 177 antibodies associated with haemolytic transfusion reactions (omitting 30 cases in which anti-A and anti-B were responsible and also omitting cases in which only cold agglutinins were found, which were unlikely to have been responsible for red cell destruction), 95, including 35 examples of anti-D, were within the Rh system. Estimates of frequencies with which other red cell alloantibodies were involved in

immediate and delayed haemolytic transfusion reactions are shown in Table 3.6.

The figures given in Table 3.6 show that the frequencies with which the different red cell alloantibodies were involved in immediate haemolytic transfusion reactions were similar to the frequencies with which the same red cell alloantibodies were found in transfusion recipients. On the other hand, the figures for delayed haemolytic transfusion reactions show one very striking difference in that antibodies of the Jk system were very much more commonly involved than expected from a frequency of these antibodies in random transfusion recipients. Possibly this discrepancy is due to the fact that red cell destruction by Kidd antibodies tends to be severe so that perhaps delayed haemolytic reactions are more readily diagnosed when these antibodies are involved, or, to put it in another way, delayed haemolytic transfusion reactions associated with other red cell alloantibodies may tend to be missed.

Perhaps a more important reason why Kidd antibodies tend to be relatively frequently involved in delayed haemolytic transfusion reactions may be that they are difficult to detect, particularly when present in low concentration. Moreover, unlike some antibodies, for example anti-D, which after having become detectable remain detectable for long periods of time, Kidd antibodies tend to disappear (see Chapter 6, p. 216).

Although examples of anti-Le[a] and some examples of anti-Le[b] are active at 37°C *in vitro*, they have very seldom been the cause of haemolytic transfusion reactions, mainly because Lewis antibodies are readily neutralized by Lewis substances which are present in the plasma of the transfused blood.

Although most antibodies that are active at 37°C *in vitro* are capable of causing red cell destruction, there are exceptions (see Chapter 11). In some cases the explanation may lie in the IgG subclass of the antibody and in others, perhaps, in the paucity of antigen sites.

Cold alloantibodies such as anti-A_1, anti-HI, anti-P_1, anti-M and anti-N are usually inactive *in vitro* at 37°C and are then incapable of bringing about red cell destruction. Occasional examples which are dubiously active at 37°C but active at 30°C or higher may bring about the destruction of small volumes of incompatible red cells given for the purpose of investigation. References to very rare examples of anti-A_1 and anti-P_1, anti-M and anti-N that have caused haemolytic transfusion reactions will be found in later chapters.

Relative potency (immunogenicity) of different antigens

An estimate of the relative potency of different red cell alloantigens can be obtained by comparing the actual frequency with which particular alloantibodies are encountered with the calculated frequency of the opportunity for immunization (Giblett 1961). For example, suppose that in transfusion recipients anti-K is found about 2.5 times more commonly than anti-Fy^a (see Table 3.6a and b). The relative opportunities for immunization to K and Fy^a can be estimated simply by comparing the frequency of the combination K-positive donor, K-negative recipient, i.e. $0.09 \times 0.91 = 0.08$, with the frequency of the combination Fy(a+) donor, Fy(a−) recipient, i.e. $0.66 \times 0.34 = 0.22$. Thus the opportunity for immunization to K is about 3.5 times less than that for Fy^a (0.08 vs. 0.22). In summary, although opportunities for immunization to K are 3.5 times less frequent than those to Fy^a, anti-K is in fact found 2.5 times more commonly than anti-Fy^a, so that overall, K is about nine times more potent than Fy^a. If a single transfusion of K-positive blood to a K-negative subject induces the formation of serologically detectable anti-K in 10% of cases (see Chapter 6) it is, therefore, predicted that the transfusion of a single unit of Fy(a+) blood to an Fy(a−) subject would induce the formation of serologically detectable anti-Fy^a in about 1% of cases.

Using earlier data, Giblett (1961) calculated that c and E were about three times less potent than K, that Fy^a was about 25 times less potent and Jk^a 50–100 times less potent.

Transfusion and pregnancy compared as a stimulus

In considering the risks of immunization by particular red cell alloantigens, the effect of transfusing multiple units of blood and the relative risks of immunization by transfusion and pregnancy must be discussed.

When an antigen has a low frequency, for example K, with a frequency of 0.09, the chance of receiving a unit containing the antigen increases directly with the number of the units transfused, up to a certain number (11 in this instance). On the other hand, when an antigen has a high frequency, for example c, frequency 0.8, the chance of exposure is high with only a single unit and increases only slightly as the number of units transfused increases. The point can be illustrated by calculating an example. For the transfusion of a single unit, the chance that the donor will be K positive and the recipient K negative is $0.09 \times 0.91 = 0.08$; the corresponding risk of incompatibility from c is $0.8 \times 0.2 = 0.16$; the relative risk from the two antigens (K/c) is thus 0.5:1.0. When 4 units are transfused, the chance of K incompatibility (at least one donor K positive and the recipient K negative) is $0.31 \times 0.91 = 0.28$ and of c incompatibility $0.997 \times 0.2 =$ approximately 0.2, so that the relative risk (K/c) is now 0.28:0.2 or 1.4:1 (Allen and Warshaw 1962). To summarize, the relative risk of exposure to K compared with c is about three times as great with a 4-unit blood transfusion as with a 1-unit transfusion.

When the antigen has a low frequency, opportunities for making the corresponding antibody are much lower from pregnancy than from blood transfusion, assuming that a woman has only one partner and that in transfusion many different donors are often involved. For example, in women who have three pregnancies the chance that in two of them the fetus will be c incompatible with its mother is about three times greater than that two of them will be K incompatible (Allen and Warshaw 1962).

These theoretical considerations are supported by actual findings: among women sensitized by blood transfusion alone, anti-K was almost three times more common than anti-c (32:12), whereas among women sensitized by pregnancy alone the incidence of the two antibodies was similar (9:7) (Allen and Warshaw 1962).

When a woman carries a fetus with an incompatible antigen, she is far less likely to form alloantibodies than when she is transfused with blood carrying the same antigen. Presumably the main reason for the difference is simply that in many pregnancies the size of transplacental haemorrhage does not constitute an adequate stimulus for primary immunization.

In two different series in which anti-c was detected in pregnant women there was a history of a previous blood transfusion in over one-third of the women (Fraser and Tovey 1976; Astrup and Kornstad 1977).

The effect of Rh D immunization on the formation of other red cell alloantibodies

Among Rh D-negative volunteers deliberately injected with D-positive red cells, those who form anti-D tend

Table 3.7 Response to K, Fy[a], Jk[a] and s in relation to Rh D compatibility of injected red cells.

Recipients making	Donor cells D-compatible	Donor cells D-incompatible	
		Recipients not making anti-D	Recipients making anti-D
Anti-K	1/12	0/20	6/12
Anti-Fy[a]	1/19	0/15	9/49
Anti-Jk[a]	0/16	0.19	16/87
Anti-s	0/21	–	3/14

For sources and for assumptions made, see Mollison (1983, p. 238).

also to form alloantibodies outside the Rh system, whereas those who do not form anti-D seldom form any alloantibodies at all. In one series of 73 subjects who formed anti-D, six formed anti-Fy[a], four formed anti-Jk[a] and four formed other antibodies; by contrast, amongst 48 subjects who failed to form anti-D, not one made any detectable alloantibodies (Archer *et al.* 1969).

An association between the formation of anti-D and that of antibodies outside the Rh system was previously noted by Issitt (1965) in women who had borne children.

Several series in which D-negative subjects have been deliberately immunized with D-positive red cells are available for analysis. In some series, donors and recipients were tested for other red cell antigens so that the numbers at risk from these other antigens are known. In other series, donors and recipients were not tested, or only donors were tested, for antigens other than D, so that it is only possible to estimate the numbers at risk from the known incidence of the relevant antigens in a random population. In Table 3.7 estimates of the immunogenicity of K, Fy[a], Jk[a] and s in three circumstances are listed: (1) in subjects receiving D-compatible red cells; (2) in D-negative recipients receiving D-positive red cells but not making anti-D; and (3) in D-negative recipients receiving D-positive red cells and making anti-D.

The data summarized in Table 3.7 emphasize the tremendously increased response to antigens outside the Rh system in subjects responding to D. In subjects who formed anti-D and had the opportunity of making other antibodies, 50% formed anti-K. The incidence of anti-Fy[a], anti-Jk[a] and anti-s in those who could respond was about 20% in each instance. In deliberately immunizing Rh D-negative subjects to

obtain anti-D, it is clearly very important to choose donors who cannot stimulate the formation of antibodies such as anti-K, -Fy[a] or -Jk[a].

The question arises whether non-responders to D are also non-responders to other red cell antigens. The data shown in Table 3.7 do not answer the question, as although no alloantibodies were formed by non-responders to D, only two such antibodies were made by recipients of D-compatible red cells, and much larger numbers are needed to discover whether there is any difference between the two categories.

Multiple alloantibodies may also be found in Rh D-positive subjects (Issitt *et al.* 1973).

Enhancing effect of 'strong' antigens: experiments in chickens

The great enhancing effect, on the immunogenicity of weak alloantigens, of a response to a strong alloantigen finds an exact parallel in experiments reported in chickens. In these animals, B is a strong antigen and A is a weak one, so that when cells carrying only one of these antigens are given, responses to B are the rule, but to A are very infrequent. However, when red cells carrying both these antigens are given, recipients make both antibodies. The effect is not found when mixed A and B red cells are given and thus depends on both antigens being carried on the same red cells (Schierman and McBride 1967).

Competition of antigens

If an animal is immunized to one antigen, X, and is subsequently re-injected with X, together with an unrelated antigen, Y, it may show a significantly lowered response to Y (see, for example, Barr and Llewellyn-Jones 1953), a phenomenon known as antigenic competition. It has been suggested that control mechanisms, designed to prevent the unlimited progression of the immune response, may be responsible and that the phrase non-specific antigen-induced suppression may be a better description of the phenomenon. It is probable that the suppression observed is due to several different mechanisms varying with the antigens used, the time sequence of immunization and other factors (Pross and Eidinger 1974).

In considering the possible interference of immunization to one red cell antigen on the response to another, the fact that both antigens may be carried on the same red cells must be taken into account. As soon as antibody has been formed to one antigen it will tend to bring about rapid destruction of the red cells and this process may interfere with the immune response to a second antigen.

There is quite extensive evidence that red cells carrying two antigens, for the first of which there is a corresponding antibody in the subject's serum, may fail to immunize against the second antigen. The best known example is the protective effect against Rh D immunization exercised by ABO incompatibility (see Chapter 5). ABO incompatibility has also been shown to protect against immunization to c (Levine 1958), K (Levine, quoted by Race and Sanger 1968, p. 283), and a number of other antigens including Fya, Jka and Dia (Stern 1975). The effect of passively administered anti-K on the response to D carried on D-positive, K-positive red cells is described on p. 81.

The following case illustrates the circumstances in which protection may be observed: a D-negative, S-positive woman was transfused with D-negative, S-negative blood. After two D-positive pregnancies she was found to have formed potent anti-s but only low-titred anti-D (Drachmann and Hansen 1969; Stern 1975). A similar phenomenon was reported by Stern and co-workers (1958). An R_1R_1 subject was injected with Be(a+), D-negative cells, and formed anti-Bea. Two weeks after the appearance of anti-Bea, anti-c was detected. After further immunization, anti-Bea reached a high titre, whereas the anti-c became weaker and was finally only just detectable. (Bea is associated with weak c and e antigens; see Race and Sanger 1975, p. 204.)

It is possible that the mechanism of protection by ABO incompatibility is different in so far as it leads to intravascular lysis of red cells and in so far as lysed red cells seem to be less antigenic than intact ones (see below).

In any case, there is a paradox to be resolved: the enhancing effect, on immunization to a weak antigen such as Jka, of a response to a strong antigen such as D and the suppressive effect, on immunization to a relatively strong antigen such as D, of ABO incompatibility. Perhaps the important difference lies in the presence or absence of alloantibody in the serum at the time when induction of immunization to a second antigen is in question. During primary immunization the induction of a response to a weak antigen may be facilitated by a response to a strong antigen but once potent antibody is present in the serum it may be difficult to induce primary immunization to another red cell antigen.

Immunogenicity of red cell stroma. There is evidence that lysed blood and stroma prepared from lysed red cells are less immunogenic than intact red cells (Schneider and Preisler 1966; Mollison 1967, p. 203; Pollack *et al.* 1968).

Autoantibodies associated with alloimmunization

The development of cold red cell autoagglutinins has been observed in animals following repeated injections of red cells (see Chapter 7) and has occasionally been observed in humans in association with delayed haemolytic transfusion reactions (see Chapter 11).

A positive direct antiglobulin test is sometimes observed during secondary immunization to D (see Chapter 5) and has been noted in about 1 in 60 subjects who are developing secondary responses to other alloantigens, such as K (PD Issitt, personal communication).

The development of autoantibodies has also been observed following an episode of red cell destruction induced by passively administered antibodies and following intensive plasma exchange (Chapter 5).

Immunological tolerance

Long-lasting immunological tolerance can be induced either by introducing into an embryo a graft that survives throughout life or by giving repeated injections of cells.

Examples of graft survival are provided by 'chimeras', i.e. individuals whose cells are derived from two distinct zygotes. Many examples of such permanent chimerism have been described in human dizygotic twins (see review in Watkins *et al.* 1980). Temporary chimerism may be observed in subjects who have received immunosuppressive therapy and have then been transfused or have received a bone marrow transplant. Occasionally, cells of two different phenotypes derived from a single zygote lineage are found, a phenomenon known as *mosaicism*. The commonest form of mosaicism encountered in blood grouping is due to somatic mutation, i.e. Tn polyagglutinability (see Chapter 7).

Examples of possible tolerance to blood cells in humans

In experiments in which weekly i.v. injections of whole heparinized blood not more than 24 h old were given from the same donors to the same recipients, in about 10% of cases there was a progressive decrease in the intensity of the antibody response to HLA antigens until humoral cytotoxic activity could no longer be demonstrated (Ferrara *et al.* 1974).

The induction of partial tolerance to skin grafts in newborn infants transfused with fresh whole blood but not stored blood was described by Fowler and co-workers (1960).

The development of fatal graft versus-host disease (GvHD) following transfusion in newborn infants in whom a previous intra-uterine transfusion had apparently induced tolerance is described in Chapter 15.

Subjects with thalassaemia to whom transfusions are given from the first year of life onwards appear to be rendered partially tolerant to red cell antigens (see p. 76).

For tolerance to grafts and neoplasia induced by transfusion, see Chapter 13.

Suppression of the immune response by passive antibody

Practical aspects of the suppression of Rh D immunization by passively administered antibody are discussed in Chapter 5. Here, some theoretical aspects of the subject are considered briefly.

Von Dungern (1900) observed that if cattle red cells saturated with antibody are injected into a rabbit, the immune response which would otherwise occur is prevented, and others found that the response to soluble antigens can be suppressed by giving 'excess' antibody (Smith 1909; Glenny and Südmersen 1921). 'Excess' in this context is usually thought of as literally an outnumbering of antigen sites by antibody molecules. The response to antigens carried on red cells can be suppressed by very much smaller amounts of antibody. For example, 20 μg of anti-D is effective in suppressing immunization when 1 ml of D-positive red cells is injected (see Chapter 5). Assuming that the antibody is distributed within a space about twice as great as the plasma volume, it can be calculated that, at equilibrium, only about 5% of antigen and about 1% of antibody will be bound. Similarly, the amount of passive antibody required to suppress the immune response in mice to SRBC was calculated to be 100 times less than the amount required to saturate the antigen sites (Haughton and Nash 1969). Evidently, in these circumstances, suppression of the immune response is not due to covering of antigen by antibody but is due to destruction of antigen-carrying cells in circumstances in which it cannot induce immunization; a possible mechanism of suppression is discussed below.

The suppressive effect of passive antibody against soluble antigen is antigen specific. In an experiment in which a molecule carrying two antigenic determinants was injected, the response to one could be suppressed without affecting the response to the other (Brody *et al.* 1967). On the other hand, discrepant results have been observed with antigens carried on red cells. In rabbits and chickens it has proved possible to suppress the response to one antigen carried on the cells without suppressing the response to another (Pollack *et al.* 1968; Schierman *et al.* 1969). However, in the only experiment reported in humans, when red cells carrying both D and K were injected together with anti-K, the response to both K and D was suppressed (Woodrow *et al.* 1975). Volunteers, all of whom were D negative, were given an injection of 1 ml of D-positive, K-positive red cells. In addition, one-half of the subjects ('treated') were given an injection of 14 μg of IgG anti-K, which was sufficient to clear the K-positive, D-positive red cells from the circulation into the spleen within 24 h. At 6 months, 7 out of 31 control subjects, but only 1 out of 31 treated subjects, had formed anti-D. After a further stimulus, four more control subjects but no more treated subjects developed anti-D.

The fact that ABO-incompatible D-positive red cells induced D immunization far less frequently than

ABO-compatible D-positive cells has been mentioned above. It should be noted that the mechanism of destruction of red cells by anti-K and anti-A is quite different. Anti-K is a non-haemolytic antibody which, when also non-complement-binding, as in the example used in the experiment described above, brings about red cell destruction predominantly in the spleen. On the other hand, anti-A and anti-B bring about destruction predominantly in the plasma by direct lysis of red cells, with sequestration of unlysed cells predominantly in the liver.

From a review of published work it was concluded that clearance of a small dose of red cells within 5 days and of a large dose within 8 days was usually associated with suppression, slower rates of clearance being associated with failure of suppression (Mollison 1984). The *rate* of destruction seems unlikely to be directly correlated with suppression. The i.m. injection of a constant amount of anti-D with varying amounts of D-positive red cells led to suppression of primary immunization when the ratio of antibody to cells was 20–25 µg antibody/ml cells but did not lead to complete suppression at ratios of 15 µg of less (Pollack *et al.* 1971; see Chapter 5). There is evidence that the rates of clearance would be only slightly greater at a ratio of 25 µg/ml than at 15 µ/ml. On the other hand, the time taken for the volume of surviving cells to fall to a given level, say 0.01 ml, too low to induce primary immunization, would increase as the ratio of antibody–cells diminished (Chapman 1996).

There is one observation which, if confirmed, would demonstrate a relationship between splenic destruction – and perhaps between rapid destruction – and suppression: in a splenectomized, D-negative subject injected with 4 ml of D-positive red cells together with 300 µg of anti-D i.v., the red cells were cleared with a $t_{1/2}$ of 14.5 days and the subject developed anti-D within 4 months (Weitzel *et al.* 1974). Thus, slow clearance was associated with failure of suppression by a normally suppressive dose of anti-D.

One model for immune suppression proposes that IgG–red cell complexes bind to the inhibitory receptor for IgG (FcγRIIB) on the surface of B lymphocytes, thereby generating signals inhibiting B-cell activation. FcγRIIB contains a cytoplasmic inhibitory motif (ITIM). The B-cell receptor (BCR) contains an activation motif (ITAM). When the ITIM is brought into proximity with ITAM, cell activation is inhibited (reviewed in Vivier and Daeron 1997). Inhibition of

B-cell activation by crosslinking FcRγIIB and BCR can be demonstrated *in vitro* (Muta *et al.* 1994). However, *in vivo* studies in FcγR-deficient mice indicate that antibodies capable of suppressing the immune response to SRBC do not do so by Fc-mediated interactions (Karlsson *et al.* 1999, 2001). These authors show that SRBC-specific IgG given up to 5 days after SRBC can induce suppression in both wild-type and FcγRIIB-deficient mice. An alternative mechanism might be that suppressive antibody binds its specific antigen, thereby preventing exposure of antigen to B cells but as Karlsson and co-workers (2001) discuss this is unlikely to be the case in man in whom it is reported that doses of anti-D insufficient to coat all D antigen sites are suppressive and IgG anti-K can suppress the immune response to D (see above). Rapid elimination of IgG–antigen complexes from the circulation by an Fc-independent process provides a third possible mechanism. In this context it is interesting to note that rapid phagocytosis of red cells from CD47-deficient mice occurs when the cells are transfused to wild-type mice, suggesting that CD47 is a marker for self-recognition and that this property is mediated by interaction with macrophage signal regulatory protein (SIRPα; Oldenborg *et al.* 2000, 2001). Direct evidence that CD47 ligation to macrophages inhibits phagocytosis is provided by Okazawa and co-workers (2005). CD47 is a component of the band 3/Rh complex in human red cells (Plate 3.1), raising the intriguing possibility that anti-D bound to red cells might indirectly inhibit self-recognition through CD47 and effect elimination of the antibody-coated cells by splenic macrophages through an as yet unidentified mechanism. Such an interaction between antibody-coated red cells and macrophages may explain the relationship between the rate of clearance and the probability that immunization will be suppressed. Macrophages that engulf antibody-coated red cells are known to be relatively ineffective presenters of antigen to the immune system, having poor expression of class II HLA antigens on their surface. In contrast, dendritic cells are responsible for the processing of antigen on red cells not coated with antibody; antigen is taken up by either pinocytosis or surface processing. Dendritic cells have very good expression of class II antigens and are the most effective cells in antigen presentation and thus in the initiation of primary immune responses (Berg *et al.* 1994). If red cells sensitized with IgG antibodies adhere to and are engulfed by macrophages, they are kept away from dendritic cells, which therefore cannot present red cell antigens to T-helper cells.

Two points of practical importance are whether immunization can be suppressed when antibody is administered at some time interval after antigen, and whether the immune response, once initiated, can be suppressed either partially or totally by passive administration of antibody. So far as D immunization is concerned, there is evidence that in a proportion of subjects the response to D can be suppressed by giving antibody as late as 2 weeks after the D-positive cells have been injected (Samson and Mollison 1975); see also Chapter 5. Passively administered anti-D is ineffective once primary D immunization has been initiated and also fails to suppress secondary responses (see Chapter 5). The latter is in contrast with results obtained in mice with SRBC (Karlsson et al. 2001).

Augmentation of the immune response by passive antibody

The term *augmentation*, applied to immune responses, has been used to describe at least three apparently different effects observed when relatively small amounts of antibody are injected together with antigen:

1 When SRBC are injected into mice, the number of plaque-forming cells (PFCs) can be increased by injecting purified IgM anti-SRBC with the SRBC (Henry and Jerne 1968). In confirming this observation, using monoclonal IgM antibody, it was found that the effect was observed only when the dose was one, i.e. 1×10^5 red cells, which ordinarily elicited a negligible immune response (Lehner et al. 1983). The effect of passive IgM antibody is thus to turn an otherwise ineffective stimulus into an effective one. Note that in this system the antigen is heterologous and that the antibody response reaches a peak at about 5 days; the response is thus more like secondary than primary immunization. In a different context, i.e. in newborn mice that have passively acquired IgG anti-malarial antibodies, passive monoclonal IgM antibody can overcome the suppressive effect of IgG antibody and induce responsiveness to malarial vaccine (Harte et al. 1983).

2 In mice injected with human serum albumin together with antibody, with antigen in slight excess, the effect of passive antibody is to accelerate primary immunization and to increase the amount of antibody formed (Terres and Wolins 1959, 1961). Similar effects

have been observed in newborn piglets (Hoerlein 1957; Segre and Kaeberle 1962).

3 The stimulus for memory (B_m) cell development appears to be the localization of antigen–antibody complexes on follicular dendritic cells, a process which, at least in mice, is C3 dependent (Klaus et al. 1980). Antigen–antibody complexes are 100-fold more effective than soluble antigen in priming virgin B cells to differentiate into B_m cells (Klaus 1978).

The relevance of the foregoing observations to possible augmentation of immune response to human red cell alloantigens is uncertain. So far as responses to D are concerned, it is unlikely that passive IgM plays any part, as the biological effects of IgM antibodies are believed to depend on complement activation and anti-D does not activate complement. Similarly, IgG D antibodies, if they can increase the formation of memory cells, must do it by a method other than that which has been shown to operate in mice. It might seem then, by exclusion, that the effect of small amounts of passively administered IgG anti-D would be to increase antibody formation in primary immunization but, in fact, this effect has not been observed. As described in Chapter 5 the only effect for which there is some evidence is the conversion of an ineffective stimulus into an effective one.

Different effects produced by different IgG subclasses

Experiments in mice indicate that one subclass of IgG when injected with antigen depresses the immune response, whereas another subclass, over a certain range of dosage, actually augments the immune response (Gordon and Murgita 1975). No information is available about possibly analogous differences between human IgG subclasses.

Tolerance effect of oral antigen

As described above, it is believed that most, if not all, naturally occurring antibodies are formed in response to bacterial antigens carrying determinants that cross-react with red cell antigens. It is likely that bacterial antigens are absorbed mainly through the gut; mechanisms for limiting the immune response to antigens absorbed in this way may therefore be relevant. It seems that at least two mechanisms are involved: (1) the production of IgA antibodies in the gut may limit the uptake of subsequently ingested antigen (André et al. 1974) and (2) oral administration of antigen induces the formation of suppressor cells (Mattingley and Waksman 1978). There is evidence that the complex of IgA antibody with antigen is tolerogenic (André et al. 1975). Under some circumstances, the administration of an antigen by mouth to mice may completely abolish the ability to respond to a subsequent parenteral dose of antigen (Hanson et al. 1979). For further references, see O'Neil et al. (2004). Transgenic mice expressing human HLA-DR15 respond to immunization with the human Rh D polypeptide. This immune response can be inhibited by nasal administration of synthetic peptides containing dominant helper T-cell epitopes (Hall et al. 2005, see also Chapter 12). In an experiment in human volunteers, the oral administration of Rh D antigen to previously unimmunized males failed to influence the subsequent primary response to D-positive red cells given intravenously (see Chapter 5).

Lectins

Although lectins are not antibodies, they share two important properties with antibodies, namely that of binding to specific structures and of causing red cells to agglutinate, and it is convenient to consider them here.

The red cell agglutinating activity of ricin, obtained from the castor bean, was described in 1888 (see reviews by Bird 1959, Boyd 1963), but the fact that plant extracts might have blood group specificity was first described 60 years later. Renkonen (1948) showed that some samples of seeds from Vicia cracca contain powerful agglutinins acting much more strongly on A than on B or O cells, and Boyd and Reguera (1949) found that many varieties of Lima beans contain agglutinins that are highly specific for group A red cells.

Lectins are sugar-binding proteins or glycoproteins of non-immune origin, which agglutinate cells and/or precipitate glycoconjugates (Goldstein et al. 1980). Although first discovered in plants, lectins have also been found in many organisms from bacteria to mammals, for example lectins for human red cell antigens are found in the albumin glands of snails and in certain fungi (animal lectins are reviewed in Kilpatrick 2000).

The simple sugars found on the red cell membrane are D-galactose, mannose, L-fucose, D-glucose, N-acetylglucosamine, N-acetylgalactosamine and N-acetylneuraminic acid. Although lectins can be classified according to their specificity for these simple sugars, it must be realized that lectin specificity is not only dependent on the presence of the reactive sugar in terminal position, but also on its anomeric configuration, the nature of the subterminal sugar, the site of its attachment to this sugar and, in cellular glycoproteins or glycolipids, on the number and distribution of receptor sites and the amount of steric hindrance caused by vicinal (neighbouring) structures. The most important factor is the outward display of the carbohydrate chain, which may depend on its 'native' configuration or on the configuration imparted to it by the structure of the protein or lipid to which it is attached (Bird 1981). Accordingly, each simple sugar may be associated with several different specificities. As there is some similarity between the various combinations of simple sugars, crossreaction is not unusual amongst lectins.

Some plant seeds contain more than one lectin; for example Griffonia simplicifolia seeds contain three lectins GS I, GS II and GS III. GS I is a family of five tetrameric isolectins, of which one, A_4, is specific for N-acetyl-D-galactosamine and another, B_4, is specific for D-galactose (Goldstein et al. 1981). GS II is specific for N-acetyl-D-glucosamine.

Examples of simple sugars found on the red cell surface which react with lectins are as follows.

D-Galactose. In α-linked position, D-galactose is the chief structural determinant of B, P_1 and p^k specificity. Lectins with this specificity include those from Fomes fomentarius, the B-specific isolectin of GS I and Salmo trutta. Many D-galactose-specific lectins, however, also react with this sugar in β-linked position and therefore agglutinate human cells regardless of blood group (e.g. the lectin from Ricinus communis). The lectins from Arachis hypogaea, Vicia cretica and V. graminea are exceptions and react specifically with certain β-galactose residues.

L-Fucose. The specific lectins for this sugar include those of Lotus tetragonolobus, Ulex europaeus and the lectin from the haemolymph of the eel Anguilla anguilla. All of these three lectins are very useful anti-H reagents.

N-Acetylgalactosamine. Lectins with a specificity for this sugar include those of Dolichos biflorus, which reacts with A_1, Tn and Cad determinants, Phaseolus lunatus (anti-A) and Helix pomatia (anti-A).

Further details about the reactions of lectins will be found in later chapters. The role of lectins in immuno-haematology is reviewed in Bird (1989).

Reaction between antigen and antibody

In blood group serology, the interaction between antigen on cells and the corresponding antibody is normally detected by observing specific agglutination of the cells concerned. Nevertheless, the fundamental reaction is simply a combination of antigen with antibody, which may or may not be followed by agglutination, and this combination must first be studied.

Combination of antigen and antibody

Antigen and antibody do not form covalent bonds. Rather, the complementary nature of the corresponding structures on antigen and antibody enable the antigenic determinants to come into very close apposition with the binding site on the antibody molecule, and antigen and antibody can then be held together by relatively weak intermolecular bonds. These bonds are believed to include opposing charges on ionic groups, hydrogen bonds, hydrophobic (non-polar) bonds and van der Waals' forces. Probably, more than one type of bond is usually involved. In one example investigated by Nisonoff and Pressman (1957), an ionic bond at one end of the molecule contributed most to the strength of the bond, but a substantial contribution was made by non-polar groups. The strength of the bond between antigen and antibody, measured as the free energy change, was calculated for examples of IgG anti-D, -c, -E and -e to lie within the range −10 200 to −12 800 cal/mol; that for IgG anti-K (−14 300 cal/mol) was rather higher (Hughes-Jones 1972) (1 cal ≡ 4.2 J). Note that these figures are all for intrinsic affinities (see below). The figures indicate that the strength of the bond between antigen and antibody-combining site for these particular antibodies is about one-tenth as great as that of a covalent bond.

The reaction between antibody (Ab) and antigen (Ag) is reversible in accordance with the law of mass action (for review, see Hughes-Jones 1963) and may be written thus:

$$Ab + Ag \underset{k_2}{\overset{k_1}{\rightleftharpoons}} AbAg \qquad (3.1)$$

where k_1 and k_2 are the rate constants for the forward and reverse reactions respectively.

According to the law of mass action, at equilibrium:

$$\frac{[AbAg]}{[Ab] \times [Ag]} = \frac{k_1}{k_2} = K \qquad (3.2)$$

where [Ab], [Ag] and [AbAg], respectively, are the concentrations of Ab, Ag and the combined product AbAg, and K is the equilibrium or association constant. Similarly, at equilibrium:

$$\frac{[AgAb]}{[Ab]} = K[Ag] \qquad (3.3)$$

That is to say, the higher the equilibrium constant, the greater will be the amount of antibody combining with antigen at equilibrium.

The *equilibrium constant* of an antibody may be looked on as a measure of the goodness of the fit of the antibody to the corresponding antigen, and of the type of bonding; for example, hydrophobic bonds generally give rise to higher affinities than do hydrogen bonds. When the equilibrium constant is high, the bond between antigen and antibody will, as a rule, be less readily broken.

IgG antibodies have two antigen-binding sites. When antigens are close together on cells, both the antigen-combining sites on an antibody may bind to the same cell, a process known as *monogamous bivalency* (Klinman and Karush 1967). IgG anti-A and anti-B appear to bind to red cells by both their binding sites (Greenbury *et al.* 1965, but see Chapter 4) and there is evidence that IgG anti-M also binds bivalently (Romans *et al.* 1979, 1980). IgG anti-D binds to red cells monovalently (Hughes-Jones 1970). Any anti-A, -B or -M which, at equilibrium, is bound to red cells by just one combining site rapidly dissociates on washing (Romans *et al.* 1979, 1980).

The strength of the bond between antigen and antibody is enormously increased when both combining sites on the antibody can bind to the red cell simultaneously. The bond between antigen and antibody is constantly being broken and, when only one site on the antibody is bound initially, the antibody molecule can drift away from the antigen. When two combining sites are bound, the breaking of one bond leaves the antibody joined to the antigen by the other combining site and there will be an increased opportunity for the first combining site to recombine with antigen before the antibody molecule drifts away. The equilibrium constant is increased approximately 1000-fold when both of the combining sites on an IgG antibody can bind to antigen (Hornick and Karush 1972).

IgM molecules have 10 binding sites, but with antigens of molecular weight greater than about 3000 they have an apparent valency of only five, owing to steric hindrance and restricted mobility between the Fab regions of each of the five main subunits (van Oss *et al.* 1973). IgM anti-D appears to bind to individual red cells by only one site, presumably because the distance between two D antigens is too great to be bridged by the combining sites on a single antibody molecule (Holburn *et al.* 1971b).

With some antigens it has been found that fewer IgM than IgG molecules will combine with a red cell. One explanation for such a finding could be that the antigen sites are so closely packed that, at saturation, IgG molecules cover virtually the whole surface; as IgM molecules are much larger, the maximum number that could bind would clearly then be less. This explanation would apply to the observations of Humphrey and Dourmashkin (1965) that with SRBC the maximum number of Forssman antibody molecules that will combine is about 600 000 for IgG and 120 000 for IgM.

Apart from differences between the average equilibrium constants of antibodies from different donors, considerable heterogeneity is always found amongst the antibody molecules of a particular specificity from any one donor (Hughes-Jones 1967).

The difference between intrinsic and functional binding constants

The term *intrinsic binding constant* is used to refer to the affinity of a single antibody-combining site for a single antigenic determinant, i.e. monovalent binding, whereas the term *functional affinity constant* refers to binding of one or more combining sites on an antibody molecule to more than one antigenic determinant on a single carrier, i.e. ignoring valency. As already mentioned, when both combining sites on an IgG antibody are bound, the functional affinity constant may be 1000 times greater than the intrinsic binding constant. For one example of IgM, the enhancement value due to multivalency was of the order of 10×10^6 indicating that multivalent binding involved three or more combining sites (Hornick and Karush 1972).

Factors affecting the equilibrium constant

The equilibrium constant (a term that includes both intrinsic and functional affinity constants) is affected by pH, ionic strength and temperature, and knowledge of the effect of these variables is helpful in predicting the optimal conditions for eluting antibodies from red cells on the one hand and for the detection of antibodies on the other.

Effect of pH. The equilibrium constant for anti-D was found to be highest between pH 6.5 and 7, although there was relatively little difference over the range 5.5–8.5 (Hughes-Jones *et al.* 1964a). A few red cell alloantibodies have been described which are detectable only when pH is reduced, for example of anti-I and anti-M (see relevant chapters).

Effect of ionic strength. The rate of association of antibody with antigen may be enormously increased by lowering ionic strength. For example, the initial rate of association of anti-D with D-positive red cells is increased 1000-fold by a reduction of ionic strength from 0.17 to 0.03 (see Hughes-Jones *et al.* 1964a). These authors pointed out that the use of a low-ionic-strength medium should be valuable in detecting antibodies with relatively low equilibrium constants. They found that, in practice, the titre of most blood group antibodies was enhanced by diluting the serum in a low-ionic-strength medium (0.2% NaCl in 7% glucose) rather than in normal saline (see also Elliott *et al.* 1964). In studying the effect of low ionic strength on the reaction between anti-D and D-positive red cells, it was noted that the enhancement observed was not additive to that observed with enzyme-treated red cells and it was concluded that in both cases the effect was due to a reduction in the electrostatic 'barrier' surrounding the red cells (Atchley *et al.* 1964).

The practical value of using a low-ionic-strength medium in the detection of blood group antibodies is discussed in Chapter 8.

Effect of temperature. Temperature affects antigen–antibody reactions in two ways: by altering the equilibrium constant and by affecting the rate of the reaction.

Antibody binds to antigen because the resulting complex has a lower free energy value than that of the two uncombined. In an uncomplicated reaction, the energy released appears as heat and the reaction is thus exothermic. According to the principle of Le Chatelier, reversible reactions that are exothermic proceed further to completion when the temperature is lowered. For example, the reactions of anti-A (Economidou *et al.* 1967) and of anti-I (Olesen 1966), which are stronger at low temperatures, are exothermic. On the other hand, the reaction between antibody and antigen may result in an increase in the disorder (entropy) of the system. The change in entropy, which may result from a release of water molecules or from structural changes in the reactants, requires energy to bring it about and this is obtained as heat from the environment. The reaction is thus endothermic. It is 'warm' antibodies that display this characteristic (Hughes-Jones *et al.* 1963a). The nature of the bond at the combining site determines whether an antibody is 'cold' or 'warm', so that the chemical nature of the antigen is the determining factor. For example, hydrogen bonding is mainly exothermic and hydrophobic bonding mainly endothermic (Hughes-Jones 1975).

In conformity with the view that antigen is the determining factor in deciding whether an antigen–antibody reaction is of a warm or cold type, seven examples of anti-s and one each of anti-S and U, although IgG, were all cold reacting; in contrast, examples of anti-D, -Fy^a and -k reacted more strongly at 37°C (Lalezari *et al.* 1973; see also p. 256). Note, however, that one kind of naturally occurring IgG anti-D is cold reacting.

Anti-I (like -i and -Pr), whether IgM or IgG, always reacts more strongly with human red cells at low temperatures. It has been suggested that the greater complementarity of I with its antibody at low temperature, justifying the description 'cold antigen' (Moore 1976), may depend on the loss of fluidity of the red cell membrane at low temperature (Cooper 1977). Although human red cells react strongly at 4°C with anti-I and, as a rule, do not react at all at 37°C, rabbit red cells are agglutinated at 37°C.

Except in the case of antibodies known to react more strongly at 4°C than at 37°C, a temperature of 37°C is recommended for antibody detection because the rate of combination with antigen is much more rapid at this temperature. For example, at 37°C anti-D combines with antigen 20 times more rapidly than at 4°C (Hughes-Jones *et al.* 1964a).

Non-specific attachment of IgG

If red cells are incubated with labelled serum proteins at a concentration of 20 g/l, about 5–15 µg of protein is taken up per millilitre of packed cells. IgG is taken up to the greatest extent (Hughes-Jones and Gardner 1962), which is not surprising as IgG is the most positively charged serum protein and red cells are negatively charged.

There is evidence that the IgG present on normal red cells interacts with anti-IgG serum. For example, in absorbing antiglobulin serum to remove heteroagglutinins, the use of untreated red cells leads to a definite fall in antiglobulin titre, whereas the use of trypsin-treated cells does not (Stratton and Jones 1955) because trypsin removes IgG from the red cells (Merry *et al.* 1982). When washed, but otherwise untreated, red cells are added to ^{125}I-labelled anti-IgG, a small amount of antiglobulin regularly binds to the cells (Rochna and Hughes-Jones 1965).

Although anti-IgG fails to agglutinate normal red cells in manual testing, positive results are obtained in an AutoAnalyzer; the specificity of the reactions is demonstrated by their inhibition by IgG but not by other proteins (Burkart *et al.* 1974).

Factors involved in red cell agglutination

Red cells normally repel one another. The electric potential (zeta potential) at the surface of red cells depends not only on the electronegative surface charge, but also on the ionic cloud that normally surrounds them.

Many human IgG antibodies fail to agglutinate red cells suspended in saline but there are certain exceptions, notably IgG anti-A, anti-B and anti-M. The reasons why IgG anti-A and IgG anti-M will agglutinate saline-suspended cells, whereas, for example, IgG anti-D will not, is likely to be related to the position of these antigens relative to the lipid bilayer of the plasma membrane. A,B and M antigens are located at the outer edge of the red cell glycocalyx, whereas D is carried on a polypeptide that does not extend greatly beyond the lipid bilayer (see Plate 3.1). The distance between A,B or M antigens on two red cells in suspension is therefore considerably less than the distance between the D antigens on two cells in suspension. Given that the known maximum distance between the two paratopes of IgG is approximately 15 nm, and knowing that IgG antibodies do not normally agglutinate red cells, the distance of closest approach between the surface glycocalyx of one red cell and the surface glycocalyx of another is likely to be of the order of 15 nm. IgM molecules (diameter 3 nm) can readily bridge the gap between antigens expressed close to the lipid bilayer and IgM anti-D can thus bring about agglutination.

Influence of number of antigen sites. The strength of agglutination is likely to be related to the number of antigen sites as well as the position of the antigen sites relative to the lipid bilayer. In experiments in which a hapten was covalently coupled to red cells in different amounts, it was found that a higher hapten density was required for agglutination by IgG antibodies than for IgM antibodies. When the hapten density fell below a certain level, the IgG antibodies behaved as incomplete antibodies and did not agglutinate untreated red cells (Leikola and Pasanen 1970).

It has also been shown that the density of epitopes on the red cell surface can influence the thermal amplitude of cold agglutinins; red cells were treated with neuraminidase to remove sialic acid and allowed to adsorb haematoside (sialyllactosylceramide). When fewer than 10^6 molecules of haematoside per cell had been absorbed, the cells were agglutinated at 0°C but not at 37°C, but when more than 10^6 molecules of haematoside were absorbed, the cells were agglutinated at both 37°C and at 0°C (Tsai *et al.* 1978).

Other factors besides site number may be the proximity of the antigen sites to one another; this will depend, first, on the number of antigen sites per red cell, second on the extent to which the sites occur normally in clusters, and finally the extent to which they are capable of forming clusters after combining with antibody.

Minimum number of antibody molecules for agglutination in saline. Some estimates of the minimum number of antibody molecules per red cell required for agglutination by IgM antibodies are as follows: anti-A, about 50 (Economidiou *et al.* 1967b); anti-D, about 120 (Holburn *et al.* 1971b); and anti-I (at 5°C), between 65 and 440 (Olesen 1966). The number of molecules required for agglutination by IgG anti-A (in saline) was found to be much higher: about 7000 (Economidou *et al.* 1967). Slightly different figures for anti-A were found by Greenbury and co-workers (1963), namely 25 for IgM and 20 000 for IgG.

Similarly, the minimum serum concentration required for agglutination was found to be approximately 0.001 µg/ml for IgM anti-A but 0.2 µg/ml for IgG anti-A (Economidou *et al.* 1967); on a molar basis, IgM anti-A is thus 100 times more effective than IgG anti-A. A similar difference was reported by Ishizaka and co-workers (1965), although the figures for the minimal concentrations of IgM and IgG anti-A for agglutination were about four times lower, presumably due to greater sensitivity of the tests employed. Incidentally, the same authors found that on a weight (and molar) basis IgG anti-A was about 10 times less effective than IgM anti-A in producing agglutination.

Effect of centrifugation. The agglutination of red cells is enhanced by centrifugation (see Chapter 8). Furthermore, some IgG antibodies that will not agglutinate saline-suspended red cells under ordinary conditions may do so if the mixtures are centrifuged. For example, IgG anti-D was found to agglutinate saline-suspended red cells after centrifugation at 12 000 rev/min, although not at 6000 rev/min (Hirszfeld and Dubiski 1954). Agglutination by anti-A from cord serum was greatly enhanced by centrifugation for 3 min at 3000 rev/min but the effect was striking only when the cells were suspended in saline (Munk-Andersen 1956).

Effect of enzyme treatment of red cells. The action of enzymes on red cells may potentiate agglutination in at least two different ways: first by reducing surface charge, thus allowing cells to come closer to one another (Steane 1982); almost all the sialic acid can be removed by treatment with neuraminidase. Although neuraminidase is the most efficient of all enzymes in reducing the surface charge of red cells (Eylar *et al.* 1962; Pollack *et al.* 1965) it is not as effective as proteases (which also remove sialic acid) in increasing red cell agglutinability with certain antibodies. For example, with papain-treated red cells the titre of incomplete anti-D is far higher than with neuraminidase-treated cells (Stratton *et al.* 1973). A second way in which enzymes may potentiate agglutination is by removing structures that sterically interfere with the access of antibody molecules (Hughes-Jones *et al.* 1964b; van Oss *et al.* 1978).

The increased agglutinability of enzyme-treated red cells is much more pronounced with IgG antibodies than with IgM antibodies. The titre of various agglutinating IgG antibodies was about 16 times higher with enzyme-treated cells than with untreated cells; by contrast, with IgM antibodies the increase was only about fourfold (Aho and Christian 1966).

Effect of polymers. Red cells suspended in various water-soluble polymers, for example serum albumin, gelatin, dextran, polyvinylpyrrolidone (PVP), are agglutinated by IgG antibodies but the way in which this effect is produced is uncertain. Pollack (1965) proposed that these polymers act by decreasing zeta potential but some of the polymers, for example dextran, actually increase zeta potential (Brooks and Seaman 1973). Although albumin does increase the dielectric constant of water (thus diminishing zeta potential), its effect seems to be too small to account for the enhancement of agglutination observed (van Oss *et al.* 1978, citing Oncley 1942). There is evidence that dextran and PVP potentiate agglutination by polymer bridging (Hummel 1962; Brooks 1973). Positively charged molecules such as polybrene potentiate agglutination by forming bridges, by virtue of their interaction with the negatively charged red cell surface.

Osmotic effects. Macromolecules, by increasing extracellular colloid osmotic pressure, even though to a much lower level than that prevailing within the red cells, may exert an influence on the shape of red cells and thus facilitate a closer approach between the surface of different cells (van Oss *et al.* 1978).

Effect of serum and plasma. A mixture of human plasma (or serum) and concentrated bovine albumin is superior to albumin alone as a medium for the agglutination of Rh D-positive red cells by 'incomplete' anti-D. Plasma greatly enhances the agglutination of A (and B) red cells by IgG anti-A (and -B). The enhancing effect of serum is negligible, suggesting that fibrinogen is responsible for the enhancing effect of plasma (Romano and Mollison 1975).

Red cell spiculation. Another factor that may be important in bringing about agglutination is the formation of red cell spicules, which undergo much less repulsion than smooth surfaces (van Oss *et al.* 1978). Spicules are induced by anti-A although not by anti-D (Salsbury and Clarke 1967). Furthermore, red cells exposed to 10% dextran (molecular weight 40 kDa) and red cells treated with a proteolytic enzyme exhibit spiculation (van Oss *et al.* 1978).

Elution of blood group antibodies from red cells

Bonds due to ionic (electrostatic) forces are expected to be dissociated at either low or high pH (Hughes-Jones *et al.* 1963b). The van der Waals' attraction between antigen and antibody can be turned into a repulsion by lowering the surface tension of the liquid medium to a value intermediate between the surface tension of the antibody-combining site and of the antigenic determinant (van Oss *et al.* 1979). Some red cell antibodies can be completely eluted from red cells by using a suitable medium in which surface tension is lowered and pH raised (van Oss *et al.* 1981).

Antibodies can also be eluted from red cells by heat (Landsteiner and Miller 1925) partly because the reaction between antigen and antibody is in general exothermic (and heat elution is therefore most successful with cold antibodies) and partly because heating denatures some antigens, for example D (NC Hughes-Jones, personal communication). However, the methods that are most widely used involve the use of organic solvents. It has been suggested that these compounds produce their effects by lowering surface tension (van Oss *et al.* 1981).

Effect of antibodies on red cells

There is a good deal of evidence to suggest that red cell antibodies do not cause any direct damage to red cells. In theory, the attachment of antibody molecules to the red cell surface might possibly interfere with the passage of substances across the red cell membrane or might alter red cell metabolism by stimulating or inhibiting enzymes situated at or near the cell surface: compare with the effect of the L antigen–antibody on potassium transport in sheep red cells (Ellory and Tucker 1969). However, so far as human red cells are concerned, there is little evidence in favour of any of these possibilities. Coating of red cells with anti-A, -B or -Rh D has no effect on dextrose consumption or on cation flux (Jandl 1965).

Red cell alloantibodies bring about red cell destruction either by activating complement to the C8/9 stage, leading to lysis, or by mediating interactions with macrophages and other phagocytic cells by which the red cell is engulfed or lysed.

Interactions of antibody-coated red cells with monocytes, other phagocytic cells and lymphocytes

Antibody-coated red cells become attached to macrophages and various other cells by an interaction between a site on the Fc fragment of either IgG1 or IgG3 molecules and an Fc receptor on the phagocytic or cytotoxic cell. The Fc receptor binding site on IgG1 and IgG3 is in the CH2 domain, near the hinge region (Radaev et al. 2001: see Plate 3.3 shown in colour between pages 528 and 529). The carbohydrate attached to As297 fills the cavity between the CH2 domains of the Fc. Removal of the carbohydrate results in a 15- to 20-fold reduction in binding of the Fc receptor to IgG1 (Radaev and Sun 2001).

As described earlier, three Fc receptors for IgG have been identified, all belonging to the immunoglobulin superfamily. FcR I(CD64) is found on monocytes and macrophages and is inducable on neutrophils and eosinophils. It has the highest affinity for IgG of all Fcγ receptors ($kd = 10^{-8}M$) and is the only Fc receptor with high affinity for monomeric IgG. It occurs in several isoforms (1a, b1, b2, c) and contains three Ig family domains. FcR II(CD32) has two Ig family domains, is found on monocytes, macrophages, neutrophils, B lymphocytes and platelets and has at least six isoforms (a1, a2, b1–b3, c). FcγRIIa and FcRγIIb have major functional differences. FcγRIIa has an immunoreceptor tyrosine-based activation motif (ITAM) in its cytoplasmic domain whereas FcγRIIb has an inhibitory motif (ITIM) in the cytoplasmic domain. There are two allotypes of FcγRIIa, high responder (HR) and low responder (LR), differing by a single amino acid, Arg131His. FcR III(CD16) also has two Ig superfamily domains. It has the lowest affinity for IgG of all the receptors and is found on macrophages, neutrophils and K lymphocytes, although not on resting monocytes (Anderson 1989). There are two forms of FcγIII (a and b). FcγRIIIa is found on T lymphocytes and natural killer (NK) cells, whereas FcγRIIIb is found on neutrophils where it expresses antigens of the HNA system (see Chapter 13). Unlike the other Fcγ receptors, FcγRIIIb does not have a cytoplasmic domain but is inserted in the plasma membrane by a glycosylphosphoinositol (GPI) tail (reviewed by Sondermann and Oosthuizen 2001).

In vitro, red cells sensitized with IgG anti-D (EA-IgG anti-D) adhere to all three Fc receptors (Klaassen et al. 1990). Only adherence to FcR I leads to lysis of EA-IgG anti-D, and adherence to this receptor is therefore probably also essential for cytotoxic lysis of IgG-sensitized cells *in vivo* (Klaassen et al. 1990; Levy et al. 1990).

Binding of antibody to the extracellular domain of Fc receptors causes a transmembrane signal resulting in phosphorylation of ITAM motifs by Src-family kinases, either on the cytoplasmic domain of the Fc receptor itself (FcγRIIa) or on associated proteins in the cases of FcγRI and FcγRIIIa. Syk kinase is recruited to the phosphorylated ITAM and becomes activated and starts a signalling cascade that may result in phagocytosis or cell-mediated killing. A key step in phagocytosis is recruitment of numerous cytoskeletal proteins and the formation of new actin filaments creating an actin network that pushes the plasma membrane of the phagocytic cell around the material to be ingested. Fusion of the plasma membrane around the material to be ingested requires remodelling of actin filaments and requires the phosphoinositide 3-kinase (PI3-K, reviewed by May and Machesky 2001).

When antigen/antibody complexes bind to the FcγRIIb receptor and co-ligate the B-cell receptor (see Plate 3.6), inhibitory signals are generated that switch off antibody production by B cells. The importance of this inhibitory cycle is clear from studies of FcγRIIb knockout mice. These mice develop autoimmune disease (Bolland and Ravetch 2000).

Binding and rosetting. Many IgG-coated red cells may become attached to the same effector cell, giving rise to the appearance of rosetting. Fewer IgG3 than IgG1 molecules bound per red cell are required to bring about attachment to effector cells. Using monoclonal anti-D, estimates for the minimum number for attachment to monocytes have ranged from 100 to 600 for IgG3, and from 2000 to 10 000 for IgG1 (Wiener et al. 1987; Merry et al. 1988, 1989). Similar results have been observed with polyclonal anti-D (Zupańska et al. 1986). The rather wide range of results is due presumably to many factors such as: heterogeneity in monocyte activity; heterogeneity of antibodies, as both IgG1 and IgG3 antibodies produced by different clones or different individuals differ in their capacity to adhere to Fc receptors (Armstrong et al. 1987; Engelfriet and Ouwehand 1990); variability of methods of scoring red cell–monocyte interaction; and a lack of standardization of methods, for example for quantifying the

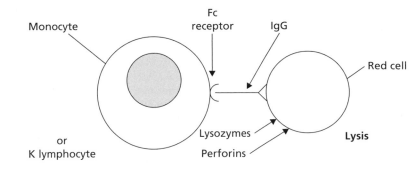

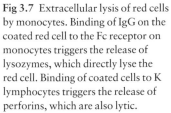

Fig 3.7 Extracellular lysis of red cells by monocytes. Binding of IgG on the coated red cell to the Fc receptor on monocytes triggers the release of lysozymes, which directly lyse the red cell. Binding of coated cells to K lymphocytes triggers the release of perforins, which are also lytic.

numbers of bound antibody molecules. Not only are fewer IgG3 than IgG1 molecules required for adherence to monocytes, but also the rate of interaction between IgG-coated red cells and monocytes is more rapid with IgG3 than with IgG1 (Brojer *et al.* 1989). It has been suggested that the more potent activity of IgG3 compared with IgG1 is due to the relatively long hinge on the IgG3 molecule, leading to the greater accessibility to the Fc-receptor binding site (Woof *et al.* 1986; Wiener *et al.* 1987) which, as stated above, is near the hinge on the Cγ2 domain of IgG.

Phagocytosis and lysis. Using polyclonal anti-D, a phagocytosis assay with monocytes was found to be no more sensitive than a rosette assay, the minimum numbers of IgG molecules per red cell for a positive result being 150–640 for IgG3 and 1230–4020 for IgG1 (Zupańska *et al.* 1986). In several other investigations, using both polyclonal and monoclonal anti-D, IgG3 antibodies have been found to be more active than IgG1 (Douglas *et al.* 1985; Hadley *et al.* 1989; Kumpel *et al.* 1989b), although in one study all of seven examples of IgG1 were more effective than seven examples of IgG3 in mediating phagocytosis (Wiener *et al.* 1988). The cause of these discrepancies is not clear but it may lie in variations in assay conditions. For example, in one investigation, at low ratios of red cells to monocytes, IgG3 was more active and, at high ratios, IgG1 was more active (Hadley and Kumpel 1989). When measuring phagocytosis, as opposed to adherence, the use of 5% CO_2 appears to be important to maintain pH at an approximately physiological level; if 5% CO_2 is not used the activity of weak antibodies may be overlooked (Branch and Gallagher 1985).

After attachment to monocytes, the red cells may be engulfed or may be lysed external to the monocyte membrane by lysosomal enzymes excreted by the monocyte (Fleer *et al.* 1978; see Fig. 3.7). The factors that determine whether the cell is engulfed or lysed are uncertain, although there is evidence that lysis is associated with relatively high concentrations of cell-bound antibody (Engelfriet *et al.* 1981). Presumably, the ratio of effector cells to red cells must be another important factor. IgG subclass and the ability to bind complement are also involved (see below). In animals, intense erythrophagocytosis is found in splenic macrophages after giving heteroimmune sera (Levaditi 1902; Dudgeon *et al.* 1909) or after transfusing incompatible red cells to an animal that has developed a corresponding alloantibody (Swisher and Young 1954). In these particular cases the antibodies were complement activating. Although red cells coated with IgG alone are also engulfed mainly by macrophages they may be engulfed by phagocytic cells other than monocytes and macrophages, for example granulocytes. Furthermore, following attachment to K lymphocytes, the red cell may be lysed by perforins excreted by the lymphocytes (Fig. 3.7), although this interaction has been studied only *in vitro*.

Erythrophagocytosis in peripheral blood. Although tissue macrophages are the chief sites of engulfment of antibody-coated incompatible red cells, erythrophagocytosis by neutrophils may sometimes be observed in samples of peripheral blood following ABO-incompatible transfusions (see Chapter 10). Erythrophagocytosis is also seen occasionally in blood films of patients with severe AIHA, cold haemagglutinin disease (CHAD) and paroxysmal cold haemoglobinuria (PCH) (see Dacie 1992, p. 400).

Role of complement. Complement-coated red cells become attached to a variety of cells through various complement receptors (CR). CR1 is expressed on red cells (see Plate 3.2b) and is also present on many other cells, including neutrophils and monocytes. CR1 binds C3b and C4b and binds weakly to iC3b. Other functions of CR1 are discussed in a later section. It is postulated that CR1 sites, with C3b molecules attached, undergo proteolytic digestion during contact with macrophages in the liver and spleen. In cold haemagglutinin disease there are only 50–200 CR1 receptors per red cell compared with the normal number of 400–1200 per cell (Ross *et al.* 1985).

CR2 is a type I transmembrane protein with an extracellular domain of 15 or 16 SCR domains, a single transmembrane domain and a short cytoplasmic domain. It is found on B lymphocytes, on which it binds mainly to C3dg and its function is to augment the antibody response to foreign antigen (see Plate 3.5); it presumably plays no significant role in red cell destruction. The structure of the first two SCRs of CR2 in complex with C3d has been determined and demonstrates that the primary site for interaction with C3d is on SCR2 (Hannan *et al.* 2001).

CR3, the beta2 integrin complement receptor 3 (CD11b/CD18), is found on neutrophils, monocytes and large granular lymphocytes, and binds primarily to iC3b. A closely related receptor, CR4, binds both iC3b and, with a much lower affinity, C3dg, and is the predominant type of C3 receptor expressed on tissue macrophages (see review by Ross 1989).

C3b and iC3b play the most active role (in collaboration with Ig) in bringing about erythrophagocytosis. C3dg is a poor opsonizer, acting only through CR4. In cold haemagglutinin disease, red cells coated with as many as 20 000 C3dg molecules per cell are present in the circulation without being cleared by the mononuclear phagocyte system (MPS) (Ross 1986).

The role of complement in erythrophagocytosis seems to be primarily to bring about attachment of red cells to macrophages. Red cells coated with C3b alone normally undergo little or no phagocytosis although they may be ingested by activated macrophages (see discussion in Chapter 10).

Red cells incubated with IgM alone bind to monocytes only if complement is present (Huber *et al.* 1968). Red cells coated with approximately 80 000 molecules of C3 per cell without Ig form abundant rosettes with monocytes but are not lysed (Kurlander *et al.* 1978).

There is a synergistic action between IgG and C3b (iC3b), and phagocytosis is enormously enhanced when both are attached to red cells (Ehlenberger and Nussenzweig 1977). Each pair of bound IgG molecules may bring about the binding of many C3b molecules. *In vivo*, the amount of bound IgG needed to produce a given rate of clearance is very much less if C3b is also bound (see Chapter 10). Most of the foregoing interactions have been used as the basis for cellular bioassays to assess the clinical significance of red cell alloantibodies.

Cellular bioassays

In trying to forecast the ability of any particular antibody to cause red cell destruction *in vivo*, measurements of antibody characteristics such as concentration have obvious limitations. Assays that involve interactions between antibody-coated red cells and effector cells, such as macrophages, may have far better predictive value.

In vivo, the main effector cells in the destruction of antibody-coated red cells are splenic and hepatic macrophages. In one assay at least (the MMA) peripheral monocytes have been shown to be as effective as splenic macrophages (Zupańska *et al.* 1995). Apart from the peripheral monocytes, cells used in assays include a cultured malignant cell line, for example 'U937' (Kumpel *et al.* 1989b), macrophages derived by culturing monocytes (Armstrong *et al.* 1987) or these cultured macrophages stimulated with γ-interferon to increase the number of IgG Fc receptors expressed on the phagocyte membrane (Wiener and Garner 1987; Wiener *et al.* 1987). There are substantial differences in activity between the monocytes of different subjects (Munn and Chaplin 1977; Douglas *et al.* 1985) and tremendous increases in phagocytic activity are noted in acute viral infections (Munn and Chaplin 1977). In practice, standardization can be achieved by using a pool of monocytes, for example derived by elutriation of mononuclear cells obtained from between 30 and 100 blood donations, each of 450 ml (for a method, see Garner *et al.* 1994). The monocytes can be mixed with dimethyl sulphoxide and stored in ampoules in the frozen state (Engelfriet and Ouwehand 1990). In two circumstances, the use of a pool is inappropriate: first, when using a bioassay to predict whether serologically incompatible red cells will be destroyed if transfused to a recipient whose serum contains an antibody of doubtful significance: in such a case, the recipient's own monocytes should be used in the assay; and second, when testing for the presence of Fc-receptor-blocking antibodies in a mother's serum, when the father's monocytes should be used.

In bioassays the method is to incubate red cells with antibody and, if appropriate, with complement, to wash the red cells, and then add them to the chosen effector cells. The degree of interaction between sensitized red cells and effector cells is taken as a measure of the ability of the antibody to cause red cell destruction *in vivo*.

Rosetting and phagocytosis

Many different assays for antibody activity, based on the ability to mediate rosetting and/or phagocytosis by monocytes or macrophages, have been devised. This type of test is often referred to as a monocyte–monolayer assay (MMA). Both adherence and phagocytosis may be measured. There are substantial differences between different laboratories in the way in which the test is done: monocytes may be taken from a single donor or from a pool; they may be fresh or stored; they may or may not be contaminated with lymphocytes; the tests may be read as the proportion of monocytes exhibiting rosetting or as the number of red cells engulfed per monocyte; or both adherence and engulfment may be measured and the result expressed as the total association index (TAI); and the laboratory may or may not use positive and negative controls.

Not surprisingly, different degrees of success have been reported in using MMA-type assays for predicting the severity of HDN and the clinical significance of particular red cell antibodies (see Chapters 10 and 12).

Antibody-dependent cell-mediated cytotoxicity assays

Antibody-dependent cell-mediated cytotoxicity (ADCC) assays are carried out either with monocytes or macrophages (ADCC(M) assay) or with K lymphocytes (ADCC(L) assay).

ADCC(M) assay. Human monocytes will lyse antiD-coated red cells *in vitro* (Kurlander *et al.* 1978). Lysis is brought about by the release of lysosomal enzymes (Fleer *et al.* 1978). An assay that has proved valuable in predicting the severity of Rh D haemolytic disease has been devised in which red cells are labelled with

^{51}Cr, coated with antibody, washed and then incubated with pooled monocytes. Lysis is measured by estimating the ^{51}Cr released into the supernatant compared with a standard (Engelfriet and Ouwehand 1990).

Red cells coated with IgG1 autoantibodies are lysed only when the number of antibody molecules bound per cell is well above the number needed to give a positive direct antiglobulin test (DAT); on the other hand, cells coated with a number of IgG3 molecules too small to give a positive DAT may be lysed in an ADCC(M) assay (Engelfriet *et al.* 1981). Similarly, using monoclonal anti-D, IgG3 has been shown to be more effective than IgG1 in mediating lysis (Wiener *et al.* 1988). In testing five IgG1 and five IgG3 monoclonal anti-D, there was some overlap in the results but, on average, IgG3 was twice as effective as IgG1 (WH Ouwehand and CP Engelfriet, unpublished observations).

ADCC(L) assay. Lymphocytes are capable of lysing antibody-coated red cells by producing 'perforins', substances similar to the terminal components of complement, which produce holes in the red cell membrane (Podack and Konigsberg 1984).

The ADCC(L) assay differs from the ADCC(M) assay not only in the use of different effector cells but also in using enzyme-treated target cells. After the latter have been prepared, they are either incubated with serum and lymphocytes together (Urbaniak 1979a, b) or the enzyme-treated red cells are first sensitized with antibody and then incubated with lymphocytes.

Results of the ADCC(L) test carried out on the serum of Rh D-immunized mothers are quite well correlated with the severity of haemolytic disease in the fetus (see Chapter 12). Only a minority of monoclonal IgG1 antibodies mediate lysis in the ADCC(L) assay (Armstrong *et al.* 1987; Kumpel *et al.* 1989a, b); three of three monoclonal IgG3 anti-D were ineffective (Kumpel *et al.* 1989a) as have been all polyclonal IgG3 anti-Ds tested so far; on the other hand, one monoclonal IgG3 anti-c mediated lysis (Second International Workshop on Red Cell Monoclonal Antibodies 1990).

Chemiluminescence assay

This assay measures the oxidative 'burst' that accompanies phagocytosis (Descamps-Latscha *et al.* 1983). Mononuclear cells are incubated at 37°C with presensitized red cells and luminol, and the chemiluminescence response is monitored for 1 h (Hadley *et al.* 1988). The results of chemiluminescence assays, carried out on the serum of Rh D-immunized mothers, have been found to be approximately as well correlated with the severity of haemolytic disease in the fetus as have the results of ADCC(M) assays; see Chapter 12.

The results of chemiluminescence assays have provided the only evidence so far of synergism between IgG1 and IgG3 antibodies. Using several examples of monoclonal anti-D, the metabolic response of monocytes was greater towards IgG3-coated cells than towards IgG1-coated cells, but was greater still towards cells coated with both subclasses (Hadley and Kumpel 1989). No evidence of synergism has been found in adherence, phagocytic or ADCC assays.

Role of complement in cellular bioassays

Some red cell alloantibodies react in bioassays only if complement is present. In tests with a phagocytosis assay, the number of examples of anti-Fy[a] and anti-Jk[a] that gave positive results was about 30% greater if complement was present in the sensitization phase (Branch *et al.* 1984). In detecting anti-Le[a] in the presence of complement, a mononuclear phagocyte assay, using cultured macrophages, was as sensitive as the antiglobulin test (Wiener and Garner 1985). Two examples of anti-Lan which had been associated with rapid destruction of ^{51}Cr-labelled incompatible red cells *in vivo* (Nance *et al.* 1987) and several other antibodies, including examples of anti-Jk[a], -Jk[b] and -Vel, gave positive results in a bioassay only if complement was present (Nance *et al.* 1988). Evidently, except when dealing with non-complement activating antibodies such as anti-Rh D, it is essential to allow complement fixation to occur in the sensitization phase of bioassays.

Comparison of different assays

ADCC assays, with the chemiluminescence assay, have the advantage that they rely on objective measurement rather than, as with tests for rosetting and phagocytosis, on visual inspection. Nevertheless, these tests have not so far been well standardized. The choice of effector cells varies between those from single donors or from pools, the cells may be fresh or stored and may be monocytes or lymphocytes. There is variation in the use of antibodies as controls and in methods of inter-

preting results. Although valid comparisons between results obtained in different laboratories are not always possible, an attempt to compare different tests in the same laboratory is described in Chapter 12. An explanation for the superiority of the ADCC(M) tests over the MMA in predicting the severity of HDN is also described there.

Complement

Complement is the name given to a system of approximately 25 soluble proteins and 10 cell surface receptors and regulatory proteins that, in response to a stimulus, interact to opsonize and clear or kill invading microorganisms or altered (e.g. apoptopic) host cells (reviewed by Sim and Tsiftsoglou (2004). Soluble complement proteins make up about 5% of the total protein content of human plasma. There are three overlapping pathways whereby the complement system can recognizes its targets. These pathways are called the classical pathway, the lectin or mannose-binding pathway and the alternative pathway (Fig. 3.8).

The products of complement activation have potent biological effects. Apart from cell destruction either directly, through activation of the whole complement cascade with the formation of the membrane attack complex (MAC), or indirectly, through a product, C3b, which mediates attachment of coated cells to effector cells, for example phagocytes, they also promote inflammation through chemotaxis and increased vascular permeability.

Activation of the classical pathway

The components involved in the activation of the classical pathway are C1, the recognition unit (a complex composed of C1q, C1r and C1s), the activation unit comprising C2, C3 and C4 and the membrane attack complex (C5, C6, C7, C8, C9). All of these components are present in plasma in their native unactivated configuration; the concentrations of most components are low with C3 and C4 being most abundant.

Immunoglobulin requirements for activation of the classical pathway

The commonest mode of activation of the classical pathway is through the binding of C1q to the C_H2

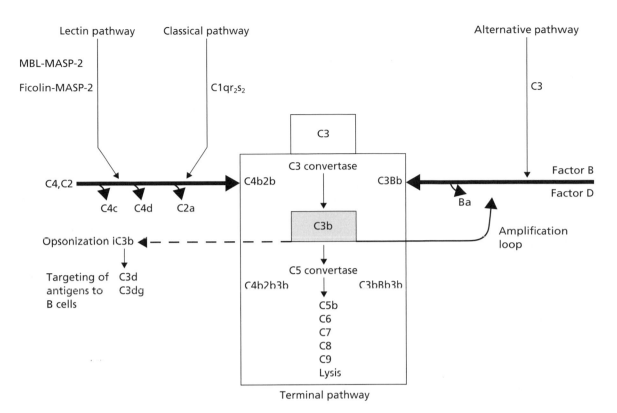

Fig 3.8 The complement system. Modified from Sim and Tsiftsoglou (2004).

domain of IgM or to the C_H2 domain of some IgG1 or IgG3 antibodies. The C1q molecule has six Fc binding sites and, in order to make a firm bond with the Ig complex, at least two of these sites must bind to Ig. In the case of IgG, two antibody molecules must be present on the antigen surface within about 20–30 nm of one another, this being the maximum span of a C1q molecule. In the case of IgM, the mechanism is different; when the molecule is in its planar or 'star' form, (with the F(ab')$_2$ pieces and the (Fc)$_5$ disc in the same plane), there is only a single binding site for C1q on each side of the (Fc)$_5$ disc and C1q cannot bind firmly. However, when combined with antigen, the IgM molecule frequently assumes a staple form with the F(ab')$_2$ at right angles to the (Fc)$_5$ disc (Feinstein et al. 1971; see Fig. 3.4). The distortion produced by this movement exposes additional C1q binding sites (Perkins et al. 1991) and a C1q molecule can thus bind to two sites on a single IgM molecule. IgM is thus considerably more efficient than IgG as an activator of C1 and the binding of a single IgM molecule to an SRBC can lead to lysis; in contrast, assuming that the red cell has 600 000 antibody binding sites, about 800 IgG molecules must be bound to provide an even chance that two will occupy closely adjacent sites and thus activate complement (Humphrey and Dourmashkin 1965). If two IgG antibodies bind to different epitopes on the same antigen, complement activation is greatly enhanced (Hughes-Jones et al. 1984).

When bound to cells, the various subclasses of IgG vary widely in their ability to bind complement: IgG3 molecules are highly active, IgG1 moderately, IgG2 slightly and IgG4 not at all. The amino acid residues Asp270, Lys322, Pro329 and Pro331 in the C_H2 domain of human IgG1 have been identified as a key binding motif for C1q (Idusogie et al. 2000). The reasons for the selective binding of complement to different IgG subclasses are not known. However, a three-dimensional model of the C1q globular domain complexed with human IgG1 indicates that binding of C1q to the critical residues in the C_H2 domain brings it into close proximity with the Fab region of the antibody molecule suggesting that the position of the Fab relative to the C1q binding site in different IgG subclasses is critical for C1q binding (Plate 3.4, shown in colour between pages 528 and 529); Gaboriaud *et al.* 2003). If this is so, the length of the hinge regions in the different IgG subclasses may be critical for C1q binding and the failure of IgG4 to bind complement explained by the short hinge region giving a rigid structure with the Fab obscuring access to the C1q binding site.

The observation that, with certain antibodies, the extent of C1q binding is not correlated with the extent of complement activity (Tao *et al.* 1993) is similar to the earlier observation that anti-Rh D can bind C1q but that C1r and C1s are not cleaved so that complement is not activated (Hughes-Jones and Ghosh 1981; see Chapter 5).

C1: The recognition unit

Complement activation occurs through binding of the recognition protein C1q to the Fc domain of IgG or IgM complexed with antigen. C1q is a large structurally complex glycoprotein of 410 kDa, present in human serum at a concentration of 70 µg/ml. C1q is often described as having a shape like a bunch of six tulips. The 'flowers' comprise three globular domains and the 'stems' are collagen triple helices (Plate 3.4, Gaboriaud *et al.* 2002). The globular domains of C1q bind relatively weakly to charged clusters on the target (on antibodies and other surfaces such as bacteria, viruses). At least two of the globular heads of C1q must be bound to the Fc of antibody for C1 activation.

The 'stems' have two C1r and two C1s molecules associated with them ($C1r_2C1s_2$). C1r and C1s are serine proteases present in unactivated C1 in the proenzyme form. The composition of C1 is thus $C1qC1r_2C1s_2$. When the globular heads of C1q bind a target surface it causes movement of the collagen 'stems', which results in autoactivation of C1r which then cleaves and activates C1s. Isolated C1 in solution slowly autoactivates, but this does not take place in the plasma owing to the presence of an inhibitory protein, C1 inhibitor (see below).

Inhibitor of C1 in serum. Serum normally contains an inhibitor of C1, C1-Inh, which has two functions: (1) it inhibits the autoactivation of native C1 in solution in the plasma by binding weakly to the C1r subcomponent of $C1r_2C1s_2$ tetramer; and (2) it inhibits activated C1r and C1s molecules.

The activation unit: formation of the C3/C5 convertase (C4b2b) and the splitting of C3

A note on discrepancies in terminology. When C3, C4 and C5 are activated, small fragments, designated C3a, C4a and C5a, are split off, leaving larger fragments, C3b, C4b and C5b. When C2 is activated, a smaller and a larger fragment are produced but at present are generally termed C2b and C2a respectively. In order to harmonize the terminology, it was proposed in 1983 that in future C2a should be used for the small fragment of C2, and C2b for the larger. Although only a few authors (e.g. Roitt *et al.* 1993; Wolpert and Lachmann 1993) have adopted the new terminology, the use of the term C2b for the larger of the two products of C2 is a very desirable change and is adopted here.

The C3/5 convertase is a bimolecular complex composed of one molecule each of activated C4 and C2. The activation of one C1 complex can generate more than 100 C3/C5 convertases attached to the cell membrane. The C4 molecule is a structural protein that has the dual function of binding to the foreign particle or to the cell surface and to C2, the molecule that carries the active enzyme site. C4 is first split by C1s into the anaphylatoxins C4a, and C4b. The splitting results in the appearance of an active but highly labile thioester bond on C4b, which enables it to bind covalently with both -OH and $-NH_2$ groups on the Fc region of Ig in the Ag/Ab complex or to the membrane of the cell itself (red cell, microbe, etc.). In the presence of Mg^{2+}, C2 then becomes attached to the bound C4b and in turn is cleaved by C1s into C2a and C2b. This cleavage results in the appearance of an active site on the C2 molecule; it is this enzyme site (on C2b) that cleaves and activates C3; see review by Hughes-Jones (1986). The C3 convertase, C4b2b, is broken down either by a C4 binding protein (C4bp) or by CR1, the cell membrane receptor for C3b, in the presence of factor I.

A small polypeptide (C3a, another anaphylatoxin) is split from the C3 molecule by C4b2b to give C3b. One molecule of C4b2b can generate hundreds of C3b molecules, thus amplifying the cascade even further. C3b carries an active site (identical to that found on C4b) that is highly labile, with a lifespan of approximately 60 µs, during which time it can diffuse

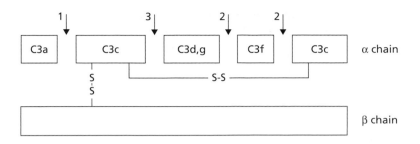

Fig 3.9 Steps in the degradation of C3. Native C3 is cleaved at site 1 on the α chain by C4b2b; a small fragment C3a is split off, leaving the $α^1$ chain of C3b, comprising C3d,g, C3f and the two moieties of C3c. The $α^1$ chain of C3b is cleaved at two closely adjacent points (site 2) by the C3b inactivator, factor I, using factor H as co-factor; a fragment, C3f, is removed, yielding iC3b (C3d,g and the two α chain-derived moieties of C3c). *In vitro*, this process takes about 1 min (Harrison and Lachmann 1980). iC3b is further cleaved by factor I at site 3; C3c, consisting of the two remaining parts of the α chain, still attached by disulphide bonds to one another and to the uncleaved β chain, is liberated, leaving C3d,g bound to the cell surface. On human red cells, carrying CR1, which acts as a co-factor for this reaction, the half-time of the cleavage is about 8 min (Medicus *et al.* 1983).

approximately 40 nm (Sim *et al.* 1981). C3b is deposited in clusters on the cell membrane around C4b2b to form the C5 splitting enzyme, C4b2b3b. Activation of complement by blood group antibodies frequently stops at this stage; only C3b can bind to C5 and C3b is very rapidly converted to iC3b (see below). Thus, unless large amounts of C3b are generated, no significant amounts are available for combination with C5, and activation of complement cannot proceed to cell lysis. C3b on the cell surface mediates adherence to phagocytic cells through CR1 (see below). The role of C3 in phagocytosis is discussed in Chapter 10.

Another factor regulating the activation of C3 is decay accelerating factor (DAF). DAF is a glycoprotein that dissociates C2b from C4b2b and Bb from C3bBb, thus preventing the formation of C3 convertases of the classical and alternative pathways (Fujita *et al.* 1987). The absence of DAF on the red cells of patients with paroxysmal nocturnal haemoglobulinuria (PNH) probably accounts, in part, for the increased binding of C3 on PNH red cells (Nicholson-Weller *et al.* 1983). For further references, see Rosse (1986 and 1989).

The degradation of C3b on the red cell membrane is described in the legend of Fig. 3.9.

Binding of C3 by bystander cells

If normal red cells in a small volume are stirred with purified C3 and trypsin is added, C3 is cleaved and a small number of C3b molecules are bound to the cells.

Similarly, if group O cells are mixed with group A_1 cells, anti-A lysin and complement, some C3 (mainly C3d) molecules can be detected on them (Salama and Mueller-Eckhardt 1985). In the foregoing circumstances, complement is very vigorously activated. It is uncertain whether the milder activation which occurs in many haemolytic transfusion reactions can account for the occasional presence of C3d on autologous red cells.

The membrane attack complex

When C3b is generated rapidly enough and in sufficient quantity, it combines with C4b2b to split C5 into an active molecule C5b and the potent anaphylatoxin C5a. This is the last of the enzymic steps; activated C5b on the membrane binds C6 and then C7, exposing hydrophobic groups on both C6 and C7 with the result that the trimolecular complex C5b67 (which appears on electron microscopy as a rod of length approximately 2530 nm) is inserted with almost 100% efficiency into the phospholipid membrane of the red cells. C8 then binds to C5b67 and is also partly inserted into the membrane with the result that a small pore is made. The presence of the C5–8 polymer then allows assembly of two or more molecules of the terminal component C9; in the fully developed polymer, up to 10–16 molecules of C9 coalesce to form a tubular structure, which has hydrophobic regions on the outer surface to allow membrane insertion and a hydrophilic region on the inner surface to allow water and solutes to pass freely in and out of the membrane (Podack 1986). Na^{2+} and H_2O get into the cell, with consequent swelling and lysis.

The lesions in the cell membrane produced by the MAC appear on electron microscopy as holes. With human complement and human red cells, the diameter of the holes is about 10 nm, irrespective of whether the antibody is anti-A, anti-I, biphasic haemolysin (anti-P) or rabbit anti-human red cell (Rosse et al. 1966).

In addition to the mechanisms described above, which accelerate the decay of C3 convertase and thus limit the formation of the MAC, there are mechanisms that inhibit the lytic potential of C5b67. C8 binding protein (C8bp) is an intrinsic membrane protein of molecular weight 65 kDa, which can bind C8 and thus inhibit the interaction of C5b67 with C8 and C9; C8bp, also known as homologous restriction factor (HRF), does not accelerate the decay of C3/5 convertases. Thus, C8bp and DAF act synergistically to minimize the self-inflicted damage by complement (Schonermark et al. 1986). Another protein, of molecular weight 18 kDa, membrane inhibitor of reactive lysis (MIRL, syn. CD59), also restricts the assembly of the MAC. DAF, C8bp and MIRL are members of a family of cell-surface molecules that is anchored to the red cell membrane via glycoinositol phospholipid (GPI) moieties rather than by membrane-spanning peptide sequences. It is the lack of this GPI anchor in PNH red cells that makes them so susceptible to complement-mediated lysis.

Reactive lysis

During the formation of the MAC complex, some C5b6 may be released into plasma from surface-bound C3b and be responsible for bystander lysis, the lysis of cells that do not have C3b bound to their surface (Thompson and Rowe 1968; Götze and Mueller-Eberhard 1970; Walpert and Lachmann 1993).

As explained earlier, activation of complement to the C5 stage, followed by formation of the MAC complex and lysis, occurs only when complement is powerfully activated. Some antibodies such as anti-Le[a] and (some) anti-Jk[a] activate complement to the C3 stage but whereas anti-Le[a] commonly produces lysis, anti-Jk[a] only occasionally does so. Antibodies of certain other specificities, such as anti-K and -Fy[a], may or may not activate complement to the C3 stage; those examples that do activate complement are not lytic.

Biological activity of split fragments

The small peptides split from the native molecules during complement activation, C3a, C5a and to a lesser extent C4a, have important biological functions. They stimulate the respiratory burst associated with the production of oxygen radicals of phagocytic cells, especially neutrophils. These split molecules stimulate the degranulation of mast cells and basophils with liberation of histamine, other vasoactive substances and cytokines, leading to increased vascular permeability, increased smooth muscle contraction and release of lysosomal enzymes from neutrophils. In addition, C5a is a potent neutrophil chemotactic agent, capable of acting directly on endothelial cells of capillaries to induce vasodilatation and increased permeability.

Activation of the lectin pathway

In the lectin pathway (see Fig. 3.8) the recognition proteins are mannan-binding lectin (MBL) and ficolins. MBL has a similar structure to C1q but its globular 'flowers' are C-type lectin domains that bind to neutral sugars (mannose and N-acetyl glucosamine). MBL forms a complex with homologues of C1r and C1s known as MASP1 and MASP2, and MASP3 an alternatively spliced product of the *MASP1* gene (MASP = MBL-associated serine protease). MASP2 acts like C1s in activating complement by cleavage of C4 and C2. Three ficolins have been described (L, H and M); L and H filocins are found in serum. M ficolin is on the surface of circulating monocytes. Ficolins are also similar in structure to C1q. They have globular 'flower' fibrinogen-like domains and bind N-acetylglucosamine but not mannose (Sim and Tsiftsoglou 2004).

MBL binds to sugar structures on bacteria, viruses, fungi and parasites (Neth et al. 2000), as well as carbohydrate structures on polymeric IgA (Roos et al. 2001). It is generally thought that IgA cannot activate complement by the classical pathway. The binding of MBL to polymeric IgA is calcium dependent (Roos et al. 2001).

Activation of the alternative pathway

The alternative pathway (see Fig. 3.9) of C3 activation can respond to both charged and neutral sugar targets and so provides an alternative to both the classical and lectin pathways of complement activation. The pathway can be activated by antibody-dependent (IgG immune complexes) or antibody-independent mechanisms (endotoxins, membranes of microorganisms).

Six proteins are involved in the alternative pathway; of these, three are concerned with activation (factors D, B and C3), one with stabilization (properdin, P) and two with inhibition (the enzyme, C3b inactivator or factor I and its co-factor, H). The function of the alternative pathway is the formation of a C3/C5 convertase, represented as C3bBb, which is different from but analogous to, the classical and lectin pathway convertase, C4b2b.

C3b brings about the destruction of foreign cells (e.g. bacteria) much more efficiently than that of host cells. The difference is due mainly to the effect of C8 binding protein and MIRL, which react much more efficiently with host than with foreign C8 and C9 (see also below). Furthermore, whereas C3b is continuously degraded to iC3b by the joint action of factors H and I, bacteria activate and stabilize C3bBb to generate large amounts of C3b on their surface.

In plasma there is a continuous but slow activation of the thioester bond on C3 by hydrolysis to form C3i. This autoactivated molecule reacts with the serine protease factor B in the presence of Mg^{2+} to form the complex C3iB. Factor B in the C3iB complex is cleaved by factor D releasing Ba and generating C3iBb. Factor D is a serine protease always present in an active state at low concentrations (about 1 µg/ml). C3bBb is a C3/C5 convertase that cleaves more C3 molecules to form C3b and C3a. These unstable C3b molecules become attached to cell surfaces and, by combination with factor B and activation by factor D, themselves become C3/C5 convertases. These convertase molecules then generate more C3b and the density of C3/C5 convertase molecules on the surface increases exponentially as a result of self-replication and amplification. This process is enhanced by the action of properdin that combines with and stabilizes C3bBb. The end result is thus both the deposition of large amounts of C3b, which brings about phagocytosis, and the activation of C5, with subsequent formation of the MAC and eventual lysis. Due to the action of factor H, the self-replication process does not take place on non-activating surfaces, such as host cells. Factor H reacts with the same binding site on C3b as factor B and so, if factor H binds before factor B, C3bBb formation is inhibited. The cell surface proteins CR1, DAF (CD55)

and membrane co-factor protein (MCP) can also bind cell- bound C3b and thereby inhibit the amplification cycle (Sim and Tsiftsoglou 2004).

Factor I enzymatically cleaves C3b to the inactive form iC3b which is recognized by the complement receptors CR3 and CR4 on phagocytic cells; iC3b is then further degraded by proteolytic enzymes in plasma to C3d or C3dg. These fragments covalently linked to antigens following complement activation are recognized by the receptor CR2(CD21) on B lymphocytes. Antigen–C3 fragment complexes can co-ligate the B-cell receptor (BCR) and CR2. This interaction can greatly amplify BCR-mediated signalling events because of the association of CR2 with CD19 and CD81 in a B cell-specific signal transduction complex (Plate 3.5) and thereby influence the adaptive immune response to target antigen (Hannan *et al.* 2001).

Other aspects of complement

Presence of C3d and C4d on normal red cells

As discussed in Chapter 7, small amounts of C3d and C4d are found on normal red cells and larger amounts are found on the red cells in many disease states. As described above, C3 contains an internal thioester bond that undergoes slow spontaneous hydrolysis or activation by trace amounts of proteolytic enzymes. There is a similar internal thioester bond in C4 which, presumably, is also hydrolysed by H_2O (Law *et al.* 1980; Janatova and Tack 1981). The spontaneous generation of activated C3 and C4 in plasma provides a mechanism for the deposition of complement components on normal red cells. The X-ray crystal structures of C3d and C4Ad have been determined (Nagar *et al.* 1998; van den Elsen *et al.* 2002). C3d and C4Ad have essentially superimposable structures despite having only about 30% sequence identity. The structure is known as an alpha-alpha six-barrel fold. This structure is characterized by six parallel alpha helices forming the core of the barrel surrounded by another set of six parallel helices running anti-parallel with the core (Plate 3.6 shown in colour between pages 528 and 529). The thioester residues are located at one side of the structure (convex surface); polymorphic residues defining the Ch/Rg blood group antigens are located on the opposite (concave) surface (see Plate 3.6 and also Chapter 6).

Complement in the infant

As measured by its power to lyse antibody-coated SRBC, the serum of newborn infants has about one-half of the activity of adults (Ewald *et al.* 1961). Estimation of individual components shows that the levels of C1q, C4 and C3 are also about 50% of the adult level; the levels of C5 and C7 are about 70% of the adult level, but that of C9 is only about 20%. Expressed as a percentage of maternal values, the figures are a little lower because the levels of some complement components are higher in pregnant women than in other adults. Adult values of the various complement components are reached within 6–12 months of birth (see review by Adinolfi and Zenthon 1984).

Species differences in complement activity

The components of complement are so similar in different species that for many purposes they can be interchanged. On the other hand, there are some striking differences in activity, one example of which is that, in bringing about haemolysis, an animal's own complement is often much less effective than that of another species. For example, there are many human alloantibodies which produce little or no haemolysis when incubated *in vitro* with appropriate red cells and with human complement, but which are strongly lytic with rabbit complement (Mollison and Thomas 1959). Rabbit complement is used routinely in tissue typing using lymphocytotoxicity tests.

Does complement affect the binding of antibody to red cells?

Possible increase in binding. Evidence that activated C1 can increase the bond between antibody and antigen was provided by Rosse and co-workers (1968). Using a partially purified preparation of C1, containing no detectable C2 or C4, they showed that activated C1 increased the binding of certain examples of human anti-I; EDTA only partially prevented this effect, suggesting that C1q may play some part in the binding of antibody. The observations suggested that only those examples of anti-I with a relatively low binding constant were bound more strongly in the presence of complement, which perhaps explains why Evans and co-workers (1965), using a potent auto-anti-I, found that the rate of association and dissociation of the antibody was unaffected by the presence of complement.

Possible interference with binding. If adult red cells are coated with complement by exposure at 25°C to serum from a patient with cold haemagglutinin disease and are then warmed to 37°C to elute anti-I they are less well agglutinated than control cells by anti-I; there is evidence that the accumulation of complement (now known to be mainly C3dg) on red cells, following exposure to anti-I, interferes with the reactivity of the cells both with anti-I and with complement (Evans *et al.* 1967). Prozones observed when certain group sera are incubated with group A red cells appear to be due to the uptake of complement (Andersen 1936; Stratton 1963), which interferes non-specifically with agglutination (Voak 1972). The uptake of complement on to red cells, mediated by one alloantibody, for example anti-Jk^a, may interfere with agglutination produced by another, for instance anti-D, introducing the possibility of misidentification or even of transfusing incompatible red cells (Lown *et al.* 1984).

Anti-complementary activity

Anticoagulants. Ca^{2+} is essential for the integrity of C1 and is therefore needed for the activation of complement by the classical pathway. Mg^{2+} is required for the formation of the C3 convertases of both the classical and alternative pathways, i.e. C4b2b and C3bBb respectively. Accordingly, all chelators of Ca^{2+} and Mg^{2+} inhibit C activity; for example the addition of 2 mg of Na_2 EDTA to 1 ml of serum completely blocks the activation of complement.

Heparin is also anti-complementary – 2.5 IU of heparin per millilitre will completely inhibit the cleavage of C4 by C1 *in vitro* (Strunk and Colten 1976), although much higher concentrations are required to prevent the uptake of C4 and C3 by antibody-coated cells. For example, if Le(a+) red cells are strongly sensitized with EDTA-treated anti-Le^a serum and then washed, they will still take up complement components from heparinized serum until the amount of heparin exceeds 100 IU/ml (seventh edition, p. 263). Similarly, in lytic tests more than 100 IU/ml are required to reduce the CH_{50} to zero (DL Brown, personal communication).

Heating serum to 56°C for 30 min completely inactivates C1 and C2 but damages C4 to a lesser extent

(Bier *et al.* 1945; Heidelberger and Mayer 1948). Factor B of the alternative pathway is inactivated by being heated to 50°C for 20 min.

Anti-complementary properties developing *in vitro* are not well understood. Ehrlich and Sachs (1905), and Bordet (1909) interpreting the work of Gay (1905), suggested that complement might be partly damaged, for example by being heated, and that the altered type of complement ('complementoid') was capable of combining with sensitized cells without producing the usual cell lysis; and that, furthermore, complementoid could block the action of normal complement. On storage, serum regularly becomes anti-complementary. The uptake of altered complement from stored serum on to sensitized red cells can be prevented by EDTA; thus if sera containing antibody and 'complementoid' were treated with EDTA and then incubated with red cells, antibody alone was taken up and the sensitized cells, after being washed, would bind complement normally (Polley and Mollison 1961).

Complement activation by blood group antibodies

In this summarizing section, almost all references are omitted but they can be found in the following chapters in which the various blood group antibodies are described in more detail.

Haemolysis

Almost all antibodies that will lyse untreated red cells have specificities within the ABO, Lewis, P or Ii systems. Anti-A and anti-B (especially anti-A,B in group O serum) will lyse untreated A and B red cells, although when the antibody is weak a high ratio of serum to cells may be required. Anti-H occurring in O_h subjects is lytic. Some examples of anti-Le^a and a very few of anti-Le^b, rare examples of anti-P$_1$, all examples of anti-PP, P^k and anti-P, many of anti-Vel and potent examples of auto-anti-I and auto-anti-i will also lyse untreated red cells. Occasional examples of anti-Jk^a will lyse untreated red cells and an example of lytic anti-D has been described.

With enzyme-treated red cells, all the aforementioned antibodies produce more rapid and more extensive lysis than with untreated red cells. Moreover, many examples of antibodies of these specificities which produce no detectable lysis of untreated red cells will readily lyse enzyme-treated red cells; for instance, although only a few examples of anti-Jk^a will lyse untreated red cells, many will lyse enzyme-treated red cells.

A few antibodies that fail to lyse red cells with human complement are lytic if rabbit complement is used; examples of antibodies behaving in this way include potent anti-P1, some examples of anti-K and of -Fya, and possibly all examples of anti-Jka (Mollison and Thomas 1959).

Coating with complement components without lysis

As explained earlier, activation of complement to the C5 stage, followed by formation of the MAC complex and lysis, occurs only when complement is powerfully activated. Some antibodies such as anti-Le^a (invariably) and anti-Jk^a (often) activate complement as far as the C3 stage, as shown by positive reactions with anti-complement reagents, but are only sometimes lytic. With antibodies of certain other specificities, such as anti-K and Fy^a, only some examples activate complement and then only to the C3 stage. Many examples of anti-I and anti-i, and those rare examples of anti-A$_1$, anti-III and anti-P$_1$ which are active at 37°C, also activate complement.

References

Adinolfi M (1965) Some serological characteristics of the normal incomplete cold antibody. Immunology 9: 31

Adinolfi M, Zenthon J (1984) Complement in infant and maternal sera. Rev Perinatal Med 5: 61–94

Adinolfi M, Polley MJ, Hunter DA et al. (1962) Classification of blood-group antibodies as β_2M or gamma globulin. Immunology 5: 566

Adinolfi A, Mollison PL, Polley MJ et al. (1966) γA blood group antibodies. J Exp Med 123: 951

Agre P, Smith BL, Baumgarten R et al. (1994). Human red cell Aquaporin CHIP. II. Expression during normal fetal development and in a novel form of congenital dyserythropoietic anemia. J Clin Invest 94: 1050–1058

Aho K, Christian CL (1966) Studies of incomplete antibodies, 1. Effect of papain on red cells. Blood 27: 662

Aird I, Bentall HH (1953) A relationship between cancer of stomach and the ABO blood groups. BMJ i: 799

Aird I, Bentall HH, Mehigan JA et al. (1954) The blood groups in relation to peptic ulceration and carcinoma of colon, rectum, breast and bronchus. An association between the ABO groups and peptic ulceration. BMJ ii: 315

Alberts B, Johnson A, Lewis J *et al.* (2002) Molecular Biology of the Cell, 4th edn. New York: Garland Science

Allen FH, Warshaw AL (1962) Blood group sensitization. A comparison of antigens K1 (Kell) and c (hr'). Vox Sang 7: 222

Alloisio N, Texier P, Denoroy L *et al.* (1996) The cisternae decorating the red blood cell membrane in congenital dyserythropoietic anaemia (type II) originate from the endoplasmic reticulum. Blood 87: 4433–4439

Andersen T (1936) Uber die Ursache der Isohaemagglutinationshemmung in frischem, unverdünnten Seren. Klin Wschr 15: 152

Anderson CL (1989) Human IgG Fc receptors. Clin Immunol Immunopath 53: 563–571

André C, Lambert R, Bazin H *et al.* (1974) Interference of oral immunization with the intestinal absorption of heterologous albumin. Eur J Immunol 4: 701

André C, Heremans JF, Vaerman JP *et al.* (1975) A mechanism for the induction of immunological tolerance by antigen feeding: antigen–antibody complexes. J Exp Med 142: 1509

Andresen PH, Henningsen K (1951) The Lewis blood system and the X-system in 5 tables. Acta Haematol (Basel) 5: 123

Anstee DJ (1990) Blood group-active surface molecules of the human red blood cell. Vox Sang 58: 1–20

Anstee DJ (1993) Minor red cell surface proteins associated with red cell dysfunction. In: Red Cell Membrane and Red Cell Antigens. MJA Tanner, DJ Anstee (eds). Baillière's Clinical Haematology 6: 445–463

Anstee DJ (1995) Blood group antigens defined by the amino acid sequences of red cell surface proteins. Transfusion Med 5: 1–13

Archer GT, Cooke BR, Mitchell K *et al.* (1969) Hyperimmunisation des donneurs de sang pour la production des gamma-globulines anti-Rh(D). Rev Fr Transfus 12: 341

Armstrong SS, Weiner E, Garner SF *et al.* (1987) Heterogeneity of monoclonal anti-Rh(D): an investigation using ADCC and macrophage binding assays. Br J Haematol 66: 257–262

Astrup J, Kornstad L (1977) Presence of anti-c in the serum of 42 women giving birth to c positive babies: serological and clinical findings. Acta Obstet Gynecol Scand 56: 185

Atchley WA, Bhagavan NV, Masouredis SP (1964) Influence of ionic strength on the reaction between anti-D and D positive red cells. J Immunol 93: 701

Avreamas S (1992) Natural antibodies. In: Encyclopedia of Immunology, vol. 3. IM Roitt, PJ Delves (eds). London: Academic Press, 1134–1135

Bacon N, Patten E, Vincent J (1991) Primary immune response to blood group antigens in burned children. Immunohematology 7: 8–11

Barandun S, Büchler H, Hässig A (1956) Das Antikörpermangelsyndrom: agammalobulinämie. Schweiz Med Wschr 86: 33

Barr M, Glenny AT (1945) Some practical applications of immunological principles. J Hyg (Lond) 44: 135

Barr M, Llewellyn-Jones M (1953) Some factors influencing the response of animals to immunization with combined prophylactics. Br J Exp Pathol 34: 12

von Beckerath N, Koch W, Mehilli J *et al.* (2004) ABO locus O1 allele and risk of myocardial infarction. Blood Coagul Fibrinolysis 15: 61–67

Benacerraf B (1981) Role of MHC gene products in immune regulation. Science 212: 1229–1238

Berg SF, Mjaaland S, Fossum S (1994) Comparing macrophages and dendritic leucocytes as antigen-presenting cells for humoral responses *in vivo* by antigen targeting. Eur J Immunol 24: 1262–1268

Bianco T, Farmer BJ, Sage RE *et al.* (2001) Loss of red cell A,B and H antigens is frequent in myeloid malignancies. Blood 97: 3633–3639

Bier OG, Leyton G, Mayer MM *et al.* (1945) A comparison of human and guinea-pig complements and their component fractions. J Exp Med 81: 445

Bird GWG (1959) Haemagglutinins in seeds. Br Med Bull 15: 165

Bird GWG (1981) Lectins. Lab–Lore 9: 683–684

Bird GWG (1989) Lectins in immunohaematology. Transfusion Med Rev 3: 55–62

Bird GWG, Wingham J (1977) Erythrocyte autoantibody with unusual specificity. Vox Sang 32: 280

Bird GWG, Wingham J, Richardson SGN (1985) Myelofibrosis, autoimmune haemolytic anaemia and Tn-polyagglutinability. Haematologia 18: 99–103

Blumberg N, Peck K, Ross K *et al.* (1983) Immune response to chronic red blood cell transfusion. Vox Sang 44: 212–217

Blumberg N, Ross K, Avila E *et al.* (1984) Should chronic transfusions be matched for antigens other than ABO and Rh$_o$(D)? Vox Sang 47: 205–208

Bolland S, Ravetch JV (2000) Spontaneous autoimmune disease in Fc(gamma)RIIB-deficient mice results from strain-specific epistasis. Immunity 13: 277–285

Bony V, Gane P, Bailly P *et al.* (1999) Time-course expression of polypeptides carrying blood group antigens during human erythroid differentiation. Br J Haematol 107: 263–274.

Bordet J (1909) Studies in Immunity. London: Chapman & Hall, p. 512

Borén T, Falk P, Roth KA *et al.* (1993) Attachment of *Helicobacter pylori* to human gastric epithelium mediated by blood group antigens. Science 262: 1892–1895

Boyd WC (1963) The lectins: their present status. Vox Sang 8: 1

Boyd WC, Reguera RM (1949) Hemagglutinating substance for human cells in various plants. J Immunol 62: 333

Boylston AW, Gardner B, Anderson RL et al. (1980) Production of human IgM anti-D in tissue culture by EB virus transformed lymphocytes. Scand J Immunol 12: 355–358

Branch DR, Gallagher MT (1985) The importance of CO_2 in short-term monocyte-macrophage assays (Letter). Transfusion 25: 399

Branch DR, Petz LD (1982) A new reagent (ZZAP) having multiple applications in immunohematology. Am J Clin Pathol 78: 161–167

Branch DR, Gallagher MT, Mison AP et al. (1984) In vitro determinations of red cell alloantibody significance using an assay of monocyte-macrophage interaction with sensitized erythrocytes. Br J Haematol 56: 19–29

Brody NI, Walker JG, Siskind GW (1967) Studies on the control of antibody synthesis: interaction of antigenic competition and suppression of antibody formation by passive antibody on the immune response. J Exp Med 126: 81

Brojer E, Merry AH, Zupańska B (1989) Rate of interaction of IgG1 and IgG3 sensitized red cells with monocytes in the phagocytosis assay. Vox Sang 56: 101–103

Brooks DE (1973) The effect of neutral polymers on the electrokinetic potential of cells and other charged particles. IV. Electrostatic effects in dextran-mediated cellular interaction. J Colloid Interface Sci 43: 714

Brooks DE, Seaman GVF (1973) The effect of neutral polymers on the electrokinetic potential of cells and other charged particles. I. Models for the zeta potential increase. J Colloid Interface Sci 43: 670

Brown DA, London E (2000) Structure and function of sphingolipid- and cholesterol-rich membrane rafts. J Biol Chem 275: 17221–17224

Buckley RH, Dees SC, O'Fallon WM et al. (1968) Serum immunoglobulins: 1. Levels in normal children and in uncomplicated allergy. Pediatrics 41: 600

Burkart P, Rosenfield RE, Hsu TCS et al. (1974) Instrumented PVP-augmented antiglobulin tests. I. Detection of allogeneic antibodies coating otherwise normal erythrocytes. Vox Sang 26: 289

Burmeister WP, Huber AH, Bjorkman PJ (1994) Crystal structure of the complex of rat neonatal Fc receptor with Fc. Nature 372: 323–324

Burnet FM, Fenner F (1949) The Production of Antibodies, 2nd edn. Melbourne: Macmillan

Callaghan TA, Fleetwood P, Contreras M et al. (1993) Human monoclonal anti-D with a normal half-life (Letter). Transfusion 33: 785–786

Chan PCY, Deutsch HF (1960) Immunochemical studies of human serum Rh agglutinins. J Immunol 85: 37

Chapman GE (1996) A pharmacokinetic/pharmacodynamic model for the action of anti-D immunoglobulin in effecting circulatory clearance of Rh D+ red cells. Transfusion Med 6: 227–233

Chattoraj A, Gilbert R Jr, Josephson AM (1968) Immunologic characterization of anti-H isohemagglutinins. Transfusion 8: 368

Chodirker WB, Tomasi TB (1963) γ globulin: quantitative relationships in human serum and non-vascular fluid. Science 142: 1080

Clarke CA, Edwards JW, Haddock DRW et al. (1956) ABO blood groups and secretor character in duodenal ulcer. Population and sibship studies. BMJ ii: 725

Cleghorn TE (1960) The frequency of the Wr^a, By and M^g blood group antigens in blood donors in the South of England. Vox Sang 5: 556

Collins JO, Sanger R, Allen FH et al. (1950) Nine blood-group antibodies in a single serum after multiple transfusions. BMJ i: 1297

Contreras M, Mollison PL (1981) Failure to augment primary Rh immunization using a small dose of 'passive' IgG anti-Rh. Br J Haematol 49: 371–381

Cooper RA (1977) Abnormalities of cell-membrane fluidity in the pathogenesis of disease. N Engl J Med 297: 371

Cooper B, Tishler PV, Atkins L et al. (1979). Loss of Rh antigen associated with acquired Rh antibodies and a chromosomal translocation in a patient with myeloid metaplasia. Blood 64: 642–647

Cossen G, Hagens D, Fukuchi R et al. (1992) Comparison of six commercial human T-cell lymphotropic virus type I (HTLV-I) enzyme immunoassay kits for detection of antibody to HTLV-I and -II. J Clin Microbiol 30: 724–725

Cox MT, Roberts M, LaJoie J et al. (1992) An apparent primary immune response involving anti-Jk^a and anti-P_1 detected 10 days after transfusion. Transfusion 32: 874

Crookston JH, Crookston MC, Burnie K et al. (1969) Hereditary erythroblastic multinuclearity associated with a positive acidified-serum test: a type of congenital dyserythropoietic anemia. Br J Haematol 17: 11

Cummins D, Contreras M, Amin S et al. (1995) Red-cell alloantibody development associated with heart and lung transplantation. Transplantation 59: 1432–1435

Dacie JV (1992) The Auto-Immune Haemolytic Anaemias, 3rd edn. Edinburgh: Churchill Livingstone, p. 40

Danielse GL, Reid ME, Anstee DJ et al. (1988) Transient reduction in erythrocyte membrane sialoglycoprotein β associated with the presence of elliptocytes. Br J Haematol 70: 477–481

Daniels GL, Cartron JP, Fletcher A et al. (2003) International Society of Blood Transfusion Committee on terminology for red cell surface antigens: Vancouver Report. Vox Sang 84: 244–247

Davies SC, McWilliam AC, Hewitt PE et al. (1986) Red cell alloimmunization in sickle cell disease. Br J Haematol 63: 241–245

De Lange GG (1988) Monoclonal antibodies against human immunoglobulin allotypes. PhD Thesis, University of London, London

Delauney J, Iolascon A (1999) The congenital dyserythropoietic anaemias. Baillière's Clin Haematol 12: 691–705

DePalma L, Criss VR, Roseff SD et al. (1991) Formation of alloanti-E in an 11-week-old infant. Transfusion 31: Suppl 52S

Descamps-Latscha B, Golub RM, Guyen AT et al. (1983) Monoclonal antibodies against T-cell differentiation antigens initiate simulation of monocyte/macrophage oxidative metabolism. J Immunol 131: 2500–2507

Dinsmore RE, Reich LM, Kapoor N et al. (1983) ABH incompatible bone marrow transplantation: removal of erythrocytes by starch sedimentation. Br J Haematol 54: 441–449

Dobson A, Ikin EW (1946) The ABO blood groups in the United Kingdom: frequencies based on a very large sample. J Pathol Bact 58: 221

Doll WRS, Drane H, Newell AC (1961) Secretion of blood group substances in duodenal, gastric and stomach ulcer, gastric carcinoma and diabetes mellitus. Gut 2: 352–359

Douglas R, Rowthorne NV, Schneider JV (1985) Some quantitative aspects of the human monocyte erythrophagocytosis and rosette assays. Transfusion 25: 535–539

Drachmann O, Hansen KB (1969) Haemolytic disease of the newborn due to anti-s. Scand J Haematol 6: 93

Dudgeon LS, Panton PN, Ross EA (1909) The action of splenotoxic and haemolytic sera on the blood and tissues. Proc R Soc Med 2: Part III, Path Section, 64

Dunsford I, Bowley CC (1955) Techniques in Blood Grouping. Edinburgh: Oliver and Boyd

von Dungern (1900) Beitrage zur Immunitätslehre. Munch Med Wschr 47: 677

Eaton BR, Morton JA, Pickles MM et al. (1956) A new antibody, anti-Ytª, characterizing a blood group of high incidence. Br J Haematol 2: 333

Economidou J, Hughes-Jones NC, Gardner B (1967) The functional activities of IgG and IgM anti-A and anti-B. Immunology 13: 227

Economidou J, Constantoulakis M, Augoustaki O et al. (1971) Frequency of antibodies to various antigenic determinants in polytransfused patients with homozygous thalassaemia in Greece. Vox Sang 20: 252

Ehlenberger AG, Nussenzweig V (1977) The role of membrane receptors for C3b and C3d in phagocytosis. J Exp Med 145: 357

Ehrlich P, Sachs H (1905) Collected Studies on Immunity. New York: John Wiley & Sons, p. 209

Elliot M, Bossom E, Dupny ME et al. (1964) Effect of ionic strength on the serologic behaviour of red cell isoantibodies. Vox Sang 9: 396

van den Elsen JMH, Martin A, Wong V (2002) X-ray crystal structure of the C4d fragment of human complement component C4. J Mol Biol 322: 1103–1115

Elson CJ, Bradley J (1970) Human peripheral blood leucocytes forming rosettes with rhesus (D) isoantigen. Lancet i: 798

Engelfriet CF, Ouwehand WH (1990) ADCC and other cellular bioassays for predicting the clinical significance of red cell alloantibodies. In: Blood Transfusion: the Impact of New Technologies. M Contreras (ed.). Baillière's Clinical Haematology 3: 321–337

Engelfriet CP, von dem Borne AEGKr, van der Meulen FW et al. (1981) Immune destruction of red cells. In: A Seminar on Immune-Mediated Cell Destruction. Chicago: American Association of Blood Banks

Epstein WV (1965) Specificity of macroglobulin antibody synthesized by the normal human fetus. Science 148: 1591

Evans RS, Turner E, Bingham M (1965) Studies with radio-iodinated cold agglutinins of ten patients. Am J Med 38: 378

Evans RS, Turner E, Bingham M (1967) Chronic hemolytic anaemia due to cold agglutinins: the mechanism of resistance of red cells to C′ hemolysis by cold agglutinins. J Clin Invest 46: 1461

Ewald RA, Williams JH, Bowden DH (1961) Serum complement in the newborn. An investigation of complement activity in normal infants and in Rh and AB hemolytic disease. Vox Sang 6: 312

Eylar EN, Madoff MA, Brody OV et al. (1962) The contribution of sialic acid to the surface charge of the erythrocyte. J Biol Chem 237: 1992

Feinstein A, Munn EA, Richardson NE (1971) The three-dimensional conformation of M and A globulin molecules. Ann NY Acad Sci 190: 104

Ferrara GB, Tosi RM, Azzolina G (1974) HL-A unresponsiveness induced by weekly transfusions of small aliquots of whole blood. Transplantation 17: 194

First International Workshop on Red Cell Monoclonal Antibodies (1987) First International Workshop on Monoclonal Antibodies against Human Red Blood Cells and Related Antigens, Paris. P Rouger, D Anstee, C Salmon (eds). Rev Fr Transf Immunohématol 30: no. 5

Fleer A, van Schaik MLJ, von dem Borne AEGKr et al. (1978) Destruction of sensitized erythrocytes by human monocytes in vitro: effects of cytochalasin B, hydrocortisone and colchicine. Scand J Immunol 8: 515

Floss AM, Strauss RG, Goeken N et al. (1986) Multiple transfusions fail to provoke antibodies against blood cell antigens in human infants. Transfusion 26: 419–422

Fowler R Jr, Schubert WK, West CD (1960) Acquired partial tolerance to homologous skin grafts in the human infant at birth. Ann NY Acad Sci 87: 403

Frame M, Mollison PL (1969) Charge differences between human IgG isoantibodies associated with specificity. Immunology 16: 277

Fraser ID, Tovey GH (1976) Observations on Rh isoimmunisation: past, present and future. Clin Haematol 5: 149

Freedman J, Masters CA, Newlands M et al. (1976) Optimal conditions for the use of sulphydryl compounds in dissociating red cell antibodies. Vox Sang 30: 231

Fujita T, Inoue T, Ogawa K et al. (1987) The mechanism of action of decay-accelerating factor (DAF). J Exp Med 166: 1221–1228

Gaboriaud C, Juanhuix J, Gruez A et al. (2003) The crystal structure of the globular head of complement protein C1q provides a basis for its versatile recognition properties. J Biol Chem 278: 46974–46982.

Gahmberg CG, Jakinen M, Andersson LC (1978) Expression of the major sialoglycoprotein (glycophorin) on erythroid cells in human bone marrow. Blood 52: 379

Garner SF, Thomson AR, Lubenko A et al. (1994) Monocyte isolation by flow cytometer-monitored centrifugal elutriation: a preparative tool for antibody-dependent cell mediated cytotoxicity assays. Br J Biomed Sci 51: 35–43

Garratty D, Petz LD (1994) Transfusing patients with autoimmune haemolytic anaemia (Letter) Lancet 341: 1220

Gay FP (1905) Observations on the single nature of haemolytic immune bodies, and on the existence of so-called 'complementoids'. Zbl Bakt (Orig) 39: 172

Giblett ER (1961) A critique of the theoretical hazard of inter- vs intra-racial transfusion. Transfusion 1: 233

Giblett ER (1977) Blood group alloantibodies: an assessment of some laboratory practices. Transfusion 17: 229

Gill JC, Endres-Brooks J, Bauer PJ et al. (1987) The effect of ABO blood group on the diagnosis of von Willebrand disease. Blood 69: 1691–1695

Gilligan DM, Bennett V (1993) The junctional complex of the membrane skeleton (Review). Semin Hematol 30: 74–83

Glenny AT, Südmersen HJ (1921) Notes on the production of immunity to diphtheria toxin. J Hyg (Camb) 20: 176

Goldstein IJ, Hughes RC, Monsigny M et al. (1980) What should be called a lectin? (Letter). Nature (Lond) 285: 66

Goldstein IJ, Blake DA, Ebisu S et al. (1981) Carbohydrate binding studies on the Bandeiraea simplicifolia I isolectins. Lectins which are mono-, di-, tri- and tetravalent for N-acetyl-D-galactosamine. J Biol Chem 256: 3890–3893

Goodrick J, Kumpel B, Pamphilon D et al. (1994) Plasma half-lives and bioavailability of human monoclonal Rh D antibodies Brad-3 and Brad-5 following intramuscular injection into Rh D-negative volunteers. Clin Exp Immunol 98: 17–20

Goosens D, Champonier F, Rouger P et al. (1987) Human monoclonal antibodies against blood group antigens. Preparation of a series of stable EBV immortalised B clones producing high levels of antibody of different isotypes and specificities. J Immunol Methods 101: 193–200

Gordon J, Murgita RA (1975) Suppression and augmentation of the primary in vitro immune response by different classes of antibodies. Cell Immunol 15: 392

Götze O, Mueller-Eberhard HJ (1970) Lysis of erythrocytes by complement in the absence of antibody. J Exp Med 132: 898

Gourdin MF, Reyes F, Lejonic JL et al. (1976) L'hétérogénéité de la distribution cellulaire des antigènes à érythrocytaires. Étude au microscope électronique. Rev Fr Transfus Immunohématol 19: 55

Green CA, Daniels GH, Khalid G et al. (1990) Monoclonal anti-S. Proc. 2nd Int. Workshop and Symposium on Monoclonal antibodies against human red blood cells and related antigens, Lund, Sweden, eds Chester MA, Johnson U, Lundblad A et al.

Greenbury CL, Moore DH, Nunn LAC (1963) Reaction of 7S and 19S components of immune rabbit antisera with human group A and AB red cells. Immunology 6: 421

Greenbury CL, Moore DH, Nunn LAC (1965) The reaction with red cells of 7S rabbit antibody, its sub-units and their recombinants. Immunology 8: 420

Griffin H, Ouwehand WH (1995) A human monoclonal antibody specific for the leucine-33 (Pl^{A1}, HPA-1a) form of platelet glycoprotein 111a from a V gene phage display library. Blood 86: 4430–4436

Grove-Rasmussen M (1964) Routine compatibility testing standards of the AABB as applied to compatibility tests. Transfusion 4: 200

Grove-Rasmussen M, Huggins CE (1973) Selected types of frozen blood for patients with multiple blood group antibodies. Transfusion 13: 124

Grubb R, Morgan WTJ (1949) The 'Lewis' blood group characters of erythrocytes and body fluids. Br J Exp Pathol 30: 198

Guest AR, Scott ML, Smythe J et al. (1992) Analysis of the structure and activity of A and A,B immunoglobulin A monoclonal antibodies. Transfusion 32: 239–245

Hadley AG, Kumpel BM, Leader K et al. (1989) An in vitro assessment of the functional activity of monoclonal anti-D. Clin Lab Haematol 11: 47–54

Hadley AG, Kumpel BM (1989) Synergistic effect of blending IgG1 and IgG3 monoclonal anti-D in promoting the metabolic response of monocytes to sensitised red cells. Immunology 67: 550–552

Hadley AG, Kumpel BM, Merry AH (1988) The chemiluminescent response of human monocytes to red cells sensitized with monoclonal anti-Rh(D) antibodies. Clin Lab Haematol 10: 377–384

Habibi B, Lecolier B (1983) Inopportunité de la prophylaxie elaborée de l'allo-immunisation transfusionelle contre les globules rouge dans l'insuffisance rénale chronique. Rev Fr Transfus Immunohématol 26: 267–277

Hakomori S (1984) Blood group glycolipid antigens and their modifications as human cancer antigens. Am J Clin Pathol 82: 635–648

Hall AM, Cairns LS, Altmann DM et al. (2005) Immune responses and tolerance to the RhD blood group protein ın HLA-transgenic mice. Blood 105: 2175–2179. Epub, 21 September 2004

Hannan J, Young K, Szakonyi G et al. (2001) Structure of complement receptor (CR) 2 and CR2-C3d complexes. Biochem Soc Trans 30: 983–989

Hanson DG, Vaz NM, Maia LCS et al. (1979) Inhibition of specific immune response by feeding protein antigens. III. Evidence against maintenance of tolerance to ovalbumin by orally induced antibodies. J Immunol 123: 2337–2343

Harrison RA, Lachmann PJ (1980) The physiological breakdown of the third component of human complement. Mol Immunol 17: 9–20

Harte PG, Cooke A, Playfair JHL (1983) Specific monoclonal IgM; a novel and potent adjuvant in murine malaria vaccination. Nature (Lond) 302: 256–258

Haughton G, Nash DR (1969) Specific immunosuppression by minute doses of passive antibody. Transplant Proc 1: 616

Heddle NM, Klama L, Frasseto R et al. (1993) A retrospective study to determine the risk of red cell alloimmunization and transfusion during pregnancy. Transfusion 33: 217–220

Heidelberger M, Mayer MM (1948) Quantitative studies on complement. Adv Enzymol 8: 71

Henry C, Jerne NK (1968) Competition of 19S and 7S antigen receptors in the regulation of the primary immune response. J Exp Med 128: 133

Hershko C, Gale RP, Ho W et al. (1980) ABH antigens and bone marrow transplantation. Br J Haematol 44: 65–73

Hirszfeld L, Dubiski S (1954) Untersuchungen über die Struktur der inkompletten Antikörper. Schweiz Z Allg Path 17: 73

Hoerlein AB (1957) The influence of colostrum on antibody response in baby pigs. J Immunol 78: 112

Holburn AM (1973) Quantitative studies with [^{125}I] IgM anti-Le^a. Immunology 24: 1019

Holburn AM, Cleghorn TE, Hughes-Jones NC (1970) Re-stimulation of anti-D in donors. Vox Sang 19: 162

Holburn AM, Frame M, Hughes-Jones NC et al. (1971a) Some biological effects of IgM anti-Rh (D). Immunology 20: 681

Holburn AM, Cartron J-P, Economidou J et al. (1971b) Observations on the reactions between D-positive red cells and ^{125}I-labelled IgM anti-D molecules and subunits. Immunology 21: 499

Hopkins DF (1969) The correlation between IgM anti-D and 'saline agglutination' of D-positive cells by anti-D sera. Br J Haematol 17: 597

Hopkins DF (1970) Saline agglutinating anti-K and anti-k in the apparent absence of IgM antibody. Br J Haematol 19: 749

Hoppe HH, Mester T, Hennig W et al. (1973) Prevention of Rh immunisation. Modified production of IgG anti-Rh for intravenous application by ion exchange chromatography (IEC). Vox Sang 25; 308–316

Hornick CL, Karush P (1972) Antibody affinity. III. The role of multivalence. Immunochemistry 9: 325

Huber H, Fudenberg HH (1968) Receptor sites of human monocytes for IgG. Int Arch Allergy 34: 18

Hughes-Jones NC (1967) The estimation of the concentration and the equilibrium constant of anti-D. Immunology 12: 565

Hughes-Jones NC (1970) Reactivity of anti-D immunoglobulin G subunits. Nature (Lond) 227: 174

Hughes-Jones NC (1972) The attachment of IgG molecules on the red cell surface. Haematologia 6: 269

Hughes-Jones NC (1975) Red-cell antigens, antibodies and their interaction. Clin Haematol 4: 29

Hughes-Jones NC (1986) The classical pathway. In: Immunobiology of the Complement System. GD Ross (ed.). London: Academic Press

Hughes-Jones NC, Gardner B (1962) The exchange of ^{131}I-labelled lipid and ^{131}I-labelled protein between red cells and serum. Biochem J 83: 404

Hughes-Jones NC, Ghosh S (1981) Anti-D-coated Rh-positive red cells will bind the first component of the complement pathway, C1q. FEBS Lett 128: 318–320

Hughes-Jones NC, Gardner B, Telford R et al. (1963a) Studies on the reaction between the blood-group antibody anti-D and erythrocytes. Biochem J 88: 435

Hughes-Jones NC, Gardner B, Telford R (1963b) Comparison of various methods of dissociation of anti-D, using ^{131}I-labelled antibody. Vox Sang 8: 531

Hughes-Jones NC, Gardner B, Telford R (1964a) The effect of pH and ionic strength on the reaction between anti-D and erythrocytes. Immunology 7: 72

Hughes-Jones NC, Gardner B, Telford R (1964b) The effect of ficin on the reaction between anti-D and red cells. Vox Sang 9: 175

Hughes-Jones NC, Gorick BD, Miller NGA et al. (1984) IgG pair formation on one antigenic molecule is the main mechanism of synergy between antibodies in complement-mediated lysis. Eur J Immunol 14: 974–978

Hummel K (1962) Quantitative Untersuchungen uber die Bindung von Polyvinylpyrrolidon an die Erythrozytenoberflache. Blut 9: 215

Humphrey JH, Dourmashkin RR (1965) Electron microscope studies of immune cell lysis. In: Ciba Foundation Symposium, Complement. GEW Wolstenholme, J Knight (eds). London: J & A Churchill

Idusogie EE, Presta LG, Gazzano-Santoro H et al. (2000) Mapping of the C1q binding site on rituxan, a chimeric antibody with a human IgG1Fc. J Immunol 164: 4178–4184

Ikin E, Kay HEM, Playfair JHI et al. (1961) P$_1$ antigen in the human foetus. Nature (Lond) 192: 4805

Inoue N, Murakami Y, Kinoshita T (2003) Molecular genetics of paroxysmal nocturnal hemoglobinuria. Int J Hematol 77: 107–12

ISBT Working Party on Terminology for Red Cell Surface Antigens (1995) Blood Group Terminology 1995. Vox Sang 69: 265–279

ISBT (1996) ISBT/ICSH Working Party on Terminology for Red Cell Surface Antigens: Makuhari Report. Vox Sang 71: 246–248

Ishizaka K, Ishizaka T, Lee EH et al. (1965) Immunochemical properties of human γA isohemagglutinin. I. Comparisons with γG- and γM-globulin antibodies. J Immunol 95: 197

Issitt PD (1965) On the incidence of second antibody populations in the sera of women who have developed anti-Rh antibodies. Transfusion 5: 355

Issitt PD, McKeever BG, Moore VK et al. (1973) Three examples of Rh-positive, good responders to blood group antigens. Transfusion 13: 316

James P, Rowe GP, Tozzo, GG (1988) Elucidation of allo-antibodies in autoimmune haemolytic anaemia. Vox Sang 54: 167–171

Janatova J, Tack BF (1981) Fourth component of human complement: studies of an amine-sensitive site comprised of a thiol component. Biochemistry 20: 2394–2402

Jandl JH (1965) Mechanisms of antibody-induced red cell destruction. Ser Haematol 9: 35

Kameh H, Landolt-Marticorena C, Charuk JH et al. (1998) Structural and functional consequences of an N-glycosylation mutation (HEMPAS) affecting human erythrocyte membrane glycoproteins. Biochem Cell Biol 76: 823–835

Karlsson MCI, Wernersson S, Diaz de Stahl T et al. (1999) Efficient IgG-mediated suppression of primary antibody responses in Fcgamma receptor deficient mice. Proc Natl Acad Sci USA 96: 2244–2249

Karlsson MC, Getahun A, Heyman B (2001) FcgammaRIIB in IgG-mediated suppression of antibody responses: different impact in vivo and in vitro. J Immunol 167: 5558–5564

Kilpatrick DC (2000) Handbook of Animal Lectins. Chichester: J Wiley and Sons

Klaassen RJL, Ouwehand WH, Huizinga TWJ et al. (1990) The Fc-receptor III on cultured human monocytes. Structural similarity with FcRIII of natural killer cells and role in the extracellular lysis of sensitized erythrocytes. J Immunol 144: 599–606

Klaus GGB (1978) The generation of memory cells. II. Generation of B memory cells with preformed antigen-antibody complexes. Immunology 34: 643

Klaus GGB, Humphrey JH, Kunkl et al. (1980) The follicular dendritic cell: its role in antigen presentation in the generation of immunological memory. Immunol Rev 53: 3–59

Klinman NR, Karush F (1967) Equine anti-hapten antibody-V. The non-precipitability of bivalent antibody. Immunochemistry, 4: 387

Köhler G, Milstein C (1975) Continuous cultures of fused cells secreting antibody of predefined specificity. Nature (Lond) 256: 495

Konugres AA (1978) Transfusion therapy for the neonate. In: A Seminar on Perinatal Blood Banking. New Orleans: American Association of Blood Banks

Kornstad L (1983) New cases of irregular blood group antibodies other than anti-D in pregnancy: frequency and clinical significance. Acta Obstet Gynecol Scand 62: 431–436

Koskimies S (1980) Human lymphoblastoid cell line producing specific antibody against Rh antigen D. Scand J Immunol 11: 73–77

Kumpel BM, Leader KA, Merry AH et al. (1989a) Heterogeneity in the ability of IgG1 monoclonal anti-D to promote lymphocyte-mediated red cell lysis. Eur J Immunol 19: 2283–2288

Kumpel BM, Wiener E, Urbaniak SJ et al. (1989b) Human monoclonal anti-D antibodies II. The relationship between IgG subclass. Gm allotype and Fc mediated function. Br J Haematol 71: 415–420

Kurlander RJ, Rosse WF, Logue GL (1978) Quantitative influence of antibody and complement coating of red cells on monocyte-mediated cell lysis. J Clin Invest 61: 1309

Lalezari P (1970) Discussion in Histocompatibility Testing. PI Teraski (ed.). Copenhagen: Munksgaard, p. 307

Lalezari P, Malamut DC, Driesiger ME et al. (1973) Anti s and anti-U cold-reacting antibodies. Vox Sang 25: 390

Landois L (1875) Die Transfusion des Blutes. Leipzig: FCW Vogel

Landsteiner K (1900) Zur Kenntnis antifermentativen, lytischen und agglutinierenden Wirkungen des Blutserums und der Lymphe. Zbl Bakt 27: 357

Landsteiner K (1901) Über Agglutinationserscheinungen normalen menschlichen Blutes. Klin Wschr 14: 1132

Landsteiner K (1931) Individual differences in human blood. Science 73: 405

Landsteiner K (1945) The Specificity of Serological Reactions, revised edn. Boston, MA: Harvard University Press, p. 132

Landsteiner K, Levine P (1927) Further observations on individual differences of human blood. Proc Soc Exp Biol (NY) 24: 941

Landsteiner K, Miller CP (1925) Serological studies on the blood of primates. II. The blood groups in anthropoid apes. J Exp Med 42: 853

Landsteiner K, Witt DH (1926) Observations on the human blood groups. Irregular reactions. Iso-agglutinin in sera of group 4. The factor A_1. J Immunol 11: 221

Landsteiner K, Wiener AS (1940) An agglutinable factor in human blood recognizable by immune sera for Rhesus blood. Proc Soc Exp Biol (NY) 43: 223

Landsteiner K, Wiener AS (1941) Studies on an agglutinogen (Rh) in human blood reacting with anti-Rhesus sera and with human iso-antibodies. J Exp Med 74: 309

Langley R, Wines B, Willoughby N *et al.* (2005) The staphylococcal superantigen-like protein 7 binds IgA and complement C5 and inhibits IgA-Fc(alpha)RI binding and stops killing of bacteria. J Immunol 174: 2926–2933

Larsen RD, Ernst LK, Nair RP *et al.* (1990) Molecular cloning, sequence and expression of a human GDP-L-fucose:Beta-D-galactoside 2-alpha-L-fucosyltransferase cDNA that can form the H blood group antiquen. Proc Natl Acad Sci USA 87: 6674

Law SK, Lichtenberg NA, Levine RP (1980) Covalent binding and hemolytic activity of complement proteins. Proc Natl Acad Sci USA 77: 7194–7198

Lechler R (ed.) (1994) HLA and Disease. London: Academic Press

Lehner P, Hutchings P, Lydyard PM *et al.* (1983) Regulation of the immune response by antibody: II. IgM mediated enhancement; dependency on antigen dose. T cell requirement and lack of evidence for an idiotype related mechanism. Immunology 50: 503–509

Leikola J, Pasanen VJ (1970) Influence of antigen receptor density on agglutination of red blood cells. Int Arch Allergy 39: 352

Levaditi (1902) État de la cytase hémolytique. Ann Inst Pasteur 16: 233

Levine P (1944) Landsteiner's concept of the individuality of human blood. Exp Med Surg 11: 36

Levine P (1958) The influence of the ABO system on hemolytic disease. Hum Biol 30: 14

Levine P, Koch E (1954) The rare human isoagglutinin anti-T$_j^a$ and habitual abortion. Science 120: 239

Levine P, Stetson R (1939) An unusual case of intragroup agglutination. JAMA 113: 126

Levine P, Bobbitt OB, Waller RK *et al.* (1951a) Isoimmunization by a new blood factor in tumor cells. Proc Soc Exp Biol (NY) 77: 403

Levy PC, Looney RJ, Shen L *et al.* (1990) Human alveolar macrophage FcR-mediated cytotoxicity. Hetero-antibody-versus conventional antibody-mediated target cell lysis. J Immunol 144: 3693–3700

Lewis M, Allen FJ Jr, Hnstee DJ *et al.* (1985) ISBT Working Party on Terminology for Red Cell Surface Antigens: Munich Report. Vox Sang 49: 171–175

Loirat MJ, Gourbil A, Frioux Y *et al.* (1992) A murine monoclonal antibody directed against the Gerbich 3 blood group antigen. Vox Sang 62: 45–48

Longster GH, Major KE (1975) Anti-Kell (K1) in ascitic fluid. Vox Sang 28: 253

Lown JAG, Holland PAT, Barr AL (1984) Inhibition of serological reactions with enzyme-treated red cells by complement binding alloantibodies. Vox Sang 46: 300–305

Lubenko A, Contreras M (1989) A review: low-frequency red cell antigens. Immunohematology 5: 7–14

Ludvigsen CW Jr, Swanson JL, Thompson TR *et al.* (1987) The failure of neonates to form red cell alloantibodies in response to multiple transfusions. Am J Clin Pathol 87: 250–251

Lukacik P, Rovers P, White J *et al.* (2004) Complement regulation at the molecular level: The structure of decay-accelerating factor. Proc Natl Acad Sci USA 101: 1279–1284

McCafferty J, Griffiths AD, Winter G *et al.* (1990) Phage antibodies: filamentous phage displaying antibody variable domains. Nature (London) 348: 552–554

McFadzean AJS, Tsang KC (1956) Antibody formation in cryptogenetic splenomegaly. I. The response to particulate antigen injected intravenously. Trans R Soc Trop Med Hyg 50: 433

Maizels M, Paterson JH (1940) Survival of stored blood after transfusion. Lancet ii: 417

Maniatis A, Theodoris H, Aravani K (1993) Neonatal immune response to red cell antigens (Letter). Transfusion 33: 90–91

Mannoni P, Bracq C, Yvart J *et al.* (1970) Anomalie de fonctionnement du locus Rh au cours d'une myélofibrose. Nouv Rev Fr Hématol 10: 381

Marks JD, Ouwehand WH, Bye JM *et al.* (1993) Human antibody fragments specific for human blood group antigens from a phage display library. BioTechnology 11: 1145–1149

Marsh WI, Jenkins WJ (1960) Anti-i: a new cold antibody. Nature (Lond) 188: 753

Mårtensson L, Fudenberg HH (1965) Gm genes and γG-globulin synthesis in the human fetus. J Immunol 94: 514

Mattingly JA, Waksman B (1978) Immunologic suppression after oral administration of antigen. I. Specific suppressor cells formed in rat's Peyer's patches after oral administration of sheep erythrocytes and their systemic migration. J Immunol 121: 1878

May RC, Machesky LM (2001) Phagocytosis and the actin cytoskeleton. J Cell Sci 114: 1061–1077

Medicus RG, Melamed J, Arnaout MA (1983) Role of human factor I and C3b receptor in the cleavage of surface-bound C3bi molecules. Eur J Immunol 13: 465–470

Melamed MD, Gordon J, Ley SJ *et al.* (1985) Senescence of a human lymphoblastoid clone producing anti-Rhesus(D). Eur J Immunol 15: 742–746

Merry AH, Brojer E, Zupańska B *et al.* (1988) Comparison of the ability of monoclonal and polyclonal anti-D antibodies to promote the binding of erythrocytes to lymphocytes, granulocytes and monocytes. Biochem Soc Trans 16: 727–728

Merry AH, Brojer E, Zupańska B *et al.* (1989) Ability of monoclonal anti-D antibodies to promote the binding of red cells to lymphocytes, granulocytes and monocytes. Vox Sang 56: 48–53

Merry AH, Thomson EE, Rawlinson v et al. (1982) A quantitative antiglobulin test for IgG for use in blood transfusion serology. Clin Lab Haematol 4: 393–402

Michaelsen TE, Kornstad L (1987) IgG subclass distribution of anti-Rh, anti-Kell and anti-Duffy antibodies measured by sensitive haemagglutination assays. Clin Exp Immunol 67: 637–645

Mollison PL (1967) Blood Transfusion in Clinical Medicine, 4th edn. Oxford: Blackwell Scientific Publications

Mollison PL (1983) Blood Transfusion in Clinical Medicine, 7th edn. Oxford: Blackwell Scientific Publications

Mollison PL (1984) Some aspects of Rh hemolytic disease and its prevention. In: Hemolytic Disease of the Newborn. G Garratty (ed.). Arlington, VA: American Association of Blood Banks

Mollison PL, Thomas AR (1959) Haemolytic potentialities of human blood group antibodies revealed by the use of animal complement. Vox Sang 4: 185

Moore BFL (1976) Biological and clinical significance of differences between RBC membrane (Rh) and non-membrane (ABH, MN, P) antigenic sites. Rev Fr Transfus Immunohématol 19: 629

Morell A, Terry WD, Waldmann TA (1970) Metabolic properties of IgG subclasses in man. J Clin Invest 49: 673

Morell A, Skvaril F, van Loghem E et al. (1971) Human IgG subclasses in maternal and fetal serum. Vox Sang 21: 481

Mosmann TR, Gallatin M, Longenecker BM (1980) Alteration of apparent specificity of monoclonal (hybridoma) antibodies recognizing polymorphic histo-compatibility and blood group determinants. J Immunol 125: 1152–1156

Mourant AE, Kopéc AC, Domaniewska-Sobczak (1976) The Distribution of the Human Blood Groups and Other Biochemical Polymorphisms, 2nd edn. Oxford: Oxford University Press

Mourant AE, Kopéc AC, Domaniewska-Sobczak K (1978) Blood Groups and Diseases. Oxford: Oxford University Press

Munk-Andersen G (1956) Demonstration of incomplete ABO-antibody with special reference to its passage through the placenta. I. The content of complete ABO-antibody in umbilical cord serum. Acta Pathol Microbiol Scand 39: 407

Munn LR, Chaplin H Jr (1977) Rosette formation by sensitized red cells – effects of source of peripheral leukocyte monolayers. Vox Sang 33: 129

Muta T, Kurosaki T, Misulovin Z et al. (1994) A 13-amino acid motif in the cytoplasmic domain of Fc gamma RIIB modulates B-cell receptor signalling. Nature 368: 70–73

Nagar B, Jones RG, Diefenbach RJ et al. (1998) X-ray crystal structure of C3d: a C3 fragment and ligand for complement receptor 2. Science 280: 1277–1281

Nance SJ, Arndt P, Garratty G (1987) Predicting the clinical significance of red cell alloantibodies using a monocyte monolayer assay. Transfusion 27: 449–452

Nance SJ, Arndt P, Garratty G (1988) The effect of fresh normal serum on monocyte monolayer assay reactivity (Letter). Transfusion 28: 398–399

Neth O, Jack DL, Dodds AW et al. (2000) Mannose-binding lectin binds to a range of clinically relevant microorganisms and promotes complement deposition. Infect Immun 68: 688–693

Neter E (1936) Observations on abnormal isoantibodies following transfusions. J Immunol 30: 255

Nicholson-Weller A, March JP, Rosenfield SI et al. (1983) Affected erythrocytes of patients with paroxysmal nocturnal hemoglobinuria are deficient in the complement regulatory protein, decay accelerating factor. Proc Natl Acad Sci USA 80: 5066–5070

Nisonoff A, Pressman D (1957) Closeness of fit and forces involved in the reactions of antibody homologous to the p-(p-azophenylazo)-benzoate ion group. J Am Chem Soc 79: 1616

O'Donnell J, Laffan MA (2001) The relationship between ABO histo-blood group, factor VIII and von Willebrand factor. Transfusion Med 11: 343–351

Okazawa H, Motegi S, Ohyama N et al. (2005) Negative regulation of phagocytosis in macrophages by the CD47-SHPS-1 system. J Immunol 174: 2004–2011

Oldenborg PA, Zheleznyak A, Fang YF et al. (2000) Role of CD47 as a marker of self on red blood cells. Science 288: 2051–2054

Oldenborg PA, Gresham HD, Lindberg FP (2001) CD47-signal regulatory protein alpha (SIRPalpha) regulates Fcgamma and complement receptor mediated phagocytosis. J Exp Med 193: 855–862

Olesen H (1966) Thermodynamics of the cold agglutinin reaction. Scand J Clin Lab Invest 18: 1

O'Neil EJ, Sundstedt A, Mazza G et al. (2004) Natural and induced regulatory T cells. Ann NY Acad Sci 1029: 180–192

Orlina AR, Unger PJ, Koshy M (1978) Post-transfusion alloimmunization in patients with sickle cell disease. Am J Hematol 5: 101

van Oss CJ, Edberg SC, Bronson PM (1973) Valency of IgM. In: Specific Receptors of Antibodies, Antigens and Cells. D Pressman, TB Tomasi Jr, AL Grossberg et al. (eds). Basel: S Karger

van Oss CJ, Mohn JF, Cunningham RK (1978) Influence of various physicochemical factors on hemagglutination. Vox Sang 34: 351

van Oss CJ, Absolom DR, Grossberg AL et al. (1979) Repulsive van der Waals forces. I. Complete dissociation of antigen-antibody complexes by means of negative van der Waals forces. Immunol Commun 8: 11–29

van Oss CJ, Beckers D, Engelfriet CP et al. (1981) Elution of blood group antibodies from red cells. Vox Sang 40: 367–371

Pappenheimer AM (1940) Anti-egg albumin antibody in the horse. J Exp Med 71: 263

Parsons SF, Jones J, Anstee DJ et al. (1994) A novel form of congenital dyserythropoietic anemia associated with deficiency of erythroid CD44 and a unique blood group phenotype [In(a–b–), Co(a–b–)]. Blood 83: 860–868

Paw BH, Davidson AJ, Zhou Y et al. (2003) Cell-specific mitotic defect and dyserythropoiesis associated with erythroid band 3 deficiency. Nature Genet 34: 59–64

Pereira A, Mazzara R, Castillo R (1990) Transfusion of racially unmatched blood (Letter). N Engl J Med 323: 1421

Perkins SJ, Nealis AS, Sutton BJ et al. (1991) Solution structure of human and mouse immunoglobulin M by synchroton X-ray scattering and molecular graphics modelling. J Mol Biol 221: 1345–1366

Perrotta S, Luzzatto L, Carella M et al. (2003) Congenital dyserythropoietic anemia type II in human patients is not due to mutations in the erythroid anion exchanger 1. Blood 102: 2704–2705

Peters LL, Lux SE (1993) Ankyrins: structure and function in normal cells and hereditary spherocytes. Semin Hematol 30: 85–118

Podack ER (1986) Assembly and functions of the terminal components. In: Immunobiology of the Complement System. GD Ross (ed.). London: Academic Press: pp. 115–137

Podack ER, Konigsberg PJ (1984) Cytolytic T cell granules. Isolation, structural, biochemical, and functional characterisation. J Exp Med 160: 695–710

Pollack W (1965) Some physicochemical aspects of hemagglutination. Ann NY Acad Sci 127: 892

Pollack W, Hager HJ, Reckel R et al. (1965) A study of the forces involved in the second stage of the hemagglutination. Transfusion 5: 158

Pollack W, Gorman JG, Hager HJ et al. (1968) Antibody-mediated immune suppression to the Rh factor; animal models suggesting mechanism of action. Transfusion 8: 134

Pollack W, Ascari WO, Kochesky RJ et al. (1971) Studies on Rh prophylaxis. I. Relationship between doses of anti-Rh and size of antigenic stimulus. Transfusion 11: 333

Polley MJ (1964) The development and use of the anti-globulin sensitization test for the study of the serological characteristics of blood-group antibodies and for the quantitive estimation of certain serum proteins. PhD Thesis, University of London, London

Polley MJ, Mollison PL (1961) The role of complement in the detection of blood group antibodies. Special reference to the antiglobulin test. Transfusion 1: 9

Polley MJ, Mollison PL, Soothill JF (1962) The role of 19S gamma globulin blood group antibodies in the antiglobulin reaction. Br J Haematol 8: 149

Polley MJ, Adinolfi M, Mollison PL (1963) Serological characteristics of anti-A related to type of antibody protein (7Sγ or 19Sγ). Vox Sang 8: 385

Porter RR (1967) The structure of immunoglobulins. Essays Biochem 3: 1–24

Pross HF, Eidinger D (1974) Antigenic competition: a review of nonspecific antigen-induced suppression. In: Advances in Immunology, vol. 18. FJ Dixon, HG Kunkel (eds). London: Academic Press

Race RR (1944) An 'incomplete' antibody in human serum. Nature (Lond) 153: 771

Race RR, Sanger R (1950) Blood Groups in Man. Oxford: Blackwell Scientific Publications

Race RR, Sanger R (1968) Blood Groups in Man, 5th edn. Oxford: Blackwell Scientific Publications

Race RR, Sanger R (1975) Blood Groups in Man, 6th edn. Oxford: Blackwell Scientific Publications

Radaev S, Sun PD (2001) Recognition of IgG by Fcgamma receptor. The role of Fc glycosylation and the binding of peptide inhibitors. J Biol Chem 276: 16478–16483

Radaev S, Motyka S, Fridman WH et al. (2001) The structure of a human type III Fcgamma receptor in complex with Fc. J Biol Chem 276: 16469–16477

Ramsey G, Larson P (1988) Loss of red cell antibodies over time. Transfusion 28: 162–165

Ramsey G, Smietana SJ (1994) Long-term follow-up testing of red cell alloantibodies. Transfusion 34: 122–124

Rearden A, Masouredis SP (1977) Blood group D antigen content of nucleated red cell precursors. Blood 50: 981

Redman M, Regan F, Contreras M (1996) A prospective study of the incidence of red cell alloimmunization following transfusion. Vox Sang 71: 216–220

Reesink HW, van der Hart Mia, van Loghem JJ (1972) Evaluation of a simple method for the determination of the IgG titre of anti-A or -B in cases of possible ABO blood group incompatibility. Vox Sang 22: 397

Reisner EC, Kostyu DD, Phillips G et al. (1987) Alloantibody responses in multiply transfused sickle cell patients. Tissue Antigens 30: 161–166

Renkonen KO (1948) Studies on hemagglutinins in seeds of some representatives of the family of Leguminosae. Ann Med Exp Fenn 26: 66

Reyes F, Lejonc JL, Gourdin MF et al. (1974) Human normoblast A antigen seen by immunoelectron microscopy. Nature (Lond) 247: 461

Riley RL (1992) Neonatal immune response. In: Encyclopedia of Immunology, vol. 3. IM Roitt, PJ Delyes (eds). London: Academic Press, pp. 1140–1143

Roberts JA (1957) Blood groups and susceptibility to disease. Br J Prev Soc Med 11: 107

Rochna E, Hughes–Jones NC (1965) The use of purified ^{125}I-labelled anti-γ globulin in the determination of the number of D antigen sites on red cells of different phenotypes. Vox Sang 10: 675

Roitt I, Brostoff J, Male D (1989) Immunology, 2nd edn. London: Gower Medical Publications

Roitt I, Brostoff J, Male D (1993) Immunology, 3rd edn. London: Gower Medical Publishing

Romano EL, Mollison PL (1975) Red cell destruction *in vivo* by low concentrations of IgG anti-A. Br J Haematol 29: 121

Romans DG, Tilley CA, Crookston MC *et al.* (1977) Conversion of incomplete antibodies to direct agglutinins by mild reduction: evidence for segmental flexibility within the Fc fragment of immunoglobulin G. Proc Natl Acad Sci USA 74: 2531

Romans DG, Tilley CA, Dorrington KJ (1979) Interactions between Fab and Fc regions in liganded immunoglobulin G. Mol Immunol 16: 859–879

Romans DG, Tilley CA, Dorrington KJ (1980) Monogamous bivalency of IgG antibodies. I. Deficiency of branched ABHI-active oligosaccharide chains on red cells of infants causes the weak antiglobulin reactions in hemolytic disease of the newborn due to ABO incompatibility. J Immunol 124: 2807–2811

Roncarolo M-G, Bigler M, Ciuti E *et al.* (1994) Immune responses by cord blood cells. Blood Cells 20: 573–586

Roos A, Bouwman LH, van Gijlswijk-Janssen DJ *et al.* (2001) Human IgA activates the complement system via the mannan-binding lectin pathway. J Immunol 167: 2861–2868

Rosenfield RE (1977) In memoriam Alexander S Wiener. Haematologia 11: 5

Rosenfield RE (1989) Who discovered Rh? A personal glimpse of the Levine–Wiener argument. Transfusion 29: 355–357

Ross GD (1986) Opsonization and membrane complement receptors. In: Immunobiology of the Complement System. GD Ross (ed.). New York: Academic Press

Ross GD (1989) Complement and complement receptors. Curr Opin Immunol 2: 50–62

Ross CR, Yount WJ, Walport MJ *et al.* (1985) Disease-associated loss of erythrocyte complement receptors (CR$_1$, C3b receptors) in patients with systemic lupus erythematosus and other diseases involving autoantibodies and/or complement activation. J Immunol 1235: 2005–2014

Rosse WF (1986) The control of complement activation by the blood cells in paroxysmal nocturnal haemoglobinuria. Blood 67: 268–269

Rosse WF (1989) Paroxysmal nocturnal hemoglobinuria: the biochemical defects and the clinical syndrome. Blood Rev 3: 192–200

Rosse WF, Dourmashkin R, Humphrey JH (1966) Immune lysis of normal human and paroxysmal nocturnal haemoglobinuria (PNH) red blood cells. III. The membrane defects caused by complement lysis. J Exp Med 123: 969

Rosse WF, Borsos T, Rapp HJ (1968) Cold-reacting antibodies: the enhancement of antibody fixation by the first component of complement (C la). J Immunol 100: 259

Rosse WF, Gallagher D, Kinney TR *et al.* (1990) Transfusion and alloimmunization in sickle cell disease. Blood 76: 1431–1437

Rowley DA (1950) The formation of circulating antibody in the splenectomized human being following intravenous injection of heterologous erythrocytes. J Immunol 65: 515

Salama A, Mueller-Eckhardt C (1985) Binding of fluid phase C3b to nonsensitised bystander human red cells. A model for in vivo effects of complement activation on blood cells. Transfusion 25: 528–534

Salama A, Berghöfer H, Mueller-Eckhardt C (1992) Red blood cell transfusion in warm-type autoimmune haemolytic anaemia. Lancet 340: 1515–1517

Salsbury AJ, Clarke JA (1967) Surface changes, in red blood cells undergoing agglutination. Rev Fr Étud Clin Biol 12: 981

Samson D, Mollison PL (1975) Effect on primary Rh immunization of delayed administration of anti-Rh. Immunology 28: 349

Sauer-Eriksson AE, Kleywegt GJ, Uhlen M *et al.* (1995) Crystal structure of the C2 fragment of streptococcal protein complex with the fc domain of human IgG. Structure 3: 265–278

Schierman LW, McBride RA (1967) Adjuvant activity of erythrocyte isoantigens. Science 156: 658

Schierman LW, Leckband E, McBride RA (1969) Immunological interaction of erythrocyte isoantigens: effect of passive antibody. Proc Soc Exp Biol (NY) 130: 744

Schleef M, Strobel E, Dick A *et al.* (2005) Relationship between ABO and Secretor genotype with plasma levels of factor VIII and von Willebrand factor in thrombosis patients and control individuals. Br J Haematol 128: 100–107

Schneider J, Preisler O (1966) Untersuchungen zur serologischen Prophylaxe der Rh-Sensibilisierung. Blut 12: 1

Schonermark S, Rauterberg EW, Shin ML *et al.* (1986) Homologous species restriction in lysis of human erythrocytes: a membrane-derived protein with C8-binding capacity functions as an inhibitor. J Immunol 136: 1772–1776

Scott ML, Guest AR, Anstee DJ (1989) Subclass dependence of reduction and alkylation of incomplete IgG monoclonal anti-D to complete anti-D (Abstract). Transfusion 29 (Suppl. 57S)

Second International Workshop on Red Cell Monoclonal Antibodies (1990) Proceedings of the Second International Workshop and Symposium on Monoclonal Antibodies against Human Red Blood Cells and Related Antigens. MA Chester, U Johnson, A Lundblad *et al.* (eds), Lund, Sweden

Segre D, Kaeberle ML (1962) The immunologic behavior of baby pigs. I. Production of antibodies in three-week-old pigs. J Immunol 89: 782

Sim RB, Tsiftsoglou SA (2004) Proteases of the complement system. Biochem Soc Trans 32: 21–27

Sim RB, Twose TW, Paterson DS *et al.* (1981) The covalent-binding reaction of complement component C3. Biochem J 193: 115–127

Sirchia G, Zanella A, Parrovicinii A et al. (1985) Red cell alloantibodies in thalassaemia major. Transfusion 25: 110–112

Smith T (1909) Active immunity produced by so-called balanced or neutral mixtures of diphtheria toxin and antitoxin. J Exp Med 11: 241

Sondermann P, Oosthuizen V (2001) X-ray crystallographic studies of IgG-Fcγ receptor interactions. Biochem Soc Trans 30: 481–486

Southcott MJ, Tanner MJ, Anstee DJ (1999) The expression of human blood group antigens during erythropoiesis in a cell culture system. Blood 93: 4425–4435

Spanos T, Krageorga M, Lapis V et al. (1990) Red cell alloantibodies in patients with thalassemia. Vox Sang 58: 50–55

Springer GF, Horton RE (1969) Blood group isoantibody stimulation in man by feeding blood group-active bacteria. J Clin Invest 48: 1280

Springer GF, Tegtmeyer H (1981) Origin of anti-Thomsen-Friedenreich (T) and Tn agglutinins in man and in white leghorn chicks. Br J Haematol 47: 453–460

Springer GF, Horton RE, Forbes M (1959) Origin of anti-human blood group B agglutinins in white leghorn chicks. J Exp Med 110: 221

Steane EA, Greenwalt TJ (1980) Erythrocyte agglutination. Prog Clin Bio Res – 'Immunobiology of the Erythrocyte', SG Sandler, J Nusbacher, MS Schanfield (eds)—43: 171–188

Steck TL (1974) The organisation of proteins in the human red cell membrane. J Cell Biol 62: 1–19

Steiner LA, Eisen HM (1967) The relative affinity of antibodies synthesised in the secondary response. J Exp Med 126: 1185

Stern K (1975) Multiple differences in red cell antigens and isoimmunization. Transfusion 15: 179

Stern K, Davidsohn I, Jensen FG et al. (1958) Immunologic studies on the Be^a factor. Vox Sang 3: 425

Stratton F (1963) Erythrocyte antibodies and autoimmunity. Lancet ii: 626

Stratton F, Jones AR (1955) The reactions between normal human red cells and antiglobulin (Coombs) serum. J Immunol 75: 423

Stratton F, Rawlinson VI, Gunson HH et al. (1973) The role of zeta potential in Rh agglutination. Vox Sang 24: 273

Strunk R, Colten HR (1976) Inhibition of the enzymatic activity of the first component of complement (C1) by heparin. Clin Immunol Immunopathol 6: 248

Swisher SN, Young LE (1954) Studies of the mechanisms of erythrocyte destruction initiated by antibodies. Trans Assoc Am Phys 67: 124

Szulman AE (1980) The ABH blood groups and development. In: Current Topics in Developmental Biology. M Friedlander (ed.). New York: Academic Press, pp. 127–145

Talmage DW (1959) Immunological specificity. Science 129: 1463

Tao M-H, Smith RIF, Morrison SL (1993) Structural features of human immunoglobulin G that determine isotype-specific differences in complement activation. J Exp Med 78: 661–667

Terres G, Wolins W (1959) Enhanced sensitization in mice by simultaneous injection of antigen and specific rabbit antiserum. Proc Soc Exp Biol Med 102: 632

Terres G, Wolins W (1961) Enhanced immunological sensitization of mice by the simultaneous injection of antigen and specific antiserum. I. Effect of varying the amount of antigen used relative to the antiserum. J Immunol 86: 361

Thompson KM, Hughes-Jones NC (1990) Production and characterization of monoclonal anti-Rh. In: Blood Transfusion; the Impact of New Technologies. M. Contreras (ed.). Baillière's Clinical Haematology 3: 243–253

Thompson RA, Rowe DS (1968) Reactive haemolysis – a distinctive form of red cell lysis. Immunology 14: 745

Thorpe S (1990) Reactivity of human monoclonal anti-body against Rh D with the intermediate filament protein vimentin. Br J Haematol 76: 116–120

Thorpe SJ (1989) Detection of Rh D-associated epitopes in human and animal tissues using human monoclonal anti-Ls antibodies. Br J Haematol 73: 527–536

Tomasi TB Jr, Tan EM, Solomon A et al. (1965) Characteristics of an immune system common to certain external secretions. J Exp Med 121: 101

Tovey GH (1974) Preventing the incompatible blood transfusion. Haematologia 8: 389

Tsai CM, Zopf DA, Ginsburg V (1978) The molecular basis for cold agglutination: effect of receptor density upon thermal amplitude of a cold agglutinin. Biochem Biophys Res Commun 80: 905

Urbaniak SJ (1979a) ADCC(K-cell) lysis of human erythrocytes with Rhesus alloantibodies. I. Investigation of in vitro culture variables. Br J Haematol 42: 303–314

Urbaniak SJ (1979b) ADCC(K-cell) lysis of human erythrocytes sensitized with alloantibodies. II. Investigation into the mechanism of lysis: Br J Haematol 42: 315–328

Vichinsky EP, Earles A, Johnson RA et al. (1990) Alloimmunization in sickle cell anaemia and transfusion of racially unmatched blood. N Engl J Med 322: 1617–1622

Vivier E, Daeron M (1997) Immunoreceptor tyrosine-based inhibition motifs. Immunol Today 18: 286–291

Voak D (1972) Observations on the rare phenomenon of anti-A prozone and the non-specific blocking of haemagglutination due to C1 complement fixation by IgG anti-A antibodies. Vox Sang 22: 408

Walker RH (1984) Relevance in the selection of serologic tests for the obstetric patient. In: Hemolytic Disease of the Newborn. G Garratty (ed.). Arlington, VA: American Association of Blood Banks, pp. 173–200

Walker W (1958) The changing pattern of haemolytic disease of the newborn (1948–1957). Vox Sang 3: 225, 336

Walker RH, Dong-Tsamn L, Hartrick MB (1989) Alloimmunization following blood transfusion. Arch Pathol Lab Med 113: 254–261

Wallhermfechtel MA, Pohl B, Chaplin H (1984) Alloimmunization in patients with warm autoantibodies: a retrospective study employing 3 donor alloabsorptions to aid in antibody detection. Transfusion 24: 482–485

Walpert MJ, Lachmann PJ (1993) Complement. In: Clinical Aspects of Immunology, 5th edn. PJ Lachmann, K Peters, FS Rosen et al. (eds). Oxford: Blackwell Scientific Publications, pp. 347–375

Warmerdam PA, van de Winkel JG, Vlug A et al. (1991) A single amino acid in the second Ig-like domain of the human Fcγ receptor II is critical for human IgG2 binding. J Immunol 147: 1338–1343

Watkins MW, Greenwell P, Yates AD et al. (1980) Blood group A and B transferase levels in serum and red cells of human chimaeras. Rev Fr Transfus Immunohématol 23: 531–544

Weitzel H, Hunerman B, Stolp W et al. (1974) Immunoclearance D-positives Erythrozyten nach Anwendung unterschiedlicher anti-D-Preparate, in Prophylaxe der Rhesus-Sensibilisierung. J Schneider and H Weitzel (eds). Frankfurt: Medizinische Verlagsgesellschaft

West CD, Hong R, Holland NH (1962) Immunoglobulin levels from the newborn period to adulthood and in immunoglobulin deficiency states. J Clin Invest 41: 2054

Wickramasinghe SN (1998) Congenital dyserythropoietic anaemias: clinical features, haematological morphology and new biochemical data. Blood Rev 12: 178–200

Wiener AS (1943) Blood Groups and Transfusion, 3rd edn. Springfield, IL: CC Thomas

Wiener AS (1944) A new test (blocking test) for Rh sensitization. Proc Soc Exp Biol (NY) 56: 173

Wiener E, Garner SF (1985) The use of cultured macrophages and anti-human globulin reagents to detect complement-fixing red cell antibodies. Abstracts, 3rd Annual Meeting of the Brish Blood Transfusion Society, Oxford

Wiener E, Garner SF (1987) The use of macrophages stimulated by immune interferon as indicator cells in the mononuclear phagocyte assay. Clin Lab Haematol 9: 397–408

Wiener AS, Peters HR (1940) Hemolytic reactions following transfusions of blood of the homologous group, with three cases in which the same agglutinogen was responsible. Ann Intern Med 13: 2306

Wiener E, Atwal A, Thompson KM et al. (1987) Differences between the activities of human monoclonal IgG1 and IgG3 subclasses of anti-Rh(D) antibodies in their ability to mediate red cell binding to macrophages. Immunology 62: 401–404

Wiener E, Jolliffe VM, Scott HCF et al. (1988) Differences between the activities of human monoclonal IgG1 and IgG3 anti-D antibodies of the Rh blood group system in their abilities to mediate effector functions of monocytes. Immunology 65: 159–163

Winkelstein JA, Mollison PL (1965) The antigen content of 'inagglutinable' group B erythrocytes. Vox Sang 10: 614

Woodrow JC, Clarke CA, Donohoe WTA et al. (1975) Mechanism of Rh prophylaxis: an experimental study on specificity of immunosuppression. BMJ 2: 57

Woof JM, Partridge LJ, Jefferis R et al. (1986) Localization of the monocyte-binding region on human immunoglobulin G. Mol Immunol 23: 319–330

Worlledge SM (1977) Red cell antigens in dyserythropoiesis. In: Dyserythropoiesis. SM Lewis, RAL Verwilghen (eds). New York: Academic Press

Yates AD, Greenwell P, Watkins WM (1983) Overlapping specification of the glycosyl-transferases specified by the blood-group A and B genes: a possible explanation for aberrant blood-group expression in malignant tissues. Biochem Soc Trans 11: 300–301

Yunis JJ, Yunis EJ (1963) Cell antigens and cell specialization. I. A study of blood group antigens on normoblasts. Blood 22: 53

Yunis JJ, Yunis EJ (1964) Cell antigens and cell specialization. II. Demonstration of some red cell antigens of human normoblasts. Blood 24: 522

Zak SJ, Good RA (1959) Immunochemical studies of human serum gamma globulins. J Clin Invest 38: 579

Zdebska E, Golaszewska E, Fabijanska-Mitek J et al. (2001) Glycoconjugate abnormalities in patients with congenital dyserythropoietic anaemia type I, II and III. Br J Haematol 114: 907–913

Zeitlin RA, Sanger R, Race RR (1958) Unpublished data cited by Race and Sanger (1975), p. 240

Zupańska B, Thomson EE, Merry AH (1986) Fc receptors for IgG1 and IgG3 on human mononuclear cells: an evaluation with known levels of erythrocyte-bound IgG. Vox Sang 50: 97–103

Zupańska B, Gronkowska A, Ziemski M (1995) Comparison of activity of peripheral monocytes and splenic macrophages in the monocyte monolayer assay. Vox Sang 68: 241–242

4

ABO, Lewis and P groups and Ii antigens

The ABH, Lewis, P and Ii antigens are carbohydrate structures. The antigens are synthesized by the sequential addition of sugar residues to a common precursor substance. The genes encode glycosyltransferases, which carry out the sequential addition of sugar residues. As a consequence, the systems interact in a number of ways. For example, single molecules may carry specificities determined by both the *ABO* and the *Le* genes. The various interactions can be understood only by studying the chemistry of the biosynthetic pathways. In this chapter, a relatively simple account of the systems is given first, and a description of the chemistry of the antigens, the biosynthetic pathways and the molecular genetics is given at the end of the chapter.

The ABO and Hh systems

The ABO blood group system, which was the first human blood group system to be discovered (see Chapter 3), remains the most important in transfusion practice. This is because of the regular occurrence of the antibodies anti-A, anti-B and anti-A,B, reactive at 37°C, in persons whose red cells lack the corresponding antigens (see Table 4.1), so that if transfusions were to be given without regard to the ABO groups, about one-third (in white people) would be incompatible.

The regular presence of anti-A and anti-B is made use of in the routine determination of ABO blood groups; in addition to testing red cells for A and B antigens, the group is checked, in serum or 'reverse' grouping, by testing the serum against red cells of known ABO groups.

Although H is encoded by a gene on a different chromosome from *ABO*, the H blood group system is considered in this chapter because H is a precursor of A and B.

Antigens of the ABO system

A brief account of the main phenotypes and genotypes of the ABO system, including the frequency of the

Table 4.1 Antigens and antibodies in the ABO system.

Group	Subgroup	Antigens on red cells	Antibodies (agglutinins) in serum
O	–	None*	Anti-A Anti-A$_1$ Anti-B Anti-A,B†
A	A$_1$ A$_2$	A + A$_1$ A	Anti-B‡
B	–	B	Anti-A Anti-A$_1$
AB	A$_1$B A$_2$B	A + A$_1$ + B A + B	Nil‡

* With very rare exceptions human red cells contain the antigen H; the amount of H is influenced by the ABO group: O cells contain most H and A$_1$B cells least (see p. 118).
† Inseparable, crossreacting anti-A,B.
‡ Also anti-A$_1$ in 1–8% of A$_2$ subjects and 22–35% of A$_2$B subjects; anti-HI is found in the serum of occasional A$_1$ and A$_1$B subjects.

Table 4.2 Frequencies of ABO groups in a few selected populations (figures from Mourant *et al.* 1976).

Population* (no. tested)	Percentage of various phenotypes						Special characteristics
	O	A_1	A_2	B	A_1B	A_2B	
South American Indians (539)	100	0	0	0	0	0	All O
Vietnamese (220)	45	21.4	0	29.1	4.5	0	No A_2B commoner than A
Australian aborigines (126)	44.4	55.6	0	0	0	0	No A_2 or B
Germans (100 000)	42.8	32.5	9.4	11.0	3.1	1.1	
Bengalese (241)	22	22.2	1.8	38.2	14.8	0.9	B commonest
Lapps (324)	18.2	36.1	18.5	4.8	6.2	6.2	Very high A_2

* The figures are for selected populations and do not necessarily apply to the racial group as a whole.

common genes in white people, has been given in the preceding chapter.

ABO phenotypes in different populations

Table 4.2 gives figures for the frequency of ABO phenotypes in selected populations. The figures have been chosen simply to illustrate a few points: for example, South American Indians all belong to group O; in Australian aborigines, only groups O and A are found; in some populations (e.g. Bengalese) the commonest group is B; and, finally, in some populations (e.g. Lapps) there is a relatively high frequency of A_2.

In Africans (black people), B is in general a much stronger antigen than in Europeans (white people) (Mourant *et al.* 1976) and black people have a higher level of B-specified glycosyltransferase in the serum (Badet *et al.* 1976). Based on quantitative agglutination, about 50% of black people have stronger B than white people (Gibbs *et al.* 1961). For a discussion of the relative frequency of ABO haemolytic disease of the newborn in group A and B infants, and in different ethnic groups, see Chapter 12.

Subgroups of A

A_1 and A_2. In Europeans, about 80% of group A individuals belong to subgroup A_1, almost all the rest being A_2. The distinction is most conveniently made by testing red cells with the lectin from *Dolichos biflorus* (Bird 1952). When diluted appropriately, the lectin agglutinates only A_1 cells (but see Table 7.3 on p. 279); if too concentrated an extract is used, some

adult A_2 samples, although not adult A_2B or cord A_2 samples, may be agglutinated (see Voak and Lodge 1968).

The distinction between A_1 and A_2 may be difficult to make in newborn infants: the red cells of some infants who can be clearly shown to be A_1 when they are older may, at the time of birth, fail to react with anti-A_1 reagents. Tests with the anti-H lectin from *Laburnum alpinum* may be helpful in distinguishing between A_1 and A_2 red cells in the first months of life, A_2 red cells reacting much more strongly than A_1 red cells: the anti-H lectin from *Ulex europaeus* does not discriminate so well (Pawlak and Lopez 1979). The lectin from *D. biflorus* is better than human anti-A_1 at distinguishing A_1 from A_2 in newborn infants (Race and Sanger 1975), especially if the cells are enzyme treated.

Some differences between A_1 and A_2 red cells. As described below, the number of A sites is substantially higher on A_1 than A_2 red cells. Both for A_1 and A_2 cells, the number of A sites per red cell varies considerably within the cell population of an individual but this heterogeneity is much greater for A_2 than for A_1 red cells (Smalley and Tucker 1983).

The immunodominant sugar is identical on A_1 and A_2 red cells, namely N-acetylgalactosamine, and in reactivity the difference between A_1 and A_2 red cells is purely quantitative. It has been estimated that a minimum of $2.5-4 \times 10^5$ A sites per red cell are needed for agglutination by anti-A_1 reagents (Lopez *et al.* 1980). Anti-A_1 may then be visualized as an antibody that reacts only with a conformation produced by a certain

115

minimum density of A sites. Nevertheless, A_1 does have qualitative differences from A_2, which is not surprising as the A_1- and A_2-specified transferases are different (see p. 148).

The difference between A_1 and A_2, and A_1B and A_2B, cannot always be made with certainty; there are some individuals who type as A_1 or A_1B with some anti-A_1 reagents and as A_2 or A_2B with others. In addition, there are subjects whose red cells type as A intermediate (A_{int}), reacting more weakly than A_1 red cells with anti-A_1, yet unexpectedly more strongly than A_2 red cells with anti-H (see Race and Sanger 1975, p. 17). A_{int} is much more common in black than white people, for example 4.8% vs. 0.3% in one investigation (Wiener et al. 1945).

Anti-A_1 is found in the serum of some A_2 and A_2B subjects (see Table 4.1) but, except in rare individuals in whom the antibody is active at 37°C, can be ignored in blood transfusion. Hence, there is no need to distinguish A_2 from A_1 donors in routine practice. Perhaps the main importance of A subgroups in clinical medicine is that A_2 infants are protected from haemolytic disease due to anti-A.

A_3 and other weaker forms of A. These phenotypes, which result from the inheritance of rare alleles of A, cannot be recognized when the rare allele is paired with A_1 or A_2.

A_3 red cells give a characteristic mixed field pattern when tested with anti-A from group B donors, consisting of small agglutinates in a sea of unagglutinated cells; with group O serum, agglutination is stronger. The frequency of A_3 subjects was found to be 1 in 1000 in Denmark (Gammelgaard 1942) but 1 in 20 000 in France (Garretta et al. 1974). A_3 is heterogeneous at the DNA level (see later).

Many other weaker forms of A have been described based on: (1) the presence or absence of reactions of the red cells with anti-A, -A_1, -H and -A,B; (2) the presence of anti-A_1 in serum; and (3) the presence of A and H substances in the saliva of ABH secretors. The following list is not comprehensive (for further information, see Daniels 2002).

A_x red cells are agglutinated weakly or not at all by serum from group B donors but are agglutinated by serum from most group O donors. Anti-A_1 is usually present in the serum of A_x people.

A_{el} red cells are either not agglutinated at all or agglutinated only very weakly by anti-A in O or B

sera, but anti-A can be adsorbed by, and eluted from, the red cells. The saliva of secretors contains a normal amount of A and H. No anti-A_1 is present in the serum.

A_{el} red cells are not agglutinated by group B or group O serum but, following incubation with anti-A, anti-A can be eluted from the cells. The saliva of secretors contains H but not A: the serum may contain anti-A_1 (Reed and Moore 1964). Like A_3 and A_x, A_{el} cells have two populations: a minor one, carrying significant amounts of A, and a major one, totally devoid of A (Poskitt and Fortwengler 1974).

A_{end} cells give a mixed field pattern of agglutination with most group O but with few B sera (Sturgeon et al. 1964). H but not A is found in the saliva of secretors: anti-A_1 is present in the serum. The frequency of A_x, A_m, A_{el} and A_{end} in the French population was in each case less than 1 in 50 000 (Garretta et al. 1974).

Using murine monoclonal anti-A reacting with all type A oligosaccharide chains, then gold-labelled goat antimouse IgG, followed by scanning electron microscopy, A antigen was found on 5% of A_m and A_{el} cells, some of which showed very strong labelling. In two A_3 subjects, A was present on 82% and 58% of the red cells, respectively, suggesting that A_3 may be heterogeneous. A was present on 75% more cells in A_x (Heier et al. 1994).

Mixtures of A and O red cells, as found in chimeras (or in group A patients transfused with O cells), may at first be mistaken for A_3 samples.

Distribution of A antigen within populations of A red cells. In A_1 subjects, most red cells have numerous A sites but in A_2 subjects there is a spectrum from heavily coated cells to cells that apparently lack A (Reyes et al. 1976). Similarly, in A_3 subjects, about one-third of the cells lack A and in A_m and in A_{el} subjects A can be detected on only about 5% of the cell population. In addition to quantitative differences between A subgroups, there are differences in the types of A chain (Heier et al. 1994) and gene structure (see below).

A, B and H antigens in relation to ageing of red cells

A, B and to a lesser extent H diminish with red cell age, as determined by red cell size; the change is thought to be due to progressive loss of red cell surface on ageing (Fibach and Sharon 1994).

Subgroups of B

There is no subgroup of B analogous to subgroup A_2 but various types of B cells reacting weakly or not at all with anti-B have been described.

Salmon (1976) suggested that terminology should parallel that of A subgroups and he proposed that the terms B_3, B_x and B_{el} should be used as follows: B_3 cells show a mixed field agglutination pattern with B in the saliva of secretors; B_x shows a weak agglutination pattern and the saliva inhibits the reaction between anti-B and B cells; weak anti-B is found in the serum. B_{el} cells are not agglutinated by anti-B but will absorb anti-B, which can subsequently be eluted: H but not B is found in the saliva of secretors.

In detecting weak B antigens, as in detecting weak A antigens, the preparation of an eluate may be helpful in two ways: first, it may be possible to prepare quite a potent eluate from cells that agglutinate only very weakly; in fact, it appears that, on the whole, the weaker the antigen the more potent the eluate; second, an eluate prepared from cells with a very weak antigen (e.g. B_x) may agglutinate the cells, even although they are not agglutinated by the whole serum used in making the eluate (Alter and Rosenfield 1964a).

Competition between A- and B-transferases

A- and B-tranferases act upon the same precursor substance and it is therefore not surprising that subjects who have both an A and a B allele show diminished expression of both A and B antigens. Thus, A_1B red cells have less A than A_1 cells and A_2B cells less A than A_2 cells. Similarly, B is slightly less strongly expressed in A_1B than in B cells. In certain pedigrees, red cells of genotype A_1B may behave as A_2B, presumably due to an interference with the expression of A_1 by a strong B allele (for references, see Alter and Rosenfield 1964b). In 5000 Black Americans only 20% of A samples typed as A_2 but almost 50% of AB samples typed as A_2B (Morel et al. 1984).

Cis AB

Occasionally, an individual passes on both A and B so that, for example, a group AB father and a group O mother have an AB child. In the cis AB phenotype, the B antigen is usually very weak so that the phenotype cannot be confused with normal AB. The serum from most cis AB individuals contains anti-B, indicating that the B in cis AB is different from normal B. The A antigen is more strongly expressed than in A_2B but less strongly expressed than in A_1B.

Two different genetic backgrounds have been demonstrated: there may be a single mutant gene, determining a transferase with both A and B activity (Yoshida et al. 1980a; Watkins et al. 1981). Sequencing of the ABO genes in several unrelated cis AB individuals showed an A_1 structure but with two single base differences, the significant one being a substitution at position 268 (Gly→Ala) representing the B-sequence (Ogasawara et al. 1996). CisAB has also been described with a Met266Leu change on the background of the B-transferase sequence (Mifsud et al. 2000). Leu266Met and Gly268Ala are the most critical residues defining A and B-transferase activity. The larger residues found in the B-transferase (Met/Ala) restrict the size of the active site preventing access to UDP-GalNac (see Plate 4.1 shown in colour between pages 528 and 529, Table 4.7 and Patenaude et al. 2002). In the case of cisAB, it would appear that substituting one or other of these critical residues in the A or B transferase allows access to both UDP-Gal and UDP-GalNAc, but reduces enzyme activity, as the phenotype has weaker A and B antigen expression than normal. In another family the A- and B enzymes were separable (Yoshida et al. 1980b), indicating that not all examples of cis AB have the same genetic origin.

B(A) and A(B)

A- and B-specified transferases are very similar and have overlapping functions. Thus, the A_1-transferase can synthesize group B determinants (Yates and Watkins 1982) and the B-transferase has the potential to synthesize blood group A-active structures, using the same donor and acceptor substrates as the A-transferase (Yates et al. 1984; Watkins 1990). Red cells are described as B(A) when, despite coming from a B subject who lacks the A gene, they are weakly agglutinated by potent anti-A monoclonals. Most B(A) subjects are black and in the serum have concentrations of B-specified enzyme that are five to six times greater than in most B subjects (Beck et al. 1987). On the other hand, A(B) individuals do not have higher levels of A-transferase but have very potent H-transferases with abundant H precursor substances, which may lead to the formation of some B determinants by the

A-transferase (see Watkins 1990). The B(A) phenotype may also result from qualitative changes in B-transferase activity. Individuals with the B(A) phenotype have been described with a Ser235Gly substitution in the B-transferase sequence (Olsson *et al.* 2001). Gly235 is found in the A-transferase. It does not have direct contact with the UDP-sugar moiety, but might influence that conformation of H-active acceptor substrates (Patenaude *et al.* 2002). Two B(A) siblings with a Pro234Ala substitution in the B-transferase sequence have also been described (Yu *et al.* 1999). It would be expected that this substitution would alter the UDP-sugar binding properties of the transferase and so account for the B(A) phenotype (see Table 4.7).

H antigen on red cells

The H determinant is found on all human red cells except those of subjects of phenotype O_h. As H is a precursor of A and B, A and B subjects have less H than O subjects. The order of reactivity of anti-H with red cells of various ABO groups tends to be $OA_2 > A_2B > B > A_1 > A_1B$. Exceptions to this order are provided by occasional subjects who are genetically A_1 or A_1B but group as A_2 or A_2B, respectively, because normal synthesis of A is hindered by a deficiency of H. In such 'A_2' or 'A_2B' subjects, H is more weakly expressed than in cells of normal A_1 or A_1B subjects.

Numbers of A, B and H antigen sites on red cells

Estimates of the numbers of sites on the red cells of adults and newborn infants of common ABO phenotypes are shown in Table 4.3. As the table shows, it has been estimated that there are approximately 800 000 A sites on adult A_1 cells, and about as many B sites on adult B cells. The only estimate for the number of H sites on the red cells of adults suggests that these are twice as numerous on O cells as are A or B sites on A or B cells. However, this apparent discrepancy is probably due simply to the method of calculation. The numbers of A and B sites are calculated from the numbers of antibody molecules combining with the red cells, on the assumption that one antibody molecule combines with one antigen site. As in fact there is evidence that, under conditions used in estimating antigen sites, the majority of anti-A and anti-B molecules bind to red cells by both their combining sites, the number of A and B sites is presumably approximately twice the

Table 4.3 Various estimates of the number of A, B and H sites on red cells of different phenotypes from adults and newborn infants.

	Sites $\times 10^6$ per red cell	Reference*
A sites[†]		
A_1 adults	0.83	(1)
A_1 adults	0.81–1.17	(2)
A_1 adults	0.85	(3)
newborn	0.25–0.37	(2)
A_2 adults	0.24–0.29	(2)
A_2 adults	0.24	(3)
newborn	0.14	(2)
A_1B adults	0.46–0.85	(2)
newborn	0.22	(2)
A_2B adults	0.14	(2)
B sites[†]		
B adults	0.75	(2)
newborn	0.2–0.32	(4)
A_1B adults	0.43	(2)
H sites		
O adults	1.7	(5)
newborn	0.325	(5)
A, B, AB newborn	0.07	(5)

* (1) Greenbury *et al.* (1963); (2) Economidou *et al.* (1967a); (3) Cartron *et al.* (1974); (4) EL Romano (personal communication); (5) Schenkel-Brunner (1980a,b).
[†] Assumes antibody molecule binds to one antigen site; even if bivalent binding is usual, at very high concentrations of antibody, as used in estimating the number of antigen sites, binding is probably univalent (NC Hughes-Jones, personal communication).

number given in the table. On the other hand, the number of H sites was estimated from the number of ^{14}C-labelled GalNAc residues transferred to red cells using *A*-specified enzyme (Schenkel-Brunner 1980a). From a consideration of estimates of the number of red cell surface molecules known to carry oligosaccharides with ABH activity, it can be inferred that the number of ABH sites on a red cell is in excess of 2.5 million (see Chapter 3).

Compared with the red cells of adults, the red cells of newborn infants have about one-third of the number of A and B sites. The numbers of antigen sites on weak A samples from adults were found to be:

A_3, 35 000; A_x, 4800; A_{end}, 3500; and A_m, 700 (Cartron 1976, and other papers in vol. 19, no.1, of the *Revue Française de Transfusion et Immunohématologie*, March 1976).

O_h, A_h and B_h red cells

In subjects of the very rare genotype *hh* (phenotype O_h), no H is made on red cells or in secretions and therefore no A or B can be made either (see section 'Biosynthesis of the P, HAB* (ABH), Ii and Lewis antigens', later in text). The serum contains anti-H as well as anti-A and anti-B. The first example of blood of this kind was found in Bombay (Bhende *et al.* 1952), hence the name 'Bombay' often given to *hh* bloods. As *Hh* and ABO are on different chromosomes, *hh* subjects may carry (unexpressed) *A* or *B* and may then be described as O_h, etc.

The red cells of almost equally rare 'paraBombay' bloods, A_h, B_h, O_h and O_{hm}, react very weakly with anti-A and anti-B, but not at all with the anti-H lectin from *Ulex europaeus*, although weak reactions have been observed with selected anti-H from O_h subjects (see Race and Sanger 1975, for details and references). A_h and B_h subjects do not secrete ABH, whereas the saliva of O_{hm}^A and O_{hm}^B subjects contains A and H or B and H respectively. The serum from A_h and B_h subjects contains anti-H but the antibody in the serum of O_{hm}^A and O_{hm}^B subjects is anti-HI. Although H in 'para-Bombay' subjects cannot be readily detected serologically, its presence has been uncovered by converting B_h cells, using suitable enzymes, into B(–), H(+) cells (Mulet *et al.* 1979).

Development of the A, B and H antigens

A and B can be detected on the red cells of 5- or 6-week-old embryos, but even at birth are not fully developed (Kemp 1930), and the number of antigen sites is less (see Table 4.3). The red cells of newborn infants also react less strongly than those of adults with anti-H.

When the reactions of the red cells of group A infants and adults with anti-A sera are compared, only slight differences are found in the agglutination of saline-suspended red cells but larger differences are observed in the indirect antiglobulin test (anti-IgG) and in tests for lysis (Crawford *et al.* 1953). In the percentage of cells lysed, adult levels are almost reached by the end of the first year of life and are fully reached by the age of 2–4 years (Grundbacher 1967).

The red cells of newborn infants who are genetically A_1 react relatively weakly with human anti-A_1 (Crawford *et al.* 1953); for the reactions with lectins, see the previous section 'Subgroups of A'. Fetal A_2 red cells behave like adult A_x red cells, i.e. they react better with O serum than with B serum (Constantoulakis *et al.* 1963). The section on biosynthesis deals with the biochemical differences between adult and fetal group A red cells.

The relative binding of anti-A to adult and cord blood group A red cells, in relation to the serological findings in ABO haemolytic disease of the newborn, is considered in Chapter 12.

Weakening of A, B and H antigens in acute leukaemia

In acute leukaemia, the A antigen may be weakened (van Loghem *et al.* 1957). Sometimes the blood appears to contain a mixture of group A and group O cells (Salmon *et al.* 1958; Gold *et al.* 1959) or of A_1 and weak A (Salmon *et al.* 1959). In other cases the red cells react weakly with anti-A, even behaving like A_3 or A_m (Salmon *et al.* 1959); Salmon and co-workers pointed out that in the course of testing some 300 000 blood samples they had encountered 22 weak A samples (10 A_x, four A_m and eight A_3). All of the 10 A_x samples came from normal subjects but two of the four A_m and two of the eight A_3 came from patients with acute leukaemia.

In a patient with erythroleukaemia, of group B, 60% of the cells were not agglutinated by anti-B and appeared to be group O, but were really very weak B: when separated from the normal B cells they would absorb anti-B (Bird *et al.* 1976).

ABH antigens may also be lost from carcinomatous tissue cells; see Chapter 3.

ABO antigens, cardiac disease and venous thromboembolism

Nydegger and co-workers (2003) report the prevalence of the B allele to be 2.5 times higher amongst patients with a history of myocardial infarction. High factor VIII levels and non-O blood groups are risk factors for venous thromboembolism (Gonzalez Ordonez *et al.* 1999; Tirrado *et al.* 2005). The rate of proteolysis ot von Willebrand factor (VWF) by the metalloprotease ADAMTS 13 is greater for group O VWF than for VWF from BA or AB (Bowen 2003). ADAMTS 13 limits platelet accumulation in microvascular thrombi by cleaving the Tyr1605–Met1606 bond in VWF. ADAMTS13 deficiency causes thrombotic thrombocytopenic purpura (Zheng *et al.* 2003a).

Acquired B antigen in A_1 subjects

In the original report of this condition, seven A_1 blood samples were described, which reacted weakly with some anti-B sera, giving the appearance of group AB with a weak expression of B. In each case, the serum contained normal anti-B. Five out of the seven subjects had cancer and six were over 60 years old (Cameron *et al.* 1959). 'Acquired B' results from the action of bacterial deacetylase, which converts N-acetylgalactosamine to α-galactosamine, which is very similar to galactose, the chief determinant of B. Some monoclonal anti-B fail to react with acquired B cells and are thus useful in discriminating between normal and acquired B. Another means of discrimination is to adjust the pH of anti-B sera to 6, as the sera will then no longer react with acquired B. A mouse monoclonal antibody specific for the acquired B group, reacting with a distinct epitope resulting from the deacetylation of the blood group A trisaccharide, was reported by Oriol and co-workers (1990).

In a case in which acquired B was mistaken for AB, and four AB units, compatible on an immediate spin, were transfused over a period of 7 days, a fatal haemolytic transfusion reaction (HTR) developed associated with immune anti-B (Garratty *et al.* 1993).

Red cells with acquired B may also show T or Tk activation (see Chapter 7), all of these changes being produced by enzymes from Gram-negative bacteria commonly associated with carcinoma of the colon or rectum, or with intestinal obstruction.

It has been suggested that the rarity of acquired B may be due to the fact that all A_2 and 95% of A_1 subjects have an antibody that can destroy B-modified cells and that most coliform organisms lack deacetylase (Gerbal *et al.* 1975). The kind of acquired B described above may be called the 'deacetylase type' and can be made only on A_1 cells. The second type of acquired B that may be called the 'passenger antigen' type is caused by adsorption of B-like bacterial products on to O or A cells but occurs only *in vitro* (Bird 1977).

Conversion of O cells to A or B

Group O cells (but not O_h) can be converted to A- or B-active red cells by incubation with the appropriate nucleotide sugar and A- or B-transferase (see p. 148).

Enzymatic conversion of A and B cells to O

Treatment of B red cells with an α-galactosidase hydrolyses away the terminal α-glycosidically linked galactose, thus removing group B activity (Harpaz *et al.* 1975). Red cells treated in this way react as group O cells and, after labelling with ^{51}Cr, have been shown to survive normally not only in the group B donor of the cells but also in a group A and a group O subject (Goldstein *et al.* 1982). In further work, 2 units of converted B cells were given to each of four group O subjects. Despite a three- to fivefold increase in anti-B titre, there was no evidence of an immediate or delayed haemolytic reaction (Lenny *et al.* 1994). A successful phase II trial using recombinant enzyme was reported by Kruskall and co-workers (2000). Comparable conversion of group A cells has proved more difficult because of the lack of suitable α-N-acetylgalactosaminidases. Candidate enzymes include those from the human fecal bacterium *Ruminococcus torques IX-70* (Hoskins *et al.* 1997; Hoskins and Boulding 2001, 2002), the marine bacterium *Arenibacter lacterius KMM426T* (Bakunina *et al.* 2002) and *Clostridium perfringens* (Hsieh and Smith 2003). Olsson (2004) reports that recombinant bacterial A- and B-degrading enzymes have been obtained with characteristics that may ultimately allow the use of this procedure in clinical practice.

Secretors and non-secretors of ABH

The fact that A and B substances are present in the saliva of most A and B individuals ('secretors') was first discovered in 1930 (for references to early papers, see Wiener 1943, p. 275). Approximately 80% of subjects are secretors of ABH.

The secretion of H, A and B is controlled by alleles, *Se* and *se*, of the secretor gene. The term *secretor* is applied to those persons (genotype *SeSe* or *Sese*) who secrete H with or without A and/or B, and does not take into account the presence of Lewis or other blood group substances in the saliva. Thus the saliva of group O secretors contains H and that of group A secretors contains A and H (Morgan and Watkins 1948). In most *non-secretors*, very small amounts of H and, according to the ABO group, of A or B are present in saliva due apparently to a low level of *H-* not *Se*-specified transferase (Betteridge and Watkins 1985); for the difference between *H-* and *Se*-specified transferases, see section on biosynthesis.

The amount of A glycoprotein in the saliva of group A secretors follows a log-normal distribution. The amounts of A and H in the saliva appear to vary independently of one another, although there is a significant correlation between the ratios of A to H amongst siblings (Clarke *et al.* 1960).

H, A and B glycoproteins in saliva are produced predominantly by the submaxillary and sublingual glands (Wolf and Taylor 1964). The greatest amounts of A glycoprotein were found in saliva from the sublingual and lip mucous glands and there was negligible activity in parotid saliva (Milne and Dawes 1973).

Group-specific glycoproteins have been found in seminal fluid, tears, sweat, urine, digestive juices, bile, milk, pleural, pericardial and peritoneal fluids, amniotic fluid and in the fluids of hydroceles and ovarian cysts (Wiener 1943, p. 271). The amounts in different secretions of the same individual vary widely.

A, B and H substances in serum

Moss (1910) showed that group A serum contains a substance that will inhibit the haemolytic properties of an anti-A serum, and Schiff (1924) demonstrated the presence of A substance in group A serum by immunization experiments in rabbits. Using a radioimmunoassay, A activity was detected in all group A sera tested, with higher levels in A_1 than in A_2, and in secretors than in non-secretors; the highest activity was found in Le(a– b–) secretors (Holburn and Masters 1974a). ABH substances in serum are glycolipids but their cellular origin is unknown. A or B substances are present in the serum of almost all group A or B newborn infants, although the concentration was lower than in adults (Høstrup 1963).

Patients with an increased amount of A or B glycoprotein in their serum have been described: most have had pseudomucinous ovarian cysts, glycoprotein from which is presumed to have entered the bloodstream (for references, see previous editions of this book).

The inhibitory power of A in plasma increases on storage (Michel 1964), due apparently to the shedding of microvesicles from the red cell surface; see Chapter 9.

Serum from group O donors inhibits occasional examples of anti-H; all such examples tested by Daniels (1984) showed a preference for type II chains. There is more H in the plasma of O and A_2 subjects than in that of A_1 and A_1B subjects (Rouger *et al.* 1979).

Uptake of A and B substances by group O red cells in vivo. This was first observed in patients of group A or B transfused with group O blood: after some days the O cells became agglutinable by certain group O sera (Renton and Hancock 1962). Similarly, group O red cells exposed *in vitro* to group A glycosphingolipid fractions become agglutinable by anti-A (Tilley *et al.* 1975).

In chimeric twins of groups O and A, it would be expected that in the twin who was genetically A (and a secretor), the 'donor' (group O) cells would have small amounts of A substance on their surface and would be agglutinated by selected O sera. Tests in one such chimeric twin showed this to be the case (Race and Sanger 1975).

A, B and H substances in amniotic fluid. Soluble A, B and H substances are found in amniotic fluid from about the ninth week of gestation onwards, and are derived from the fetus; according to several authors they are found only when the fetus is a secretor (e.g. Przestwor 1964; Harper *et al.* 1971), although small amounts have been found in non-secretors (Høstrup 1964). Blood group substances corresponding to the maternal ABO group may be found if care is not taken to exclude cells from the fluid examined.

A, B and H on leucocytes, platelets, other cells and bacteria

Granulocytes. Despite earlier reports to the contrary, it seems that A, B and H cannot be detected on human granulocytes (Dunstan *et al.* 1985a).

Lymphocytes. A and B are present on lymphocytes and are detectable by lymphocytotoxicity tests. These antigens, like Lewis antigens, are acquired from the plasma, and thus are most readily detected on the lymphocytes of individuals whose plasma contains relatively large amounts of A or B glycolipid (Rachkewich *et al.* 1978).

Platelets. At least part of the A, B and H antigens detectable on platelets is acquired by adsorption of glycolipids from plasma (Kools *et al.* 1981; Kelton *et al.* 1982). However, in addition to type 1 H, representing passively acquired antigen, type 2 H can also be detected on platelets and is presumably synthesized by the cells themselves (Dunstan *et al.* 1985b). The distribution of ABH antigens on platelets was shown to be heterogeneous by fluorescence flow cytometry (Dunstan and Simpson 1985). Antigen A expression on platelets is found in donors with the A_1 phenotype on red cells and the intensity of expression varies considerably between donors but is constant for a given donor. Individuals with an A_2 red cell phenotype lack A and H antigens on their platelets (Cooling *et al.* 2004).

Other cells. The presence of A and B antigens has been demonstrated on epidermal cells, cells of amniotic fluid, sinusoidal cells of the spleen and spermatozoa, as well as in the cell walls of the endothelium of capillaries, veins and arteries. In non-secretors, A and B are demonstrable only in the deeper layers of the gastric mucosa, but in secretors they are also demonstrable in glands, goblet cells and secreting surface epithelia (for references, see eighth edition).

The amount of ABH-active glycolipids in parenchymatous organs (liver, spleen, kidney) is about the same as in red cells, whereas the amount in glandular tissues (pancreas, gastric mucosa) is larger (see Watkins 1980). Some cells, such as vascular endothelial and biliary cells, are rich in ABH as well as in HLA antigens, whereas other cells such as the hepatocytes are totally devoid of them. These differences in antigen distribution may be important in graft rejection (Rouger *et al.* 1982).

In embryos of 5- to 60-mm crown–rump length, A, B and H have been found on all epithelial cells except those of the central nervous system, and on all endothelial cells (Szulman 1965).

A and B antigens on bacteria. Schiff (1934) first showed unequivocally that a bacterium (*Shigella shigae*) had blood group activity, after growing it in a medium free from blood group substances. Springer and co-workers (1962) tested approximately 300 strains of bacteria and found that about half of them had A, B or H activity.

Antibodies of the ABO system

The common occurrence of naturally occurring antibodies reacting with antigens of the ABO, Hh, Ii, Lewis and P systems is doubtless related to the fact that these antigens are widely distributed in nature, for example in animals other than humans and in bacteria. The antibodies tend to be IgM cold agglutinins; they activate complement and, when active at 37°C, are often lytic.

Anti-A and anti-B

If A is absent from a person's red cells, anti-A agglutinins are found in the serum, and if B is absent from a person's red cells the serum contains anti-B agglutinins (see Table 4.1). The titre of the agglutinins varies considerably in different sera and appears to have a lognormal distribution. The titre recorded is affected by the red cell phenotype (e.g. A_1 or A_2), by the concentration of red cells in the final mixture, by the time and temperature of incubation and by the technique of reading the endpoint. There is usually a wider range of titres for anti-A (e.g. 8–2048) than for anti-B (e.g. 8–256).

In white people, anti-A titres tend to be higher than anti-B titres, either when comparing group B with group A subjects or when comparing the titres of the two antibodies in group O subjects. The anti-A titre tends to be higher in group O subjects than in group B subjects, and the anti-B titre to be higher in O than in A (Ichikawa 1959). In black people, anti-A and anti-B titres tend to be higher than in white people, and anti-B titres are almost as high as anti-A titres (Grundbacher 1976). In a series of Nigerian donors, although anti-A agglutinin titres were higher than those of anti-B, haemolytic activity was more commonly anti-B than anti-A (Worlledge *et al.* 1974). It is possible that the differences in strength and haemolytic characteristics of ABO antibodies are more strongly correlated with environmental factors than with race; a recent study of donors living in the UK failed to show any significant differences between black, white and Asian people (Redman *et al.* 1990).

Except in AB subjects, complete absence of anti-A and anti-B is very rare in healthy subjects. Race and Sanger (1975) refer to only three cases of missing anti-A or anti-B for which no cause could be found. Extremely weak anti-B was presumably present in the three healthy group A subjects described by van Loghem and colleagues (1965), as, although no antibody could be detected serologically, the survival of group B cells was shortened: $T_{50}Cr$ of 10, 20 and 21 days compared with 29 ± 3.5 days in normal subjects.

Anti-A and anti-B are often present in very low concentration in patients with hypogammaglobulinaemia and are absent in the rare X-linked Wiskott–Aldrich syndrome. Boys with this syndrome are unable to mount an immune response to polysaccharide antigens and thus have no ABO antibodies; responses to protein antigens are often unimpaired (see Miescher and Müller-Eberhard 1978). The gene affected in Wiskott–Aldrich syndrome encodes WASP, a protein involved in the regulation of cytoskeletal assembly in blood cells. Defects in WASP affect T-lymphocyte function and may also result in impaired T- and B-lymphocyte maturation, thereby accounting for the immune deficiency found in these patients (Park et al. 2004). Anti-A and anti-B may also be present in very low concentration in patients immunosuppressed by therapy or disease and in patients undergoing intensive plasma exchange.

In chimeras, the presence of a population of red cells of different ABO group may lead to the absence of the corresponding alloantibody; for example, in a chimera that is genetically group O but has a population of A cells, anti-A is absent (see Race and Sanger 1975, p. 526).

Development of anti-A and anti-B

As described in Chapter 3, the only immunoglobulin synthesized in relatively large amounts by the fetus is IgM, and the level of this protein in cord serum is about one-tenth to one-twentieth of that in adult serum.

Anti-A and anti-B present in cord sera are usually IgG and are of maternal origin but, occasionally, they are IgM, synthesized by the fetus. For example, 8 out of 192 unselected infants had an agglutinin in cord serum, which could not have been of maternal origin, for example anti-B in the cord serum of an infant born to a group B mother (Thomaidis et al. 1967). In another series, in 33 selected cases, in all of which it would have been possible to have detected anti-A or anti-B of non-maternal origin, such antibodies were found in seven cases (Chattoraj et al. 1968). In a third series, agglutinins incompatible with maternal red cells were found in 8 out of 44 neonatal sera (Toivanen and Hirvonen 1969).

The production of ABO agglutinins in fetal life appears to be more common in Nigeria: of 50 cord bloods tested using a 'sensitive technique', 40% had IgM anti-A and/or anti-B, which, on the basis of specificity, could not have been of maternal origin (Worlledge et al. 1974).

In most infants, anti-A and anti-B agglutinins (presumably IgM) produced by the infant can first be demonstrated at 3–6 months. In one series of 900 infants, levels at 3 months were 25% as high as those of adults (Godzisz 1979). In another series, 85% of infants had the expected agglutinins at the age of 6 months (Yliruokanen 1948). In a series of 150 group O children, the median anti-A titre was 4 at 3–6 months, 16 at 6–9 months and 64 at 12–18 months. The maximum value (128) was reached in the fifth year. Anti-B titres tended to lag behind, particularly in the first year of life, so that by the age of 12 months, although 30% of O and B children had anti-A titres equal to the adult median value, only 4% of group A children had anti-B titres equal to the median adult level. These findings show that reverse ABO grouping in infants is not worth performing before 6 months of age (Fong et al. 1974).

The titre of anti-A and anti-B agglutinins reaches its maximum at the age of 5–10 years and the level of haemolysins follows a similar pattern, reaching a maximum at 7–8 years. Levels are higher in girls than in boys (Grundbacher 1967).

Several studies have shown a progressive decrease in anti-A and -B agglutinin titres with age, with low levels (titre 4 or less) being common in subjects aged 80 or more (Thomsen and Kettle 1929; Somers and Kuhns 1972; Baumgarten et al. 1976). In more recent studies, on the other hand, agglutinin titres have been found to fall slightly or not at all with age, with median values as high as 64–128 in the tenth decade of life (Petzl and Tanew 1985; Auf der Maur et al. 1993).

The influence of genetic factors on agglutinin titres is unclear. In one series it was found that the difference between dizygotic twins was no greater than that between monozygotic twins (Nijenhuis and Bratlie 1962), although in another, it was concluded that genetic factors played some part (Grundbacher 1976).

Murine monoclonal anti-A and anti-B

Numerous monoclonal anti-A and anti-B have been produced and have proved entirely suitable as blood grouping reagents (see Chapter 8). Anti-H has also been produced (see p. 136). However, some ABO monoclonals cannot be used in absorption/elution tests to classify weak subgroups of A (Zelenski 1986). Also, inhibition tests have shown that monoclonal anti-A varies according to the source of the A immunogen.

IgM, IgG and IgA anti-A and anti-B

In a given serum anti-A may be wholly IgM or partly IgM and partly IgG (Fudenberg et al. 1959), partly IgM and partly IgA or may be made of all three immunoglobulins (Kunkel and Rockey 1963), even in subjects who have had no identifiable stimulus. IgG anti-A and anti-B are found far more commonly in group O than in B or A subjects (Rawson and Abelson, 1960a).

In mixtures containing IgG and IgM anti-A, the IgM antibody can be inactivated by treatment with 2-mercaptoethanol (2-ME) or dithiothreitol (DTT); see Chapter 3. The serological activity of IgA anti-A is reduced but not destroyed by treatment with 2-ME (for references, see eighth edition).

IgG subclasses. Of 42 sera containing IgG anti-A and anti-B, obtained from group O mothers of A or B infants, 39 reacted with subclass antisera; of these, one was solely IgG2 and the remaining 38 were all partly IgG2; the other subclasses present were as follows: IgG1 (19); IgG1 + IgG3 (3); IgG1 + IgG3 + IgG4 (12); and IgG1 + IgG4 (4) (Brouwers et al. 1987).

Complement binding. Both IgM and IgG anti-A may be haemolytic (Rawson and Abelson 1960b). In one investigation all examples of IgG anti-A and about 90% of examples of IgM anti-A were readily haemolytic; the remaining examples of IgG anti-A would haemolyse cells if the test was made sensitive enough (Polley et al. 1963). On the other hand, IgA anti-A is not haemolytic (for references, see eighth edition). Similar results are obtained if complement binding is detected by the use of specific antiglobulin sera (Polley et al. 1963; Adinolfi et al. 1966).

The minimum number of IgM anti-A molecules that, when bound to a group A red cell will activate complement, is not known, but on theoretical grounds might be one (see Chapter 3). The minimum number of IgG anti-A molecules for complement binding is expected to be substantial. Using an anti-C3c reagent

to demonstrate complement binding by the antiglobulin test, a minimum of 14 µg of IgG anti-A /ml red cells was required, corresponding to approximately 7000 molecules of anti-A per cell or very approximately 1% of the maximum number that could be bound (Romano and Mollison 1975). An approximate estimate of the minimum number of IgG anti-A molecules that will cause lysis can be calculated from the data of Ishizaka and co-workers (1968). Making various assumptions about the equilibrium constant of the antibody and the number of antigen sites, the number of antibody molecules required for lysis is of the order of 30 000 per cell (NC Hughes-Jones, personal communication).

Factors affecting haemolysis. Three factors are known to affect antibody-mediated lysis of red cells *in vitro*.
1 *Storage.* Red cells stored as a saline suspension for 1–4 days or as whole blood mixed with ACD for 3 weeks are more easily lysed (e.g. by anti-A) than are fresh cells (Thomsen and Thisted 1928a; Chaplin et al. 1956).
2 *The ratio of serum to red cells.* With a ratio of 20:1 (i.e. two volumes of serum to one volume of a 10% suspension of cells) 58% of group O sera would lyse A_1 cells; with a ratio of 40:1, 90% were lytic; and with a ratio of 200:1 (using a ^{51}Cr-release method), all were lytic (Polley et al. 1963).
3 *The freshness of the serum.* Haemolytic activity diminishes within 1–2 h of taking blood (Thomsen and Thisted 1928b; Kabat and Meyer 1961, p. 136). The highly unusual anti-Rh D serum 'Ripley' was often observed to lyse D-positive red cells only when freshly taken (Waller and Lawler 1962).

Ethnic differences in frequencies of haemolysins. The frequency of strong anti-A lysins (sera giving complete lysis of a 2% red cell suspension) was found to be slightly higher in one series of white people (USA) than in one of black people (Nigeria): 32% vs. 24%. On the other hand, for anti-B the figures were lower in white people: 10% vs. 27% for the Nigerians (Chaplin et al. 1956; Kulkarni et al. 1985). Amongst the Nigerians there were large differences between different ethnic groups. The overall frequency of sera with anti-A or -B lysins or both was 20.4% in Hausas (over 2000), but 60.2% in Yorubas (980) (Kulkarni et al. 1985).

Enhancement by specific antiglobulin serum. If a serum fraction containing only IgG anti-A is titrated, the greatest dilution in which the anti-A can be detected by the indirect antiglobulin technique after adding anti-IgG is found to be about five doubling dilutions greater than the dilution which will agglutinate red cells suspended in saline; for example, a fraction that agglutinates red cells to a titre of 64 will, at a dilution of 2048, sensitize red cells to agglutination by anti-IgG (Polley *et al.* 1965). The use of anti-IgA increases the titre of IgA anti-A by about two doubling dilutions but anti-IgM scarcely enhances agglutination by IgM anti-A at all (Ishizaka *et al.* 1965; Adinolfi *et al.* 1966).

Enhancement of agglutination by serum or plasma. Agglutination produced by IgG anti-A is enhanced in a medium of serum compared with saline, and plasma is considerably more effective than serum. When group A red cells were coated with varying amounts of IgG anti-A, the least amount of anti-A detectable by agglutination in plasma was about 0.5 μg/ml of cells, which was about the same as when they were tested with antiglobulin serum; however, the least amount detectable by agglutination in serum was 2.2–3.0 μg/ml of cells (Romano and Mollison 1975).

Inhibitory effect of A substance. As a rule, IgM anti-A is more readily inhibited than IgG anti-A (Witebsky 1948; Kochwa *et al.* 1961). To obtain an equivalent reduction in agglutinin titre the amount of purified human A substance required to inhibit IgG anti-A was found to be 20 times that required to inhibit IgM anti-A, although occasional exceptions were encountered by Polley and co-workers (1963). The difference between IgM and IgG antibodies seems to be due to the fact that, when reacting with A and B glycoproteins in solution, IgM anti-A and anti-B have higher binding constants than corresponding IgG antibodies, presumably because IgM combines multivalently with a single glycoprotein molecule in solution (Holburn and Masters 1974b). In the ease with which it is inhibited by A glycoprotein IgA is intermediate between IgM and IgG anti-A (Rawson and Abelson 1964; Adinolfi *et al.* 1966).

Thermal optimum. Naturally occurring anti-A and anti-B react more strongly at 4°C than at 37°C. By contrast, immune sera react equally well at 37°C and at 4°C (Wiener 1941). IgG anti-A (in 2-ME-treated serum) agglutinates untreated or papain-treated red cells as well at 37°C as at 4°C (Voak *et al.* 1973).

Effect of heating. Heating a serum at 56°C for 3 h has no measurable effect on the titre of IgG or IgA anti-A but leads to a distinct fall in IgM anti-A titre (Adinolfi *et al.* 1966).

Anti-A and anti-B in colostrum and saliva. The titre of anti-A and anti-B tends to be higher in colostrum than in plasma from the same woman; alloagglutinins in colostrum are often wholly IgA but some IgM antibody may be present (for references, see eighth edition).

Anti-A in low concentrations is present in the saliva of most group O and group B subjects (Adinolfi *et al.* 1966). Anti-B is found a little less commonly than anti-A and is less common in group A than in group O subjects (Denborough and Downing 1969).

Concentration and equilibrium constants of IgM and IgG anti-A and anti-B

Concentrations needed to produce agglutination. It has been concluded that to bring about 50% agglutination of a suspension of group A red cells, only 25 IgM anti-A molecules per cell are required, but for IgG anti-A the number is 20 000 (Greenbury *et al.* 1963). The minimal concentration of anti-A required for agglutination (i.e. at the endpoint of a titre) has been estimated to be, for IgG, 0.2 μg/ml, and for IgM, 0.01 μg/ml (Economidou *et al.* 1967a); taking into account that the molecular weight of IgM is five times that of IgG, the agglutinating effect of IgM is thus approximately 100 times as great as that of IgG.

Equilibrium constants. Examples of both human and rabbit IgM and IgG anti-A were investigated by Economidou and co-workers (1967a). Equilibrium constants ranged from 0.6 to 13.0×10^8 l/mol, but on average were approximately the same for IgM antibodies as for IgG. Monomers prepared from IgM anti-B were tested by Economidou and co-workers (1967b) and found to have an equilibrium constant 36–170 times lower than that of the whole IgM molecule, providing further support for the idea that native IgM anti-B (and anti-A) is attached to red cells by at least two binding sites. The authors concluded that with both IgM and IgG anti-B more than one antigen–antibody bond must be broken simultaneously to permit dissociation of the antibody.

The question whether IgG anti-A and anti-B normally bind to A and B sites bivalently or univalently does not seem to have been resolved. There is evidence for bivalent binding (Greenbury *et al.* 1965; Romans *et al.* 1980) and for univalent binding (Romano *et al.* 1983). Antibody concentration may determine which mode of binding predominates (see comment in footnote to Table 4.3). In any case, some IgG antibody molecules must bind univalently to each cell or there would be no agglutination.

The association constant of rabbit IgG anti-A was found to have the following values: with A_1 cells, 7.4×10^8 l/mol; with A_1B cells, 5.1×10^8 l/mol; and with A_2 cells, 2.1×10^8 l/mol. Anti-A was found to dissociate three times more rapidly from A_2 than from A_1 cells (Economidou and Hughes-Jones 1967).

The binding constant of human IgG anti-A for cord A_1 red cells was found to be 3.3×10^7 l/mol compared with $5.7–8.7 \times 10^7$ l/mol for adult A_1 red cells and that for cord A_1B red cells to be 2.1×10^7 l/mol compared with $3.2–7.0 \times 10^7$ l/mol for adult A_1B red cells (Economidou 1966).

Exposure to A and B antigens in early life. The mother's ABO group was found to have no influence on the serological characteristics (agglutinin titre, haemolytic activity, etc.) of anti-A in her offspring (Kennell and Muschel 1956).

Crossreacting anti-A,B

Moss (1910) found that absorption with A or B cells could reduce the titre of group O serum against both A and B cells, and Landsteiner and Witt (1926) showed that some of the antibody in group O serum behaved as anti-AB; thus, the eluate made from A cells previously incubated with group O serum agglutinated both B and A cells. Similarly, the reaction of group O serum with B cells is inhibited by the saliva of A or B secretors and the reaction with A cells is inhibited by the saliva of B or A secretors.

Anti-A,B in group O serum is presumably an antibody directed against a structure common to A and B (Owen 1954). This conclusion is supported by the observation that the antibody can be completely inhibited with either D-galactose or *N*-acetylgalactosamine (Holburn 1976), which are structurally similar (see section on biosynthesis).

Crossreacting anti-A,B can be either IgG or IgM and can probably also be IgA: very little anti-A,B can be demonstrated in the serum of an unimmunized group O subject (Yokoyama and Fudenberg 1964). Crossreacting anti-A,B increased in concentration in all six group O subjects who were immunized with blood group substances (Contreras *et al.* 1983) and it was easier to demonstrate its presence if the cells used for absorption and elution were of a different specificity from that of the glycoprotein used for immunization (Dodd *et al.* 1967; Contreras *et al.* 1983). The role of anti-A,B in haemolytic disease of the newborn is discussed in Chapter 12.

Crossreacting anti-A,B may be cytotoxic for the lymphocytes of group A secretors (for references, see seventh edition, p. 281). Many monoclonal antibodies with anti-A,B specificity have been described (Messeter *et al.* 1984; Moore *et al.* 1984; Guest *et al.* 1992).

Anti-A_1

If serum from a B or O person is absorbed once or twice with A_2 cells it will no longer agglutinate A_2 cells but will still agglutinate A_1 cells. On the other hand if B or O serum is absorbed with A_1 cells it will no longer react with A_1 or with A_2 cells. Accordingly, B (or O) serum is regarded as containing two separate populations of antibody molecules: anti-A reacting both with A_2 and with A_1 cells, and anti-A_1 reacting only with A_1 cells. The anti-A_1 has a lower thermal range than the anti-A (Friedenreich 1931). If an excess of A_2 cells is used in absorbing group B serum, anti-A_1 as well as anti-A may be absorbed (Lattes and Cavazutti 1924).

When tested at room temperature, anti-A_1 was found in 1–2% of A_2 bloods and in 25% of A_2B bloods in one study (Taylor *et al.* 1942); in 22% of A_2B bloods in another (Juel 1959), and in 7.9% in A_2 bloods and 35% in A_2B bloods in another (Speieser *et al.* 1951). Anti-A_1 in A_2 and A_2B subjects is usually inactive at 37°C.

Anti-A_1 is very rare in infants; only one example was found in examining 10 000 blood samples (Speiser 1956).

As expected, anti-A_1 in an A_2B serum proved to be wholly IgM but, perhaps surprisingly, anti-A_1 separated from group O serum by absorption with A_2 cells was found to be wholly IgG (Plischka and Schäfer 1972). An example of anti-A_1 that became active at 37°C after a series of transfusions was partly IgG and partly IgM (Lundberg and McGinniss 1975).

Two kinds of anti-A_1 can be recognized: the first, which is the commoner, reacts with A_1 red cells independently of their Ii group and is inhibited by the saliva of group A secretors; the second is anti-AI, which does not react with A_1i cells and is not inhibited by the saliva of group A secretors.

Clinical significance of anti-A_1. Most examples of anti-A_1 found in A_2 or A_2B subjects agglutinate A_1 cells only up to a temperature of 25°C or so and are of no clinical significance. Antibodies which are active *in vitro* at about 30°C but only dubiously active at 37°C will bring about the destruction of a proportion of A_1 cells *in vivo* when a small dose of cells is injected (see Chapter 10). Those antibodies that are only dubiously active at 37°C would almost certainly fail to produce detectable red cell destruction following the transfusion of therapeutic quantities of blood. On the other hand, in several instances in which anti-A_1 has been quite clearly active at 37°C, extensive destruction of A_1 cells *in vivo* has been recorded (see below). Such cases are extremely rare.

It appears that following the transfusion of A_1 cells to patients whose serum contains anti-A_1, there is usually no increase in the thermal range of the anti-A_1 (see Stratton 1955), but a few examples of the development of anti-A_1, active at 37°C, have been described (e.g. Jakobowicz *et al.* 1961; Lundberg and McGinniss 1975). References to haemolytic transfusion reactions due to anti-A_1 are given in Chapter 11.

Anti-A_1 passively transferred to A_2 or A_2B recipients by the transfusion of group O blood may cause the destruction of subsequently transfused A_1 or A_1B red cells; see Chapter 11.

Anti-A_1 may develop in the serum of group A_2 subjects who have received a tissue graft from a group O donor 1 week or so previously; see Chapter 11.

Anti-A and anti-B as autoantibodies

Anti-A and anti-B are sometimes found as autoantibodies (see Chapter 7). Anti-A or anti-B 'pseudo-autoantibodies' may be found in A, B or AB subjects who have recently received a group O bone marrow or solid organ transplant (see Chapter 11).

Anti-A_1 has been found as an autoantibody, reacting weakly at room temperature, in a patient of group A_1 without haemolytic anaemia. The auto-anti-A_1 reacted with adult A_1i red cells and was inhibited by group A secretor saliva (Wright *et al.* 1980).

Anomalous occurrence of anti-A and anti-B. Occasionally, anti-A and anti-B are found in A or B subjects, respectively, but not as autoagglutinins, i.e. with a specificity which differs from normal anti-A or anti-B. A few examples of anti-A of this kind have been found in A_1 subjects (M Stroup, personal communication). As mentioned above, the serum from most cis AB people contains allo-anti-B.

In a group A_1B subject whose serum agglutinated group B red cells, although not her own cells, the B-specified transferase was shown to be abnormal (Yoshida *et al.* 1981).

Anti-H and anti-HI

'Pure' anti-H is a very uncommon antibody; it is found in subjects of the very rare phenotype O_h as a haemolysin, and as an agglutinin which is almost as active at 37°C as at O°C. Although usually IgM, it may be partly IgG (Haddad 1974). In rare cases, anti-H may also be found in A_1 subjects (Gouge *et al.* 1977).

The 'normal incomplete cold antibody' has anti-H specificity and is neutralized by secretor saliva; see Chapter 7.

The name 'anti-H' used to be applied to an alloagglutinin found not uncommonly in sera from A_1 and A_1B donors (see Morgan and Watkins 1948), but the name was changed to anti-HI after it had been shown that the antibody reacted only with red cells carrying both H and I specificities (Rosenfield *et al.* 1964). Anti-HI, like anti-H, reacts most strongly with O red cells and most weakly with A_1B cells. Voak and co-workers (1968) mentioned that all examples of anti-HI that they had found were in women, most of whom were pregnant. Their findings were made impressive by their mention of the fact that more than 90 000 samples from males were tested each year.

Potent anti-HI is found invariably in the serum of O_{hm}^A and O_{hm}^B people.

An example of anti-H (possibly -HI), which in the presence of sodium azide (0.1% w/v) reacted strongly at 37°C, but in the absence of azide reacted only weakly and only in the cold, has been encountered (P Watson, personal communication, 1981). The effect of the azide appeared to be due to some interaction with plasma protein rather than with the red cell membrane. An autoagglutinin enhanced by azide is mentioned in Chapter 7.

Anti-A, -A$_1$, -B and -H lectins

A highly potent anti-A can be extracted from the albumin gland or the eggs of various species of snail, for example *Helix aspersa, Helix hortensis, Helix pomatia, Otala lactea* and *Cepaea nemoralis* (for references, see eighth edition).

Some snail anti-A extracts react equally well with A$_1$ and A$_2$ red cells, although others do not and still others react equally well with A$_1$ and A$_2$ cells but less strongly with A$_2$B. The different specificities of the anti-A from different snails can be indicated by referring to them, for example, as anti-A$_{HP}$, for *H. pomatia*. Anti-A purified from the albumin gland of *H. pomatia* was found to be a fairly homogeneous protein with a molecular weight of 100 kDa; from the point of view of specificity, it was more homogeneous than human anti-A (Hammarström and Kabat 1969). Snail anti-A reactions are enormously enhanced with bromelin-treated red cells.

Useful anti-B can be prepared from the fungus *Fomes fomentarius* (Mäkelä *et al.* 1959).

Reagents with the specificity anti-H can be obtained from four plants: *Ulex europaeus, Cytisus sessilifolius, Laburnum alpinum* and *Lotus tetragonolobus. Ulex* extract is the most commonly used reagent for determining secretor status by testing inhibition by saliva. The extract reacts about equally well with HI as with Hi red cells, whereas extracts from the other three plants mentioned tend to react more strongly with HI cells (Voak and Lodge 1971). The extract from *L. tetragonolobus* does not react with type I chains and is therefore unsuitable for testing for H in secretions (Pereira and Kabat 1974).

Immune responses to A and B antigens

Incompatible transfusions

If A blood is injected intravenously into a person of group B or group O, or B blood is injected into a person of group A or group O, the titre of anti-A or anti-B increases after an initial fall due to absorption of antibody (Wiener 1941).

An immune response following the transfusion of ABO-incompatible blood can be inferred from a case in which a boy aged 6 years received two transfusions from his father at an interval of 18 days. The first transfusion was without incident but the second

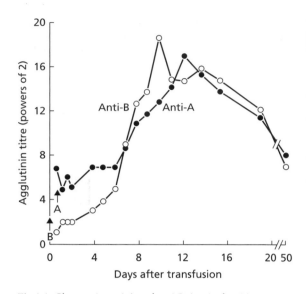

Fig 4.1 Changes in anti-A and anti-B titre (as log$_2$) in a group O patient after the transfusion of 360 ml of group B blood (at 'B') and of group A serum (at 'A'). These titrations and those recorded in Fig. 4.2 were performed by the standard technique of making doubling dilutions, using the same unrinsed pipette, and were not checked by making direct dilutions (from the data of Mollison and Young 1941).

produced a severe haemolytic reaction. It was now found that the father was group B and the child group O. Direct matching before the first transfusion had not revealed incompatibility, and it may be presumed that at that time the child had only a low titre of anti-B. Because of the success of the first transfusion, it was considered unnecessary to carry out a direct matching test before the second transfusion, although had the test been repeated the incompatibility would presumably have been obvious (Thalheimer 1921).

In a case illustrated in Fig. 4.1, the patient (group O) received 360 ml of group B blood; 8 h after transfusion, the anti-B titre was only 2 compared with an anti-A titre of 128. After 48 h the anti-B titre started to increase, and between the sixth and tenth days it rose very rapidly to a peak. It then fell slowly and had still not reached a stable level 3 weeks after transfusion. After the transfusion of incompatible blood the peak titre of anti-A or anti-B is usually reached after about 9–12 days (Boorman *et al.* 1945; Fig. 4.2). Although an increase in agglutinin titre is common after the transfusion of ABO-incompatible blood it is by no means invariable; it was noted in only 6 out of 15

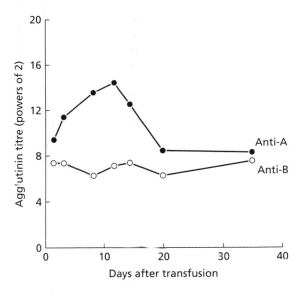

Fig 4.2 Changes in anti-A and anti-B agglutinin titre in a group O patient after the transfusion of 45 ml of group A blood (data from Mollison 1943).

group O subjects after the i.v. injection of 25 ml of A_1 or A_2 blood (Wiener et al. 1953a).

An initial decrease in titre, after the transfusion of ABO-incompatible blood was observed in several of the subjects receiving only 25 ml of blood, referred to above, and has even been noted after the injection of as little as 4 ml of incompatible red cells (see Chapter 10).

Intramuscular injections of incompatible blood. In a series in which subjects received four to six injections, each of 10–15 ml of a 50% suspension of twice-washed red cells, some group O or B subjects who had received A red cells developed powerful anti-A haemolysins, although no changes in agglutinin titre were observed (Thomsen 1930). The development of haemolysins has also been noted following i.m. injections of blood (Rapoport and Stokes 1937).

During an epidemic of poliomyelitis, the prophylactic value of i.m. injections of blood was investigated; 60 ml of blood were taken from one or other of a child's parents and injected into the child's buttocks. Among 1341 children, 52 showed a reaction that followed a characteristic pattern: some 6 days after the injection the child became acutely ill and febrile; the sites of injection became hot, red and painful. The reaction subsided after 3–4 days. In 17 cases the blood

groups of the child and its parents were investigated; in every case the parent's cells were incompatible with the child's serum. In 13 out of 17 cases in which the test was made within 4 weeks of injection, the child's serum haemolysed the parent's cells. In one case, a child who had had a reaction was given a second injection of blood some months later; in this case, the second reaction developed only 28 h after the injection (Rapoport and Stokes 1937).

Solid organ transplants. Except for bone marrow transplantation, where ABO incompatibility can be dealt with by depleting the donor bone marrow of red cells or by lowering the titre of anti-A and anti-B in the recipient by plasma exchange, organ transplantation across the ABO barrier often leads to vascular or humoral hyperacute graft rejection (Cooper 1990; for further discussion, see Chapter 14).

Injections of human blood group substances

The A and B group-specific substances are present in the plasma and serum. Even when the substances cannot be detected serologically, they may provoke an immune response following the transfusion of serum to a suitable recipient (e.g. A to O). The peak of the immune response is usually reached at about 10–15 days after the transfusion (Aubert et al. 1942; see also Fig. 4.1). Immune responses to A have also been produced by injecting saliva (Wiener et al. 1953b) and urine (Freda et al. 1957).

Cryoprecipitates and factor IX concentrates may also stimulate the production of 'immune' anti-A and anti-B (McShine and Kunst 1970).

Using a purified preparation of human A substance, substantial increases in titre and avidity of anti-A were found after injecting 1.5-mg doses of the preparation; 0.1 mg appeared to be a suboptimal dose (Polley et al. 1963; Contreras et al. 1983).

Alloimmunization by A and B antigens during pregnancy

The term 'ABO-incompatible' may conveniently be used to describe a pregnancy in which the infant's red cells carry A or B, and the mother's serum contains the corresponding antibody. Dienst (1905) first observed that, following such pregnancies, after delivery there might be a rise in the mother's anti-A or anti-B agglutinin titre. In an investigation in which tests were made only for anti-A or anti-B haemolysins, the incidence in recently delivered group O women was 14.5%, compared with 3.5% in a control series of group O males. In relation to the group of infants born to the mothers, the incidence of haemolysins was as follows: O infants, 7.1%; B infants, 20.8%; and A infants, 28.1% (Jonsson 1936).

After delivery, most commonly between 10 and 20 days, there is a rise in the titre of anti-A or anti-B agglutinins in most women who have given birth to an infant with ABO-incompatible red cells (Boorman et al. 1945). There is evidence that those infants who fail to stimulate an immune response are non-secretors (Smith 1945).

Injections of purified group-specific substances of animal origin

An experiment made by Forssman (1911) revealed the existence of serologically related substances in animals widely separated in the zoological system: the injection of extracts of guinea pig organs into rabbits provoked the formation of lysins active against sheep red cells. Subsequently, the name 'Forssman antigen' was used for any substance that would stimulate the formation of sheep haemolysin. The sheep antibody produced in this way is an example of a 'heterophil' antibody; the cardinal feature of such an antibody is that it is produced by an animal in response to contact with an antigen from a different species. It is the antibody that is heterophil, not the antigenic determinant; the antigens are identical or related (Franks and Coombs 1969).

Human A antigen is closely related to the Forssman antigen; in both, the terminal sugar is N-acetylgalactosamine. A proposed structure of the Forssman antigen (Siddiqui and Hakomori 1971) is included in the footnote to Fig. 4.3. on p. 131).

In the past, hog A substance and equine AB substance were used for stimulating the production of potent anti-A or anti-B in human volunteers and for neutralizing anti-A and anti-B in group O plasma, but animal group-specific substances are no longer considered suitable for use in humans.

Injections of vaccines containing hog pepsin. Increases in anti-A or anti-B concentration following the injection of diphtheria or tetanus toxoid are due to the presence of hog pepsin in the preparation. Tetanus

toxoid prepared in a medium free from peptone of animal origin does not cause rises in anti-A or anti-B titre (Hendry and Sickles 1951).

Injections of pneumococcal or influenza vaccine. Substantial rises in anti-A titre have been found in patients receiving certain batches of pneumococcal vaccine. The effect appeared to be due to A-like substances from culture media tightly bound to bacterial polysaccharide (Noël 1981; Siber et al. 1982). Similarly, injections of influenza virus vaccine may stimulate anti-A, due to the incorporation of A-like substances present in the cytoplasm of the chick embryo on which the virus is grown (Springer and Tritel 1962; Springer and Schuster 1964).

Clinical significance of stimulation of anti-A and anti-B by vaccines, etc.

The practical importance of injections of vaccine containing hog pepsin in rendering group O donors 'dangerous' was shown by Dausset and Vidal (1951); they described six haemolytic reactions following the transfusion of O blood to A recipients; in every case the donor had received injections of vaccine known to contain hog pepsin. In most cases the donors had received the injections within the previous 3 months, but in two instances it was shown that the immune characteristics of the donor's anti-A persisted for at least 7 years after the last injection. In a case described in Chapter 11 of a severe haemolytic transfusion reaction in a group A patient following the transfusion of group O blood, 1 month before giving blood the donor had received an injection of anti-tetanus serum prepared by digestion with hog pepsin. It seems logical to conclude that stimulation of anti-A in group O women following the injection of vaccines, etc. containing A-like substances must also lead to the production of potent IgG anti-A and thus increase the risk that any A infants born subsequently will be affected by haemolytic disease of the newborn. In fact, there is virtually no evidence of the magnitude of the risk. One survey suggested that the offspring of women who had received injections of tetanus toxoid during the last trimester of pregnancy had an increased risk of developing ABO haemolytic disease (Gupte and Bhatia 1980) but the control group was not strictly comparable.

In a study of 11 moderately severe cases of haemolytic disease of the newborn due to ABO

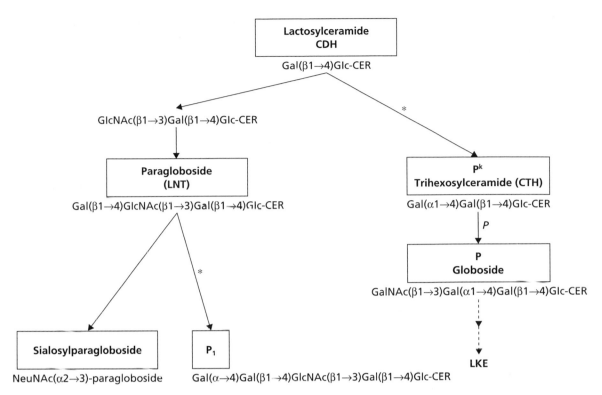

Fig 4.3 Biosynthetic pathways of the p^k, P and P_1 glycolipid antigens (adapted from Watkins 1980). Abbreviations: CER (ceramide), N-acylsphingosine; Gal, D-galactose; GalNAc, N-acetyl-D-galactosamine; Glc, D-glucose; GlcNAc, N-acetyl-D-glucosamine; NeuNAc, N-acetylneuraminic acid.

The Forssman antigen is globoside with a terminal αGalNAc linked to the βGalNac. *An α-galactosyl-transferase is required (or possibly two transferases) for the synthesis of p^k and P_1 antigens from different precursors.

incompatibility, not one of the mothers gave a history of having had injections of bacterial vaccines or toxoids (Crawford *et al.* 1953).

Toxocara infection. Emulsified toxocara worms inhibit anti-A and anti-B; infected children commonly have high titres of these antibodies (Heiner and Kevy 1956; Shrand 1964).

ABH antigens acquired by viruses. Measles virus cultured *in vitro* will take on the ABH status of the host cell in which it is grown. These ABH-active virus particles can then be neutralized by natural ABO antibodies in a complement-dependent manner (Preece *et al.* 2002). These results suggest that virus particles produced in infected group A individuals would be susceptible to neutralization by the natural anti-A of group B and O individuals.

IgM, IgG and IgA anti-A and anti-B in relation to immune responses

In group B subjects, before and after stimulation with A substance, IgM anti-A predominates. In group O subjects, even before stimulation, some of the anti-A may be IgG; after stimulation, IgG anti-A as well as IgM anti-A is produced in most subjects (Abelson and Rawson 1961; Kochwa *et al.* 1961).

In an investigation of the effect of injecting purified human A substance into five normal B subjects, no IgG anti-A could be detected before antigenic stimulation; after two injections, each of 1.5 mg, at an interval of 1 week, low-titre IgG anti-A was produced in three out of the five subjects, but in no case was this antibody readily haemolytic. In four out of the five the titre of IgM anti-A increased. Of five O subjects who were stimulated in the same way, three had IgG anti-A

131

before stimulation and all five had IgG anti-A after stimulation (Polley *et al.* 1963).

Most sera containing IgA anti-A have come from subjects who have recently received an antigenic stimulus (Kunkel and Rockey 1963; lshizaka *et al.* 1965), although in a few group O subjects IgA anti-A or anti-B are found before immunization (Contreras *et al.* 1983).

Persistence of immune anti-A. After an injection of hog A substance or horse A and B substances, the peak level of antibody tended to be maintained for many months. There was then a steady fall, but even after 12 months the level was still about 50% of the peak (Allen and Kabat 1958). In blood donors whose serum contained anti-A or anti-B haemolysins, repeated tests during a 2-year period showed that these antibodies persisted in 80% of subjects (Tovey 1958).

The Lewis system

The Lewis blood group system differs from most of the other human blood group systems in some important ways. First, it is a system of soluble antigens present in saliva and plasma (Grubb 1951) and red cells acquire their Lewis phenotype by adsorbing Lewis substances from the plasma (Sneath and Sneath 1955). Second, the Lewis phenotype of the red cells is influenced by the ABH secretor status (although the Lewis genes and secretor genes are inherited independently); subjects who inherit *Le* will have the red cell phenotype Le(a+ b–) if they are a non-secretor (*sese*), but the phenotype Le(a– b+) if they are secretors (*Sese* or *SeSe*) (Grubb 1951; Ceppellini 1955). Third, as the products of *ABH* and *Le* share the same precursor substrate, the Lewis phenotype may be modified by the ABO phenotype;

for example, A_1 may decrease the expression of Le^b (Andresen 1948) and also of Le^a (Cutbush *et al.* 1956). The biochemical basis of the Lewis system and the relationship between the Lewis and ABH antigens are described in later sections.

The Lewis groups of adults

For details, see Table 4.4.

The phenotype Le(a– b+)

Subjects with the phenotype Le(a– b+) have the alleles *Se* and *Le* and their secretions contain H, Le^a and Le^b glycoproteins (and A or B, if the subject is group A or B).

The plasma of Le(a– b+) persons contains predominantly Le^b glycosphingolipid but also some Le^a. The amount of Le^a in the saliva of Le(a– b+) subjects is substantially less than in that of Le(a+ b–) subjects.

The amount of Le^b-active glycolipid in the plasma of 35 group O, Le(a– b+) subjects was estimated to be 0.9 μg/ml; no Le^b was present in the plasma of group O, Le(a+ b–) and Le(a– b–) subjects. About one-third of the total Le^b-active glycolipid in whole blood was associated with the red cells, the rest being in the plasma (Rohr *et al.* 1980).

As discussed later, there are two main types of anti-Le^b: anti-Le^{bH} (anti-HLe^b), reacting preferentially with cells carrying Le^b and abundant H (i.e. group O and A_2 Le(a– b+) cells); and anti-Le^{bL}, reacting with Le(b+) cells regardless of ABH groups.

The phenotype Le(a+ b+)

In white people, the red cells of O and A_2 subjects who have the alleles *Se* and *Le* react not only with anti-Le^b,

Red cell phenotype	Genotype	Lewis substance in saliva	H substance in saliva	Frequency in white people (approx.)
Le(a–b+)	*Se, Le*	$Le^b + Le^a$	+	75
Le(a+b–)	*sese, Le*	Le^a	–	20
Le(a–b–)*	*Se, lele*	–	+	4
Le(a–b–)[†]	*sese, lele*	–	–	1

Table 4.4 Lewis groups of adults.

* Apart from intrinsic type 2 H, red cells carry type 1 H (previously called Le^d), taken up from the plasma and also present in the saliva.
[†] Red cells carry Le^c, taken up from the plasma and also present in the saliva.

but also, although only weakly, with some examples of anti-Le^a; this latter reaction may be demonstrable only by the indirect antiglobulin test (IAT). If the Le(b+) cells are first enzyme treated, most if not all samples of O and A_2 cells appear to be Le(a+ b+) (Cutbush et al. 1956). The reaction between anti-Le^a and group O, Le(a+ b+) red cells can be inhibited by Le(a+ b–) plasma in vitro (Cutbush et al. 1956) and in vivo (Mollison et al. 1963). In AI Le(b+) adults no reaction of the red cells with anti-Le^a can be demonstrated, probably because less Le^a substance is made as the result of competition between the A_1- and Le-transferases for substrate.

The phenotype Le(a+ b+), with strong Le^a, is common in Australian Aborigines, Indonesians, Japanese, Polynesians and Taiwanese (for references, see Yu et al. 1955; Henry et al. 1996a). In these subjects, Le^b can be detected only with certain potent anti-Le^b reagents (mainly monoclonal antibodies). The weak expression of Le^b is due to the presence in double dose of a weak Se (FUT2) allele, Se^w, characterized by a missense mutation at nucleotide 385 (Yu et al. 1955; Henry et al. 1996b).

The phenotype Le(a+ b–)

Persons belonging to this phenotype have Le^a substance in their plasma and in their saliva, and their red cells are agglutinated by anti-Le^a. They are non-secretors of ABH.

Great variation is found between the reactions of Le(a+ b–) cells from different O donors, as judged by their degree of agglutination in an antiglobulin test after exposure to anti-Le^a at 37°C (Mollison and Cutbush 1955). Agglutination tests at room temperature apparently fail to detect these differences.

Le(a+ b–) red cells do not react with anti-Le^b either in vitro or in vivo, showing that they have no Le^b antigen. Thus in a patient of group AB, Le(a– b–) with potent anti-Le^b in her serum who was given test injections of O, Le(a– b+) and O, Le(a+ b–) red cells, more than 80% of the Le(b+) red cells were destroyed within 6 min of injection, but the Le(a+ b–) red cells underwent no destruction (see fourth edition, p. 274).

The phenotype Le(a– b–)

Subjects of genotype lele have red cells of the phenotype Le(a– b–) that react either with anti-Le^c or with

anti-type I H (previously anti-Le^d). The genotype lele is more than three times commoner in black than in white people.

Subjects of phenotype Le(a– b–) were previously subdivided into Le(c+ d–) or Le(c– d+), according to whether they had Le^c or Le^d in their saliva and plasma. The status of Le^c and Le^d is described below, under anti-Le^c and -Le^d.

Subjects of the genotype lele have traces of Le^a in their serum (Holburn 1973) and saliva (Grubb 1951; Arcilla and Sturgeon 1973), and have traces of readily detectable Lewis antigens in tissues such as colon and bladder (Ørntoft et al. 1991).

Phenotype frequencies in races other than white people

The phenotype Le(a– b–) is substantially commoner in black people than in white people: approximately 25% compared with 8%; and the phenotype Le(a– b+) is less common in black than in white people: 54% compared with 71% (see Daniels, 1995). The frequency of ABH secretors in Australian Aborigines and Polynesians is 98% and the Le(a+ b–) phenotype is absent or rare. On the other hand, many subjects have a weak secretor gene, Se^w (see above); evidently, conversion of Le^a to Le^b is incomplete and both racial groups have a high frequency of the red cell phenotype Le(a+ b+) (Vos and Comley 1967; Henry et al. 1990). Findings in Chinese are similar (Broadberry and Lin-Chu 1991; Lin and Shieh 1994).

Lewis groups in pregnant women

The agglutinability of red cells by anti-Le^a and anti-Le^b is reduced during pregnancy (Brendemoen 1952; Taylor et al. 1974). This effect does not seem to be due primarily to the slight decrease in Lewis glycolipid in plasma during pregnancy, but rather to the increased ratio of lipoprotein to red cell mass that occurs during pregnancy and which results in a repartitioning of glycolipids between plasma and red cells (Hammar et al. 1981).

Lewis groups and bladder cancer

The higher frequency of the phenotype Le(a– b–) in patients with cancer of the bladder seems to be due to the conversion of Le-positive to Le-negative with

133

advanced disease. The true Le phenotype can be determined by measuring fucosyltransferase in saliva (Langkilde *et al.* 1990).

The Lewis groups of infants

Cord red cells do not react with anti-Le^b and are not agglutinated by anti-Le^a. However, using the IAT, Le^a can be demonstrated on the red cells of about 50% of cord blood samples (Cutbush *et al.* 1956).

The red cells of an infant which is destined to become an Le(a– b+) adult may react successively as Le(a– b–), Le(a+ b–) and finally Le(a– b+) during the first 15 months of its life (Cutbush *et al.* 1956).

The weak reactions of the red cells of newborn infants seem to be due to the very low concentration of Lewis glycolipids in the plasma. The plasma of newborn infants will not 'transform' red cells, although the red cells of newborn infants can be transformed by plasma from adults (Mäkelä and Mäkelä 1956) or by glycosphingolipid fractions of plasma from adults (Tilley *et al.* 1975).

The frequency of the Le(a+) phenotype is much higher in infants under the age of 1 year than it is in adults. In one study, the frequency was 90% at 1–2 months, 45% at 12 months, and 22%, i.e. about the same as in adults, at 2–3 years (Jordal 1956). Those Le(a+ b–) infants who are going to retain this phenotype as adults can be distinguished by their failure to secrete ABH substances.

The term Le^x was originally used to describe a hypothetical antigen present on the red cells of 90% of newborn infants, i.e. presumably all those with an *Le* gene, and whose red cells carry a low density of Le antigens (Schenkel-Brunner and Hanfland, 1981). Le^x is now used to describe a quite unrelated stage-specific embryonic antigen (SSEA), carried on a fucosylated unbranched type II chain (Hakomori 1984), and the original use of Le^x has been abandoned.

Uptake of Lewis substances on to red cells

Sneath and Sneath (1955) found that when Le(a+ b–) cells were transfused to an Le(a– b+) recipient, the cells adsorbed Le^b substance from the recipient's plasma and then reacted as Le(a+ b+). The transformation could also be produced *in vitro* by incubating Le(a+ b–) cells in Le(a– b+) plasma at 35°C for 24 h. Le(a+ b–) or Le(a– b+) cells incubated with Le(a– b–)

plasma lost their antigen to the plasma. Nevertheless, Lewis substances on red cells are relatively firmly attached; even after washing Le(a+) cells 20 times in saline they still react just as well with anti-Le^a sera (Cutbush *et al.* 1956); similarly, Le(a– b–) cells that have taken up Le^a or Le^b from glycosphingolipid fractions are not affected by repeated washing in saline (Tilley *et al.* 1975). It is now established that there is a continuous exchange of glycosphingolipids between plasma and the red cell membrane (Cooper 1977).

Confirmation of the view that the Lewis phenotype depends entirely on uptake of antigens from the plasma is provided by findings in twins displaying red cell chimerism. One of a pair of chimeric twins had 49% O cells and 51% A$_1$ cells. The 'true' genotype of this twin was shown to be OO by the finding of H substance but not A substance in the saliva; all the red cells in this twin behaved as Le(a– b+). In the other twin, 61% of the cells were A$_1$ and 39% O. The saliva of this twin contained Le^a substance but not A or H; all the red cells behaved as Le(a+ b–). Thus, red cells of the non-secretor twin behaved as Le(a+ b–) in that twin, but as Le(a– b+) in the secretor twin. The red cells from the secretor twin behaved as Le(a– b+) in that twin and as Le(a+ b–) in the circulation of the non-secretor twin (Nicholas *et al.* 1957).

Two other chimeric twins provided evidence that a complex, ALe^b, is present in the plasma of subjects who carry *Se*, *A$_1$* and *Le* alleles. When such a subject receives O cells, by graft or transfusion, the O cells become coated with ALe^b; these coated cells are agglutinated by anti-A$_1$Le^b (Crookston *et al.* 1970; Swanson *et al.* 1971).

Rate of uptake or loss of Lewis substance from red cells in vivo

In a case in which group O, Le(b+) red cells were transfused to an A$_1$,Le(b+) recipient and the O cells were extracted for testing, no uptake of ALe^b substance was found at 48 h; on days 4 and 5 the cells reacted weakly and on days 7 and 11 more strongly with anti-A$_1$Le^b (Crookston *et al.* 1970).

In a case in which the loss rather than the uptake of Lewis substance was investigated, O,Le(b+) red cells were transfused to an A$_1$Lc(a– b–) patient and the transfused red cells separated by agglutinating out the patient's cells. The extracted O cells still reacted strongly with anti-Le[b] after 48 h but at 7 days gave a scarcely detectable reaction (Mollison *et al.* 1963).

Lewis antigens on leucocytes and platelets

Using a cytotoxicity test, Lewis antigens have been demonstrated on lymphocytes (Dorf *et al.* 1972; Oriol *et al.* 1980) and, using fluorescence flow cytometry, have been demonstrated both on lymphocytes (Dunstan 1986) and on platelets, where their distribution was found to be heterogeneous (Dunstan and Simpson 1985). Lewis antigens could not be demonstrated on granulocytes or monocytes (Dunstan 1986).

Molecular genotyping

In the *FUT3* gene, various point mutations are associated with *le*, making it possible to distinguish this allele from *Le* (Elmgren *et al.* 1996; for a review, see Daniels 2002).

Antibodies of the Lewis system

Systematic work on the Lewis blood group system stemmed from the discovery by Mourant in 1946 of an antibody that was subsequently given the name anti-Le[a]. There is little doubt that isolated examples of human anti Le[a] had been encountered by earlier workers. Landsteiner and Levine (1929) described five sera that gave parallel reactions and agglutinated about 16% of samples. The agglutination reactions were 'of a special sort' – a few rather large clumps, but mostly free cells. Parr and Krischner (1932) described an antibody which at 36°C failed to agglutinate red cells but caused slow lysis; Neter (1936) described an antibody that showed agglutinating and haemolysing activity, acting on about 25% of blood samples. Levine and Polayes (1941) also described an antibody that agglutinated 25% of red cell samples at 20°C and caused lysis at 37°C. As described below, anti-Le[a] sera react with about 20% of samples in white people and, unlike most other human blood group antibodies, cause haemolysis *in vitro*.

The second antibody belonging to the Lewis blood group system was discovered by Andresen in 1948 and was subsequently named anti-Le[b]. Both anti-Le[a] and anti-Le[b] are found mainly in Le(a– b–) people.

Anti-Le[a]

Anti-Le[a] occurs relatively commonly in human sera. For example, it was present in 57 (0.3%) out of 17 000 samples in one series (Kissmeyer-Nielsen *et al.* 1955), and in 249 (0.35%) out of 72 000 in another (Salmon *et al.* 1984). Anti-Le[a] is found only in persons who are Le(a– b–) and secrete ABH substances (Miller *et al.* 1954; Pettenkofer and Hoffbauer 1954). In 121 adults of this phenotype, there were 14 examples of anti-Le[a] and nine of anti-X (anti-Le[x], see below). This is an overall frequency of about 20% in Le(a– b–) subjects and would correspond to about 1% in the population as a whole. This is significantly higher than figures reported by others (Kissmeyer-Nielsen *et al.* 1955; Salmon *et al.* 1984), but the difference may be partially explained by the fact that in Jordal's series a special search was being made for Lewis antibodies.

Donors of anti-Le[a] belong more frequently to groups A, B or AB than would be expected in a random distribution (Jordal 1956; third edition, p. 290). In one series of 548 donors of Lewis antibodies, approximately 30% were group O compared with 44% of group O subjects in a random sample of the population (Kissmeyer-Nielsen 1965).

A single example of 'auto-anti-Le[a]' has been reported in a multitransfused Le(a– b+) patient with carcinoma of the oesophagus. The patient's own red cells partially adsorbed the antibody (Judd *et al.* 1978).

Anti-Le[b]

Anti-Le[b] can often be demonstrated as a weak antibody in serum which contains a relatively potent anti-Le[a]. Anti-Le[b] occurs on its own relatively infrequently; for example, Pettenkofer and Hoffbauer (1954) tested the sera of 12 000 unselected pregnant or recently delivered women and found 52 examples of anti-Le[a] but only two of anti-Le[b] (i.e. without anti-Le[a]). Most sera which contain potent anti-Le[b] do not contain anti-Le[a].

Subjects who make anti-Le[b] without anti-Le[a] are usually of the phenotype Le(a– b–) although they may be le(a+ b–). In such cases, the subjects are sometimes A$_1$, Le(a+), and the antibody is anti-HLe[b].

Some anti-Le[b] sera fail to react with A$_1$ cells, although they react strongly with cells of group O or A$_2$. As mentioned above, there are in fact two kinds of anti-Le[b]: (1) more commonly, those that are inhibited by the saliva of all ABH secretors (i.e. including those of Le(a– b–) subjects); these anti-Le^b sera, called anti-Le^{bH} (i.e. anti-HLe^b), react only with O and A$_2$ samples; and (2) those that are not inhibited by the saliva of Le(a– b–) secretors of ABH but are inhibited by the saliva of Le(a– b–) persons. These anti-Le^b sera react with A$_1$ Le(a– b+) samples almost as well as with those of other ABO groups, and are called anti-Le^{bL} (i.e. true anti-Le^b). Of 72 000 individuals, 29 were found to have anti-Le^{bH} and only two anti-Le^{bL} (Salmon *et al.* 1984).

Anti-Le^{bH} occurring as an autoantibody active only at 4°C with the patient's own red cells or at 18°C with other Le(b+) red cells was described by Giles and Poole (1979).

Other Lewis or Lewis-related antibodies

Anti-A1Le^b and anti-BLe^b. Anti-A$_1$Le^b reacts with A$_1$, Le(b+) red cells but not with A$_2$Le(b+), A$_1$, Le(b–) or O, Le(b+) cells (Seaman *et al.* 1968; Crookston *et al.* 1970); anti-Ble^b reacts only with B, Le(b+) cells.

Anti-Le^x. Anti-Le^x was described (as anti-X) by Andresen and Jordal (1949); it reacted with all blood samples except those of the phenotype Le(a– b–). According to Jordal (1956) anti-Le^x reacts with more than 90% of cord samples and, moreover, reacts almost as well with cord red cells as with adult red cells – a claim upheld by Sturgeon and Arcilla (1970) (see also Arcilla and Sturgeon 1974).

There is some evidence that the structure with which anti-Le^x reacts is in fact Le^a, and that anti-Le^x is capable of reacting with red cells carrying only a very low density of Le^a receptors (Schenkel-Brunner and Hanfland 1981).

As already mentioned, the Le^x described here is quite different from the SSEA antigen for which the same name has subsequently been used (see p. 133).

Anti-Le^c. Anti-Le^c reacts with the red cells of Le(a– b–) non-secretors, i.e. from individuals of genotype *lele, sese*; the antibody is inhibited by saliva from individuals of the same genotypes. The first example of anti-Le^c was found in a group O,Le(a– b+) woman (Gunson and Latham 1972). Le^c is not a product of an allele at the *Le* locus (Watkins 1980), but is a non-fucosylated type 1 chain and is sometimes referred to as type 1 precursor.

Anti-Le^d. Anti-Le^d reacts with the red cells of Le(a– b–) secretors, i.e. from individuals of genotype *lele, Se* (Potapov 1970); the strongest reactors are of group O or A$_2$. The structure of the Le^d antigen is type I H (see section on biosynthesis); hence Le^d cannot be part of the Lewis system.

Anti-type 1 A. Anti-type 1 A was first observed in an A$_2$, Le(a– b+) subject; the antibody reacted only with the red cells of Le(a– b–) secretors who were group A$_1$ or A$_2$ and was originally described as 'Magard' (Andersen 1958). The antibody is specific for type 1 A, previously termed ALe^d, which is taken up from the plasma by red cells and lymphocytes and which is present in the greatest concentrations in A, Le(a– b–) secretors (Hirsch *et al.* 1975).

Monoclonal and polyclonal Lewis antibodies produced in animals

Excellent monoclonal anti-Le^a and anti-Le^b reagents are available commercially. Monoclonal anti-Le^a sera crossreact with type 1 precursor (see p. 144). Monoclonal anti-Le^b may be anti-Le^{bL}, -Le^{bH} or -Le^{H,L} (intermediate). This last type and anti-Le^{bL} crossreact with type 1 (Le^{d}H) and Le^y, and all anti-Le^{bL} and anti-Le^{bH,L} crossreact with Le^a (Good *et al.* 1992). Nevertheless, provided that suitable methods are used, monoclonal anti-Lewis reagents are very satisfactory.

Polyclonal anti-Le^a, -Le^b, -Le^d and -Le^{dH} have been produced after injecting Lewis glycoproteins in different forms into rabbits or goats (for references, see eighth edition, p. 305). Monoclonal anti-type 1 H (-Le^d), -type 2 H, -type 1 A and -type 1 B have also been described.

Serological characteristics of Lewis antibodies

Sera containing anti-Le^a usually agglutinate Le(a+) cells suspended in saline and react more strongly at 4°C and at room temperature than at 37°C. Red cells agglutinated by anti-Le^a have a 'stringy' appearance (Dunsford and Bowley 1955). In some cases the serum may fail to agglutinate cells at 37°C (Grubb and Morgan 1949), and occasionally may not agglutinate saline-suspended cells at all and be detectable only by the indirect antiglobulin test, especially if the cells and serum have been incubated at temperatures below 37°C.

Lewis antibodies seem almost always to bind complement. Most examples of anti-Le^a will bring about some lysis of red cells at 37°C (Andresen and Henningsen 1951; Rosenfield and Vogel 1951); Le(a+) cells from infants lyse more readily than Le(a+) cells from adults even though they are not agglutinated and react weakly in the IAT (Cutbush *et al.* 1956). Sera that fail to lyse untreated test cells almost always lyse enzyme-treated cells.

Lewis antibodies are most conveniently detected by an IAT, using a reagent containing anti-complement. The reactions are enhanced if the test is carried out in a medium of low ionic strength or using enzyme-treated cells. In detecting anti-Le^a in those occasional samples of fresh serum that are anti-complementary or in samples of stored serum, which are frequently anti-complementary, the two-stage antiglobulin test described in Chapter 8 should be used.

In general, Lewis antibodies, especially anti-Le^{bH}, react more strongly with group O cells than with A or B cells.

Lewis antibodies and type of immunoglobulin

Potent Lewis antibodies will sensitize red cells to agglutination by anti-IgM but very seldom to agglutination by anti-IgG.

One example of anti-Le^a that appeared to be solely IgG has been reported (fourth edition, pp. 281–283); the antibody bound complement only weakly. An example of anti-Le^b that was solely IgG was found by G Garratty (personal communication) in a man who said he had never been transfused; the antibody was potent and did not bind complement.

In tests with ^{125}I-labelled Le^a or Le^b substances in solution, IgG anti-Le^a was demonstrated in five of five potent anti-Le^a sera. The IgG anti-Le^a had a significantly lower binding constant than the accompanying IgM anti-Le^a, and the difference was thought to account for the failure to detect IgG anti-Le^a by the indirect antiglobulin test. An IgG concentrate of the anti-Le^a serum, treated with 2-ME to inactivate any IgM antibody present, agglutinated ficin-treated Le(a+b–) red cells (Holburn 1984, cited in seventh edition p. 310) and sensitized red cells to agglutination by anti-IgG (seventh edition, p. 310).

Using an enzyme-linked immunosorbent assay, IgG anti-Le^a was demonstrable in 13 out of 13 samples from mothers with anti-Le^a and in 12 out of 13 of the infants (Spitalnik *et al.* 1985).

Studies with ^{125}I-labelled IgM anti-Le^a

In studies with ^{125}I-labelled IgM anti-Le^a, the maximum number of molecules bound was found to be 4500–7300 per red cell (group O or A). The amounts of Le^a in the plasma and on the red cells of the same individual were not well correlated. The binding constant of intact (i.e. pentameric) IgM antibody molecules was 8.4×10^9 l/mol, but that of the monomeric fragments (IgMs) prepared from the antibody was very low. It was concluded that anti-Le^a normally binds multivalently to clusters of Le^a sites on the cell surface, thus accounting for both the good complement-binding properties and the poor agglutinating properties of the antibody. With IgM anti-Le^a an agglutinin titre of 1 corresponded to an antibody concentration of 1.1 µg/ml with 5900 molecules of antibody bound per cell; using a tile test, an indirect antiglobulin titre of 1 with an anti-IgM serum corresponded to an antibody concentration of 0.42 µg/ml, with 500 molecules bound per cell; an indirect antiglobulin titre of 1 with an anti-complement serum corresponded to an antibody concentration of 0.04 µg/ml, with 50 molecules of antibody bound per cell (Holburn 1973).

Immune responses to Lewis substances

In subjects whose serum already contains Lewis antibodies, significant rises in titre can be produced either by transfusion of Lewis-incompatible blood (Hossaini 1972) or by the i.m. injection of 5 mg of purified Lewis glycoprotein (Holburn 1973). In a case in which Lewis-incompatible blood and plasma were transfused after giving injections of purified Le^a and Le^b substance, the titre of anti-Le^a rose from 2 to 8000, and that of anti-Le^b from 1 to 250 (Mollison *et al.* 1963) (see Chapter 10).

The appearance of IgG Lewis antibodies in the plasma after massive transfusion, in patients in whom no Lewis antibodies could be detected before transfusion, has been described (Cheng and Lukomsky 1989).

Clinical significance of Lewis antibodies

HTR. Lewis antibodies, particularly anti-Le^a, can cause rapid destruction of small volumes of injected washed incompatible red cells but, for reasons discussed in Chapter 10, very rarely cause haemolytic transfusion reactions. The only risk arises if Le(a+) red cells of group O, which have more Lewis antigens than A or B cells, are selected for a patient whose serum contains potent anti-Le[a]; in these circumstances Le(a–) red cells should be transfused. When screening patients of group A, B or AB whose serum contains Lewis antibodies, the antibodies will react with Lewis-positive cells in the panel, as these cells are group O. However, when donor red cells of the patient's ABO group are crossmatched, most samples will be found to be compatible, as Lewis antigens are more weakly expressed on A, B and AB cells than on O cells (see also section on Chemistry of HAB, and Lewis antigens, later in text). In these circumstances, compatible red cells untyped for Lewis can be transfused in the knowledge that they will survive normally.

In countries in South-East Asia, Lewis antibodies are said to be significantly more potent than in Europe and to cause severe haemolytic transfusion reactions (D Chandanayingyong, personal communication).

HDN. Lewis antibodies are found more commonly in women in the reproductive period (Kissmeyer-Nielsen 1965), a fact possibly related to the weakening of Le antigens on red cells in pregnancy.

Lewis antibodies are not known to cause haemolytic disease of the newborn; this outcome is to be expected because Lewis antibodies are predominantly IgM and also because the red cells of newborn infants react only very weakly or not at all with Lewis antibodies.

Renal grafts. In a prospective study involving 70 donor–recipient pairs of cadaveric renal allografts, no significant differences in 1-year graft survival were found between Le-matched and Le-mismatched pairs (Posner *et al.* 1986).

The P_1 system and globoside collection

The P blood group system was discovered by Landsteiner and Levine (1927) by testing immune sera prepared by injecting human red cells into rabbits.

For several reasons, the terminology is confusing. The antigen described by Landsteiner and Levine (1927) is now called P_1, not P. The gene encoding CD77 synthase on chromosome 22q13.2 is thought to be responsible for the synthesis of P_1 and P^k antigens (Iwamura *et al.* 2003), but the antigens called P and LKE, which have close serological and biochemical relationships to P_1 and P^k, are controlled by genes other than the one that controls P_1 and P^k. The P antigen is the only antigen in a separate blood group system denoted GLOB and the LKE antigen is placed in a blood group collection denoted the Globoside collection (Daniels *et al.* 2003).

Antigens

For details, see Table 4.5.

P_1. Almost all individuals are either P_1 (about 75% of the English population) or P_2; P_2 simply implies P_1 negative: there is no P_2 antigen; P_2 subjects frequently have anti-P_1 in their serum as a cold agglutinin which is only occasionally active at 20°C or higher. Among P_1 subjects there is considerable variation in the strength of the P_1 antigen and this variation is inherited (Henningsen 1952).

Frequency* (%)	Phenotype	Antigens on red cells	Antibodies in serum
75	P_1	$P_1P(P^k)$[†]	None
25	P_2	$P(P^k)$[†]	Anti-P_1[‡]
Very rare	P_1^k	P_1P^k	Anti-P
	P_2^k	P^k	Anti-P
	p	None	Anti-PP_1P^k

Table 4.5 P_1 and related antigens and antibodies.

* Frequency in the English population.
[†] P^k has been detected on P_1 and P_2 cells (Tippett 1975; Naiki and Marcus 1975), although this antigen is not detected routinely on such cells.
[‡] Not present in all P_2 subjects.

P and P^k. Almost all P$_1$ and P$_2$ individuals have the antigen P on their red cells. Very rarely, P is lacking and such individuals have the p^k antigen, or P$_1$ and p^k, or neither on their red cells; in these last subjects, of phenotype p, the serum contains anti-PP$_1$P^k (originally described as anti-Tj^a by Levine *et al.* 1951). P^k and p cells can be identified either by their failure to react with anti-P or by their failure to react with B19 capsids (Davey *et al.* 1994). The P antigen is the receptor for parvovirus B19 and subjects who lack P are naturally resistant to infection with the virus (Brown *et al.* 1994).

When measured by fluorescence flow cytometry, the distribution of P$_1$ and P antigens on red cells was shown to be heterogeneous, the amounts varying from cell to cell within a given red cell population (see Dunstan 1986). P$_1$ and P were found on platelets and their distribution was also heterogeneous (Dunstan *et al.* 1985c). P$_1$ and P are present on lymphocytes and fibroblasts. P^k is present on fibroblasts of normal P$_1$ and P$_2$ people (Fellous *et al.* 1974).

P$_1$ of non-human origin

Echinococcus cyst fluid. Scolices in hydatid cyst fluid contain P$_1$ and occasionally stimulate the production of anti-P$_1$ in humans with hydatid disease (Cameron and Staveley 1957; Ben-Ismail *et al.* 1980).

Bovine liver flukes. In an outbreak of bovine liver fluke disease (fascioliasis), all of five P$_2$ subjects had powerful anti-P$_1$ in their serum (Bevan *et al.* 1970). Liver flukes contain P^k antigen (CD77) in their tegument (Wuhrer *et al.* 2001).

Clonorchiasis. In South-East Asia, infestation with *Clonorchis sinensis* is common. In a study of refugees from Kampuchea and Laos, countries in which the frequency of the phenotype P$_2$ happens to be as high as 80%, it was found that about 50% of P$_2$ subjects had an IgM anti-P$_1$ active at room temperature (Petit *et al.* 1981).

Pigeon protein. Pigeon red cells and serum contain an antigen similar to, but not identical with, human P$_1$ (Brocteur *et al.* 1975). In pigeon breeders who are P$_2$ there is an increased incidence of anti-P$_1$ (Radermecker *et al.* 1975).

Antibodies

For details see Table 4.5.

Anti-P$_1$. In an early investigation, anti-P agglutinins (now called anti-P$_1$) were found in the serum of approximately two out of three unselected P$_2$ individuals; the agglutinins were usually very weak and were active only at low temperatures. In pregnant P$_2$ women, the frequency of anti-P$_1$ was almost 90% but no evidence was obtained that this was connected with alloimmunization in pregnancy. Moreover, some of the most potent anti-P$_1$ sera came from men who had never had injections or transfusions of blood (Henningsen 1949).

Relatively few examples of anti-P will agglutinate red cells at 25°C and fewer still are active at 37°C. Those sera that agglutinate cells at or near 37°C may fix complement, as shown by an indirect antiglobulin test and by the lysis of ficin-treated cells (Cutbush and Mollison 1958).

In most patients whose serum contains anti-P$_1$ no increase in anti-P$_1$ titre is observed following the i.v. injection of P$_1$ red cells, even when the anti-P is active at 37°C before injection (PL Mollison, unpublished observations), although the development of anti-P$_1$ after a series of transfusions has been described (Wiener and Unger 1944).

The only really clear-cut immediate haemolytic transfusion reaction due to anti-P$_1$ seems to be that reported by Moureau (1945). A patient with acquired haemolytic anaemia became increasingly jaundiced after the transfusion of P$_1$ blood and was found to have an anti-P$_1$ agglutinin with a titre of 32 at 37°C; *in vitro*, the addition of guinea pig serum resulted in the lysis of P$_1$ cells by the patient's serum. Anti-P$_1$ was undoubtedly responsible for a delayed haemolytic transfusion reaction, characterized by a fall in packed cell volume (PCV) and a substantial rise in serum bilirubin concentration, in a patient whose plasma contained a potent lytic IgG anti-P$_1$ active over a wide thermal range (DiNapoli *et al.* 1977). In another case, haemoglobinuria occurring on the second day after massive transfusion was attributed to red cell destruction by anti-P$_1$ (Chandeysson *et al.* 1981), but this conclusion has been questioned (seventh edition, p. 317).

The effect of anti-P$_1$ on the survival of small volumes of transfused P$_1$ red cells is described in Chapter 10.

Production of anti-P_1 in animals

Anti-P_1 has been produced in rabbits by injecting human (P_2) or rabbit red cells, tanned and coated with *Echinococcus* cyst fluid (Levine *et al*. 1958), and by injecting pig hydatid cyst fluid alone into goats (Kerde *et al*. 1960).

Two murine monoclonal anti-P_1, both IgM, reacting in high dilution at 4°C were obtained from hybridomas after immunization of mice with turtle dove ovomucoid, which carries the immunodominant trisaccharide of the P_1 antigen (Bailly *et al*. 1986).

Anti-PP_1P^k (anti-Tj^a)

Anti-PP_1P^k is found only in subjects of the very rare phenotype p. According to Race and Sanger (1975, p. 154), the frequency of the p phenotype is 5.8 per million in most parts of the world (and slightly greater in parts of north Sweden). Most anti-PP_1P^k contain separable antibody specificities but in some sera it is not possible to isolate anti-P^k by absorption of anti-PP_1P^k with P_1 cells.

Anti-PP_1P^k is not present at birth in the serum of p infants but develops early in life without exposure to foreign red cells (Obregon and McKeever 1980).

Anti-PP_1P^k is associated with abortion early in pregnancy (Levine and Koch 1954). Although some women found to have the antibody in their serum have a history of several live births without any abortions (Race and Sanger 1975, p. 170), the overall frequency of abortion is highly suggestive of a causal relationship. Among p women with anti-PP_1p^k in their serum, abortions are no commoner when the partner is P_1 than when he is P_2 (Sanger and Tippett 1979). Moreover, some examples of anti-PP_1P^k, at least, react as well with P_2 cells as with P_1 cells (Levene 1979). The effect of anti-PP_1p^k on the fetus seems to be closely related to the IgG subclass of the antibody (see below) and to the presence of P antigen in the placenta with the same carbohydrate structure as P in red cells (Hansson *et al*. 1988).

In two women with IgG anti-P in their plasma and a history of repeated abortions (one had lost all of six previous fetuses between 3 and 5 months), large amounts of anti-P were removed during a succeeding pregnancy. Starting as early as the seventh week of pregnancy, plasma was withdrawn at frequent intervals, absorbed with P-positive red cells and returned to the patient. The red cells were separated by centrifugation and the plasma was passed through a micropore filter to remove any residual cells. The total amounts of plasma treated were 135–215 l. The titre of anti-P fell appreciably and remained at a low level as long as treatment was continued. Both women gave birth to healthy infants (Yoshida *et al*. 1984, 1994). Haemolytic disease of the newborn due to anti-PP_1P^k is mentioned in Chapter 12.

Anti-PP_1P^k is haemolytic *in vitro* and is capable of causing rapid destruction of transfused red cells. In the first subject (Mrs 'Jay') in whom the antibody was found, a test injection of 25 ml of incompatible blood was followed by an immediate severe reaction with haemoglobinaemia. Subsequently the antibody titre rose from 8 to 512 (Levine *et al*. 1951).

'Anti-Tj^a-like' refers to the specificity of a haemolytic activity found at one time or another in 89% of pregnant 'habitual aborters'. The activity might be present one week and absent the next, or even disappear within 9 h, but was present only during pregnancy (Vos 1965). *In vitro*, the serum lysed the patient's own washed red cells at 37°C; haemolysis was not complement dependent; the haemolytic factor was apparently not an immunoglobulin. This strange activity, found in the serum of habitual aborters living in Perth, Australia, has not been found in habitual aborters in the USA or Canada (Vos *et al*. 1964; Vos 1965, 1966).

Anti-P found in all P^k people

Anti-P differs from anti-PP_1P^k in not reacting with P_1^k or P_2^k cells. However, this kind of anti-P behaves serologically like anti-PP_1P^k, that is to say as an agglutinin at room temperature and as a haemolysin at 37°C. In contrast, anti-P occurring as an autoantibody behaves as a biphasic haemolysin (Donath–Landsteiner antibody), producing lysis only when allowed to act first at a relatively low temperature and subsequently at a higher temperature (see Chapter 7). The P^k phenotype is even rarer than p (Race and Sanger 1975). Both anti-P and anti-P^k have been produced as monoclonal antibodies in mice.

'Anti-p'

Examples of antibodies reacting preferentially with p cells have been described but, for reasons given later, the designation anti-p for these antibodies is inappropriate.

Immunoglobulin classes and IgG subclasses of antibodies of the P_1 system and globoside collection

Examples of potent anti-P_1 and of anti-PP_1P^k that appeared to be solely IgM have been described (Adinolfi *et al.* 1962) but anti-PP_1P^k, as mentioned above, may be partly IgG, predominantly IgG or wholly IgG (Wurzel *et al.* 1971; Lopez *et al.* 1983). Biphasic haemolysins are always IgG. An exceptional case of anti-P found in a patient with cold haemagglutinin disease was IgM; see Chapter 7.

In a study of 29 p subjects, anti-P or anti-P^k was detected in every case. Almost all the antibodies were partly IgM and partly IgG, the latter being almost solely IgG3. Of the 29 subjects, 17 were parous women; of these 17, three had had only normal pregnancies and in two of these no IgG3 anti-P or anti-P^k was found. All of the remaining women had had one or more spontaneous abortions and 13 out of these 14 had IgG3 antibodies, suggesting a causal relationship between anti-PP_1p^k of IgG3 subclass and abortions (Söderström *et al.* 1985). In a smaller series, a relationship was found between early abortions and cytotoxic IgG anti-P^k (Lopez *et al.* 1983). Evidence that anti-pk(CD77) can induce apoptosis in Burkitt's lymphoma cells (Tetaud *et al.* 2003) may be relevant to explaining the impact these antibodies have on placental tissue.

The Ii antigens and antibodies

Antigens

Antigens on red cells

The red cells of almost all healthy adults have I determinants and lesser numbers of i determinants. I and i are not determined by the alleles of a single gene but by different genes encoding distinct glycosyltransferases. The I antigen is the only antigen of the I blood group system. The i antigen is in blood group collection 207 (Daniels *et al.* 2003). Very rare normal adults of phenotype i have little or no I antigen (Jenkins *et al.* 1960).

Red cells that fail completely to react with anti-I are very rare; they usually come from white people; red cells that have a small amount of I (and a large amount of i) are usually from black people, and are slightly less rare. The adult i phenotype is inherited (see Race and Sanger 1975).

Cord red cells react weakly with anti-I and strongly with anti-i. During the first 18 months of life the red cells gradually come to react strongly with anti-I and weakly with anti-i. This phenotype (strong I, weak i) is retained by healthy persons throughout life.

Among adults, there is a wide normal range of reactivity of the red cells with anti-i and with anti-I (both auto- and allo-anti-I). The i reactivity of the red cells of normal subjects can be increased by repeated phlebotomy, suggesting that there is an inverse relationship between i reactivity and marrow transit time (Hillman and Giblett 1965). There is evidence that as red cells age in the circulation they become progressively less reactive with anti-i (Testa *et al.* 1981).

I^T is an antigen which is expressed strongly on cord red cells, more weakly on normal adult cells and more weakly still on adult i cells; because the antigen appeared to be best expressed during the transition from i to I, the name I^T was chosen (Booth *et al.* 1966). However, the description 'transitional' is now considered to be inappropriate, as I^I is more strongly expressed on fetal than on newborn red cells.

The number of I and i sites on red cells

Estimates of the number of I sites on adult cells have varied from 5×10^5 (normal red cells, Evans *et al.* 1965; paroxysmal nocturnal haemoglobinuria red cells, Rosse *et al.* 1966) to 1×10^5 with one example of anti-I and half this number with another (Doinel *et al.* 1976), and an even lower number, 0.3×10^5, with yet another (Olesen 1966). The number of i sites on cord red cells was found to be between 0.2 and 0.65×10^5 (Doinel *et al.* 1976).

The I antigen has been found on the red cells of many species, for example rabbit, sheep, cattle and kangaroo (Curtain 1969).

I and i on other cells and in secretions

Leucocytes and platelets. The presence of I and i on leucocytes can be demonstrated in agglutination tests or in cytotoxicity tests (Lalezari 1970). I was more weakly expressed on cord lymphocytes than on adult lymphocytes, but i is almost as strongly expressed on adult lymphocytes as on cord lymphocytes (Shumak *et al.* 1971).

I antigens on platelets show a heterogeneous distribution when tested by flow cytometry (Dunstan and Simpson 1985).

Saliva and milk. Only a minority of anti-I agglutinins are strongly inhibitable by saliva, milk and extracts of stroma from OI red cells (Feizi and Marsh 1970). Inhibition studies have emphasized the heterogeneity of anti-I sera, as, for example, the glycoprotein from milk inhibited only 2 out of 21 anti-I sera (Feizi *et al.* 1971). The amount of I in secretions is not correlated with that on red cells, indicating that the two may be under separate genetic control (Salmon *et al.* 1984).

Plasma. Samples of plasma from all of 39 adults, after treatment with 2-ME to inactivate any anti-I present, inhibited one example of anti-I. There was no relationship between the amounts of I and i in the plasma of the different samples (Rouger *et al.* 1979).

Changes in Ii antigens in disease

An increased agglutinability by anti-i was found with the red cells of all patients with thalassaemia major tested (excluding those recently transfused) and with the cells of some patients with hypoplastic anaemia, sideroblastic anaemia, megaloblastic anaemia, chronic haemolytic states and acute leukaemia (Giblett and Crookston 1964; Cooper *et al.* 1968). The red cells of patients with hereditary erythroblastic multinuclearity with a positive acidified serum (HEMPAS) test give a very high agglutination score with anti-i and are usually susceptible to lysis both by anti-i and by anti-I (Crookston *et al.* 1969a).

The amount of i on lymphocytes of patients with chronic lymphocytic leukaemia is greatly reduced even in the early stages of the disease, whereas the amount is normal on the blasts of patients with acute lymphocytic leukaemia and on the lymphocytes of some patients with lymphosarcoma cell leukaemia (Shumak *et al.* 1979).

In Asians there is a marked association between the adult i phenotype and autosomal recessive congenital cataracts (see Page *et al.* 1987; Yu *et al.* 2003). The association is not so apparent in white people but this has been explained by Yu and co-workers (2003) and is discussed in the section on biosynthesis of Ii antigens below.

Anti-I. Anti-I was first described as a potent cold autoagglutinin in the serum of a patient with acquired haemolytic anaemia (Wiener *et al.* 1956) and later, as a weak cold autoagglutinin in the serum of most normal subjects (Tippett *et al.* 1960). The monoclonal antibody found in patients with cold haemagglutinin disease has anti-I specificity in the vast majority of cases; compared with auto-anti-I found in normal subjects, the antibody has a far higher titre (usually much greater than 1000 at 4°C), and has a much wider thermal range, often reacting at 30°C or more. Auto-anti-I is described in more detail in Chapter 7.

Anti-I is found as an alloagglutinin, acting best at 4°C (titre 16–32) and sometimes at room temperature, in the serum of most i subjects. A typical example is solely IgM; it agglutinates red cells at temperatures up to 30°C; in tests carried out strictly at 37°C the serum sensitizes the cells to agglutination by anti-IgM and, provided that complement is present, to agglutination by anti-complement. Murine monoclonal anti-I have been described (Messeter and Johnson 1990).

Anti-i. Anti-i was first described by Marsh and Jenkins (1960) as a cold autoagglutinin in the serum of a patient with reticulosis; auto-anti-i is not uncommon in the serum of patients with infectious mononucleosis (see Chapter 7). No example of allo-anti-i has been described.

The difficulty of classifying potent cold autoagglutinins as anti-I or anti-i was emphasized by a study of 13 such sera by Cooper and Brown (1973). The ratio of antibody removed by cord cells to that removed by adult cells varied from 2.4 to 0.0, i.e. there was a spectrum from those sera that clearly had anti-i specificity to those which were clearly anti-I, with many in between that reacted slightly more strongly with cord cells than with adult cells or vice versa.

Anti-I^T. Anti-I^T may occur as a harmless cold autoagglutinin, rarely in white people (see Chapter 7) but commonly in certain Venezuelans (Layrisse and Layrisse 1968); or as a warm autoantibody associated with autoimmune haemolytic anaemia (AIHA) (Chapter 7), and has been described as warm IgG alloantibody in a subject with Hodgkin's disease (Garratty *et al.* 1972).

Anti-HI, -AI, -BI, Hi, Bi, -P_1I, -$P_1$$I^T$ and -HILe^b

Of this list of antibodies that react only with red cells carrying I (or i) and a second antigen, anti-HI is the commonest. Antibodies with this specificity often cause problems when pre-transfusion tests are carried out at room temperature. Most patients who make anti-HI are group A_1; when the patient's serum is screened against a panel of group O red cells, it will be found to contain an antibody (i.e. anti-HI) but when it is crossmatched with A_1 red cells, the result will be negative. References for other antibodies are as follows: anti-AI (Tippett *et al.* 1960); anti BI (Tegoli *et al.* 1967); anti-Hi (Bird and Wingham 1977); anti-Bi (Pinkerton *et al.* 1977); anti-P_1I (Issitt *et al.* 1968); anti-$P_1$$I^T$ (Booth 1970); and anti-HILe^b (Tegoli *et al.* 1971).

Anti-P_1I and -$P_1$$I^T$ are only slightly inhibited by hydatid cyst fluid, in contrast to anti-P_1, which is readily inhibited.

Anti-HILe^b was found to agglutinate only red cells which were O,I,Le(a– b+) or A_2,I,Le(a– b+). The antibody (which can also be described as anti-ILe^{bH}) was inhibited by saliva containing I, H and Le^b but was not inhibited by serum from the donor of the saliva.

Biosynthesis of the P, HAB* (ABH), Ii and Lewis antigens

* The sequence HAB, rather than ABH, is used in this section because, in biosynthesis, the formation of H precedes that of A and B (Watkins and Morgan 1959).

As mentioned at the beginning of this chapter, the antigens of all of these blood group systems are synthesized by the sequential addition of sugar residues to a common precursor substance. As the antigenic determinants are not proteins, but oligosaccharides, they cannot be the direct gene products. The gene products are glycosyltransferases that transfer a specific sugar to a specific oligosaccharide chain.

On red cells, the oligosaccharide chain may be bound by D-glucose through sphingosine to fatty acid moieties, in which case the blood group substance is a glycosphingolipid (or glycolipid). More commonly, the oligosaccharide chain is bound to a peptide chain, usually through N-acetyl-D-glucosamine to asparagine and the blood group substance is then a glycoprotein. In glycoproteins in secretions the oligosaccharide chains

are bound through N-acetyl-D-galactosamine to serine or threonine. HAB, Lewis and P antigens in plasma are carried on glycosphingolipids and the oligosaccharide chain is bound by D-glucose to ceramide.

The P antigens are discussed first because the relevant genes act early in the biosynthetic pathway (see Fig. 4.5 on p. 147).

Chemistry of the P antigens

As stated above, the terminology used so far is confusing because it implies that all the P antigens belong to the same genetic system. However, as Fig. 4.3 shows, two biosynthetic pathways are involved, one leading to the production of P and the other to the production of P_1.

P, which is globoside, is present on the red cells of almost all individuals; in those rare subjects who lack P, P^k (trihexosylceramide) cannot be converted to globoside and is therefore found on the red cells. As the P_1 gene is independent of P, p^k subjects may be P_1^k or P_2^k.

The P gene encodes a glycosyltransferase that converts p^k to P by adding N-acetylgalactosamine to trihexosylceramide (Hellberg *et al.* 2002). The p^k gene encodes an α-galactosyltransferase (CD77 synthase), which synthesizes trihexosylceramide (Furukawa *et al.* 2000; Steffensen *et al.* 2000); hence P and p^k are not alleles. Several examples of the rare phenotypes P1k,P2k and p have been examined at the DNA level and shown to result from a diverse array of inactivating mutations in the P and pk genes (Hellberg *et al.* 2003, 2004; Yan *et al.* 2004).

As P_1 and p^k possess the same terminal non-reducing disaccharides Gal(α1→4)Galβ (see Fig. 4.3), the nature of the P_1-specified transferase has posed a problem. However, Iwamura and co-workers (2003) have provided evidence that the pk transferase (CD77 synthase) is also the P_1 transferase. They observed that P_1-negative red cells have lower levels of CD77 synthase mRNA than P_1-positive red cells and were able to find two homozygous mutations upstream of the CD77 synthase coding region in P_1-negative individuals. They concluded that differences in transcriptional regulation of the CD77 synthase gene in P_1-positive and P_1-negative individuals may account for the differences in P_1 antigen expression.

P, P^k and P_1 antigens on red cells are on glycosphingolipids (Marcus *et al.* 1981). P and p^k also occur in plasma as glycosphingolipids. None of these substances has been found in secretions.

It has been shown that the terminal disaccharide Gal(α1→4)Galβ shared by P_1 and p^k is a receptor on epithelial cells for one of the adhesins of most strains of uropathogenic *Escherichia coli*. Strains with adhesins specific for this disaccharide agglutinate red cells from individuals of blood groups P_1, P_2 and p^k but not p (Källenius *et al.* 1981; Leffler and Svanborg-Edén 1981; Lomberg *et al.* 1986). Cellular injury in post-diarrhoeal haemolytic-uraemic syndrome is linked to *E. coli*-derived shigatoxin (syn. Verotoxin) binding to p^k (CD77, Hughes *et al.* 2002).

LKE and its proposed biosynthetic relationship to P

The Luke antigen was discovered by finding that the serum of a patient with Hodgkin's lymphoma agglutinated all red cells tested except those of the rare p or p^k phenotypes and about 2% of P+ samples (Tippett *et al.* 1965). The incidence of the Luke-negative phenotype in one white population was 0.0017 (Bruce *et al.* 1988). For details of the possible structure of the Luke antigen, see Daniels (2002). Luke antibodies appear to be of no clinical significance.

Inhibition studies

Anti-P_1. Anti-P_1 is inhibited by sheep hydatid cyst fluid (Cameron and Staveley 1957). The inhibiting substance is a glycoprotein with a terminal trisaccharide (Cory *et al.* 1974) that has the same structure (Gal(α1→4)Gal(β1→4)GlcNAc) as the terminal trisaccharide of the P_1 glycolipid isolated from red cells (Naiki *et al.* 1975). Anti-P_1 is highly specific for the terminal trisaccharide and is not inhibited by the terminal disaccharide shared with P^k (see Watkins 1980). Egg whites from pigeons and turtle doves are powerful inhibitors of anti-P_1 (François-Gérard *et al.* 1980).

Anti-P^k. Anti-P^k is obtained either by absorption of anti-PP$_1$p^k with globoside or by absorption of some anti-PP$_1$P^k with P_1 red cells. Anti-P^k is inhibited by both hydatid cyst fluid and trihexosylceramide isolated from red cells. The inhibition of anti-P^k and of anti-P_1 by hydatid cyst fluid is not surprising, as both p^k and P_1 have the same terminal disaccharide (Gal(α1→4)Gal).

Anti-P. Anti-P, whether occurring as an autoantibody (biphasic haemolysin) or as an alloantibody in P_1^k

and P_2^k individuals, is inhibited by globoside. Many examples of anti-P, whether allo- or autoantibodies, are also inhibited by Forssman glycosphingolipid, indicating that P antibodies represent a heterogeneous response to globoside and Forssman glycolipids, present in many animal tissues, as well as to crossreacting microbial antigens (Marcus *et al.* 1981).

'Anti-p'. 'Anti-p' is a cold agglutinin that reacts best with p red cells, but also reacts, although less well, with P_2 cells and only very weakly with P_1 cells (Engelfriet *et al.* 1972). The antibody is inhibited by sialosylparagloboside (Schwarting *et al.* 1977) and more strongly inhibited by glycolipids containing the same terminal structure as sialosylparagloboside (see Fig. 4.3) but with two or three repeating Gal(β1→4) GlcNAc units (Marcus *et al.* 1981); these compounds also inhibited two examples of anti-Gd (see Chapter 7).

Sialosylparagloboside is expected to accumulate in p people due to blocking of the synthesis of P_1 and trihexosylceramide (see Fig. 4.3) which would lead to accumulation of paragloboside, which would then be available for other biosynthetic pathways (Schwarting *et al.* 1977).

Chemistry of HAB and Lewis antigens

For details, see Table 4.6 and Fig. 4.4.

Expression of H, A and B antigens is determined by the attachment of specific monosaccharides to various precursor disaccharides at the non-reducing end of a carbohydrate chain. The main precursor structures are as follows:

1 Type 1 Galβ1→3GlcNAcβ1-R;
2 Type 2 Galβ1→4GlcNAcβ1-R;
3 Type 3 Galβ1→3GalNAcα1-R;
4 Type 4 Galβ1→3GalNAcβ1-R.

An important difference between HAB and Lewis antigens is that HAB occur on all four types of precursor structure, whereas Le^a and Le^b antigens occur only on type 1 chains. As only type 2, 3 and 4 chains are synthesized on red cells, the presence of Le^a and Le^b on red cells depends on uptake from the plasma.

Secretions and plasma

HAB and Lewis antigens occur in plasma as glycosphingolipids and in secretions as glycoproteins. The products of the *Se*, *A*, *B* and *Le* alleles are glycosyl-

Table 4.6 Products of *Le*, *A* and *B* genes in secretions.

Genes	Gene product	Sugar attached by enzyme	Terminal structure of oligosaccharide chain	Serological specificity
Se (FUT 2)	α1→2-L-fucosyl-transferase (1)	Fuc	Gal(β,1→3)GlcNAc-R Gal(β1→3)GlcNAc-R | (α1→2) Fuc	* H†
Le (FUT 3)	α1→4-L-fucosyl-transferase (2)	Fuc	Gal(β1→3)GlcNAc-R | (α1→4) Fuc	Le^a
Se and *Le*	α-L-fucosyl-transferases (2 and 3)	Fuc	Gal(β1→3)GlcNAc-R | (α1→2) | (α1→4) Fuc Fuc	Le^b
A	α-N-acetyl-D-galactosaminyltransferase	GalNAc	GalNAc(α1→3)Gal(β1→3)GlcNAc-R | (α1→2) Fuc	A
B	α-D-galactosyltransferase	Gal	Gal(α1→3)Gal(β1→3)GlcNAc-R | (α1→2) Fuc	B

* Type 1 chain.
Abbreviations: Gal, D-galactose; GlcNAc, N-acetyl-D-glucosamine; Fuc, fucose; GalNAc, N-acetyl-D-galactosamine; R, remainder of chain.
For products of *FUT 1* (the *H*-specified fucosyl transferase) and the *A* and *B*-specified transferases on type 2 chains on red cells, see text.

transferases, which transfer the immunodominant epitope for H, A, B or Lewis specificity to an acceptor chain. The H antigen Fuc (α1β2)Galβ-R is the structure expressed in group O individuals (who lack A- or B- transferases). *Se* (FUT2) encodes an α-1,2-fucosyltransferase which uses a type 1 structure as an acceptor, but can also use a type 2 structure (Le Pendu *et al.* 1982). In secretions and plasma, in which only type 1 chains occur, the *Se* (FUT2)-specified transferase catalyses the synthesis of type 1 H but, as described later, on red cells the production of type 2, 3 and 4 H is catalysed by H (FUT1).

A and B are formed by addition of specific sugars to H and can therefore be synthesized in plasma and secretions only in subjects with an *Se* allele. The *A*-transferase adds N-acetyl-D-galactosamine in α1→3 linkage to the terminal D-galactose of H; the *B*-transferase adds D-galactose in α1→3 linkage to H. The product of the *Le* gene (FUT3) is an α-L, 3/4 L-fucosyltransferase that adds L-fucose in α1→4 to the subterminal N-acetyl-D-glucosamine of a type 1 acceptor, making the Le^a and Le^b epitopes of plasma and

secretions in non-secretors and secretors respectively. Although FUT3 uses preferentially type 1 chains, it can also use type 2 chains, giving rise to Le^x and Le^y epitopes (type 2 isomers of Le^a and Le^b).

The Le-transferase adds L-fucose to a type 1 chain to form Le^a, to type 1 H to form Le^b, to A to form ALe^b and to B to form BLe^b (see Fig. 4.4); hence, the same structural allele *Le* codes for the expression of both Le^a and Le^b antigens. The addition of L-fucose to N-acetyl-D-glucosamine would act as a chain-stopper; once L-fucose is added, no other sugar can be added to the chain (Kobata *et al.* 1968). Therefore, it is generally accepted that Le^a cannot be converted to Le^b.

In an individual with *H* (FUT1), *Se* (FUT2), *A*, *B* and *Le* (FUT3) alleles, not all of the acceptor is converted to H, A or B, or to Le^b; thus, the secretions and plasma of such an individual will contain some acceptor and H as well as A, B and Le^b. In addition, some Le^a will be present, as even in the presence of *Se*, the *Le*-transferase converts some type 1 acceptor to Le^a.

The Le-specified transferase can use only type 1 chains as acceptors to join L-fucose to the C-4 position

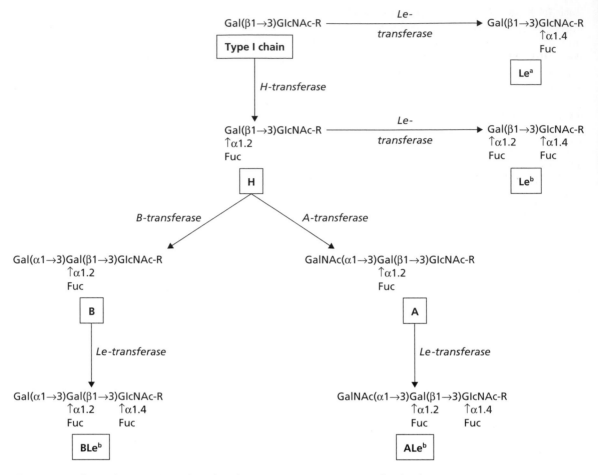

Fig 4.4 Biosynthesis of Lewis, HAB and combined antigens in secretions. R, rest of molecule.

of the subterminal N-acetylglucosamine. As red cells only synthesize type 2 chains where the C-4 position of the subterminal N-acetylgucosamine is occupied by the terminal β-galactosyl residue, it is not possible to form Le^a or Le^b structures on these chains.

'Le^c' in plasma is an unfucosylated type I precursor chain in glycosphingolipids and is adsorbed onto red cells (Hirsch and Graham 1980; Oriol 1990). Le^d is type 1 H.

Interactions between blood group substances and micro-organisms

The glycosyltransferases involved in the biosynthesis of HAB and Lewis antigens provide a mechanism for generating enormous diversity in the structures

of glycans at mucosal surfaces. These diverse glycan structures are thought to provide an important protective mechanism against microbial infection (see for example, Marionneau *et al.* 2001 and discussion of Sd^a antigen in Chapter 6). 'Helicobacter pylori colonises the stomachs of about half of the world's population' Bjorkholm and co-workers (2001). The infection correlates with the occurrence of peptic ulcers, atrophic gastritis and gastric adenocarcinoma in a proportion of infected individuals. Most clinical isolates of *H. pylori* express adhesins that bind to Le^b structures produced by gastric pit and surface mucous cells of secretors (Ilver *et al.* 1998). In a high proportion of *H. pylori* isolates, the bacteria themselves express Le^b antigen but this does not interfere with the ability of the organism to bind Le^b antigen on gastric mucosal cells (Zheng *et al.* 2003b). Treatment of *H. pylori* infection with lansoprazole, amoxicillin and clarithromycin was more successful in individuals with the *le* allele (Matsuo *et al.* 2003). A study of dyspeptic patients showed that Le^b-positive patients had a higher *H. pylori* density than Le^b-negative patients and that *H. pylori* density increased with a higher Le^b intensity (Sheu *et al.* 2003).

The frequency of non-secretors of HAB is significantly increased in patients with infections due to *Candida albicans*, meningococci or pneumococci (Blackwell *et al.* 1986). When pneumococci and *Haemophilus influenzae* are incubated with milk glycocompounds, known to contain HAB antigens, their attachment to epithelial cells decreases considerably (Andersson *et al.* 1986). Two mechanisms have been proposed by which glycoproteins in secretions might influence the adherence of micro-organisms to epithelial cells: (1) A, B or H substances in saliva of secretors inhibit binding of the yeast or bacterium to epithelial cells; and (2) the Le^a antigen in secretions recognizes an adhesin on the surface of the micro-organism and subsequently binds to the epithelium along with the attached microbe (see Blackwell *et al.* 1986).

An investigation following an outbreak of *E. coli* O157 in Scotland in 1996 showed a greater susceptibility of group O to the bacterium (Blackwell *et al.* 2002). Noroviruses, common causes of non-bacterial acute gastroenteritis, use glycans containing Le and HAB structures on intestinal epithelial cells as receptors for infection (Huang *et al.* 2003; Hutson *et al.* 2003).

Blood group A and B antigens have been demonstrated as coreceptors in *Plasmodium falciparum* rosetting (Barragan *et al.* 2000). Consistent with this, group O appears to confer relative protection against cerebral malaria (Hill 1992).

The HAB and Lewis antigens on red cells

Most H, A and B antigen sites are on glycoproteins, mainly on band 3 but also on other major glycoproteins such as the glucose transporter (GLUT 1), RhAG and the water transporter (aquaporin 1). A small amount of HAB sites are on simple glycolipids and the remainder are on polyglycosyl ceramide (Koscielak 2001). All subjects, except for those of the very rare Bombay type (*hh*), express ABH antigens on their red cells. H adds fucose in α-1,2 linkage to type 2 β-D-galactosyl residues to form H, and A and B then add their specific sugars as in the synthesis of A and B in plasma and secretions.

In Fig. 4.5, the biosynthetic relationship of the glycolipid H, A and B antigens in plasma is compared with those on red cells. Type I, H and A and B antigens are not synthesized by red cell precursors but can be passively adsorbed from plasma. These structures (type 1 H, type 1 A and type 1 B) were previously termed Le^d, ALe^d and BLe^d. The new terms are logical

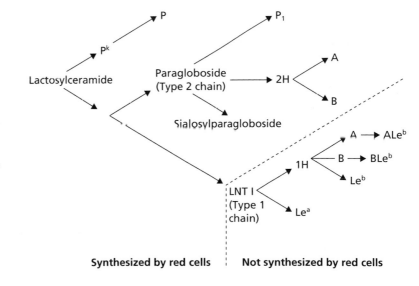

Fig 4.5 Biosynthesis of P, HAB and Lewis antigens. Structures within the area indicated by the broken line are present in plasma: they are not made by the red cells. Details of these pathways and structures can be seen in Figs 4.3 and 4.4 and Table 4.6. Abbreviations: 1 H, type 1 H chain; 2 H, type 2 H chain; LNT, lacto-N-tetraose or basic type 1 chain, Gal(β1→3) GlcNAc(β1→3) Gal(β1→4) Glc-CER.

because neither *le* nor *Le* is involved in the production of these antigens. H, A and B antigens synthesized by red cell precursors are type Il.

Ulex europaeus and several murine monoclonal anti-H react well with red cells because they are specific for H type 2 (Young *et al.* 1981; Knowles *et al.* 1982).

A_1 and A_2

A^1- and A^2-transferases in serum differ quantitatively as well as qualitatively. The level of A-transferase in the serum of A_2 donors is only about 10% of the level in A_1 donors. The A^1- and A^2-transferases differ in their pH optima, cation requirements and Michaelis constants (Schachter *et al.* 1971, 1973). In a donor of the genotype A_1A_2, the A^1- and A^2-transferases in serum can be separated using isoelectric focusing (Topping and Watkins 1975).

As the A^2-transferase is less efficient than the A^1-transferase, there are fewer A sites on A_2 red cells than on A_1 red cells. In addition to quantitative differences, there are qualitative differences. A^1 but not A^2 can convert type 3 H and type 4 H chains to type 3 A and type 4 A, which have repetitive A chains and are found on A_1 but not on A_2 red cells. As A^2 cannot convert type 3 H and type 4 H, A_2 red cells (compared with A^1) not only lack repetitive A chains but have more H and less A. It seems, then, that anti-A_1 reagents may recognize repetitive A structures, as may certain monoclonal anti-A which react with A_1 but not A_2 red cells (Clausen *et al.* 1985).

The molecular bases of A_2 and other variants of A, such as A_3 and A_m, are discussed below.

Conversion of O red cells to A or B cells. In the presence of the appropriate nucleotide sugar and the A- (or B-) transferase, group O red cells are readily converted to A- (or B-) active red cells (Schenkel-Brunner and Tuppy 1969; Race and Watkins 1972); O_h red cells are not converted (Race and Watkins 1972).

Group O red cells have been used to demonstrate the presence of B-transferase in saliva; the transferase was present both in secretors and non-secretors (Kogure and Furukawa 1976).

Aberrant expression of ABO, H and Lewis antigens in tumours

As discussed in Chapter 3, neoplastic change may be accompanied by changes in cell surface antigens, with loss of antigenic expression in some types of carcinoma and appearance of new antigens (neoantigens) in others. In carcinoma of the bladder, deletion of A and B antigens occurs frequently; the loss of A activity is associated with a failure of expression of the A-transferase with the consequent accumulation of Le^b due to the fucosylation of the excess H antigen formed. On the other hand, although the A antigen is not normally expressed in the adult distal colon, in group A patients with carcinoma of the colon A is 'neo-expressed'. In normal distal colon, the levels of H-transferase are very low, but in colonic tumour there is a significant elevation of this enzyme, allowing synthesis of H, which leads to the neo-expression of A (for references, see Watkins 1990).

Structure of ABO, H and Se genes and transferases

Table 4.7 shows some of the differences in predicted amino acid (aa) sequences, based on observed differences in nucleotides, for various alleles of the ABO gene; Plate 4.1 (shown in colour between pages 528 and 529) shows the three-dimensional structure of the catalytic domain (residues 63–354) of the B-transferase. The catalytic domains of the A- and B-transferases are organized in two subdomains separated by a cleft that contains the active site. One subdomain comprises the N-terminal region and recognizes the UDP-sugar donor. The other, C-terminal, subdomain provides the acceptor binding site. The A- and B-transferases differ by only four amino acid residues (see Table 4.7). The amino acid differences (Arg176Gly and Gly235Ser) are not in direct contact with the UDP-sugar, although Gly235Ser may influence the nature of the acceptor to be glycosylated. The other amino acids (Leu266Met and Gly268Ala) are situated in the active sites of the enzymes. In the B-transferase, residues Met266 and Ala268 are bulkier than the corresponding residues in the A-transferase and restrict the size of the active site cleft to exclude UDP-GalNAc (Patenaude *et al.* 2002).

The common kind of O (O^1) allele has a deletion at nucleotide 261, leading to a frameshift that alters the protein sequence after amino acid 88 and results in a truncated protein product, with only 117 amino acids compared with 354 for A and B. The product of this gene would therefore be enzymatically inactive. A

Table 4.7 Differences in amino acids (aa) between various alleles of the ABO gene. The insertion of brackets around four of the aa in A^1 and B indicates that these are the same in the two alleles, although they differ from those found in some rare alleles.

Amino acid	156	176	216	235	266	268	291	352
A^1	(Pro)	Arg	(Phe)	Gly	Leu	Gly	(Asp)	(Arg)
B	(Pro)	Gly	(Phe)	Ser	Met	Ala	(Asp)	(Arg)
O^{1*}								
O^2		Gly				Arg		
A^2	Leu							
A^3							Asn	
A^x			Ile					
B^3								Trp
$B^{(A)}$		Gly		Gly	Met	Ala		
$cisAB$	Leu			Ser		Ala		

* Truncated product.

For further details, see text (data from Yamamoto 1995).

variant of O^1, having the same truncated product but differing in having many point mutations (Yamamoto et al. 1990), has been termed O^{1v} and has been shown to be common, accounting for 40% of all O^1 samples (Olsson and Chester 1996). A second type of O allele (O^2) has no deletion at nucleotide 261 and, like A^1 and B, specifies a protein of 354 amino acids. The product resembles B in having glycine rather than arginine at residue 176 but (unlike A or B) it has arginine at residue 268. The presence of a large amino acid such as arginine in the active site of the enzyme is likely to account for the absence of transferase activity in this gene product (Table 4.7; Plate 4.1). This second type of O allele comprises 2–5% of O alleles in white people but appears to be rare in other populations (Chester and Olsson 2001). Several other rare O alleles have been described (Hosseini-Maaf et al. 2005). Hosseini Maaf and co-workers point out that the occurrence of unusual O alleles lacking the common deletion of nucleotide 261 or the presence of Arg268 is a considerable concern when ABO typing is carried out using DNA-based methods because there is a serious risk that the wrong information concerning the ABO phenotype of the red cells will be deduced (for further discussion of DNA-based blood typing see Chapter 8).

The A^2 transferase differs from A^1 in having leucine instead of proline at amino acid 156, and in having an extended carboxyl terminus due to a frameshift mutation (Yamamoto et al. 1992). A^3 is heterogeneous at the DNA level; in two A_3B subjects, the A-transferase differed from A^1 in having aspartic acid instead of asparagine at 291, but in two A^3O subjects, there was

no evidence that the A allele differed from A^1 within the regions of the gene (exons 6 and 7) encoding the catalytic domain (Yamamoto et al. 1993a). A^x differs from A^1 in having isoleucine instead of pheny-lalanine at 216 (Yamamoto et al. 1993b). A single example of B^3 differed from normal B in having tryptophan instead of arginine at 352 but no other examples showed any differences from B, indicating that B^3 is heterogeneous (Yamamoto et al. 1993a). An example of $B^{(A)}$ was identical to B at residues 176, 266 and 268 but at residue 235 resembled A in having glycine instead of the serine found in B (Yamamoto et al. 1993c). Two examples of cis AB had leucine at 156, as in A^2 but were like B at residues 235 and 268 (Yamamoto et al. 1993b). See also p. 117. For further information on the molecular bases of weak A, B and O variants see Daniels (2002); see also the Blood Group Antigen Gene Mutation Database [at http://www.bioc.aecom.yu.edu/bgmut/abo.htm)].

The H gene has been cloned and sequenced (Rajan et al. 1989; Larsen et al. 1990). The cDNA predicted a protein of 365 amino acids with the same overall structure as the A-transferase but lacking significant sequence homology with it. The secretor gene product was cloned by Kelly and co-workers (1995). The secretor transferase has substantial sequence homology with the H-transferase in its carboxy-terminal domain. The H- and Se-specified enzymes are two distinct fucosyl transferases, now named FUT1 and FUT2. Numerous different inactivating mutations in FUT1 have been described in DNA from individuals with the rare Bombay phenotype. Similarly, several different inactivating mutations in FUT2 result in the secretornegative

149

phenotype (reviewed in Daniels 2002). In the Far East and South Pacific, a mutation Ile129Phe in *FUT2* encodes a secretor transferase with a fivefold lower activity. This allele (Se^w) results in reduced levels of H antigen in secretions and the red cell phenotype Le(a+ b+) (Henry *et al.* 1996a,b).

I and i

I and i determinants are carbohydrate structures of

i: Gal(β1→4)GlcNAc(β1→3)Gal(β1→4)GlcNAc(β1→3)Gal(β1→4)Glc-R

I: Gal(β1→4)GlcNAc(β1→3)Gal(β1→4)GlcNAc(β1→3)Gal(β1→4)Glc-R

$$\diagup (β1→6)$$

Gal(β1→4)GlcNAc

These structures may carry, on their non-reducing end, other antigenic determinants such as ABH, Lewis and P$_1$.

The combined action of β1→3 GlcNAc-transferase and β1→4 Gal-transferase is required for the biosynthesis of i antigenic structures (Piller and Cartron 1983). The *I* gene is located on chromosome 6p24. It encodes a β6-*N*-acetylglucosaminyltransferase (*IGnT* syn.*GCNT2*). There are three isoforms of *IGnT* (*A,B* and *C*). Each isoform utilises a different open reading frame in exon 1 with the same exons 2 and 3. The isoform responsible for the human *I* gene is *IgnTC*, as this is the only isoform expressed in reticulocytes (Yu *et al.* 2003). Inactivating mutations in *IGnT* in Asians with the adult i phenotype and associated congenital cataracts affect all isoforms, whereas mutations giving rise to the adult i phenotype in white people without congenital cataracts affect only the isoform *IGnTC*. As the only isoform found in lens-epithelium cells is *IGnTB* there is no enzyme deficiency in the lens epithelium of the white people and consequently no congenital cataracts (Yu *et al.* 2003).

It seems that the heterogeneity of anti-I depends upon recognition of different parts of the above structure. Using analogues of the branched glycolipid on red cells, Feizi and co-workers (1979) found three patterns of reaction: some examples of anti-I recognized the 1→4, 1→6 branch; others recognized the 1→4, 1→3 sequence in the presence of branching; and others required both branches to be intact. However, it seems clear that the immunodominant group of the I antigen is GlcNAc linked 1→6 to a galactose of the 3 position

HAB-active oligosaccharides. i specificity is determined by a straight polylactosamine chain containing repeating Gal(β1→4)GlcNAc(β1→3) sequences, attached to ceramide or protein (R below). In normal development, i antigen is converted to I antigen by a glycosyltransferase which adds a branch by β1→6 linkage to the middle galactose of the unbranched i-active structure, as shown in the structure below; up to five branches can be added per chain (see review by Hakomori 1981).

of this galactose is necessary for the expression of the I activity detected with most anti-I sera, but not for all. Substitution of other positions of the GlcNAc sequence will either depress or enhance I activity and this effect will be different for different examples of anti-I.

In general, ABH determinants of red cells are carried on branched type 2 chains linked to lipids (ceramide) or to intrinsic membrane glycoproteins (predominantly band 3 and the glucose transporter, GLUT1, see Chapter 3) in adults, whereas red cells of the fetus and newborn have unbranched type 2 molecules. The Ii determinants available for reactivity with anti-I and anti-i can be regarded as uncompleted ABH-active chains (for review, see Hakomori 1981; 1984). The process of branching through GlcNAc(β1→6) linkage is related to the ontogenic development of red cells, and the total quantity of type 2 chains increases during differentiation of erythroblasts or erythrocytes (Hakomori 1984).

The i antigen occurs in plasma as glycoprotein (Cooper and Brown 1973).

References

Abelson NM, Rawson AJ (1961) Studies of blood group antibodies. V. Fractionation of examples of anti-B, anti-A, B, anti-M, anti-P, anti-Jk^a, anti-Le^a, anti-D, anti-CD, anti-K, anti-Fy^a and anti-Good. Transfusion 1: 116

Adinolfi M, Polley MJ, Hunter DA *et al.* (1962) Classification of blood-group antibodies as β$_2$M or gamma globulin. Immunology 5: 566

Adinolfi A, Mollison PL, Polley MJ et al. (1966) γA blood group antibodies. J Exp Med 123: 951

Allen PZ, Kabat EA (1958) Persistence of circulating antibodies in human subjects immunized with dextran, levan and blood group substances. J Immunol 80: 495

Alter AA, Rosenfield RE (1964a) B_x: subtype of B. Blood 23: 600

Alter AA, Rosenfield RE (1964b) The nature of some subtypes of A. Blood 23: 605

Andersen J (1958) Modifying influence of the secretor gene on the development of the ABH substance. Vox Sang 3: 251

Andersson B, Porras O, Hanson LÅ et al. (1986) Inhibition of attachment of Streptococcus pneumoniae and Haemophilus influenzae by human milk and receptor oligosaccharides. J Infect Dis 153: 232–237

Andresen PH (1948) The blood group system L. A new blood group L_2. A case of epistasy within the blood groups. Acta Pathol Microbiol Scand 25: 728

Andresen PH, Jordal K (1949) An incomplete agglutinin related to the L-(Lewis) system. Acta Pathol Microbiol Scand 26: 636

Arcilla MB, Sturgeon P (1973) Studies on the secretion of blood group substances. II. Observations on the red cell phenotype Le(a– b– x–). Vox Sang 25: 72

Arcilla MB, Sturgeon P (1974) Le^x, the spurned antigen of the Lewis blood group system. Vox Sang 26: 425

Aubert EF, Boorman KE, Dodd BE et al. (1942) The universal donor with high titre iso-agglutinins: the effect of anti-A iso-agglutinins on recipients of group A. BMJ i: 659

Auf der Maur C, Hodel M, Nydegger UE et al. (1993) Age dependency of ABO histo-blood group antibodies: reexamination of an old dogma. Transfusion 33: 915–918

Badet J, Ropars C, Cartron JP et al. (1976) Groups of α-D-galactosyltransferase activity in sera of individuals with normal B phenotype. II. Relationship between transferase activity and red cell agglutinability. Vox Sang 30: 105

Bailly P, Sondag D, Chevaleyre J et al. (1986) Monoclonal antibodies directed against the human P blood group glycolipid antigen (Abstract), 19th Congress of the International Society of Blood Transfusion, Sydney, p. 503

Bakunina IY, Kuhlmann RA, Likhosherstov LM et al. (2002) Alpha-N-acetylgalactosaminidase from marine bacterium Arenibacter latericius KMM 426T removing blood type specificity of A erythrocytes. Biochemistry (Mosc) 67: 689–695

Barragan A, Kremsner PG, Wahlgren M et al. (2000) Blood group A antigen is a coreceptor in Plasmodium falciparum rosetting. Infect Immun 68: 2971–2975

Baumgarten A, Kruchok AH, Weirich F (1976) High frequency of IgG anti-A and -B antibody in old age. Vox Sang 30: 253

Beck ML, Yates ASD, Hardman JT et al. (1987) Consequences of overlapping substrate specificity of glycosyltransferases (Abstract). Transfusion 27: 535

Ben-Ismail R, Rouger P, Carme B et al. (1980) Comparative automated assay of anti-P_1 antibodies in acute hepatic distomiasis (fascioliasis) and in hydatidosis. Vox Sang 38: 165–168

Betteridge A, Watkins WM (1985) Variant forms of alpha-2-L fucosyltransferase in human submaxillary glands from blood group ABH 'secretor' and 'non-secretor' individuals. Glycoconj J 2: 61–78

Bevan A, Hammond W, Clarke RL (1970) Anti-P_1 associated with liver-fluke infection. Vox Sang 18: 188

Bhende YM. Despande CK, Bhatia HM et al. (1952) A 'new' blood-group character related to the ABO system. Lancet i: 903

Bird GWG (1952) Relationship of the blood sub-groups A_1, A_2 and A_1B, A_2B to haemagglutinins present in the seeds of Dolichos biflorus. Nature (Lond) 170: 674

Bird GWG (1977) Erythrocyte polyagglutination. In: CRC Handbook Series in Clinical Laboratory Science, Section D: Blood Banking. TJ Greenwalt and EA Steane (eds), vol. 1. Cleveland, OH: CRC Press, p. 443

Bird GWG, Wingham J (1977) Erythrocyte autoantibody with unusual specificity. Vox Sang 32: 280

Bird GWG, Wingham J, Chester GH et al. (1976) Erythrocyte membrane modification in malignant disease of myeloid and lymphoreticular tissues. II. Erythrocyte 'mosaicism' in acute erythroleukaemia. Br J Haematol 33: 295

Bjorkholm B, Lundin A, Sillen A et al. (2001) Comparison of genetic divergence and fitness between two subclones of Helicobacter pylori. Infect Immun 69: 7832–7838

Blackwell CC, Jóndsóttir K, Hanson M et al. (1986) Non-secretion of ABO antigens predisposing to infection by Neisseria meningitidis and Streptococcus pneumoniae. Lancet ii: 284–285

Blackwell CC, Dundas S, James VS et al. (2002) Blood group and susceptibility to disease caused by Escherichia coli 0151. J Infect Dis 185: 393–396

Boorman KE, Dodd BE, Mollison PL (1945) Iso-immunisation to the blood-group factors A, B and Rh. J Pathol Bacteriol 57: 157

Booth PB (1970) Anti-I^TP_1: an antibody showing a further association between the I and P blood group system. Vox Sang 19: 85

Booth PB, Jenkins WJ, Marsh WL (1966) Anti-I^T: A new antibody of the I blood group system occurring in certain Melanesian sera. Br J Haematol 12: 341

Bowen DJ (2003) An influence of ABO blood group on the rate of proteolysis of von Willebrand factor by ADAMTS13. J Thromb Haemost 1: 33–40

Brendemoen OJ (1952) A cold agglutinin specifically active against stored red cells. Acta Pathol Microbiol Scand 31: 574

Broadberry RE, Lin-Chu M (1991) The Lewis blood group system among Chinese in Taiwan. Hum Hered 41: 290–294

Brocteur J, Francois-Gerard C, André A *et al.* (1975) Immunization against avian proteins. Haematologia 9: 43

Brouwers HAA, Overbeeke MAM, Gemke RJBJ *et al.* (1987) Sensitive methods for determining subclasses of IgG anti-A and anti-B in sera of blood-group-O women with a blood-group-A or -B child. Br J Haematol 66: 267–70

Brown KE, Hibbs JR, Gallinella G *et al.* (1994) Resistance to parvovirus B19 infection due to lack of virus receptor (erythrocyte P antigen). N Engl J Med 330: 1192–1196

Bruce M, Watt A, Gabra GS *et al.* (1988) LKE red cell antigen and its relationship to P_1 and P^k: serological study of a large family. Vox Sang 55: 237–240

Cameron GL, Staveley JM (1957) Blood group P substance in hydatid cyst fluids. Nature (Lond) 179: 147

Cameron C, Dunsford I, Sickle GR *et al.* (1959) Acquisition of a B-like antigen by red blood cells. BMJ ii: 29

Cartron JP (1976) Étude quantative et thermodynamique des phénotypes érythrocytaires 'A faible'. Rev Fr Transfus Immunohématol 19: 35

Cartron JP, Gerbal A, Hughes-Jones NC *et al.* (1974) 'Weak A' phenotypes. Relationship between red cell agglutinability and antigen site density. Immunology 27: 723

Ceppellini R (1955) On the genetics of secretor and Lewis characters: a family study. Proceedings of the 5th Congress of the International Society of Blood Transfusion, Paris

Chandeysson PL, Flye MW, Simpkins SM *et al.* (1981) Delayed hemolytic transfusion reaction caused by anti-P_1 antibody. Transfusion 21: 77–82

Chaplin H Jr, Wallace MG, Chang E *et al.* (1956) A study of iso-agglutinin and hemolysin screening procedures for universal donors. Am J Clin Pathol 26: 721

Chattoraj A, Gilbert R Jr, Josephson AM (1968) Serological demonstration of fetal production of blood group isoantibodies. Vox Sang 14: 289

Cheng MS, Lukomsky J (1989) Lewis antibody following a massive blood transfusion. Vox Sang 57: 155–156

Chester MA, Olsson ML (2001) The ABO blood group gene – a locus of considerable genetic diversity. Transfusion Med Rev 11: 295–313

Clarke CA, McConnell RB, Sheppard PM (1960) A genetical study of the variations in ABH secretion. Ann Hum Genet 24: 295

Clausen H, Levery SB, Nudelman SS *et al.* (1985) Repetitive A epitope (Type 3 chain A) defined by blood group A_1-specific antibody TH-1: chemical basis of qualitative A_1 and A_2 distinction. Proc Natl Acad Sci USA 82: 1119–1203

Constantoulakis M, Kay HEM, Giles *et al.* (1963) Observations on the A_2 gene and H antigen in foetal life. Br J Haematol 9: 63

Contreras M, Armitage SE, Hewitt PE (1983) Response to immunization with A and B human glycoproteins for the procurement of blood grouping reagents. Vox Sang 47: 224–235

Cooling LL, Kelly K, Barton J *et al.* (2005) Determinants of ABH expression on human blood platelets. Blood 105: 3356–3364. Epub, 21 December 2004

Cooper DKC (1990) A clinical survey of cardiac transplantation between ABO blood group-incompatible recipients and donors. Transplant Proc 22: 1457

Cooper RA (1977) Abnormalities of cell-membrane fluidity in the pathogenesis of disease. N Engl J Med 297: 371

Cooper AG, Brown MC (1973) Serum i antigen: a new human blood group glycoprotein. Biochem Biophys Res Commun 55: 297

Cooper AG, Hoffband AV, Worlledge SM (1968) Increased agglutinability by anti-i of red cells in sideroblastic and megaloblastic anaemia. Br J Haematol 15: 381

Cory HT, Yates AD, Donald ASR *et al.* (1974) The nature of the human blood group P_1 determinant. Biochem Biophys Res Commun 61: 1289

Crawford H, Cutbush M, Mollison PL (1953) Hemolytic disease of the newborn due to anti-A. Blood 8: 620

Crookston MC, Tilley CA, Crookston JH (1970) Human blood chimaera with seeming breakdown of immune tolerance. Lancet ii: 1110

Curtain CC (1969) Anti-I agglutinins in non-human sera. Vox Sang 16: 161

Cutbush M, Mollison PL (1958) Relation between characteristics of blood-group antibodies *in vitro* and associated patterns of red cell destruction *in vivo*. Br J Haematol 4: 115

Cutbush M, Giblett ER, Mollison PL (1956) Demonstration of the phenotype Le(a+ b+) in infants and in adults. Br J Haematol 2: 210

Daniels GL (1984) Studies on anti-H reagents. Rev Fr Transfus Immunohématol 27: 603–612

Daniels G (1995) Human Blood Groups. Oxford: Blackwell Science

Daniels GL (2002) Human Blood Groups, 2nd edn. Oxford: Blackwell Science, pp. 7–67

Daniels GL, Cartron JP, Fletcher A (2003) International Society of Blood Transfusion Committee on terminology for red cell surface antigens: Vancouver Report. Vox Sang 84: 244–247

Dausset J, Vidal G (1951) Accidents de la transfusion chez des receveurs de groupe A ayant reçu du sang de groupe O: rôle de la vaccination par l'anatoxine diphtérique et tétanique. Sang 22: 478

Davey RJ, Procter JL, Brown KE (1994) Identification of P antigen-negative red cells using parvovirus B19 capsids. Vox Sang 67 (Suppl.): 2–8

Denborough MA, Downing HJ (1969) The incidence of anti-A and anti-B isoagglutinins in cord blood and maternal saliva. Br J Haematol 16: 111

Dienst A (1905) Das Eklampsiegift. Zbl Gynäk 29: 353 and 651

DiNapoli JB, Nichols ME, Marsh WL et al. (1977) Hemolytic Transfusion Reaction caused by IgG anti-P_1. Atlanta, GA: Commun Am Assoc Blood Banks

Dodd BE, Lincoln PJ, Boorman KE (1967) The cross-reacting antibodies of group 0 sera: immunological studies and a possible explanation of the observed facts. Immunology 12: 39

Doinel C, Ropars C, Salmon C (1976) Quantitative and thermodynamic measurements on I and i antigens of human red blood cells. Immunology 30: 289

Dorf ME, Eguro SY, Cabrera G et al. (1972) Detection of cytotoxic non-HL-A antisera I. Relationship to anti-Le^a. Vox Sang 22: 447

Dunstan RA (1986) Status of major red cell blood group antigens on neutrophils, lymphocytes and monocytes. Br J Haematol 62: 301–309

Dunstan RA, Simpson MB (1985) Heterogeneous distribution of antigens on human platelets demonstrated by fluorescence flow cytometry. Br J Haematol 61: 603–609

Dunstan RA, Simpson MB, Borowitz M (1985a) Absence of ABH antigens on neutrophils. Br J Haematol 60: 651–657

Dunstan RA, Simpson MB, Knowles RW et al. (1985b) The origin of ABH antigens on human platelets. Blood 65: 615–619

Dunstan RA, Simpson MB, Rosse WF (1985c) Presence of P blood group antigens on human platelets. Am J Clin Pathol 83: 731–735

Economidou J (1966) A study of the reactions between certain human blood group antigens and their respective antibodies with special reference to the ABO system. PhD Thesis, London University, London

Economidou J, Hughes-Jones NC (1967) Quantitative measurements concerning A and B antigen sites. Vox Sang 12: 321

Economidou J, Hughes-Jones NC, Gardner B (1967a) The functional activities of IgG and IgM anti-A and anti-B. Immunology 13: 227

Economidou J, Hughes-Jones NC, Gardner B (1967b) The reactivity of subunits of IgM anti-B. Immunology 13: 235

Elmgren A, Börjeson C, Svensson L et al. (1996) DNA sequencing and screening for point mutations in the human Lewis (FUT3) gene enables molecular genotyping of the human Lewis blood group system. Vox Sang 70: 97–103

Engelfriet CP, Beckers D, von dem Borne AEGKr et al. (1972) Haemolysins probably recognising the antigen p. Vox Sang 23: 176

Evans RS, Turner E, Bingham M (1965) Studies with radio-iodinated cold agglutinins of ten patients. Am J Med 38: 378

Feizi T, Marsh WL (1970) Demonstration of I–anti-I interaction in a precipitin system. Vox Sang 18: 379

Feizi T, Kabat EA, Vicari G et al. (1971) Immunochemical studies on blood groups, XLVII. The I antigen complex–precursors in the A, B, H, Le^a and Le^b, blood group system–hemagglutination-inhibition studies. J Exp Med 133: 39

Feizi T, Childs RA, Watanabe K et al. (1979) Three types of blood group I specificity among monoclonal anti-I autoantibodies revealed by analogues of a branched erythrocyte glycolipid. J Exp Med 149: 975–980

Fellous M, Gerbal A, Thessier C et al. (1974) Studies on the biosynthetic pathway of human P erythrocyte antigens using somatic cells in culture. Vox Sang 26: 516–536

Fibach E, Sharon R (1994) Changes in ABH antigen expression on red cells during in vivo aging: a flow cytometric analysis. Transfusion 34: 328–332

Fong SW, Qaqundah BY, Taylor WF (1974) Developmental patterns of ABO isoagglutinins in normal children correlated with the effects of age, sex and maternal isoagglutinins. Transfusion 14: 551

Forssman J (1911) Die Herstellung hochwertiger spezifischer Schafhämolysine ohne Verwendung von Schafblut. Ein Beitrag zur Lehre von heterologer Antikörperbildung. Biochem Z 37: 78

François-Gérard C, Brocteur J, André A (1980) Turtledove: a new source of P_1-like material cross-reacting with the human erythrocyte antigen. Vox Sang 39: 141–148

Franks D, Coombs RRA (1969) General aspects of heterophil antibody systems. In: Infectious Mononucleosis. RL Carter, HG Penman (eds). Oxford: Blackwell Scientific Publications

Freda VJ, Wiener AS, Gordon EB (1957) An unsuspected source of ABO sensitization. Am J Obstet Gynecol 73: 1148

Friedenreich V (1931) Ueber die Serologie der Untergruppen A_1 und A_2. Z Immun-Forsch 71: 283

Fudenberg HH, Kunkel HG, Franklin EC (1959) High molecular weight antibodies. Acta Haematol (Basel) Fasc 10: 522

Furukawa K, Iwamura K, Uchikawa M et al. (2000) Molecular basis for the p phenotype. Identification of distinct and multiple mutations in the alpha 1,4-galactosyltransferase gene in Swedish and Japanese individuals. J Biol Chem 275: 37752–37756

Gammelgaard A (1942) Om Sjaeldne Svage A-receptorer (A_3, A_4, A_5, og A_x), Haos Mennesket. Copenhagen: Nyt Nordisk Forlag. [English translation published in 1964 by Walter Reed Army Institute of Medical Research, Washington, DC]

Garratty G, Haffleigh B, Dalziel J et al. (1972) An IgG anti-I^T detected in a caucasian American. Transfusion 12: 325

Garratty G, Arndt P, Co S et al. (1993) Fatal ABO hemolytic transfusion reaction resulting from acquired B antigen only detectable by some monoclonal anti-B reagents. Transfusion 33 (Suppl.): 47S

Garretta M, Muller A, Gener J et al. (1974) Reliability in automatic determination of the ABO group by the groupamatic system. Vox Sang 27: 141

Gerbal A, Maslet C, Salmon C (1975) Immunological aspects of the acquired B antigen. Vox Sang 28: 398

Gibbs MB, Akeroyd JH, Zapf JJ (1961) Quantitative sub-groups of the B antigen in man and their occurrence in three racial groups. Nature (Lond) 192: 1196–1197

Giblett ER, Crookston MC (1964) Agglutinability of red cells by anti-i in patients with thalassaemia major and other haematological disorders. Nature (Lond) 201: 1138

Giles CM, Poole J (1979) Auto-anti-Le^b in the serum of a renal dialysis patient. Clin Lab Haematol 1: 239–242

Godzisz J (1979) La synthèse des allohémagglutinines naturelles du système ABO chez les enfants sains âgés de 3 mois à 3 ans. Rev Fr Transfus Immunohématol 22: 399–412

Gold ER, Tovey GH, Benney S et al. (1959) Changes in the group A antigen in a case of leukemia. Nature (Lond) 183: 892

Goldstein J, Siviglia G, Hurst R et al. (1982) Group B erythrocytes enzymatically converted to group O survive normally in A, B, and O individuals. Science 215: 168–170

Gonzalez Ordonez AJ, Medina Rodriguez JM, Martin L et al. (1999) The O blood group protects against venous thromboembolism in individuals with the factor V Leiden but not the prothrombin (factor II G20210A) mutation. Blood Coagul Fibrinolysis 10: 303–307

Good AH, Yau O, Lamontagne et al. (1992) Serological and chemical specificities of twelve monoclonal anti-Le^a and anti-Le^b antibodies. Vox Sang 62: 180–189

Gouge JJ, Boyce F, Peterson P et al. (1977) A puzzling problem due to a harmless cold auto-antibody: unpublished observations

Greenbury CL, Moore DH, Nunn LAC (1963) Reaction of 7S and 19S components of immune rabbit antisera with human group A and AB red cells. Immunology 6: 421

Greenbury CL, Moore DH, Nunn LAC (1965) The reaction with red cells of 7S rabbit antibody, its sub-units and their recombinants. Immunology 8: 420

Grubb R (1951) Observations on the human group system Lewis. Acta Pathol Microbiol Scand 28: 61

Grundbacher FJ (1967) Quantity of hemolytic anti-A and anti-B in individuals of a human population: correlations with isoagglutinins and effects of the individual's age and sex. Z Immun Forsch 134: 317

Grundbacher FJ (1976) Genetics of anti-A and anti-B levels. Transfusion 16: 48

Guest AR, Scott ML, Smythe J et al. (1992) Analysis of the structure and activity of A and A,B immunoglobulin A monoclonal antibodies. Transfusion 32: 239–245

Gunson HH, Latham V (1972) An agglutinin in human serum reacting with cells from Le(a–b–) non-secretor individuals. Vox Sang 22: 344

Gupte SC, Bhatia HM (1980) Increased incidence of haemolytic disease of the new-born caused by ABO-incompatibility when tetanus toxoid is given during pregnancy. Vox Sang 38: 22–28

Haddad SA (1974) A serological study of an O$_h$ woman and her newborn infant. Can J Med Technol 36: 373

Hakomori S-I (1981) Blood group ABH and Ii antigens of human erythrocytes: chemistry, polymorphism, and their developmental change. Semin Hematol 18: 39–62

Hakomori SI (1984) Monoclonal antibodies directed to cell-surface carbohydrates. In: Monoclonal Antibodies and Functional Cell Lines. RH Kennett, KB Bechtol, TJ McKearn (eds). New York: Plenum Press, pp. 67–100

Hammar L, Mansson S, Rohr T et al. (1981) Lewis phenotype of erythrocytes and Le^b-active glycolipid in serum of pregnant women. Vox Sang 40: 27–33

Hammarström S, Kabat EA (1969) Purification and characterization of a blood-group A reactive hemagglutinin from the snail Helix pomatia and a study of its combining site. Biochemistry 8: 2696

Hansson GC, Wazniowska K, Rock JA et al. (1988) The glycosphingolipid composition of the placenta of a blood group P fetus delivered by a blood group P$_1^k$ woman and analysis of the anti-globoside antibodies found in maternal serum. Arch Biochem Biophys 260: 168–176

Harpaz N, Flowers HN, Sharon N (1975) Studies on B-antigenic sites of human erythrocytes by use of coffee bean α-galactosidase. Arch Biochem Biophys 170: 676

Harper P, Bias WB, Hutchinson JK et al. (1971) ABH secretor status of the fetus: a genetic marker identifiable by amniocentesis. J Med Genet 8: 438

Heier HE, Namork E, Ualkovská Z (1994) Expression of A antigens on erythrocytes of weak blood group A subgroups. Vox Sang 66: 231–236

Heiner DC, Kevy SV (1956) Visceral larva migrans: report of the syndrome in three siblings. N Engl J Med 254: 629

Hellberg A, Poole J, Olsson ML (2002) Molecular basis of the globoside-deficient P(k) blood group phenotype. Identification of four inactivating mutations in the UDP-N-acetylgalactosamine: globotriaosylceramide 3-beta-N-acetylgalactosaminyltransferase gene. J Biol Chem 277: 29455–29459

Hellberg A, Steffensen R, Yahalom V et al. (2003) Additional molecular bases of the clinically important p blood group phenotype. Transfusion 43: 899–907

Hellberg A, Ringressi A, Yahalom V et al. (2004) Genetic heterogeneity at the glycosyltransferase loci underlying GLOB blood group system and collection. Br J Haematol 125: 528–536

Hendry JL, Sickles GR (1951) Ann Rep of Division of Labs and Res NY State Dept of Health

Henningsen K (1949) Investigations on the blood factor P. Acta Pathol Microbiol Scand 26: 639

Henningsen K (1952) Om Blodtypesystemet P. MD Thesis, Dansk Videnskabs Forlag A/S, Copenhagen (cited by Race and Sanger, 1954)

Henry SM, Benny AG, Woodfield DG (1990) Investigation of Lewis phenotypes in polynesians. Vox Sang 58, 61–66

Henry S, Mollicone R, Fernandez P *et al.* (1996) Molecular basis for erythrocyte Le(a+ b+) and salivary ABH partial-secretor phenotypes: expression of a FUT2 secretor allele with an A→T mutation at nucleotide 385 correlates with reduced alpha(1,2) fucosyltransferase activity. Glycoconj J 13: 985–993

Henry SM, Mollicone R, Fernandez P *et al.* (1996b) Homozygous expression of a missense mutation at nucleotide 385 in the FUT2 gene associates with the Le(a+ b+) partial-secretor phenotype in an Indonesian family. Biochem Biophys Res Commun 219: 675–678

Hill AVS (1992) Malarial resistance genes: a natural selection. Trans R Soc Trop Med Hyg 86: 225–226, 232

Hillman RS, Giblett ER (1965) Red cell membrane alteration associated with 'marrow stress'. J Clin Invest 44: 1730

Hirsch HF, Graham HA (1980) Adsorption of Le^c and Le^d from plasma onto red blood cells. Transfusion 20: 474–475

Hirsch HF, Graham HA, Davies DM (1975) The relationship of the Le^c and Le^d antigens to the Lewis, Secretor and ABO systems (Abstract). Transfusion 15: 521

Holburn AM (1973) Quantitative studies with [^{125}I] IgM anti-Le^a. Immunology 24: 1019

Holburn AM (1976) Radioimmunoassay studies of the cross-reacting antibody of human group O sera. Br J Haematol 32: 589

Holburn AM, Masters CA (1974a) The radioimmunoassay of serum and salivary blood group A and Le^a glycoproteins. Br J Haematol 28: 157

Holburn AM, Masters CA (1974b) The reactions of IgG and IgM anti-A and anti-B blood group antibodies with ^{125}I-labelled blood group glycoproteins. Vox Sang 27: 115

Hoskins LC, Boulding ET (2001) Changes in immunologic properties of group A RBCs during treatment with an A-degrading exo-alpha-N-acetylgalactosaminidase. Transfusion 41: 908–916

Hoskins LC, Boulding ET, Larson G (1997) Purification and characterization of blood group A-degrading isoforms of alpha-N-acetylgalactosaminidase from *Ruminococcus torques* strain IX-70. J Biol Chem 272: 7932–7939

Hossaini AA (1972) Neutralization of Lewis antibodies *in vivo* and transfusion of Lewis incompatible blood. Am J Clin Pathol 57: 489

Hosseini-Maaf B, Irshaid NM, Hellborg A *et al.* (2005) New and unusual O alleles at the ABO locus are implicated in unexpected blood group phenotypes. Transfusion 45: 70–81

Høstrup H (1963) A and B blood group substances in the serum of the newborn infant and the foetus. Vox Sang 8: 557

Høstrup H (1964) Influence of foetal A and B blood-group substances on the immunization of pregnant women. Vox Sang 9: 301

Hsieh HY, Smith D. (2003) *Clostridium perfringens* alpha-N-acetylgalactosaminidase blood group A2-degrading activity. Biotechnol Appl Biochem 37(Pt 2):157–163

Huang P, Farkas T, Marionneau S *et al.* (2003) Noroviruses bind to human ABO, Lewis, and secretor histo-blood group antigens: identification of 4 distinct strain-specific patterns. J Infect Dis 188: 19–31

Hughes AK, Ergonul Z, Stricklett PK *et al.* (2002) Molecular basis for high renal cell sensitivity to the cytotoxic effects of shigatoxin-1: upregulation of globotriaosylceramide expression. J Am Soc Nephrol 13: 2239–2245

Hutson AM, Atmar RL, Marcus DM *et al.* (2003) Norwalk virus-like particle hemagglutination by binding to h histo-blood group antigens. J Virol 77: 405–415

Ichikawa Y (1959) A study of the iso-agglutinin titres in the sera of Australian subjects (white). Jap J Med Sci Biol 12: 1

Ilver D, Arnqvist A, Ogren J *et al.* (1998) *Helicobacter pylori* adhesin binding fucosylated histo-blood group antigens revealed by retagging. Science 279: 373–377

Ishizaka K, Ishizaka T, Lee EH *et al.* (1965) Immunochemical properties of human γA isohemagglutinin. I. Comparisons with γG- and γM-globulin antibodies. J Immunol 95: 197

Ishizaka T, Tada T, Ishizaka K (1968) Fixation of C' and C'Ia by rabbit γG- and γM-antibodies with particulate and soluble antigens. J Immunol 100: 1145

Issitt PD, Tegoli I, Jackson V *et al.* (1968) Anti-IP$_1$; antibodies that show an association between the I and P blood group systems. Vox Sang 14: 1

Iwamura K, Furukawa K, Uchikawa M *et al.* (2003) The blood group P1 synthase gene is identical to the Gb3/CD77 synthase gene. A clue to the solution of the P1/P2/p puzzle. J Biol Chem 278:44429–44438

Jakobowicz R, Simmons RT, Carew JP (1961) Group A blood incompatibility due to the development of apparent anti-A$_1$ antibodies in a patient of subgroup A$_2$. Vox Sang 6: 320

Jenkins WJ, Marsh WL, Noades J *et al.* (1960) The I antigen and antibody. Vox Sang 5: 97

Jonsson B (1936) Zur Frage der heterospezifischen Schwangerschaft. Acta Pathol Microbiol Scand 13: 424

Jordal K (1956) The Lewis blood groups in children. Acta Pathol Microbiol Scand 39: 399

Judd WJ, Steiner EA, Friedman BA *et al.* (1978) Anti-Le^a as an autoantibody in the serum of a Le(a− b+) individual. Transfusion 18: 436

Juel E (1959) Anti-A agglutinins in sera from A$_2$B individuals. Acta Pathol Microbiol Scand 46: 91

Kabat EA, Mayer MM (1961) Experimental Immuno-chemistry, 2nd edn. Springfield, IL: Charles C Thomas

Källenius G, Svenson SB, Möllby R *et al.* (1981) Structure of carbohydrate part of receptor on human uroepithelial cells for pyelonephritogenic *Escherichia coli*. Lancet ii: 604–606

Kelly RJ, Rouquier S, Giorgi D *et al.* (1995) Sequence and expression of a candidate for the human Secretor blood group alpha(1,2)fucosyltransferase gene (FUT2). Homozygosity for an enzyme-inactivating nonsense mutation commonly correlates with the non-secretor phenotype. J Biol Chem 270: 4640–4649

Kelton JG, Hamid C, Aker S *et al.* (1982) The amount of blood group A substance on platelets is proportional to the amount in the plasma. Blood 59: 980–985

Kemp T (1930) Über den Empfindlichkeitsgrad der Blutkörperchen gegenüber Isohämagglutinen im Fötalleben und im Kindesalter beim Menschen. Acta Pathol Microbiol Scand 7: 146

Kennell CB, Muschel LH (1956) Effect of mothers' ABO blood group on isoantibody levels of group O children. US Army Med Forces Med J 7: 1313

Kerde C, Fünfhausen G, Brunk Re *et al.* (1960) Über die Gewinnung von hochwertigen Anti-P-Immunserun durch Immunisierung mit Echinokokken-zysten Flüssigkeit. Z Immun-Forsch 119: 216

Kissmeyer-Nielsen F (1965) Irregular blood group antibodies in 200,000 individuals. Scand J Haematol 2: 331

Kissmeyer-Nielsen F, Bastrup-Madsen K, Stenderup A (1955) Irregular blood-group antibodies. Incidence and clinical significance. Dan Med Bull 2: 202

Knowles RW, Bai Y, Daniels GL *et al.* (1982) Monoclonal anti-Type 2 H: an antibody detecting a precursor of the A and B blood group antigens. J Immunogenet 9: 69–76

Kobata A, Grollman EF, Ginsburg V *et al.* (1968) An enzymatic basis for blood type A in humans. Arch Biochem Biophys 124: 609

Kochwa S, Rosenfeld RE, Tallal L *et al.* (1961) Isoagglutinins associated with erythroblastosis. J Clin Invest 40: 874

Kogure T, Furukawa K (1976) Enzymatic conversion of human group O red cells into group B active cells by α-D-galactosyltransferases of sera and salivas from group B and its variant types. J Immunogenet 3: 147

Kools A, Collins J, Aster RH (1981) Studies of the ABO antigens of human platelets (Abstract). Transfusion 21: 615–616

Koscielak J (2001) ABH blood group active glycoconjugates from human red cells. Transfusion Med 11: 267–279

Kruskall MS, AuBuchon JP, Anthony KY *et al.* (2000) Transfusion to blood group A and O patients of group B RBCs that have been enzymatically converted to group O. Transfusion 40: 1290–1298

Kulkarni AG, Ibazeke R, Fleming AF (1985) High frequency of anti-A and anti-B haemolysins in certain ethnic groups of Nigeria. Vox Sang 48: 39–41

Kunkel HG, Rockey JH (1963) β_2A and other immunoglobulins in isolated anti-A antibodies. Proc Soc Exp Biol (NY) 113: 278

Landsteiner K, Levine P (1927) Further observations on individual differences of human blood. Proc Soc Exp Biol (NY) 24: 941

Landsteiner K, Levine P (1929) On isoagglutinin reactions of human blood other than those defining the blood groups. J Immunol 17: 1

Landsteiner K, Witt DH (1926) Observations on the human blood groups. Irregular reactions. Iso-agglutinin in sera of group 4. The factor A_1. J Immunol 11: 221

Langkilde NC, Wolf H, Orntoft TF (1990) Lewis negative phenotype and bladder cancer (Letter). Lancet i: 926

Larsen GL, McCarthy K, Webster RV *et al.* (1980 – date correct?) A differential effect of $C5^a$ and $C5^a$ des Arg. in induction of pulmonary inflammation. Am J Pathol 100: 179–192

Lattes L, Cavazutti A (1924) Sur l'existence d'un troisième élément d'isogglutination. J Immunol 9: 407

Layrisse Z, Layrisse M (1968) High incidence cold auto-agglutinins of anti-I^T specificity in Yanomama Indians of Venezuela. Vox Sang 14: 369

Leffler H, Svanborg-Edén C (1981) Glycolipid receptors for uropathogenic *Escherichia coli* on human erythrocytes and uroepithelial cells. Infect Immun 34: 920–929

Lenny LL, Hurst R, Goldstein J *et al.* (1994) Transfusions to group O subjects of 2 units of red cells enzymatically converted from group B to group O. Transfusion 34: 209–214

Le Pendu J, Lemieux RU, Lambert F *et al.* (1982) Distribution of H Type 1 and Type 2 antigenic determinants in human sera and saliva. Am J Hum Genet 34: 402–415

Levene C (1979) Live children and abortions of p mothers (Letter). Transfusion 19: 224

Levine P, Polayes SH (1941) An atypical hemolysin in pregnancy. Ann Intern Med 14: 1903

Levine P, Bobbitt OB, Waller RK *et al.* (1951) Isoimmunization by a new blood factor in tumor cells. Proc Soc Exp Biol (NY) 77: 403

Levine P, Celano M, Staveley JM (1958) The antigenicity of P-substance in echinococcus cyst fluid coated onto tanned red cells. Vox Sang 3: 434

van Loghem JJ, Dorfmeier H, van der Mart M (1957) Two A antigens with abnormal serologic properties. Vox Sang 2: 16

van Loghem JJ, van der Hart M, Moes M *et al.* (1965) Increased red cell destruction in the absence of demonstrable antibodies *in vitro*. Transfusion 5: 525

Lin M, Shieh S-H (1994) Postnatal development of red blood cell he[a] and he[b] antigens in Chinese infants. Vox Sang 66: 137–140

Lomberg H, Cedergren B, Leffler H *et al.* (1986) Influence of blood group on the availability of receptors for attachment of uropathogenic *Escherichia coli*. Infect Immun 51: 919–926

Lopez M, Benali J, Cartron JP et al. (1980) Some notes on the specificity of anti-A_1 reagents. Vox Sang 39: 271–276

Lopez M, Cartron J, Cartron JP et al. (1983) Cytotoxicity of anti-PP_1P^k antibodies and possible relationship with early abortions of p mothers. Clin Immunol Immunopathol 28: 296–303

Lundberg WB, McGinniss MH (1975) Hemolytic transfusion reaction due to anti-A_1. Transfusion 15: 1

McShine RL, Kunst VAJM (1970) The stimulation of immune antibodies anti-A and anti-B in patients after treatment with cryoprecipitate and factor IX concentrate (PPSB according to Soulier). Vox Sang 18: 435

Mäkelä O, Mäkelä P (1956) Le^b antigen: studies on its occurrence in red cells, plasma and saliva. Ann Med Exp Fenn 34: 157

Mäkelä O, Mäkelä P, Krüppe M (1959) Zur Spezifität der anti-B Phythämagglutinine. Z Immun-Forsch 117: 220

Marcus DM, Kundu SK, Suzuki A (1981) The P blood group system: recent progress in immunochemistry and genetics. Semin Haematol 18: 63–71

Marionneau S, Cailleau-Thomas A, Rocher J et al. (2001) ABH and Lewis histo-blood group antigens, a model for the meaning of oligosaccharide diversity in the face of a changing world. Biochimie 83: 565–573

Matsuo K, Hamajima N, Ikehara Y et al. (2003) Smoking and polymorphisms of fucosyltransferase gene Le affect success of H. pylori eradication with lansoprazole, amoxicillin, and clarithromycin. Epidemiol Infect 130: 227–33

Messeter L, Johnson U (1990) Preface to the proceedings on monoclonal antibodies against human red blood cells and related antigens. J Immunogenet 17: 213–215

Messeter L, Brodin T, Chester MA et al. (1984) Mouse monoclonal antibodies with anti-A, anti-B and anti-A,B specificities; some superior to human polyclonal ABO reagents. Vox Sang 46: 185–194

Michel FW (1964) The occurrence of blood-group specific material in the plasma and serum of stored blood. Vox Sang 9: 471

Miescher PA, Müller-Eberhard HJ (eds) (1978) Seminars in Immunopathology, vol 1: Immunodeficiency Diseases. Berlin: Springer-Verlag

Mifsud NA, Watt JM, Condon JA et al. (2000) A novel cis-AB variant allele arising from a nucleotide substitution A796C in the B transferase gene. Transfusion 40: 1276–1277

Miller EB, Rosenfield RE, Vogel P et al. (1954) The Lewis blood factors in American Negroes. Am J Phys Anthropol 12: 427

Milne RW, Dawes C (1973) The relative contributions of different salivary glands to the blood group activity of whole saliva in humans. Vox Sang 25: 298

Mollison PL (1943) The investigation of haemolytic transfusion reactions. BMJ i: 529, 559

Mollison PL (1961) Blood Transfusion in Clinical Medicine, 3rd edn. Oxford: Blackwell Scientific Publications

Mollison PL (1967) Blood Transfusion in Clinical Medicine, 4th edn. Oxford: Blackwell Scientific Publications

Mollison PL (1983) Blood Transfusion in Clinical Medicine, 7th edn. Oxford: Blackwell Scientific Publications

Mollison PL, Cutbush M (1955) The use of isotope-labelled red cells to demonstrate incompatibility in vivo. Lancet i: 1290

Mollison PL, Young IM (1941) Iso-agglutinin changes after transfusion of incompatible blood and serum. Lancet ii: 635

Mollison PL, Polley MJ, Crome P (1963) Temporary suppression of Lewis blood-group antibodies to permit incompatible transfusion. Lancet i: 909

Moore S, Chirnside A, Micklem LR et al. (1984) A mouse monoclonal antibody with anti-A,(B) specificity which agglutinates Ax cells. Vox Sang 47: 427–434

Morel PA, Watkins WM, Greenwell P (1984) Genotype A^1B expressed as phenotype A_2B in a Black population (Abstract). Transfusion 24: 426

Morgan WTJ, Watkins WM (1948) The detection of a product of the blood group O gene and the relationship of the so-called O-substance to the agglutinogens A and B. Br J Exp Pathol 29: 159

Moss WL (1910) Studies on isoagglutinins and isohemolysins. Bull Johns Hopkins Hosp 21: 63

Mourant AE (1946) A 'new' human blood group antigen of frequent occurrence. Nature (Lond) 158: 237

Mourant AE, Kopéc AC, Domaniewska-Sobczak K (1976) The Distribution of the Human Blood Groups and Other Biochemical Polymorphisms, 2nd edn. Oxford: Oxford University Press

Moureau F (1945) Les réactions post-transfusionnelles. Rev Belge Sci Méd 16: 258

Mulet C, Cartron J-P, Schenkel-Brunner H et al. (1979) Probable biosynthetic pathway for the synthesis of the B antigen from B_h variants. Vox Sang 37: 272–280

Naiki M, Marcus DM (1975) An immunochemical study of the human blood group P_1, P and P^k glycosphingolipid antigens. Biochemistry 14: 4837

Naiki M, Fong J, Ledeen R et al. (1975) Structure of the human erythrocyte blood group P_1. Biochemistry 14: 4831

Nicholas JW, Jenkins WJ, Marsh WL (1957) Human blood chimeras. BMJ i: 1458

Nijenhuis LE, Bratlie K (1962) ABO antibodies in twins. Vox Sang 7: 236

Noël A (1981) Anti-A isoagglutinins and pneumococcal vaccine. Lancet ii: 687–688

Nydegger UE, Wuillemin WA, Julmy F et al. (2003) Association of ABO histo-blood group B allele with myocardial infarction. Eur J Immunogenet 30: 201–206

Obregon E, McKeever BG (1980) Studies in offspring of pp mothers (Abstract). Transfusion 20: 621–622

Ogasawara K, Yabe R, Uchikawa M et al. (1996) Molecular genetic analysis of variant phenotypes of the ABO blood group system. Blood 88: 2732–2737

Olesen H (1966) Thermodynamics of the cold agglutinin reaction. Scand J Clin Lab Invest 18: 1

Olsson ML (2004) New developments in immunohaematology. Vox Sang 87(Suppl. 2): S66–S71

Olsson ML, Chester MA (1996) Frequent occurrence of a variant O gene at the blood group ABO locus. Vox Sang 70: 26–30

Olsson ML, Irshaid NM, Hosseini-Maaf B et al. (2001) Genomic analysis of clinical samples with serological ABO blood grouping discrepancies: identification of fifteen novel A and B subgroup alleles. Blood 98: 1585–1593

Oriol R (1980) Genetic control of the fucosylation of ABH precursor chains. Evidence for new epistatic interactions in different cells and tissues. J Immunogenet 17: 235–245

Oriol R, Danilovs J, Lemieux R et al. (1980) Lymphocytoxic definition of combined ABH and Lewis antigens and their transfer from sera to lymphocytes. Hum Immunol 3: 195–205

Oriol R, Samuelsson BE, Messeter L (1990) ABO antibodies – serological behaviour and immuno-chemical characterization. J Immunogenet 17: 279–299

Ørntoft TF, Holmes EH, Johnson P et al. (1991) Differential tissue expression of the Lewis blood group antigens: enzymatic, immunohistologic, and immunochemical evidence for Lewis a and b antigen expression in Le(a– b –) individuals. Blood 77: 1389–1396

Owen RD (1954) Heterogeneity of antibodies to the human blood groups in normal and immune sera. J Immunol 73: 29

Page PL, Langevin S, Petersen RA et al. (1987) Reduced association between the Ii blood group and congenital cataracts in white patients. Am J Clin Pathol 87: 101–102

Park JY, Kob M, Prodeus AP et al. (2004) Early deficit of lymphocytes in Wiskott–Aldrich syndrome: possible role of WASP in human lymphocyte maturation. Clin Exp Immunol 136: 104–110. [Erratum in Clin Exp Immunol 137: 223]

Parr LW, Krischner H (1932) Hemolytic transfusion fatality with donor and recipient in the same blood group. JAMA 98: 47

Patenaude SI, Seto NOL, Borisova SN et al. (2002) The structural basis for specificity in human ABO(H) blood group biosynthesis. Nature Struct Biol 9: 685–690

Pawlak Z, Lopez M (1979) Développement des antigènes ABH et Ii chez les enfants de O à 16 ans. Rev Fr Transfus Immunohématol 22: 253–263

Pereira MEA, Kabat EA (1974) Specificity of purified hemagglutinin (lectin) from Lotus tetragonolobus. Biochemistry 13: 3184

Petit A, Duong TH, Brémond JL et al. (1981) Alloanticorps irréguliers anti-P₁ et Clonorchiase à clonorchis sinensis. Rev Fr Transfus Immunohématol 24: 197–210

Pettenkofer HJ, Hoffbauer H (1954) Über die Bedeutung des Lewis-Blutgruppen-systems für die Entstehung eines Morbus haemolyticus neonatorum. Zbl Gynäk 76: 576

Petzl DH, Tanew A (1985) Blutgruppenisoagglutinin und Immunglobuline (IgG, IgM) im hohen Alter. Wien Klin Wsch 97, 595–602

Piller F, Cartron JP (1983) Biosynthesis of antigenic structures. In: Red Cell Membrane Glycoconjugates and Related Genetic Markers. JP Cartron, P Rouger, C Salmon (eds). Paris: Lib Arnette, pp. 175–181

Pinkerton PH, Tilley CA, Crookston MC (1977) cited by Bird and Wingham (1977)

Plischka H, Schäfer E (1972) A study on the immunoglobulin class of the anti-A₁ isoagglutinin. J Immunol 108: 782

Polley MJ, Adinolfi M, Mollison PL (1963) Serological characteristics of anti-A related to type of antibody protein (7Sγ or 19Sγ). Vox Sang 8: 385

Polley MJ, Mollison PL, Rose J et al. (1965) A simple serological test for antibodies causing ABO-haemolytic disease of the newborn. Lancet i: 291

Poskitt TR, Fortwengler HP (1974) A study of weak subgroups of A with an antiglobulin-latex test. Transfusion 14: 158

Posner MP, McGeorge MB, Mendez-Picon G et al. (1986) The importance of the Lewis system in cadaver renal transplantation. Transplantation 41: 474–477

Potapov MI (1970) Detection of the antigen of the Lewis system, characteristic of the erythrocytes of the secretory group Le(a– b–). Probl Hematol Blood Transfus 15: 45

Preece AF, Strahan KM, Devitt J et al. (2002) Expression of ABO or related antigenic carbohydrates on viral envelopes leads to neutralisation in the presence of serum containing specific natural antibodies and complement. Blood 99: 2477–2482

Przestwor E (1964) Distribution of ABH group substances in amniotic fluid. Poznanski Towarzystwo Przjaciol Nauk 29: 197

Race RR, Sanger R (1975) Blood Groups in Man, 6th edn. Oxford: Blackwell Scientific Publications

Rachkewich RA, Crookston MC, Tilley CA et al. (1978) Evidence that blood-group A antigen on lymphocytes is derived from the plasma. J Immunogenet 5: 25

Radermecker M, Bruwier M, François C et al. (1975) Anti-P₁ activity in pigeon breeders' serum. Clin Exp Immunol 22: 546

Rajan VP, Larsen RD, Ajmera S et al. (1989) A cloned human DNA restriction fragment determines expression of a GDP-L-fucose: β-D-galactoside 2-α-L-fucosyltransferase in transfected cells. J Biol Chem 264: 11158–11167

Rapoport M, Stokes J (1937) Reactions following the intramuscular injection of whole blood. Am J Dis Childh 53: 471

Rawson AJ, Abelson NM (1960a) Studies of blood group antibodies. III. Observations on the physicochemical properties of isohemagglutinins and isohemolysins. J Immunol 85: 636

Rawson AJ, Abelson NM (1960b) Studies of blood group antibodies. IV. Physico-chemical differences between iso-anti-A,B and iso-anti-A or iso-anti-B. J Immunol 85: 640

Rawson AJ, Abelson NM (1964) Studies of blood group antibodies. VI. The blood group isoantibody activity of γ_{1A} globulin. J Immunol 93: 192

Redman M, Malde R, Contreras M et al. (1990) Comparison of IgM and IgG anti-A and anti-B levels in Asian, Caucasian and Negro donors in the north-west Thames region. Vox Sang 59: 89–91

Reed TE, Moore BPL (1964) A new variant of blood group A. Vox Sang 9: 363

Renton PH, Hancock JA (1962) Uptake of A and B antigens by transfused group O erythrocytes. Vox Sang 7: 33

Reyes F, Gourdin MF, Lejonc JL et al. (1976) The heterogeneity of erythrocyte antigen distribution on human normal phenotypes: an immunoelectron microscopy study. Br J Haematol 34: 613

Rohr TE, Smith DF, Zopf DA et al. (1980) Le^b-active glycolipid in human plasma: measurement by radioimmunoassay. Arch Biochem Biophys 199: 265–269

Romano EL, Mollison PL (1975) Red cell destruction in vivo by low concentrations of IgG anti-A. Br J Haematol 29: 121

Romano EL, Zabner-Oziel P, Soyano A et al. (1983) Studies on the binding of IgG and F(ab) anti-A to adult and newborn group A red cells. Vox Sang 45: 378–383

Romans DG, Tilley CA, Dorrington KJ (1980) Monogamous bivalency of IgG antibodies. I. Deficiency of branched ABHI-active oligosaccharide chains on red cells of infants causes the weak antiglobulin reactions in hemolytic disease of the newborn due to ABO incompatibility. J Immunol 124: 2807–2811

Rosenfield RE, Vogel P (1951) The identification of hemagglutinins with red cells altered with trypsin. Trans NY Acad Sci 13: 213

Rosenfield RE, Schroeder R, Ballard R et al. (1964) Erythrocyte antigenic determinants characteristic of H, I in the presence of H[IH], or H in the absence of i [H(− i)]. Vox Sang 9: 415

Rosse WF, Dourmashkin R, Humphrey JH (1966) Immune lysis of normal human and paroxysmal nocturnal haemoglobinuria (PNH) red blood cells. III. The membrane defects caused by complement lysis. J Exp Med 123: 969

Rouger P, Riveau D, Salmon C (1979) Detection of the H and I blood group antigens in normal plasma. A comparison with A and i antigens. Vox Sang 37: 78–83

Rouger P, Goossens D, Gane P et al. (1982) Antigens common to blood cells and tissues: from red cell antigens

to tissue antigens. In: Blood Groups and Other Red Cell Surface Markers in Health and Disease. C Salmon (ed.). Paris: Masson Publishing, pp. 101–109

Salmon Ch (1976) Les phénotypes B faibles B$_3$, B$_x$, B$_{el}$. Classification pratique proposée. Rev Fr Transfus Immunohématol 19: 89

Salmon C, Dreyfus B, André R (1958) Double population de globules, différant seulement par l'antigène de groupe ABO, observée chez un malade leucémique. Rev Hématol 13: 148

Salmon C, André R, Dreyfus B (1959) Existe-t-il des mutations somatiques du gène de groupe sanguin A au cours de certaines leucemies aiguës? Rev Fr Étud Clin Biol 4: 468

Salmon C, Cartron JP, Rouger P (1984) The Human Blood Groups. Paris: Masson Publishing

Sanger R, Tippett P (1979) Live children and abortions of p mothers (Letter). Transfusion 19: 222

Schachter H, Michaels MA, Crookston MC et al. (1971) A quantitative difference in the activity of blood group A-specific N-acetylgalactosaminyl-transferase in serum from A$_1$ and A$_2$ human subjects. Biochem Biophys Res Commun 45: 1011

Schachter H, Michaels MA, Tilley CA et al. (1973) Qualitative differences in the N-acetyl-D-galactosaminyl-transferases produced by human A^1 and A^2 genes. Proc Natl Acad Sci USA 70: 220

Schenkel-Brunner H (1980a) Blood-group-ABH antigens of human erythrocytes. Quantitative studies on the distribution of H antigenic sites among different classes of membrane components. Eur J Biochem 104: 529–534

Schenkel-Brunner H (1980b) Blood group ABH antigens on human cord red cells. Number of A antigenic sites and their distribution among different classes of membrane constituents. Vox Sang 38: 310–314

Schenkel-Brunner H, Hanfland P (1981) Immunochemistry of the Lewis blood group system. III. Studies on the molecular basis of the Le^x property. Vox Sang 40: 358–366

Schenkel-Brunner H, Tuppy H (1969) Enzymatic conversion of human O into A erythrocytes and of B into AB erythrocytes. Nature (Lond) 223: 1272

Schiff F (1924) Über gruppenspezifische Serumpräcipitine. Klin Wschr 3: 679

Schiff F (1934) Zur Kenntnis der Blutantigene des Shigabazillus. Z Immun-Forsch 82: 46

Schwarting GA, Marcus DM, Metaxas M (1977) Identification of sialosylparagloboside as the erythrocyte receptor for an 'anti-p' antibody. Vox Sang 32: 257

Seaman MJ, Chalmers DG, Franks D (1968) Siedler: an antibody which reacts with A$_1$ Le(a− b+) red cells. Vox Sang 15: 25

Sheu BS, Sheu SM, Yang HB et al. (2003) Host gastric Lewis expression determines the bacterial density of Helicobacter pylori in babA2 genopositive infection. Gut 52: 927–932. [Erratum in Gut (2005) 54: 442]

Shrand J (1964) Visceral larva migrans: Toxacara canis infection. Lancet i: 1357

Shumak KH, Rachkewich RA, Crookson MC et al. (1971) Antigens of the Ii system on lymphocytes. Nature New Biol 231: 148

Shumak KH, Beldotti LE, Rachkewich RA (1979) Diagnosis of haematological disease with anti-i. Br J Haematol 41: 399–405

Siber GR, Ambrosino DM, Gorgon BC (1982) Blood group A-like substance in a preparation of pneumococcal vaccine. Ann Intern Med 96: 580–586

Siddiqui B, Hakomori S (1971) A revised structure for the Forssman glycolipid hapten. J Biol Chem 246: 5766

Smalley CE, Tucker EM (1983) Blood group A antigen site distribution and immunoglobulin binding in relation to red cell age. Br J Haematol 54: 209–219

Smith GH (1945) Isoagglutinin titres in hetero-specific pregnancy. J Pathol Bacteriol 57: 113

Sneath JS, Sneath PHA (1955) Transformation of the Lewis groups of human red cells. Nature (Lond) 176: 172

Söderström T, Enskog A, Samuelsson BE et al. (1985) Immunoglobulin subclass (IgG3) restriction of anti-P and anti-P^k antibodies in patients of the rare p blood group. J Immunol 134: 1–3

Somers H, Kuhns WJ (1972) Blood group antibodies in old age. Proc Soc Exp Biol Med (NY) 141: 1104

Speiser P (1956) Zur Frage der Vererbbarkeit des irregulaeren Agglutinins Anti-A_1 (α_1). Acta Genet Med (Roma) 3: 192

Speiser P, Schwarz J, Lewkin D (1951) Statistische Ergebnisse von 10,000 Blutgruppen- und Blutfaktorenbestimmungen in der Wiener Bevölkerung 1948 bis 1950. Klin Med (Wien) 6: 105

Spitalnik S, Cowles J, Cox MT et al. Detection of IgG anti-Lewis (a)antibodies in cord sera by kinetic ELISA. Vox Sang 48: 235–238

Springer GF, Schuster R (1964) Stimulation of isohemolysins and isohemagglutinins by influenza virus preparations. Vox Sang 9: 589

Springer GF, Tritel H (1962) Influenza virus vaccine and blood group A-like substances. JAMA 182: 1341

Springer GF, Williamson P, Readler BL (1962) Blood group active gram-negative bacteria and higher plants. Ann NY Acad Sci 97: 104

Steffensen R, Carlier K, Wiels J et al. (2000) Cloning and expression of the histo-blood group Pk UDP-galactose: Ga1beta-4G1cbeta1-cer alpha1, 4-galactosyltransferase. Molecular genetic basis of the p phenotype. J Biol Chem 275: 16723–16729

Stratton F (1955) Iso-immunization to blood group antigens. In: Modern Trends in Blood Diseases. JF Wilkinson (ed.). London: Butterworth

Sturgeon P, Arcilla MB (1970) Studies on the secretion of blood group substances. 1. Observations on the red cell phenotype Le(a+ b+ x+). Vox Sang 18: 301

Sturgeon P, Moore BPL, Weiner W (1964) Notations for two weak A variants: A_{end} and A_{el}. Vox Sang 9: 214

Szulman AE (1965) The ABH antigens in human tissues and secretions during embryonal development. J Histochem Cytochem 13: 752

Taylor GL, Race RR, Prior AM et al. (1942) Frequency of the isoagglutinin α_1 in the serum of the sub-groups A_2 and A_2B. J Pathol Bacteriol 54: 514

Taylor PA, Rachkewich Ra, Gane DJ et al. (1974) Effect of pregnancy on the reactions of lymphocytes with cytotoxic antisera. Transplantation 17: 142

Tegoli J, Harris JP, Issitt PD et al. (1967) Anti-IB, an expected 'new' antibody detecting a joint product of the I and B genes. Vox Sang 13: 144

Tegoli J, Cortez M, Jensen L et al. (1971) A new antibody, anti-ILe^{bH}, reacting with an apparent interaction product of the I, Le, Se and H genes. Vox Sang 21: 397

Testa U, Rochant H, Henri A et al. (1981) Change in i-antigen expression of erythrocytes during in vivo aging. Rev Fr Transfus Immunohématol 24: 299–305

Tetaud C, Falguieres T, Carlier K et al. (2003) Two distinct Gb3/CD77 signaling pathways leading to apoptosis are triggered by anti-Gb3/CD77 mAb and verotoxin-1. J Biol Chem 278: 45200–45208

Thalheimer W (1921) Hemoglobinuria after a second transfusion with the same donor. JAMA 76: 1345

Thomaidis T, Fouskaris G, Matsaniotis N (1967) Isohemagglutinin activity in the first day of life. Am J Dis Child 113: 654

Thomsen O (1930) Immunisierung von Menschen mit Antigenem Gruppenfremden Blute. Z Rassenphysiol 2: 105

Thomsen O, Kettel K (1929) Die Stärke der menschlichen Isoagglutinine und entsprechenden Blutkörperchenrezeptoren in verschiedenen Lebensaltern. Z lmmun-Forsch 63: 67

Thomsen O, Thisted A (1928a) Untersuchungen über Isohämolysin in Menschenserum. I. Reaktivierung. Z Immun-Forsch 59: 479

Thomsen O, Thisted A (1928b) Untersuchungen über Isohämolysin in Menschenserum. II. Die relative Stärke des α und β-lysins. Z Immun-Forsch 59: 491

Tilley CA, Crookston MC, Brown BL et al. (1975) A and B and A_1Le^b substances in glycosphingolipid fractions of human serum. Vox Sang 28: 25

Tippett P (1975) Antibodies in the sera of p and P^k people. Abstracts, 14th Congress of the International Society of Blood Transfusion, Helsinki, p. 94

Tippett P, Noades J, Sanger R et al. (1960) Further studies of the I antigen and antibody. Vox Sang 5: 107

Tippett P, Sanger R, Race RR et al. (1965) An agglutinin associated with the P and the ABO blood group systems. Vox Sang 10: 269–280

Tirrado I, Mateo J, Soria JM *et al.* (2005) The ABO blood group genotype and factor VIII levels as independent risk factors for venous thromboembolism. Thromb Haemost 93: 468–474

Toivanen P, Hirvonen T (1969) Iso- and heteroagglutinins in human fetal and neonatal sera. Scand J Haematol 6: 42

Topping MD, Watkins WM (1975) Isoelectric points of the human blood group A^1, A^2, and *B* gene-associated glycosyltransferases in ovarian cyst fluids and serum. Biochem Biophys Res Commun 64: 89

Tovey AD (1958) The incidence, distribution and life history of the anti-A and anti-B haemolysins in the general population. Vox Sang 3: 363

Voak D, Lodge TW (1968) The role of H in the development of A. Vox Sang 15: 345

Voak D, Lodge TW (1971) The demonstration of anti-HI/HI-H activity in seed anti-H reagents. Vox Sang 20: 36

Voak D, Lodge TW, Hopkins J *et al.* (1968) A study of the antibodies of the H'O'I-B complex with special reference to their occurrence and notation. Vox Sang 15: 353

Voak D, Abu-Sin AY, Downie DM (1973) Observations on the thermal optimum, saline agglutinating activity and partial neutralization characteristics of IgG anti-A antibodies. Vox Sang 24: 246

Vos GH (1965) A comparative observation of the presence of anti-Tj^a-like hemolysins in relation to obstetric history, distribution of the various blood groups and the occurrence of immune anti-A or anti-B hemolysins among aborters and nonaborters. Transfusion 5: 327

Vos GH (1966) The serology of anti-Tj^a-like hemolysins observed in the serum of threatened aborters in Western Australia. Acta Haematol (Basel) 35: 272

Vos GH, Comley P (1967) Red cell and saliva studies among the Caucasian and Aboriginal populations of Western Australia. Acta Genet 17: 495

Vos GH, Celano MJ, Falkowski F *et al.* (1964) Relationship of a hemolysin resembling anti-Tj^a to threatened abortion in Western Australia. Transfusion, 4: 87

Waller M, Lawler SD (1962) A study of the properties of the Rhesus antibody (Ri) diagnostic for the rheumatoid factor and its application to Gm grouping. Vox Sang 7: 591

Watkins WM (1980) Biochemistry and genetics of the ABO, Lewis, and P blood group systems. In: Advances in Human Genetics. H Harris, K Hirschhorn (eds). New York: Plenum Publishing Corporation

Watkins WM (1990) Monoclonal antibodies as tools in genetic studies on carbohydrate blood group antigens. J Immunogenet 17: 259–276

Watkins WM, Morgan WTJ (1959) Possible genetical pathways for the biosynthesis of blood group mucopolysaccharides. Vox Sang 4: 97

Watkins WM, Greenwell P, Yates AD (1981) The genetic and enzymic regulation of the synthesis of the A and B

determinants in the ABO blood group system. Immunol Commun 10: 83–100

Wiener AS (1941) Subdivisions of group A and group AB. II Isoimmunization of A_2 individuals against A_1 blood: with special reference to the role of the subgroups in transfusion reactions. J Immunol 41: 181

Wiener AS (1943) Blood Groups and Transfusion, 3rd edn. Springfield, IL: CC Thomas

Wiener AS, Unger LJ (1944) Isoimmunization to factor P by blood transfusion. Am J Clin Pathol 14: 616

Wiener AS, Sonn EB, Belkin RB (1945) Distribution and heredity of the human blood properties, A, B, M, N, P and Rh. J Immunol 50: 341

Wiener AS, Samwick AA, Morrison H *et al.* (1953a) Studies on immunization in man. I. The blood group substances A and B. Exp Med Surg 11: 267

Wiener AS, Samwick AA, Morrison H *et al.* (1953b) Studies on immunization in man. II. The blood factor C. Exp Med Surg 11: 276

Wiener AS, Unger LJ, Cohen L *et al.* (1956) Type-specific cold auto-antibodies as a cause of acquired hemolytic anemia and hemolytic transfusion reactions: biologic test with bovine red cells. Ann Intern Med 44: 221

Witebsky E (1948) Interrelationship between the Rh system and the ABO system. Blood 3: 66

Wolf RO, Taylor LL (1964) The concentration of blood group substances in the parotid, sublingual and submaxillary salivas. J Dent Res 43: 272

Worlledge S, Ogiemudia SE, Thomas CO *et al.* (1974) Blood group antigens and antibodies in Nigeria. Ann Trop Med Parasitol 68: 249

Wright J, Lim FC, Freedman J (1980) An example of auto-anti-A_1 agglutinins. Vox Sang 39: 222–224

Wuhrer M, Berkefeld C, Dennis RD *et al.* (2001) The liver flukes *Fasciola gigantica* and *Fasciola hepatica* express the leucocyte cluster of differentiation marker CD77 (globotriaosylceramide) in their tegument. J Biol Chem 382: 195–207

Wurzel HA, Gottlieb AJ, Abelson NM (1971) Immunoglobulin Characterization of anti-Tj^a Antibodies. Chicago, IL: Commun Am Assoc Blood Banks

Yamamoto F-I (1995). Molecular genetics of the ABO histo-blood ABO system. Vox Sang 69: 1–7

Yamamoto F, Clausen H, White T *et al.* (1990) Molecular genetic basis of the histo-blood group ABO system. Nature (Lond) 345: 229–233

Yamamoto F, McNeill PD, Hakomori S *et al.* (1992) Human histo-blood group A^2 transferase coded by A^2 allele, one of the subtypes, is characterized by a single base deletion in the coding sequence, which results in an additional domain at the carboxyl terminal. Biochem Biophys Res Commun 187: 366–374

Yamamoto F-I, McNeill PD, Kominato Y *et al.* (1993a) Molecular genetic analysis of the ABO blood group system: 2. *cis*AB alleles. Vox Sang 64: 120–123

Yamamoto F-I, McNeill PD, Yamamoto M *et al.* (1993b) Molecular genetic analysis of the ABO blood group system: A^x and B$^{(A)}$ alleles. Vox Sang 64: 171–174

Yan L, Zhu F, Xu X *et al.* (2004) Molecular basis for p blood group phenotype in China. Transfusion 44: 136

Yates AD, Watkins WM (1982) Biosynthesis of blood group B determinants by the blood group A gene specified anti-3-N-acetyl-D-galactosaminyl-transferase. Biochem Biophys Res Commun 109: 958–965

Yates AD, Feeney J, Donald ASR *et al.* (1984) Characterisation of a blood-group A-active tetrasaccharide synthesized by a blood group *B* gene-specified glycosyltransferase. Carbohydrate Res 130: 251–260

Yliruokanen A (1948) Blood transfusions in premature infants. Ann Med Exp Biol Fenn 26(Suppl.): 6

Yokoyama M, Fudenberg HH (1964) Studies on 'cross-reacting' isoagglutinins. J Immunol 92: 966

Yoshida A, Yamaguchi H, Okuto Y (1980a) Genetic mechanism of cis AB inheritance. II. Cases associated with structural mutation of blood group glycosyltransferases. Am J Hum Genet 32: 645–650

Yoshida A, Yamaguchi H, Okubo Y (1980) Genetic mechanism of *cis* AB inheritance. I. A case associated with unequal chromosomal crossing over. Am J Hum Genet 32:332–338

Yoshida A, Dave V, Tregellas WM *et al.* (1981) Abnormal blood group galactosyltransferase in blood type B subjects whose serum contains anti-B agglutinin (Abstract). Blood 58 (Suppl. 1): 92a

Yoshida H, Ito K, Emi N *et al.* (1984) A new therapeutic antibody removal method using antigen-positive red cells. II. Application to a P-incompatible pregnant woman. Vox Sang 47: 216–223

Yoshida H, Ito K, Kusakari T *et al.* (1994) Removal of maternal antibodies from a woman with repeated fetal loss due to P blood group incompatibility. Transfusion 34: 702–705

Young WW Jr, Portoukalian J, Hakomori S (1981) Two monoclonal anticarbohydrate antibodies directed to glycosphingolipids with a lacto-N-glycosyl type II chain. J Biol Chem 256: 10967–10972

Yu L-C, Yang Y-H, Broadberry RB *et al.* (1955) Correlation of a missense mutation in the human *Secretor* α1,2-fucosyltransferase gene with the Lewis(a+ b+) phenotype: a potential molecular basis for the weak *Secretor* allele (*Se^w*). Biochem J 312: 329–332

Yu L-C, Lee H-L, Chan Y-S *et al.* (1999) The molecular basis for the B(A) allele: an amino acid alteration in the human histoblood group B alpha(1–3) galactosyltransferase increases its intrinsic alpha(1–3)-N-acetylgalactosaminyltransferase activity. Biochem Biophys Res Commun 262: 487–493

Yu LC, Twu YC, Chou ML *et al.* (2003) The molecular genetics of the human I locus and molecular background explain the partial association of the adult i phenotype with congenital cataracts. Blood 101: 2081–2088

Zelenski KR (1986) Serologic characterization of monoclonal anti-A and anti-B blood group antibodies. Abstracts, 19th Congress of the International Society of Blood Transfusion, Sydney, p. 502

Zheng X, Nishio K, Majerus EM *et al.* (2003a) Cleavage of von Willebrand factor requires the spacer domain of the metalloprotease ADAMTS13. J Biol Chem 278: 30136–30141

Zheng PY, Hua J, Ng HC *et al.* (2003b) Expression of Lewis(b) blood group antigen in *Helicobacter pylori* does not interfere with bacterial adhesion property. World J Gastroenterol 9: 122–124

The Rh blood group system (and LW)

The clinical importance of the Rh blood group system stems from the fact that the antigen D of the system is highly immunogenic: if a unit of D-positive blood is transfused to a D-negative recipient, the recipient forms anti-D in some 90% of cases and thereafter cannot safely be transfused with D-positive red cells. Moreover, if a D-negative woman becomes pregnant with a D-positive (ABO-compatible) infant, the passage of red cells across the placenta from fetus to mother induces primary immunization to D in about one in six cases, unless the mother receives anti-D Ig. In a subsequent pregnancy with a D-positive infant, secondary immunization may be induced, leading to haemolytic disease in the infant. Rh is also involved in the specificity of some of the warm autoantibodies of autoimmune haemolytic anaemia.

In this chapter, the antigens and antibodies of the Rh system, and of the closely related LW system, are considered, together with immune responses to transfused red cells carrying foreign Rh alloantigens and the suppression of the response to D by passively administered anti-D. Molecular methods of Rh typing are discussed in Chapter 12. The mechanism of the destruction of incompatible red cells by anti-D and other antibodies of the Rh system is considered in Chapter 10 and haemolytic reactions caused by Rh antibodies in Chapter 11. In Chapter 12, Rh immunization of women during pregnancy following transplacental haemorrhage from an incompatible fetus is described, together with haemolytic disease of the fetus resulting from the development of maternal alloantibodies.

Rh antigens and genes

CDE nomenclature

For clinical purposes, at least, the CDE nomenclature is now used almost universally. Five main antigens, D, C, c, E and e can be distinguished, as well as certain combinations such as ce, rarer antigens such as C^w and variant phenotypes such as the partial D phenotype D^{VI}.

D is by far the most immunogenic of the Rh antigens, being at least 20 times more immunogenic than c, the next most potent antigen. Because D is so much more immunogenic than other Rh antigens, it is common in clinical practice to equate D with Rh and to use the terms Rh positive and Rh negative to describe D positive and D negative. Nevertheless, since the introduction of immunosuppressive therapy with anti-D immunoglobulin, the frequency of anti-D in comparison with other Rh antibodies has greatly declined. In this book, therefore, Rh is not used as a synonym for D but the more specific terms D or Rh D are used.

C is antithetical to c and E to e. That is to say, each parent hands on either C or c and either E or e. There is no antigen antithetical to D. Although d does not exist, it is in practice useful to use the symbol to indicate that D is absent.

Other nomenclatures

A numerical nomenclature

As will be described later, the assumption that Rh gene structure could be reliably predicted from the Rh phenotype proved to be wrong and led to difficulties in

Table 5.1 Rh antigens in three nomenclatures.

No.	CDE	Rh–Hr	No.	CDE	Rh–Hr	No.	CDE	Rh–Hr
1	D	Rh_o	22	CE	–	41	Ce-like	rh_i-like
2	C	rh′	23	Wiel, D^w	–	42	Ce^s	hr^H-like
3	E	rh″	24	E^T	–	43	Crawford	–
4	c	hr′	26	Deal, c-like	–	44	Nou	–
5	e	hr″	27	cE	–	45	Riv	–
6	f, ce	hr	28	–	hr^H	46	Sec	–
7	Ce	rh_i	29	'Total Rh'	–	47	Dav	–
8	C^w	rh^{w1}	30	Go^a	–	48	JAL	–
9	C^x	rh^x	31	e-like	hr^B	49	STEM	
10	V, ce^s	hr^v	32	‡		50	FPTT	
11	E^w	rh^{w2}	33	§		51	MAR	
12	G	rh^G	34	Bas	Hr^B	52	BARC	
17	*	Hr_o	35	1114¶	–	53	JAHK	
18	†	Hr	36	Be^a	–	54	DAK	
19	–	hr^s	37	Evans	–	55	LOCR	
20	VS, e^s	–	39	C-like	Hr_o-like	56	CENR	
21	C^G	–	40	Tar	–			

* High-frequency antigen reacting with antibodies made by D––/D–– subjects.

† Anti-Rh18 is part or all of the immune response made by hr^s-negative subjects; the antibody reacts with all cells except hr^s and D––.

‡ Low-incidence antigen determined by $\bar{\bar{R}}^N$.

§ Low-incidence antigen determined by R_o^{Har}.

¶ D (C) (E) cells positive with 1114 antibody.

For omission of nos 13–16, 25 and 38, see text.

terminology. To meet this problem, a numerical nomenclature 'divorced from speculative implications' was introduced. The system proposed was essentially a description of the reactions of red cells with particular antisera, which give equal importance to positive and negative findings. D is Rh1, anti-D is anti-Rh1, etc. Table 5.1 gives the equivalent terms for Rh antigens in the CDE and numerical nomenclatures. A sample that reacts with anti-Rh1 and anti-Rh2, but fails to react with anti-Rh3 is described as Rh: 1, 2, –3 (Rosenfield *et al.* 1962).

Although numbers up to 56 are included in Table 5.1, some are omitted: 13–16, because they were given to Rh^A, etc., no longer regarded as distinct antigens; and 25, because it was allotted to LW, now known to belong to a system independent of Rh and 38 (Duclos) because this antigen is also not part of Rh (Daniels *et al.* 2004).

Of the antigens listed in Table 5.1, Rh 9, 10, 11, 20, 22, 23, 28, 30, 32, 33, 35, 36, 37, 40, 42, 43, 45, 48, 49, 50, 52, 53, 54, 55 and 56 are found in fewer than 1% of white people; Rh 17, 29, 34, 39, 44, 46, 47 and 51 are found in more than 99%.

Wiener's nomenclature (Rh-hr)

Although this nomenclature is almost obsolete, some short symbols based upon it are still in use; those for antigens (seldom used) are included in Table 5.1 and those for haplotypes (quite frequently used) are in Table 5.2.

Rh genes

In 1943, RA Fisher proposed that there were three closely linked genes, *Cc*, *Dd* and *Ee*, which determined corresponding antithetical antigens (Race 1944) and he later proposed that the order of the genes was *DCE* (Fisher and Race 1946). Experience soon showed that d did not occur and it was presumed that *d* was an amorphic allele. Application of the techniques of

Table 5.2 Approximate frequencies of common haplotypes in selected populations.

Short symbol*	CDE nomenclature	Approximate frequencies[†]		
		English	Nigerians	Chinese
R^1	*DCe*	0.421	0.060	0.730
r	*dce*	0.389	0.203	0.023
R^2	*DcE*	0.141	0.115	0.187
R^0	*Dce*	0.026	0.591	0.033
r″	*dcE*	0.012	0	0
r′	*dCe*	0.010	0.031	0.019
R^z	*DCE*	0.002	0	0.004
r^y	*dCE*	0	0	0.004

* Based partly on Wiener (1949) and partly on Race (1944); R implies that D is formed and r that it is not.
[†] Based on data cited by Daniels (1995, p. 261).

molecular biology has since shown that there are only two genes: *D*, which has no allele and a second gene, *CeEe* (Colin *et al.* 1991), which has many alleles. It is convenient to use *d* to indicate the absence of *D*. Further details of the genetics of Rh and of the molecular biology of Rh antigens are given in a later section.

Rh phenotypes

The completeness with which the Rh phenotype can be determined depends on the antisera available; if anti-c is available but not anti-C, samples can be classified as c positive (i.e. cc or Cc) and c negative (i.e. CC). If anti-C is also available, Cc can be distinguished from cc.

A convenient notation for Rh phenotypes is that introduced by Mourant (1949). Suppose a sample is tested with anti-D, anti-C, anti-c and anti-E and gives positive reactions with all four antisera: the phenotype is written DCcE. If positive reactions are obtained with anti-D, anti-C and anti-c, but the reaction with anti-E is negative, the phenotype is written as DCcee, as an absence of E implies a double dose of e. Similarly, red cells that fail to react with anti-D are described as dd. Mourant's notation is occasionally misleading; for example, although a negative reaction with anti-E usually implies that the cells are ee, they may be e^se. Perhaps a more important objection to the notation is that it is very clumsy in speech; for this reason, the short symbols shown in Table 5.2 are often used for both phenotypes and genotypes.

Phenotypes are often symbolized as the most probable genotype. For example, use of the term R_1r to represent the phenotype DEcee implies that the genotype is R^1r (*DCe/dce*) but it may be R^1R^0 (*DCe/Dce*). When a given blood sample is described in this way, the symbols should not be italicized, as they do not describe true genotypes.

One of the advantages of the numbered nomenclature is that the sera used in testing a sample are always indicated. Thus the description Rh: −1, −2, −3 indicates that the sample does not react with anti-D, anti-C and anti-E.

Determination of the genotype

When a woman has anti-D in her serum it is important to know whether her partner is *Dd* or *DD*. If he is *DD* he can father only D-positive offspring but if he is *Dd* there will be a 50% chance that any child which he fathers will be D negative and so be unaffected by anti-D in his/her mother's plasma. Routine serological tests do not distinguish reliably between red cells of *DD* and *Dd* individuals; indeed, there is an overlap between the numbers of antigen sites on the cells of the two genotypes. If relatives are available for serological testing, it may be possible to establish the genotype of a D-positive subject with certainty. For example, anyone with a D-negative parent cannot be *DD*.

A variety of molecular methods for the determination of the Rh D genotype of D-positive subjects have been described and are discussed in Chapter 12 (reviewed in Van der Schoot *et al.* 2003).

Common Rh genotypes and phenotypes

As Table 5.1 shows, in white people the commonest Rh haplotypes are *DCe* and *dce* and the commonest three genotypes are thus (1) *DCe/dce* with an approximate frequency of (0.42 × 0.39) × 2 = 0.32, or 32%: the × 2 is accounted for by the fact that *DCe* can combine with *dce* and *dce* with *DCe*; (2) *Dce/DCe* with a frequency of (0.42 × 0.42) = 0.18, or 18%; and (3) *dce/dce* with a frequency of (0.39 × 0.39) = 0.15, or 15%. D negatives comprise *dCe/dce*, *dCE/dce*, etc., as well as *dce/dce* and total 17%.

The frequencies given in the foregoing paragraph are for an English population, in whom the overall frequency of the phenotype DCcee is about 35%; the approximate frequencies of the next commonest phenotypes in order are: DCCee 18.5%; ddccee 15%; DCcEe 13.5% and DccEe 11.5%. These together account for approximately 94% of the total Rh phenotypes of English white people (Race *et al.* 1948a). Phenotype frequencies in most other European white people are similar, although in Basques 20–40% of the population are D negative. The frequency of D negatives is only 0–1% in Burmese, Chinese, Japanese, Maoris, Melanesians, American Indians and Inuit, (Mourant *et al.* 1976).

Numbers of D sites on red cells of different phenotypes

Using polyclonal IgG anti-D, followed by purified ^{125}I-labelled anti-IgG, the numbers of available D antigen sites on intact red cells of various phenotypes (probable genotypes in parentheses) were as follows (Rochna and Hughes-Jones 1965):

- Dccee (D*Ce*/*dce*) 9900–14 600;
- Dccee (*Dce*/*dce*) 12 000–20 000;
- DccEe (*DcE*/*dce*) 14 000–16 000;
- DCCee (*DCe*/*DCe*) 14 500–19 300;
- vvDccEe (*DCe*/*DcE*) 23 000–31 000;
- DccEE (*DcE*/*DcE*) 15 800–33 300.

Similar figures, also using polyclonal IgG anti-D, have been published by others (Edgington 1971; Masouredis *et al.* 1976). Although estimates with monoclonal IgG anti-D have given broadly similar results, a considerable variation has been found, depending on the particular antibody used: some examples gave 10 000–12 000 sites, others 25 000–30 000 sites with yet others giving intermediate values (Gorick *et al.* 1988).

Four examples of D– –/D– – red cells were found to have between 110 000 and 202 000 sites per cell (Hughes-Jones *et al.* 1971) and a sample of D• •/D• • cells was found to have 56 000 sites per cell (Contreras *et al.* 1979).

Numbers of c, e and E antigen sites per red cell

In one investigation, the figures were as follows (Hughes-Jones *et al.* 1971):

- *c sites:* cc cells, 70 000–85 000; cC cells, 37 000–53 000;
- *e sites:* ee cells, 18 200–24 000; eE cells, 13 400–14 500;
- *E sites:* 450–25 600, depending on the source of anti-E and the red cell phenotype.

In another investigation, using different methodology but also using polyclonal IgG antibodies, substantially different figures (for various probable genotypes) were obtained (Masouredis *et al.* 1976):

- *c sites: dce*/*dee* cells, 31 500; *DcE*/*DcE* cells, 24 000;
- *e sites: DCe*/*DC*^{w}*E* cells, 20 000;
- *E sites: DcE*/*DcE* cells, 27 500; *DcE*/*dce* cells, 17 900.

Results with single examples of IgG monoclonal anti-c and anti-E gave the following results: on *DcE*/*DcE* cells, c sites 32 000 and E sites 38 000 (Bloy *et al.* 1988).

Quantitative binding studies using monoclonal antibodies to Rh proteins

Quantitative binding studies with radioiodinated murine monoclonal antibodies (R6A-type) reactive with red cells of normal Rh phenotype but not with Rh$_{null}$ red cells identified 100 000–200 000 binding sites on normal red cells (Gardner *et al.* 1991). Monoclonal antibodies reactive with the Rh-related glycoprotein RhAG (2D10 type, Mallinson *et al.* 1990) see a similar number of binding sites (Gardner *et al.* 1991). These results suggest that data obtained with blood group antibodies specific for D, Cc and Ee antigens (see above) are the result of binding to a subset of the Rh polypeptides expressed at the red cell surface. It is known that the Cc and Ee antigens are encoded by the same gene and expressed on the same polypeptide (Smythe *et al.* 1996). Therefore, it might be anticipated that the number of Cc and Ee sites on a given cell would be the same. However, this assumes that the Cc and Ee antigens are equally accessible at the red cell surface and independent of one another. This is clearly not the case for C and E as expression of cDNA encoding CE antigens in the erythroid cell line K562 results in a cell surface Rh polypeptide reactive with anti-E, but poorly or not at all with anti-C (Smythe and Anstee 2001).

Weak D (D^u)

A weakly reacting form of D was described as D^u (Stratton 1946) and came to be considered as a definable phenotype. The original kind of D^u was shown to be inherited (Stratton 1946; Race *et al.* 1948b). However, most 'high-grade' D^u samples are due to an interaction between normal *D* in one chromosome and *C* in the subject's other chromosome ('*C* in trans'), for example, red cells from a person of genotype *DcE*/*dCe* react relatively weakly with anti-D (Ceppellini *et al.* 1955).

The number of D antigen sites on cells classified as D^uCe/D^ucE was found to be 540 per cell; four siblings classified as D^uce/dce had 290–470 sites per cell, and two siblings classified as D^uCe/dce had 110–174 sites per cell (Bush *et al.* 1974). Evidently, C in cis also interferes with the expression of *D*.

The term D^u is now redundant and should not be used. It has been replaced by the term weak D, which defines any D phenotype where the expression of D antigen is quantitatively weaker than normal (Agre *et al.* 1992). Weak D is distinguished from partial D, which defines a D phenotype qualitatively different from normal D. As red cells expressing qualitatively different D antigens may also give weak reactions with some anti-D reagents (partial weak D), this whole area of blood grouping has been a source of great confusion over many years. Many examples of weak D and partial D have been examined at the DNA level (see below). This has allowed the correlation of sequence variation in *RHD* with topological models of the D polypeptide and led to the conclusion that mutations changing the amino acid sequence of D in regions of the protein predicted to be in either membrane-spanning domains or intracellular domains are a general feature of weak D, whereas mutations changing the amino acid sequence in regions of the protein predicted to be extracellular are a general feature of partial D (Wagner *et al.* 1999). It has been considered important to distinguish weak D from partial D in clinical practice because of the assumption that a weak D patient would not produce anti-D if transfused with D-positive blood (because the D antigen they express is weak but normal), whereas a partial D patient would have the potential to produce anti-D (against the part of D antigen they lack) and so should be given D-negative blood. However, the validity of this assumption is challenged by the demonstration of nucleotide substitutions in *RHD* encoding amino acid changes in different weak D samples (i.e. the D polypeptide is not normal) and by evidence that patients with weak D phenotype can produce allo-anti-D (Flegel *et al.* 2000). It is therefore a moot point as to whether or not subdividing D variants between weak D and partial D is of any practical value. Comprehensive databases describing the molecular bases of the most common D variants in different populations are developing rapidly (see below). Ultimately, one can envisage the design of

molecular methods to identify demonstrably immunogenic D variants that are common in a given population as an alternative, more reliable route to transfusion safety. Using flow cytometry, 35 samples classified as weak D were found to have at least 10 times lower expression of D than normal D-positive samples (Tazzari *et al.* 1994). Wagner and colleagues (2000a) examined 18 weak D types using flow cytometry and concluded that the number of D antigen sites varied from 70–4000 per red cell.

Current practice requires red cells from first-time donors to be tested for D using two potent agglutinating anti-D reagents and a sensitive automated method. Subsequent donations need to be confirmed with only a single potent anti-D. In a survey in which 15 000 samples from donors were tested in the Groupamatic, using potent anti-DC and anti-DE, the frequency of weak D, i.e. samples that were classified as D negative in the Groupamatic but which reacted with anti-D in the antiglobulin test, was 0.23% (Contreras and Knight 1989).

D_{el} is a weak form of D common in Far Eastern populations detectable by demonstrating that anti-D can be adsorbed onto, and eluted from, red cells that do not give other positive serological reactions with anti-D (Okubo *et al.* 1984). D_{el} has never been encountered in association with the LE phenotype, probably because the expression of D is enhanced by E in cis (see data above on the number of D sites on red cells of different Rh genotypes). In the Japanese population studied, some 10% of apparently D-negative samples were considered to be D_{el}. In Hong Kong Chinese, the figure was about 30% (Mak *et al.* 1993). The molecular basis of Del is discussed in a later section.

Partial D (D variants; categories of D)

The D antigen is unlike other blood group antigens as it comprises an entire polypeptide rather than structural changes within a polypeptide arising from single nucleotide substitutions (as is the case for most of the other blood group antigens, see Chapter 6). Because D and CE are encoded by two separate but highly homologous genes adjacent on the same chromosome (see later section) it is possible for exchange of DNA between the genes to occur during meiosis with the creation of hybrid genes encoding variant D polypeptides containing part of the normal D sequence replaced by CE polypeptide sequence. The red cells of individuals with such hybrid *RHD* may type as D positive because of the normal D sequence that is present, while at the same time making an antibody against normal D-positive red cells corresponding to the part of the D polypeptide that they lack. This antibody will have the specificity anti-D so the individuals will appear to be D positive with allo-anti-D. In the first study that recognized the existence of missing parts of D antigen, the red cells were described as Rh variants; originally, three, Rh[A], Rh[B] and Rh[C] were defined (Unger and Wiener 1959) and a fourth (Rh[D]) was soon added (Sacks *et al.* 1959). The collection of original sera defining these four variants is no longer available.

In the second classification, D-positive subjects who have made anti-D were divided into seven categories (Tippett and Sanger 1962, 1977; Lomas *et al.* 1986). Antibodies made by different members of the same category may not be identical but, by definition, red cells and sera of members of the same category are mutually compatible. Several categories are characterized by having a particular low-incidence antigen, in addition to lacking certain parts of D. Classification by categories is likely to fall out of use eventually, because the sera used originally are scarce and rather weak (reviewed by Tippett *et al.* 1996).

A third classification became possible when large numbers of monoclonal anti-D reagents became available. In this classification different partial D antigens are distinguished by their pattern of reactivity with a large panel of monoclonal anti-Ds and allo-anti-D made by D-positive individuals is not employed. Using this approach, 30 different patterns of reactivity were observed (Table 5.3). This dramatic increase in the number of partial D phenotypes is a reflection of the experimental method (i.e. use of monoclonal antibodies), which allows detection of partial D in D-positive individuals who have not made allo-anti-D.

Partial E

There is evidence of the existence of several variants of E. Of 58 250 Japanese samples that reacted with polyclonal anti-E, eight failed to react with a monoclonal anti-E; three out of these eight that were tested with anti-E[W] were all negative, indicating that the new variant was different from E[W]. None of the eight had anti-E in their serum. Most, but not all, anti-E IgM monoclonals reacted with E variant cells; all but one

reacted with papain-treated cells. This aberrant expression of E was shown to be inherited; the variant was shown to be different from another described by Lubenko and colleagues (1991) (Okubo *et al.* 1994). Sera recognizing other variants such as E[T] are no longer available (Daniels 2002). The genetic bases of four patterns of reactivity observed with a panel of monoclonal anti-Es were determined by Noizat-Pirenne and colleagues (1998). The molecular bases of three E variants found in Japanese are described by Kashiwase and colleagues (2001).

Structure of Rh D, C, c, E and e

Rh polypeptides were first characterized biochemically by immune precipitation with Rh antibodies from intact red cells labelled with [125]I. The radiolabelled Rh proteins were visualized by sodium dodecyl sulphate-polyacrylamide gel electrophoresis (SDS-PAGE) followed by autoradiography. The results revealed strongly labelled bands with an approximate molecular weight of 30 kDa (Gahmberg 1982; Moore *et al.* 1982). Subsequent studies indicated the presence of two polypeptides, one corresponding to the D polypeptide and the other to the CE polypeptide. Isolation and sequencing of cDNA encoding these polypeptides predicted that they encoded proteins of 417 amino acids, from which the translation-initiating methionine is post-translationally cleaved to give 416 amino acids in the mature protein (Le Van Kim *et al.* 1992; Anstee and Tanner 1993). These proteins lacked *N*-glycosylation sites and had a calculated molecular weight of 45.5 kDa. It is believed that the lower estimate for molecular weight (30 kDa) mentioned above, derived from mobility by SDS-PAGE, was aberrant because of anomalous binding of Rh polypeptide to SDS (Agre and Cartron 1991).

Hydropathy plots indicated that D and CE polypeptides have 12 transmembrane domains with the amino and carboxyl termini in the cytoplasm (Anstee and Tanner 1993; compare with Plate 3.1, Fig. 5.1.

The D and CcEe antigens are carried by proteins that are distinct but with 92% homology. In all, the CE polypeptide differs from the D polypeptide by only 35/36 amino acid substitutions, suggesting that the corresponding genes have evolved by duplication of a common ancestor gene (Le Van Kim *et al.* 1992; Fig. 5.1).

Both *D* and *CE* have 10 exons (Mouro *et al.* 1994). *C* and *c* differ by one nucleotide change in exon 1 and

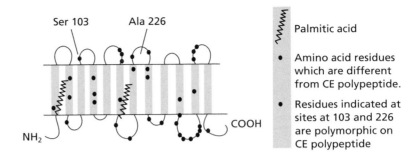

Fig 5.1 Structure of D polypeptide.

by 5 nucleotide changes in exon 2 (Colin *et al*. 1994). However, C/c polymorphism appears to depend primarily on a mutation at position 103 (in exon 2): serine determines C and proline c (Anstee and Mallinson 1994; see also Colin *et al*. 1994). E/e polymorphism is determined by a single amino acid substitution at position 226 (in exon 5): proline determines E and alanine, e (Mouro *et al*. 1993). Initially, it was believed that different splicing isoforms are transcribed from *CE*, which has four main alleles, *Ce*, *CE*, *ce* and *cE*, each of which is 'read' to produce a *C/c* and an *E/e* mRNA, which are translated into substantially different polypeptides (Mouro *et al*. 1993), However, expression of the *D* and *CE* genes in the K562 erythroid cell line demonstrated that Cc and Ee antigens are carried on the same protein (Smythe *et al*. 1996).

Fatty acylation of Rh polypeptides

The serological activity of Rh proteins depends on the presence of phospholipid (Green 1968; Hughes-Jones *et al*. 1975). Palmitic acid appears to be covalently attached to Rh polypeptides by thioester linkages onto free sulphydryls on certain cysteine residues within the molecule (De Vetten and Agre 1988). Mutation of these cysteine residues to alanine does not prevent expression of D polypeptide in K562 cells, but the resulting polypeptide has altered expression of some epitopes of D, suggesting that palmitoylation may be important for the correct folding of the polypeptide (Smythe and Anstee 2000).

Genetic basis of the D-negative phenotype in different races

The organisation of the *Rh* genes was investigated in detail by Wagner and Flegel (2000). These authors

reported that the *D* and *CE* genes are in opposite orientation on chromosome 1 (5′RHD3′–3′RHCE5′) with *D* centromeric of *CE*. The genes are separated by a stretch of around 30 kb, which includes another gene (*SMP1*). The *D* gene is flanked by two 9-kb regions of homology denoted rhesus boxes by Wagner and Flegel (Fig. 5.2) and these authors suggest that the deletion of *D*, the common cause of the D-negative phenotype in white people, results from chromosomal misalignment at meiosis and subsequent unequal crossing over between the rhesus boxes (see Fig. 5.2).

In black Africans the D-negative phenotype commonly results not from the absence of *RHD* but from inheritance of an altered *RHD*, which contains a duplicated 37-bp sequence comprising the last 19 nucleotides of intron 3, the first 18 nucleotides of exon 4 and a nonsense mutation in exon 6, which creates a stop signal (Tyr269stop). As a result of these changes, no D polypeptide reaches the surface of the red cell (Singleton *et al*. 2000). Of 82 D-negative black African samples studies by Singleton and colleagues, 67% had this altered *RHD* (referred to as the *RHD* pseudogene), 18% had a deletion of *RHD* and 15% had a hybrid gene (*RHD–CE–D*ˢ) that produces no D antigen.

The D-negative phenotype accounts for less than 1% of Asian individuals (see Table 5.2). In a study of 204 D-negative Taiwanese, the most common cause of the phenotype (150 individuals) was a deletion of *RHD*. In 41 individuals, a deletion of 1013 bp between introns 8 and 9 (including exon 9) of *RHD* was found corresponding to the Del phenotype (as reported by Chang *et al*. 1998). In the remaining 13 individuals, a hybrid *RHD–CE–D* was found with exons 1, 2 and 10 deriving from *RHD* (Peng *et al*. 2003). In a study of 264 D-negative Koreans, 74% had a deletion of *RHD*, 9% had a hybrid *RHD–CE–D* and the remainder had a silent mutation G1227A in *RHD*. The G1227A allele

169

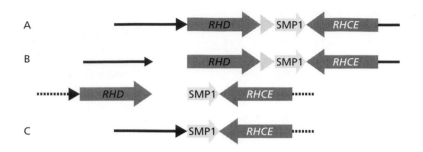

A

B

C

Fig 5.2 Structure of RH genes (from Wagner and Flegel 2000).

was also found in 26Del and two weak D samples in Chinese (Shao *et al.* 2002) and in Japanese Del samples. G1227A alters RNA splicing with the result that transcripts are generated with exon 9 spliced out (Zhou *et al.* 2005).

The very different molecular backgrounds of D-negative phenotype in different racial groups become of considerable significance when DNA-based methods of D typing are contemplated. Clearly, a method that is very reliable in white people will not necessarily be reliable in other racial groups. It is essential to analyse the Rh genes of any given population in detail so that an appropriate molecular method can be devised for routine typing (see Chapter 12 for further discussion).

Structure of D variant antigens

Once the structure of *D* and *CE* had been elucidated, Rh genes from individuals expressing different Rh blood group phenotypes could be sequenced in order to elucidate the molecular bases of the numerous Rh antigens. Essentially, two general mechanisms for generating antigenic diversity have been found, nucleotide substitutions and gene conversion. Nucleotide substitution resulting in a single amino acid change in the protein sequence is the commonest mechanism for generating antigenic change in all systems other than Rh and the MNS system (see Chapter 6). Rh and MNS differ from all the other systems in that the antigens are encoded by the products of two highly homologous adjacent genes (*RHD/RHCE* and *GYPA/GYPB* respectively). The occurrence of two adjacent, highly homologous genes predisposes to misalignment between the genes when chromosomes pair at meiosis (for example, *D* with *CE* rather than *D* with *D*), a process which can result in the insertion or deletion of stretches of DNA sequence in the misaligned genes with the creation of novel DNA sequences, which,

when translated, result in novel protein sequences and thereby novel antigens. This gene conversion mechanism explains why there are many more antigens in the RH and MNS blood group systems than in other blood group systems. Understanding the structure of Rh antigens is further complicated because different antigens encoded by *RHD* are referred to as partial D antigens, rather than having more distinctive names (see Table 5.3 and section above for discussion of partial D). In many cases, partial D antigens result from gene conversion events creating D polypeptides with substantial regions where D polypeptide sequence is replaced by CE polypeptide sequence. Many partial D phenotypes (DIIIa, DVa, DVI, DAR, DFR, DBT) have in common the substitution of sequence in exon 5 of *RHD* with sequence from exon 5 of *RHCE*. Exon 5 encodes that portion of the polypeptide predicted to form the fourth extracellular loop of the D polypeptide. Others (DIV) have substitution of sequence in exon 7 corresponding to the protein sequence predicted to form the sixth extracellular loop of D polypeptide (Fig. 5.3). The molecular bases of red cells expressing weak D antigens have been studied by Wagner and colleagues (1999). Comprehensive databases listing the molecular bases of weak D (over 40 different types) and partial D antigens can be found at http://www.uni-ulm.de/%7Efwagner/RH/RB/. In contrast with partial D antigens, where the genetic changes frequently involve exchange of large portions of *D* for *CE* and affect regions of the D polypeptide predicted to be exposed on the outside of the red cell, weak D generally derives from point mutations in *RHD* changing single amino acids in the D polypeptide. Of the many different weak D mutations described most, if not all, encode amino acid substitutions in the predicted transmembrane and cytosolic domains of the D polypeptide (Fig. 5.4). These amino acid substitutions frequently cause substantial changes in the protein sequence, for

Table 5.3 Division of monoclonal anti-Ds into reaction patterns using D variant red cells (from Scott 2002).

	DII	DIII	DIVa	DIVb	DVa1	DVa2	DVa3	DVa4	DVa5	DVI	DVII	DFR	DBT	DHA	DHMi	DNB	DAR	DNU	DOL	DYO
1.1	+	+	–	–	–	–	–	–	–	–	+	+	–	–	+	+	V	V	V	–
1.2	+	+	–	–						–	+	–	–	–	+					
2.1	+	+	–	–	+	+	+	+	+	–	+	+	–	–	+	+	+	+	+	V
2.2	+	+	–	–	+	+	+	+	–	–	+	–	–	–	–	+	–	+	+	V
3.1	+	+	–	–	+	+	+	+	+	+	+	+	–	–	+	V	+	+	+	+
4.1	–	+	+	–	+	+	+	+	+	+	+	–	–	–	+	+	+	+	+	+
5.1	+	+	+	+	–	–	–	–	–	–			–	+	–	+	+	+	+	
5.2	+	+	+	+	+	+	–	–	–	–	+	–	–	–	+	+	–	+	+	–
5.3	+	+	+	+	–	–	–	–	–	–	+	–	+	–	+	+	–	+	–	
5.4	+	+	+	+	+	–	–	–	–	–	–	–	–	–	+	+	+	+	V	–
5.5	+	+	+	+	–					–	+	–	–	–	–					
6.1	+	+	+	+	+	+	+	+	+	–	+	+	+	+	+	+	+	+	+	+
6.2	+	+	+	+	+	+	+	+	+	–	+	+	+		+	+	+	+	+	V
6.3	+	+	+	+	+	+	+	+	+	–	+	+	–		+	+	+	+	+	V
6.4	+	+	+	+	+	+	+	+	+	–	+		+		+	+	+		+	V
6.5	+	+	+	+	+	+	+	+	+	–	+	+	–	+	+	+		+	+	+
6.6	+	+	+	+	+	+	–	–	–	–	+		–		V	+	+	+	+	V
6.7	+	+	+	+	+	+	+	+	–	–	+				+	+	+	+	+	V
8.1	+	+	+	+	+	+	+	+	+	–			–	–	V	+	–	–	+	V
8.2	+	+	+	+	+	+	+	+	+	–			+		+	+	+	+	+	+
8.3	+	+	+	+	+	+	+	–	–	–	+		+		–				+	+
9.1	–	+	–	–	+	+	+	+	+	+	+	–	–	+	+	+			+	+
10.1	+	+	–	–	–					–	–	–	–	–	–					
11.1	+	+	+	+	–					–	–	–	–	–	–					
12.1	+	+	+	+	+					–	+	+	+	–	–					
13.1	+	+	+	–	+	+	+	+	+	–	+	+	+		–	+		+	+	nt
14.1	+	+	+	–	+					–	+	+	–	–	+					
15.1	+	+	+	–	+	+	+	+	+	+	+	+	–	+		+	+	+	+	–
16.1	+	+	+	+						+	+	+	+	–	+					

+, positive; –, negative; V, variable; nt, not tested.

example by introduction of charged or bulky residues, and presumably impede the transport and assembly of the D polypeptide to the red cell membrane, hence weak expression of D.

Clinical relevance of D variant (partial D and weak D) phenotypes

The importance of determining whether a D variant phenotype is present on the red cells of a donor relates to whether or not the red cells will be immunogenic if transfused to a D-negative patient (or a patient with a different D variant). For a patient with a D variant phenotype the question is whether or not they will make anti-D if transfused with red cells of normal D phenotype. In addition, anti-D in women with partial D antigens has been the cause of haemolytic disease of the newborn (HDN) (Okubo *et al.* 1991; Beckers *et al.* 1996; Wallace *et al.* 1997).

Common D variants in white people

D^{VI} is the most abundant serologically defined partial D variant occurring among weak D samples from white people. D^{VI} is reported to constitute about 6–10% of weak D samples and has a phenotype frequency of 0.02–0.05% in white people (Leader *et al.* 1990; van Rhenen *et al.* 1994). Almost all subjects with the genotype *DCe/dce* have an antigen, BARC. The majority of Rh D-positive individuals with allo-anti-D encountered by Jones and colleagues (1995) were D^{VI}. Severe HDN has been reported in Rh D-positive babies born

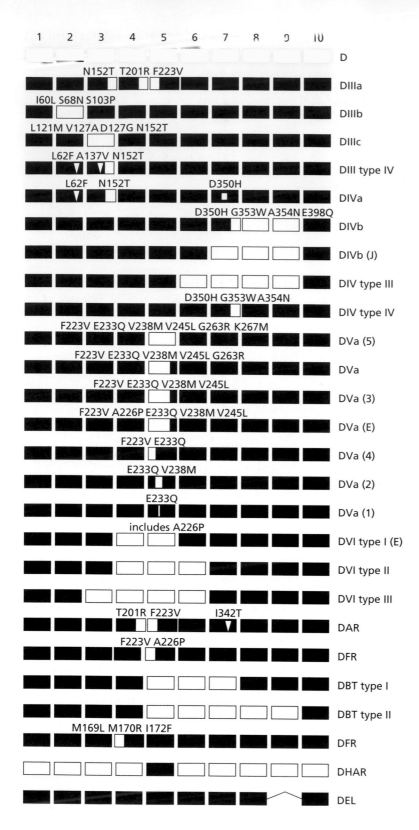

Fig 5.3 Gene structure of D variants (from Daniels 2002). Exons derived from D gene in black. Exons derived from CE gene in white.

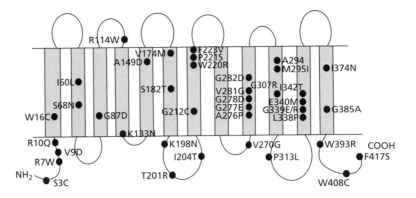

Fig 5.4 Weak D antigens. Position of amino acid substitutions associated with different weak D phenotype is indicated using the single letter code for amino acids with the wild-type amino acid on the left.

to D^{VI} mothers with anti-D (Lacey *et al.* 1983). D^{VI} can arise from three different genetic backgrounds (see Fig. 5.3). The common feature of all three types is the replacement of exons 4 and 5 of *RHD* with exons 4 and 5 of *RHCE*. In type II, exon 6 is also replaced by *RHCE* and in type III exons 3 and 6 are also replaced by *RHCE* (Wagner *et al.* 1998). The number of D sites/red cell on D^{VI} type I was found to be 500, 2400 on type II and 12 000 on type III (Wagner *et al.* 1998). Most monoclonal anti-D do not react with D^{VI} red cells, and D^{VI} red cells react with only about 35% of anti-D made by D-negative subjects (Lomas *et al.* 1989). From this it can be deduced that the amino acid sequence encoded by exons 4 and 5 of the D polypeptide is the most immunogenic region of the D polypeptide (Plate 5.1, cat VI model, shown in colour between pages 528 and 529).

Monoclonal anti-D reactive with D^{VI} red cells should not be used to D type patients because of the risk that a D^{VI} patient would then be typed as D positive and might be transfused with D-positive blood.

Sixty-eight out of 60 000 German blood donors had the D variant D^{VII} (Flegel *et al.* 1996). This variant results from a Leu110Pro substitution in the D polypeptide (Rouillac *et al.* 1995). D^{VII} is characterized serologically by its reaction with anti-Tar (Lomas *et al.* 1986).

DNB is a D variant with a frequency of up to 1 in 292 in white people. Anti-D is found in individuals with the DNB phenotype, which results from a Gly355Ser (predicted to be in extracellular loop 6) substitution in the D polypeptide. No adverse consequences as a result of pregnancy or transfusion have been attributed to the DNB phenotype. Almost all monoclonal anti-D used for routine blood typing would be reactive with DNB cells, so current serological practice would not avoid

exposure of DNB-positive individuals to D-positive blood if transfusion were required (Wagner *et al.* 2002a). An analogous D variant, DWI, was described in an Austrian patient with allo-anti-D. In this case the amino acid substitution Met358Thr was found (Kormoczi *et al.* 2004).

Most white people with D variants described as weak D have weak D type 1 (Val270Gly), type 2 (Gly385Ala) or type 3 (Ser3Cys; Cowley *et al.* 2000; Wagner *et al.* 2000a). Production of anti-D in a D-negative patient transfused with weak D type 2 red cells (450 D antigen sites/cell) has been recorded (Flegel *et al.* 2000). Anti-D alloimmunization by weak D type 1 red cells has also been reported (Mota *et al.* 2005).

Common D variants in black people

D variants appear to be more common in black people than in white people or Asians; 11% of anti-D in pregnancies in the Cape Town area, South Africa, occurred in D-positive women (du Toit *et al.* 1989). The D variants found in black people fall into three clusters known as the DIVa, DAU and weak D type 4 clusters (Wagner *et al.* 2002b).

DIVa is defined by the presence of the low-frequency antigen Go^a, an antigen found in 2% of black people (Lovett and Crawford 1967). Anti-Go^a has caused HDN. DIVa differs from D at three amino acids (Leu62Phe, Asn152Thr and Asp350His; Rouillac *et al.* 1995). The DIVa cluster is characterized by Asn152Thr and also includes DIII type 4 and Ccde^s.

Five DAU alleles are recognized (DAU-0 occurs in white people and Asians). All DAU types share a Thr379Met substitution predicted to be within the twelfth transmembrane domain. In addition, the amino acid substitutions distinguishing DAU 1–4 are Ser230Ile in DAU-1 and Glu233Gln in DAU-4, both predicted to be located in exofacial loop 4. The substitutions Arg70Gln and Ser333Asn in DAU-2 and the Val279Met substitution of DAU-3 are predicted to be located in intramembranous regions. Anti-D immunization was recorded in DAU-3. DAU-1, DAU-2 and DAU-4 were not agglutinated by most commercial monoclonal IgM anti-D and so patients would be typed as D negative and receive D-negative transfusions. DAU-1 cells had 2113 antigen sites per cell, DAU-2 cells 373 sites per cell, DAU-3 cells 10 879 sites per cell and DAU 4 1909 antigen sites per cell (Wagner *et al.* 2002b).

The weak D type 4 cluster is characterized by Phe223Val in the D polypeptide and includes DOL and many alleles sharing Phe223Val and Thr201Arg. DAR is a partial D variant functionally the same as weak D type 4.2. Five out of 326 black South Africans (1.5%) had the DAR phenotype. DAR differs from D at three amino acids (Thr201Arg, Phe223Val and Ile342Thr). One out of four Dutch African black people with the DAR phenotype produced anti-D after multiple transfusions with D-positive blood (Hemker *et al.* 1999). The D variant, DIIIa, falls into this cluster (the phenotype results from three amino acid substitutions in the D polypeptide, Asn152Thr, Thr201Arg, Phe223Val). Eight out of 130 patients with sickle cell disease were found to have one of the phenotypes DIIIa, DAR or DIIIa/DAR. Three of these patients (one DAR phenotype and two DIIIa/DAR) had made anti-D (Castilho *et al.* 2005). Castilho and colleagues suggest that DIIIa and DAR typing should be considered prior to transfusion for sickle cell patients who are likely to require multiple transfusions over a long period.

Common D variants in Asians

The commonest D variant found in Asian populations is Del (see previous section for discussion of this phenotype).

Antigens of the Rh system other than C, c, D, E and e

G

Almost all red cells that carry D and all cells that carry C also carry an antigen G (Allen and Tippett 1958).

Amongst the findings that this observation helps to explain is that about 30% of D-negative subjects who are deliberately immunized with Dccee red cells make an antibody that reacts with D-negative, C-positive red cells, the explanation being that the donor cells elicit the formation of anti-G which, as implied above, reacts with all C-positive red cells. The G antigen seems to be defined by Ser103, which is common to both the D and the CE polypeptide when C is expressed (Faas *et al.* 1996).

Very rarely, a sample may be D positive but G negative (Stout *et al.* 1963), or C and D negative but G positive, when it is called r^G (Race and Sanger 1975, p. 202). The number of G sites on red cells of various Rh phenotypes was estimated, using an eluate made from G-positive *cE/ce* cells previously incubated with ^{125}I-labelled IgG anti-DC. Results were as follows: *DCe/DcE*, 9900–12 200; *dCe/dCe*, 8200–9700; and *DcE/DcE* 3600–5800 (Skov 1976). If r^{G}r cells are not available, anti-G can be made by eluting anti-DC from *dCe/dce* cells and then re-eluting from *Dce/dce* cells. However, not all non-hyperimmune anti-DC sera contain anti-G (Issitt and Tessel 1981).

C^w, C^x and *MAR* can be regarded as forming an allelic subsystem. C^w and C^x are low-frequency antigens that behave as if they are antithetical to a high-frequency antigen, MAR (Sistonen *et al.* 1994). The CE polypeptide amino acid substitutions Gln41Arg and Ala36Thr define C^w and C^x respectively (Mouro *et al.* 1995). The frequency of C^w in most white populations is less than 2% and that of C^x less than 1%, although both are substantially commoner in Finns. Anti-C^w has caused HTR and HDN and anti-C^x, HDN. The only example of anti-Mar described so far did not cause HDN.

'Joint products' of the CDE genes

Ce is a product of *C* and *e* in cis. Most anti-C sera contain separable anti-Ce (or -rh$_i$), which reacts with cells from subjects of the genotype *DcE/Ce* but not with those of *DCE/ce* (Issitt and Tessel 1981). A simple explanation for the high frequency of anti-Ce is offered by structural models of the CE polypeptide, which suggests that the amino acids defining C and e specificity are in close proximity (Plate 5.2 shown in colour between pages 528 and 529). Anti-Ce has been the cause of HDN requiring exchange transfusion (Malde *et al.* 2000; Wagner *et al.* 2000b;

Ranasinghe *et al.* 2003). An IgA autoantibody with anti-Ce specificity has been the cause of autoimmune haemolytic anaemia (Lee and Knight 2000).

ce or f. When *c* and *e* are in cis, they determine a compound antigen ce(f); for example, ce is determined by *DCE/dce* but not by *DCe/DcE* and can distinguish between these two genotypes. Anti-ce is a common component of anti-c and anti-e sera and has been implicated as the cause of HDN (Spielmann *et al.* 1974) and delayed haemolytic transfusion reaction (O'Reilly *et al.* 1985).

CE and cE. Antibodies to these compound antigens have also been found though much less frequently than antibodies of specificity anti-Ce and anti-ce (see Race and Sanger 1975).

V and VS. V(ce^s) is an antigen found in about 27% of black people in New York and 40% of West Africans but only very rarely in white people. VS and V typing of 100 black South African blood donors revealed 34 of phenotype VS+V+, 9 VS+V– and 4 VS–V+ with weak V (Daniels *et al.* 1998). These authors concluded that anti-VS and anti-V recognize conformational changes in the Rh polypeptide resulting from a Leu245Val substitution and that anti-V was also affected by an additional substitution (Gly336Cys). Clinically significant anti-V and anti-VS have not been reported.

Other Rh antigens. These are listed in Table 5.1. As already mentioned, some 20 Rh antigens have a frequency in white people of less than 1%; most of these low-frequency antigens are associated with altered expression of the main Rh antigens (see Daniels 2002).

The low-frequency antigen HOFM, associated with depressed C, has not yet been proven to be part of Rh (Daniels *et al.* 2004). Another rare antigen, OL^a, associated with weakened expression of C or E or both, is determined by a gene that segregates independently from *Rh* (Kornstad 1986).

Red cells lacking some expected Rh antigens

D– – is a very rare phenotype in which there is no expression of C, c, E or e. In subjects who are homozygous for the relevant allele, the red cells appear to have an abnormally large amount of D antigen, as judged by

their agglutination in a saline medium by most sera containing incomplete anti-D. As mentioned above, the red cells have an increased number of D sites. With one sample, the amount of lysis produced by the complement-binding anti-D serum 'Ripley' (Waller and Lawler 1962) was found to be 50–70% compared with not more than 5% for cells of common Rh phenotypes (Polley 1964).

D• • is another very rare phenotype in which D is expressed without C, c, E or e. The red cells, unlike those of the phenotype D– –, carry a low-incidence antigen, 'Evans' (Contreras *et al.* 1978). Red cells that are homozygous for the relevant allele have more D sites than *DcE/DcE* cells but less than those of subjects who are homozygous for the allele determining D– –.

Dc– is a haplotype that determines increased D, decreased c and some f (Tate *et al.* 1960). Not all *Dc–* haplotypes express f (Race and Sanger 1975). Two individuals homozygous for DC^w– have been reported. This phenotype expresses elevated D antigen and depressed C^w but lacks C and c antigens (Tippett *et al.* 1962; Huang 1996).

Several examples of D– –, D• •, Dc– and DC^w– have been analysed at the DNA level. It has been reported generally, although not exclusively, that the phenotype results from a normal *RHD* in tandem with an altered *RHCE*, in which several CE exons are substituted for exons from D (reviewed by Daniels 2002).

Rh$_{null}$

A sample of blood that completely failed to react with all Rh antibodies was described by Vos and colleagues (1961) and given the name Rh$_{null}$ by R Ceppellini (cited by Levine *et al.* 1964). A second example was described by Levine and colleagues (1964); in this case, the parents and one offspring had normal Rh phenotypes, although the Rh antigens had diminished reactivity; the authors suggested that the Rh$_{null}$ phenotype was due to the operation of a suppressor gene ($X^O r$) in double dose, and that the relatives with diminished Rh reactivity were heterozygous for the suppressor gene.

A second type of Rh$_{null}$ phenotype, apparently due to an amorphic Rh haplotype (in double dose) was described later (Ishimori and Hasekura 1967). This kind is referred to as the amorph type of Rh-null to distinguish it from the 'regulator' type described above

(Race and Sanger 1975, p. 220). Most examples of Rh$_{null}$ described are of the 'regulator' type.

Rh$_{null}$ cells lack not only Rh polypeptides (D and CE) but are also deficient in the Rh-associated glyco-protein (RhAG), glycophorin B, CD47 and LW glyco-protein. In addition to lacking Rh antigens, Rh$_{null}$ cells lack LW and Fy5, and have a marked depression of U and Duclos and, to a lesser extent, of Ss. Glycophorin B levels are approximately 30% of normal (Dahr *et al.* 1987). Rh$_{null}$ cells of the 'regulator' type have defects in the gene encoding RhAG. When *RHAG* is not expressed normally, the Rh polypeptides are not trans-ported to the red cell surface and so the red cells have the Rh$_{null}$ phenotype (Cherif-Zahar *et al.* 1996). Some mutations in *RHAG* result in low-level expression of Rh polypeptides and give rise to the Rh$_{mod}$ phenotype. Rh$_{mod}$ cells have very greatly weakened Rh antigens and, like Rh$_{null}$ cells, have a reduced lifespan (Chown *et al.* 1972) and bind anti-U, –S and –s only weakly.

Individuals with Rh$_{null}$ of the amorph type lack *RHD* and have inactivating mutations in *RHCE* (reviewed in Daniels 2002).

Rh$_{null}$ red cells exhibit spherocytosis and stomatocy-tosis and have a diminished lifespan, associated with a mild haemolytic state (Schmidt and Vos 1967; Sturgeon 1970). The red cells have an increased content of HbF and react more strongly with anti-i; the cells also have an increased osmotic fragility and an increased Na$^+$–K$^+$ pump activity (Lauf and Joiner 1976).

In Rh$_{null}$ subjects the commonest antibody formed in response to transfusion or pregnancy reacts with all cells except Rh$_{null}$ and is called anti-Rh29.

Transient weakening of Rh antigens in autoimmune haemolytic anaemia. This has been observed in an infant; when recovery occurred and the direct anti-globulin test became negative, the antigens became normally reactive (Issitt *et al.* 1983).

Absence of D from tissues other than red cells

D has not been demonstrated in secretions or in any tissues other than red cells (for references, see seventh edition, p. 343; see also Dunstan *et al.* 1984; Dunstan 1986). Crossreactivity of some monoclonal anti-D with vimentin in tissues is mentioned in Chapter 3.

RhAG expression appears very early during ery-thropoiesis and before the appearance of Rh polypep-tides (Southcott *et al.* 1999).

Other Rh-associated proteins

Rh-associated glycoprotein (RhAG)

When Rh polypeptides (molecular weight approximately 30 kDa) are precipitated by Rh antibodies, ABH-active glycoprotein (denoted Rh-associated glycoprotein or RhAG) is co-precipitated (Moore and Green 1987). A cDNA encoding RhAG was isolated and sequenced and found to encode a protein of 409 amino acids with 12 predicted transmembrane domains and cytoplas-mic amino and carboxyl termini. The protein has one extracellular N-glycosylation site on the first predicted extracellular loop, which is the presumed location of ABH antigen activity (Ridgwell *et al.* 1992). RhAG has a similar overall structure to the D and CcEe polypep-tides but is not sequence related. The gene for RhAG is on a different chromosome (6) from that (1) for Rh polypeptides. It is the Rh polypeptides that determine Rh antigen specificity while RhAG is required for the efficient transport of Rh polypeptides to the red cell membrane (Cherif-Zahar *et al.* 1996).

In intact red cells, Rh polypeptides, RhAG, LW gly-coprotein, Glycophorin B and CD47 are associated as an Rh membrane complex, which is absent or greatly reduced in Rh$_{null}$ red cells (see Fig. 3.1) (reviewed by Cartron 1999). Analysis of the red cell membranes of an individual with almost complete deficiency of band 3 (band 3, Coimbra – see also Chapter 6) showed absence or gross reduction of the proteins of the Rh complex in addition to deficiency of band 3, gly-cophorin A and protein 4.2. These results suggest that the Band 3 complex (band 3, Glycophorin A and pro-tein 4.2) is associated with the Rh complex in the red cell membrane (Bruce *et al.* 2003). Further support for this model is provided from the analysis of patients with hereditary spherocytosis resulting from inactivat-ing mutations in the protein 4.2 gene. These individuals have a gross reduction of CD47 and abnormal glyco-sylation of RhAG suggesting that interaction occurs between CD47 in the Rh complex and protein 4.2 in the band 3 complex (Bruce *et al.* 2002). Evidence for a direct interaction between the Rh complex and the red cell skeleton component ankyrin is provided by Nicolas and colleagues (2003).

CD47

CD47 (synonym: integrin-associated protein, IAP)

contains 305 amino acids, has a heavily N-glycosylated amino-terminal extracellular immunoglobulin superfamily domain and five transmembrane domains with a cytoplasmic carboxyl terminus. It is encoded by a gene on chromosome 3q13.1–q13.2 (Campbell et al. 1992; Lindberg et al. 1994; Mawby et al. 1994). CD47 on murine red cells appears to act as a marker for self as, unlike normal murine red cells, red cells from CD47 'knockout' mice are rapidly cleared from the circulation by macrophages. In the case of normal murine red cells, CD47 on the red cells interacts with the inhibitory signal regulatory protein alpha (SIRPalpha) on macrophages to prevent clearance (Oldenborg et al. 2000). Increased adhesiveness of sickle red cells to thrombospondin may be mediated through CD47 (Brittain et al. 2001).

Poss and colleagues (1993) describe a murine monoclonal antibody, UMRh, which reacts with a wide range of tissues, such as stem cells, mononuclear cells, granulocytes and platelets, but appears to be different from anti-CD47. UMRh reacts less well with Rh_{null} and D–– than with cells of common D-positive phenotypes.

LW glycoprotein (ICAM-4)

As already mentioned, LW glycoprotein appears to be part of the Rh complex; with anti-LW, D-positive red cells react more strongly than D-negative red cells. Nevertheless, LW is a blood group system genetically independent of Rh, LW being on chromosome 19 and Rh on chromosome 1.

The first example of anti-LW was obtained by injecting rhesus monkey red cells into rabbits and guinea pigs (Landsteiner and Wiener 1940, 1941). The resulting antiserum, after partial absorption with certain samples of human red cells (later described as D negative) reacted only weakly with the same cells but reacted strongly with other samples (later described as D positive). Although for a time it appeared that the antibody produced was identical with human anti-D, it was later shown to be directed against a different specificity to which the name LW (Landsteiner/Wiener) was given (Levine et al. 1963).

The first evidence that anti-LW was different from anti-D was the finding that the antibody produced in guinea pigs reacted equally strongly with D-negative and D-positive cord blood red cells (Fisk and Foord 1942). Other evidence soon followed: it was found that the injection of extracts of D-negative red cells

into guinea pigs induced the formation of an antibody which, although it was not the same as anti-D, resembled it (Murray and Clark 1952; Levine et al. 1961); this antibody was later identified as anti-LW.

The first two examples of anti-LW ('anti-D like') in humans were identified in 1955 (Race and Sanger 1975, p. 228); the antibodies gave the same reactions as the animal sera and were later shown to give negative reactions with Rh_{null} cells. The cells of one of the antibody makers and her brothers were then found to be negative with the guinea pig anti-LW (Levine et al. 1963). A distinction can easily be made between anti-D and anti-LW with the use of pronase, which, unlike other proteolytic enzymes, destroys LW (Lomas and Tippett 1985).

LW antigens may disappear temporarily from the cells of LW-positive people, who can then transiently make anti-LW. The number of LW sites on D-positive red cells was found to be 4400 and on D-negative cells to be 2835–3620 (Mallinson et al. 1986).

Subdivision of LW. The LW antigen and antibody described above are known as LW[a] and anti-LW[a]. An antigen, LW[b], antithetical to LW[a], is found on the red cells of about 1% of the population in most parts of Europe. Anti-LW[b] has been found rarely in LW (a+ b–) subjects, and anti-LW[ab] has been found in LW (a– b–) subjects, in some of whom LW antigens have been lost transiently (see later). All LW antibodies react more strongly with D-positive than with D-negative red cells and fail to react with Rh_{null} cells. Auto-anti-LW is mentioned on p. 179 and in Chapter 7. For the effect of anti-LW on the survival of incompatible red cells, see Chapter 10.

Structure and function of LW glycoprotein

LW encodes a mature protein of 241 amino acids with an amino-terminal extracellular segment comprising two Ig superfamily domains, a single transmembrane domain and a short cytoplasmic domain (fig. 3.2 in Bailly et al. 1994). The LW glycoprotein shows considerable sequence homology with the family of intercellular adhesion molecules (ICAMs) and has also been denoted ICAM-4. The protein is a ligand for several different integrins including LFA-1 Mac-1 on leucocytes (Bailly et al. 1995), GpIIbIIIa on platelets (Hermand et al. 2003) and VLA-4 and alpha v-type integrins (Spring et al. 2001). These interactions suggest that this red cell protein may play a role in erythropoiesis and in haemostasis (reviewed in Parsons *et al.* 1999).

The function of Rh proteins

Rh polypeptides and particularly RhAG share homology with a family of ammonium transporters found in bacteria, yeast and plants (Marini *et al.* 1997) and there is experimental evidence interpreted as indicating RhAG can function as an ammonia transporter (Marini *et al.* 2000; Westhoff *et al.* 2002; Hemker *et al.* 2003; Ripoche *et al.* 2004). Others provide evidence that Rh-related proteins in the green alga *Chlamydomonas reinhardtii* are involved in carbon dioxide transport (Soupene *et al.* 2002). The structure of a bacterial ammonia transporter (AmtB) has been elucidated and the mechanism of ammonia transport determined (Khademi *et al.* 2004; Knepper and Agre 2004.

Rh antibodies

In this section, the specificities of Rh antibodies are briefly considered together with some of their serological characteristics; Rh immunization by transfusion and pregnancy is considered in later sections.

Naturally occurring Rh antibodies

Anti-D

When the sera of normal D-negative subjects are screened in an AutoAnalyzer, using a low-ionic-strength method, cold-reacting IgG anti-D is found in occasional samples. In one series, the frequency was 2.8% in D-negative pregnant women and 3% in males (Perrault and Högman 1972). In another series, the frequency was substantially lower, namely 0.16% in pregnant women and 0.15% in blood donors; in this series the antibodies were detected in the AutoAnalyzer but identified using a manual polybrene test; cold-reacting anti-D could be demonstrated in cord serum and on the red cells of newborn D-positive infants born to mothers whose serum contained the antibody (Nordhagen and Kornstad 1984).

Of four males with cold-reacting anti-D who were given repeated injections of D-positive red cells, two formed immune anti-D; when ^{51}Cr-labelled D-positive red cells were injected into the two subjects who had failed to form anti-D, a diminished survival time was found in one but a strictly normal survival in the other (Lee *et al.* 1984).

Rarely, anti-D detectable by the indirect antiglobulin test (IAT) at 37°C is found in previously unimmunized subjects; in two men described by Contreras *et al.* (1987) the antibodies were mainly IgG in one case and wholly IgG in the other; a small dose of D-positive red cells was destroyed at an accelerated rate in both cases (50–99% destruction in the first 24 h; see Chapter 10). In the same series there was one subject with anti-D detectable at 37°C only with enzyme-treated cells in whom the survival of D-positive cells was normal.

Rh antibodies other than anti-D

Anti-E is found not infrequently in patients who have not been transfused or been pregnant. Often the antibody can be detected only by the agglutination of enzyme-treated cells; at one centre, 60 out of 146 examples of anti-E found in pregnant women were of this kind (Harrison 1970). The highest incidence was in primigravidae whose partners were no more frequently E positive than in a random sample of the population. In the whole series, only 60% of partners were E positive, reinforcing the conclusion that most examples of anti-E encountered in pregnant women are naturally occurring.

In sera from more than 200 000 individuals (prospective recipients of transfusion, antenatal patients, etc.), the incidence of anti-E in D-positive subjects was greater than 0.1% (Kissmeyer-Nielsen 1965). Most of the antibodies were very weak, however, and the detection of so many examples was perhaps partly due to the use of papain-treated ddccEE cells; only 20% were reactive by the indirect antiglobulin technique. In another investigation, of 218 examples of anti-E detected in a single year, using papain-treated ccEE cells from a single donor, only 14% gave a positive indirect antiglobulin reaction; 21% of the subjects had never had a previous transfusion or pregnancy (Dybkjaer 1967).

Some examples of naturally occurring anti-E are detectable by the IAT at 37°C. In two such cases, E-positive red cells were destroyed at an accelerated rate, although in another subject in whom anti-E could be detected (at 37°C) only with enzyme-treated cells, the survival of E-positive cells was normal. All of the three examples of anti-E were wholly, or mainly, IgG (Contreras *et al.* 1987).

Examples of naturally occurring anti-C, -C^w and -C^x have been described (for references, see previous editions of this book). The antibodies have been agglutinins tending to react more strongly at 20°C than at 37°C, and to react more strongly with enzyme-treated red cells; one anti-C was shown to be IgM. Other examples of antibodies within the Rh system that may be naturally occurring are anti-Rh 30 and anti-Rh 32. A very low incidence of cold-reacting Rh antibodies with specificities other than anti-D has been reported (Nordhagen and Kornstad 1984).

Cold-reacting auto-anti-LW

In screening 45 000 blood samples in the AutoAnalyzer using a low-ionic-strength polybrene method, 10 examples of auto-anti-LW were found. The sera reacted as well at 18°C as at lower temperatures but did not react at 31–35°C. The titre, as determined in the AutoAnalyzer in eight of the cases, was 8 or less. Three sera were fractionated by DEAE-cellulose chromatography; two of the antibodies appeared to be solely IgG and one to be partly IgM and partly IgG. The cold anti-LW was found to be less positively charged than the bulk of the IgG, unlike immune IgG anti-LW, which resembled IgG anti-D in being more positively charged (Perrault 1973).

Immune Rh antibodies

As it has long been a routine practice to transfuse D-negative subjects only with D-negative blood, the formation of anti-D as a consequence of transfusion is now uncommon. When an antibody within the Rh system is formed as a consequence of transfusion, it is quite likely to be of a different specificity, such as anti-c, as c is not normally taken into account when selecting blood for transfusion (unless, of course, the recipient is known to have formed anti-c). By contrast, in women immunized to Rh antigens by pregnancy, anti-D was, until the introduction of immunoprophylaxis in about 1970, easily the commonest antibody to be found. At one US centre, 94% of immune antibodies within the Rh system found in pregnant women were anti-D (Giblett 1964). At an English centre the figure (for 1970) was substantially lower, namely 82% (LAD Tovey, personal communication), possibly because examples of non-immune anti-E were included among the Rh antibodies. At this centre the figure for anti-D,

as a percentage of all Rh antibodies found in pregnant women, had fallen to 35% by 1989 (GJ Dovey, personal communication).

Of sera containing anti-D, about 30% will also react with C-positive, D-negative red cells and about 2% will react with E-positive, D-negative red cells (Medical Research Council 1954).

In tests on 50 single donor sera containing anti-DC or anti-DCE, 37 were found to react with r^G red cells, at first suggesting that these sera contained anti-G. However, after sequential elutions from Ccee and Dccee cells, only three of the original sera contained potent anti-G and a further 12 contained weak anti-G. The reactions of many of the original sera with r^G red cells were presumed to be due to the presence of anti-Cc (Issitt and Tessel, 1981). [Anti-C^G is a term used for those anti-C sera that react with r^G cells (Issitt 1985).]

In sera from immunized patients who have formed Rh antibodies other than anti-D, the antibodies most commonly found are anti-c and anti-E; anti-c reacts with approximately 80% of random samples from white people and anti-E with approximately 30%. Figures for the prevalence of these antibodies are given in Chapter 3.

Anti-ce is present in most sera containing anti-c and in most sera containing anti-e. Anti-CE is sometimes found with anti-D (Race and Sanger 1968, p. 164) or with anti-C (Dunsford 1962).

Anti-C without anti-D is rare. Even in D-negative subjects, C in the absence of D is poorly immunogenic (see below). In sera containing 'incomplete' anti-D, anti-C is not uncommonly present as an agglutinin (IgM); such sera are often used as anti-C reagents in blood grouping. The finding of anti-C in a C^W-positive person (Leonard et al. 1976) is very rare indeed. Most anti-C sera are mixtures of anti-C and anti-Ce.

Anti-V and anti-VS (e^s) react with corresponding antigens found most commonly in black people. 'Anti-non-D' (Rh 17) is made by D– –, DC^W–, Dc– and D• • subjects (Contreras et al. 1979). 'Anti-total Rh' (Rh 29) is made by some Rh_{null} subjects.

Because of the outstanding importance of anti-D, this antibody has been far more thoroughly studied than any other antibodies of the Rh system and the following sections deal exclusively with it. Immune responses to Rh antigens other than D are discussed later.

Characteristics of anti-D

Most examples of anti-D are IgG and, in a medium of saline, unless present in high concentration will not agglutinate untreated D-positive red cells but can be detected using a colloid medium, polybrene or enzyme-treated red cells, or by the IAT.

A minority of anti-D sera contain some IgM antibody, almost always accompanied by IgG antibody; provided the IgM antibody is present in sufficient concentration these sera agglutinate red cells suspended in saline. Occasional anti-D sera contain some IgA antibody but, in all examples encountered so far, antibody of this Ig class has occurred as a minor component in a serum containing predominantly IgG antibody.

IgM anti-D. As mentioned above, sera that contain a sufficient amount of IgM anti-D agglutinate untreated D-positive red cells suspended in saline. In a medium of recalcified plasma, diluted up to 1:32 in saline, the titre of purified IgM anti-D is enhanced four-fold; the titre is also slightly enhanced by using enzyme-treated red cells (Holburn *et al.* 1971a). Several examples of IgM anti-D detectable only with enzyme-treated red cells have been described.

In the early stages of Rh D immunization, it is common to be able to detect anti-D only by a test with enzyme-treated red cells. The finding gives no indication of the Ig class of the antibody. A positive result with enzyme-treated cells is usually soon followed by a positive IAT due to a reaction with anti-IgG.

The number of IgM molecules that can be taken up by a particular sample of D-positive red cells is considerably smaller than the number of IgG anti-D molecules that can be taken up by the same sample. For instance, a particular sample of *DCe/dce* red cells would take up about 31 000 IgG molecules per cell, but only 11 500 molecules of IgM anti-D (Holburn *et al.* 1971a).

IgG anti-D. Undiluted anti-D serum containing only IgG anti-D not uncommonly agglutinates D-positive red cells suspended in saline and, occasionally, with potent IgG anti-D, agglutination may be observed even when the serum is diluted in saline as much as 1 in 100 (M Contreras, personal observations).

Although, apart from the exceptions just mentioned, IgG anti-D in a medium of saline will not agglutinate untreated D-positive red cells of 'normal'

phenotype, some examples will agglutinate red cells which are heterozygous for the very rare haplotype D– – and most examples will agglutinate D– –/D– – cells (Race and Sanger 1975, p. 214).

IgG anti-D will agglutinate red cells in a variety of colloid media, for example 20–30% bovine albumin will agglutinate enzyme-treated cells suspended in saline and will sensitize red cells to agglutination by an anti-IgG serum.

IgG subclasses and anti-D. IgG Rh antibody molecules are predominantly of the subclasses IgG1 and IgG3 (Natvig and Kunkel 1968), although occasional examples are partly IgG2 or IgG4. In testing the serum of 96 Rh D-immunized male volunteers, IgG1 anti-D was present in all cases with, or without, anti-D of other subclasses: IgG3 anti-D was present in many cases, moderately potent IgG2 in eight cases and moderately potent IgG4 anti-D in three (CP Engelfriet, personal observations,). An example of anti-D that was wholly or mainly IgG2 has been described. The donor had been immunized many years previously and the antibody concentration was only 1 µg/ml (Dugoujon *et al.* 1989).

In demonstrating the presence of different IgG subclasses amongst anti-D molecules it is important to use red cells with a 'strong' D antigen (DDccEE rather than Ddccee or DdCcee) as otherwise minor subclass components may be overlooked (CP Engelfriet, personal observations). It may sometimes be helpful to fractionate sera on DEAE cellulose before testing them. For example, an anti-D found to be partly IgG4 by Frame and colleagues (1970) was tested by Erna van Loghem (personal communication), who found the IgG4 component difficult to demonstrate in whole serum but readily demonstrable in a fraction relatively rich in IgG4.

In women immunized by pregnancy, it is common to find that anti-D is composed predominantly of a single subclass; on the other hand, most subjects who have been hyperimmunized by repeated injections of D-positive cells have both IgG1 and IgG3 anti-D (Devey and Voak 1974). The findings in another series were similar, anti-D being composed of more than one IgG subclass more commonly in immunized male volunteers than in women immunized by pregnancy (CP Engelfriet, personal observations).

The different effects produced by IgG1 and IgG3 anti-D in monocyte assays *in vitro* and in causing red cell destruction *in vivo* are referred to in Chapters 3, 10 and 12.

Different IgG subclass composition of anti-D in individual donors and in immunoglobulin preparations from pooled donations. After incubating D-positive red cells with anti-D sera, the amounts of IgG1 and IgG3 anti-D bound to the cells can be determined using monoclonal anti-IgG1 and anti-IgG3 in a procedure involving flow cytometry. Using sera from 12 hyperimmunized subjects, the mean amount of IgG3 bound was 16% of the total (Shaw *et al.* 1988). In another series, an almost identical figure (17%) was obtained, with a range of 0–60% (Gorick and Hughes-Jones 1991). In this second investigation, 17 IgG anti-D preparations for immunoprophylaxis were also tested and, unexpectedly, found to deposit less IgG3 on red cells: the mean was 8% of the total, with a range of 1–18%. It was suggested that certain methods of IgG production might result in preferential loss of IgG3.

Anti-D in relation to Gm allotypes. In those subjects who make anti-D and who are heterozygous for G1m(f) and G1m(a) there is a preferential production of anti-D molecules bearing G1m(a) (Litwin 1973). Gm allotypes are described in Chapter 13.

In one reported case, an example of anti-D examined in 1957 contained both G3m(b) and G1m(f) molecules, but in a sample taken from the subject 8 years later the antibody carried only G1m(f) (Natvig 1965).

IgA anti-D can be demonstrated by the antiglobulin test, using a suitably diluted anti-IgA, in some sera that contain at least moderately potent IgG anti-D. Although many sera containing IgA anti-D do not agglutinate D-positive red cells in saline, one example containing IgA anti-D with a titre of 128 agglutinated saline-suspended red cells after centrifugation (PL Mollison, unpublished observations). Fractionation of plasma from this later sample confirmed that the agglutinating activity was present in the IgA but not in the IgM fraction (W Pollack, personal communication).

The production of IgA anti-D seems to be associated with hyperimmunization. In one case, following boosting of an already immunized subject, the titre of IgG anti-D rose first and IgA anti-D became detectable only some months later (Adinolfi *et al.* 1966). Estimates of the frequency with which IgA anti-D is found in hyperimmunized subjects vary. In one series, of 52 sera with IgG anti-D titres of 1024 or more,

50 gave positive results with one anti-IgA serum and 47 gave positive results with another (J James and MG Davey, personal communication). In another series, of 11 hyperimmunized donors, IgA anti-D was found in six, with IgG anti-D concentrations varying from 29 to 75 µg/ml, but no IgA anti-D could be demonstrated in the remaining five donors, including one with an IgG anti-D concentration of 272 µg/ml. No discrepancies were found between tests made with two different anti-IgA sera (seventh edition, p. 351). In another series of hyperimmunized subjects, IgA anti-D was detected in 14 out of 19 (Morell *et al.* 1973).

Failure of anti-D to activate complement

The vast majority of anti-D sera do not activate complement. If untreated red cells, or cells treated with a proteolytic enzyme, are incubated with fresh serum containing potent incomplete anti-D, no lysis is observed, even using a sensitive benzidine method (Mollison 1956, p. 217). Similarly, in testing red cells sensitized with anti-D, positive results with anti-complement have scarcely ever been reported; the most fully studied example came from a donor 'Ripley': freshly taken serum lysed D-positive red cells (Waller and Lawler 1962); the serum also sensitized D-positive red cells to agglutination by anti-C4 and anti-C3 as well as by anti-IgG (Harboe *et al.* 1963). D-positive red cells take up twice as much antibody when incubated with 'Ripley' as when incubated with a normal anti-D serum (NC Hughes-Jones, personal communication).

A mysterious example of a complement-binding anti-D was described by Ayland and colleagues (1978). The donor had a weakly reacting partial D and the anti-D was therefore of restricted specificity; although the antibody was not potent it sensitized red cells to agglutination by anti-complement as well as by anti-IgG.

The usual explanation for the failure of almost all examples of anti-D to bind complement is that only a single anti-D molecule can bind to each D polypeptide and that D sites are too far apart from one another on the red cell surface. As discussed in Chapter 3, two IgG molecules must be present on the red cell surface within the maximum span (20–30 nm) of a C1q molecule if C1q is to be bound. When there are 10 000 D antigen molecules per red cell and if the molecules are uniformly distributed on the red cell surface, the average distance between two molecules may be about

0.13 µm or 130 nm (Mollison 1983, p. 337). On the average then, two bound IgG molecules will be too far apart to activate complement. On the other hand, if the antigen sites are randomly distributed a certain fraction of the sites will be within the span of a C1q molecule so that, particularly when red cells are heavily coated with anti-D, the binding of a certain number of C1q molecules is expected. Using ^{125}I-labelled C1q and ^{131}I-labelled IgG anti-D, it has been shown that in fact C1q molecules can bind to anti-D on the red cell surface; the number of C1q molecules bound is relatively low (about 100 per cell) when the number of anti-D molecules per cell is 10 000, but when the number of anti-D molecules per cell rises to 20 000, approximately 600 C1q molecules per cell are bound. In experiments in which D-positive red cells were very heavily coated with anti-D as many as 1600 C1q molecules per cell were bound (Hughes-Jones and Ghosh 1981). Nevertheless, when purified labelled C1 is added to red cells coated with anti-D, C1r and C1s are not activated, as shown by absence of cleavage (NC Hughes-Jones, personal communication).

At first sight it is perplexing that although the number of K antigen molecules per red cell is even lower than that of D molecules, some examples of anti-K activate complement. The explanation might be that the K antigen unlike D is at some distance from the lipid bilayer, making it easier for two or more IgG molecules to come into close apposition (see Fig. 6.1).

Quantification of Rh antibodies

Methods of estimating the concentration of anti-D are described in Chapter 8. The approximate minimum concentrations of anti-D detectable by different techniques are as follows: AutoAnalyzer, 0.01 µg/ml; 'Spin' IAT, 0.02 mg/ml; two-stage papain test, 0.01 mg/ml; and manual polybrene test, 0.001 µg/ml.

The maximum concentration of IgG anti-D found in serum is about 1000 µg/ml. The lowest concentration of IgM anti-D detectable in a medium of saline is about 0.03 µg/ml (Holburn et al. 1971a), although in a medium of recalcified plasma a concentration of 0.008 µg/ml can be detected (Holburn et al. 1971a,b).

Affinity constants of Rh antibodies

The affinity constant of Rh antibodies are heterogeneous both among examples of antibodies of the same specificity from different donors and within the population of antibody molecules of a particular specificity from a single donor (Hughes-Jones et al. 1963, 1964). In 24 examples of IgG anti-D the constant varied from 2×10^7 to 3×10^9 l/mol, with an average of approximately 2×10^8 l/mol (Hughes-Jones 1967). The affinity constants of some other IgG antibodies were as follows: anti-E, 4×10^8 l/mol; anti-e, 2.5×10^8 l/mol; and anti-c, $3.2–5.6 \times 10^7$ l/mol (Hughes-Jones et al. 1971). In anti-D immunoglobulin prepared from pooled plasma, the range as expected was less: 18 out of 25 preparations had constants within the range 2×10^8 to 4×10^8 l/mol (Hughes-Jones and Gardner 1970). The affinity constants of monoclonal IgG anti-D tend to be higher than those of polyclonal antibodies: seven monoclonals had values ranging from 2×10^8 to 2×10^9 (Gorick et al. 1988), compared with an average of 2×10^8 for polyclonals.

In a study of 14 monoclonal anti-D, the affinities of the four IgM antibodies ($1–4 \times 10^7$/M) were found to be lower than those of the 10 IgG antibodies ($2.3–3.0 \times 10^8$/M). The difference was correlated with the genetic origin and extent of mutation of the rearranged V_H and V_L germline genes responsible for the variable regions of the Fab pieces. The rearranged genes of three out of the four IgM antibodies (characteristic of the primary response) were all derived from the same V_H and V_L germline genes and had undergone relatively few point mutations; the V_H of the fourth antibody had undergone only a single point mutation compared with the germline. The increased affinity of the 10 IgG antibodies (characteristic of the secondary response) was achieved by two mechanisms. First, by an increase in the number of point mutations in the same genes used by the IgM antibodies, resulting in a better fit between antibody-combining site and antigen; and second, by a recruitment of other highly mutated V_H and V_L genes, which also resulted in a binding site with a better fit for the antigen. Recruitment of other genes in this way is known as a *repertoire shift*. Affinity generally increased with increasing somatic hypermutation (Bye et al. 1992).

An ELISA method for measurement of the affinity of monoclonal anti-D gave affinity constants ranging from $1.3–7.4 \times 10^8$/M. The authors argue that measurement of affinity constants using radioiodinated antibodies underestimates the value obtained because of inactivation of the antibody during radiolabelling (Debbia and Lambin 2004).

Gene usage by Rh antibodies

Antibodies to D antigen use a restricted set of V and J gene segments (Perera *et al.* 2000). Using a single chain Fv phage antibody library based on the germline gene segment DP50 and light chain shuffling it was shown that the CDR1 and CDR2 sequences of the DP50-based antibodies were common to both anti-D and anti-E and that specificity was conferred by the VHCDR3 sequences and their correct pairing with an appropriate L chain (Hughes-Jones *et al.* 1999). In another study light chain shuffling was used to prepare six D-specific Fab phages paired with the H chain of an anti-D (43F10). The L chains of the six D-specific 43F10(Fab) clones used five different germline genes from three Vkappa families and three different Jkappa segments. The three F(ab)s most reactive with D had light chains with a Ser-Arg amino acid substitution in CDR1 (St-Amour *et al.* 2003). A similar Ser to Arg substitution in kappa L chains utilized by anti-D has been observed by others (Chang and Siegel 1998; Meischer *et al.* 1998). Some monoclonal anti-D recognize a c polypeptide in which Arg145 was substituted by Thr; Thr154 is not found in the D polypeptide (Wagner *et al.* 2003). This observation and the frequent occurrence of so-called mimicking anti-Rh in the serum of patients with warm-type autoimmune haemolytic anaemia (Issitt and Anstee 1998, p. 962) may be a reflection of the gross homology between the two polypeptides, which stimulates the formation of anti-bodies with similar structural properties.

Rh D immunization by transfusion

The response to large amounts of D-positive red cells

When a relatively large amount of D-positive red cells (200 ml or more) is transfused to D-negative subjects, within 2–5 months anti-D can be detected in the plasma of some 85% of the recipients. In about one-half of those D-negative subjects who fail to make serologically detectable anti-D after a first relatively large transfusion of D-positive red cells, further injections of D-positive red cells fail to elicit the formation of anti-D (see section Responders and non-responders, below).

Evidence that some 85% of D-negative subjects will make serologically detectable anti-D after a single transfusion of D-positive red cells is as follows. In one series, following the transfusion of 500 ml of D-positive blood, 18 out of 22 D-negative subjects developed anti-D within 5 months; none of the remaining four subjects made anti-D within 14 days of a further injection of D-positive red cells (Pollack *et al.* 1971). However, the red cells of this second injection were labelled with ^{51}Cr, and in two of the four subjects without serologically demonstrable anti-D the $T_{1/2}$Cr was diminished, to 4.8 and 12.1 days respectively (Bowman 1976). The number of subjects primarily immunized was thus 20 out of 22. In another series in which D-negative subjects received 200 ml of red cells, previously stored in the frozen state, 24 out of 28 produced anti-D within 6 months (average time 120 days), and two of the remaining four produced anti-D after a further injection of D-positive red cells (Urbaniak and Robertson 1981). The overall incidence of primary Rh D immunization following an injection of about 200 ml of D-positive red cells in these two series seems therefore to have been over 90% (46 out of 50).

In a follow-up of D-negative patients who had received an average of 19.4 units of D-positive blood during open heart surgery, anti-D was detected in 19 out of 20 cases (Cook and Rush 1974), but this report is made a little less impressive by the fact that in seven of the subjects the antibody was detected only in tests with enzyme-treated cells and in two of these seven the antibody was detectable only on a single occasion and could not be detected subsequently. In a study of 78 D-negative patients who received D-positive blood, anti-D was detected in only 16 patients. The patients belonged to the following diagnostic categories: abdominal surgery, including gynaecological and urological interventions (42%); cardiosurgery (33%); trauma (14%); disseminated intravascular coagulation (5%); and miscellaneous (6%). Most patients received a single-unit transfusion (Frohn *et al.* 2003). These authors conclude that the probability of making anti-D in response to a D-positive transfusion is much lower in patients than in healthy volunteers.

None of eight D-negative AIDS patients receiving 2–11 units of D-positive red cells developed anti-D; in contrast, all of six D-negative patients with other diagnoses receiving 1–9 units of D-positive red cells developed anti-D within 7–19 weeks of transfusion (Boctor *et al.* 2003). These observations may relate to the immunosuppression occurring in AIDS patients.

183

Table 5.4 Formation of anti-D after injections of 1 ml of red cells of different Rh genotypes.

Donors		Recipients		
		No. with anti-D		
Probable Rh genotype	Total no.	Within 6 months of 1st injection	Within a few weeks of 2nd injection	Reference
DCe/dce	10	1	4	Mollison *et al.* (1969)
DCe/dce	31	7	11	Woodrow *et al.* (1975)
DCe/DcE	12	5	9	Samson and Mollison (1975)
DcE/DcE	12	4	6	Contreras and Mollison (1981)
DCe/dce	20*		6	⎰ B Bevan, personal
DcE/dce	19*		16	⎱ communication

* These subjects received an initial injection of 2 ml of whole blood, then two further injections of 1.5 ml of whole blood at monthly intervals; after a 4-month rest, three further injections of 1.5 ml of blood were given at monthly intervals. The other subjects in the table received two injections of red cells at an interval of about 6 months.

The response to small amounts of D-positive red cells

Following a single injection of 0.5–1.0 ml of D-positive red cells, anti-D has been detected in less than 50% of the recipients in many series; see Table 5.4. The table also shows that if a second injection of D-positive red cells is given at 6 months to the subjects without detectable anti-D, some of them form readily detectable antibody within a few weeks, indicating that the original injection of D-positive cells evoked primary immunization.

Following an injection of D-positive red cells or a pregnancy with a D-positive fetus, a D-negative subject can be primarily immunized to D without having detectable anti-D in the plasma. For example, in some D-negative subjects injected with 2–4 ml of D-positive red cells, a second injection of D-positive cells given after 6 weeks was rapidly cleared and in these subjects anti-D became detectable later (Krevans *et al.* 1964; Woodrow *et al.* 1969). Similarly in 13 D-negative subjects who were injected with 1 ml of D-positive red cells and tested at 6 months, only two had detectable anti-D but five more showed accelerated clearance of a small dose of D-positive red cells and four of these formed serologically detectable anti-D within the following month (Mollison *et al.* 1969; see Fig. 5.5).

The fact that a D-negative subject can be primarily immunized to D without having serologically detectable

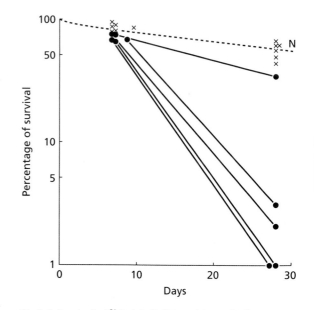

Fig 5.5 Survival of ^{51}Cr-labelled D-positive red cells in 11 D-negative subjects, each of whom had received an injection of 1 ml of D-positive red cells 6 months previously. In five subjects (●), survival was below normal from 7–10 days onwards; all of these subjects formed anti-D. Two other subjects (not shown) developed serologically demonstrable anti-D a few months after their first injection. In the remaining six subjects (×), the survival of D-positive red cells was normal and, despite further injections of D-positive red cells, anti-D was never formed (data from Mollison *et al.* 1969). N, normal survival of ^{51}Cr-labelled red cells.

anti-D in the plasma was first recognized by Nevanlinna (1953), who described the condition as 'sensibilization'. As just described, sensibilization is observed more commonly after the injection of small doses of D-positive cells than of large ones; it is observed commonly in women primarily immunized by a pregnancy.

Responders and non-responders

As already mentioned, of D-negative subjects transfused with 200 ml of D-positive red cells, about 15% fail to make anti-D within the following few months; about one-half of these subjects fail to make anti-D after further injections of D-positive red cells and are termed *non-responders*.

The terms *responder* and *non-responder* were originally used to describe the ability, or inability, of particular strains of guinea pigs to produce antibodies against hapten–polylysine conjugates, a characteristic which was shown to be under genetic control (Levine *et al.* 1963b; see also Chapter 3). There must be a strong presumption that responsiveness to Rh D is genetically determined, although this has not been demonstrated. No consistent differences between the HLA groups of responders and non-responders have been found. Although a non-significant increase of DRw6 in responders has been reported by two groups (see Darke *et al.* 1983), in another series no differences in HLA groups were found between high and low responders to Rh D (Teesdale *et al.* 1988).

When small amounts of D-positive red cells are injected into D-negative subjects and the subjects are subsequently given a second small injection of D-positive red cells, the cells may survive normally on both occasions. When this occurs, the subject invariably fails to form anti-D, even when further injections of small amounts of D-positive red cells are given (Krevans *et al.* 1964; Mollison *et al.* 1969; Woodrow *et al.* 1969; Samson and Mollison 1975; Contreras and Mollison 1981). The survival of D-positive red cells may continue to be normal even after seven injections given over a period of 21 months (for examples, see Mollison *et al.* 1970 and previous editions of this book). These subjects are clearly non-responders to small amounts of D-positive red cells. However, as the frequency of non-responders seems to be significantly higher when small amounts of D-positive red cells are given, it seems likely that there are intermediate grades

of responder. The probability that this concept is correct is reinforced by the observation that the proportion of responders can almost certainly be increased by giving a very small amount of IgG anti-D together with a small dose of D-positive red cells; see later.

Poor responders

Although most D-negative responders produce serologically detectable anti-D after two injections of D-positive red cells, given at an interval of 3–6 months, a few do not; such subjects can be classified as responders or non-responders only if the survival of D-positive red cells is measured or if several further injections of D-positive cells are given. Details of one such case are shown in Fig. 5.6.

Two similar cases were encountered in a long-term follow-up of the 'series I' of Archer and colleagues (1969) in which subjects received 10 ml of D-positive blood initially, followed by 5 ml every 5 weeks. Of 124 subjects, 73 developed anti-D within 18 months. In two further subjects who received regular injections for about 1 year and then, after a further year, two small injections in one case and one small injection followed by a 3-unit transfusion in the other, anti-D was detected for the first time 2.5 years after the start of the experiment; in both cases the antibody was present in relatively low titre.

A few subjects produce a trace of anti-D after a few injections of D-positive cells, but no increase in antibody level occurs after further injections. The antibody may even become undetectable (see Fig. 5.7).

Subjects who take a long time to produce anti-D tend to produce low-titre antibody; in subjects in whom anti-D was first detected only 12 months or more after a first injection of red cells, the titre reached a maximum of 128 or less in 8 out of 18 cases after further injections; in contrast, in 116 subjects who produced anti-D within 9 months of their first injection, the titre eventually reached 512 or more in every case after further injections (Fletcher *et al.* 1971).

Similarly, in D-negative subjects in whom antibody was first detected only after three or more injections of D-positive cells, the titre never exceeded 8, whereas in those subjects who formed detectable anti-D after a single injection of cells, titres of 128 or more were reached in all cases (Lehane 1967).

185

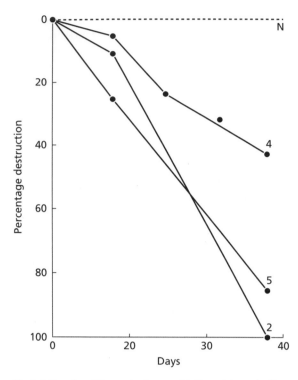

Fig 5.6 Results of Cr survival tests with D-positive red cells in a 'poor responder'. In order to express the extent of red cell destruction due to antibody, results on any particular day (*n*) have been expressed as

$$100 - \left(\frac{\text{Observed Cr survival, day } n}{\text{Expected Cr survival, day } n} \right) \times 100$$

so that, if survival had been normal, a horizontal line (N) would have been obtained. The serial number of each injection of red cells is shown against the appropriate curve. Injection 2 was given 6 months after injection 1; injection 3 (not shown) was given 5 months later; injection 4, 3 months after that; and injection 5, after a further 5 months. Anti-D was detected for the first time approximately 2 months after the fourth injection (from Mollison *et al.* 1970).

Other aspects of primary Rh D immunization

Effect of donor's Rh genotype

Table 5.4 shows that of 41 subjects injected with 1 ml of *DCe/ce* red cells, eight (20%) made anti-D within 6 months of the first injection and a total of 15 (37%) made anti-D after two injections. By contrast, of 24 subjects receiving 1 ml of *DCe/DcE* or *DcE/DcE* red

cells, nine (38%) made anti-D within 6 months of the first injection and a total of 15 (63%) made anti-D after two injections. Again, among subjects receiving approximately 1 ml of blood at monthly intervals, after 1 year only 30% of those injected with *DCe/dce* red cells but 84% of those injected with *DcE/dce* red cells had detectable anti-D in their plasma. The data set out in Table 5.4 cannot be considered to establish decisively that red cells of the probable Rh genotype *DCe/dce* are less immunogenic than red cells of other Rh genotypes because the studies were not carried out in a properly controlled fashion; for example, the sensitivity of serological tests may have varied, the subjects may not have been strictly comparable, etc. Nevertheless, they supply suggestive evidence of the poor immunogenicity of *Dce/dce* red cells when given in small volumes. It should be noted that *DCe/dce* red cells, when transfused in relatively large volumes, do not appear to be less immunogenic than those of other genotypes; see the results of Pollack and colleagues (1971a) referred to above.

Immunogenicity of D variant (partial D and weak D (Dᵘ)) red cells

There have been two reports of the formation of anti-D in D-negative subjects after repeated injections of red cells originally believed to be *ddCcee* but later recognized as Dᵘ. In both, injections of *ddCcee* cells were given twice weekly. In the first case, anti-C was detected after 13 injections and anti-D after 17 (van Loghem 1947). The donor was then found to be 'low on the scale of grades of Dᵘ antigens' (RR Race in a footnote to the same paper). In the second report, three of four subjects made anti-D after 7, 11 and 18 injections respectively (Ruffie and Carrière 1951). In a case in which a weak D sample appeared to have caused primary immunization to D, the donor's red cells were found to have 820–1470 D sites per red cell. In two cases, red cells with 390–1400 D sites caused secondary responses (Gorick *et al.* 1993).

In a follow-up of 45 D-negative subjects who had been transfused with weakly reacting D (D′) red cells (68 transfusions, 50 of DᵘccE and 18 Dᵘccee blood), none developed anti-D, although one developed anti-E and one developed anti-K. In 34 of the recipients, D-positive red cells could be detected for up to 100 days after transfusion (Schmidt *et al.* 1962). The transfused red cells were described as low-grade Dᵘ and the

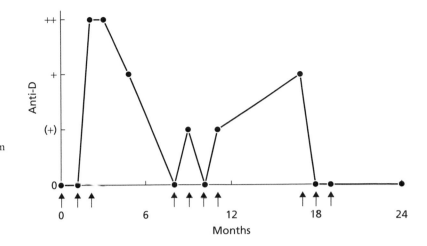

Fig 5.7 Disappearance of anti-D from the serum despite repeated injections (↑) of D-positive cells (data kindly supplied by T Gibson). The amount of anti-D detectable by a test with papainized red cells is shown on an arbitrary scale.

frequency of such cells in the relevant donor population was 0.4%. Among the 45 recipients there were 15 who were receiving drugs (6-mercaptopurine or steroids) known to suppress immune responses but, even if these 15 are excluded, the failure of 30 D-negative subjects to develop anti-D after transfusion suggests that weak D (D^u) is far less immunogenic than normal D.

A single case has been described in which partial D red cells (D^{Va}) stimulated the production of normal, although very weak, anti-D (Mayne *et al.* 1990). Production of anti-D in a D-negative patient transfused with weak D type 2 red cells (450 D antigen sites/cell) has been recorded (Flegel *et al.* 2000). Anti-D alloimmunization by weak D type 1 red cells has also been reported (Mota *et al.* 2005).

There is one report of immunization of a D-negative Japanese woman by a red cell unit from a donor of Del phenotype with the G1227A allele (Ohto, cited in Wagner *et al.* 2005). One out of four Dutch African black people with the DAR phenotype produced anti-D after multiple transfusions with D-positive blood (Hemker *et al.* 1999).

The minimum dose of D-positive red cells for primary immunization

Very few observations have been made with doses less than 0.5 ml. In one series, five injections each of 0.1 ml of D-positive cord blood (approximately 0.05 ml of red cells) of unstated Rh phenotype were given at 6-weekly intervals to D-negative subjects; four out of 15 formed anti-D (Zipursky *et al.* 1965). In another series, injections of 0.01 ml of blood (about 0.005 ml

red cells) of phenotype R$_2$r were given at 2-weekly intervals to eight D-negative subjects. Six of the subjects were parous women and only the data for the two male subjects can be used to decide whether such a dose can induce primary immunization. Of the two, one formed anti-D after six injections, i.e. after a total of about 0.03 ml of red cells. Two other men were given injections of about 0.05 ml of red cells at 2-week intervals and one of these formed anti-D after 10 injections, equivalent to a total of 0.5 ml of red cells. These findings suggest that a cumulative dose of not more than about 0.03 ml of red cells is capable of inducing primary D immunization, but they do not go very far towards defining the frequency with which such a dose is effective.

Earliest time at which anti-D can be detected in primary immunization

In a series in which 22 D-negative subjects were transfused with a unit of D-positive blood, all still had detectable D-positive red cells in their circulation at 1 month; 2 months after transfusion, nine of the subjects had detectable anti-D in their serum, and at 3 months, 16; anti-D was detected for the first time at 4 months in one subject and at 5 months in another (Pollack *et al.* 1971a).

In six subjects receiving 5 ml of DcE/DcE red cells, one had detectable anti-D at 37 days, although in four other responding subjects antibody was first detected at 63–119 days (Gunson *et al.* 1970).

In another series in which 12 subjects were injected with 1 ml of DcE/DcE red cells, and in which the subjects were tested at 2-weekly intervals, the earliest time at which anti-D was detected was 4 weeks; all four subjects who made serologically detectable anti-D after the first injection had detectable antibody in their plasma by the end of 10 weeks (Contreras and Mollison 1981).

In previously unimmunized D-negative subjects anti-D cannot be produced more rapidly by giving a series of injections of D-positive red cells rather than a single injection. For example, among 121 subjects given an initial injection of 5 ml of positive blood, followed by 2 ml every 5 weeks, eight formed anti-D within 10 weeks, and 27 within 15 weeks (Archer et al. 1969).

Apparent discrepancies between different series in the earliest time at which antibody is detected are doubtless due partly to differences in the sensitivity of testing.

Production of anti-D within a few weeks of a first stimulus has been observed after the injection of specially treated D-positive red cells. The cells were incubated in a low-ionic-strength medium at 37°C and at the time of injection reacted strongly with anti-C4, -C3 and -C5. No observations were made on the rate of disappearance of the cells after injection into D-negative volunteers. Of seven subjects, one first developed anti-D at 15 days and five others developed antibody between 41 and 71 days after injection. It was considered that the time before the appearance of antibody was not significantly shorter than that observed following the injection of untreated cells (Gunson et al. 1971).

Influence of ABO incompatibility on primary Rh D immunization

The effect of ABO incompatibility in protection against Rh D immunization was first discovered from an analysis of the ABO groups of the parents of infants with Rh D haemolytic disease (see Chapter 12) and was first demonstrated experimentally by Stern and colleagues (1956). These investigators gave from two to ten intravenous injections of D-positive red cells at intervals of 6–10 weeks (sometimes 5 months). The amounts injected were at first 5 ml, then 2.5 ml. If anti-D developed, only one further injection of 1 ml was given. Only one adverse reaction was noted (flushing of the face and faintness), and this was in a subject receiving ABO-incompatible cells. Of 17 subjects

injected with ABO-compatible cells, 10 developed anti-D; in five subjects the titre rose to between 16 and 128, and reached from 256 to 512 in the remainder. By contrast, anti-D developed in only two out of 22 subjects receiving ABO-incompatible D-positive cells, and the titre was only 2–8. In one of these two cases seven further injections of D-positive cells failed to produce any increase in titre.

In a later study (Stern et al. 1961), the series was extended slightly and the total figures for the production of anti-D became: after ABO-compatible D-positive cells, 17 out of 24 (anti-D titre 16 or more); after ABO-incompatible cells, 5 out of 32 (anti-D titre 8 or less in four of five subjects). Ten subjects who failed to form anti-D after receiving ABO-incompatible D-positive cells were subsequently injected with ABO-compatible D-positive cells and four produced anti-D.

ABO incompatibility also protects against immunization to c and other red cell antigens; see Chapter 3 for references.

Effect of cytotoxic drugs on primary immunization to D

Of 19 D-negative patients who were transfused with many units of D-positive red cells during liver or heart transplant surgery, only three made anti-D, in each case at 11–15 days. In two out of these three, the response was assumed to be secondary (both were women with previous pregnancies); in the third, the response was possibly primary. Of the remaining 16 patients, not one made anti-D within the following 2.5–51 months; 13 of the 16 were followed for more than 11.5 months. The low rate of primary immunization was assumed to be due to immunosuppressive therapy with ciclosporin and corticosteroids (Ramsey et al. 1989). In another series, recipients of heart or lung, or heart–lung transplants receiving immunosuppressive therapy including ciclosporin, both primary and secondary responses to Rh D appeared to be suppressed. Of 51 D-negative recipients of D-positive grafts, only one developed anti-D and this was a multiparous woman in whom the response was presumed to be secondary. Of six D-negative patients transfused with D-positive red cells, only two developed anti-D and then only transiently (Cummins et al. 1995). Non-myeolablative conditioning containing fludarabine and/or Campath 1 with ciclosporin A given post haemopoietic stem cell transplantation prevented anti-D formation in D-negative recipients of a D-positive graft. However, anti-D developed in one of seven D-positive recipients of a D-negative graft, who was exposed to D-positive blood products before and after transplant (Mijovic 2002).

Rh D immunization by red cells present as contaminants

Platelet concentrates

In a retrospective study of 102 D-negative patients, all of whom had diseases associated with impaired immunological reactivity (mainly acute leukaemia), and all of whom were receiving immunosuppressive drugs, who were transfused with numerous units of platelets from D-positive donors, eight patients (7.8%) developed anti-D within an average of about 8 months from the first platelet transfusion. It was estimated that each platelet concentrate contained approximately 0.37 ml of red cells (Goldfinger and McGinniss 1971). In another series, of patients with a variety of malignancies, only 2 out of 115 developed anti-D (Lichtiger and Hester 1986). In another study, 3 out of 78 D-negative patients with haematological malignancies who received a D-negative transplant developed anti-D after receiving D-positive platelet transfusions (Asfour et al. 2004).

In 22 D-negative patients, mostly with malignant disease, receiving a mean of 8 D-positive platelet concentrates and 50 µg of anti-D intravenously and in 20 D-negative patients, all with malignant disease, receiving a mean of 10 concentrates and 20 µg of anti-D intravenously, no instance of Rh D immunization was observed. In the second series, the volume of red cells was found to be less than 0.8 ml in 99.4% of all concentrates (Zeiler et al. 1994). When platelet concentrates from D-positive donors are transfused to D-negative women who have not yet reached the menopause, an injection of anti-D immunoglobulin should be given to suppress primary Rh D immunization. Such an injection is not expected to impair the survival of platelets from D-positive donors, as platelets do not carry Rh antigens.

Plasma transfusion

Liquid-stored plasma may contain small numbers of red cells, and plasma transfusions have been shown to be capable of causing both primary and secondary responses to red cell alloantigens. In one case, primary immunization was observed in a patient with systemic lupus erythematosus, who had received liquid-stored plasma from 104 D-positive donors during the course of several plasma exchanges. It was estimated that between 0.1 and 0.5 ml of D-positive red cells were introduced; anti-D was found in the plasma 6 weeks after the last plasma exchange (McBride et al. 1978). In another case, the transfusion of a single unit of liquid-stored plasma from a D-positive donor apparently induced primary immunization, although red cell counts on other units of similarly prepared plasma suggested that each unit contained not more than about 0.05 ml of packed red cells; in four further cases, the transfusion of a small number of units of stored plasma induced secondary responses: in two cases to D and in two to Fy^a (KL Burnie and RM Barr, personal communication).

The use of fresh-frozen plasma (FFP) from D-positive donors for plasma exchange may be followed by substantial increases in anti-D (Barclay et al. 1980). It is very suggestive that the rise in anti-D titre starts after a few days and reaches a peak at about 14 days (Wensley et al. 1980). In a case in which 4 units of FFP from D-positive donors were transfused (without plasma exchange) there was an obvious secondary response (de la Rubia et al. 1994).

Renal transplantation

Anti-D developed in a D-negative male 3 months after the transplantation of a cadaver kidney from a D-positive donor, despite the fact that the kidney had been immediately perfused with saline after removal from the donor (Kenwright et al. 1976). Of 42 D-negative patients on immunosuppressive therapy who received a kidney from D-positive donors, two were found to have anti-D not detectable before transplantation (Quan et al. 1996) These authors suggest that all D-negative women of childbearing age receiving a D-positive kidney should be given prophylactic anti-D at the time of transplantation.

Liver transplantation

Severe haemolysis resulted from transplantation of a D-negative liver from a donor with anti-D, anti-C and anti-K into a D-positive recipient. The patient required

189

two separate red cell exchange transfusions and intermittent red cell transfusions over the course of a year and underwent a variety of immunosuppressive therapies; a normalization of haemoglobin levels was not achieved until splenectomy on day 321 (Fung *et al.* 2004).

Bone grafts

In two women of childbearing age, bone allografts appear to have been the cause of Rh immunization. One of the women (evidently partial D) was typed as ccD^{u}ee. She made anti-D and 13 years after receiving the graft her first infant was born with haemolytic disease (Hill *et al.* 1974). The second woman was D negative, and made anti-C and anti-G, which were detected on routine antibody screening after a blood donation (Johnson *et al.* 1985).

Contaminated syringes

Cases have been reported in which young women have been immunized to D by sharing syringes for the i.v. injection of 'hard' drugs. In one such case, the patient received an injection of cocaine to which blood from her sexual partner had deliberately been added in a 'ritualistic mingling'. She received further injections from shared syringes, contaminated with her partner's blood, over the next few months; 11 months from the time of the first injection she had an anti-D titre of 1000 (Vontver 1973). In another case, a young woman was immunized by sharing a syringe for i.v. morphine injections with her sexual partner and with other people. The partner was not only R_1R_2 but also K positive and the patient developed not only potent anti-D, but also anti-K (McVerry *et al.* 1977).

Secondary Rh D immunization

In subjects who had been primarily immunized to D by being given a first injection of 1 ml of D-positive red cells but at 6 months had made no detectable anti-D, a second injection of D-positive red cells at that time often produced a relatively slow and weak secondary response. In six such subjects, who had been given two doses of 1 ml of D-positive red cells at an interval of 6 months, anti-D was first detected in four at 2–5 weeks and in two more at 10–20 weeks after a second injection; in no case did the antibody concentration exceed 0.3 µg/ml (Samson and Mollison 1975; Contreras and

Mollison 1981). On the other hand, when anti-D was made after a first injection of 1 ml of D-positive red cells and a second injection was given at 6 months, antibody levels rose rapidly and in one case reached a level of 92 µg/ml (Samson and Mollison 1975).

In subjects immunized to D by transfusion or pregnancy some years previously, with low levels of anti-D in the plasma, the injection of 0.2–2.0 ml of D-positive red cells often produced a maximal or near-maximal increase in anti-D concentration within 3 weeks; in 9 out of 30 subjects, the level rose from less than 4 µg/ml to more than 40 µg/ml, and it ultimately reached this level in about one-half of the subjects (Holburn *et al.* 1970). In another series in which six out of ten subjects had pre-injection levels of 4 µg or less and in which eight of the ten subjects received only one injection of about 0.5 ml of R_0r cells (two injections in the other two cases), the average antibody level reached 112 µg/ml, sometimes within 2 weeks and in all cases by 4 months (J Bowman, personal communication). In other subjects, antibody levels may continue to rise for many months when injections are given at intervals of 5–8 weeks (Archer *et al.* 1971).

When no further injections of red cells are given, there is usually a progressive decline in antibody concentration; for example, in five subjects in one series, the values fell to 50% of the maximum after 5–13 months (Holburn *et al.* 1970). In another series there was a more rapid initial fall, titres falling to 50% of their maximum value in 11–40 days in some subjects, although not until 100 days in others (Gunson *et al.* 1974). Some subjects maintain anti-D concentrations above 50 µg/ml for 1–2 years without further injections of red cells (M Contreras, unpublished observations).

Antibody concentrations tend to be higher in re-stimulated subjects than in women immunized by pregnancy; anti-D levels of 21 µg/ml or more were found in 96% of re-stimulated donors but in only 7% of previously pregnant women (Moore and Hughes-Jones 1970); 42% of the re-stimulated donors had levels of 101 µg/ml or more.

In a case referred to in Chapter 11, in which a subject with a faint trace of anti-D (0.004 µg/ml) was transfused with 4 units of D-positive blood and developed a delayed haemolytic transfusion reaction, the anti-D concentration on day 9 was estimated to be 512 µg/ml.

In the secondary response it is common for the serum to agglutinate saline-suspended red cells. For example, in one series before re-stimulation, only four of 30 Rh D-immunized subjects had anti-D saline agglutinins, but after stimulation the proportion was 20 out of 30; in 10 cases the agglutinin titre exceeded 4 (Holburn *et al.* 1970). In another series in which male donors who had been immunized some years previously were re-stimulated, about 1 week after re-injection most had agglutinin titres vs. saline-suspended red cells of 16–128 (Gibson 1979). Similarly, in a series of about 100 women immunized by previous pregnancy the injection of 1 ml of D-positive red cells provoked the appearance of anti-D agglutinins in 30% of cases (Hotevar and Glonar 1972). The agglutination of saline-suspended cells by the serum of re-immunized subjects appears to be due to IgG anti-D, as the property is not diminished by treatment of the serum with dithiothreitol (M Contreras, unpublished observations).

In stimulating secondary responses, R_1r cells seem to be as effective as R_2R_2 cells (Gunson *et al.* 1974) and i.m. injections of D-positive cells as effective as i.v. injections (PL Mollison, personal observations), although after i.m. injection the peak titre may be reached as late as 28 days compared with 7–14 days after i.v. injection (Gunson *et al.* 1974).

Persistence of antibodies

Anti-D can sometimes be detected in the serum a very long time after the last known stimulus; for example, it has been found in a woman 38 years after her last pregnancy (Stratton 1955). In cases in which anti-D can no longer be demonstrated serologically, a transfusion given 20 years or so after the last known stimulus may evoke a powerful secondary response, leading to a delayed haemolytic transfusion reaction (see Chapter 11).

Because immunization to D persists indefinitely, D-negative blood should always be used for transfusion to D-negative women, even when the menopause has been reached and there is no history of pregnancy. One must always consider the possibility that the patient has been immunized by a pregnancy which she does not choose to reveal or by an abortion of which she is unaware.

Whereas, in subjects immunized to Rh D, incomplete (IgG) antibodies may persist for very long periods, complete ('saline') agglutinins disappear comparatively rapidly: in women found to have saline agglutinins shortly after their last pregnancy, the titre was found to decline very rapidly during the following 12 months,

so that at the end of this time only one-third of the women had a saline agglutinin titre of 8 or more, and after 4 years less than one-tenth of the women had a saline agglutinin titre of 8 or more. In women whose serum contained incomplete anti-D, the rate of decline was much slower: 6 years after the last pregnancy incomplete antibody could still be demonstrated in 460 out of 478 cases (Ward 1957; see also Hopkins 1969).

Anti-D saline agglutinins are occasionally demonstrable in subjects who have not received an antigenic stimulus for a long period (44 years in one reported case: Hutchison and McLennan 1966). In one subject, a persistent Rh agglutinin (titre 5000) was shown to be IgM (MC Contreras, unpublished observations). In a single case, in which anti-D had been shown to be partly IgA as well as partly IgG, the titre of IgA anti-D actually rose over a period of 12 years after the last known stimulus (PL Mollison, unpublished observations).

Cyclical fluctuations in anti-D level have been observed; daily samples were taken from eight female and two male Rh D-immunized subjects for several weeks; all samples were tested at the same time. In 6 out of the 10 subjects, values fell for 3–5 days then rose more rapidly so that the total cycle from one low point to another was exactly 7 days. The difference between the highest and the lowest levels was 25–30% (Rubinstein 1972).

Production of anti-D by human lymphocytes transplanted to mice

Human lymphocytes can be successfully transplanted to mice with severe combined immunodeficiency. If lymphocytes from a recently re-stimulated human donor are injected, anti-D appears in the mouse's serum and persists for 8 weeks or more, indicating that long-lived B lymphocytes, or memory B lymphocytes, have been transferred (Leader *et al.* 1992). This model seems to have potential value for experiments on Rh immunization.

Immunization to Rh antigens other than D

G, C and E

The formation of anti-G, anti-C and (far less frequently) anti-E in subjects immunized to D is relatively common, but the formation of these antibodies in subjects who are D positive and therefore do not form anti-D is very rare. Presumably, this difference is simply an example of the augmenting effect of strong antigens on weak antigens, discussed in Chapter 3.

The formation of anti-G (at first mistaken for anti-D) after the transfusion of ddCcee blood to a ddccee recipient has been reported only once (Smith *et al*. 1977).

Anti-C alone, i.e. without anti-D, is rare. Some evidence of the low immunogenicity of C is as follows. In one series in which either C-negative or E-negative, D-positive recipients were given frequent i.v. injections of C-positive or E-positive red cells over a period of 1–1.5 years, not one of the 32 subjects formed the desired antibody (Jones *et al*. 1954). In a study in which 74 C-negative, D-negative subjects were transfused with one or more units of C-positive, D-negative blood (and in some cases also with E-positive, D-negative blood) only two formed anti-C. Of 66 C-negative, D-positive patients transfused with 136 units of C-positive blood, none made antibody (Schorr *et al*. 1971). And of four ddccee subjects who had been transfused with 2, 4, 7 and 17 units of dCe blood, respectively, none made anti-C (Huestis 1971).

Anti-E is much commoner than anti-C but, as explained above, is often naturally occurring. Immune anti-E is uncommon. Of 47 E-negative, D-negative patients transfused with a total of 89 units of E-positive blood, not one made anti-E and of 44 E-negative, D-positive patients transfused with 71 units of E-positive blood, only one made anti-E (Schorr *et al*. 1971).

Issitt (1979), reviewing data from the literature and comparing them with his own experience in Cincinnati, showed that the frequency with which anti-C and anti-E were found in D-negative subjects was virtually the same whether they were transfused with D-negative blood, which was also C negative and E negative, or with D-negative blood that was either C positive or E positive. With either practice, the frequency of anti-C was about 1 in 10 000 and of anti-E about 1 in 1000. Moreover, of four examples of anti-C and 44 examples of anti-E detected in Cincinnati every example was found in a D-positive patient.

Of 100 patients with anti-E, 32 also had anti-c (Shirey *et al*. 1994).

C^w

Of three volunteers who were given twice-weekly injections of 0.5 ml of C^w blood, one produced anti-CW after 21 injections (van Loghem *et al*. 1949).

c

Two attempts to produce anti-c by giving repeated injections of c-positive blood to c-negative volunteers have been recorded: in one, none of 19 subjects responded (Wiener 1949), but in the other antibody was produced in two out of nine (Jones *et al*. 1954).

After anti-D, anti-c is (in white people) the most important Rh antibody from the clinical point of view. Although anti-E is commoner than anti-c, as mentioned above anti-E is frequently a naturally occurring antibody; on the other hand, anti-c (like anti-e) is found only as an immune antibody. Anti-c is relatively often involved in delayed haemolytic transfusion reactions and in HDN.

The risk of forming anti-c in DCCee subjects who already have anti-E in their serum and are transfused with blood untyped for c is substantial. Out of 27 such subjects who were transfused with 2–14 (mean 8) units, five formed anti-c within 13–193 days. Although no delayed haemolytic transfusion reactions (DHTRs) were observed, the authors concluded that the selection of c-negative red cells for DCCee patients with anti-E may be justified (Shirey *et al*. 1994). A better case may be made for selecting c-negative red cells for CC women who have not yet reached the menopause, to minimize the risk of HDN due to anti-c, although the costs of such a policy are bound to limit its implementation (see Chapter 8).

e

Two successful attempts at producing anti-e in DDccEE subjects have been reported. In the first, repeated injections of e-positive blood were given to a single volunteer over a period of 6 years before the antibody was detected (Jones *et al*. 1954). In the second, weekly injections of 0.5 ml of blood were given to three subjects for 8 weeks; after 2 months' rest, the weekly injections were resumed and, after the third injection, anti-a was detected in one subject (van Loghem *et al*. 1953).

Development of a positive direct antiglobulin test following Rh D immunization

Positive direct antiglobulin test following secondary immunization

As described in Chapters 3 and 11, the direct antiglobulin

test (DAT) may become positive following secondary immunization. The positive DAT persists long after the stimulating red cells have been cleared from the circulation. Two examples are as follows: in a D-negative patient who developed potent anti-D after a transfusion of 4000 ml of D-positive red cells, the DAT was positive at 6 months, although negative at 1 year. It is probably not relevant that, after the transfusion, the patient was given 7000 µg of anti-D in the hope of suppressing Rh D immunization before it was realized that she was already primarily immunized (Beard et al. 1971). A D-negative woman with anti-D in her serum developed severe haemolysis 2 weeks after the transfusion of 4 units of D-negative red cells. The DAT was found to have become positive and an autoantibody of a specificity mimicking anti-D was eluted. The DAT was still positive 1 year later (Dzik et al. 1994).

In a patient of group Rh^d who had developed anti-Rh^d, D-positive red cells were transfused and rapidly destroyed. The DAT was positive at 4 days and more strongly positive 4 months later; the reaction was weaker at 6 months and negative at 7 months (Lalezari et al. 1975).

Anti-LW developing in subjects who are transiently LW negative

In two D-negative, LW-positive pregnant women, anti-LW was detected as well as anti-D. At this time the patients' red cells behaved as LW negative. One of the two patients then developed a positive DAT and the anti-LW could no longer be demonstrated in the plasma. Ten weeks later the patient was clearly LW positive. It was postulated that the anti-LW was responsible for the positive DAT and that the anti-LW was probably produced only when the patient was functionally LW negative and was therefore not really an autoantibody. From the time when the patient became LW positive again, the antibody was like a passively acquired incompatible antibody (Chown et al. 1971). In a very similar case, a D-negative woman was found to have developed anti-D 3 weeks before her first delivery. In addition her plasma reacted with all D-negative samples. Just before delivery, her DAT became positive. It was still positive 6 months later but was negative at 1 year. The patient's cells were LW negative at the time of delivery but positive 1 year later. At the time of delivery the serum contained anti-LW as well as anti-CD, but at 1 year only anti-CD

(Giles and Lundsgaard 1967). The development of anti-LWa with concurrent depression of LW^a has also been described in a 10-month-old infant (Devenish 1994).

Anti-LW may also develop transiently in D-positive patients who have a chronic, often terminal, illness, possibly with some underlying immunological disorder. These subjects do not develop anti-D (Perkins et al. 1977; Giles 1980).

D-negative subjects of undetermined LW status

In a series in which male D-negative subjects were immunized to provide anti-D for immunoprophylaxis, it was found that pooled plasma obtained from them reacted weakly with bromelin-treated D-negative cells. Samples from 11 out of 18 subjects when tested separately showed the same reaction and the red cells of two more subjects gave a positive DAT. Five months later all reactions had become negative and no clinical signs of red cell destruction were observed at any time (Cook 1971). Although the specificity of the autoantibody was anti-LW (P Tippett, personal communication) the LW status of the subjects during the period when the DAT was positive was not determined. In several other series this phenomenon has been looked for but not found (e.g. Contreras and Mollison 1981, 1983).

Association with intensive plasma exchange

In two women who had had previous infants with hydrops fetalis, intensive plasma exchange was carried out in a subsequent pregnancy between about the 11th and 24th weeks. The total amount of plasma exchanged in this period was about 95 l. In one of the two cases, despite this treatment, the antibody titre rose from 512 at 17 weeks to about 60 000 at 24 weeks, and in both cases the mothers had a stillbirth at about the 25th week, in one case following an intrauterine transfusion. In both women, at the conclusion of the course of plasma exchange, it was found that the patient's red cells had acquired a positive DAT and that the plasma reacted with D-negative red cells. An IgG antibody of apparent specificity anti-G was eluted from the red cells. In one of the patients who was followed up for 1 year, the DAT remained positive, but there were no signs of a haemolytic process. The reaction of the patient's own red cells with anti-LW was not determined (Isbister et al. 1977).

Auto-anti-D in a D-positive subject with weak D

In the first case of this kind to be reported, a man with the phenotype DCCEe and a 'very low grade' partial D developed anti-D and anti-c following transfusion, and also developed a positive DAT. The strength of this reaction varied directly with the amount of anti-D in his serum at any particular time; anti-D could be eluted from his red cells (Chown *et al*. 1963).

A positive direct antiglobulin test in a D-positive subject following a massive dose of anti-D

In an experimental study, plasma containing potent anti-DC was transfused to an R_2R_2 subject, producing a severe haemolytic episode. Between 70 and 229 days after the transfusion, an eluate prepared from the recipient's red cells contained specific anti-E and this eluate reacted with the recipient's pre-transfusion red cells. It was concluded that an autoantibody had been produced, possibly due to an alteration to the Rh site by an interaction of transfused anti-DC with the D antigen (Mohn *et al*. 1964).

Suppression of primary Rh D immunization by passively administered anti-D

For a general discussion of the suppression of primary immunization by passively administered antibody, see Chapter 3.

Early work

The first experiments showing that passively administered anti-D could interfere with primary Rh D immunization were performed by Stern and colleagues (1961), who found that if D-positive red cells were coated *in vitro* with anti-D before being injected into D-negative subjects, there might be no antibody response. Of 16 subjects given a course of injections (in most cases five) of coated D-positive cells, not one produced anti-D; 10 of the subjects were later given injections of uncoated D-positive cells and five produced anti-D. These experiments were not pursued further and it was left to others to consider the possibility that Rh D immunization, which would otherwise occur as a result of pregnancy, could be suppressed by a timely injection of anti-D.

In a brief report of a meeting of the Liverpool Medical Institution, Finn (1960) was quoted as saying '. . . It might be possible to destroy any fetal red cells found in the maternal circulation following delivery by means of a suitable antibody. If successful, this would prevent the development of erythroblastosis, so mimicking the natural protection afforded by ABO incompatibility'.

The Liverpool group at first assumed that treatment would have to be given during pregnancy; accordingly, their first experiments were made with IgM antibody, as, following injection into the mother's circulation, this type of antibody would not cross the placenta to cause harm to the fetus (Finn *et al*. 1961). At much the same time, Freda and Gorman (1962) referred to experiments which they had started in male volunteers, and discussed the possibility that it might be necessary, in treating pregnant women, to use either 19S antibody or 3.5S fragments of antibody, neither of which was expected to cross the placenta.

Suppression of Rh D immunization by 'incomplete' (IgG) anti-D was demonstrated by Clarke and colleagues (1963) and also by Freda and colleagues (1964, 1966), who were the first to use an immunoglobulin concentrate of IgG anti-D, given intramuscularly. Shortly afterwards, it was realized that transplacental haemorrhage occurred chiefly at the time of delivery and both groups showed that anti-D given soon after delivery would suppress Rh D immunization, which would otherwise have occurred (Combined Study 1966; Pollack *et al*. 1968b).

In this chapter, the suppression of Rh D immunization following the i.v. injection of D-positive red cells is discussed; the suppression of Rh D immunization that would otherwise follow pregnancy is discussed in the chapter on HDN (Chapter 12).

Minimum amount of IgG anti-D that will suppress immunization

Intramuscular administration of anti-D

Although there is relatively little evidence about the minimum amount of IgG anti-D required to suppress Rh D immunization when different volumes of D-positive red cells are injected, and although it seems quite possible that the amount varies with different preparations of anti-D immunoglobulin, the rule of thumb that 20 µg of anti-D/ml of D-positive red cells is sufficient to suppress Rh D immunization is a very useful one. Some of the evidence on which this rule is based is as follows.

Less than 10 ml of red cells. A dose of 50 µg of anti-D appears to be sufficient to suppress Rh D immunization completely when 2.5 ml of *DcE/DcE* red cells (approximately 5 ml of blood) are injected. Of 39 treated subjects who received the anti-D 72 h after the D-positive cells and who received a second injection of 0.1 ml of D-positive cells at 6 months (without anti-D), none had anti-D in their serum 2 weeks later. In control subjects who received the same doses of D-positive cells but no anti-D, 11 out of 36 made anti-D during the 6 months after the first injection of red cells and three more made anti-D within 2 weeks of the second injection (Crispen 1976).

In an earlier series it was reported that when 40 µg of anti-D were injected with 2.0–2.5 ml of red cells, i.e. approximately 18 µg of anti-D/ml of cells, immunization was not suppressed (Pollack *et al.* 1968b). However, it seems not unlikely that the dose of anti-D given was overestimated; the same anti-D preparation produced apparent augmentation of the immune response at an approximate dosage of 4.5 µg of antibody/ml of cells, which is substantially higher than later estimates of the probable augmenting dose (see below). The estimates in the series of Pollack and colleagues were made very shortly after the method for quantifying anti-D was first described.

A dose of 10 µg of anti-D/ml of red cells (5 µg of anti-Rh with 0.5 ml of *DcE/DcE* red cells) failed to suppress Rh D immunization (Gunson *et al.* 1971). In another series, in which 5 µg of anti-D were given with 1 ml of *DcE/DcE* red cells, there was suggestive evidence of partial suppression of primary immunization (Contreras and Mollison 1981).

10–40 ml of red cells. Following the injection of about 12 ml of D-positive red cells to 10 subjects and about 25 ml to 10 others, given in each case with an injection of 260 µg of IgG anti-D, no anti-D could be detected at 6–9 months in any subject. Between 6 and 30 months after the first injection of red cells, 2.5 ml of red cells were injected, followed by a further injection of 260 µg of anti-D. (This second injection of anti-D was given to suppress primary Rh D immunization and was not expected to interfere with secondary immunization.) No subjects formed anti-D (Bartsch 1972).

In easily the most valuable experiment yet described on defining the dose of anti-D required to suppress Rh D immunization, a fixed amount of IgG anti-D, namely 267 µg, was given to groups of D-negative subjects who received doses of D-positive red cells varying from 11.6 to 37.5 ml. Control subjects received the same dose of red cells without anti-D. All of the subjects were given a challenge dose of 0.2 ml of whole blood at 6 months and tested 1 week later. Of the controls, 49 out of 86 (57%) formed anti-D. There was suggestive but not decisive evidence of a relation between the dose of D-positive red cells and the incidence of Rh D immunization. From the results in the treated group (Table 5.5), it was concluded that 267 µg of this particular preparation of anti-D was completely effective against about 13 ml of red cells and was partially effective against larger amounts (Pollack *et al.* 1971).

Table 5.5 An estimate of the maximum amount of D-positive red cells against which a fixed amount of anti-D will protect from immunization (from Pollack *et al.* 1971b).

Average amount of red cells (ml) injected						
	11.6	13.4	18.1	21.2	30.1	37.5
Proportions immunized						
Treated	0/19	0/18	3/18	2/8	4/12	6/17
Control	7/16	6/12	11/19	5/8	7/11	13/20

Treated subjects received 267 µg of anti-D intramuscularly; control subjects received 'inert' immunoglobulin.
The totals for the numbers immunized are for subjects who developed detectable anti-D either 6 months after the first injection of cells or 1 week after that, after having received a challenge dose of 0.2 ml of D-positive red cells.

Table 5.6 Administration of anti-D immunoglobulin i.v. to four D-negative women inadvertently transfused with D-positive blood.

D-positive blood transfused (units)	Anti-D (μg) given		Time to clear D-positive red cells (days)	Reaction	Follow-up
	Total	Per ml red cells			
1	3000	15	6	Nil	No anti-D at 6 and 12 months
2	5625	14	3	Nil	No anti-D at 4 years
2	4000	10	2	Haemoglobinuria	No anti-D after 2nd D-positive pregnancy
3	7750	13	8	Pyrexia	No anti-D at 8 months

Sooner or later, an attempt is likely to be made to repeat an experiment of this kind using monoclonal anti-D. It is therefore worth pointing out that, at least after primary immunization with 1 ml of red cells, if subjects are tested only 1 week after a second dose of D-positive red cells, given 6 months after the first, there is a serious risk of failing to detect some secondary responses (see p. 190).

200 ml of red cells. In an experiment in which 22 D-negative subjects were transfused with 500 ml of blood, eight were given 14.6 μg of anti-D/ml cells and 14 received 20 μg/ml of cells. None of the 22 subjects formed anti-D within 5 months (Pollack *et al.* 1971a). When challenged with a small dose of D-positive cells at 5 months, many of the subjects showed accelerated clearance (Bowman 1976) but this was probably due to the persistence of passively administered anti-D.

Intravenous administration of IgG anti-D

As described in Chapters 10 and 14, following the i.m. administration of anti-D, the maximum level in the plasma is reached only after about 48 h. Moreover, the maximum concentration reached is equivalent to only about 40% of the level expected if the anti-D were injected intravenously. If the suppression of Rh D immunization is related to the degree of antibody coating of red cells at the time of clearance, the amount of anti-D required for suppression when given intravenously should be less than one-half of the amount required when given intramuscularly.

The only direct evidence of the superiority of the i.v. route in suppressing Rh D immunization comes from a single experiment: D-negative subjects were injected with 5 ml of *DcE/DcE* blood and with 15 μg of anti-D, given either intramuscularly or intravenously. At 5 months, when none of the subjects had formed antibody, a second injection of *DcE/DcE* blood (2 ml) was given. Five months later, anti-D was present in four out of six subjects who had received the anti-D intramuscularly but in none of eight subjects who had received anti-D intravenously (Jouvenceaux 1971). The probability of getting such a difference by chance is only 0.015.

In D-negative women who have inadvertently been transfused with D-positive blood, and particularly when more than 1 unit has been transfused, it is advantageous to give the anti-D immunoglobulin intravenously, mainly to avoid the discomfort of injecting large amounts of the material intramuscularly, but also because the dose needed for suppression when given intravenously is probably smaller. Table 5.6 shows some results in four cases (seventh edition, p. 385). The results of the serological follow-up suggest, but do not prove, that a dose of 10–15 μg of anti-D/ml of red cells, given intravenously, is sufficient to prevent primary Rh D immunization when 1 or more units of D-positive blood are transfused.

The effect of delayed administration of anti-D

D-negative volunteers were given 1 ml of ^{51}Cr-labelled, D-positive red cells, followed 13 days later by an intramuscular injection of 100 μg of anti-D. Control subjects received only D-positive cells. At 6 months, 5 out of 12 control subjects, but no treated subjects, had anti-D in their serum. Both treated and control subjects were now given second injections of 1 ml of labelled D-positive red cells. After a further 6 months, a third injection of labelled D-positive red cells was given to those subjects in the treated group in whom the survival of the second injection had been normal. From these experiments it was concluded that Rh D immunization was completely suppressed in one-half of the responders in the treated group; that is to say, in these subjects the survival of the red cells injected on the second occasion was normal but the survival of those injected on the third occasion was grossly curtailed and was followed by the production of anti-D (Samson and Mollison 1975).

In a case in which a woman, who said she had never been pregnant, was transfused with 1000 ml of D-positive blood and was given 3000 μg of anti-D within 24 h and had a further 8400 μg 6–7 days after transfusion (7.7 and 20 μg anti-D/ml of red cells), anti-D with a titre of 256 was present at 4 and 9 months (Branch et al. 1985). If primary immunization by an undisclosed abortion can be excluded, it seems that failure of suppression was due to the interval of 7 days between transfusion and the administration of a normally adequate dose of anti-D.

The suppressive effect of monoclonal anti-D

Evidence of immunosuppression by monoclonal anti-D was obtained in an experiment in which 26 D-negative men were injected intramuscularly with different amounts of either an IgG1 or an IgG3 monoclonal followed, 3 days later, by an i.v. injection of 3 ml of (previously frozen) D-positive red cells. Of the 16 subjects who received the IgG1 monoclonal, eight were injected with 100 μg and the remaining eight with 300 μg. Of the 10 who received the IgG3 monoclonal, seven were injected with 300 μg and three with 100–200 μg. None of the subjects developed anti-D within 6 months. After a second injection of red cells at 9 months, two subjects produced anti-D and, after a third injection at 12 months, three more produced antibody. Of 19 of the remaining subjects who were now given an injection of ^{51}Cr-labelled D-positive red cells, 18 exhibited normal survival (Goodrick et al. 1994). The high proportion of non-responders (18 out of 26) was not explained.

Can Rh D immunization be switched off once it has been initiated?

In a series of pregnant D-negative women in whom

anti-D was detected only with enzyme-treated red cells, the injection of anti-D immunoglobulin failed to prevent the development of a progressive increase in anti-D concentration. Moreover, in some women injected with anti-D immunoglobulin at a time when they had no detectable antibody, immunization subsequently developed, suggesting that once primary Rh D immunization has been initiated the process cannot be reversed by passively administered antibody (Bowman and Pollock 1984).

Failure of passively administered anti-D to affect secondary responses

In subjects with relatively low concentrations of IgG anti-D in their plasma, the i.m. injection of 500 μg of anti-D failed to modify the response to 0.3 ml of red cells (De Silva et al. 1985).

Possible augmentation by passive antibody

Rh D immunization facilitated by small amounts of 'passive' IgG anti-D?

There is suggestive evidence that when D-positive red cells are injected with a relatively small dose of IgG anti-D into D-negative subjects, the probability of Rh D immunization is increased. This effect was first noted in experiments in which a fixed amount of red cells (approximately 2.25 ml) was injected intravenously, together with varying amounts of IgG anti-D (1–40 μg) intramuscularly. As judged by the formation of anti-D within 3 months, subjects receiving 10 μg of anti-D (at an approximate ratio of 4.5 μg of anti-D/ml of red cells) had an increased chance of responding, i.e. 8 out of 11 made anti-D compared with 1 out of 6 receiving no anti-D and with 7 out of 25 who received either 1 μg or 20 μg of anti-Rh (Pollack et al. 1968b).

These results, although suggestive, were not statistically significant. In two later studies the administration of a small dose of IgG anti-D with D-positive red cells has also resulted in a suggestive increase in the proportion of responders:

1 In a trial carried out at five different centres, 83 out of 113 (73%) subjects injected with 7 ml of red cells and 10 μg of anti-D (1.4 μg of anti-D/ml red cells) became immunized compared with 53 out of 98 (54%) subjects receiving only 7 ml of red cells (WQ

Ascari, personal communication, 1984). Although these results are very suggestive of augmentation, the data were somewhat heterogeneous.

2 Subjects who were injected with 0.8 ml of red cells and 1 µg of anti-D: 9 out of 13 subjects made anti-D within 6 months and two more made anti-D after a second injection of red cells (Contreras and Mollison 1983). These results were compared with those observed earlier in subjects given 1 ml of red cells alone from the same donor; amongst these subjects 4 out of 12 made anti-D after a single injection of red cells and two more after a second injection. Apart from the fact that this was not a strictly controlled experiment, the difference observed between the numbers making anti-D after a first stimulus (9 out of 13 vs. 4 out of 12) was only just significant ($P < 0.05$). Nevertheless, the dose (1.25 µg of anti-D/ml red cells) that produced suggestive augmentation was very close to that used in Ascari's study. In both studies, the dose that appeared to produce an increase in the proportion of responders was appreciably lower than that (4.5 µg/ml of cells) found by Pollack and colleagues (1968b) to be augmenting but, as discussed above, it is likely that the anti-D content of the preparation used by Pollack and colleagues was overestimated. In another series in which D-negative subjects were given 1 ml of D-positive cells with 5 µg of anti-D there was mild suppression of the immune response as judged by the anti-D concentration of plasma after a second injection of red cells, namely a mean of 0.55 µg/ml compared with 8.6 µg/ml in a control series (Contreras and Mollison 1981).

Effect of IgM anti-D

As described in Chapter 3, there is convincing evidence derived from animal experiments that passively administered IgM antibody can augment immunization. It is probable that all the IgM antibodies that have been shown to have this effect are capable of activating complement and it is very doubtful whether the same effect can be produced by a non-complement-binding IgM antibody such as anti-D. As discussed in Chapter 10, evidence that IgM anti-D alone can destroy red cells is very meagre. If it cannot mediate red cell–macrophage interaction, it is doubtful whether it can affect immunization.

In an often-quoted experiment, of 11 D-negative volunteers who were given two i.v. injections of D-

positive red cells alone, only one became immunized, whereas of 13 who were given two i.v. injections of cells with an i.v. dose of plasma containing agglutinating anti-D, eight became immunized (Clarke et al. 1963). This result certainly suggests that the effect of the agglutinating anti-D was to increase the probability of Rh D immunization, but this may not be the correct interpretation. It is possible that the effect was due instead to the relatively small amount of IgG anti-D that was present in the plasma (in addition to the IgM anti-D).

Experiments with purified IgM anti-D appeared to show that the antibody could clear D-positive red cells (Holburn et al. 1971b) but it has subsequently been pointed out that the anti-D preparation may have contained enough IgG antibody to have produced the effect (Mollison 1986). Accordingly, it now seems unsafe to draw conclusions from these results about the possible augmenting effect of IgM anti-D.

In another experiment, D-negative volunteers injected with D-positive red cells weakly agglutinated by being mixed with plasma containing IgM anti-D formed anti-D after a mean interval of 5.4 weeks compared with 10.75 weeks in subjects injected with untreated D-positive red cells (Lee et al. 1977). Three points may be made: the difference in time interval between the two groups was not significant; earlier formation of antibody after immunization is not a recognized effect of immune augmentation; and, if an effect was produced, it could have been due to the presence of small amounts of IgG anti-D in the plasma used for agglutinating the D-positive red cells.

Treatment of inadvertent D-positive transfusion

In any D-negative woman who is not already immunized to Rh D, and who may have further children, the inadvertent transfusion of D-positive blood should be treated by giving a suitable dose of anti-D. In D-negative post-menopausal women or in men who have been transfused with D-positive blood, it does not seem worth trying to suppress Rh D immunization; first, because the consequences to the subject of becoming immunized are not likely to be serious, and second, because treatment with large amounts of anti-D is wasteful and can produce unpleasant effects.

When the decision is taken to try to suppress Rh D immunization in a subject whose circulation contains large amounts of red cells, various questions arise:

How much anti-D should be given? Should it be given in a single dose or in divided doses, and by what route should it be given? When anti-D is given intramuscularly the total dose should be about 25 µg/ml of red cells (WHO 1971). When it is given intravenously it is probable that a lesser dose will suffice, i.e. 10–15 µg/ml red cells. The main advantage of i.v. injection is that it avoids a large and therefore painful i.m. injection. In the past, the chance of transmitting viral infections was higher with preparations for i.v. use but these preparations can now be treated to make them safe (see Chapter 16). When anti-D is injected intramuscularly, to minimize pain the dose should not all be injected into the same site. However, there is no need to separate the doses in time, as the material is absorbed slowly from the site of injection and the peak concentration in the plasma is not reached for about 48 h. On the other hand, when anti-D is injected intravenously, several different types of reaction may be produced, two of which may be caused by injecting too much anti-D within a given period. First, there may be rapid red cell destruction resulting in shivering and fever as in patients described by Huchet and colleagues (1970); in two cases of massive transplacental haemorrhage equivalent to about 75 ml of red cells, 600 µg of anti-D was injected intravenously, resulting in clearance of the red cells with a $T_{1/2}$ of about 85 min. Second, haemoglobinuria may develop; see Table 5.6 and Chapter 11.

Apart from reactions due to red cell destruction, the i.v. injection of anti-D immunoglobulin may cause immediate hypersensitivity-type reactions. These may be due to the activation of complement by aggregated IgG in the preparation or, very rarely, to an interaction between IgA in the immunoglobulin preparation and anti-IgA in the recipient's plasma.

Although the i.v. injection of IgG is potentially hazardous, very low reaction rates have been observed following the i.v. injection of anti-D immunoglobulin purified on DEAE-Sephadex (see Chapter 12). In practice, when large amounts of immunoglobulin are being administered at one time, it seems wise to give a dose of hydrocortisone (100 µg i.v.) immediately before the injection of anti-D immunoglobulin. To avoid reactions due to the rapid destruction of large volumes of D-positive cells, it is suggested that the initial dose of anti-D should be limited to about 5 µg/ml of D-positive red cells and should be administered, diluted in saline, over a period of 1 h. In the cases recorded in Table 5.6,

the anti-D immunoglobulin was always given in divided doses, with no more than 2500 µg being given on a single occasion. Provided that no adverse reaction develops after the first injection of anti-D, a further dose of 5 µg/ml of red cells may be given after 12 h. Thereafter, a suitable test (e.g. rosetting) should be made to see that the D-positive cells are being cleared reasonably rapidly from the circulation. If all the cells have not been cleared after 2–3 days, a further dose of anti-D should be given.

Preliminary exchange transfusion with D-negative red cells

In D-negative subjects who have been transfused with very large volumes of D-positive red cells, the dose of anti-D needed for the suppression of primary Rh D immunization can be greatly reduced by carrying out a preliminary exchange transfusion with D-negative blood, a possibility discussed by Bowman and colleagues (1972). This manoeuvre is particularly worthwhile in D-negative infants who have inadvertently been transfused with D-positive blood. If an exchange transfusion is now given with D-negative blood, the amount of D-positive red cells remaining in the circulation can be reduced to an amount of the order of 5 or 10 ml (a formula for calculating the amount is given in Chapter 1). It will then be necessary to give only a relatively small dose of anti-D immunoglobulin to ensure that primary Rh D immunization is suppressed. It should be added that evidence of the frequency with which newborn infants become immunized to red cell antigens by transfusion is meagre. Exchange transfusion followed by administration of anti-D was used successfully to prevent anti-D production in two cases (both young D-negative girls) of patients who had been transfused with D-positive red cells (Nester et al. 2004). In the first case, a 16-kg 16-year-old girl involved in a road traffic accident received 4 units of D+ red cells and underwent total red cell exchange, 36 h after hospital admission, with 10 units of D-negative red cells, followed by 2718 µg of i.v. anti-D over 32 h. In the second case, a 39-kg 10-year-old girl with aplastic anaemia received 1 unit of D-positive red cells and underwent exchange with 5 units of D-negative red cells on the same day, followed by 900 µg of i.v. anti-D. Anti-D was not detected in the serum of either girl 6 months later.

Failure of D antigen, given orally, to induce tolerance

As described in Chapter 3, antigen given orally may induce tolerance; however, there is no evidence that tolerance can be induced to Rh D in this way. In an experiment in male volunteers the administration of D antigen daily by mouth for 2 weeks had no apparent effect on subsequent Rh D immunization, the percentage of subjects forming anti-D after a single i.v. injection of D-positive red cells being virtually the same as in a control group (Barnes *et al.* 1987).

References

Adinolfi A, Mollison PL, Polley MJ *et al.* (1966) γA blood group antibodies. J Exp Med 123: 951

Agre P, Cartron JP (1991) Molecular biology of the Rh antigens. Blood 78: 1–5

Agre PC, Davies DM, Issitt PD *et al.* (1992) A proposal to standardize terminology for weak D antigen. Transfusion 32: 86

Allen FH Jr, Tippett PA (1958) A new Rh blood type which reveals the Rh antigen G. Vox Sang 3: 321

Anstee DJ, Mallinson G (1994) The biochemistry of blood group antigens: some recent advances. Vox Sang 67 (Suppl.) 3: 1–6

Anstee DJ, Tanner MJA (1993) Biochemical aspects of the blood group Rh(Rhesus) antigens. In: Red Cell Membrane and Red Cell Antigens. MJA Tanner, DJ Anstee (eds). Baillière's Clinical Haematology 6: 401–422

Archer GT, Cooke BR, Mitchell K *et al.* (1969) Hyperimmunisation des donneurs de sang pour la production des gamma-globulines anti-Rh(D). Rev Fr Transfus 12: 341

Archer GT, Cooke BR, Mitchell K *et al.* (1971) Hyperimmunisation of blood donors for the production of anti-Rh(D) gamma globulin. Proc 12th Congr Int Soc Blood Transfusion, Moscow

Asfour M, Narvios A, Lichtiger B (2004) Transfusion of RhD-incompatible blood components in RhD-negative blood marrow transplant recipients. Med Gen Med 13: 22

Ayland J, Horton MA, Tippett P *et al.* (1978) Complement binding anti-D made in a D^u variant woman. Vox Sang 34: 40

Bailly P, Hermand P, Callebaut I *et al.* (1994) The LW blood group glycoprotein is homologous to intercellular adhesion molecules. Proc Natl Acad Sci USA 91: 5306–5310

Bailly P, Tontti E, Hermand P *et al.* (1995) The red cell LW blood group protein is an intercellular adhesion molecules which binds to CD11/CD18 leukocyte integrins. Eur J Immunol 25: 3316–3320

Barclay GR, Greiss MA, Urbaniak SJ (1980) Adverse effect of plasma exchange on anti-D production in rhesus immunization owing to removal of inhibitory factors. BMJ ii: 1569

Barnes RMR, Duguid JKM, Roberts FM *et al.* (1987) Oral administration of erythrocyte membrane antigen does not suppress anti-Rh(D) antibody responses in humans. Clin Exp Immunol 67: 220–226

Bartsch FK (1972) Fetale Erythrozyten im mütterlichen Blut und Immunprophylaxe der Rh-Immunisierung. Klinische und experimentelle Studie. Acta Obstet Gynecol Scand 20 (Suppl.):

Beard MEJ, Pemberton J, Blagdon J *et al.* (1971) Rh immunization following incompatible blood transfusion and a possible long-term complication of anti-D immunoglobulin therapy. Med Genet 8: 317

Beckers EAM, Porcelijn P, Lightart P *et al.* (1996) The R₀^Har antigenic complex is associated with a limited number of D epitopes and alloanti-D production: a study of three unrelated persons and their families. Transfusion 36: 104–108

Bloy C, Blanchard D, Dahr W *et al.* (1988) Determination of the N-terminal sequence of human red cell Rh(D) polypeptide and demonstration that the Rh(D), (c) and (E) antigens are carried by distinct polypeptide chains. Blood 72: 661–666

Boctor FN, Ali NM, Mohandas K *et al.* (2003) Absence of D-alloimmunisation in AIDS patients receiving D-mismatched RBCs. Transfusion 43: 173–176

Bowman HS (1976) Effectiveness of prophylactic Rh immunosuppression after transfusion with D-positive blood. Am J Obstet Gynecol 124: 80

Bowman JM, Pollock JM (1984) Reversal of Rh immunization. Fact or fancy? Vox Sang 47: 209–215

Bowman HS, Mohn JF, Lambert RM (1972) Prevention of maternal Rh immunisation after accidental transfusion of D (Rh₀)-positive blood. Vox Sang 22: 385–396

Branch DR, Gallagher MT (1985) The importance of CO_2 in short-term monocyte-macrophage assays (Letter). Transfusion 25: 399

Brittain JE, Mlinar KJ, Anderson CS *et al.* (2001) Integrin-associated protein is an adhesion receptor on sickle red blood cells for immobilized thrombospondin. Blood 97: 2159–2164

Bruce LJ, Ghosh S, King M-J *et al.* (2002) Absence of CD47 in protein 4.2-deficient hereditary spherocytosis in man: an interaction between the Rh complex and the band 3 complex. Blood 100: 1878–1885

Bruce LJ, Beckmann R, Ribeiro ML *et al.* (2003) A band 3-based macrocomplex of integral and peripheral proteins in the RBC membrane. Blood 101: 4180–4188

Bush M, Sabo B, Stroup M *et al.* (1974) Red cell D antigen sites and titration scores in a family with weak and normal

D^u phenotypes inherited from a homozygous D^u mother. Transfusion 14: 433

Bye JM, Carter C, Cui Y et al. (1992) Germline variable region gene segment derivation of human monoclonal anti-Rh (D) antibodies. J Clin Invest 90: 2481–2490

Campbell IG, Freemont PS, Foulkes W et al. (1992) An ovarian tumor marker with homology to vaccinia virus contains an IgV-like region and multiple transmembrane domains. Cancer Res 52: 5416–5420

Cartron J-P (1999) Rh blood group system and molecular basis of Rh-deficiency. In: Baillières Clinical Haematology. MJA Tanner, DJ Anstee (eds). London: Bailière Tindall, pp. 655–689

Castilho L, Rios M, Rodrigues A et al. (2005) High frequency of partial DIIIa and DAR alleles found in sickle cell disease patients suggests increased risk of alloimmunization to RhD. Transfusion Med 15: 49–55

Ceppellini R, Dunn LC, Turri M (1955) An interaction between alleles at the Rh locus in man which weakens the reactivity of the Rh$_o$ factor (D^u). Proc Natl Acad Sci USA 41: 283

Chang TY, Siegel DL (1998) Genetic and immunological properties of phage-displayed human anti-RhD antibodies: implications for RhD epitope topology. Blood 91: 3066–3078

Chang JG, Wang JC, Yang TY et al. (1998) Human RhDel is caused by a deletion of 1013 bp between introns 8 and 9 including exon 9 of RHD gene. Blood 92: 2602–2604

Chérif-Zahar B, Raynal V, Gane P et al. (1996) Candidate gene acting as a suppressor of the RH locus in most cases of Rh-deficiency. Nature Genet 12: 168–173

Chown B, Kaita H, Lewis M et al. (1963) A 'D-positive' man who produced anti-D. Vox Sang 8: 420

Chown B, Kaita H, Lowen R et al. (1971) Transient production of anti-LW by LW-positive people. Transfusion 11: 220

Chown B, Lewis M, Hiroko K et al. (1972) An unlinked modifier of Rh blood groups: effects when heterozygous and when homozygous. Am J Hum Genet 24: 623

Clarke CA, Donohoe WTA, McConnell RB et al. (1963) Further experimental studies on the prevention of Rh haemolytic disease. BMJ i. 979

Colin Y, Chérif-Zahar B, Le van Kim C et al. (1991) Genetic basis of the Rh-D positive and Rh-D negative blood group polymorphism as determined by Southern analysis. Blood 78: 1–6

Colin Y, Bailly P, Cartron J-P (1994) Molecular genetic basis of Rh and LW blood groups. Vox Sang 67 S3: 67–72

Combined Study (1966) Prevention of Rh-haemolytic disease: results of the clinical trial. A combined study from centres in England and Baltimore. BMJ 2: 907

Contreras M, Knight RC (1989) The Rh-negative donor. Clin Lab Haematol 11: 317–322

Contreras M, Mollison PL (1981) Failure to augment primary Rh immunization using a small dose of 'passive' IgG anti-Rh. Br J Haematal 49: 371–381

Contreras M, Mollison PL (1983) Rh immunization facilitated by passively-administered anti-Rh? Br J Haematol 53: 153–159

Contreras M, Stebbing B, Blessing M et al. (1978) The Rh antigen Evans. Vox Sang 34: 208–211

Contreras M, Amitage S, Daniels GL et al. (1979) Homozygous D. Vox Sang 36: 81–84

Contreras M, De Silva M, Teeesdale P et al. (1987) The effect of naturally occurring Rh antibodies on the survival of serologically incompatible red cells. Br J Haematol 65: 475–478

Cook IA (1971) Primary rhesus immunisation of male volunteers. Br J Haematol 20: 369

Cook K, Rush B (1974) Rh (D) immunisation after massive transfusion of Rh (D) positive blood. Med J Aust 1: 166

Cowley NM, Saul A, Hyland CA (2000) RHD gene mutations and the weak D phenotype: an Australian blood donor study. Vox Sang 79: 251–252

Crispen J (1976) Immunosuppression of small quantities of Rh-positive blood with MICRhoGAM in Rh-negative male volunteers. Proceedings of Symposium on Rh Antibody Mediated Immunosuppression, Ortho Research Institute, Raritan, NJ

Cummins D, Contreras M, Amin S et al. (1995) Red-cell alloantibody development associated with heart and lung transplantation. Transplantation 59: 1432–1435

Dahr W, Kordowicz M, Moulds J et al. (1987) Characterization of the Ss sialoglycoprotein and its antigens in Rh$_{null}$ erythrocytes. Blut 54: 13–24

Daniels GL (1995) Human Blood Groups. Oxford: Blackwell Science

Daniels GL (2002) Human Blood Groups. Oxford: Blackwell Science

Daniels GL, Faas BH, Green CA et al. (1998) The VS and V blood group polymorphisms in Africans: a serologic and molecular analysis. Transfusion 38: 951–958

Daniels GL, Fletcher A, Garratty G et al. (2004) Blood group terminology 2004: from the International Society of Blood Transfusion committee on terminology for red cell surface antigens. Vox Sang 87: 304–316

Darke C, Street J, Sargeant C et al. (1983) HLA-DR antigens and properdin factor B allotypes in responders and non-responders to the Rhesus-D antigen. Tissue Antigens 21: 333–335

Debbia M, Lambin P (2004) Measurement of anti-D intrinsic affinity with unlabeled antibodies. Transfusion 44: 399–406

De Silva M, Contreras M, Mollison PL (1985) Failure of passively administered anti-Rh to prevent secondary Rh responses. Vox Sang 48: 178–180

Devenish A (1994) An example of anti-LW^a in a 10-month-old infant. Immunohematology 10: 127–129

De Vetten MP, Agre P (1988) The Rh polypeptide is a major fatty acid acylated erythrocyte membrane protein. J Biol Chem 263: 18193–18196

Devey ME, Voak D (1974) A critical study of the IgG subclasses of Rh anti-D antibodies formed in pregnancy and in immunized volunteers. Immunology 27: 1073

Dugoujon JM, De Lange GG, Blancher A et al. (1989) Characterization of an IgG2, G2m(23) anti-Rh-D antibody. Vox Sang 57: 133–136

Dunsford I (1962) A new Rh antibody-anti-CE. Proceedings of the 8th Congress of the European Society of Haematology, Vienna, 1961

Dunstan RA (1986) Status of major red cell blood group antigens on neutrophils, lymphocytes and monocytes. Br J Haematol 62: 301–309

Dunstan RA, Simpson MB, Rosse WF (1984) Erythrocyte antigens on human platelets. Absence of the Rhesus, Duffy, Kell, Kidd, and Lutheran antigens. Transfusion 24: 243–246

Dybkjaer E (1967) Anti-E antibodies disclosed in the period 1960–1966. Vox Sang 13: 446

Dzik W, Blank J, Lutz P et al. (1994) Autoimmune hemolysis following transfusion: a mimicking autoanti-D in a D-patient with alloanti-D. Immunohematology 10: 117–119

Edgington TS (1971) Dissociation of antibody from erythrocyte surfaces by chaotropic ions. J Immunol 106: 673

Faas BHW, Beckers EAM, Simsek S et al. (1996) Involvement of Ser103 of the Rh polypeptides in G epitope formation. Transfusion 36: 506–511

Finn R (1960) In: Report of the Liverpool Medical Institution. Lancet i: 526

Finn R, Clarke CA, Donohoe WTA et al. (1961) Experimental studies on the prevention of Rh haemolytic disease. BMJ i: 1486

Fisher RA, Race RR (1946) Rh gene frequencies in Britain. Nature (Lond) 157: 48

Fisk RT, Foord AG (1942) Observations on the Rh agglutinogen of human blood. Am J Clin Pathol 12: 545

Flegel WA, Hillesheim B, Kerowgan M et al. (1996) Lack of heterogeneity in the molecular structure of RHD category VII. Transfusion 36 (Suppl.): 50S

Flegel WA, Khull SR, Wagner FF (2000) Primary anti-D immunisation by weak D type 2 RBCs. Transfusion 40: 428–434

Fletcher G, Cooke BR, McDowall J (1971) Attempts to immunize Rh(D) negative volunteers against the D antigen. Proceedings of the 2nd Meeting of the Asian and Pacific Division of the International Society of Haematology, Melbourne, p. 69

Frame M, Mollison PL, Terry WD (1970) Anti-Rh activity of human γG4 proteins. Nature (Lond) 225: 641

Freda VJ, Gorman JG (1962) Current concepts. Antepartum management of Rh haemolytic disease. Bull Sloane Hosp Women, NY 8: 147

Freda VJ, Gorman JG, Pollack W (1964) Successful prevention of experimental Rh sensitization in man with an anti-Rh gamma$_2$-globulin antibody preparation: a preliminary report. Transfusion 4: 26

Freda VJ, Gorman JG, Pollack W (1966) Rh factor: prevention of immunization and clinical trial on mothers. Science 151: 828

Frohn C, Dumbgen L, Brand JM et al. (2003) Probability of anti-D development in D-patients receiving D+ RBCs. Transfusion 43: 893–898

Fung MK, Sheikh H, Eghtesad B et al. (2004) Severe haemolysis resulting from D incompatibility in a case of ABO-identical liver transplant. Transfusion 44: 1635–1639

Gahmberg CG (1982) Molecular identification of the human $Rh_0(D)$ antigen. FEBS Lett 140: 93–97

Gardner B, Anstee DJ, Mawby WJ et al. (1991) The abundance and organisation of polypeptides associated with antigens of the Rh blood group system. Transfusion Med 1: 77–85

Giblett ER (1964) Blood group antibodies causing hemolytic disease of the newborn. Clin Obset Gynecol 7: 1044

Gibson T (1979) Providing saline reacting anti-D cell typing reagent. Clin Lab Haematol 1: 321–323

Giles CM (1980) The LW blood group: a review. Immunol Commun 9: 225–242

Giles CM, Lundsgaard A (1967) A complex serological investigation involving LW. Vox Sang 13: 406

Goldfinger D, McGinniss MH (1971) Rh-incompatible platelet transfusions: risks and consequences of sensitizing immunosuppressed patients. N Engl J Med 284: 942

Goodrick J, Kumpel B, Pamphilon D et al. (1994) Plasma half-lives and bioavailability of human monoclonal Rh D antibodies Brad-3 and Brad-5 following intramuscular injection into Rh D-negative volunteers. Clin Exp Immunol 98: 17–20

Gorick BD, Hughes-Jones NC (1991) Relative functional binding activity of IgG1 and IgG3 anti-D in IgG preparations. Vox Sang 62: 251–254

Gorick BD, Thompson KM, Melamed MD et al. (1988) Three epitopes on the human Rh antigen D recognised by ^{125}I-labelled human monoclonal IgG antibodies. Vox Sang 55: 165–170

Gorick B, McDougall DCJ, Ouwehand WH et al. (1993) Quantitation of D sites on selected 'weak D' and 'partial D' red cells. Vox Sang 65: 136–140

Green FA (1968) Phospholipid requirement of Rh antigenic activity. J Biol Chem 243: 5519

Gunson HH, Stratton F, Cooper DG (1970) Primary immunization of Rh-negative volunteers. BMJ i: 593

Gunson HH, Stratton F, Phillips PK (1971) The use of modified cells to induce an anti-Rh response. Br J Haematol 21: 683

Gunson HH, Stratton F, Phillips PK (1974) The anti-Rh$_O$(D) responses of immunized volunteers following spaced antigenic stimuli. Br J Haematol 27: 171

Harboe M, Müller-Eberhard HJ, Fudenberg H et al. (1963) Identification of the components of complement participating in the antiglobulin reaction. Immunology 6: 412

Harrison J (1970) The 'naturally occurring' anti-E. Vox Sang 19: 123

Hemker MB, Lightart PC, Berger L et al. (1999) DAR, a new RhD variant involving exons 4,5 and 7, often in linkage with ceAR, a new Rhce variant frequently found in African blacks. Blood 94: 4337–4342

Hemker MB, Cheroutre G, van Zweiten R et al. (2003) The Rh complex exports ammonium from human red blood cells. Br J Haematol 122: 333–340

Hermand P, Gane P, Huet M et al. (2003) Red cell ICAM-4 is a novel ligand for platelet-activated alpha IIb/beta3 integrin. J Biol Chem 278: 4892–4898

Hill Z, Vacl J, Kalasova E et al. (1974) Haemolytic disease of the newborn in a D^u positive mother. Vox Sang 27: 92–94

Holburn AM, Cleghorn TE, Hughes-Jones NC (1970) Re-stimulation of anti-D in donors. Vox Sang 19: 162

Holburn AM, Frame M, Hughes-Jones NC et al. (1971a) Some biological effects of IgM anti-Rh (D). Immunology 20: 681

Holburn AM, Cartron JP, Economidou J et al. (1971b) Observations on the reactions between D-positive red cells and ^{125}I-labelled IgM anti-D molecules and subunits. Immunology 21: 499

Hopkins DF (1969) The decline and fall of anti-Rh(D). Br J Haematol 17: 199

Hotevar M, Glonar L (1972) Re-immunization of sensitized women. Vox Sang 22: 532

Huang C-H (1996) Alteration of RH gene structure and expression in human dCCee and DCw-red blood cells: phenotypic homozygosity versus genotypic heterozygosity. Blood 88: 2326–2333

Huchet J, Crégut R, Pinon F (1970) Immuno-globulines anti-D. Efficacité comparée des voies intra-musculaire et intra-veineuse. Rev Fr Transfus 13: 231

Huestis DW (1971) In: International Forum: What constitutes adequate routine Rh typing on donors and recipients? Vox Sang 21: 183

Hughes-Jones NC (1967) The estimation of the concentration and the equilibrium constant of anti-D. Immunology 12: 565

Hughes-Jones NC, Gardner B (1970) The equilibrium constants of anti-D immunoglobulin preparations made from pools of donor plasma. Immunology 18: 347

Hughes-Jones NC, Ghosh S (1981) Anti-D-coated Rh-positive red cells will bind the first component of the complement pathway, C1q. FEBS Lett 128: 318–320

Hughes-Jones NC, Gardner B, Telford R et al. (1963) Studies on the reaction between the blood-group antibody anti-D and erythrocytes. Biochem J 88: 435

Hughes-Jones NC, Gardner B, Telford R (1964) The effect of pH and ionic strength on the reaction between anti-D and erythrocytes. Immunology 7: 72

Hughes-Jones NC, Gardner B, Lincoln P et al. (1971) Observations of the number of available c, D, e and E antigen sites on red cells. Vox Sang 21: 210

Hughes-Jones NC, Green EJ, Hunt VAM (1975) Loss of Rh antigen activity following the action of phospholipase A$_2$ on red cell stroma. Vox Sang 29: 184–191

Hughes-Jones NC, Bye JM, Gorick BD et al. (1999) Synthesis of Rh Fv phage-antibodies using VH and VL germline genes. Br J Haematol 105: 811–816

Hutchison HE, McLennan W (1966) Long persistence of rhesus antibodies. Vox Sang 11: 517

Isbister JP, Ting A, Seeto KM et al. (1977) Development of Rh specific maternal autoantibodies following intensive plasmapheresis for Rh immunization during pregnancy. Vox Sang 33: 353

Ishimori T, Hasekura H (1967) A Japanese with no detectable Rh blood group antigens due to silent Rh alleles or deleted chromosomes. Transfusion 7: 84

Issitt PD (1979) Serology and Genetics of the Rhesus Blood Group System. Cincinnati, OH: Montgomery Scientific Publications

Issitt PD (1985) Applied Blood Group Serology, 3rd edn. Miami, FL: Montgomery Scientific Publications

Issitt PD, Anstee DJ (1998) Applied Blood Group Serology, 4th edn. Miami, FL: Montgomery Scientific Publications

Issitt PD, Tessel JA (1981) On the incidence of antibodies to the Rh antigens G, rh$_i$ (Ce), C, and C^G in sera containing anti-CD or anti-C. Transfusion 21: 412–418

Issitt PD, Wilkinson SL, Gruppo RA et al. (1983) Depression of Rh antigen expression in antibody-induced haemolytic anaemia (Letter). Br J Haematol 53: 688

Johnson CA, Brown BA, Lasky LC (1985) Rh immunization caused by osseous allograft (Letter). N Engl J Med 312: 121–122

Jones AR, Diamond LK, Allen FH Jr (1954) A decade of progress in the Rh blood-group system. N Engl J Med 250: 283 and 324

Jones J, Scott ML, Voak D (1995) Monoclonal anti-D specificity and Rh D structure: Criteria for selection of monoclonal anti-D reagents for routine typing of patients and donors. Transfusion Med 5: 171

Jouvenceaux A (1971) Prévention de l'immunisation anti-Rh. Rev Fr Transfus 14: 39

Kashiwase K, Ishikawa Y, Hyodo H et al. (2001) E variants found in Japanese and c antigenicity alteration without substitution in the second extracellular loop. Transfusion 41: 1408–1412

Kenwright MG, Sangster JM, Sachs JA (1976) Development of RhD antibodies after kidney transplantation. BMJ 2: 151

Khademi S, O'Connell J III, Remis J et al. (2004) Mechanism of ammonia transport by Amt/MEP/Rh: structure of AmtB at 1.35A. Science 305: 1587–1594

Kissmeyer-Nielsen F (1965) Irregular blood group antibodies in 200 000 individuals. Scand J Haematol 2: 331

Knepper MA, Agre P (2004) Structural biology. The atomic architecture of a gas channel. Science 305: 1573–1574

Kormoczi GF, Legler TJ, Daniels GL et al. (2004) Molecular and serological characterisation of DWI, a novel 'high-grade' partial D. Transfusion 44: 575–580

Kornstad L (1986) A rare blood group antigen, Ol^a (Oldeide), associated with weak Rh antigens. Vox Sang 50: 235–239

Krevans JR, Woodrow JC, Nosenzo C et al. (1964) Patterns of Rh-immunization. Communication from the 10th Congress of the International Society of Haematology, Stockholm

Lacey PA, Caskey CR, Werner DJ et al. (1983) Fatal hemolytic disease of a newborn due to anti-D in an Rh-positive D^u variant mother. Transfusion 23: 91

Lalezari P, Talleyrand NP, Wenz B et al. (1975) Development of direct antiglobulin reaction accompanying alloimmunization in a patient with Rh^d (D, category III) phenotype. Vox Sang 28: 19

Landsteiner K, Wiener AS (1940) An agglutinable factor in human blood recognizable by immune sera for Rhesus blood. Proc Soc Exp Biol (NY) 43: 223

Landsteiner K, Wiener AS (1941) Studies on an agglutinogen (Rh) in human blood reacting with anti-Rhesus sera and with human iso-antibodies. J Exp Med 74: 309

Lauf PK, Joiner CH (1976) Increased potassium transport and ouabain binding in human Rh$_{null}$ red blood cells. Blood 48: 457

Leader KA, Kumpel BM, Poole GD et al. (1990) Human monoclonal anti-D with reactivity against category D^{VI} cells used in blood grouping and determination of the incidence of the category D^{VI} phenotype in the D^u population. Vox Sang 58: 106–111

Leader KA, Macht LM, Steers F et al. (1992) Antibody responses to the blood group antigen D in SCID mice reconsituted with human blood mononuclear cells. Immunology 76: 229–234

Lee D, Flowerday MHE, Tomlinson J (1977) The use of IgM anti-D coated cells in the deliberate immunization of Rh-negative male volunteers. Vox Sang 32: 189

Lee D, Remnant M, Stratton F (1984) 'Naturally occurring' anti-Rh in Rh(D) negative volunteers for immunization. Clin Lab Haematol 6: 33–38

Lee E, Knight RC (2000) A case of autoimmune haemolytic anaemia with an IgA ant-Ce autoantibody. Vox Sang 78 (Suppl.1): p. 130

Lehane D (1967) Production of plasma for making anti-D γ-globulin (Abstract). Br J Haematol 13: 800

Leonard GL, Ellisor SS, Reid ME et al. (1976) An unusual Rh immunization. Vox Sang 31: 275

Le Van Kim C, Mouro I, Chérif-Zahar B et al. (1992) Molecular cloning and primary structure of the human blood group RhD polypeptide. Proc Natl Acad Sci USA 89: 10925–10929

Levine P, Gelano M, Fenichel R et al. (1961) A 'D-like' antigen in rhesus monkey, human Rh positive and human Rh negative red blood cells. J Immunol 87: 6

Levine P, Celano MJ, Wallace J et al. (1963a) A human 'D-like' antibody. Nature (Lond) 198: 596

Levine BB, Ojeda A, Benacerraf B (1963b) Studies of artificial antigens. III. The genetic control of the immune response to hapten-poly-L-lysine conjugates in guinea pigs. J Exp Med 118: 953

Levine P, Celano MJ, Falkowski F et al. (1964) A second example of –/– blood or Rh$_{null}$. Nature (Lond) 204: 892

Lichtiger B, Hester JP (1986) Transfusion of Rh-incompatible blood components to cancer patients. Haematologia 19: 81–88

Lindberg FP, Lublin DM, Telen MJ et al. (1994) Rh-related antigen CD47 is the signal-transducer integrin-associated protein. J Biol Chem 269: 1567–1570

Litwin SD (1973) Allotype preference in human Rh antibodies. J Immunol 110: 717

van Loghem JJ (1947) Production of Rh agglutinins anti-C and anti-E by artificial immunization of volunteer donors. BMJ ii: 958

van Loghem JJ, Bartels HLJM, van der Hart M (1949) La production d'un anticorps anti-C^w par immunization artificielle d'un donneur bénévole. Rev Hématol 4: 173

van Loghem JJ, Harkink H, van der Hart M (1953) Production of the antibody anti-e by artificial immunization. Vox Sang (OS) 3: 22

Lomas CG, Tippett P (1985) Use of enzymes in distinguishing anti-LW^a and anti-LW^{ab} from anti-D. Med Lab Sci 42: 88–89

Lomas C, Bruce M, Watt A et al. (1986) TAR+ individuals with anti-D, a new category D^{VII} (Abstract). Transfusion 26: 560

Lomas C, Tippett P, Thompson KM et al. (1989) Demonstration of seven epitopes on the Rh antigen D using human monoclonal anti-D antibodies and red cells from D categories. Vox Sang 57: 261–264

Lovett DA, Crawford MN (1967) Js^b and Go^a screening of Negro donors. Transfusion 7: 442

Lubenko A, Burslem SJ, Fairclough LM et al. (1991) A new qualitative variant of the RhE antigen revealed by heterogeneity among anti-E sera. Vox Sang 60: 235–240

McBride JA, O'Hoski P, Blajchman MA et al. (1978) Rhesus alloimmunisation following intensive plasmapheresis. Transfusion 18: 626–627

McVerry BA, O'Connor MC, Price A et al. (1977) Isoimmunisation after narcotic addiction. BMJ i: 1324

Mak KH, Yan KF, Cheng SS et al. (1993) Rh phenotypes of Chinese blood donors in Hong Kong, with special reference to weak D antigens. Transfusion 33: 348–351

Malde R, Stanworth S, Patel S et al. (2000) Haemolytic disease of the newborn due to anti-Ce. Transfusion Med 10: 305–306

Mallinson G, Martin PG, Anstee DJ et al. (1986) Identification and partial characterization of the human erythrocyte membrane component(s) which express the antigens of the LW blood group system. Biochem J 234: 649–652

Mallinson G, Anstee DJ, Avent ND et al. (1990) Murine monoclonal antibody MB-2D10 recognises Rh-related glycoproteins in the human red cell membrane. Transfusion 30: 222–225

Marini AM, Urrestarazu A, Beauwens R et al. (1997) The Rh (rhesus) blood group polypeptides are related to NH4+ transporters. Trends Biochem Sci 22: 460–461

Marini AM, Matassi G, Raynal V et al. (2000) The human Rhesus-associated RhAG protein and a kidney homologue promote ammonium transport in yeast. Nature Genet 26: 341–344

Masouredis SP, Sudora EJ, Mahan L et al. (1976) Antigen site densities and ultrastructural distribution patterns of red cell Rh antigens. Transfusion 16: 94

Mawby WJ, Holmes CH, Anstee DJ et al. (1994) Isolation and characterization of CD47 glycoprotein; a multispanning membrane protein which is the same as integrin-associated protein (IAP) and the ovarian tumour marker OA3. Biochem J 304: 525–530

Mayne K, Bowell P, Woodward T et al. (1990) Rh immunization by the partial D antigen of category D^{Va}. Br J Haematol 76: 537–539

Meischer S, Vogel M, Biaggi C et al. (1998) Sequence and specificity analysis of recombinant human Fab anti-RhD isolated by phage display. Vox Sang 75: 278–287

Mijovic A (2002) Alloimmunisation to RhD antigen in RhD-incompatible haemopoietic cell transplants with non-myeloablative conditioning. Vox Sang 83: 358–362

Mohn JF, Bowman HS, Lambert RM et al. (1964) The formation of Rh specific autoantibodies in experimental isoimmune hemolytic anemia in man. Communication from the 10th Congress of the International Society of Blood Transfusion, Stockholm

Mollison PL (1956) Blood Transfusion in Clinical Medicine, 2nd edn. Oxford: Blackwell Scientific Publications

Mollison PL (1970) The effect of isoantibodies on red-cell survival. Ann NY Acad Sci 169: 199

Mollison PL (1983) Blood Transfusion in Clinical Medicine, 7th edn. Oxford: Blackwell Scientific Publications

Mollison PL (1986) Survival curves of incompatible red cells. An analytical review. Transfusion 26: 43–50

Mollison PL, Hughes-Jones NC, Lindsay M et al. (1969) Suppression of primary Rh immunization by passively-administered antibody. Experiments in volunteers. Vox Sang 16: 421

Mollison PL, Frame M, Ross ME (1970) Difference between Rh(D) negative subjects in response to Rh(D) antigen. Br J Haematol 19: 257

Moore BPL, Hughes-Jones NC (1970) Automated assay of anti-D concentration in plasmapheresis donors. In: Advances in Automated Analysis. Chicago, IL: Technicon

Moore S, Green C (1987) The identification of specific Rhesus polypeptide blood group ABH active glycoprotein complexes in the human red cell membrane. Biochem J 244: 735–741

Moore S, Woodrow CF, McClelland BL et al. (1982) Isolation of membrane components associated with human red cell antigens Rh(D), (`), (E) and Fy^a. Nature (Lond) 295: 529–531

Morell A, Skvaril F, Rufener JL (1973) Characterization of Rh antibodies for Med after incompatible pregnancies and after repeated booster injections. Vox Sang 24: 323

Mota M, Fonseca NL, Rodrigues A et al. (2005) Anti-D alloimmunisation by weak D type 1 red blood cells with a very low antigen density. Vox Sang 88: 130–135

Mourant AE (1949) Rh phenotypes and Fisher's CDE notation. Nature (Lond) 163: 913

Mourant AE, Kopéc AC, Domaniewska-Sobczak K (1976) The Distribution of the Human Blood Groups and Other Biochemical Polymorphisms, 2nd edn. Oxford: Oxford University Press

Mouro I, Colin Y, Chérif-Zahar B et al. (1993) Molecular genetic basis of the human Rhesus blood group system. Nature Genet 5: 62–65

Mouro I, Le Van Kim C, Rouillac C et al. (1994) Rearrangements of the blood group D gene associated with the D^{VI} category phenotype. Blood 83: 1129–1135

Mouro I, Colin Y, Sistonen P et al. (1995) Molecular basis of the RhC^w (Rh8) and RhC^x (Rh9) blood group specificities. Blood 86: 1196–1201

MRC (1954) The Rh blood groups and their clinical effects. Memorandum Med Res Coun (Lond) 27

Murray J, Clark EC (1952) Production of anti-Rh in guinea pigs from human erythrocyte extracts. Nature (Lond) 169: 886

Natvig JB (1965) Incomplete anti-D antibody with changed Gm specificity. Acta Pathol Microbiol Scand 65: 467

Natvig JB, Kunkel HG (1968) Genetic markers of human immunoglobulins: the Gm and Inv systems. Ser Haematol 1: 66

Nester TA, Rumsey DM, Howell CC et al. (2004) Prevention of immunization to D+ red blood cells with red blood cell exchange and intravenous immunoglobulin. Transfusion 44: 1720–1723

Nevanlinna HR (1953) Factors affecting maternal Rh immunization. Ann Med Exp Fenn 31 (Suppl 2):

Nicolas V, Le Van Kim C, Gane P et al. (2003) RhAG/ankyrin-R, a new interaction site between the membrane bilayer and the red cell skeleton, is impaired by Rh(null)-associated mutation. J Biol Chem 278: 25526–25533

Noizat-Pirenne F, Mouro I, Gane P et al. (1998) Heterogeneity of blood group RhE variants revealed by serological analysis and molecular alteration of the RHCE gene and transcript. Br J Haematol 103: 429–436

Nordhagen R, Kornstad L (1984) The manual polybrene test in relation to low concentration red cell antibodies. Abstracts, 18th Congress of the International Society of Blood Transfusion, Munich, p. 218

Okubo Y, Yamaguchi H, Tomita T et al. (1984) A D-variant, Del? Transfusion 24: 542

Okubo Y, Seno T, Yamano H et al. (1991) Partial D antigens disclosed by a monoclonal anti-D in Japanese blood donors. Transfusion 31: 782

Okubo Y, Yamano H, Nagao N et al. (1994) A partial E antigen in the Rh system? (Letter). Transfusion 34: 183

Oldenborg PA, Zheleznyak A, Fang YF et al. (2000) Role of CD47 as a marker of self on red blood cells. Science 288: 2051–2054

O'Reilly RA, Lombard CM, Azzi RL (1985) Delayed hemolytic transfusion reaction associated with Rh antibody anti-f: first reported case. Vox Sang 49: 336–339

Parsons SF, Spring FA, Chasis JA et al. (1999) Erythroid cell adhesion molecules Lutheran and LW in health and disease. Baillières Best Pract Res Clin Haematol 12: 729–45

Peng CT, Shih MC, Liu TC et al. (2003) Molecular basis for the Rh D negative phenotype in Chinese. Int J Mol Med 11: 515–521

Perera WS, Moss MT, Urbaniak SJ (2000) V D J germline gene repertoire analysis of monoclonal D antibodies and the implications for D epitope specificity. Transfusion 40: 846–855

Perkins HA, McIlroy M, Swanson J et al. (1977) Transient LW-negative red blood cells and anti-LW in a patient with Hodgkin's disease. Vox Sang 33: 299

Perrault R (1973) 'Cold' IgG autologous anti-LW. Vox Sang 24: 150

Perrault RA, Högman CF (1972) Low concentration red cell antibodies. III. 'Cold' IgG anti-D in pregnancy: incidence and significance. Acta Univ Uppsaliensis, no. 120

Pollack W, Gorman JG, Hager HJ et al. (1968a) Antibody-mediated immune suppression to the Rh factor; animal models suggesting mechanism of action. Transfusion 8: 134

Pollack W, Gorman JG, Freda VJ et al. (1968b) Results of clinical trials of RhoGAM in women. Transfusion 8: 151

Pollack W, Ascari WO, Kochesky RJ et al. (1971a) Studies on Rh prophylaxis. I. Relationship between doses of anti-Rh and size of antigenic stimulus. Transfusion 11: 333

Pollack W, Ascari WQ, Crispen JF et al. (1971b) Studies on Rh prophylaxis. II. Rh immune prophylaxis after transfusion with Rh-positive blood. Transfusion 11: 340

Polley MJ (1964) The development and use of the antiglobulin sensitization test for the study of the serological characteristics of blood-group antibodies and for the quantitive estimation of certain serum proteins. PhD Thesis, University of London, London

Poss MT, Green C, Telen MJ et al. (1993) Monoclonal antibody recognising a unique Rh-related specificity. Vox Sang 64: 231–239

Quan VA, Kemp LJ, Payne A et al. (1996) Rhesus immunisation after renal transplantation. Transplantation 61: 149–150

Race RR (1944) An 'incomplete' antibody in human serum. Nature (Lond) 153: 771

Race RR, Mourant AE, Lawler SD et al. (1948a) The Rh chromosome frequencies in England. Blood 3: 689

Race RR, Sanger R, Lawler SD (1948b) The Rh antigen D^u. Ann Eugen (Camb) 14: 171

Race RR, Sanger R (1968) Blood Groups in Man, 5th edn. Oxford: Blackwell Scientific Publications

Race RR, Sanger R (1975) Blood Groups in Man, 6th edn. Oxford: Blackwell Scientific Publications

Ramsey G, Hahn LF, Cornll FW et al. (1989) Low rate of rhesus immunization from Rh-incompatible blood transfusions during liver and heart transplant surgery. Transplantation 47: 993–995

Ranasinghe E, Goodyear E, Burgess G (2003) Anti-Ce complicating two consecutive pregnancies with increasing severity of haemolytic disease of the newborn. Transfusion Med 13: 53–55

van Rhenen DJ, Thijssen PMHJ, Overbeeke MAM (1994) Serological characteristics of partial D antigen category VI in 8 unrelated blood donors. Vox Sang 66: 133

Ridgwell K, Spurr Nk, Laguda B et al. (1992) Isolation of cDNA clones for a 50 kDa glycoprotein of the human erythrocyte membrane associated with Rh (rhesus) blood-group antigen expression. Biochem J 287: 223–228

Ripoche P, Bertrand O, Gane P et al. (2004) Human Rhesus-associated glycoprotein mediates facilitated transport of NH3 into red blood cells. Proc Natl Acad Sci USA 101: 17222–17227

Rochna E, Hughes–Jones NC (1965) The use of purified ^{125}I-labelled anti-γ globulin in the determination of the number of D antigen sites on red cells of different phenotypes. Vox Sang 10: 675

Rosenfield RE, Allen FH Jr, Swisher SN et al. (1962) A review of Rh serology and presentation of a new terminology. Transfusion 2: 287

Rouillac C, Colin Y, Hughes-Jones NC et al. (1995) Transcript analysis of D category phenotypes predicts hybrid Rh D-CE-D proteins associated with alteration of D epitopes. Blood 85: 2937–2944 de la Rubia J, Garcia R, Arriaga F *et al.* (1994) Anti-D immunization after transfusion of 4 units of fresh frozen plasma. Vox Sang 66: 297–298

Rubinstein P (1972) Cyclical variations in anti-Rh titer detected by automatic quantitative hemagglutination. Vox Sang 23: 508

Ruffie J, Carriere M (1951) Production of a blocking anti-D antibody by injection of D^u red cells. BMJ ii: 1564

Sacks MS, Wiener AS, Jahn EF *et al.* (1959) Isosensitization to a new blood factor, Rh^D, with special reference to its clinical importance. Ann Intern Med 51: 740

Samson D, Mollison PL (1975) Effect on primary Rh immunization of delayed administration of anti-Rh. Immunology 28: 349

Schmidt PJ, Morrison EG, Shohl J (1962) The antigenicity of the Rh$_o$(D^u) blood factor. Blood 20: 196

Schmidt PJ, Vos GH (1967) Multiple phenotypic abnormalities associated with Rh$_{null}$ (. . . / . . .). Vox Sang 13: 18–20

Schorr JB, Schorr PT, Francis R *et al.* (1971) The antigenicity of C and E antigens when transfused into Rh-negative (rr) and Rh-positive recipients. Chicago, IL: Commun Am Assoc Blood Banks

Scott ML (2002) Rh serology: co-ordinator's report. 4th International Workshop Monoclonal Antibodies against Human Red Cell Surface Antigens, Paris. Transfusion Clin Biol 9: 23–29

Shao CP, Maas JH, Su YQ *et al.* (2002) Molecular background of RhD positive, D-negative, D(el) and weak D phenotypes in Chinese. Vox Sang 83:156–161

Shaw DR, Conley ME, Knox FJ *et al.* (1988) Direct quantitation of IgG subclasses 1, 2, and 3 bound to red cells by Rh1 (D) antibodies. Transfusion 28: 127–131

Shirey RS, Edwards RE, Ness PM (1994) The risk of alloimmunization to c (Rh4) in R$_1$R$_1$ patients who present with anti-E. Transfusion 34: 756–758

Singleton BK, Green CA, Avent ND *et al.* (2000) The presence of an RHD pseudogene containing a 37 base pair duplication and a nonsense mutation in Africans with the RhD-negative blood group phenotype. Blood 95: 12–18

Sistonen P, Saraneva H, Pirkola A *et al.* (1994) Mar, a novel high-incidence Rh antigen revealing the existence of an allelic sub-system including C^W (Rh8) and C^x (Rh9) with exceptional distribution in the Finnish population. Vox Sang 66: 287–292

Skov F (1976) Observations of the number of available G (rh^G, Rh 12) antigen sites on red cells. Vox Sang 31: 124

Smith TR, Sherman S, Nelson C *et al.* (1977) Formation of anti-G by the transfusion of D-negative blood. Atlanta, GA: Commun Am Assoc Blood Banks

Smythe JS, Anstee DJ (2000) The role of palmitoylation in RhD expression. Transfusion Med 10 (Suppl. 1): 30

Smythe JS, Anstee DJ (2001) Expression of C antigen in transduced K562 cells. Transfusion 41: 24–30

Smythe JS, Avent PA, Judson SF *et al.* (1996) Expression of RHD and RHCE gene products using retroviral transduction of K562 cells establishes the molecular basis of Rh blood group antigens. Blood 87: 2968–2973

Soupene E, King N, Field E *et al.* (2002) Rhesus expression in a green alga is regulated by CO(2). Proc Natl Acad Sci USA 99: 7769–7773

Southcott MJ, Tanner MJA, Anstee DJ (1999) The expression of human blood group antigens during erythropoiesis in a cell culture system. Blood 93: 4425–4435

Spielmann W, Seidl S, von Pawel J (1974) Anti-ce(f) in a CDe–cD– mother, as a cause of haemolytic disease of the newborn. Vox Sang 27: 473–477

Spring FA, Parsons SF, Ortlepp S *et al.* (2001) Intercellular adhesion molecule-4 binds alpha(4)beta(1) and alpha(V)-family integrins through novel integrin-binding mechanisms. Blood 98: 458–66

St-Amour I, Proulx C, Lemieux R *et al.* (2003) Modulations of anti-D affinity following promiscuous binding of the heavy chain with naïve light chains. Transfusion 43: 246–253

Stern K, Davidsohn I, Masaitis L (1956) Experimental studies on Rh immunization. Am J Clin Pathol 26: 833

Stern K, Goodman HS, Berger M (1961) Experimental isoimmunization to hemo-antigens in man. J Immunol 87: 189

Stout TD, Moore BPL, Allen FH Jr *et al.* (1963) A new phenotype D+ G– (Rh: 1, –12). Vox Sang 8: 262

Stratton F (1946) A new Rh allelomorph. Nature (Lond) 158: 25

Stratton F (1955) Rapid Rh-typing: a sandwich technique. BMJ i: 201

Sturgeon P (1970) Hematological observations on the anemia associated with blood type Rh$_{null}$. Blood 36: 310

Tate H, Cunningham C, McDale MG *et al.* (1960) An Rh gene complex Dc–. Vox Sang 5: 398

Tazzari PL, Bontadini A, Belletti D *et al.* (1994) Flow cytometry: a tool in immunohematology for D+w (D^u) antigen evaluation? Vox Sang 67: 382–386

Teesdale PW, de Silva PM, Fleetwood P *et al.* (1988) Responsiveness to Rh(D) and its association with HLA, red cell and serum markers. Abstracts, 20th Congress of the International Society of Blood Transfusion, London

Tippett P, Sanger R (1962) Observations on subdivisions of the Rh antigen D. Vox Sang 7: 9

Tippett P, Sanger R (1977) Further observations on subdivisions of the Rh antigen D. Arztl Lab 23: 476–480

Tippett P, Gavin J, Sanger R (1962) The antigen C^w produced by the gene complex CwD–. Vox Sang 7: 249–250

Tippett P, Lomas-Francis C, Wallace M (1996) The Rh antigen D: partial D antigens and associated low incidence antigens. Vox Sang 70: 123–131 du Toit ED, Martell RW, Botha I *et al.* (1989) Anti-D antibodies in Rh-positive mothers. S Afr Med J 75: 452

Unger LJ, Wiener AS (1959) Observations on blood factors Rh^A, Rh$^\alpha$, Rh^B and Rh^C. Am J Clin Pathol 31: 95

Urbaniak SJ, Robertson AE (1981) A successful program of immunizing Rh-negative male volunteers for anti-D production using frozen/thawed blood. Transfusion 21: 64–69

Van der Schoot CE, Tax GHM, Rijnders RJP *et al.* (2003) Prenatal typing of Rh and Kell blood group system antigens: the edge of a watershed. Transfusion Med Rev 17: 31–44

Vontver LA (1973) Rh sensitization associated with drug use. JAMA 226: 469

Vos GH, Vos D, Kirk RL *et al.* (1961) A sample of blood with no detectable Rh antigens. Lancet i: 14

Wagner FF, Flegel WA (2000) RHD gene deletion occurred in the Rhesus box. Blood 95: 3662–3668

Wagner FF, Gassner C, Muller TH *et al.* (1998) Three molecular structures cause rhesus D category VI phenotypes with distinct immunohaematological features. Blood 91: 2157–2168

Wagner FF, Gassner C, Muller TH *et al.* (1999) Molecular basis of weak D phenotypes. Blood 93: 385–393

Wagner FF, Frohmajer A, Ladewig B *et al.* (2000a) Weak D alleles express distinct phenotypes. Blood 95: 2699–2708

Wagner FF, Eicher NI, Jorgensen JR *et al.* (2002a) DNB: a partial D with anti-D frequent in Central Europe. Blood 100: 2253–2256

Wagner FF, Ladewig B, Angert KS *et al.* (2002b) The DAU allele cluster of the RHD gene. Blood 100: 306–311

Wagner FF, Ladewig B, Flegel WA (2003) The RHCE allele ceRT: D epitope 6 expression does not require D-specific amino acids. Transfusion 43: 1248–1254

Wagner T, Resch B, Legler TJ *et al.* (2000b) Severe HDN due to anti-Ce that required exchange transfusion. Transfusion 40: 571–574

Wagner T, Kormoczi GF, Buchta C *et al.* (2005) Anti-D immunisation by DEL red blood cells. Transfusion 45: 520–526

Wallace M, Lomas-Francis C, Beckers E *et al.* (1997) DBT: a partial D phenotype associated with the low incidence antigen RL 32. Transfus Med 7: 233–238

Waller M, Lawler SD (1962) A study of the properties of the Rhesus antibody (Ri) diagnostic for the rheumatoid factor and its application to Gm grouping. Vox Sang 7: 591

Ward HK (1957) The persistence of antibodies in the absence of antigenic stimulus. Aust J Exp Biol Med Sci 35: 499

Wensley RT, Snape TJ (1980) Preparation of improved cryoprecipitated Factor VIII concentrate: a controlled study of three variables affecting the yield. Vox Sang 38: 222–228

Westhoff CM, Ferreri-Jacobia M, Mak DO *et al.* (2002) Identification of the erythrocyte Rh blood group glycoprotein as a mammalian ammonium transporter. J Biol Chem 277: 12499–12502

WHO (1971) Prevention of Rh Sensitization. Technical Report Series 468. Geneva: WHO

Wiener AS (1949) Further observations on isosensitization to the Rh factor. Proc Soc Exp Biol (NY) 70: 576

Woodrow JC, Finn R, Krevans JR (1969) Rapid clearance of Rh positive blood during experimental Rh immunization. Vox Sang 17: 349

Woodrow JC, Clarke CA, Donohoe WTA *et al.* (1975) Mechanism of Rh prophylaxis: an experimental study on specificity of immunosuppression. BMJ 2: 57

Zeiler Th, Wittman G, Zingsem J *et al.* (1994) A dose of 100 IU intravenous anti-D gammaglobulin is effective for the prevention of RhD immunisation after RhD-incompatible single donor platelet transfusion. Vox Sang 66: 243

Zhou Y-Y, Xiong W, Shao CP (2005) Multiple isoforms excluding normal RHD mRNA detected in Rh blood group Del phenotype with RHD 1227A allele. Athens: ISBT, Abstract 10

Zipursky A, Pollock J, Chown B *et al.* (1965) Transplacental isoimmunization by foetal red blood cells. Birth Defects, Original Article Series 1: 84

6

Other red cell antigens

In this chapter, various other red cell antigens are described in the order in which they were given the status of 'systems'. Then, a list is given of 'collections' of antigens (see below), followed by a description of other high- and low-frequency antigens. Corresponding antibodies, both naturally occurring and immune, are also described but only brief notes are included about their clinical significance, which is considered in more detail in Chapters 7, 10, 11 and 12.

The Kell (K) and Kx systems

Kell antigens

A list of the antigens of the Kell system is given in Table 6.1. K (K1) is by far the most important from a clinical point of view, as the corresponding antibody is involved in haemolytic transfusion reactions (HTRs) and in haemolytic disease of the newborn (HDN) more frequently than any other antibody outside the ABO and Rh systems.

K is expressed on red cells by about the tenth week of life (Marsh and Redman 1990). Nine per cent of the English population are K (K1) positive, having the genotype KK or Kk; the frequency of K is 0.046 and that of k (K2), 0.954. (Throughout this chapter, frequencies of alleles in white people are taken from Race and Sanger 1975.) In black people in the USA the frequency of K positives is about 1.5% (Stroup et al. 1965) and in Japanese is only about 0.02% (Hamilton and Nakahara 1971).

Four other sets of alleles are closely linked to K1 and K2 but only two of these sets, Kp^a, Kp^b and Kp^c (K3, K4, K21) and Js^a and Js^b (K6, K7) are known to be

Table 6.1 Notations and frequencies of antigens in the Kell blood group system (slightly modified from Marsh and Redman 1990, Daniels et al. 2004).

Notation			Antigen
Name	Letter	Number	frequency (%)
Kell	K	K1	9.1
Cellano	k	K2	99.8
Penney	Kp^a	K3	2.0
Rautenberg	Kp^b	K4	>99.9
	Ku	K5	>99.9
Sutter	Js^a	K6	< 1.0 in white people
			19.5 in black people
Matthews	Js^b	K7	>99.9 in white people
			99.9 in black people
Karhula	Ul^a	K10	2.6 in Finns
			> 0.1 in others
Côté		K11	>99.9
Bockman		K12	>99.9
Sgro		K13	>99.9
Santini		K14	>99.9
	k-like	K16	99.8
Weeks	Wk^a	K17	0.3
Marshall		K18	>99.9
Sublett		K19	>99.9
	Km	K20	>99.9
Levay	Kp^c	K21	< 0.1
Ikar		K22	>99.9
Centauro	Cent	K23	< 0.1
Callois	Cls	K24	< 2.0
	VLAN	K25	low
	TOU	K26	high
	RAZ	K27	high
	VONG	K28	low

Kw (previously K8), KL (previously K9) and Kx (previously K15) are now known not to belong to the Kell system.

clinically important. (The other sets are K11, K17, K14 and K24.) In white people, Kp^b and Js^b have a very high frequency. Although Js^a is rare in white people, it is not uncommon in black people. In the extremely rare null phenotype K_0, no Kell system antigens are present on red cells. Ku (K5) is found on all red cells except those that are K_0, as are the other high-frequency antigens, K12, K13, K14, K18, K19, K22, K26 and K27. There are *three* other low-frequency antigens: K10, K23 and K25.

In the numerical notation for Kell, as for Rh and other systems, phenotypes are designated according to reactions with particular antibodies; for example, a sample reacting negatively with anti-K is designated K: −1; if the sample has also reacted positively with anti-k, it is designated K: −1, 2.

Numbers of K and k antigen sites

Using both polyclonal and monoclonal radio-iodinated anti-K, the number of K sites on *KK* red cells was found to be 4000–6100 and on *Kk* cells 2500–3500 (Hughes-Jones and Gardner 1971; Jaber *et al.* 1989). Using four monoclonal antibodies reacting with epitopes absent from K_0 red cells, 2000–4000 epitopes were detected per red cell; with Fab fragments of the same monoclonals, estimates were higher, namely 4000–8000 sites in three out of four cases and 18 000 in the fourth (Parsons *et al.* 1993). Using ferritin-labelled anti-IgG and polyclonal IgG anti-k, the number of k sites, on both *Kk* and *kk* cells, was found to be 2000–5000 (Masouredis *et al.* 1980a).

Molecular biology and chemistry of Kell antigens

The glycoprotein that carries Kell system antigens (CD238) is encoded by a gene on chromosome 7 at 7q33. It has a molecular weight of 93 kDa and comprises 732 amino acids. It is a type II membrane protein with its amino-terminal domain in the cytosol, a single membrane-spanning domain and a large extracellular carboxy-terminal domain of 665 amino acids. The extracellular domain contains 15 cysteine residues, suggesting that this part of the molecule is highly folded, consistent with its sensitivity to reducing agents. One of these residues (Cys72) forms a disulphide bond with the Xk protein. There are five potential glycosylation sites in the extracellular domain. The molecule is a member of the M13 group of zinc endopeptidases and its preferred substrate is big endothelin-3. Proteolytic cleavage of big endothelins releases bioactive peptides with diverse physiological functions including vasodilatation effects. The molecular bases of most Kell system antigens are known and all result from single amino acid substitutions (Table 6.1; Redman *et al.* 1999; Daniels 2002). The K_0 and K_{mod} phenotypes result from a diverse array of inactivating mutations in the *KEL* gene (Lee *et al.* 2001; Lee *et al.* 2003a). A model of the Kell protein based on the crystal structure of neutral endopeptidase 24.11 (NEP) indicates that the extracellular domain of the protein has two globular domains rich in alpha helix. The domain closest to the lipid bilayer encompasses the enzyme active site, whereas the domain furthest from the membrane contains all the amino acids whose substitution is related to the expression of blood group antigens (Lee *et al.* 2003b; Plate 6.1 shown in colour between pages 528 and 529).

K/k polymorphism is determined by methionine at position 193 in K rather than threonine, as in k (Plate 6.1). The ability to distinguish K from k in a polymerase chain reaction (PCR) method that can be applied to DNA samples obtained from amniotic fetal cells is proving useful in predicting haemolytic disease in pregnant women with anti-K (Lee *et al.* 1995; Van der Schoot *et al.* 2003; see also Chapter 12).

Using the monoclonal antibody-specific immobilization of erythrocyte antigens (MAIEA) technique (see Chapter 8), at least five spatially distinct regions could be distinguished on the Kell glycoprotein; for instance, one containing K, k, Ul^a, K22 and, possibly, Js^a and Js^b, and another containing Kp^a, K^b and Kp^c (Petty *et al.* 1994). Kell antigens are destroyed by treating red cells with a reagent 'ZAPP', containing 0.1 mol/l of dithiothreitol (DTT) and 0.1% papain (Branch and Petz 1980), or by treatment with 2-aminoethyliso-thiouronium bromide (AET). K_0 red cells, occurring naturally or produced by treating red cells of common groups with AET, may be useful in demonstrating that antibodies are or are not recognizing antigens within the Kell blood group system and may also be useful in recognizing antibodies outside the Kell system when these are present together with Kell antibodies (Advani *et al.* 1982). However, some antigens outside the Kell system are also inactivated by AET (see Chapter 8).

Kell antigens are inactivated after the combined treatment of red cells with trypsin and chymotrypsin;

treatment with either of these enzymes separately enhances the expression of Kell antigens (Judson and Anstee 1977).

Red cells can acquire K-like antigens; the red cells of a K-negative patient with *Streptococcus faecium* septicaemia were shown to react with anti-K. K-negative red cells became agglutinable by anti-K when treated *in vitro* with the streptococcus isolated from the patient. Jk(b–) cells also became agglutinable by anti-Jk^b when this organism was disrupted and used to treat the cells (McGinniss *et al.* 1984).

Kell antigens on other cells. Using immunofluorescence flow cytometry, K and k antigens were not detected on lymphocytes, monocytes or granulocytes (Dunstan 1986) or on platelets (Dunstan *et al.* 1984). However, Kell protein could be detected in testis, skeletal muscle and lymphoid tissues and was co-isolated with Kx protein in skeletal muscle (Russo *et al.* 2000).

The antigen Kx

Kx is expressed most strongly on red cells that lack Kell antigens, i.e. K_0 red cells. Similarly, red cells treated with AET (see above) have a high expression of Kx (Advani *et al.* 1982).

Kx is the only antigen in the Kx system; its inheritance is determined by an X-borne recessive gene Xk at Xp21. The gene encodes a protein of 444 amino acids of a molecular weight of 51 kDa with 10 putative transmembrane domains, a very short (four amino acids) cytosolic amino-terminal domain and a larger (71 amino acids) cytosolic carboxy-terminal domain (Ho *et al.* 1994). A single extracellular cysteine residue (Cys 347) on the fifth extracellular loop forms a disulphide bond with Cys72 of the Kell protein. The function of Kx protein is unknown but its structure and covalent linkage to a type II membrane protein (Kell protein) is very reminiscent of the family of heterodimeric amino acid transporters (Southcott 1999; Palacin and Kanai 2004).

Kx is present on all red cells except those belonging to the very rare McLeod phenotype, on which all Kell antigens are depressed. Subjects with this phenotype have various other characteristics, which together constitute the McLeod syndrome: acanthocytic red cells, elevated serum creatine kinase and various muscular and neurological defects (Marsh *et al.* 1981; for a recent review, see Danek *et al.* 2001). Consistent with this the Xk gene is expressed in skeletal muscle and brain (Ho *et al.* 1994).

The McLeod phenotype can result from deletion of that part of the X chromosome that carries *Xk* but other inactivating mutations have also been described (Russo *et al.* 2002). A minority of patients with the X-linked type of chronic granulomatous disease also have the McLeod phenotype and in these the region of X that is deleted includes the locus for X-linked CGD as well as the Xk locus (reviewed in Daniels 2002).

Antibodies of the Kell and Kx systems

Anti-K

Naturally occurring anti-K is rare. Although an example that was IgG has been described (fourth edition, p. 344), most examples of naturally occurring anti-K are IgM, usually reacting best at room temperature and, in some cases, first found after an illness and disappearing following the patient's recovery (Tegoli *et al.* 1967; Kanel *et al.* 1978; Judd *et al.* 1981). In one case, the antigenic stimulus was an infection with an uncommon strain of *Escherichia coli* O125: B15. A cell-free filtrate of a culture of the organisms inhibited the anti-K (and the anti-A) in the serum of the patient, who was a newborn infant. Both the anti-K and the anti-A had disappeared by the time the infant was 3 months old (Marsh *et al.* 1978). One patient had pulmonary lesions suggestive of tuberculosis and in another the relevant organisms were unidentified (Tegoli *et al.* 1967; Kanel *et al.* 1978). Some strains of *Campylobacter jejuni* and *Campylobacter coli*, major aetiological agents of gastrointestinal infections in humans, carry surface sites reactive with anti-K (Wong *et al.* 1985).

Immune anti-K is the commonest immune red cell antibody outside the ABO and Rh systems, accounting for almost two-thirds of non-Rh immune red cell alloantibodies (see Table 3.6, p. 76). An estimate of the frequency with which it is formed in K-negative subjects transfused with at least 1 unit of K-positive blood was made by Kornstad and Heistö (1957). In a series of 130 such subjects, 53 were tested at 4–12 months and five had anti-K; of the remaining 77 subjects, tested at 13–37 months, only one had anti-K. The authors concluded that the probability that a K-negative subject transfused with a unit of K-positive blood would develop anti-K was about 1 in 10. If this estimate were correct, K would be eight times less immunogenic than D, but it may be even less immunogenic than this.

Other evidence of the immunogenicity of K comes from two series of experiments: in the first, three spaced injections of K-positive red cells were given to 16 subjects, at least 10 of whom were K negative; none formed anti-K (Wiener *et al.* 1955). In the second, a series of injections of K-positive, D-positive red cells was given to 31 K-negative, D-negative subjects (FM Roberts, personal communication). Of the 19 subjects who failed to form anti-D, none formed anti-K. Of the 12 who formed anti-D, six formed anti-K but it is well known that subjects who make anti-D have a greatly increased chance of making antibodies to other antigens carried by the immunizing D-positive red cells (see Chapter 3).

Opportunities for alloimmunization to K as a result of pregnancy are relatively common but, assuming that K is 10 times less immunogenic than D, it can be shown that the incidence of HDN due to anti-K in second pregnancies would be expected to be only about 1 in 3500 (seventh edition, p. 405). Data on the frequency with which anti-K is found in pregnancy are given in Chapter 12.

In screening samples for anti-K, Kk red cells are almost always used; as some samples of anti-K can be detected only with KK red cells, the estimates given above for the frequency of anti-K must be too low.

The woman in whose serum anti-K was first discovered (Coombs *et al.* 1946) had been transfused previously with blood from her husband (information not in the original paper), as had the woman investigated by Chown (1949) who emphasized the moral 'never transfuse a woman with her husband's blood'.

Several monoclonal antibodies with K specificity have been produced.

Anti-k

Anti-k was first found in the serum of a recently delivered woman whose infant was mildly affected with haemolytic disease of the newborn (Levine *et al.* 1949). The rarity of the antibody is accounted for by the rarity of k-negative (i.e. *KK*) subjects: 0.04–2% in white people in various parts of Europe, 0.005% in black people in the USA and very much rarer in

Japanese (see Daniels 1995). A murine monoclonal anti-k has been described (Sonneborn *et al.* 1983).

Other antibodies of the K system and anti-Kx

Anti-Kp^a, anti-Kp^b, anti-Js^a and anti-Js^b are all rare. The original example of anti-Kp^a appeared to be naturally occurring (Allen and Lewis 1957); this antibody and anti-Kp^b may also occur as autoantibodies (see Chapter 7); the other antibodies mentioned in this section have been described only as immune alloantibodies. Anti-Ku reacts with all samples except K_0 and is found only in K_0 subjects (Corcoran *et al.* 1961).

Subjects with the McLeod phenotype may make two alloantibodies following transfusion, anti-Kx and anti-Km. Km is an antigen present on red cells of common Kell phenotypes but not on K_0 red cells or on cells of McLeod phenotype.

Four monoclonal antibodies recognize high-frequency epitopes absent from K_0 cells; all four identify the Kell glycoprotein (molecular weight 95.6 kDa); the four epitopes recognized fall into two non-overlapping groups: the first includes Kp^{bc} and K14 and the second, k (Parsons *et al.* 1993).

An antibody found in patients with the McLeod syndrome, previously known as anti-KL, is a mixture of anti-Kx and anti-Km and is found only after transfusion. Anti-Km reacts with all samples except those that are K_0 or Kx negative; anti-Kx, on the other hand, reacts strongly with K_0 red cells, which, as already mentioned, possess greatly increased amounts of Kx. Anti-Kx can cause rapid destruction of Kx-positive red cells, associated with haemoglobinuria, but does not interfere with the successful transfusion of granulocytes (Taswell *et al.* 1976), implying an absence of Kx from such cells.

Serological characteristics of immune anti-K and anti-k

Anti-K and anti-k are usually IgG. Kell antibodies were found to be solely IgG1 in seven out of eight and 12 out of 14 cases respectively (Engelfriet 1978; Hardman and Beck 1981). As with anti-D, sera containing only IgG anti-K may, when undiluted, agglutinate saline-suspended cells. Many examples of IgG anti-K activate complement but only to the C3 stage, and are non-lytic.

Anti-K may be IgM but only the most potent examples agglutinate red cells suspended in saline; weaker examples sensitize red cells to agglutination by anti-IgM and sometimes to anti-complement.

Anti-K tends to react poorly in low-ionic-strength solution (LISS) and may be relatively difficult to detect with the LISS-IAT, or the low-ionic-strength polybrene method, with or without the IAT, and in the Auto-Analyzer (see Chapter 8) .

Studies with ^{125}I-labelled anti-K

The equilibrium constants of several examples of IgG anti-K ranged from 0.6 to 4.5×10^{10} l/mol, figures that are 100 times greater than those found with IgG anti-D, indicating that, if anti-K binds monovalently, its intrinsic affinity for K must be much higher than that of anti-D for D. The concentration of anti-K corresponding to an indirect antiglobulin titre of 1 is about the same as for anti-D (Hughes-Jones and Gardner 1971).

Clinical aspects

Anti-K and much less frequently anti-k can cause severe haemolytic transfusion reactions; anti-Js[a] and -Js[b] have been known to cause a delayed haemolytic transfusion reaction (DHTR) (for references, see Daniels 1995). Anti-Kp[a], and far more rarely -Kp[b] and -Js[b], have caused severe HDN and milder disease due to anti-Js[a] and -Ku has been reported (for references, see Chapter 12). Anti-K has several times been the cause of haemolytic transfusion reactions due to inter-donor incompatibility (see Chapter 11 and West et al. 1986). Antibodies of the Kell system, particularly anti-Kp[b], may be found as autoantibodies in autoimmune haemolytic anaemia (AIHA); there may be concomitant depression of the patient's own Kell antigens (see Chapter 7).

Transient depression of Kell antigens, with the development of alloantibodies reacting with a high-incidence Kell antigen or with all but K_0 cells has been observed in association with autoimmune thrombocytopenic purpura (Vengelen-Tyler et al 1987; Williamson et al. 1994). In the second of the two cases, in a subsequent relapse of autoimmune thrombocytopenic purpura (AITP) the red cells became Lu(a– b–) and an antibody against a high-incidence Lu antigen appeared in the serum. In both relapses,

antigen changes persisted for many months; LW[a] and CD44 were also markedly weakened.

The Duffy (Fy) system

The red cells of about 66% of the English population are Fy(a+), belonging to the genotype Fy^aFy^a or Fy^aFy^b, the remainder being Fy^bFy^b (Cutbush and Mollison 1950).

In white people, the alleles Fy[a] and Fy[b] have frequencies of 0.425 and 0.557 respectively; a further allele, Fy[x], which makes a weak form of Fy[b], has a frequency of 0.016. The frequency of the gene Fy, which produces neither Fy[a] nor Fy[b], is only 0.002 but in black people in the USA is about 0.7. In parts of tropical Africa the frequency of Fy is 1.0, all the native inhabitants having the phenotype Fy(a– b–) (Mourant et al. 1976). Fy(a– b–) is extremely rare in white people and other races.

The Fy locus is on chromosome 1q21–q25; it was the first blood group gene to be assigned to an autosome in humans (Donahue et al. 1968).

A monoclonal antibody produced in mice by injecting pooled human red cells was found to recognize a unique epitope on the Duffy glycoprotein and was named anti-Fy6 (Nichols et al. 1987).

Fy[a] and Fy[b] sites on red cells and nature of the Fy[a] and Fy[b] antigens

The number of Fy[a] sites on Fy^aFy^a red cells and of Fy[b] sites on Fy^bFy^b red cells was estimated to be 17 000; the number of Fy[a] sites on Fy^aFy^b was estimated to be 6900 (Masouredis et al. 1980b). Using flow cytometry, Woolley et al. (2000) report that Fy antigen expression is significantly higher (by $49 \pm 19\%$) on reticulocytes than on mature red cells.

Using an immunoaffinity technique for isolating antigens in the form of soluble antigen–antibody complexes, the Fy[a] and Fy[b] antigens were shown to be associated with membrane components of apparent molecular weight of 40 kDa (Moore 1983). Similarly, using immunoblotting of red cell ghosts with a potent anti-Fy[a], the Fy[a] antigen was located on a glycoprotein of 35–43 kDa, migrating between bands 5 and 6 (Hadley et al. 1984).

Sequencing of cDNA encoding the Duffy glycoprotein (synonym: DARC, Duffy antigen chemokine receptor) revealed a protein of 338 amino acids with an apparent molecular weight of 35 733 (Chaudhuri *et al.* 1993; Iwamoto *et al.* 1996). The protein would be predicted to have seven membrane-spanning domains with an amino-terminal extracellular domain of 65 amino acids and a small carboxy-terminal cytoplasmic domain. Of three potential N-glycosylation sites in the extracellular amino-terminal domain, *N16SS* is utilized (Tournamille *et al.* 2003). The Fy^a/Fy^b polymorphism is due to a point mutation at amino acid 44, there is Asp in Fy^b instead of Gly in Fy^a (Mallinson *et al.* 1995). The Fy6 epitope has been mapped to a region in the extracellular domain involving residues 22 (Phe), 23 (Glu) and 25 (Val), whereas Fy3 is influenced by residues in extracellular domains 1, 2 and 4 (Tournamille *et al.* 2003). The Fy^x (synonym: weak Fy^b expression) results from a nucleotide substitution (C265T) resulting in Arg89Cys in the first intracellular loop of the Duffy glycoprotein. The replacement of arginine appears to adversely affect the insertion of the protein into the plasma membrane and the reduced levels of surface protein that result account for the weak expression of Fy^b antigen (and Fy3, Fy5 and Fy6) on the red cells (Olsson *et al.* 1998; Tournamille *et al.* 1998).

The Fy^a antigen is destroyed by crude preparations of proteolytic enzymes although not by crystalline trypsin (or neuraminidase); it is destroyed by chymotrypsin (Morton 1962). Fy3, 4 and 5 are not destroyed by papain. Treatment of membrane components with endoglycosidase F (Endo F) sharpened the diffuse band, carrying Fy^a activity, obtained by immunoblotting to a band of molecular weight 26 kDa; it was concluded that the Fy^a protein is heavily glycosylated, with 40–50% of its mass consisting of N-glycan (Tanner *et al.* 1988).

Fy^a and Fy^b tend to elute from red cells stored in a low pH low-ionic-strength medium, leading to the appearance of substances with specific inhibitory activity for anti-Fy^a or anti-Fy^b in the supernatant fluid. Duffy antigens also elute from red cells after prolonged storage, or mixing, in saline at pH 7.0 (Williams *et al.* 1981).

The structure of Fy glycoprotein (seven membrane spans) is characteristic of the G protein-coupled receptor family which includes chemokine receptors, and the Fy glycoprotein is a promiscuous chemokine receptor, binding to both CXC and CC families. However, it lacks the intracellular G protein binding domain (Murphy 1994). Fy glycoprotein is a receptor for IL-8 and melanoma growth stimulatory activity (MGSA);

these two chemokines block the invasion of red cells by *Plasmodium knowlesi* (Horuk *et al.* 1993). IL-8 binding involves residues on extracellular domains 1 and 4 and requires the presence of intact intrachain disulphide bonds (Tournamille *et al.* 2003). The Fy glycoprotein is expressed on capillaries and post-capillary venular endothelial cells as well as red cells, and it has been suggested that the Fy glycoprotein has a role in enhancing leucocyte recruitment to sites of inflammation by facilitating the movement of chemokines across the endothelium (Lee *et al.* 2003). Fukuma and co-workers (2003) suggest that the Duffy antigen delays the disappearance of chemokines from plasma.

Fy antigens on other cells. Using a sensitive radioimmunoassay, Fy antigens were shown to be absent from platelets (Dunstan *et al.* 1984). Using immunofluorescence flow cytometry, Fy^a, Fy^b and Fy5 were not detected on lymphocytes, monocytes or granulocytes (Dunstan 1986).

Duffy groups and malaria

Fy(a– b–) subjects are protected from infection by *Plasmodium vivax* (Miller *et al.* 1976). In parts of Africa, the frequency of *Fy* is 1.0 and in these areas *P. vivax* malaria is absent (Welch *et al.* 1977). The Fy(a– b–) phenotype in these individuals results from a mutation in the binding site for GATA-1, which is upstream of the Fy gene. GATA-1 is a transcription factor that regulates the expression of erythroid genes. The mutation in Fy(a– b–) prevents GATA-1 binding so that the Fy gene is not transcribed and Fy glycoprotein is not expressed in the erythroid cells. Expression in non-erythroid cells is not affected (Tournamille *et al.* 1995). In Africa, the Fy(a– b–) phenotype occurs on an Fy^b genetic background. In Papua New Guinea, the Fy null allele occurs on an Fy^a genetic background (Zimmerman *et al.* 1999). The antigen responsible for the susceptibility of red cells to penetration by *P. vivax* appears to be Fy6 (Barnwell *et al.* 1989).

For *P. falciparum* infection, there is no association with Duffy groups, so that black people are as susceptible as white people. The specific ligands concerned in binding the parasites to red cells are the glycophorins and especially the N-acetylneuraminic acid linked in an α2,3 configuration on them, although some strains of *P. falciparum* may use alternative ligands for invasion (Pasvol *et al.* 1993; Maier *et al.* 2003).

Duffy groups and HIV

Lachgar and co-worker (1998) report that Duffy gly-coprotein on red cells binds HIV and that this binding is inhibited by the chemokine RANTES, which binds the Duffy glycoprotein, but not by MIP-1-α, which does not bind Duffy glycoprotein. They suggest that red cells may be a reservoir for HIV and transmit the virus to leucocytes.

Antibodies of the Duffy system

Anti-Fy^a

This antibody is found mainly following transfusion and, much less commonly, following pregnancy; it is almost never naturally occurring. Anti-Fy^a occurs about three times less frequently than anti-K (see Table 3.6 on p. 76). Most examples are IgG; about 50% activate complement up to the C3 stage.

Anti-Fy^a (and -Fy^b) are predominantly IgG1; in three series they were solely of this subclass in six out of seven, 12 out of 14 and 11 out of 16 cases respect-ively (Engelfriet 1978; Hardman and Beck 1981; Szymanski et al. 1982). In the last of these series, three anti-Fy^a had an IgG2 component and four were partly IgM; two anti-Fy^b were entirely IgG1.

Occasionally, anti-Fy^a agglutinates Fy(a+) red cells suspended in saline and may react with Fy(a+ b–) cells more strongly than with Fy(a+ b+) cells (Race et al. 1953). Some anti-Fy^a fail to react in manual poly-brene and polybrene antiglobulin tests (Malde et al. 1986).

Fy^a is significantly more immunogenic in Fy(a– b+) white people than it is in Fy(a– b–) black people. In two series, of 25 and 130 patients with anti-Fy^a, four and 11, respectively, were Fy(a– b–) black people (Kosanke 1983; Vengelen-Tyler 1983); in the second series, none of 11 patients with anti-Fy^b was black.

Anti-Fy^b

Anti-Fy^b is about 20 times less common than anti-Fy^a (Marsh 1975); it is usually found, not on its own, but in sera containing other red cell alloantibodies. A few examples agglutinate red cells suspended in saline. An example of naturally occurring anti-Fy^b reacting by the indirect antiglobulin technique has been described by Issitt (1985).

Anti-Fy3, -Fy4 and -Fy5

Anti-Fy3 reacts with all human red cells except those of the phenotype Fy(a– b–). As the latter phenotype is enormously commoner in black people than in white people, it was somewhat unexpected that the antibody is about as rare in black people as in white people. This is probably because the common mutation giving rise to the Fy(a– b–) phenotype in black people (a GATA-1 site mutation, see above) does not affect Duffy glyco-protein expression in non-erythroid tissues, whereas in other races the Fy(a– b–) phenotype has generally had a different genetic background involving inactivating mutations in the Duffy gene itself (Mallinson et al. 1995; Rios et al. 2000). It should be noted that the GATA-1 mutation has also been found in white people (Rios et al. 2000; Pisacka et al. 2001).

The only example of anti-Fy4 reacted with all Fy(a– b–) cells from black people and with most Fy(a+ b–) and Fy(a– b+) cells from black people, i.e. of presumed genotypes Fy^{a}Fy and Fy^{b}Fy respectively (Behzad et al. 1953). Anti-Fy5 is made by black patients and is often found in sera that contain other immune antibodies; it reacts with most red cells except with Fy(a– b–) cells from black people, with Rh$_{null}$ cells or with cells carrying variant forms of the c antigen regardless of their Fy status (Meredith 1985).

Clinical aspects

Duffy antibodies seldom cause severe haemolytic transfusion reactions and only occasionally cause HDN, which is then usually mild (Goodrick et al. 1997). They have been implicated in delayed haemolytic transfusion reactions in multi-transfused black patients with sickle cell disease. Of five patients with anti-Fy3 or anti-Fy5, four had evidence of DHTRs; anti-Fy^a preceded the appearance of anti-Fy3 or anti-Fy5 (Vengelen-Tyler 1985). In another series, five Fy(a–b–3–) patients with sickle cell disease experienced DHTRs or failed to show the desired HbA increment after transfusion; they all had anti-Fy^a and other alloantibodies in the serum (Le Pennec et al. 1987).

The development of allo-anti-Fy^a (and anti-Jk^b) 14 months after an allogenic bone graft, which had previously been frozen, has been described in a patient who had not been transfused and not been pregnant (Cheek et al. 1995).

Mimicking anti-Fy[b] has been found in autoimmune haemolytic anaemia (see Chapter 7).

The Kidd (Jk) system

About 76% of white people possess the Jk[a] antigen; 26% have the genotype Jk^aJk^a, phenotype Jk(a+ b–), and 50% have the genotype Jk^aJk^b, phenotype Jk(a+ b+). The remaining 24% have the genotype Jk^bJk^b, phenotype Jk(a– b+). Gene frequencies in white people: Jk^a, 0.514; Jk^b, 0.486 (Race and Sanger 1975). The frequency of Jk^a is as high as 0.75 in parts of Africa and as low as about 0.25 in some Chinese and Japanese populations (for references, see Daniels 2002).

The type Jk(a– b–) has been found in Filipinos, South-East Asians, Chinese and others and is least uncommon in Polynesians, in whom the frequency is about 1%; it is extremely rare in white people. Two different genetic backgrounds seem to be responsible for the Jk(a– b–) phenotype: a silent recessive gene Jk (Race and Sanger 1975) or a dominant inhibitor gene, $In(Jk)$, which depresses the expression of Kidd antigens (Okubo et al. 1986). Whereas the recessive type completely lacks Jk[a], Jk[b] and also Jk3, an antigen which is found in all Jk(a+) and Jk(b+) subjects, traces of these three antigens can be demonstrated in subjects of the inhibitor gene type (Okubo et al. 1986). Jk is less common than $In(Jk)$.

Number of Jk[a] and Jk[b] sites and nature of Kidd protein

The number of Jk[a] sites on Jk^aJk^a red cells has been estimated to be 14 000 per red cell (Masouredis et al. 1980).

Red cells carrying Jk[a] or Jk[b], when exposed to 2 mol/l of urea in water, rapidly become swollen and spherocytic before lysing, but Jk(a– b–) red cells exhibit shrinkage and crenation and lyse relatively slowly (Heaton and McLoughlin 1982). This behaviour relates to the fact that Kidd antigens are located on a urea transporter protein. It has been estimated that the passage of urea across the red cell membrane is 1000 times slower in Jk(a– b–) red cells than in normal cells (Fröhlich et al. 1991). Individuals with the Jk(a– b–) phenotype have a urine-concentrating defect (Sands et al. 1992).

The Kidd glycoprotein (synonym: hUT-B1) comprises 389 amino acids and has 10 membrane-spanning domains with its amino and carboxyl termini in the cytoplasm. A single extracellular N-glycosylation site is located at Asn211 on the third predicted extracellular loop. The Jk[a]/Jk[b] polymorphism results from an Asp280Asn transition located in the fourth predicted extracellular loop of the protein (Lucien et al. 2002). The Jk(a– b–) phenotype can result from a variety of different mutations in the gene (reviewed in Daniels 2002).

Kidd antigens were found to be absent from platelets when using a sensitive radioimmunoassay (Dunstan et al. 1984) and from lymphocytes, monocytes and granulocytes when using immunofluorescence flow cytometry (Dunstan 1986).

Antibodies

The first example of anti-Jk[a] was discovered in the serum of a woman who had given birth to an infant with HDN (Allen et al. 1951). Anti-Jk[b] is rarer than anti-Jk[a], and is usually found in sera that contain other immune blood group antibodies. The antibody anti-Jk[a]Jk[b] (i.e. inseparable), also known as anti-Jk3, was present in the serum of the first Jk(a– b–) patient described (Pinkerton et al. 1959).

Anti-Jk[a] and anti-Jk[b] occur only as immune antibodies; they seldom agglutinate saline-suspended red cells and are mainly IgG but may be at least partly IgM (Polley et al. 1962). Although the paper just quoted reported that all of 15 examples of anti-Jk[a] bound complement, a later study of a larger number of Kidd antibodies (55 anti-Jk[a] and 15 anti-Jk[b]) showed that only about 50% were complement-binding (G Garratty, personal communication). Yates and co-workers (1998) report that Kidd antisera bind complement only when at least a trace of IgM antibody is present and that serum fractions containing only IgG antibody do not bind complement. This observation may explain the fact that the pattern of destruction of incompatible red cells by Kidd antibodies is often characteristic of that produced by non-complement-binding antibodies (see Chapter 10). Anti-Jk[a] reacts far more strongly with Jk^aJk^a than with Jk^aJk^b cells and may be undetectable with the latter.

Anti-Jk[a] and anti-Jk[b] were found to be predominantly IgG3 in three out of three cases (Engelfriet 1978). In another series, of 17 cases, most antibodies were a mixture of IgG1 and IgG3 but some were partly IgG2, some partly IgG4 and some partly IgM (Hardman and Beck 1981).

Three IgM human monoclonal anti-Jk^b and one IgM anti-Jk^a have been produced. The antibodies agglutinate red cells, even of phenotype Jk(a+ b+), in saline after an immediate spin (Thompson *et al.* 1991).

Clinical aspects

Both anti-Jk^a and anti-Jk^b can cause haemolytic transfusion reactions. Kidd antibodies are particularly associated with DHTR, being responsible for about one-third of all cases (see Chapter 11). This association is due, at least in part, to the fact that it is not uncommon for Kidd antibodies to become undetectable within a few months of first being detected. Kidd antibodies only rarely cause HDN, a fact for which there is no obvious explanation.

Anti-Jk^a has occasionally been found as an autoantibody in autoimmune haemolytic anaemia (see Chapter 7). A transient auto-anti-Jk^b was apparently stimulated by proteus urinary tract infection; Jk(b–) red cells pre-incubated with *Proteus mirabilis* became agglutinable by anti-Jk^b (McGinniss *et al.* 1979).

Temporary suppression of Jk^a was observed in a patient of phenotype Jk(a+ b–), in association with the development of anti-Jk^{a}Jk^b (anti-Jk3); the antibody appeared to be responsible for a haemolytic reaction following the transfusion of Jk(a+ b–) blood (Issitt *et al.* 1990).

The MNSs system

Antigens

The antigens M and N were discovered by injecting human red cells into rabbits, absorbing the resulting immune serum with one sample of human cells and showing that it would still react with other samples (Landsteiner and Levine 1927).

M and N are alleles giving rise to three genotypes, *MM*, *MN* and *NN*, with frequencies in white people of about 28%, 50% and 22% respectively. The corresponding phenotypes are written M+ N–, M+ N+ and M– N+. When tested with most anti-M, M+ N– red cells react more strongly than M+ N+ cells. Red cells of the phenotype M+ N– show some reaction with anti-N except when they come from a subject who is S negative, s negative, because the Ss glycoprotein (syn. glycophorin B) also carries an amino-terminal determinant with N specificity, sometimes written 'N' (see below).

As described in more detail below, in the section on the chemistry of MN and Ss blood group systems, M and N are carried on glycophorin A (GPA, MN glycoprotein) and the antigens S and s are carried on glycophorin B (GPB, Ss glycoprotein). The inheritance of S and s is closely associated with that of M and N, i.e. the Ss locus is very close to the *MN* locus. The antigen S is found about twice as frequently in *MM* as in *NN* subjects. Among white people, about 55% are S positive and 89% are s positive (Race and Sanger 1975). Haplotype frequencies in white people are approximately as follows: *MS*, 0.247; *Ms*, 0.283; *NS*, 0.080; *Ns*, 0.390. About 1.5% of black people are S– s– but this phenotype has not been found in white people.

Rare genetic variants associated with MN and Ss

There are many rare genetic variants associated with the MNSs blood group system. Some are due to absence of glycophorin A (GPA) or glycophorin B (GPB) or both, namely (1) complete absence of GPA, as in some types of En(a–) red cells; (2) complete absence of GPA and GPB, as in the extremely rare genotype M^kM^k; and (3) complete absence of GPB, as in subjects with red cells of the phenotype S– s–.

Numerous low-frequency antigens have been identified; some of these result from amino acid substitutions or glycosylation changes, or both, in *GPA* or *GPB*; most are associated with abnormal hybrid glycophorin molecules (partly GPA and partly GPB: for reviews, see Issitt and Anstee 1998; Daniels 2002). It has been suggested that the high rate of structural change in the glycophorins provides a means of evasion of *P. falciparum* (Wang *et al.* 2003) or that the variant glycophorins act as more general decoy receptors attracting pathogens to the anucleated red cell and away from their target tissues (Baum *et al.* 2002).

En(a–). There are at least two kinds of En(a–) red cells: (1) total absence of GPA but a normal GPB and therefore some trypsin-resistant 'N' activity (Furuhjelm *et al.* 1969); and (2) total absence of N and 'N' but a weak trypsin-resistant M (Darnborough *et al.* 1969); it has been shown that this represents a hybrid molecule of a normal M-active GPA aminoterminal segment with the carboxy-terminal segment from a normal S-active GPB, i.e. a GP(A-B) hybrid (Dahr *et al.* 1978).

Both kinds of En(a–) red cells have a greatly reduced sialic acid content and electrophoretic mobility. The

217

red cells (if Rh D positive) are agglutinated in saline by IgG anti-D.

Sialic acid deficiency per se does not seem to affect red cell survival, as the En(a–) condition is not associated with a haemolytic anaemia. Moreover, Tn red cells, which are also sialic acid deficient, may survive normally (see Chapter 7). On the other hand, sialic acid deficiency of red cells induced experimentally with neuraminidase in animals is associated with gross shortening of red cell survival (Jancik and Schauer 1974; Durocher et al. 1975).

The use of the terms En^a antigen and anti-En^a is inappropriate, as what is being observed is the inherited deficiency of GPA and the antibody response of GPA-deficient individuals to the surface of normal red cells (Anstee 1981).

M^k is regarded as a silent allele resulting, in homozygotes, with the absence of MN and Ss antigens. Two M^kM^k individuals had red cells which completely lacked the GPA and GPB and had a sialic acid content of between 25% and 31% of normal; both subjects were normal haematologically (Tokunaga et al. 1979). Very few other M^kM^k propositi have been found but M^k heterozygotes, whose red cells, such as those of En(a–) heterozygotes, have reduced sialic acid levels, are commoner (approximate frequency of M^k, 0.0005). For references, see Daniels (2002). GPA associates with the anion transport protein band 3 in the red cell membrane (see also Diego blood groups in this chapter) and absence of GPA in En(a–) and M^kM^k red cells results in band 3 adopting a structure with lower anion transport activity than when GPA is present (Bruce et al. 2003).

S– s–. This phenotype occurs mainly in black people; it has been found in one Indian family but not yet in white people. S– s– red cells lack 'N' and M+ N– S– s red cells are thus the only ones that are completely N negative. S– s– American black people either completely lack the U antigen or have a weak variant form of it (Issitt and Anstee 1998).

U. The U antigen is found in all white people and in about 99% of black people. U-negative subjects are always S– s–.

In some Rh$_{null}$ cells the Ss and U antigens may be difficult to detect, especially when using the IAT. The amount of GPB was found to be reduced to one-third in Rh$_{null}$ cells. It is believed that, during biosynthesis, Rh proteins form a complex with GPB facilitating its incorporation into the red cell membrane (Dahr et al. 1987; see also Chapter 5).

The Miltenberger (Mi.) series of antigens are all carried on glycophorins A or B on hybrid molecules composed of both glycophorins. It has been proposed that these antigens, which formerly had a wide variety of names (Vw, Hut, Mur, etc.) and were also termed Mi.I–XI, should no longer be regarded as belonging to a subsystem of MNSs. Instead they should be termed GP. Vw, GP. Hut, etc. (GP standing for glycophorin). For a fuller description, see Tippett and co-workers (1992); for a review of the chemistry of the antigens, see Dahr (1992) and Daniels (2002). The existence of antibodies of specificity anti-Mi^a has been questioned but such a specificity has been reported for a monoclonal antibody (Chen et al. 2001).

In white people, the frequency of each of the various Mi antigens is less than 1 per 1000 but the Mi.III phenotype (predominantly GP.Mur) is relatively common in South-East Asia, with a frequency reaching 10% in Thailand, 7% in Chinese and 88% in the Ami mountain people of Taiwan (Broadberry and Lin 1996). Anti-'Mi^a', that is to say an antibody reacting with Mi.III red cells but not tested with other Mi cells (probably anti-Mur), has a frequency of 0.28% in Chinese patients in Taiwan and is, in that region, the commonest alloantibody of clinical significance. It may be responsible for both HDN and, in all probability, HTR (Broadberry and Lin 1994; Lin and Broadberry 1994). The high frequency of this antibody in Asian populations necessitates the inclusion of Mur-positive red cells in antibody screening panels. GP.Mur is an altered GPB molecule which results from splicing a small segment of exon 3 of the GPA gene into the GPB gene to create a GP(B – A – B) hybrid protein with residues 1–48 from GPB, residues 49–57 from GPA and residues 58–103 from GPB (Huang and Blumenfeld 1991). The resultant hybrid glycoprotein is more heavily sialylated than GPB (Anstee et al. 1979). Human IgM monoclonal anti-Mur has been produced (Uchikawa et al. 2000).

Numbers of S, s and U antigen sites

The number of available s sites on ss red cells was found to be approximately 12 000 and of available U sites on U-positive red cells to be about 17 000 (Masouredis et al. 1980). These numbers are clearly far less than the number of potential sites; it has been estimated that each red cell has about 2.5×10^5 copies of GPB and, incidentally, about 1×10^6 copies of GPA (see review by Anstee *et al.* 1982).

MNSs antigens on other cells

M, N, S, s and U antigens were not detected on lymphocytes, monocytes or granulocytes by immuno-fluorescence flow cytometry (Dunstan 1986). Using a sensitive radioimmunoassay, MNSs antigens could not be detected on platelets (Simpson *et al.* 1987).

Chemistry of the MN and Ss antigens

As described above, MN and Ss antigens are found respectively on glycophorins A and B of the red cell membrane (Fig. 6.1).

The glycoproteins of the red cell membrane can be separated by SDS-PAGE (see Chapter 3); glycopro-teins rich in sialic acid (glycophorins) can be stained with PAS (periodic–acid Schiff).

The only difference between M and N is that the polypeptide chain determining M has the amino-terminal sequence ser–ser–thr–thr–gly– and that the

chain determining N has the amino-terminal sequence: leu–ser–thr–thr–glu–. Some examples of monoclonal anti-M react with the 'ser' region of the determinant and others with the 'gly' region (Nichols *et al.* 1985).

S and s are carried on glycophorin B and differ from one another in a single amino acid substitution, i.e. at position 29 there is a methionine in S and a threonine in s (Dahr *et al.* 1980a,b). The Ss glycoprotein on intact red cells is not affected by trypsin treatment but is inactivated by pronase, by high concentrations of chy-motrypsin (Judson and Anstee 1977) and by bromelin, ficin and papain.

The first 26 residues of the Ss and the N-specific MN glycoproteins are identical (Dahr *et al.* 1980a,b), thus explaining the fact that red cells of M+ subjects, unless they are S– s–, react with anti-N. Nevertheless, with anti-N the reactions of 'N' (see above) and N are not identical: with anti-N, MM red cells react less strongly than MN red cells, which, in turn, react less strongly than NN red cells.

It seems that oligosaccharides (sialic acid residues) attached to terminal amino acids of the MN glyco-protein, as well as the amino acids themselves, are involved in M and N specificity (Uhlenbruck *et al.* 1976; see also Judd *et al.* 1979).

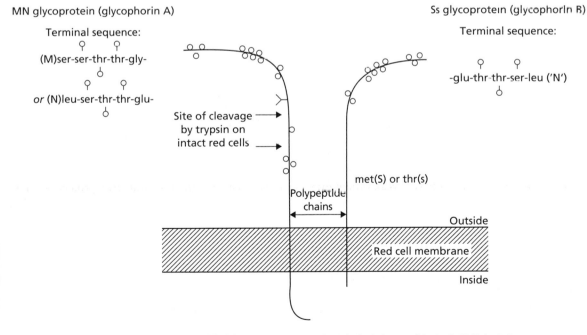

Fig 6.1 The MN and Ss glycoproteins (modified from Anstee 1980). ○, O-linked glycans; Υ, single N-linked glycan on GPA.

Antibodies of the MNSs system

Anti-M

In adults, anti-M is a relatively common naturally occurring antibody reacting optimally at 4°C; it usually reacts weakly or not at all at 37°C. In blood donors, the prevalence of naturally occurring anti-M, detectable in microplates with saline-suspended cells at room temperature, is 1 in 2500 with M+ N– cells, and 1 in 5000 with M+ N+ cells (A Lubenko, personal communication). A higher incidence has been found using an AutoAnalyzer and a low-ionic-strength polybrene method (Perrault 1973).

Anti-M is distinctly commoner in infants than in adults (Strahl et al. 1955). In infants in hospital in Toronto, approximately 4% of agglutinins active at room temperature were anti-M, whereas in adults the figure was approximately 1% (personal communication reported in previous editions of this book).

The development of anti-M in Rh D-immunized subjects following a series of boosting injections has been reported (Wiener 1950; Teesdale et al. 1991). In the latter publication, anti-M developed in 3 out of 25 NN subjects, but in two of the three the antibody was very weak and reactive only at room temperature.

Although almost all examples of anti-M occur in M– N+ subjects, a few have been found in M+ N+ subjects, although not as autoantibodies (e.g. Konugres et al. 1966). Anti-M occurring as an autoantibody in M+ N+ subjects has also been described (e.g. Fletcher and Zmijewski 1970).

Anti-M *detectable only at reduced pH.* Some examples of anti-M can be detected only after the serum has been acidified. Twenty-one such examples were found in testing the plasma of 1000 group N donors (Beattie and Zuelzer 1965). The presence of anti-M should be suspected when an agglutinin is found in the plasma of an ACD (or CPD) sample from a donor whose unacidified serum has no abnormal antibodies.

Anti-M *reacting only with glucose-treated red cells.* This was described by Reid and colleagues (1981). The antibody agglutinated M-positive red cells that had been incubated in 2% glucose for a minimum of 2 h at 37°C or for substantially longer periods at low temperatures. It also agglutinated red cells from patients with diabetes mellitus. Red cells that had become agglutinable following glycosylation could be rendered unagglutinable by incubation in saline. The anti-M activity was totally inhibited by adding an equal volume of 1% glucose to the serum. Fourteen other examples of human anti-M were not inhibited by glucose. Another anti-M agglutinin reacted with red cells incubated with either glucose or galactose and was inhibited by 2% glucose, mannose or maltose (Morel et al. 1981).

Anti-M_1 is found as an additional specificity in about one in three sera containing anti-M; it has only rarely been found on its own. M_1 is commoner in black than in white people (Race and Sanger 1975).

*Immunoglobulin class of anti-*M. Of 10 examples of human anti-M, all were at least partly IgM (P Rubinstein personal communication), although naturally occurring anti-M may be solely IgG (Mollison 1972, fifth edn, p. 332). In a series of 45 cases, anti-M was at least partly IgG in 34, being solely IgM in the remainder (Smith and Beck 1977).

Most anti-M react more strongly in albumin than in saline: one example associated with HDN reacted as well at 37°C as at 4°C (Stone and Marsh 1959) and was subsequently shown to be IgG (Adinolfi et al. 1962).

Apart from one case of allo-anti-M (see Chapter 10) and one of auto-anti-N (see below), no examples of anti-M or anti-N have been shown to bind complement using ordinary serological methods. However, in an investigation with ^{125}I-labelled anti-Cad, a small amount of complement appeared to be bound by one example of IgM anti-M; two examples of IgG anti-M did not bind complement (Freedman et al. 1980).

Murine monoclonal antibodies to M and N are available. Two examples of anti-M were shown to react with different epitopes (see above); at room temperature, the antibodies had titres of 128–256 with M+ N– red cells and of eight with M– N+ cells (Nichols et al. 1985).

The reactions of monoclonal anti-M and anti-N, such as those of some polyclonal anti-M (see above), are greatly affected by pH. Testing the pH dependency of MN monoclonals is important because, in some instances, the specificity of agglutination reactions can be greatly improved by selection of the proper pH (Lisowska 1987).

Other non-human sources of anti-M

Good anti-M sera can be produced in rabbits (see Menolasino *et al.* 1954). The anti-M lectin prepared from the seeds of *Iberis amara* (candytuft) does not seem to be a useful reagent.

Allo-anti-N

Anti-N is rarer than anti-M; in a series of 86 000 (excluding patients on renal dialysis, see below), only two examples were found (B Croucher, personal communication).

Although naturally occurring, anti-N is typically an IgM cold agglutinin, inactive above a temperature of 20–25°C; one naturally occurring IgG anti-N has been encountered (ER Giblett, personal communication). It is very rare for anti-N to be formed as an immune antibody. The first example was described by Callender and Race (1946). In another case, IgG anti-N developed after multiple transfusions in a subject of phenotype M+ N– S– s– U– (Ballas *et al.* 1985).

The demonstration that the Ss glycoprotein carries 'N' antigen (see above) explains the fact that anti-N agglutinates M+ cells and also agglutinates trypsin-treated M+ cells, as the 'N' antigen on Ss glycoprotein is not destroyed by trypsin. As expected, anti-N does not react with M+ N–, S– s– red cells. Similarly, potent anti-N is found almost exclusively in S– s– subjects (Telischi *et al.* 1976; see also above).

Anti-N reacting only with glucose-treated red cells was found in three different sera (Morel *et al.* 1975). The reactions were inhibited by adding glucose to the serum. Glucose-dependent anti-N requires a determinant resulting from the reaction of glucose with the N-terminal amino acid of glycophorin A, but no sialic acid, for binding (Dahr *et al.* 1981; Morel *et al.* 1981).

Cold-reacting auto-anti-N

In screening 45 000 blood samples against M– N+ (or M+ N+) cells in the AutoAnalyzer, using a low-ionic-strength polybrene method, low-titre anti-N not detectable by manual methods was found in six M+ N+ subjects and in one M+ N subject; a more potent example was found in one M– N+ subject (Perrault 1973). The last example was remarkable in that it was IgG and could be detected by manual methods

only by using a 10–20% cell suspension, no agglutination being obtained with a 2% cell suspension. The antibody was active at 4°C but not at 12°C or at higher temperatures.

Anti-Nf developing in patients on chronic haemodialysis

Patients undergoing regular haemodialysis, irrespective of their MN phenotype, may develop anti-N, usually active at 20°C as well as 4°C, but never active at 37°C (Howell and Perkins 1972). The stimulus for anti-N production comes from small amounts of red cells left in dialysis equipment previously sterilized by formaldehyde treatment: an antigen 'Nf' develops. Exposure of M+ N– red cells to 0.06% formaldehyde induces Nf specificity after only 30 s at 37°C; at room temperature exposure to a concentration as low as 0.002% is sufficient to induce Nf specificity in 20 h (Gorst *et al.* 1977). In one series, anti-Nf was found in 68 out of 325 patients on renal dialysis, all of whom had been treated with a formaldehyde-sterilized dialyser (Fassbinder *et al.* 1978).

Although anti-Nf, being inactive at 37°C, is not expected to destroy transfused red cells, a case has been described in which the antibody appeared to be responsible for the rejection of a chilled transplanted kidney. When a second kidney from the same cadaver was perfused with warm saline before transplantation, grafting was successful (Belzer *et al.* 1971).

Anti-N lectins

Anti-N is present in the seeds of *Vicia graminea* and of *Bauhinea purpurea* var. *alba*. Of the two, the lectin of *V. graminea* is the more potent. The anti-N lectin from *V. graminea* reacts not only with N+ red cells but also with neuraminidase-treated red cells of all MN phenotypes; the receptor with which the lectin reacts is known as N_{vg}.

The lectin from *Moluccella laevis* carries anti-A and anti-N on the same molecule (Bird and Wingham 1970). The lectin also reacts strongly with T and Tn cells (Bird 1978).

Anti-N lectin from *V. graminea* reacts with both normal N and 'formaldehyde N' red cells but the lectin from *M. laevis* reacts only with normal N (of group B or O subjects) (Bird and Wingham 1977).

Anti-S, anti-s, anti-U

Anti-S has occasionally been found as a naturally occurring antibody, but is more commonly found as an immune antibody in patients who have received many transfusions.

Some examples of 'incomplete' anti-S can be detected much more readily by incubating serum and red cells at room temperature rather than at 37°C (Lalezari *et al.* 1973, see below). Although most examples of 'immune' anti-S are incomplete IgG antibodies, two examples behaving as saline agglutinins were found to be IgM (Adinolfi *et al.* 1962).

Antibodies to low-frequency antigens are commonly found in anti-S sera; of nine anti-S investigated with a collection of S-negative cells with rare phenotypes, seven were found to react with one or more cells and two sera contained 15 specificities each (A Lubenko and M Contreras, personal observations).

Anti-s is rare; it may be IgG or IgM.

In tests in an AutoAnalyzer, all of seven examples of anti-s and one of anti-U (all IgG) reacted more strongly at low temperatures. Similarly, using the IAT, three examples of anti-s and one of anti-S gave stronger reactions at low temperatures, whereas examples of anti-D, -K and -Fy^a reacted more strongly at 37°C (see also Chapter 8).

Anti-U is also rare; as a rule it is a non-complement-binding IgG antibody (Issitt 1981). The antibody is found exclusively in black people. There are two kinds of anti-U, one reacting with about 1.25% of black people and one with about 0.25%, i.e. 1% of black people have a U variant antigen (see Issitt 1990). Anti-U is occasionally encountered in frequently transfused patients with sickle cell disease.

Anti-S and anti-U were found to be IgG1 with or without other subclasses in 13 out of 17 examples tested. On the other hand, anti-s was found to be solely IgG3 in four out of five cases (Hardman and Beck 1981).

Other antibodies of the MNSs system

Anti-Vw and anti-M^g have frequencies of 1–2% and most commonly occur as agglutinins reacting more strongly at room temperature than at 37°C. Anti-Vw, which reacts only with Miltenberger class I cells (MLI), occasionally develops immune characteristics and its specificity then broadens to become anti-Mi^a

(reacting with Mi.I, II, III, IV and VI cells) (TE Cleghorn, personal communication).

As mentioned above, in Taiwan the frequency of Mi.III was found to be 7.3% and 'anti-Mi^a', i.e. an antibody reacting with Mi.III red cells but not tested with other Mi antigens, was found to be the most frequently occurring immune alloantibody (Broadberry and Lin 1994).

'Anti-En^a'

As mentioned above, there is no such antigen as En^a, although subjects who lack glycophorin A ['En (a–)'] may make a spectrum of antibodies, 'anti-En^a', which are directed against different portions of the glycophorin A molecule (Pavone *et al.* 1981; Vengelen-Tyler *et al.* 1981). Anti-En^a has only once been found as a naturally occurring antibody (Taliano *et al.* 1980), the other examples having been found following transfusion or pregnancy.

The term 'auto-anti-En^a' has been used to describe a heterogeneous group of related but not identical specificities, several of which recognize different portions of the MN sialoglycoprotein (Pavone *et al.* 1981). Auto-anti-En^a is found in certain patients with the warm antibody type of autoimmune haemolytic anaemia.

Clinical aspects

Most antibodies of the MNSs system are not active at 37°C and are thus of no clinical significance. Isolated examples of wider thermal amplitude have been shown to destroy test doses of incompatible red cells or cause HTRs, e.g. anti-M (Wiener 1950; see also Chapters 10 and 11); anti-Mi^a (Cutbush and Mollison 1958); anti-N (Ballas *et al.* 1985); anti-S (Cutbush and Mollison 1949) and anti-s (Fudenberg and Allen 1957; see also Chapter 10). Anti-U can cause immediate haemolytic transfusion reaction (IHTR) (Wiener *et al.* 1953) and DHTR, particularly in frequently transfused patients with sickle cell disease (Davies *et al.* 1986). HDN caused by MNSs antibodies is described in Chapter 12.

Antibodies to low-frequency antigens such as Vw are of negligible importance in blood transfusion because of the rarity of the corresponding antigen. One of the very few haemolytic transfusion reactions associated with antibodies to low-frequency antigens occurred in a patient who happened to be transfused more than once with blood from the same donor: a carrier of the low-frequency antigen Kamhuber (Speiser *et al.* 1966), later shown to be identical with Far (Giles 1977). Some examples of antibodies to the low-frequency antigens of the MNSs system, for example anti-M^g, -Vw, -Ri^a, -Dantu, -Hop and -Nob, have been naturally occurring; other examples, such as anti-Vw, Mt^a, Mit and -M^v, have been discovered in the serum of women whose infants have been affected with HDN. Whereas in blood transfusion the chance of receiving more than one unit carrying one of these antigens is very low when random blood donors are used, in women who have several children by a man who carries one of the antigens, the chance of allo-immunization is obviously far higher.

Mi.III is not a low-frequency antigen in Chinese in Taiwan and, there, a corresponding antibody is the commonest alloantibody encountered in patients (Broadberry and Lin 1994).

Cold-reacting anti-N and warm-reacting anti-U have been found as autoantibodies (see Chapter 7).

Venom from the Loxosceles spider induces intravascular haemolysis by rendering red cells susceptible to lysis by human complement. The mechanism by which this occurs appears to involve activation of an endogenous metalloproteinase, which cleaves glycophorins (GPA, B and C) from the red cell surface (Tambourgi *et al.* 2000, 2002). Evidence that GPA is an inhibitor of red cell lysis by autologous complement was reported by others (Okada and Tanaka 1983; Tomita *et al.* 1993).

The lutheran (Lu) system

The first example of an antibody revealing the existence of this system was found in a transfused patient (Callender *et al.* 1945).

About 8% of Europeans, Africans and North Americans are Lu(a+), but the antigen is rare or absent in other populations. Almost all Lu(a+) subjects have the genotype *Lu^{a}Lu^b*, the overall frequency of the genotype *Lu^{a}Lu^a* being only 0.15%. Virtually all other subjects (approximately 92% of the population) have the phenotype Lu(a– b+) (gene frequencies: Lu^a, 0.039; Lu^b, 0.961). Very rarely, subjects have the phenotype Lu(a– b–) (Crawford *et al.* 1961); the first example to be detected was found to be due to a dominant inhibitor gene, *In (Lu)*, which is the least uncommon genetic background of Lu(a– b–). Other examples of

this phenotype are due to a double dose of a recessive gene *Lu* or to an X-borne recessive inhibitor, XS2, of expression of the Lu antigens; *XS1* is the common allele permitting expression of Lu (see review by Crawford 1988). *In (Lu)* also inhibits the production of P$_1$, i, In^b and the high-incidence antigen, AnWj. Thus, antibodies which fail to react with Lu(a– b–) samples may not always belong to the Lutheran system.

Subjects with an *In (Lu)* gene are reported to have some red cell abnormalities. On incubation in plasma for 24 h, osmotic fragility decreases, owing to a reduction in total cation content (Udden *et al.* 1987). Although survival *in vivo* of autologous red cells is normal, lysis *in vitro* after 7 days' storage in Alsever's solution was five times that of normal red cells, and the subjects are presumably unsuitable as donors (Ballas *et al.* 1992).

With anti-Lu^b, Lu(a–b+) samples from newborn infants react more weakly than those from adults (Kissmeyer-Nielsen 1960), and Lu(a+b+) samples from newborn infants react very weakly indeed (Greenwalt *et al.* 1967).

Transient depression of Lu^a with the production of an antibody against a high-frequency Lu antigen has been observed in a patient with AITP (see Chapter 7).

In the numbered nomenclature, Lu^a is Lu1 and Lu^b is Lu2; Lu3 is an antigen present on all except Lu(a–b–) red cells. There are three pairs of antithetical antigens in addition to Lu1 and Lu2 which have been shown to be inherited at the Lu locus: Lu6 and Lu9; Lu8 and Lu14; Lu18 (Au^b) and Lu19 (Au^b). Only the latter pair are polymorphic; Lu6 and Lu8 are high-frequency antigens and Lu8 and Lu14, low. In addition to the aforementioned antigens, there are 10 high-frequency antigens (Lu4, Lu5, Lu7, Lu11, Lu12, Lu13, Lu16, Lu17, Lu20 and Lu21).

Using a sensitive radioimmunoassay, the main Lu antigens could not be detected on platelets (Dunstan *et al.* 1984) and, using immunofluorescence flow cytometry, Lu^b could not be detected on lymphocytes, monocytes or granulocytes (Dunstan 1986). On the other hand, the Lutheran glycoprotein is widely expressed in human tissues (Parsons *et al.* 1995).

Chemistry of Lutheran antigens

Using a murine monoclonal anti-Lu^b, two glycoproteins, a major protein of apparent mol. wt. 85 kDa and a minor protein of 78 kDa carrying Lu^b activity have been identified (Parsons *et al.* 1987). The 85-kDa form of the Lutheran glycoprotein comprises 597 amino acids with a large amino-terminal extracellular domain of 518 residues, a single membrane traverse and a small cytoplasmic domain of 59 residues (Parsons *et al.* 1995). The 78-kDa form has an alternatively spliced cytoplasmic domain of 19 residues and corresponds to a protein previously described as B-CAM (Rahuel *et al.* 1996). The extracellular domain of the Lutheran glycoprotein comprises five immunoglobulin superfamily domains (V– V– C2– C2– C2) and contains five potential sites for N-glycosylation, one on domain three and four on domain four (Parsons *et al.* 1995). The polymorphic antigens Lu^a/Lu^b and Au^a/Au^b are located on domains one and five, respectively, and arise from nucleotide substitutions that change a single amino acid (Lu^a/Lu^b, His77Arg; Au^a/Au^b,Thr539Ala: Parsons *et al.* 1997). Analysis of the location and structure of the other antigens in the Lutheran system has shown there are antigens on each of the five Ig domains and each is defined by nucleotide substitutions that encode single amino acid substitutions (Crew *et al.* 2003).

Lu^b activity has been reported in human red cell gangliosides, most of which contain the lactoneotetraosyl structure, as found in P_1 and Ii. This observation suggested that the inhibitor type of Lu(a– b–) might result from the action of a glycosyltransferase that adds an extraneous sugar to the backbone structure shared by the Lu, P_1, i antigens (Marcus *et al.* 1981) as well as by AnWj, In^a and In^b. These results are not readily explained given the dependence of Lu^a and Lu^b on amino acid sequence (see above). Nevertheless, altered glycosylation remains one of the more attractive explanations for the pleiotropic effect of *In(Lu)*.

Using a murine monoclonal anti-Lu^b the number of Lu^b sites per red cell was estimated to be about 2000–4000 on *Lu^bLu^b* cells and 1000–2000 on *Lu^aLu^b* cells (Merry *et al.* 1987).

The Lu^a antigen is destroyed by trypsin, chymotrypsin and pronase (Judson and Anstee 1977). Lutheran antigens are destroyed when red cells are treated with thiol reagents (DTT or AET: Levene *et al.* 1987), an observation consistent with antigenic structures located on Ig domains whose structures are defined by intrachain disulphide bonding.

Antibodies of the Lutheran system

Anti-Lu^a

This antibody usually occurs as an agglutinin, reacting more strongly at room temperature than at 37°C. Typically, although large agglutinates are formed, many cells are unagglutinated (Callender and Race 1946). Anti-Lu^a is most commonly IgM but may be IgG or a mixture of IgM and IgG, and may also be partly IgA. Of 19 examples, only three failed to agglutinate red cells suspended in saline and these three appeared to be solely IgG; of the remaining 16, at least nine were partly IgG and at least two partly IgA, as judged by the fact that agglutinating titres were enhanced by anti-IgG or anti-IgA respectively (A Lubenko, personal communication).

In a deliberate search for anti-Lu^a, only three examples were found in more than 18 000 donors (Greenwalt and Sasaki 1957). Attempts to stimulate the formation of the antibody by injecting Lu(a+) red cells have given apparently conflicting results. In one series, two out of eight patients developed anti-Lu^a 2–4 weeks after the transfusion of a single unit of blood, although the antibody was detectable only transiently (Mainwaring and Pickles 1948). In another series, in which four injections of relatively small amounts of blood were given at 3-monthly intervals to 12 subjects, none formed antibody (Race and Sanger 1954, p. 208). Perhaps the apparent discrepancy is explained by the fact that large amounts of red cells are required to induce immunization to Lu^a.

Anti-Lu^b

The first example of this antibody was found in an Lu(a+ b–) woman who had never been transfused but had had three previous pregnancies (Cutbush and Chanarin 1956). Anti-Lu^b is rare, as expected from the rarity of the Lu(a+ b–) phenotype; all examples have been found in patients who have either been pregnant or been transfused.

Most examples of anti-Lu^b appear to be mixtures of IgM and IgG. In one laboratory, 14 out of 16 examples agglutinated red cells in saline, the remaining two being solely IgG; of the 14 agglutinins all were enhanced by anti-IgG but only four were enhanced by anti-IgA (A Lubenko, personal observations). In another laboratory, all examples were at least partly

IgG although some may have been partly IgM; none was IgA (WL Marsh, personal communication).

Of 11 IgG anti-Lu[b], all were believed to be at least partly IgG4 (Hardman and Beck 1981). However, as most anti-Lu[b] are agglutinins and as IgG subclasses cannot be determined reliably on DTT-treated sera, the finding is difficult to confirm.

Anti-Lu[a]Lu[b] (anti-Lu3)

An antibody with this specificity in which the anti-Lu[a] and anti-Lu[b] activities were inseparable was found by Darnborough and colleagues (1963) in a woman of the rare phenotype Lu(a– b–). The antibody may have been immune as it was absent from the woman's serum before she had a transfusion 13 years previously and was also absent during a pregnancy that she had borne 6 years previously. This, and subsequently described examples of anti-Lu[a]Lu[b] reacted more strongly by IAT than by agglutination tests. The antibody seems to be made by subjects of the recessive type and not by those of the dominant type of Lu(a– b–).

Other Lutheran antibodies

Many other antibodies against high-frequency antigens, for example anti-Lu4, etc., have been described; all fail to react with Lu(a– b–) red cells but react with the red cells of other rare Lutheran phenotypes (Daniels 2002).

Two monoclonal antibodies detecting high-frequency antigens absent from red cells of the dominant type of Lu(a– b–) were later identified as anti-AnWj (Knowles et al. 1982).

Clinical aspects

Anti-Lu[a] has not been clearly incriminated as a cause of increased red cell destruction. In a patient whose plasma contained relatively potent anti-Lu[a], active at 37°C, ^{51}Cr-labelled Lu(a+) red cells (approximately 10 ml) survived normally (Greendyke and Chorpenning 1962); perhaps the antibody was solely IgM (non-complement binding) or IgG4. Anti-Lu[b] has very rarely caused a DHTR (see Chapter 11) but is not known to have caused HDN (Lu[b] is weakly expressed at birth). Examples of anti-Lu[b] that were at least partly IgG have destroyed test doses of Lu(a+ b+) cells only slowly (Cutbush and Mollison 1958; Tilley et al.

1977), with more rapid destruction of Lu(a– b+) cells (Cutbush and Mollison 1958; Peters et al. 1978). An IgG1 anti-Lu6 destroyed 80% of a test dose of incompatible red cells in 1 h; results with ^{51}Cr and flow cytometry agreed closely (Issitt et al. 1990).

An autoantibody to a high-frequency Lu antigen was associated with AIHA; the transfusion of 150 ml of least-incompatible blood caused chills, fever, dyspnoea and haemoglobinuria (Fitzsimmons and Caggiano 1981).

The Lutheran glycoprotein binds the basement membrane protein laminin 10/11. This interaction involves a binding site within the three amino-terminal Ig domains on Lutheran glycoprotein and the alpha 5 chain of laminin (Parsons et al. 2001; Kikkawa et al. 2002). Elevated levels of Lutheran glycoprotein are found on red cells from sickle cell patients (Udani et al. 1998) and, as sickle red cells adhere to alpha 5 chain containing laminin preparations (Hillery et al. 1996), it is possible that adherence of sickle red cells to laminin may be relevant to the vaso-occlusion occurring in vivo in patients with sickle cell disease.

The Di, Yt, Xg, Sc, Do, Co, Ch/Rg, Ge, Cr, Kn, In, Ok, Raph, JMH and GIL systems

Diego (Di)

The Diego system consists of two pairs of antithetical antigens, Di[a] and Di[b], and Wr[a] and Wr[b], and several low-frequency antigens, Wd[a], Rb[a], WARR, ELO, Wu, Bp[a], Mo[a], Hg[a], Vg[a], Sw[a], BOW, NFLD, Jn[a], KREP, Tr[a], Fr[a] and SW1, all carried on band 3 and the result of single amino acid substitutions in the protein sequence (reviewed in Daniels 2002).

Di[a] and Di[b]. The antibody revealing the existence of the antigen Di[a] was found in a woman whose infant was affected with HDN (Layrisse et al. 1955). It soon became apparent that Di[a] is relatively common (frequency 5–15%) in South American Indians and in most Mongoloid populations but is very rare in white people. Surprisingly, it has been found in about 0.5% of Poles, possibly reflecting invasion by Tartars (Kusnierz-Alejska and Bochenek 1992). More than 99.9% of white people are Di(b+); no Di(a– b–) subjects have been recognized through blood grouping studies but one individual is known who is homozygous for a band 3 mutation Val488Met (Band 3 Coimbra) that results in almost complete deficiency of band 3. Repeated blood transfusion was required during early childhood because of severe anaemia (Ribiero *et al.* 2000). Extensive analysis of the red cell membranes of this child revealed, in addition to band 3 deficiency, deficiency of protein 4.2, GPA, GPB, RhAG, Rh polypeptides, CD47 and LW glycoprotein (Bruce *et al.* 2003).

The number of Di^b sites on Di^bDi^b red cells was estimated to be 15 000 per cell (Masouredis *et al.* 1980b), although there are about 1×10^6 copies of band 3 per red cell. The substitution of Pro for Leu at amino acid 854 determines Di^b rather than Di^a (Bruce *et al.* 1994). Di^b was not detected on lymphocytes, monocytes or granulocytes (Dunstan 1986).

Most examples of anti-Di^a and anti-Di^b are found in association with pregnancy; both antibodies are often IgG1 + IgG3 (Zupanska *et al.* 1990). A naturally occurring example of anti-Di^a has been described (Steffey 1983) but anti-Di^b seems always to be immune; the first two examples could be detected only by IAT and, apparently, their reactions were not enhanced by complement (Thompson *et al.* 1967).

Clinical aspects

Anti-Di^a is known to have been responsible for many cases of HDN but has not been definitely shown to have caused an HTR. Anti-Di^b has only once been shown to have caused serious HDN (Ishimori *et al.* 1976), and infants may be completely unaffected (Habash *et al.* 1991). Only one HTR (delayed) has been described (Thompson *et al.* 1967).

Wr^a and Wr^b

Wr^a and Wr^b are antithetical antigens (Wren and Issitt 1988). Wra has an incidence of about 0.1% in white people; its incidence in other populations has not been extensively studied. All Wr(a–) subjects are Wr(b+), with the exception of those subjects who are GPA deficient. Wr^b is a site of interaction between band 3 and GPA. A mutation at amino acid 658 (Glu→Lys) on band 3 defines Wr^b and Wr^a respectively (Bruce *et al.* 1995). Mutations Gln63Lys (Jarolim *et al.* 1996) and Ala65Pro (Poole *et al.* 1999) in GPA cause abnormal Wr^b expression. It is not known whether GPA is required for the expression of Wr^a. About 70 000 Wr^a sites were found on Wr(a+ b–) and Wr(a+ b+) red cells; the number of Wr^b sites on Wr(a+ b+) cells was

150 000–350 000 and on Wr(a– b+) cells was 500 000 (Ring 1992).

Anti-Wr^a is a relatively common naturally occurring antibody, being found in about 1% of all blood samples. It is often found in subjects who have formed other blood group antibodies and in patients with AIHA. Anti-Wr^a often agglutinates red cells in saline, reacting more strongly at room temperature than at 37°C, but is frequently incomplete. Of 44 examples of anti-Wr^a, 16 were solely IgM, nine were partly IgM and 19 were solely IgG (Lubenko and Contreras 1992). The antibody was solely IgG1 in nine out of nine examples (Hardman and Beck 1981). For a description of murine monoclonal anti-Wr^a, see Ring and co-workers (1994).

Anti-Wr^b was first described in a Wr(a+ b–) subject (Adams *et al.* 1971). The antibody has also been found as a separable specificity, together with 'anti-En^a', in the serum of En(a–) subjects who were also Wr(a– b–) (Pavone *et al.* 1978). Anti-Wr^b occurs relatively commonly as an autoantibody in AIHA (see Chapter 7). Many examples of murine monoclonal anti-Wr^b have been described (see Daniels 2002).

Clinical aspects

Anti-Wr^a has caused haemolytic transfusion reactions (van Loghem *et al.* 1955; Metaxas and Metaxas-Bühler 1963) and HDN (Holman 1953). A mild DHTR has been described in an En(a–) patient with anti-Wr^b and 'anti-En^a' (Furuhjelm *et al.* 1973). Auto-anti-Wr^b has been responsible for fatal haemolysis (Dankbar *et al.* 1987).

Cartwright (Yt)

Yt^a is a very common antigen, being found on the red cells of all but 2 per 1000 white people; an allelic antigen, Yt^b, is present in about 8% of white people; approximate gene frequencies: Yt^a, 0.956; Yt^b, 0.044 (Daniels 2002).

Yt^a and Yt^b are found on the GPI-linked red cell glycoprotein acetylcholinesterase (AChE). The difference between the two antigens is determined by a single amino acid substitution at position 322: histidine for Yt^a and asparagine for Yt^b (Bartels *et al.* 1993).

Yt^a was found to be absent from lymphocytes, monocytes and granulocytes (Dunstan 1986).

Many examples of anti-Yt^a have been described but anti-Yt^b is rare. Both antibodies may be found following transfusion or pregnancy; naturally occurring examples have not been described.

Anti-Yt^a may be partly IgG (Bergvalds *et al.* 1965) or wholly IgG. Some examples bind complement (e.g. Bettigole *et al.* 1968); others do not (e.g. Göbel *et al.* 1974). Of 4 out of 14 examples of anti-Yt^a that could be typed with subclass antisera, all were solely IgG4 (Vengelen-Tyler and Morel 1983). Of 16 other examples, 13 could be typed and of these two were solely IgG4 and three partly IgG4; 11 were partly IgG1 but none was IgG3 (Pierce *et al.* 1980).

Only a few examples of anti-Yt^b have been reported.

Clinical aspects

Some examples of anti-Yt^a can destroy test doses of Yt(a+) red cells (Bettigole *et al.* 1968) but others cannot (Dobbs *et al.* 1968). In patients in whom the antibody had first been detected less than 6 weeks previously, the MMA was positive (more than 3% reactive monocytes) in 24 out of 30; of eight who were transfused with Yt(a+) blood, three with a negative MMA had no adverse reaction; of five with a positive MMA, two had a mild DHTR. A positive MMA was significantly less common (6 out of 33) in patients in whom anti-Yt^b had been detected more than 6 weeks previously. Of 10 of these who were transfused with Yt(a+) blood, the only patient with a positive MMA had a mild DHTR (Eckrich *et al.* 1995). Yt antibodies are not known to have caused HDN.

Xg

The great interest of this blood group system lies in the fact that the relevant genes are carried on the X chromosome so that males have only one gene for this system instead of the pair of genes that they have for all the other known blood group systems. Up to the present only one antigen, determined by the allele Xg^a, has been described. An allele, Xg, which may be amorphic, is postulated.

Females may be Xg^aXg^a, Xg^aXg or $XgXg$ but males can only be Xg^a or Xg. Thus males who are Xg(a+) pass on Xg^a to all their daughters but cannot transmit an Xg gene to their sons; the mating of an Xg(a+) man with an Xg(a–) woman must produce all Xg(a+) daughters and Xg(a–) sons. The frequency of the phenotype Xg(a+) is about 89% in females and 67% in males (Race and Sanger 1968, p. 523). Gene frequencies: Xg^a 0.659; Xg, 0.341. In males these are also the genotype and phenotype frequencies; in females genotype frequencies are: Xg^aXg^a, 0.434; Xg^aXg, 0.450; $XgXg$, 0.116.

The Xg^a antigen, which is probably a sialoglycoprotein, is inactivated by treatment with proteases (Habibi *et al.* 1979). Immunoblotting indicates a molecular weight of 22.5–28 kDa (Herron and Smith 1989). DNA sequencing predicts that the Xg^a glycoprotein has 180 amino acids with a signal sequence, an extracellular amino terminal domain containing several potential O-glycosylation sites but no potential N-glycosylation sites, a single transmembrane domain and a small cytoplasmic carboxy-terminal domain (Ellis *et al.* 1994). The glycoprotein appears late in erythropoiesis after band 3 and glycophorin A (Daniels and Green 2000).

X-inactivation or 'lyonization' is the phenomenon occurring in very early embryonic life in which one of the two X chromosomes (maternal or paternal) is inactivated in a given cell and in all the subsequent progeny of that cell. However, the *Xg* locus is not subject to inactivation, (for references, see Race and Sanger 1975), suggesting that it is on the pseudoautosomal region of the X chromosome (but see below). During meiosis, the X and Y chromosomes undergo pairing although only a limited length of the chromosomes is involved. Most of the human genes known to escape X-inactivation have a homologue on the Y chromosome. These genes may be of autosomal origin and are referred to as pseudoautosomal (see review by Rappold 1993). Cloning of *Xg* has shown that exons 1–3 are on the pseudoautosomal region of X and exons 4–10 are on the X-specific region, i.e. *Xg* spans the pseudoautosomal boundary (Ellis *et al.* 1994). The Xg protein shares considerable sequence homology with CD99, the product of the *MIC2* gene. *MIC2* is pseudoautosomal and situated upstream of *Xg*. In order to explain a phenotypic relationship between CD99 and Xg^a, Goodfellow and co-workers (1987) proposed that *MIC2* and *Xg* are regulated by the same locus. Uchikawa and co-workers (1995) described the presence of anti-CD99 in two female unrelated Japanese blood donors.

Xg^a develops late in fetal life (Toivanen and Hirvonen 1973). It has been estimated that in adults there are about 9000 sites per red cell in one study

(Szabo *et al.* 1977) and 159 sites per red cell in another (Fouchet *et al.* 2000). The expression of Xg^a was found to decline exponentially with red cell age, with a $T_{1/2}$ of 47 days (Campana *et al.* 1978).

Most examples of anti-Xg^a have been found in males, presumably because the frequency of Xg(a–) is three times higher than in females; some examples of anti-Xg^a activate complement (Mann *et al.* 1962). A potent example of a complement-binding anti-Xg^a was found to be of IgG1 and IgG2 subclasses (Devenish *et al.* 1986). An example of anti-Xg^a capable of agglutinating red cells suspended in saline has been described (Metaxas and Metaxas-Bühler 1970).

Up to 1986, 36 examples of anti-Xg^a were known to Ruth Sanger (personal communication) and at least 10 of these were naturally occurring. One example of anti-Xg^a has been shown not to cause red cell destruction (Sausais *et al.* 1964). Anti-Xg^a has never been incriminated as a cause of a HTR or HDN; it has once been described as an autoantibody.

Scianna (Sc)

Three antigens are recognized: Sc1, which has a very high frequency, an allelic antigen Sc2, which has a frequency of about 0.01 in northern Europe, and Sc3, which is absent only from red cells of the null phenotype Sc: –1, –2, –3. Gene frequencies in white people are: *Sc1*, 0.992; *Sc2*, 0.008 (Daniels 1995).

Sc1 and Sc2 are carried on a red cell membrane glycoprotein of 60 kDa. Intact disulphide bonds are necessary for full expression of the antigens and the presence of one or more complex *N*-glycans is needed for the expression of Sc2 (Spring *et al.* 1990). Sc alloantibodies do not fix complement and are not known to occur naturally. The *Radin (Rd)* antigen was suspected of belonging to the Sc system, partly because it is on a protein of molecular weight of about 60 kDa, closely resembling the Sc glycoprotein (Spring 1993) and partly because of genetic linkage evidence (Lewis *et al.* 1980). Anti-Rd has caused mild to moderate HDN (Rausen *et al.* 1967). It is now clear that Sc antigens and Rd are carried on ERMAP (erythrocyte membrane-associated protein) and that Sc2 results from a Gly57Arg substitution, whereas Rd results from a Pro60Ala substitution (Wagner *et al.* 2003). The high incidence antigen STAR results from Glu 47 Lys in ERMAP (Hue-Roye *et al.* 2004).

There is only a little evidence about the immuno-

genicity of Sc2. The original example of anti-Sc2 (which was detectable by IAT) was found in a man who had been transfused on a single occasion with 3 units of blood. Amongst 14 Sc: –2 subjects injected with Sc2 red cells four made anti-Sc2 (Seyfried *et al.* 1966). Sc2 appears to be very much less immunogenic than D: of 19 D-negative, Sc: –2 subjects given two or more injections from a D-positive, Sc: 2 donor, eight formed anti-D and only one of these also made anti-Sc2 (Mollison, unpublished results). Of the 11 who failed to make anti-D, none made anti-Sc2.

The phenotype Sc: –1,–2,–3 is very rare, although a cluster of eight subjects with this phenotype was found in Papua New Guinea (Woodfield *et al.* 1986). An example of IgG anti-Sc3 was found in a transfused thalassaemic child; the antibody disappeared after splenectomy and was not stimulated by transfusion with Sc:1,–2 blood (Woodfield *et al.* 1986). Naturally occurring antibodies within the Sc system have not been described.

Sc1 is absent from lymphocytes, monocytes and granulocytes (Dunstan 1986).

Clinical aspects

Sc antibodies have never been known to cause an HTR; an example of anti-Sc3 cleared a test dose of Sc1 red cells with a $T_{1/2}$ of less than 3 days but the antibody soon disappeared and did not become detectable again after further stimulation (McCreary *et al.* 1973). One example of an IgG3 anti-Sc1, detected in a pregnant woman, led to a positive direct antiglobulin test (DAT) in the infant but not to HDN (Kaye *et al.* 1990) and an example of anti-Sc2 caused mild HDN (DeMarco *et al.* 1995). Anti-Sc1 has been found as an autoantibody in a healthy donor (McDowell *et al.* 1986) and, possibly, in a patient with Evans-like syndrome (Steane *et al.* 1982).

Dombrock (Do)

Approximately 66% of northern Europeans are Do(a +) and 82% are Do(b+). Gene frequencies: *Do^a*, 0.42; *Do^b*, 0.58. The frequency of Do^a is somewhat lower in black people and much lower in mongoloids.

The antigens Gy^a (Gregory), Hy (Holley) and Jo^a, all with an incidence of more than 99%, also belong to the Do system. Gy(a–) is inherited as a recessive character; Gy(a–) red cells also lack Hy and Jo^a and are Do(a– b–), i.e. they are Dombrock-null (Banks *et al.*

1995), Gy^a, Hy and Jo^a, like Do^a and Do^b, are carried on the same GPI-linked glycoprotein with a molecular weight of approximately 50 kDa (Banks *et al*. 1992). The Dombrock glycoprotein is a member of the ADP-ribosyltransferase gene family and encoded by a gene on chromosome 12p (Gubin *et al*. 2000). The molecular bases of Dombrock antigens are described by Reid (2003).

No naturally occurring antibodies within the Do system have been described. Anti-Do^a, -Dob, -Gy^a and -Hy are all IgG and fail to bind complement (for references, see Daniels 2002).

Clinical aspects

The antibodies of this system are rare and usually weak, although examples of anti-Do^a have been shown to shorten the survival of a test dose of incompatible red cells (Polesky and Swanson 1966) and to cause immediate HTRs (Judd and Steiner 1991) and anti-Do^b has been the cause of both immediate and delayed haemolytic reactions (Moheng *et al*. 1985; Halverson *et al*. 1994). Anti-Gy^a has caused severe transfusion reactions, although without definite evidence of red cell destruction (Moulds *et al*. 1975). One example of anti-Hy (which did not bind complement) cleared 50% of a test dose of red cells with a half-time of 3.5 days and the remainder with a half-time of 15 days (Hsu *et al*. 1975); another caused a severe IHTR (Beattie and Castillo 1975). There is no evidence about the clinical significance of anti-Jo^a (see Issitt 1985, pp. 400 and 405). It is doubtful if Dombrock system antibodies cause HDN, although one suspicious case (involving anti-Do^a) has been reported (Roxby *et al*. 1994).

Colton (Co)

About 99.8% of white people are Co(a+) and about 8% are Co(b+), although in a Latin American population the frequency of Co(b+) was 4.6% (Issitt *et al*. 1987). Gene frequencies in most white people are: Co^a, 0.959; Co^b, 0.041. The antigen Co3 is present on all except Co(a– b–) red cells. In black people, no Co(a–) sample was found among 1706 subjects (Race and Sanger 1975).

Colton antigens are carried on the water transporter protein, aquaporin1 (AQP-1, synonym: channel-forming integral protein, CHIP) (Smith *et al*. 1994). The unglycosylated protein has a molecular weight of 28 kDa and the glycosylated protein one of 40–60 kDa (Denker *et al*. 1988). Colton polymorphism is determined by an amino acid difference at position 45 of the protein: alanine for Co^a and valine for Co^b (Smith *et al*. 1994). AQP-1 is one of the few mammalian transport proteins for which the three-dimensional structure has been resolved (Mitsuoka *et al*. 1999); it occurs in the membrane as a tetramer, with one monomer in each tetramer having an N-glycan. Individuals with the rare Co(a– b–) phenotype have mutations preventing expression of an active protein (Preston *et al*. 1994; Chretien and Cartron 1999; Joshi *et al*. 2001) and impaired urinary concentrating ability (King *et al*. 2001).

Monosomy of chromosome 7 (on which *Co* genes are located) is associated with acute myeloid leukaemia and pre-leukaemia and is often associated with weakening or absence of Co^a and Co3 (De la Chapelle *et al*. 1975; Boetius *et al*. 1977).

The Co^a antigen was not detected on lymphocytes, monocytes or granulocytes (Dunstan 1986).

Anti-Co^a is usually IgG although an IgM example has been reported (Kurtz *et al*. 1982); anti-Co^b is rarer and may be found in sera containing other alloantibodies. Anti-Co3 is found only in Co(a– b–) subjects. Both anti-Co^b (Lee and Bennett 1982) and anti-Co3 (Lacey *et al*. 1987) may bind complement; the latter antibody was lytic.

Clinical aspects

Anti-Co^a has been responsible for a DHTR, with haemoglobinuria (Kitzke *et al*. 1982) and for severe HDN (Simpson 1973), and anti-Co^b for an IHTR (Lee and Bennett 1982) and a DHTR (see Chapter 11). The example of anti-Co3 mentioned above, which was haemolytic *in vitro*, caused severe HDN (Lacey *et al*. 1987). A patient with a novel form of congenital dyserythropoietic anaemia with persistent embryonic and fetal globins and absence of CD44 had less than 10% of normal AQP-1 levels and very low osmotic water permeability but no mutation in *AGP-1* (Agre *et al*. 1994).

Chido/Rodgers (Ch/Rg)

Ch and Rg are antigenic determinants on the complement C4 component (O'Neill *et al*. 1978) and are thus antigens of plasma adsorbed on to red cells. Ch and Rg determinants can be demonstrated on a tryptic C4d fragment (Plate 3.6; Tilley *et al.* 1978). The C4 poly-morphism is controlled by two genes, *C4A* and *C4B*, which are thought to have arisen by duplication. Most Rg antigens are encoded by *C4A* and most Ch antigens by *C4B*. *Chido*, *Rodgers* and *HLA* are closely linked on chromosome 6 (Middleton *et al.* 1974; Giles *et al.* 1976). Rg-negative individuals are almost always HLAAl-B8-DR3 (Giles *et al.* 1976; James *et al.* 1976).

Red cells normally carry only small amounts of C4d passively adsorbed from plasma and it is therefore not surprising that reactions of anti-Ch and anti-Rg with normal red cells are usually weak. Conversely, if red cells and serum are incubated at low ionic strength, for example by adding ACD blood to a relatively large volume of 10% sucrose, which causes large amounts of C4 (and C3) to be deposited on the red cell surface, the resulting cells are strongly agglutinated by anti-Ch and anti-Rg provided that the corresponding antigens are present in the plasma (Tilley *et al.* 1978). The reactions of anti-Ch and anti-Rg with Ch-positive and Rg-positive red cells are inhibited by the addition of Ch-positive and Rg-positive plasma respectively. The antigenic determinants of C4 are very stable in stored plasma and serum and can be used to determine Ch/Rg groups in inhibition assays (Swanson *et al.* 1971; Middleton and Crookston 1972).

In patients with cold haemagglutinin disease, the red cells carry increased amounts of C4d and therefore react strongly with anti-Ch and anti-Rg when both Ch and Rg are present in the patient's plasma (Tilley *et al.* 1978).

All normal individuals are either Ch positive and/or Rg positive: 95% are Ch+ Rg+, 3% are Ch+ Rg– and 2% are Ch– Rg+ (Middleton and Crookston 1972; Longster and Giles 1976); $C4_{null}$ individuals are Ch–Rg– (O'Neil *et al.* 1978) and $C4_{null}$ genes are found in most patients with systemic lupus erythematosus (SLE) (see review by Moulds 1993).

Anti-Ch and anti-Rg are found only as immune anti-bodies, in the plasma of Ch- or Rg-negative subjects. Anti-Ch is found twice as commonly as anti-Rg (Giles 1985). Neither anti-Ch nor anti-Rg can cause red cell destruction. Of four anti-Ch tested in an automated antiglobulin test, all had a strong IgG4 component and three were partly IgG2; one was partly IgG1 and partly IgM (Szymanski *et al.* 1982).

Two mouse monoclonal anti-C4d reagents were found to have specificities related to Rgl and Chl rather than C4A and C4B (see Giles 1989).

Clinical aspects

Small volumes of ^{51}Cr-labelled Ch+ red cells have been shown to survive normally in subjects with anti-Ch (Tilley *et al.* 1975; Silvergleid *et al.* 1978). Even if anti-Ch and anti-Rg were capable of causing red cell destruction, they would not be expected to cause haemolytic transfusion reactions except when washed red cells were transfused, because the antigens are present in the plasma as well as on the red cells and thus neutralize the antibodies. Ch+ blood has been transfused to patients with potent anti-Ch without producing signs of haemolysis (Nordhagen and Aas 1979). On the other hand, there are two reports of acute anaphylactic reactions, characterized by severe hypotension and dyspnoea, following transfusions of plasma or platelet concentrates, one in a patient with precipitating IgG anti-Rg and one in a patient with an IgG4 anti-Ch. Both patients had had many previous transfusions (Lambin *et al.* 1984; Westhoff *et al.* 1992).

Gerbich (Ge)

There are eight antigens in the Ge system: Ge2, Ge3 and Ge4 have a very high frequency; Ge5 (Wb), Ge6 (Ls^a), Ge7 (An^a), Ge8 (Dh^a) and GEIS have a low frequency (Daniels *et al.* 2004). The antigens are carried on glycophorins (GP) C or D, or both. GPC and GPD are products of a single gene, but GPD is a truncated product, resulting from translation of the gene at an alternative initiation site later than the normal site of initiation (Le Van Kim *et al.* 1987; High *et al.* 1989). Consequently, GPD lacks the terminal 21 amino acids of GPC. The molecular weights of GPC and GPD have been estimated to be about 40 kDa and 30 kDa respectively (see Reid 1989). There are 143 000 molecules of GPC per red cell and 225 000 of GPC + GPD (Smythe *et al.* 1994). Ge5, Ge7 and Ge8 result from point mutations in GPC, and Ls^a from duplication of exon 3 of GPC (for references, see Daniels 2002).

Three different types of the Ge-negative pheno-type occur (Leach, Yus and Gerbich); all three are characterized by absence of normal GPC and GPD, and absence of one of the high-incidence antigens. Glycophorin C gene is encoded by 4 exons; in the Leach phenotype, absence of glycophorins C and D is due to absence or marked alteration of exons 3 and 4 of glycophorin C gene (Telen *et al.* 1991; Winardi *et al.*

1993). In the Yus gene, exon 2 is missing and in Gerbich, exon 3 (High *et al.* 1989). In the Leach phenotype, some of the red cells are elliptocytes (for references, see review by Reid 1989).

Although Ge-negative subjects are excessively rare amongst white people, they are common in some parts of Papua New Guinea (Booth and McLoughlin 1972). The first three examples of anti-Ge came from pregnant or recently delivered women and were detected by the IAT. The infants born to all three women had a positive DAT but no evidence of haemolytic disease (Rosenfield *et al.* 1960). Of 15 examples of anti Ge, six were immune and nine naturally occurring; one of the latter, encountered in a previously untransfused male, agglutinated red cells at room temperature and had an indirect antiglobulin titre of 64 (McLoughlin and Rogers 1970). The high incidence of the Ge-negative phenotype in Papua New Guinea is likely to be the result of selection against malaria, as *Plasmodium falciparum* erythrocyte binding antigen 140(EBA-140) binds glycophorin C on normal red cells (Lobo *et al.* 2003; Maier *et al.* 2003).

Clinical aspects

Anti-Ge has not been known to cause a HTR, although an IgG1 example that gave positive reactions in a monocyte bioassay caused mild HDN (Sacks *et al.* 1985). Of 10 other examples of anti-Ge that could be typed with subclass antisera, nine were solely IgG1 (Vengelen-Tyler and Morel 1983). Anti-Ge has been described as an autoantibody involved in autoimmune haemolytic anaemia. In the third case to be reported, the antibody was IgA (Göttsche *et al.* 1990).

Murine monoclonal anti-Ge has been described (Rouger *et al.* 1983; Anstee *et al.* 1984). These antibodies react with determinants on GPC and, although not true anti-Ge, distinguish between Ge positives and negatives in agglutination tests.

The Ge antigen has not been detected on granulocytes (Gaidulis *et al.* 1985), or on lymphocytes or monocytes (Dunstan 1986).

Cromer (Cr)

The antigens Cr[a], Tc[a], Tc[b], Tc[c], Dr[a], WES[a], WES[b], Es[a], UMC, IFC, GUT1 and SERF are all carried on the decay-accelerating factor (DAF, CD55; Lublin *et al.* 2000; Storry *et al.* 2003; Banks *et al.* 2004; see also Chapter 3). Three of the antigens (Tc[b], Tc[c] and WES[a]) are of low frequency. All eleven antigens are destroyed by chymotrypsin but not by other proteolytic enzymes. Dr[a]-negative red cells have weak expression of all the other Cromer antigens because the mutation giving rise to the phenotype (Ser165Leu) also creates a new splice site so that two transcripts are produced, only one of which translates into a viable protein, which is itself expressed at low abundance (Lublin *et al.* 1994). Cromer antigens are present in urine and, possibly, plasma (Daniels 1983). The null phenotype, Inab, is devoid of all Cromer-related antigens. Inab cells completely lack DAF but other GPI-linked membrane proteins are present; the red cells are more susceptible than normal cells, but less susceptible than PNH red cells, to lysis by complement (Merry *et al.* 1989). Individuals with the Inab phenotype do not show signs of increased red cell destruction, although such signs are characteristic of individuals with PNH whose red cells lack not only DAF but also several other molecules of the family of glycoproteins, all of which are anchored to the cell membrane through glycosylated phosphatidylinositol (GPI) molecules (Rosse 1989). This property of PNH red cells is most likely to be attributable to the absence of CD59, as a Japanese individual with inherited deficiency of CD59 and normal DAF also had PNH-like symptoms (Yamashina *et al.* 1990). Three of five Inab individuals described had intestinal disorders, which may be related to the absence of DAF on the epithelial surface of intestinal mucosa in these individuals (Daniels 2002). Such a link is not proven but may reflect a greater susceptibility to cell damage as a result of infection when DAF is absent. Dr[a] is a receptor for 075X fimbria-like adhesin of uropathogenic *Escherichia coli* (Nowicki *et al.* 1988). DAF is also a receptor for echoviruses and coxsackieviruses (Powell *et al.* 1998).

Inab-negative individuals can make anti-IFC, which reacts with all except Inab cells. Several monoclonal antibodies have been found to react with all cells tested except Inab; the antibodies react weakly with Dr(a–) cells (Spring *et al.* 1987).

Clinical aspects

Antibodies to Cr antigens are mostly IgG and predominantly IgG1. The first example of anti-Cr[a] (Stroup and McCreary 1975), like all subsequently recognized examples, was found in a black person. In two cases, anti-Cr^a caused only dubious destruction of a test dose of incompatible red cells: in the first the T_{50}Cr was 14 days but the subject had rheumatoid arthritis (Smith *et al.* 1983); in the second, Cr survival at 96 h was 73%; survival was not followed further and the subject was transfused uneventfully 2 months later with Cr(a+) red cells (Ross and McCall 1985). In a third case, more than 40% of a test dose of Cr(a+) cells was destroyed within 4 h (McSwain and Robins 1988). In one patient with anti-Tc^a, the survival of a test dose of incompatible red cells at 24 h was probably within normal limits and a monocyte monolayer assay (MMA) was negative; at this time the antibody was a mixture of IgG2 and IgG4, although some years previously it had also been partly IgG1 and the results of an MMA had been higher than normal (Anderson *et al.* 1991). In another patient anti-Tc^a was thought to be the cause of a HTR (Kowalski *et al.* 1999). An example of anti-IFC destroyed about 60% of a test dose of incompatible red cells in 24 h (Walthers *et al.* 1983). Although some Cromer system antibodies have the capacity to destroy red cells, they are not known to have caused cases of HTR or HDN.

Knops (Kn)

The antigens Kn^a/Kn^b, McC^a/McC^b, Sl^a/Vil and Yk^a are located on the complement receptor CRl (CD35) and comprise the Knops system. The antigens vary in strength from one individual to another in relation to CR1 levels (Moulds *et al.* 1992). Approximate frequencies of the antigens in American black and white people are as follows: Kn^a, 0.988 and 0.980; McC^a, 0.936 and 0.985; Yk^a, 0.983 and 0.899 (Molthan 1983) and Sl^a, 0.606 and 0.977 (Lacey *et al.* 1980). McC^b is found only in black people, in whom the frequency of the antigen is about 0.45, and Kn^b is found only in white people (Daniels 2002). Kn^a, McC^a, Yk^a and Sl^a type as absent from red cells of the Helgeson phenotype, which have only about 10% of the normal number of CR1 molecules per cell (Moulds *et al.* 1992); the phenotype has a frequency of about 1%, in both black and white people. The molecular bases of McC^a/McC^b and Sl^a/Vil were determined by Moulds and co-workers (2001) and the antigens shown to result from single amino acid substitutions (Lys1590Glu and Arg1601Gly respectively) in the 24th complement control repeat domain in the fourth long homologous repeat of CR1.

Antibodies of the Knops system are usually found in transfused patients but can be evoked by pregnancy alone. They are IgG and non-complement binding (Molthan 1983). They have never been known to cause HTRs or HDN, or to shorten the survival of a test dose of incompatible red cells (see, for example, Tilley *et al.* 1977; Silvergleid *et al.* 1978; Daniels 1995). The antibodies are reported to give false-positive results in *in vitro* functional assays utilizing monocytes because they crosslink CR1 on red cells with CR1 on the monocytes (Hadley *et al.* 1999).

The term high-titre, low-avidity (HTLA) has in the past been applied to the antibodies of the Knops system and to certain other antibodies, also of no clinical significance but the description is not useful as not all of the antibodies concerned have high titres and not all have 'low avidity', a term which is, in any case, imprecise.

The Sl^a– phenotype is common in West Africa, where it appears to confer a selective advantage against *Plasmodium falciparum*. Sl^a– red cells are far less able to form rosettes around parasitized red cells than Sl^a+ red cells, and so the risk of vasocclusion and consequent cerebral malaria is reduced in individuals with the Sl^a– phenotype (Rowe *et al.* 1997; Cockburn *et al.* 2004).

Indian (In)

The In^a antigen has a frequency in Bombay Indians of about 3% (Badakere *et al.* 1974) but is almost unknown in races other than Indians and some Arabs. In the latter, the frequency of In^a may reach 10% or more (Badakere *et al.* 1980). In other populations, the allelic antigen In^b has an incidence of virtually 100%. In^a and In^b are located on CD44, a widely occurring glycoprotein with a molecular weight of 80 kDa, which acts as a cellular adhesion molecule and binds the extracellular matrix molecule hyaluron (Spring *et al.* 1988). In^a/In^b polymorphism depends on a point mutation at nucleotide 252 (Washington *et al.* 1994), which produces proline in In^a and arginine in In^b at amino acid 46.

In^b is one of the antigens regulated by In(Lu) (see p. 223) and its expression is reduced in Lu$_{null}$ cells from subjects with an *In (Lu)* gene (Spring *et al.* 1988).

Anti-In^a and anti-In^b often agglutinate untreated red cells but do not agglutinate enzyme-treated cells; reactions are strongest in the IAT (for references, see Daniels 2002).

Clinical aspects

In[a] is a potent immunogen: of 39 D–,In(a–) subjects who were immunized with D+,In(a+) red cells for anti-D production, 30 made anti-In[a] (Bhatia *et al.* 1980). An In(a– b+) multiparous woman with an In(a– b+) husband and In(a– b+) children made anti-In[a] after the transfusion of a single unit of In(a+) blood (Joshi *et al.* 1993).

Both anti-In[a] and anti-In[b] have caused the destruction of test doses of incompatible red cells (Bhatia *et al.* 1980; Ferguson and Gaal 1988). An immediate reaction (chills, breathlessness) after the transfusion of 50 ml of blood was ascribed to anti-In[b] but no evidence of increased red cell destruction was given (Joshi 1992). Neither anti-In[a] nor anti-In[b] is known to have caused HDN.

CD44 on macrophages binds *Mycobacterium tuberculosis* (Leemans *et al.* 2003). The chemokine RANTES which blocks HIV-1 infectivity by binding to the Duffy glycoprotein also binds to CD44 and can under certain conditions enhance HIV-1 infectivity through this pathway (Roscic-Mrkic *et al.* 2003).

Anton (AnWj)

AnWj is a high-frequency antigen that is either located on an isoform of CD44 or closely associated with it (Telen *et al.* 1993). For this reason, it is convenient to mention it here, even although it does not belong in the Indian system.

The AnWj–phenotype is usually acquired although it may also be inherited (Poole *et al.* 1991). All newborn infants are AnWj– (see below). AnWj is expressed only very weakly on red cells of individuals with the dominant gene *In (Lu)*.

AnWj has been shown to be a red cell receptor for *Haemophilus influenzae*, the main agent for bacterial meningitis in infants (van Alphen *et al.* 1986). This receptor and the AnWj antigen appear between 3 and 46 days after birth; conversion takes only 24 h (Poole and van Alphen 1988).

Anti-AnWj may occur as an autoantibody (Marsh *et al.* 1983) or as an alloantibody; one allo-anti-AnWj was a mixture of IgG1, weak IgG3, IgM and IgA; it fixed complement and reacted equally well with untreated and with papain-treated red cells (Harris *et al.* 1986); another (an apparent alloantibody) was described in a patient with a transient loss of the AnWj antigen (Mannessier *et al.* 1986).

Clinical aspects

In one patient, anti-AnWj caused chills and haemoglobinuria (De Man *et al.* 1992). If patients with anti-AnWj need transfusion, In(Lu) Lu_null red cells are most suitable (Daniels 1995). As expected from the fact that the AnWj antigen is not present at birth, the antibody is not known to have caused HDN.

Ok[a]

The Ok[a] antigen is located on CD147, also known as EMMPRIN. This glycoprotein, a member of the immunoglobulin (Ig) superfamily, is encoded by a gene on chromosome 19pter–p13.2. It has a glycosylated amino-terminal extracellular domain of 187 amino acids, comprising two Ig domains, a single transmembrane domain and a cytosolic domain of 40 amino acids. The glycoprotein has a wide tissue distribution and is reported to function in a wide variety of adhesive interactions and to regulate matrix metalloproteinase production and function (Spring *et al.* 1997; Toole 2003). There is evidence that HIV-1 entry into cells depends on an interaction between virus-associated cycophilin A and CD147 on the target cell (Pushkarsky *et al.* 2001). Treatment of mice with F(ab')2 fragments of anti-CD147 causes selective trapping of erythrocytes in the spleen and anaemia (Coste *et al.* 2001). Three Ok(a–) individuals had a Glu92Lys substitution in the amino-terminal Ig domain of the glycoprotein (Spring *et al.* 1997). The corresponding antibody has been shown to be capable of clearing incompatible red cells (Morel and Hamilton 1979) but is not known to have caused an HTR or HDN.

Raph

The MER 2 antigen of the Raph system is located on the tetraspanin CD151. This protein is encoded by a gene on chromosome 11p15.5. Tetraspanins function as facilitators for the assembly of protein complexes in cell membranes. CD151 forms strong associations in kidney with the laminin-binding integrins α3β1 in glomerulus and α6β1 in tubules. CD151-integrin association is mediated by the second extracellular loop on CD151. A Turkish blood donor who typed as MER2 negative and had allo-anti-MER2 in her serum had a single amino acid substitution (Arg178His) in the second extracellular loop. Three Indian Jews with MER2-negative red cells and allo-anti-MER2 in their serum had a nucleotide insertion (G383) in *CD151*, which introduced a premature stop signal at codon 140. The resultant protein would lack the integrin binding region of CD151. All three had end-stage renal failure with defects in glomerular and renal tubular basement membranes (Crew *et al.* 2004).

JMH

The JMH antigen is located on CDw108, also known as semaphorin 7A. This GPI-linked glycoprotein, encoded by a gene on chromosome 15q23–24, has a large cysteine-rich extracellular domain of 606 amino acids with five potential glycosylation sites. The semaphorin family of proteins is involved in a wide variety of functions including cell migration and adhesion. Semaphorin 7A is a potent monocyte activator. It also appears to be involved in lymphocyte development and activation. Its function on red cells is unknown (Yamada *et al.* 1999; Holmes *et al.* 2002). The corresponding antibody is found mainly in old people in whom the antigen has been lost from the red cells. The antibody is of no clinical significance (see, for example, Sabo *et al.* 1978); all of 14 examples were at least partly IgG4 (Tregellas *et al.* 1980).

GIL

The high-incidence GIL antigen is located on aquaporin 3, a glycerol transporter encoded by a gene on chromosome 9 at 9p13. The GIL-negative phenotype results from an inactivating mutation in the *AQP3* gene (Roudier *et al.* 2002).

Collections of antigens

This term has been introduced to describe specificities that are connected in one of the following ways (Daniels *et al.* 2004): (1) *serological*, i.e. dosage results supporting a genetic relationship; or altered expression of some, if not all, of the antigens in certain phenotypes; or antigen absence in apparent 'null' phenotypes; (2) *biochemical*, i.e. studies of epitope structures; and (3) *genetic*, i.e. family or population studies.

Collections that have already been described are I (collection 207), Glob (collection 209) and Le^c, Le^d (collection 210), see Chapter 4. Two more are described here.

Cost (Cs, Collection 205)

The antigens Cs^a and Cs^b have long been thought to be related to the antigens of the Kn system discussed above, mainly because corresponding antibodies have similar serological properties, described as high titre, low avidity (see above). However, there is no evidence that the Cost antigens are genetically related to the Knops system, and they could not be demonstrated on CR1 (Petty 1993).

Cs^a has a frequency of about 0.988 in American black people and of about 0.952 in American white people (Molthan 1983). Anti-Cs^a has never been shown to destroy red cells (see Issitt 1985).

Er (Collection 208)

Er^a has a frequency of more than 99.9% and Er^b, its apparent allele, one of less than 1% (Daniels 1995). Examples of anti-Er^a have been IgG and have not activated complement (Daniels *et al.* 1982; Thompson *et al.* 1985). Anti-Er^a has no clinical significance: it failed to shorten the survival of a test dose of incompatible red cells (Thompson *et al.* 1985) and failed to cause HTR in one case and to cause HDN in another (Daniels *et al.* 1982).

Other antigens with a very high or very low incidence

Antigens with a very high incidence

Many antigens that occur on the red cells of almost all human subjects (i.e. H, Rh29, LW, k, Kp^b, Lu^b, Yt^a and Scl) belong to one of the systems or (P) to one of the collections of antigens, and have already been described. Further antigens, not known to be related to any others, and in most cases found in more than 999 of every 1000 individuals (Sd^a is an exception), are described here. AnWj, a member of the series, has been described in the section on the Indian system.

If a patient in need of a blood transfusion is found to have an antibody reacting with a high-incidence antigen, the specificity should be identified, as it may then be possible to find an antigen-negative blood for transfusion from a panel of donors of rare groups (e.g. WHO, American Red Cross) or a bank of frozen red cells (American Red Cross, Council of Europe). A simpler way of searching for compatible red cells is to test siblings and close relatives. It should be added that, of the antigens described below, only two (anti-Vel and anti-Lan) are known to have caused an HTR and none is known to have caused HDN that is severe enough to need treatment.

Vel

Of the first two examples of anti-Vel described, one was an agglutinating antibody and the other haemolytic (Sussman and Miller 1952; Levine *et al.* 1955). Another haemolytic example had apparently been formed as an immune response to transfusion. A later transfusion provoked a rigor, lumbar pain and anuria. Six relatives of the propositus were also Vel negative (Ve(a–)); none of them had anti-Vel in their serum (Levine *et al.* 1961). Anti-Vel may be partly IgG but has not been associated with HDN (Stiller *et al.* 1990); it has been found as an autoantibody (Szalóky and van der Hart 1971).

The Vel antigen was not detected on lymphocytes, monocytes or granulocytes (Dunstan 1986).

Sid (Sd^a) and Cad

About 91% of English people have Sd(a+) red cells. Anti-Sd^a, when mixed with Sd(a+) cells, gives a characteristic pattern of agglutination with compact agglutinates in a sea of unagglutinated cells. Only about 1% of samples react strongly; about 80% show distinct small agglutinates and about 10% react very weakly with only occasional tiny agglutinates (Pickles and Morton 1977). Sd^a is not demonstrable on cord blood red cells and begins to be detectable only at about the age of 10 weeks. In pregnancy there is a weakening of the Sd^a antigen (Pickles and Morton 1977).

The Sd^a antigen is present in most secretions, with the greatest concentration in urine. Approximately 50% of the people with Sd(a–) red cells secrete Sd^a in the urine (Morton *et al.* 1970), i.e. 96% of English people are Sd(a+).

In urine, the Sd^a determinants are on Tamm–Horsfall glycoprotein, carrying 1–2% terminal N-acetylgalactosamine linked β1→4 to Gal. In Sd(a–) subjects, GalNAc is virtually absent from this glycoprotein (Soh *et al.* 1980).

Anti-Sd^a. Of the 4% of people who are Sd(a–), about one-half (i.e. about 1–2% of the population) have demonstrable anti-Sd^a in their serum (Renton *et al.* 1967; Morton *et al.* 1970); the antibody is generally IgM. Most examples of anti-Sd^a react with saline suspensions of red cells at 20°C and 37°C, and may fix complement. The antibody can also be detected with enzyme-treated cells (occasional sera, when fresh, haemolyse enzyme-treated cells) and by the antiglobulin test (Pickles and Morton 1977).

Anti-Sd^a is of no clinical significance although one example caused some destruction of a small sample of red cells with a very strongly expressed Sd^a antigen (Petermans and Cole-Dergent 1970).

Cad is an antigen of very low frequency associated with polyagglutinability (Cazal *et al.* 1968), due to the presence of anti-Cad in almost all samples of human serum (Gerbal *et al.* 1976).

Cad red cells react very strongly with anti-Sd^a, which led to the conclusion that Cad is simply a strong form of Sd^a (Sanger *et al.* 1971). However, although Sd^a and Cad determinants have the same terminal trisaccharide, this sequence is differently linked in the two determinants. Cad red cells have strongly expressed Sd^a in addition to the specific Cad pentasaccharide (see review by Watkins 1995).

Cad red cells and cells which are moderately strongly Sd^a+, even when group O, are agglutinated by *Dolichos bifiorus* lectin. Although this reaction of the lectin and that with group A$_1$ red cells are both inhibited by N-acetylgalactosamine (GalNAc), the specificities are not identical since in Sd^a the GalNAc is β-linked and in A is α-linked (see review by Watkins 1995). A candidate gene encoding the glycosyltransferase (Sd(a) beta1, 4GalNAc transferase), which adds a terminal GalNAc residue to alpha2,3-sialylated acceptor substrates to create Sd^a and Cad antigen, was cloned by Montiel and co-workers (2003). The gene is highly expressed in colon and to a lesser extent in kidney, stomach, ileum and rectum. Renal tubular cells synthesize Tamm–Horsfall glycoprotein (THP), the most abundant glycoprotein in urine. THP expresses Sd^a antigen activity (see review by Watkins 1995) and binds to type 1 fimbriated *E. coli* to prevent the bacteria from binding to the urinary tract causing urinary tract infection (Pak *et al.* 2001). In the gut Sd^a activity increases from the ileum to the colon, in contrast with ABH activity, which decreases from ileum to colon. The extreme diversity of carbohydrate structures on mucins in the gut is thought to provide binding sites for a wide range of micro-organisms, preventing the organisms from infecting the underlying epithelia (Robbe *et al.* 2003).

Cad-positive(Sd^a+++) red cells are relatively resistant

to invasion by *P. falciparum* (Cartron *et al.* 1983). As the Sd^a gene would add GalNAc to sialylated *O*-glycans on glycophorins A, B, C and D, all of which are known to be receptors for the parasite, it seems reasonable to suppose that the additional glycosylation impedes access to the glycophorins and hence entry.

Other high-incidence antigens
(see Daniels 2002)

Lan. The corresponding antibody has caused a severe HTR (van der Hart *et al.* 1961) and mild HDN (Smith *et al.* 1969).

At^a. The corresponding antibody has destroyed test doses of incompatible red cells (Sweeney *et al.* 1995; Ramsey et al. 1995) but is not known to have caused an HTR or HDN.

Jr^a. The corresponding antibody has been shown to clear a small dose of incompatible red cells from the circulation in 24 h (Kendall 1976) but has not caused an HTR and has caused only mild HDN (Nakajima and Ito 1978).

Duclos. This is possibly located on RhAG, as the antigen is absent only in Rh$_{null}$ or Rh$_{mod}$ subjects who are also U negative and also in the subject, Mme Duclos, in whom anti-Duclos was found.

Emm PEL, ABTI and MAM. These are the other high-incidence antigens belonging to the 901 series. Anti-MAM caused HDN (Montgomery *et al.* 2000). Antibodies to the other antigens have not been shown to be clinically significant.

Antigens with a very low incidence

Antigens with a low incidence are found in several blood group systems, for example Rh, MNSs, Lu, In, etc. but the term 'low-frequency antigens' is applied to those with a frequency of less than 1%, which are neither part of a recognized blood group system nor related closely enough to any other antigens to merit 'collection' status. About 20 such antigens, with a frequency of less than one in 400 in white people, are included in the 700 series (Daniels 2002). Some have frequencies greater than one in 400 in certain non-Caucasian populations or even in isolated Caucasian populations. The list (in ISBT number order) is as follows: By, Chr^a, Bi, Bx^a, To^a, Pt^a, Rea, Je^a, Hey, Li^a, Milne, RASM, Ol^a, JFV, Kg, JONES, HJK, HOFM, SARA, LOCR, REIT and SHIN (Daniels 2002)

Some low-frequency antigens stimulate the production of maternal antibodies, leading to a positive DAT in the fetus or to HDN. An example of hydrops fetalis due to anti-HJK, treated successfully by intrauterine transfusion, has been reported (Rouse *et al.* 1990).

In general, low-frequency antigens are unimportant in blood transfusion, as it is so easy to find compatible donors for patients with the corresponding antibodies. The antibodies pose a potential hazard when blood is selected simply on the basis of screening the patient's serum against red cells carrying all common antigens, followed by abbreviated crossmatch or a computer crossmatch. In an infant receiving a series of transfusions from a single donor, the consequences are theoretically more serious but, in practice, the hazard from antibodies to low-frequency antigens is a very small one.

Antibodies to low-frequency antigens tend to be present in sera used for blood grouping, as these sera may be derived from hyperimmunized donors in whom such antibodies are often present (see below). Sera containing anti-E and anti-S are notorious for having antibodies to low-frequency antigens, but even polyclonal anti-A and anti-B may have them. The presence of these unwanted antibodies may have serious consequences; for example, an antibody to a low-frequency antigen in an anti-Rh D reagent might lead to a D-negative woman who was positive for the antigen concerned being misgrouped as D positive. Of course, problems of this kind do not arise when monoclonal reagents are used.

In sera from patients with autoimmune haemolytic anaemia, it is not uncommon to find antibodies to several low-frequency antigens. Cleghorn (1960) noted that anti-Sw^a, -Wr^a and -By, as well as -Vw, -Mi^a, -M^g and -C^x, might be present. In another series, one or more antibodies to low-frequency antigens were found in 30% of patients with AIHA (Salmon and Holmberg 1971).

Antibodies to low-frequency antigens were found more commonly in D-negative donors hyperimmunized to Rh D than in control subjects, suggesting that such antibodies may be made when the immune system is stimulated by alloantigens as well as by autoantigens (Contreras *et al.* 1979). Multiple antibodies to low-frequency antigens are also not uncommon in normal donors. One donor was found to have as many as 27 such antibodies and many other normal donors to have between 6 and 15 (M Contreras, personal observations).

HLA antigens detectable on red cells

HLA antigens were first demonstrated on reticulocytes by showing that these cells, but not mature red cells, would adsorb cytotoxic antibodies (Harris and Zervas 1969). It seems likely that HLA antigens on mature red cells represent the remnant of antigens present in greater amount on nucleated red cells, using monoclonal antibodies to common determinants of HLA class I and II, by either radioimmunoassay or flow cytometry, red cells of 50% of donors bound HLA-A, -B and -C but not HLA-DR antibodies (Rivera and Scornik 1986). The number of HLA sites on mature red cells was found to be 40–550 per cell, with a median value of 78 (Botto et al. 1990); in contrast, the number on T lymphocytes was about 100 000 per cell and on B lymphocytes about 260 000 per cell (Trucco et al. 1980).

Of the HLA antigens regularly present on red cells, A28 and B7 are the most strongly expressed, followed by B8 and B17 (Nordhagen 1978). HLA-A10 (Morton et al. 1971) as well as A9, B12 and B15 (Nordhagen 1977) are also sometimes recognizable.

The first leucocyte antigen to be demonstrated unequivocally on the red cells was HLA-B7 (Seaman et al. 1967) and it has subsequently become apparent that individuals with B7 on their lymphocytes always express measurable amounts of this antigen on their red cells (Rivera and Scornik 1986). HLA-B7 subjects also have about four times as many HLA class I sites as are found in other subjects (Botto et al. 1990). A weakly reacting red cell antigen, Bg[a], is intimately related to HLA-B7 (Morton et al. 1969). Bg[b] (much less common in white people than Bg[a]) corresponds to HLA-B7 and Bg[c] with HLA-A28 (Morton et al. 1971). Subsequent work showed that red cells carrying Bg[c] also reacted with anti-HLA-A2, a not unexpected observation, as the antigens A2 and A28 are known to crossreact (Norhagen and Ørjasaeter 1974). The molecular basis of this crossreactivity is the presence of glycine at position 62 on the α-domain of the heavy chain (Takemoto et al. 1992).

HLA class I antigens can be removed from the red cell membrane by chloroquine treatment (Swanson and Sastamoinen 1985); the procedure may be useful in identifying antibodies or grouping red cells when using sera containing Bg antibodies.

Increased expression of HLA antigens on red cells

Occasional normal subjects with strongly expressed HLA antigens on the red cells have been described. In one such subject, when the red cells were crossmatched with serum containing HLA antibody, the antiglobulin test (anti-IgG only) was strongly positive. The HLA antigens detectable were A2, B7 and BW40. If the red cells were incubated with cytotoxic HLA antibodies of more than one specificity, complement as well as IgG was bound (van der Hart et al. 1974). In the first of two other cases, with HLA groups A1,2; B8,17, all but HLA A1 could be recognized on the red cells by IAT. In the second donor (HLA A2,11; B5,40), B5 and B40 were particularly strongly expressed on the red cells (Nordhagen 1979).

In healthy subjects, red cells with strongly expressed HLA antigens must be very rare. In a deliberate search only five examples were discovered over a period of several years (P Rubinstein, personal communication).

Increased expression of HLA antigen on red cells in disease. In SLE, the mean number of HLA sites on red cells is almost three times as high as in normal subjects (Botto et al 1990). Bg antigens (see above) are more reactive in patients with leukaemia, lymphoma, polycythaemia, megaloblastic anaemia and haemolytic anaemia; other HLA-related antigens that are of low incidence on the red cells of normal donors are found in much higher incidence in these patients (Morton et al. 1980).

Following an attack of infectious mononucleosis the red cells of HLA-B7 patients may show a greatly increased reactivity with the corresponding antibody; the increase is found from about the third week of the illness and thereafter decreases slowly over a period of months or years. The cause of this phenomenon is not yet known. There is no evidence that the less dense, i.e. youngest, red cells in the circulation react any more strongly than the rest (Morton et al. 1977).

Agglutination due to HLA antigens on red cells

Unwanted positive results in crossmatching due to HLA are common because HLA-A28 and -B7 are so commonly present on red cells and because the corresponding antibodies are frequently present in sera: anti-HLA-B7 (anti-Bg[a]) has been found in the serum of about 1.5% of the general patient population (Marshall 1973; Eska and Grindon 1974) and in more than 10% of multiply transfused patients (M Contreras, personal observations). It is important to ensure that typing sera, particularly polyclonal anti-D, are free of anti-HLA (Pavone and Issitt 1974).

Clinical aspects

HLA antibodies have not often been incriminated as a cause of HTRs or of HDN. Some examples of HLA antibodies do not affect the survival of red cells on which corresponding antigens are expressed (Silvergleid *et al.* 1978), although in a few instances accelerated destruction has been found. After injecting red cells on which HLA antigens were exceptionally strongly expressed into the circulation of a patient with an incompatible cytotoxic HLA antibody, a two-component curve of elimination was observed, about 60% of the cells being removed with a $T_{1/2}$ of about 100 min and the rest with a $T_{1/2}$ of 20 h (van der Hart *et al.* 1974). A two-component curve of elimination was also observed when red cells with very strongly expressed HLA-28 were injected into a patient whose serum contained anti-HLA-28: 20% of the cells were removed with a $T_{1/2}$ of 1.5 days, the rest having a more or less normal survival (Nordhagen and Aas 1978; see Fig. 10.11). Similarly, the data published by Panzer and co-workers (1984), relating to their cases 1 and 2, show about 25% destruction in the first 24 h, with more or less normal survival of the remaining cells, although the data were not interpreted in this way by the authors. Benson and co-workers (2003) describe a case of DHTR followed by acute HTR they attributed to the presence of anti-HLA (anti-HLA-A2, A28, B7, B7 crossreactive group) in the patient's serum. Subsequent transfusion with one irradiated unit from an HLA-compatible donor was uneventful. The full red cell antigen phenotype of the patient and the units transfused was not provided.

Membrane abnormalities involving red cell antigens

Sialic acid deficiency

En(a–) and M^kM^k red cells have been described earlier in this chapter; T and Tn red cells are described in Chapter 7.

An abnormality detected in some Melanesians in Papua New Guinea with South-East Asian ovalocytosis

In about 15% of Melanesians in coastal areas of Papua New Guinea, there is hereditary ovalocytosis (South-East Asian ovalocytosis, SAO) and the following red cell antigens are depressed: I^T, I^F, C, D, e, LW, Kp^b, Jk^a, Jk^b, S, s, En^a, Di^b, Wr^b, Xg^a and Scl; the following are not depressed: A_1, I^D, i, P1, k, Fy^a, MN, Lu^b, Co^a, Ge and Vel (Booth *et al.* 1977). The phenotype results from a small deletion encoding nine residues in band 3 at the point of insertion of the first transmembrane domain. The result of this mutation is an abnormally folded band 3, which does not function as an anion transport protein (for a review, see Bruce and Tanner 1999). Subjects with SAO are heterozygous for the mutant band 3 gene. Individuals homozygous for this mutation have not been described and it is likely to be lethal in the absence of regular transfusion therapy (Liu *et al.* 1994). SAO confers resistance to cerebral falciparum malaria (Allen *et al.* 1999). The cause of the depression of so many red cell antigens is unknown but may be related to the effect of the abnormal band 3 protein on other associated proteins in the red cell membrane. SAO cells contain linear arrangements of intramembranous particles (probably band 3 aggregates) not found in normal cells (Che *et al.* 1993). SAO is not confined to Melanesians and has been found in a Mauritian family of Indian descent, an African-American family, two South African kindreds and a white family (Bruce and Tanner 1999).

HEMPAS red cells

Patients with hereditary erythroblastic multinuclearity with a positive acidified serum test (HEMPAS) have red cells which, at 15–20°C, are agglutinated (and lysed) by an IgM antibody present in the serum of most normal subjects. The red cells exhibit various other abnormalities such as a greatly increased reactivity with anti-i and an increased sensitivity to complement (Crookston *et al.* 1969a,b). H is depressed (Bird and Wingham 1976). For reviews, see Crookston and Crookston (1982) and Delaunay and Iolascon (1999). Band 3 and GPA have aberrant glycosylation in HEMPAS (Mawby *et al.* 1983; Zdebska *et al.* 2000). Altered glycosylation of band 3 may account for the elevated expression of i antigen (Fukuda *et al.* 1990) and altered glycosylation of GPA the increased sensitivity to complement (Tomita and Parker 1994).

Paw and co-workers (2003) describe a zebrafish mutant with an erythroid-specific defect in cell division resulting in dyserythropoiesis similar to that seen in human congenital dyserythropoietic anaemia type II (HEMPAS). The erythroblasts were binuclear and had 'double membranes' in around 11% of binucleated cells. The defect giving rise to this phenotype was shown to result from mutations in the band 3 gene. The authors conclude that band 3 is required for proper segregation of the chromosomes during anaphase. In man, band 3 is encoded by a gene (*SLC4A1*) on chromosome 17q12-q21 but most cases of HEMPAS map to chromosome 20q11.2 (Delaunay and Iolascon 1999) suggesting that additional genes are involved.

Rh null, Kx negative (McLeod syndrome), Ge negative (Leach phenotype). These red cell abnormalities, which are associated with the absence of normal red cell membrane proteins, have been described earlier.

Other abnormalities involving red cell antigens

See Chapter 3.

References

Adams J, Broviac M, Brooks W *et al.* (1971) An antibody, in the serum of a Wr(a+) individual, reacting with an antigen of very high frequency. Transfusion 11: 290

Adinolfi M, Polley MJ, Hunter DA *et al.* (1962) Classification of blood-group antibodies as β_2M or gamma globulin. Immunology 5: 566

Advani H, Zamor J, Judd WJ *et al.* (1982) Inactivation of Kell blood group antigens by 2-amino-ethylisothiouronium bromide. Br J Haematol 51: 107–115

Agre P, Smith BL, Baumgarten R *et al.* (1994) Human red cell Aquaporin CHIP. II. Expression during normal fetal development and in a novel form of congenital dyserythropoietic anemia. J Clin Invest 94: 1050–1058

Allen FH, Lewis SJ (1957) Kp^a(Penney), a new antigen in the Kell blood group system. Vox Sang 2: 81

Allen FH Jr, Diamond LK, Niedziela B *et al.* (1951) A new blood-group antigen. Nature (Lond) 167: 482

Allen SJ, O'Donnell A, Alexander ND *et al.* (1999) Prevention of cerebral malaria in children in Papua New Guinea by southeast Asian ovalocytosis band 3. Am J Trop Med Hyg 60: 1056–60

van Alphen L, Poole J, Overbeeke M *et al.* (1986) The Anton blood group antigen is the erythrocyte receptor for *Haemophilus influenzae*. FEMS Microbiol Lett 37: 69–71

Anderson G, Gray LS, Mintz PD (1991) Red cell survival studies in a patient with anti-Tc^a. Am J Clin Pathol 95: 87–90

Anstee DJ (1980) Blood group MNSs-active sialoglycoproteins of the human erythrocyte membrane. In: Immunobiology of the Erythrocyte. SG Sandler, J Nusbacher, MS Schanfield (eds). Progress in Clinical and Biological Research 43: 67–98. New York: Alan R. Liss

Anstee DJ (1981) The blood group MNSs-active sialoglycoproteins. Semin Hematol 18: 13–31

Anstee DJ, Mawby WJ, Tanner MJA (1979) Abnormal blood-group-Ss-active sialoglycoproteins in the membrane of Miltenberger class III, IV and V human erythrocytes. Biochem J 183: 193–203

Anstee DJ, Mawby WJ, Tanner MJ (1982) Structural variations in human erythrocyte sialoglycoproteins. In: Membranes and Transport, a Critical Review. A. Martonosi (ed.). New York: Plenum Press

Anstee DJ, Ridgwell K, Tanner MJA *et al.* (1984) Individuals lacking the Gerbich blood group antigen have alterations in the human erythrocyte membrane sialoglycoproteins β and γ. Biochem J 221: 97–104

Badakere SS, Parab BB, Bhatia HM (1974) Further observations on the In^a (Indian) antigen in Indian populations. Vox Sang 26: 400–403

Badakere SS, Vasantha K, Bhatia HM *et al.* (1980) High frequency of In^a antigen among Iranians and Arabs. Hum Hered 30: 262–263

Ballas SK, Dignam C, Harris M *et al.* (1985) A clinically significant anti-N in a patient whose red cells were negative for N and U antigens. Transfusion 25: 377–380

Ballas SK, Marcolina MJ, Crawford MN (1992) *In vitro* storage and *in vivo* survival studies of red cells from persons with the In(Lu) gene. Transfusion 32: 607–611

Banks JA, Parker N, Poole J (1992) Evidence to show that Dombrock (Do) antigens reside on the Gy^a/Hy glycoprotein (Abstract). Transfus Med 2 (Suppl. 1): 68

Banks JA, Hemming N, Poole J (1995) Evidence that the Gy^a, Hy and Jo^a antigens belong to the Dombrock system. Vox Sang 68: 177–182

Banks J, Poole J, Ahrens N *et al.* (2004) SERF: a new antigen in the Cromer blood group system. Transfusion Med 14: 31318

Barnwell JW, Nichols ME, Rubinstein P (1989) *In vitro* evaluation of the role of the Duffy blood group in erythrocyte invasion by *Plasmodium vivax*. J Exp Med 169: 1795–1802

Bartels CF, Zelinski T, Lockridge O (1993) Mutation at codon 322 in human cholinesterase (ACHE) gene accounts for YT blood group polymorphism. Am J Hum Genet 52: 928–936

Baum J, Ward RH, Conway DJ (2002) Natural selection on the erythrocyte surface. Mol Biol Evol 19: 223–229

Beattie KM, Castillo S (1975) A case report of a hemolytic transfusion reaction caused by anti-Holley. Transfusion 15: 476

Beattie KM, Zuelzer WW (1965) The frequency and properties of pH-dependent anti-M. Transfusion 5: 322

Behzad O, Lee CL, Gavin J et al. (1973) A new anti-erythrocyte antibody in the Duffy system: anti-Fy4. Vox Sang 24: 337–342

Belzer FO, Kountz SL, Perkins HA (1971) Red cell cold autoagglutinins as a cause of failure of renal transplantation. Transfusion 11: 422

Benson K, Agosti SJ, Latoni-Benedetti GE et al. (2003) Acute and delayed hemolytic transfusion reactions secondary to HLA alloimmunization. Transfusion 43: 753–757

Bergvalds H, Stock A, McClure PD et al. (1965) A further example of anti-Yt^a. Vox Sang 10: 627

Bettigole R, Harris JP, Tegoli J et al. (1968) Rapid in vivo destruction of Yt(a+) red cells in a patient with anti-Yt^a. Vox Sang 14, 143

Bhatia HM, Badakere SS, Mokashi SA et al. (1980) Studies on the blood group antigen In^a. Immunol Commun 9: 203–215

Bird GWG (1978) The application of lectins to some problems in blood group serology. Rev Fr Transfus Immunohématol 21: 103

Bird GWG, Wingham J (1976) The action of seed and other reagents on HEMPAS erythrocytes. Acta Haematol 55: 174

Bird GWG, Wingham J (1977) Anti-N antibodies in renal dialysis patients. Lancet i: 1218

Bird GWG, Wingham J (1970) Agglutinins for antigens of two different human blood group systems in the seeds of Moluccella laevis. Vox Sang 18: 235

Boetius G, Hustinx TWJ, Smits APT et al. (1977) Monosomy 7 in two patients with a myeloproliferative disorder. Br J Haematol 37: 101–109

Booth PB, McLoughlin K (1972) The Gerbich blood group system, especially in Melanesians. Vox Sang 22: 73

Booth PB, Serjeantson S, Woodfield DG et al. (1977) Selective depression of blood group antigens associated with hereditary ovalocytosis among Melanesians. Vox Sang 32: 99

Botto M, So AK-L, Giles CM et al. (1990) HLA class I expression on erythrocytes and platelets from patients with systemic lupus erythematosus, rheumatoid arthritis and from normal subjects. Br J Haematol 75: 106–111

Branch DR, Petz LD (1980) A new reagent having multiple applications in immunohematology (Abstract). Transfusion 20: 642

Broadberry RE, Lin M (1994) The incidence and significance of anti-Mi^a in Taiwan. Transfusion 34: 349–352

Broadberry RE, Lin M (1996) The distribution of the MiIII (Gp.Mur) phenotype among the population of Taiwan. Transfusion Med 6: 145–148

Bruce LJ, Tanner MJA (1999) Erythroid band 3 variants and disease. Baillière's Clin Haematol 12: 637–654

Bruce LJ, Anstee DJ, Spring FA et al. (1994) Band 3 Memphis variant II. Altered stilbene disulfonate binding and the Diego (Di^a) blood group antigen are associated with the human erythrocyte band 3 mutation Pro854→Leu. J Biol Chem 269: 16155–16158

Bruce LJ, Ring SM, Anstee DJ et al. (1995) Changes in the blood group Wr (Wright) antigens are associated with a mutation at amino acid 658 in human erythrocyte band 3: a site of interaction between band 3 and glycophorin A in the red cell membrane under certain conditions. Blood 85: 541–547

Bruce LJ, Beckmann R, Ribiero ML et al. (2003) A band 3-based macrocomplex of integral and peripheral proteins in the RBC membrane. Blood 101: 4180–4188

Bruce LJ, Pan RJ, Cope DL et al. (2004) Altered structure and anion transport properties of band 3 (AE1, SLC4A1) in human red cells lacking glycophorin A. J Biol Chem 279: 2414–2420

Callender STE, Race RR (1946) A serological and genetical study of multiple antibodies formed in response to blood transfusion by a patient with lupus erythematosus diflusus. Ann Eugen (Camb) 13: 102

Callender S, Race RR, Paykoç ZV (1945) Hypersensitivity to transfused blood. BMJ ii: 83

Campana T, Szabo, Piomelli S et al. (1978) The Xg^a antigen on red cells and fibroblasts. Cytogenet Cell Genet 22: 524

Cartron JP, Prou O, Luilier M et al. (1983) Susceptibility to invasion by Plasmodium falciparum of some human erythrocytes carrying rare blood group antigens. Br J Haematol 55: 639–647

Chaudhuri A, Polyakova J, Zbrzezna V et al. (1993) Cloning of glycoprotein D cDNA, which encodes the major subunit of the Duffy blood group system and the receptor for the Plasmodium vivax malaria parasite. Proc Natl Acad Sci USA 90: 10793–10797

Cazal P, Monis M, Caubel J et al. (1968) Polyagglutinabilité héréditaire dominante: antigène privé (Cad) correspondant à un anticorps public et à une lectine de Dolichos biflorus. Rev franç Transfus 11: 209

Che A, Cherry RJ, Bannister LH et al. (1993) Aggregation of band 3 in hereditary ovalocytic red blood cell membranes. Electron microscopy and protein rotational diffusion studies. J Cell Sci 105 (Pt 3):655–660

Cheek RF, Harmon JV, Stoewll CP (1995) Red cell alloimmunization after a bone allograft. Transfusion 35: 507–509

Chen V, Halverson G, Wasniowska K et al. (2001) Direct evidence for the existence of Miltenberger antigen. Vox Sang 80: 230–233

Chown B (1949) Never transfuse a woman with her husband's blood. Can Med Assoc J 61: 419

Chretien S, Cartron JP (1999) A single mutation inside the NPA motif of aquaporin-1 found in a Colton-null phenotype. Blood 93: 4021–4023

Cleghorn TE (1960) The frequency of the Wr[a], By and M[g] blood group antigens in blood donors in the South of England. Vox Sang 5: 556

Cockburn IA, Mackinnon MJ, O'Donnell A et al. (2004) A human complement receptor 1 polymorphism that reduces *Plasmodium falciparum* rosetting confers protection against severe malaria. Proc Natl Acad Sci USA 101: 272–277

Contreras M, Barbolla A, Lubenko A et al. (1979) The incidence of antibodies to low frequency antigens (LFA) in plasmapheresis donors with hyperimmune Rh antisera. Br J Haematol 41: 413

Coombs RRA, Mourant AE, Pace RR (1946) *In vivo* isosensitization of red cells in babies with haemolytic disease. Lancet i: 264

Corcoran PA, Allen FH, Lewis M et al. (1961) A new antibody, anti-Ku (anti-Peltz) in the Kell blood-group system. Transfusion 1: 181

Coste I, Gauchat JF, Wilson A et al. (2001) Unavailability of CD147 leads to selective erythrocyte trapping in the spleen. Blood 97: 3984–3988

Crawford MN (1988) The Lutheran blood group system: serology and genetics. In: Blood Group Systems: Duffy, Kidd and Lutheran. Arlington, VA: Am Assoc Blood Banks

Crawford MN, Greenwalt TJ, Sasaki T et al. (1961) The phenotype Lu(a–b) together with unconventional Kidd groups in one family. Transfusion 1: 228

Crew VK, Green C, Daniels G (2003) Molecular bases of the antigens of the Lutheran blood group system. Transfusion 43: 1729–1737

Crew VK, Burton N, Kagan A et al. (2004) CD151, the first member of the tetraspanin (TM4) superfamily detected on erythrocytes, is essential for the correct assembly of human basement membranes in kidney and skin. Blood 104: 2217–2223

Crookston JH, Crookston MC (1982) HEMPAS: clinical, hematologic and serologic features. In: Blood Groups and Other Red Cell Surface Markers in Health and Disease. C. Salmon (ed.). New York: Masson Publishing

Crookston JH, Crookston MC, Burnie K et al. (1969a) Hereditary erythroblastic multinuclearity associated with a positive acidified-serum test: a type of congenital dyserythropoietic anaemia. Brit J Haematol 17: 11

Crookston JH, Crookston MC, Rosse WF (1969b) Red cell membrane abnormalities in hereditary erythroblastic multinuclearity. Blood 34: 844

Cutbush M, Chanarin I (1956) The expected blood-group antibody anti-Lu[b]. Nature (Lond) 178: 855

Cutbush M, Mollison PL (1949) Haemolytic transfusion reaction due to anti-S. Lancet ii: 102

Cutbush M, Mollison PL (1950) A new human blood group. Nature (Lond) 165: 188

Cutbush M, Mollison PL (1958) Relation between characteristics of blood-group antibodies *in vitro* and associated patterns of red cell destruction *in vivo*. Br J Haematol 4: 115

Dahr W (1992) The Miltenberger subsystem of the MNSs blood group system. Review and outlook. Vox Sang 62: 129–135

Dahr W, Uhlenbruck G, Leikola J et al. (1978) Studies on the membrane glycoprotein defect of En(a–) erythrocytes: III. N-terminal amino acids of sialoglycoproteins from normal and En(a–) erythrocytes. J Immunogenet 5: 117

Dahr W, Gielen W, Beyreuther K et al. (1980a) Structure of the Ss blood group antigens. I. Isolation of Ss-active glycopeptides and differentiation of the antigens by modification of methionine. Hoppe-Seyler's Z Physiol Chem 361: 145–152

Dahr W, Beyreuther K, Steinbach H et al. (1980b) Structure of the Ss blood group antigens. II. A methionine/threonine polymorphism within the N-terminal sequence of the Ss glycoprotein. Hoppe-Seyler's Z Physiol Chem 361: 895–906

Dahr W, Metaxas-Bühler M, Metaxas MN et al. (1981) Immunochemical properties of M[g] erythrocytes. J Immunogenet 8: 79–87

Dahr W, Kordowicz M, Moulds J et al. (1987) Characterization of the Ss sialoglycoprotein and its antigens in Rh[null] erythrocytes. Blut 54: 13–24

Danek A, Rubio JP, Rampoldi L et al. (2001) McLeod neuroacanthocytosis: genotype and phenotype. Ann Neurol 50: 755–764

Daniels GL (1983) Characteristics of Cromer related antibodies (Abstract). Transfusion 23: 410

Daniels G (1995) Human Blood Groups. Oxford: Blackwell Science

Daniels GL (2002) Human Blood Groups, 2nd edn. Oxford: Blackwell Science

Daniels GL, Fletcher A, Garratty G et al. (2004) Blood group terminology 2004: from the International Society of Blood Transfusion committee on terminology for red cell surface antigens. Vox Sang 87: 304–316

Daniels GL, Green C. (2000) Expression of red cell surface antigens during erythropoiesis. Vox Sang 78 (Suppl. 1): 149–153

Daniels GL, Judd WJ, Moore BPL et al. (1982) A 'new' high frequency antigen Er[a]. Transfusion 22: 189–193

Dankbar DT, Pierce SR, Issitt et al. (1987) Fatal intravascular hemolysis associated with auto anti-Wr[b] (Abstract). Transfusion 27: 534

Darnborough J, Firth R, Giles CM et al. (1963) A 'new' antibody anti-Lu[a]Lu[b] and two further examples of the genotype Lu(a–b–). Nature (Lond) 198: 796

Darnborough J, Dunsford I, Wallace JA (1969) The En[a] antigen and antibody: a genetical modification of human red cells affecting their blood grouping reactions. Vox Sang 17: 241

Davies SC, McWilliam AC, Hewitt PE et al. (1986) Red cell alloimmunization in sickle cell disease. Br J Haematol 63: 241–245

De la Chapelle A, Vuopio P, Sanger R et al. (1975) Monosomy-7 and the Colton blood groups (Letter). Lancet ii: 817

Delaunay J, Iolascon A (1999) The congenital dyserythropoietic anaemias. Baillière's Clin Haematol 12: 691–705

De Man AJM, van Dijk BA, Daniels GL (1992) An example of anti-AnWj causing haemolytic transfusion reaction. Vox Sang 63: 238

DeMarco M, Uhl L, Fields L et al. (1995) Hemolytic disease of the newborn due to the Scianna antibody, anti-Sc2. Transfusion 35: 58–60

Denker BM, Smith BL, Kuhadja FP et al. (1988) Identification, purification, and partial characterization of a novel M 28,000 integral membrane protein from erythrocytes and renal tubules. J Biol Chem 263: 15634–15642

Devenish A, Burslem MF, Morris R et al. (1986) Serologic characteristics of a further example of anti-Xg[a] and the frequency of Xg[a] in North London blood donors. Transfusion 26: 426–427

Dobbs JV, Prutting DL, Adebahr ME et al. (1968) Clinical experience with three examples of anti-Yf[a]. Vox Sang 15: 217

Donahue RP, Bias W, Renwick JH et al. (1968) Probable assignment of the Duffy blood group locus to chromosome 1 in man. Proc Natl Acad Sci USA 61: 949

Dunstan RA (1986) Status of major red cell blood group antigens on neutrophils, lymphocytes and monocytes. Br J Haematol 62: 301–309

Dunstan RA, Simpson MB, Rosse WF (1984) Erythrocyte antigens on human platelets. Absence of the Rhesus, Duffy, Kell, Kidd, and Lutheran antigens. Transfusion 24: 243–246

Durocher JR, Payne RC, Conrad ME (1975) Role of sialic acid in erythrocyte survival. Blood 45: 11

Eckrich RJ, Mallory D, Sandler SG (1995) Correlation of monocyte monolayer assays and posttransfusion survival of Yt(a+) red cells in patients with anti-Yt[a]. Immunohematology 11: 81–84

Ellis NA, Tippett P, Petty A et al. (1994) PBDX is the XG blood group gene. Nature Genet 8: 285–289

Engelfriet CP (1978) Unpublished observations cited in the 7th edn of this book

Eska PL, Grindon AJ (1974) The high frequency of anti-Bg[a]. Br J Haematol 27: 613

Fassbinder W, Seidl S, Koch KM (1978) The role of formaldehyde in the formation of haemodialysis-associated anti-N-like antibodies. Vox Sang 35: 41

Ferguson DJ, Gaal GD (1988) Some observations on the In[b] antigen and evidence that anti-In[b] causes accelerated destruction of radiolabeled red cells. Transfusion 28: 479–482

Fitzsimmons J, Caggiano V (1981) Autoantibody to a high-frequency Lutheran antigen associated with immune hemolytic anaemia and a hemolytic transfusion episode (Abstract). Transfusion 21: 612

Fletcher JL, Zmijewski CM (1970) The first example of auto-anti-M and its consequences in pregnancy. Int Arch Allergy 37: 586

Fouchet C, Gane P, Cartron JP et al. (2000) Quantitative analysis of XG blood group and CD99 antigens on human red cells. Immunogenetics 51: 688–694

Freedman J, Massey A, Chaplin H et al. (1980) Assessment of complement binding by anti-D and anti-M antibodies employing labelled antiglobulin antibodies. Br J Haematol 45: 309–318

Fröhlich O, Macey RI, Edwards-Moulds J et al. (1991) Urea transport deficiency in Jk(a-b-) erythrocytes. Am J Physiol 260: C778–C783

Fudenberg HH, Allen FH Jr (1957) Transfusion reactions in the absence of demonstrable incompatibility. N Engl J Med 256: 1180

Fukuda MN, Masri KA, Dell A et al. (1990) Incomplete synthesis of N-glycans in congenital dyserythropoietic anaemia type II caused by a defect in the gene encoding alpha-mannosidase II. Proc Natl Acad Sci USA 87: 7443–7447

Fukuma N, Akimitsu N, Hamamoto H et al. (2003) A role of the Duffy antigen for the maintenance of plasma chemokine concentrations. Biochem Biophys Res Commun 303: 137–139

Furuhjelm U, Myllylä G, Nevanlinna HR et al. (1969) The red cell phenotype En(a-) and anti-En[a]: serological and physicochemical aspects. Vox Sang 17: 256

Furuhjelm U, Nevanlinna HR, Pirkola A (1973) A second Finnish En(a–) propositus with anti-En[a]. Vox Sang 24: 545–549

Gaidulis L, Branch DR, Lazar GS et al. (1985) The red cell antigens A, B, D, U, Ge, Jk 3 and Yt[a] are not detected on human granulocytes. Br J Haematol 60: 659–668

Gerbal A, Lopez M, Maslet C et al. (1976) Polyagglutinability associated with the Cad antigen. Haematologia 10: 383

Giles CM (1977) The identity of Kamhuber and Far antigens. Vox Sang 32: 269

Giles CM (1985) 'Partial inhibition' of anti-Rg and anti-Ch reagents. II. Demonstration of separable antibodies for different determinants. Vox Sang 48: 167–173

Giles CM (1989) An update on Rodgers and Chido, the antigenic determinants of human C4. Immunohematology 5: 1–6

Giles CM, Gedde-Dahl T Jr, Robson EB et al. (1976) Rg[a] (Rodgers) and the HLA region: Linkage and associations. Tissue Antigens 8: 143

Göbel U, Drescher KH, Pöttgen W *et al.* (1974) A second example of anti-Yt^a with rapid *in vivo* destruction of Yt(a+) red cells. Vox Sang 27: 171

Goodfellow PJ, Pritchard C, Tippett P *et al.* (1987) Recombination between the X and Y chromosomes: implications for the relationship between MIC2, XG and YG. Ann Hum Genet 51 (Pt 2): 161–7

Goodrick MJ, Hadley AG, Poole G (1997) Haemolytic disease of the fetus and newborn due to anti-Fy^a and the potential value of Duffy genotyping in pregnancies at risk. Transfusion Med 7: 301–304

Gorst DW, Riches RA, Renton PH (1977) Formaldehyde induced anti-N: a possible cause of renal graft failure. J Clin Pathol 30: 956

Göttsche B, Salama A, Mueller-Eckhardt C (1990) Auto-immune hemolytic anemia associated with an IgA autoantiGerbich. Vox Sang 58: 211–214

Greendyke RM, Chorpenning FW (1962) Normal survival of incompatible red cells in the presence of anti-Lu^a. Transfusion 2: 52

Greenwalt TJ, Sasaki T (1957) The Lutheran blood groups: a second example of anti-Lu^b and three further examples of anti-Lu^a. Blood 12: 998

Greenwalt TJ, Sasaki TT, Steane EA (1967) The Lutheran blood groups: A progress report with observations on the development of the antigens and characteristics of the antibodies. Transfusion 7: 189

Gubin AN, Njoroge JM, Wojda U *et al.* (2000) Identification of the dombrock blood group glycoprotein as a polymorphic member of the ADP-ribosyltransferase gene family. Blood 96: 2621–2627

Habash J, Devenish A, Macdonald A *et al.* (1991) A further example of anti-Di^b not causing haemolytic disease of the newborn. Vox Sang 61: 77

Habibi B, Tippett P, Lebesnerais M *et al.* (1979) Protease inactivation of the red cell antigen Xg^a. Vox Sang 36: 367–368

Hadley TJ, David PH, McGinniss MH *et al.* (1984) Identification of an erythrocyte component carrying the Duffy blood group Fy^a antigen. Science 223: 597–599

Hadley AG, Wilkes A, Poole J *et al.* (1999) A chemiluminescence test for predicting the outcome of transfusing incompatible blood. Transfusion Med 9: 337–342

Halverson G, Shanahan E, Santiago I *et al.* (1994) The first reported case of anti-Do^b causing an acute hemolytic transfusion reaction. Vox Sang 66: 206–209

Hamilton HB, Nakahara Y (1971) The rare blood group phenotype Ko in a Japanese family. Vox Sang 20: 24–28

Hardman JT, Beck ML (1981) Hemagglutination in capillaries: correlation with blood group specificity and IgG subclass. Transfusion 21: 343–346

Harris R, Zervas JD (1969) Reticulocyte HL-A antigens. Nature (Lond) 221: 1062

Harris T, Steiert S, Marsh WL *et al.* (1986) A Wj-negative patient with anti-Wj (Letter). Transfusion 26: 117

van der Hart M, Szaloky A, van der Berg-Loonen EM *et al.* (1974) Présence d'antigènes HL-A sur les hématies d'un donneur normal. Nouv Rev Fr Hématol 14: 555

Heaton DC, McLoughlin K (1982) Jk(a– b–) red cells resist urea lysis. Transfusion 22: 70–71

Herron R, Smith GA (1989) Identification and immunochemical characterization of the human erythrocyte membrane glycoproteins that carry the Xg^a antigen. Biochem J 262: 369–371

High S, Tanner MJA, Macdonald EB *et al.* (1989) Rearrangements of the red cell membrane glycophorin C (sialoglycoprotein β gene). Biochem J 262: 47–54

Hillery CA, Du MC, Montgomery RR *et al.* (1996) Increased adhesion of erythrocytes to components of the extracellular matrix: isolation and characterization of a red blood cell lipid that binds thrombospondin and laminin. Blood 87: 4879–4886

Ho M, Chelly J, Carter N *et al.* (1994) Isolation of the gene for McLeod syndrome that encodes a novel membrane transport protein. Cell 77: 869–880

Holman CA (1953) A new rare human blood-group antigen. Lancet ii: 119

Holmes S, Downs AM, Fosberry A *et al.* (2002) Sema7A is a potent monocyte stimulator. Scand J Immunol 56: 270–275

Horuk R, Chitnis CE, Darbonne WC *et al.* (1993) A receptor for the malarial parasite *Plasmodium vivax*: the erythrocyte chemokine receptor. Science 261: 1182–1184

Howell ED, Perkins HA (1972) Anti-N-like antibodies in the sera of patients undergoing chronic hemodialysis. Vox Sang 23: 291

Hsu TCS, Jagathambal K, Sabo BH *et al.* (1975) Anti-Holley (Hy): characterization of another example. Transfusion 15: 604

Huang CH, Blumenfeld OO (1991) Molecular genetics of human erythrocyte MiIII and MiVI glycophorins. Use of a pseudoexon in construction of two delta-alpha-delta hybrid genes resulting in antigenic diversification. J Biol Chem 266: 7248–7255

Hue-Roye K, Chaudhuri A, Veliquette RW *et al.* (2004) A novel high prevalence antigen in the Scianna blood group system. Vox Sang 87 (Suppl. 3): 40

Hughes-Jones NC, Gardner B (1971) The Kell system studied with radioactively-labelled anti-K. Vox Sang 21: 154

Ishimori T, Fukomoto Y, Abe K *et al.* (1976) Rare Diego blood group phenotype Di (a+ b–). I. Anti-Di^b causing hemolytic disease of the newborn. Vox Sang 31: 61

Issitt PD (1981) The MN Blood Group System. Cincinnati, OH: Montgomery Scientific Publications

Issitt PD (1985) Applied Blood Group Serology, 3rd edn. Miami, FL: Montgomery Scientific Publications

243

Issitt PD (1990) Heterogeneity of anti-U. Vox Sang 58: 70–71

Issitt PD, Anstee DJ (1998) Applied Blood Group Serology, 4th edn. Miami, FL: Montgomery Scientific Publications

Issitt PD, Tessel JA (1981) On the incidence of antibodies to the Rh antigens G, rh_i (Ce), C, and C^G in sera containing anti-CD or anti-C. Transfusion 21: 412–418

Issitt PD, Wren MR, Rueda E et al. (1987) Red cell antigens in Hispanic blood donors. Transfusion 27: 117

Issitt PD, Obarski G, Hartnett PL et al. (1990) Temporary suppression of Kidd system expression accompanied by transient production of anti-Jk3. Transfusion 30: 46–50

Iwamoto S, Li J, Omi T et al. (1996) Identification of a novel exon and spliced form of Duffy mRNA that is the predominant transcript in both erythroid and postcapillary venule endothelium. Blood 87: 378–385

Jaber A, Blanchard D, Goosens D et al. (1989) Characterization of the Kell (K1) antigen with a human monoclonal antibody. Blood 73:1597–1602

James J, Stiles P, Boyce F et al. (1976) The HL-A type of Rg(a–) individuals. Vox Sang 30: 214

Jancik J, Schauer R (1974) Sialic add—a determinant of the life-time of rabbit erythrocytes. Hoppe-Seyler's Z Physiol Chem 355: 395

Jarolim P, Murray JL, Rubin HL et al. (1996) Characterization of 13 novel band 3 gene defects in hereditary spherocytosis with band 3 deficiency. Blood 88: 4366–4374

Joshi SR (1992) Immune haematological transfusion reaction due to anti-In^b. Vox Sang 63: 232–233

Joshi SR, Gupta D. Choudhury RK et al. (1993) Transfusion —induced anti-In^a following a single transfusion. Transfusion 33: 444

Joshi SR, Wagner FF, Vasantha K et al. (2001) An AQP1 null allele in an Indian woman with Co(a–b–) phenotype and high-titer anti-Co3 associated with mild HDN. Transfusion 41: 1273–1278

Judd WJ, Steiner EA (1991) Multiple hemolytic transfusion reactions caused by anti-Do^b (Letter). Transfusion 31: 477–478

Judd WJ, Issitt PD, Pavone BG et al. (1979) Antibodies that define NANA-independent MN-system antigens. Transfusion 19: 12–18

Judd WJ, Walter WJ, Steiner EA (1981) Clinical and laboratory findings on two patients with naturally-occurring anti-Kell agglutinins. Transfusion 21: 184–188

Judson PA, Anstee DJ (1977) Comparative effect of trypsin and chymotrypsin on blood group antigens. Med Lab Sci 34: 1

Kanel GC, Davis I, Bowman JE (1978) 'Naturally-occurring' anti-K1: possible association with mycobacterium infection. Transfusion 18: 472

Kaye T, Williams EM, Garner SF et al. (1990) Anti-Sc1 in pregnancy. Transfusion 30: 439–440

Kendall AG (1976) Clinical importance of the rare erythrocyte antibody anti-Jr^a. Transfusion 16: 646

Kikkawa Y, Moulson CL, Virtanen I et al. (2002) Identification of the binding site for the Lutheran blood group glycoprotein on laminin alpha 5 through expression of chimeric laminin chains in vivo. J Biol Chem 277: 44864–44869

King LS, Choi M, Fernandez PC et al. (2001) Defective urinary-concentrating ability due to a complete deficiency of aquaporin-1. N Engl J Med 345: 175–179

Kissmeyer-Nielsen F (1960) A further example of anti-Lu^b as a cause of a mild haemolytic disease of the newborn. Vox Sang 5: 517

Kitzke HM, Julius H, Delaney M et al. (1982) Anti-Co^a implicated in delayed hemolytic transfusion reaction (Abstract). Transfusion 22: 407

Knowles RW, Bai Y, Lomas C et al. (1982) Two monoclonal antibodies detecting high frequency antigens absent from red cells of the dominant type of Lu(a– b–) Lu:–3. J Immunogenet 9: 353–357

Konugres AA, Brown LS, Corcoran PA (1966) Anti-M^A, and the phenotype M^{A}N, of the MN blood group system (a new finding). Vox Sang 11: 189

Kornstad L, Heistö H (1957) The frequency of formation of Kell antibodies in recipients of Kell-positive blood. Proceedings of the 6th Congress of the European Society of Haematology, Copenhagen, p. 754

Kosanke J (1983) Production of anti-Fy^a in Black Fy(a– b–) individuals. Red Cell Free Press 8: 4–5

Kowalski MA, Pierce SR, Edwards RL et al. (1999) Hemolytic transfusion reaction due to anti-Tc(a). Transfusion 39: 948–950

Kurtz SR, Kuszaj T, Ouellet R et al. (1982) Survival of homozygous Co^a (Colton) red cells in a patent with anti-Co^a. Vox Sang 43: 28–30

Kusnierz-Alejska G, Bochenek S (1992) Haemolytic disease of the newborn due to anti-Di^a and incidence of the Di^a antigen in Poland. Vox Sang 62: 124–126

Lacey P, Laird-Fryer B, Block U et al. (1980) A new high incidence blood group factor, Sl^a; and its hypothetical allele (Abstract). Transfusion 20: 632

Lacey PA, Robinson J, Collins ML et al. (1987) Studies on the blood of a Co(a– b–) proposita and her family. Transfusion 27: 268–271

Lachgar A, Jaureguiberry G, Le Buenac (1998) Binding of HIV-1 to RBCs involves the Duffy antigen receptors for chemokines (DARC). Biomed Pharmacother 52: 436–439

Lalezari P, Malamut DC, Driesiger ME et al. (1973) Anti-s and anti-U cold-reacting antibodies. Vox Sang 25: 390

Lambin P, LePennec PY, Hauptmann G et al. (1984) Adverse transfusion reactions associated with a precipitating anti-C4 antibody of anti-Rodgers specificity. Vox Sang 47: 242–249

Landsteiner K, Levine P (1927) Further observations on individual differences of human blood. Proc Soc Exp Biol (NY) 24: 941

Layrisse M, Arends T, Sisco RD (1955) Nuevo grupo sanguineo encontrado en descendientes de Indios. Acta Med Venez 3: 132

Lee EL, Bennett C (1982) Anti-Co[b] causing acute hemolytic transfusion reaction. Transfusion 22: 159–160

Lee JS, Frevert CW, Wurfel MM et al. (2003) Duffy antigen facilitates movement of chemokine across the endothelium in vitro and promotes neutrophil transmigration in vitro and in vivo. J Immunol 170: 5244–5251

Lee S, Russo DC, Reiner AP et al. (2001) Molecular defects underlying the Kell null phenotype. J Biol Chem 276: 27281–27289

Lee S, Russo DC, Reid ME, Redman CM (2003a) Mutations that diminish expression of Kell surface protein and lead to the Kmod RBC phenotype. Transfusion 43: 1121–1151

Lee S, Debnath AK, Redman CM (2003b) Active amino acids of the Kell blood group protein and model of the ectodomain based on the structure of neutral endopeptidase 24.11. Blood 102: 3028–3034

Lee S, Wu X, Reid M et al. (1995) Molecular basis of the Kell (K1) phenotype. Blood 85: 912–916

Leemans JC, Florquin S, Heikens M et al. (2003) CD44 is a macrophage binding site for Mycobacterium tuberculosis that mediates macrophage recruitment and protective immunity against tuberculosis. J Clin Invest 111: 681–689

Le Pennec Py, Rouger P, Klein MT et al. (1987) Study of anti-Fy[a] in five black Fy[a] patients. Vox Sang 52: 246–249

Le Van Kim C, Colin Y, Blanchard D et al. (1987) Gerbich blood group deficiency of the Ge:-1,-2,-3 and Ge:-1,-2,3 types. Immunochemical study and genomic analysis with cDNA probes. Eur J Biochem 165: 571–579

Levene C, Karniel Y, Sela R (1987) 2-Aminoethylisothiouronium bromide-treated red cells and the Lutheran antigens Lu[a] and Lu[b]. Transfusion 27: 505–506

Levine P, Backer M, Wigod M et al. (1949) A new human hereditary blood property (Cellano) present in 99.8% of all bloods. Science 109: 464

Levine P, Robinson EA, Herrington LB et al. (1955) Second example of the antibody for the high-incidence blood factor Vel. Am J Clin Pathol 25: 751

Levine P, White JA, Stroup M (1961) Seven Ve[a] (Vel) negative members in three generations of a family. Transfusion 1: 111

Lewis M, Kaita H, Philipps S et al. (1980) The position of the Radin blood group locus in relation to other chromosome 1 loci. Ann Hum Genet 44: 179–184

Lin M, Broadberry RE (1994) An intravascular hemolytic transfusion reaction due to anti-'Mi[a]' in Taiwan (Letter). Vox Sang 67: 320

Lisowska E (1987) MN monoclonal antibodies as blood group reagents. In: Monoclonal Antibodies Against Human Red Blood Cell and Related Antigens. P Rouger, C Salmon (eds). Paris.

Liu SC, Jarolim P, Rubin HL et al. (1994) The homozygous state for the band 3 protein mutation in Southeast Asian Ovalocytosis may be lethal. Blood 84: 3590–3591

Lobo CA, Rodriguez M, Reid M et al. (2003) Glycophorin C is the receptor for the Plasmodium falciparum erythrocyte binding ligand PfEBP-2 (baebl). Blood 101: 4628–4631

Longster G, Giles CM (1976) A new antibody specificity, anti-Rg[a], reacting with a red cell and serum antigen. Vox sang 30: 175

van Loghem JJ, van der Hart M, Land ME (1955) Polyagglutinability of red cells as a cause of severe haemolytic transfusion reaction. Vox Sang (OS) 5: 125

Lubenko A, Contreras M (1992) The incidence of HDN attributable to anti-Wr[a] (Letter). Transfusion 32: 87–88

Lublin DM, Mallinson G, Poole J et al. (1994) Molecular basis of reduced or absent expression of decay-accelerating factor in Cromer blood group phenotypes. Blood 84: 1276–1282

Lublin DM, Kompelli S, Storry JR et al. (2000) Molecular basis of Cromer blood group antigens. Transfusion 40: 208–213

Lucien N, Sidoux-Walter F, Roudier N et al. (2002) Antigenic and functional properties of the human red blood cell urea transporter hUT-B1. J Biol Chem 277: 34101–34108

McCreary J, Vogler AL, Sabo B et al. (1973) Another minus-minus phenotype: Bu(a–) Sm(a+). Two examples in one family (Abstract). Transfusion 13: 350

McDowell MA, Stocker I, Nance S et al. (1986) Auto anti-Scl associated with autoimmune hemolytic anemia (Abstract). Transfusion 26: 578

McGinniss MH, Leiberman R, Holland PV (1979) The Jk[b] red cell antigen and gram-negative organisms. Transfusion 19: 663

McGinniss JD, MacLowry JD, Holland PV (1984) Acquisition of K: 1-like antigen during terminal sepsis. Transfusion 24: 28–30

McLoughlin K, Rogers J (1970) Anti-Ge[a] in an untransfused New Zealand male. Vox Sang 19: 94

McSwain B, Robins C (1988) A clinically significant anti-Cr[a] (Letter). Transfusion 28: 289–290

Maier AG, Duraisingh MT, Reeder JC et al. (2003) Plasmodium falciparum erythrocyte invasion through glycophorin C and selection for Gerbich negativity in human populations. Nature Med 9: 87–92

Mainwaring UR, Pickles MM (1948) A further case of anti-Lutheran immunization, with some studies on its capacity for human sensitization. J Clin Pathol 1: 292

Malde R, Kelsall G, Knight RC et al. (1986) The manual low-ionic strength polybrene technique for the detection of red cell antibodies. Med Lab Sci 43: 360–363

Mallinson G, Soo KS, Schall TJ et al. (1995) Mutations in the erythrocyte chemokine receptor (Duffy) gene: the molecular basis of the Fy^a/Fy^b antigens and identification of a deletion in the Duffy gene of an apparently healthy individual with the Fy(a–b–) phenotype. Br J Haematol 90: 823–829

Mann JD, Cahan A, Gelb AG et al. (1962) A sex-linked blood group. Lancet i: 8

Mannessier L, Rouger P, Johnson CL et al. (1986) Acquired loss of red-cell Wj antigen in a patient with Hodgkin's disease. Vox Sang 50: 240–244

Marcus DM, Kundu SK, Suzuki A (1981) The P blood group system: recent progress in immunochemistry and genetics. Semin Haematol 18: 63–71

Marsh WL (1975) Present status of the Duffy blood group system. CRC Clin Rev Clin Lab Sci 5: 387–412

Marsh WL, Redman CM (1990) The Kell blood group system: a review. Transfusion 30: 158–167

Marsh WL, Nichols ME, Øyen R et al. (1978) Naturally-occurring anti-Kell stimulated by E. coli enterocolitis in a 20-day-old child. Transfusion 18: 149

Marsh WL, Marsh NJ, Moore A et al. (1981) Elevated serum creatine phosphokinase in subjects with McLeod syndrome. Vox Sang 40: 403–411

Marsh WL, Brown PJ, DiNapoli J et al. (1983) Anti-Wj: an autoantibody that defines a high-incidence antigen modified by the In(Lu) gene. Transfusion 23: 128–130

Marshall JV (1973) The Bg antigens and antibodies. Can J Med Technol 35: 26

Masouredis SP, Sudora E, Mahan LC et al. (1980a) Immunoelectron microscopy of Kell and Cellano antigens on red cell ghosts. Haematologia 13: 59–64

Masouredis SP, Sudora E, Mahan L et al. (1980b) Quantitative immunoferritin microassay of Fy^a, Fy^b, Jk^a, U and Di^b antigen site numbers on human red cells. Blood 56: 969–977

Mawby WJ, Tanner MJA, Anstee DJ et al. (1983) Incomplete glycosylation of erythrocyte membrane proteins in congenital dyserythropoietic anaemia type II (CDA II). Br J Haematol 55: 357–368

Menolasino NJ, Davidsohn I, Lynch DE et al. (1954) A simplified method for the preparation of anti-M and anti-N typing sera. J Lab Clin Med 44: 495

Meredith LC (1985) Anti-Fy5 does not react with e variants (Abstract). Transfusion 25: 482

Merry AH, Gardner B, Parsons SF et al. (1987) Estimation of the number of binding sites for a murine monoclonal anti-Lu^b on human erythrocytes. Vox Sang 53: 57–60

Merry AH, Rawlinson VI, Uchikawa M et al. (1989) Studies on the sensitivity to complement-mediated lysis of erythrocytes (Inab phenotype with a deficiency of decay acceleration factor). Br J Haematol 73: 248–251

Metaxas MN, Metaxas-Bühler M (1963) Studies on the Wright blood group system. Vox Sang 8: 707

Metaxas MN, Metaxas-Bühler M (1970) An agglutinating example of anti-Xg^a and Xg^a frequencies in 559 Swiss blood donors. Vox Sang 19: 527

Middleton J, Crookston M (1972) Chido-substance in plasma. Vox Sang 23: 256

Middleton J, Crookston MC, Falk JA et al. (1974) Linkage of Chido and HL-A. Tissue Antigens 4: 366

Miller LH, Mason SJ, Clyde DF et al. (1976) The resistance factor to Plasmodium vivax in blacks. The Duffy blood group genotype, FyFy. N Engl J Med 295: 302

Mitsuoka K, Murata K, Walz T et al. (1999) The structure of aquaporin-1 at 4.5-A resolution reveals short alpha-helices in the center of the monomer. J Struct Biol 128: 34–43

Moheng MC, McCarthy P, Pierce SR (1985) Anti-Do^b implicated as the cause of a delayed hemolytic transfusion reaction. Transfusion 25: 44–46

Mollison PL (1967) Blood Transfusion in Clinical Medicine, 4th edn. Oxford: Blackwell Scientific Publications

Mollison PL (1972) Blood Transfusion in Clinical Medicine, 5th edn. Oxford: Blackwell Scientific Publications

Mollison PL (1983) Blood Transfusion in Clinical Medicine, 7th edn. Oxford: Blackwell Scientific Publications

Molthan L (1983) The serology of the York-Cost-McCoy-Knops red blood cell system. Am J Med Technol 49: 49–55

Montgomery WM Jr, Nance SJ, Donnelly SF et al. (2000) MAM: a 'new' high-incidence antigen found on multiple cell lines. Transfusion 40: 1132–1139

Montiel MD, Krzewinski-Recchi MA, Delannoy P et al. (2003) Molecular cloning, gene organization and expression of the human UDP-GalNAc:Neu5Acalpha2–3Galbeta-R beta1,4-N-acetylgalactosaminyltransferase responsible for the biosynthesis of the blood group Sd^a/Cad antigen: evidence for an unusual extended cytoplasmic domain. Biochem J 373(Pt 2): 369–379

Moore S (1983) Identification of red cell membrane components associated with rhesus blood group antigen expression. In: Red Cell Membrane Glycoconjugates and Related Genetic Markers. JP Cartron, P Rouger, C Salmon (eds), pp. 97–106. Paris: Lib Arnette

Morel PA, Hamilton HB (1979) Ok^a: an erythrocytic antigen of high frequency. Vox Sang 36: 182–185

Morel P, Hill V, Bergren M et al. (1975) Sera exhibiting hemagglutination of N red blood cells stored in media containing glucose (Abstract). Transfusion 15: 522

Morel PA, Bergren MO, Hill V et al. (1981) M and N specific hemagglutinins of human erythrocytes stored in glucose solutions. Transfusion 21: 652–662

Morton JA (1962) Some observations on the action of blood-group antibodies on red cells treated with proteolytic enzymes. Br J Haematol 8: 134

Morton JA, Pickles MM, Sutton L (1969) The correlation of the Bg^a blood group with the HL-A7 leucocyte group:

demonstration of antigenic sites on red cells and leucocytes. Vox Sang 17: 536

Morton JA, Pickles MM, Terry AM (1970) The Sd^a blood group antigen in tissues and body fluids. Vox Sang 19: 472

Morton JA, Pickles MM, Sutton L et al. (1971) Identification of further antigens on red cells and lymphocytes. Association of Bg^b with W17 (Te57) and Bg^c with W28 (Da15, Ba*). Vox Sang 21: 141

Morton JA, Pickles MM, Darley JH (1977) Increase in strength of red cell Bg^a antigen following infectious mononucleosis. Vox Sang 32: 26

Morton JA, Pickles MM, Turner JE et al. (1980) Changes in red cell Bg antigens in haematological disease. Immunol Commun 9: 173–190

Moulds JM (1993) Association of blood group antigens with immunologically important proteins. In: Immunobiology of Transfusion Medicine. G Garratty (ed.). New York: Marcel Dekker

Moulds JJ, Polesky HF, Reid M et al. (1975) Observations on the Gy^a and Hy antigens and the antibodies that define them. Transfusion 15: 270

Moulds JM, Moulds JJ, Brown M et al. (1992) Antiglobulin testing for CR1-related (Knops/McCoy/Swain-Langley/York) blood group antigens: negative and weak reactions are caused by variable expression of CR1. Vox Sang 62: 230–235

Moulds JM, Zimmerman PA, Doumbo OK et al. (2001) Molecular identification of Knops blood group polymorphisms found in long homologous region D of complement receptor 1. Blood 97: 2879–2885

Mourant AE, Kopéc AC, Domaniewska-Sobczak (1976) The Distribution of the Human Blood Groups and Other Biochemical Polymorphisms, 2nd edn. Oxford: Oxford University Press

Murphy PM (1994) The molecular biology of leukocyte chemoattractant receptors. Annu Rev Immunol 12: 593–633

Nakajima H, Ito K (1978) An example of anti-Jr^a causing haemolytic disease of the newborn and frequency of Jr^a antigen in the Japanese population. Vox Sang 35: 265–267

Nichols ME, Rosenfield RE, Rubinstein P (1985) Two blood group M epitopes disclosed by monoclonal anti-bodies. Vox Sang 49: 138–148

Nichols ME, Rubinstein P, Barnwell J et al. (1987) A new human Duffy blood group specificity defined by a murine monoclonal antibody. J exp Med 166: 776–785

Nordhagen R (1977) Association between HLA and red cell antigens. IV. Further studies of haemagglutinins in cytotoxic HLA antisera. Vox Sang 32: 82

Nordhagen R (1978) Association between HLA and red cell antigens. V. A further study of the nature and behaviour of the HLA antigens on red blood cells and their corresponding haemagglutinins. Vox Sang 35: 49

Nordhagen R (1979) HLA antigens on red blood cells. Two donors with extraordinarily strong reactivity. Vox Sang 37: 209–215

Nordhagen R, Aas M (1978) Association between HLA and red cell antigens. VII. Survival studies of incompatible red cells in a patient with HLA-associated haemagglutinins. Vox Sang 35: 319

Nordhagen R, Aas M (1979) Survival studies of ^{51}Cr Ch(a+) red blood cells in a patient with anti-Ch^a, and massive transfusion of incompatible blood. Vox Sang 37: 179–181

Nordhagen R, Ørjasaeter H (1974) Association between HL-A and red cell antigens. An AutoAnalyzer study. Vox Sang 26: 97

Nowicki B, Moulds J, Hull R et al. (1988) A hemagglutinin of uropathogenic Escherichia coli recognises the Dr blood group antigen. Infect Immunol 56: 1057–1060

Okada H, Tanaka H (1983) Species-specific inhibition by glycophorins of complement activation via the alternative pathway. Mol Immunol 20: 1233–1236

Okubo Y, Yamaguchi H, Nagao N et al. (1986) Heterogeneity of the phenotype Jk(a− b−) found in Japanese. Transfusion 26: 237–239

Olsson ML, Smythe JS, Hansson C et al. (1998) The Fy(x) phenotype is associated with a missense mutation in the Fy(b) allele predicting Arg89Cys in the Duffy glycoprotein. Br J Haematol 103: 1184–1191

O'Neill GJ, Yang SY, Tegoli J et al. (1978) Chido and Rodgers blood groups are distinct antigenic components of human complement C4. Nature (Lond) 273: 668

Pak J, Pu Y, Zhang ZT et al. (2001) Tamm-Horsfall protein binds to type 1 fimbriated Escherichia coli and prevents E. coli from binding to uroplakin Ia and Ib receptors. J Biol Chem 276: 9924–30

Palacin M, Kanai Y (2004) The ancillary proteins of HATs:SLC3 family of amino acid transporters. Pflugers Arch 447: 490–494

Panzer S, Mueller-Eckhardt G, Salama A et al. (1984) The clinical significance of HLA antigens on red cells. Survival studies in HLA-sensitized individuals. Transfusion 24: 486–489

Parsons SF, Mallinson G, Judson PA et al. (1987) Evidence that the Lu^b blood group antigen is located on red cell membrane glycoproteins of 85 and 78 kd. Transfusion 27: 61–63

Parsons SF, Gardner B, Anstee DJ (1993) Monoclonal antibodies against Kell glycoprotein: serology, immunochemistry and quantification of antigen sites. Transfusion Med 3: 137–142

Parsons SF, Mallinson G, Holmes CH et al. (1995) The Lutheran blood group glycoprotein, another member of the immunoglobulin superfamily, is widely expressed in human tissues and is developmentally regulated in human liver. Proc Natl Acad Sci USA 92: 5496–5500

Parsons SF, Mallinson G, Daniels GL et al. (1997) Use of domain-deletion mutants to locate Lutheran blood group antigens to each of the five immunoglobulin superfamily domains of the Lutheran glycoprotein: elucidation of the molecular basis of the Lu(a)/Lu(b) and the Au(a)/Au(b) polymorphisms. Blood 89: 4219–4225

Parsons SF, Lee G, Spring FA et al. (2001) Lutheran blood group glycoprotein and its newly characterized mouse homologue specifically bind alpha5 chain-containing human laminin with high affinity. Blood 97: 312–320

Pasvol G, Carlsson J, Clough B (1993) The red cell membrane and invasion by malarial parasites. In: Red Cell Membranes and Red Cell Antigens. MJA Tanner, DJ Anstee (eds). Baillière's Clinical Haematology 6: 513–534

Pavone BG, Issitt PD (1974) Anti-Bg antibodies in sera used for red cell typing. Br J Haematol 27: 607

Pavone BG, Pirkola A, Nevanlinna HR et al. (1978) Demonstration of anti-Wr^b in a second serum containing anti-En^a. Transfusion 18: 155

Pavone BG, Billman R, Bryani J et al. (1981) An auto-anti-En^a, inhibitable by MN sialoglycoprotein. Transfusion 21: 25–31

Paw BH, Davidson AJ, Zhou Y et al. (2003) Cell-specific mitotic defect and dyserythropoiesis associated with erythroid band 3 deficiency. Nature Genet 34:59–64

Perrault R (1973) Naturally-occurring anti-M and anti-N with special case: IgG anti-N in a NN donor. Vox Sang 24: 134

Petermans ME, Cole-Dergent J (1970) Haemolytic transfusion reaction due to anti-Sd^a. Vox Sang 18: 67

Peters B, Reid ME, Ellisor SS et al. (1978) Red cell survival studies of Lu^b incompatible blood in a patient with anti-Lu^b (Abstract). Transfusion 18: 623

Petty AC (1993) Direct confirmation of the relationship between the Knops-system antigens and the CR1 protein using the MAIEA technique (Abstract). Transfusion Med 3(Suppl. 1): 84

Petty AC, Daniels GL, Tippett P (1994) Application of the MAIEA assay to the Kell blood group system. Vox Sang 66: 216–224

Pickles MM, Morton JA (1977) The Sd^a blood group. In: Human Blood Groups. JF Mohn, RW Plunkett, RK Cunningham et al. (eds). Basel: S Karger, pp. 277–286

Pierce SR, Hardman JT, Hunt JS et al. (1980) Anti-Yt^a: characterization by IgG subclass composition and macrophage assay (Abstract). Transfusion 20: 627–628

Pinkerton FJ, Mermod LE, Liles BA et al. (1959) The phenotype Jk(a– b–) in the Kidd blood group system. Vox Sang 4: 155

Pisacka M, Vytiskova J Latinakova A et al. (2001) Molecular background of the Fy(a–b–) phenotype in a gypsy popula-tion living in the Czech and Slovak Republics. Transfusion 41: 15S

Polesky HF, Swanson JL (1966) Studies on the distribution of the blood group antigen Do^a (Dombrock) and the characteristics of anti-Do^a. Transfusion 11: 162

Polley MJ, Mollison PL, Soothill JF (1962) The role of 19S gamma globulin blood group antibodies in the antiglobulin reaction. Br J Haematol 8: 149

Poole J, van Alphen L (1988) Haemophilus influenzae receptor and the AnWj antigen (Letter). Transfusion 28: 289

Poole J, Levene C, Bennett M et al. (1991) A family showing inheritance of the Anton blood group antigen AnWj and independence of AnWj from Lutheran. Transfusion Med 1: 245–251

Poole J, Banks J, Bruce LJ et al. (1999) Glycophorin A mutation Ala65→Pro gives rise to a novel pair of MNS alleles ENEP (MNS39) and HAG (MNS41) and altered Wr^b expression: direct evidence for GPA/band 3 interaction necessary for normal Wr^b expression. Transfusion Med 9: 167–174

Powell RM, Schmitt V, Ward T et al. (1998) Characterization of echoviruses that bind decay accelerating factor (CD55): evidence that some haemagglutinating strains use more than one cellular receptor. J Gen Virol 79: 1707–1713

Preston GM, Smith BL, Zeidel ML et al. (1994) Mutations in aquaporin-1 in phenotypically normal humans without functional CHIP water channels. Science 265: 1585–1587

Pushkarsky T, Zybarth G, Dubrovsky L et al. (2001) CD147 facilitates HIV-1 infection by interacting with virus-associated cyclophilin A. Proc Natl Acad Sci USA 98: 6360–6365

Race RR, Sanger R (1954) Blood Groups in Man, 2nd edn. Oxford: Blackwell Scientific Publications

Race RR, Sanger R (1968) Blood Groups in Man, 5th edn. Oxford: Blackwell Scientific Publications

Race RR, Sanger R (1975) Blood Groups in Man, 6th edn. Oxford: Blackwell Scientific Publications

Race RR, Sanger R, Lehane D (1953) Quantitative aspects of the blood-group antigen Fy^a. Ann Eugen (Camb) 17: 255

Rahuel C, Le Van Kim C, Mattei MG et al. (1996) A unique gene encodes spliceoforms of the B-cell adhesion molecule cell surface glycoprotein of epithelial cancer and of the Lutheran blood group glycoprotein. Blood 88: 1865–1872

Ramsey G, Sherman LA, Zimmer AM et al. (1995) Clinical significance of anti-At^a. Vox Sang 69: 1135–1137

Rappold GA (1993) The pseudoautosomal regions of the sex chromosomes (Review). Hum Genet 92: 315–324

Rausen AR, Rosenfield RE, Alter AA et al. (1967) A 'new' infrequent red cell antigen, Rd (Radin). Transfusion 7: 336–342

Redman CM, Russo D, Lee S (1999) Kell, Kx and the McLeod syndrome. Baillière's Clin Haematol 12: 621–635

Reid ME (1989) Biochemistry and molecular cloning analysis of human red cell sialoglycoproteins that carry Cerbich blood group antigens. In: Blood Group Systems: MN and Gerbich. PJ Unger, B Laird-Fryer (eds). Arlington, VA: Am Assoc Blood Banks

Reid ME (2003) The Dombrock blood group system: a review. Transfusion 43: 107–114

Reid ME, Ellisor SS, Barker JM et al. (1981) Characteristics of an antibody causing agglutination of M-positive non-enzymatically glycosylated human red cells. Vox Sang 41: 85–90

Renton PH, Howell P, Ikin EW et al. (1967) Anti-Sd^a, a new blood group antibody. Vox Sang 13: 493

Ribiero ML, Alloisio N, Almeida H et al. (2000) Severe hereditary spherocytosis and distal renal tubular acidosis associated with the total absence of band 3. Blood 96: 1602–1604

Ring SM (1992) An immunochemical investigation of the Wr^a and Wr^b blood group antigens. PhD Thesis, University of London, London

Ring SM, Green CA, Swallow DM et al. (1994) Production of a murine monoclonal antibody to the low-incidence red cell antigen Wr^a: characterisation and comparison with human anti-Wr^a. Vox Sang 67: 222–225

Rios M, Chaudhuri A, Mallinson G et al. (2000) New geno-types in Fy(a–b–) individuals: nonsense mutations (Trp to stop) in the coding sequence of either FY A or FY B. Br J Haematol 108: 448–454

Rivera R, Scornik JC (1986) HLA antigens on red cells. Implications for achieving low HLA antigen content in blood transfusion. Transfusion 26: 375–381

Robbe C, Cappon C, Maes E et al. (2003) Evidence of regio-specific glycosylation in human intestinal mucins: presence of an acidic gradient along the intestinal tract. J Biol Chem 278: 46337–46348

Roscic-Mrkic B, Fischer M, Leeman C et al. (2003) RANTES (CCL5) uses the proteoglycan CD44 as an auxiliary recep-tor to mediate cellular activation signals and HIV-1 enhancement. Blood 102:1169–1177

Rosenfield RE, Haber GV, Kissmeyer-Nielson F et al. (1960) Ge, a very common red-cell antigen. Br J Haematol 6: 344

Ross DG, McCall L (1985) Transfusion significance of anti-Cr^a. Transfusion 25: 84

Rosse WF (1989) Paroxysmal nocturnal hemoglobinuria: the biochemical defects and the clinical syndrome. Blood Rev 3: 192–200

Roudier N, Ripoche P, Gane P et al. (2002) AQP3 deficiency in humans and the molecular basis of a novel blood group system, GIL. J Biol Chem 277: 45854–45859

Rouger P, Lee H, Juszczak G (1983) Murine monoclonal antibodies against Gerbich antigens. J Immunogenet 10: 333–335

Rouse D, Weiner C, Williamson R (1990) Immune hydrops fetalis attributable to anti-HFK. Obstet Gynecol 76: 988–990

Rowe JA, Moulds JM, Newbold CI et al. (1997) P. falci-parum rosetting mediated by a parasite-variant erythrocyte membrane protein and complement-receptor 1. Nature 388: 292–295

Roxby DJ, Paris JM, Stern DA et al. (1994) Pure anti-Do^a stimulated by pregnancy. Vox Sang 66: 49–50

Russo D, Wu X, Redman CM et al. (2000) Expression of Kell blood group protein in nonerythroid tissues. Blood 96: 340–346

Russo DC, Lee S, Reid ME et al. (2002) Point mutations caus-ing the McLeod phenotype. Transfusion 42: 287–293

Sabo B, Moulds JJ, McCreary J (1978) Anti-JMH: another high titer-low avidity antibody against a high frequency antigen (Abstract). Transfusion 18: 387

Sacks DA, Johnson CS, Platt LD (1985) Isoimmunization in pregnancy to Gerbich antigen. Am J Perinatol, 2: 208–210

Salmon C, Homberg JC (1971) Les anticorps associés au cours des anémies hémolytiques acquises avec autoanticorps. In: Les Anémies Hémolytiques. Rapports présentés au 38e Congrès de Medécine, Beyrouth, p. 83. Paris: Masson.

Sands JM, Gargus JJ, Frohlich O et al. (1992) Urinary con-centrating ability in patients with Jk(a–b–) blood type who lack carrier-mediated urea transport. J Am Soc Nephrol 2: 1689–1696

Sanger R, Gavin J, Tippett P et al. (1971) Plant agglutinin for another human blood-group (Letter). Lancet i: 1130

Sausais L, Krevans JR, Townes AS (1964) Characteristics of a third example of anti-Xg^a (Abstract) Transfusion 4: 312

Seaman MJ, Benson R, Jones MN et al. (1967) The reactions of the Bennett-Goodspeed group of antibodies tested with the AutoAnalyzer. Br J Haematol 13: 464

Seyfried H, Frankowska K, Giles CM et al. (1966) Further examples of anti-Bu^a found in immunized donors. Vox Sang 11: 512

Silvergleid AJ, Wells RF, Hafleigh EB et al. (1978) Com-patibility test using ^{51}chromium-labelled red blood cells in crossmatch positive patients. Transfusion 18: 8

Simpson WKH (1973) Anti-Co^a and severe haemolytic dis-ease of the newborn. S Afr Med J 47: 1302–1304

Simpson MB, Dunstan RA, Rosse WF et al. (1987) Status of the MNSs antigens on human platelets. Transfusion 27: 15–18

Smith BL, Preston GM, Spring F et al. (1994) Human red cell Aquaporin CHIP. I. Molecular characterization of ABH and Colton blood group antigens. J Clin Invest 94: 1043–1049

Smith DS, Stratton F, Johnson T et al. (1969) Haemolytic dis-ease of the newborn caused by anti-Lan antibody. BMJ 3: 90

Smith KJ, Coonce LS, South SF et al. (1983) Anti-Cr^a: family study and survival of chromium-labeled incompatible red cells in a Spanish-American patient. Transfusion 23: 167–169

Smith ML, Beck ML (1977) The immunoglobulin class of antibodies with M specificity. Atlanta, GA: Commun Am Assoc Blood Banks

Smythe J, Gardner B, Anstee DJ (1994) Quantitation of the number of molecules of glycophorins C and D on normal red cells using radioiodinated Fab fragments of monoconal antibodies. Blood 83: 1668–1672

Soh CPC, Morgan WTJ, Watkins WM et al. (1980) The relationship between the N-acetylgalactosamine content and the blood group Sd^a activity of Tamm and Horsfall urinary glycoprotein. Biochem Biophys Res Commun 93: 1132–1139

Sonneborn HH, Uthemann H, Pfeffer A (1983) Monoclonal antibody specific for human blood group k (cellano). Biotest Bull 4: 328–330

Southcott M (1999) Expression of blood group antigens on erythroid progenitor cells during differentiation using an in vitro culture system. PhD thesis, University of Bristol, Bristol

Speiser P, Kühböck J, Mickerts D et al. (1966) 'Kamhuber' a new human blood group antigen of familial occurrence, revealed by a severe transfusion reaction. Vox Sang 11: 113

Spring FA (1993) Characterization of blood-group-active erythrocyte membrane glycoproteins with human antisera. Transfusion Med 3: 167–178

Spring FA, Judson PA, Daniels GL et al. (1987) A human cell-surface glycoprotein that carries Cromer-related blood group antigens on erythrocytes and is also expressed on leucocytes and platelets. Immunology 62: 307–313

Spring FA, Dalchau R, Daniels GL et al. (1988) The In^a and In^b blood group antigens are located on a glycoprotein of 80 000 Mw (the CD$_w$ 44 glycoprotein) whose expression is influenced by the In (hu) gene. Immunology 64: 37–43

Spring FA, Herron R, Rowe G (1990) An erythrocyte glycoprotein of apparent M_r 60 000 expresses the Sc1 and Sc2 antigens. Vox Sang 58: 122

Spring FA, Holmes CH, Simpson KL et al. (1997) The Ok^a blood group antigen is a marker for the M6 leukocyte activation antigen, the human homolog of OX-47 antigen, basigin and neurothelin, an immunoglobulin superfamily molecule that is widely expressed in human cells and tissues. Eur J Immunol 27: 891–897

Steane EA, Sheehan RG, Brooks BA et al. (1982) Therapeutic plasmapheresis in patients with antibodies to high frequency red cell antigens, in Therapeutic Apheresis and Plasma Perfusion, ed RSA Tindall, Progress in Clinical and Biological Research 106: 347–353. Alan R Liss, New York

Steffey NB (1983) Investigation of a probable non-red cell stimulated anti-Di^a. Red Cell Free Press 8: 24

Stiller RJ, Lardas O, Haynes de Regt R (1990) Vel isoimmunisation in pregnancy. Am J Obstet Gynecol 162: 1071–1072

Stone B, Marsh WL (1959) Haemolytic disease of the newborn caused by anti-M. Br J Haematol 5: 344

Storry JR, Sausais L, Hue-Roye K et al. (2003) GUTI: a new antigen in the Cromer blood group system. Transfusion 43: 340–344

Strahl M, Pettenkofer HJ, Hasse W (1955) A haemolytic transfusion reaction due to anti-M. Vox Sang (OS) 5: 34

Stroup M, McCreary J (1975) Cr^a, author high frequency blood group factor. Transfusion 15: 522

Stroup M, MacIlroy M, Walker R et al. (1965) Evidence that Sutter belongs to the Kell blood group system. Transfusion 5: 309–314

Sussman LN, Miller EB (1952) Un nouveau facteur sanguin 'Vel'. Rev Hématol 7: 368

Swanson JL, Sastamoinen R (1985) Chloroquine stripping of HLA AB antigens from red cells. Transfusion 25: 439–440

Swanson J, Olsen J, Azar MM et al. (1971) Serological evidence that antibodies of Chido-York-Cs^a specificity are leukocyte antibodies (Abstract). Fed Proc 30: 248

Sweeney JD, Holme S, McCall L et al. (1995) At(a–) phenotype: description of a family and reduced survival of At(a+) red cells in a proposita with anti-At^a. Transfusion 35: 63–67

Szabo P, Campana T, Siniscalco M (1977) Radioimmune assay for the Xg(a) surface antigen at the individual cell level. Biochem Biophys Res Commun 78: 655

Szalóky A, van der Hart M (1971) An auto-antibody anti-Vel. Vox Sang 20: 376

Szymanski IO, Huff SR, Delsignore R (1982) An auto-analyzer test to determine immunoglobulin class and IgG subclass of blood group antibodies. Transfusion 22: 90–95

Takemoto S, Gjertson DW, Terasaki PI (1992) HLA matching: a comparison of conventional and molecular approaches. In: Clinical Transplants. PI Terasaki, JM Cecka (eds). Los Angeles, CA: UCLA Tissue Typing Laboratory

Taliano V, Guévin R-M, Hébert D et al. (1980) The rare phenotype En(a–) in a French-Canadian family. Vox Sang 38: 87–93

Tambourgi DV, Morgan BP, de Andrade RM et al. (2000) Loxosceles intermedia spider envenomation induces activation of an endogenous metalloproteinase, resulting in cleavage of glycophorins from the erythrocyte surface and facilitating complement-mediated lysis. Blood 95: 683–691

Tambourgi DV, De Sousa Da Silva M, Billington SJ et al. (2002) Mechanism of induction of complement susceptibility of erythrocytes by spider and bacterial sphingomyelinases. Immunology 107: 93–101

Tanner MJA, Anstee DJ, Mallinson G et al. (1988) Effect of endoglycosidase F preparations on the surface components of the human erythrocyte. Carbohydrate Res 178: 203–212

Taswell HG, Pineda AA, Brzica SM (1976) Chronic granulomatous disease: successful treatment of infection with granulocyte transfusions resulting in subsequent hemolytic transfusion reaction. San Francisco, CA: Commun Am Assoc Blood Banks

Teesdale P, de Silva M, Contreras M *et al.* (1991) Development of non-Rh antibodies in volunteers stimulated for the production of hyperimmune anti-D. Vox Sang 61: 37–39

Tegoli J, Sausais L, Issitt PD (1967) Another example of a 'naturally-occurring' anti-K1. Vox Sang 12: 305

Telen MJ, Le van Kim C, Chung A *et al.* (1991) Molecular basis for elliptocytosis associated with glycophorin C and D deficiency in the Leach phenotype. Blood 78: 1603–1606

Telen MJ, Rao N, Udani M *et al.* (1993) Relationship of the AnWj blood group antigen to expression of CD44 (Abstract). Transfusion 33 (Suppl.): 485

Telischi M, Behzad O, Issitt PD *et al.* (1976) Hemolytic disease of the newborn due to anti-N. Vox Sang 31: 109

Thompson PR, Childers DM, Hatcher DE (1967) Anti-Di[b]: first and second examples. Vox Sang 13: 314

Thompson HW, Skradski KJ, Thoreson JR *et al.* (1985) Survival of Er(a+) red cells in a patient with alloanti-Er[a]. Transfusion 25: 140–141

Thompson K, Barden G, Sutherland J *et al.* (1991) Human monoclonal antibodies to human blood group antigens Kidd Jk[a] and Jk[b]. Transfusion Med 1: 91–96

Tilley CA, Crookston MC, Brown BL *et al.* (1975) A and B and A$_1$Le[b] substances in glycosphingolipid fractions of human serum. Vox Sang 28: 25

Tilley CA, Crookston MC, Haddad SA *et al.* (1977) Red blood cell survival studies in patients with anti-Ch[a], anti-Yk[a], anti-Ge and anti-Vel. Transfusion 17: 169

Tilley CA, Romans DG, Crookston MC (1978) Localisation of Chido and Rodgers determinants to the C4d fragment of human C4. Nature (Lond) 276: 713

Tippett P, Reid ME, Poole J *et al.* (1992) The Miltenberger subsystem: is it obsolescent? Transfus Med Rev 6: 170–182

Toivanen P, Hirvonen T (1973) Antigens Duffy, Kell, Kidd, Lutheran and Xg[a] on fetal red cells. Vox Sang 24: 372

Tokunaga E, Sasakawa S, Tamaka K *et al.* (1979) Two apparently healthy Japanese individuals of type M^kM^k have erythrocytes which lack both the blood group MN and Ss-active sialoglycoproteins. J Immunogenet 6: 383–390

Tomita A Parker CJ (1994) Aberrant regulation of complement by the erythrocytes of hereditary erythroblastic multinuclearity with a positive acidified serum lysis test (HEMPAS). Blood 83: 250–259

Tomita A, Radike EL, Parker CJ (1993) Isolation of erythrocyte membrane inhibitor of reactive lysis type II. Identification as glycophorin A. J Immunol 151: 3308–3323

Toole BP (2003) Emmprin (CD147), a cell surface regulator of matrix metalloproteinase production and function. Curr Topics Dev Biol 54: 371–389

Tournamille C, Colin Y, Cartron JP (1995) Disruption of a GATA motif in the Duffy gene promoter abolishes erythroid gene expression in Duffy-negative individuals. Nature Genet 10: 224–228

Tournamille C, Le Van Kim C, Gane P *et al.* (1998) Arg89Cys substitution results in very low membrane expression of the Duffy antigen/receptor for chemokines in Fy(x) individuals. Blood 92: 2147–2156 [Erratum in Blood 2000; 95: 2753]

Tournamille C, Filipe A, Wasniowska K, *et al.* (2003) Structure-function analysis of the extracellular domains of the Duffy antigen/receptor for chemokines: characterization of antibody and chemokine binding sites. Br J Haematol 122: 1014–1023

Tregallas WM, Pierce SR, Hardman JT *et al.* (1980) Anti-JMH: IgG subclass composition and clinical significance. Transfusion 20: 628

Trucco M, de Petris S, Garrotta G *et al.* (1980) Quantitative analysis of cell surface HLA structures by means of monoclonal antibodies. Hum Immunol 3: 233–243

Uchikawa M, Tsuneyama H, Tadokoro K *et al.* (1995) An alloantibody to 12E7 antigen detected in 2 healthy donors. Transfusion 35: 23S

Uchikawa M, Suzuki Y, Onodera Y *et al.* (2000) Monoclonal anti-Mi[a] and anti-Mur. Vox Sang 78(Suppl. 1): P021

Udani M, Zen Q, Cottman M *et al.* (1998) Basal cell adhesion molecule/lutheran protein. The receptor critical for sickle cell adhesion to laminin. J Clin Invest 101: 2550–2558

Udden MM, Umeda M, Hirano Y *et al.* (1987) New abnormalities in the morphology, cell surface receptors. and electrolyte metabolism of In(Lu) erythrocytes. Blood 69: 52–57

Uhlenbruck G, Dahr W, Schmalisch R *et al.* (1976) Studies on the receptors of the MNSs blood group system. Blut 32: 163

Van der Hart, Moes M, VD Veer M *et al.* (1961): Ho and Lan: two new blood groups antigens. VIIIth Europ Congr Haematol

Van der Schoot CE, Tax GHM, Rijnders RJP *et al.* (2003) Prenatal typing of Rh and Kell Blood Group System Antigens: The edge of a watershed. Transfusion Med Rev 17: 31–44

Vengelen-Tyler V (1983) Letter to the Editor. Red Cell Free Press 8: 14

Vengelen-Tyler V (1985) Anti-Fy[a] preceding anti-Fy3 or -Fy5: a study of five cases (Abstract). Transfusion 25: 482

Vengelen-Tyler V, Morel PA (1983) Serologic and IgG subclass characterization of Cartwright (Yt) and Gerbich (Ge) antibodies. Transfusion 23: 114–116

Vengelen-Tyler V, Anstee DJ, Issitt PD *et al.* (1981) Studies on the blood of an Mi^v homozygote. Transfusion 21: 1–14

Vengelen-Tyler V, Gonzalez B, Garratty G *et al.* (1987) Acquired loss of red cell Kell antigens. Br J Haematol 65: 231–234

Wagner FF, Poole J, Flegel WA (2003) Scianna antigens including Rd are expressed by ERMAP. Blood 101: 752–757

Walthers L, Salem M, Tessel J *et al.* (1983) The Inab phenotype: another example found (Abstract). Transfusion 23: 423

Wang HY, Tang H, Shen CK *et al* (2003) Rapidly evolving genes in human. I. The glycophorins and their possible role in evading malaria parasites. Mol Biol Evol 20: 1795–1804

Washington MK, Udani M, Rao N *et al.* (1994) Molecular genetic basis of the In$^{a/b}$ polymorphism (Abstract). Transfusion 34, Suppl 1: 62S

Watkins W (1995) Sd^a and Cad antigens. In: Molecular Basis of Major Human Blood Group Antigens. J-P Cartron, P Rouger (eds). New York: Plenum Press

Welch SG, McGregor IA, Williams K (1977) The Duffy group and malaria prevalence in Gambian West Africans. Trans R Soc Trop Med Hyg 71: 295–296

West NC, Jenkins JA, Johnston BR *et al.* (1986) Inter-0donor incompatability due to anti-Kell antibody undetectable by automated antibody screening. Vox Sang 50: 174–176

Westhoff CM, Sipherd BD, Wylie BD *et al.* (1992) Severe anaphylactic reactions following transfusions of platelets to a patient with anti-Ch. Transfusion 32: 576–579

Wiener AS (1950) Reaction transfusionnelle hémolytique due à une sensibiliation anti-M. Rev Hématol 5: 3

Wiener AS, Unger LJ, Gordon EB (1953) Fatal hemolytic transfusion reaction caused by sensitization to a new blood factor U. JAMA 153: 1444

Wiener AS, Samwick AA, Morrison H *et al.* (1955) Studies on immunization in man. III. Immunization experiments with pooled human blood cells. Exp Med Surg 13: 347

Williams D, Johnson CL, Marsh WL (1981) Duffy antigen changes on red blood cells stored at low temperature. Transfusion 21: 357–359

Williamson LM, Poole J, Redman C *et al.* (1994) Transient loss of proteins carrying Kell and Lutheran red cell antigens during consecutive relapses of autoimmune thrombocytopenia. Br J Haematol 87: 805–812

Winardi R, Reid M, Conboy J *et al.* (1993) Molecular analysis of glycophorin C deficiency in human erythrocytes. Blood 81: 2799–2803

Wong KH, Skelton SK, Feeley JC (1985) Interaction of *Campylobacter jejuni* and *Campylobacter coli* with lectins and blood group antibodies. J Clin Microbiol 22: 134–135

Woodfield G, Giles C, Poole J *et al.* (1986) A further null phenotype (Sc-1-2) in Papua New Guinea. Proceedings of the 19th Congress of the International Society of Blood Transfusion, Sydney, p. 651

Woolley IJ, Hotmire KA, Sramkoski RM *et al.* (2000) Differential expression of the duffy antigen receptor for chemokines according to RBC age and FY genotype. Transfusion 40: 949–953

Wren MR, Issitt PD (1988) Evidence that Wr^a and Wr^b are antithetical. Transfusion 28: 113–118

Yamada A, Kubo K, Takeshita T *et al.* (1999) Molecular cloning of a glycosylphosphatidylinositol-anchored molecule CDw108. J Immunol 162: 4094–4100

Yamashina M, Ueda E, Kinoshita T *et al.* (1990) Inherited complete deficiency of 20-kilodalton homologous restriction factor (CD59) as a cause of paroxysmal haemoglobinuria. N Engl J Med 323: 1184–1189

Yates J, Howell P, Overfield J *et al* (1998) IgG anti-Jk^a/Jk^b antibodies are unlikely to fix complement. Transfusion Med 8: 133–140

Zdebska E, Wozniewicz B, Adamowicz-Salach A *et al.* (2000) Short report: erythrocyte membranes from a patient with congenital dyserythropoietic anaemia type I (CDA-I) show identical, although less pronounced, glycoconjugate abnormalities to those from patients with CDA-II (HEMPAS). Br J Haematol 110: 998–1001

Zimmerman PA, Woolley I, Masinde GL (1999) Emergence of FY*A(null) in a *Plasmodium vivax*-endemic region of Papua New Guinea. Proc Natl Acad Sci USA 96: 13973–13977

Zupanska B, Brojer E, McIntosh J *et al.* (1990) Correlation of monocyte-monolayer assay results, number of erythrocyte-bound IgG molecules: and IgG subclass composition in the study of red cell alloantibodies other than D. Vox Sang 58: 276–280

7 Red cell antibodies against self-antigens, bound antigens and induced antigens

Antibodies to self-antigens result from a breakdown of immune tolerance causing B or T lymphocytes (or both) to respond to the host's own cells and tissues. The causes of this breakdown are complex and involve genetic predisposition with, in some cases, linkage to a particular HLA type, and environmental factors. There is a large body of evidence suggesting that the trigger for the autoimmune response is frequently bacterial and/or viral infection (reviewed by Oldstone 1998). Murakami and co-workers (1997) used a transgenic mouse model in which the mice carry immunoglobulin genes encoding an anti-red cell autoantibody (4C8) to show that autoimmune disease in these animals does not develop when the animals are kept in pathogen-free conditions. Goverman and co-workers (1993) used a transgenic mouse model constructed to express a rearranged T-cell receptor specific for myelin basic protein and showed that the mice developed spontaneous experimental allergic encephalomyelitis when kept in a non-sterile facility, but not when maintained in a sterile pathogen-free facility.

In immunohaematology, the term *red cell auto-antibody* is used for any antibody that reacts with an antigen on the subject's own red cells, whether or not any pathological effects are produced *in vivo*. The most important antibodies considered here are those that react with self-antigens, intrinsic to red cells. In addition, various other antibodies that may react with a subject's own red cells are described, for example antibodies against bound penicillin. Autoantibodies and drug-dependent antibodies may seem to have little to do with blood transfusion, but they may be detected in pre-transfusion testing and must then be investigated.

Moreover, some of them cause destruction of transfused red cells.

Red cell autoantibodies

Most red cell autoantibodies can be classified as 'cold' or 'warm'.

Cold antibodies, by definition, are those that react more strongly at 0°C than at higher temperatures. The thermal range of particular cold autoantibodies varies widely; at one extreme there are the harmless cold autoagglutinins found in all normal subjects, which are active only up to a temperature of 10–15°C; at the other extreme there are cold autoagglutinins active *in vitro* up to a temperature of 30°C or more, which are associated with such harmful effects as blocking of small vessels in the hands and feet on exposure to cold, due to red cell agglutination, and the production of haemolytic anaemia. In between, there are many examples of cold autoagglutinins that are active up to a temperature of 25°C or so, and which are found in association with disease. For instance, many patients with mycoplasma infection transiently develop anti-I in their serum, but usually this antibody is active only at low temperatures and is harmless. For cold antibodies, the distinction between harmless and harmful depends solely on the maximum temperature at which they are active. Cold autoantibodies that are harmless, because they are active only up to a temperature of about 25°C, may nevertheless be very troublesome in the laboratory, especially if tests are carried out at room temperature or the antiglobulin test is carried out in an albumin-containing solution or in a low-ionic-strength medium.

Warm autoantibodies react as strongly at 37°C, or more strongly at 37°C, than at lower temperatures. These autoantibodies, too, may be classified as harmful or harmless, according to whether or not they are associated with red cell destruction. In these cases the property of harmlessness is clearly not related to thermal range, but depends rather on the biological properties of the particular immunoglobulin molecules as well as on the number of antibody molecules that bind to the red cells and therefore also on the number and distribution of the corresponding antigen sites.

Whereas in patients with cold autoagglutinins the bulk of the antibody is in the serum, in patients with warm incomplete autoantibodies most is on the red cells.

Harmless cold autoantibodies

(see Table 7.1)

Normal cold autoagglutinins

Landsteiner (1903) observed that if the serum of an animal was mixed with a sample of its own red cells at a temperature near 0°C, agglutination occurred. He later showed that serum from most human subjects would agglutinate autologous red cells at 0°C (Landsteiner and Levine 1926).

The titre of normal autoagglutinins at 0–2°C does not usually exceed 64 using a tube technique with a 2% cell suspension and reading the results microscopically (Dacie 1962, p. 460), but is much higher with more sensitive methods, or when using microplates. In about one in four cases the titre of normal cold autoagglutinins is enhanced two- to four-fold if the serum is titrated in 22% bovine serum albumin instead of saline (Haynes and Chaplin 1971).

Normal cold autoagglutinins almost always have the specificity anti-I (Tippett *et al.* 1960) but, occasionally, may have other specificities: a mixture of anti-I and anti-i (Jackson *et al.* 1968); anti-I^T (Booth *et al.* 1966); anti-Pr (Garratty *et al.* 1973; Roelcke and Kreft 1984); anti-A, -B, -A$_1$I and -BI (for references, see seventh edition, p. 292); anti-M and -N (Moores *et al.* 1970; Tegoli *et al.* 1970; Sacher *et al.* 1989). Anti-LW occurring as a cold autoantibody is described in Chapter 5.

Anti-i was found in 10 out of 47 patients with cirrhosis of the liver, but active only at low temperatures and with a titre of 32 or less in 7 out of the 10 cases (Rubin and Solomon 1967).

Table 7.1 Some cold autoantibodies.

Description	Specificity	Notes
Harmless		
Normal cold autoagglutinins	anti-I	Present in all normal sera, occasionally accompanied by anti-i
	anti-Pr, etc.	Very rare
Normal incomplete cold 'antibody'	anti-H	Present in all normal sera, not an immunoglobulin but fixes complement to cells *in vitro*
Harmful		
Pathological cold autoagglutinins	anti-I	Usual specificity in chronic cold haemagglutinin disease (CHAD); also found transiently after mycoplasma infection
	anti-i	Rare alternative to anti-I in CHAD; also sometimes found transiently after infectious mononucleosis
	anti-Pr, etc.	See text
Biphasic haemolysins (Donath–Landsteiner antibody)	anti-P	Usual specificity in paroxysmal cold haemoglobinuria
	other	Very rare

Anti-I cold agglutinins can usually be demonstrated in cord blood (second edition, p. 252). They are IgM and presumed to be synthesized by the fetus *in utero* (Adinolfi 1965a).

An exceptional high-titre cold agglutinin that agglutinated cells at 37°C, but which was not associated with red cell destruction *in vivo*, has been described (Sniecinski *et al*. 1988).

Autoagglutinins inhibited by ionized calcium

Some examples of cold autoagglutinins react only in the absence of ionized calcium. The first example was described by Parish and Macfarlane (1941) as an autoagglutinin reacting in citrate but not in saline. Many examples have since been published, most with anti-HI or anti-H specificity. In all cases agglutination has been inhibited by Ca^{2+} and has depended on the presence of citrate or EDTA (for references, see previous editions of this book). Yasuda and colleagues (1997) describe an auto-anti-B whose reactivity depended on the concentration of ionized calcium being inhibited in concentrations of calcium chloride above 0.5 mM.

An autoagglutinin demonstrable only against borate-suspended red cells, with anti-A specificity, has been described (Strange and Cross 1981).

An autoagglutinin enhanced by sodium azide, with anti-I specificity, has been reported (Reviron *et al*. 1984).

Normal incomplete cold 'antibody' (n.i.c. antibody), which binds complement to red cells at low temperatures (Dacie 1950; Dacie *et al*. 1957), has anti-H specificity (Crawford *et al*. 1953) but is not an immunoglobulin (Adinolfi *et al*. 1963) and, in its properties, has some resemblance to properdin (Adinolfi 1965b).

Harmful cold autoantibodies
(see Table 7.1)

By definition, harmful cold autoantibodies are those associated with increased red cell destruction and/or vascular occlusion on exposure to cold. Autoimmune haemolytic anaemia (AIHA) is less commonly associated with cold autoantibodies than with warm ones. In several published series, each of more than 100 cases of AIHA, about 15–20% have been due to cold autoantibodies (Dausset and Colombani 1959; Dacie 1962; van Loghem *et al*. 1963; Petz and Garratty 1975).

A similar percentage (16%) was found in a series of 2000 patients with red cell autoantibodies (Engelfriet *et al*. 1982). A slightly higher percentage (about 35%) was observed in two other series (Vroclans-Deiminas and Boivin 1980; Sokol *et al*. 1981).

Harmful cold autoantibodies may be (1) cold autoagglutinins and haemolysins or (2) biphasic haemolysins (Donath–Landsteiner antibodies).

Cold haemagglutinin disease with autoimmune haemolytic anaemia

Two clinical syndromes may be distinguished, one chronic and one transient. In both, the pathological effects of the autoantibodies – vascular occlusion and accelerated red cell destruction – are exacerbated when the patient is exposed to cold. Vascular occlusion is seen particularly in the exposed parts of the body; accelerated red cell destruction may lead to haemoglobinuria.

The chronic syndromes are nearly always, if not always, associated with IgM paraproteins (monoclonal) with cold agglutinin activity. Only a small proportion of IgM paraproteins have cold agglutinin activity, for example 11 out of 99 in the series of Pruzanski and co-workers (1974). Of patients in whose serum IgM paraproteins are found, the majority have chronic lymphocytic leukaemia or some form of lymphoma and a minority have so-called Waldenström's macroglobulinaemia (Mackenzie and Fudenberg 1972); intermediate disease states are not uncommon (Tubbs *et al*. 1976). In some of the patients the paraproteinaemia is of the benign kind. Sometimes the cold autoagglutinins are detected before the paraproteinaemia becomes manifest.

In the transient syndromes, the cold haemagglutinins are polyclonal. The syndromes occur following infectious diseases, particularly mycoplasma infection and, less commonly, infectious mononucleosis. When the antibodies are active at 30°C or higher there may be an associated immune haemolytic anaemia.

In children, following infectious disease, high-titre cold agglutinins are only rarely observed (Habibi *et al*. 1974). A striking inverse correlation has been found between the titre of IgG anti-F(ab')2 antibodies and the titre of anti-I cold agglutinins in cold haemagglutinin disease (CHAD) not associated with infection ($P < 0.0001$) but not in CHAD associated with infection. An important role of IgG anti-F(ab')2 in the regulation of the production of cold anti-anti-I in patients with CHAD unassociated with infection is postulated (Terness *et al.* 1995).

Thermal range of autoantibody

Some examples of pathological cold autoagglutinins have titres of 1×10^6 or more at $0-4°C$. At higher temperatures they are markedly less active and often will not agglutinate red cells *in vitro* above a temperature of about $31°C$ (Dacie 1962, p. 468). Less commonly, the titre at low temperatures is only moderately increased but the antibody has a very wide thermal range and may then cause moderately severe anaemia (Schreiber *et al.* 1977; Rousey and Smith 1990). It should be emphasized that the clinical significance of a cold antibody is determined entirely by its ability to combine with red cells at, or near, body temperature rather than by its titre at some lower temperature.

Factors enhancing agglutination

In many cases the titre of cold autoagglutinins is enhanced by using an albumin solution rather than saline as a medium; 22% albumin is distinctly better than 12% (Haynes and Chaplin 1971).

In testing 28 examples of anti-I associated with AIHA, at $30°C$ 14 failed to agglutinate cells suspended in saline but all 28 agglutinated them in albumin. In tests at $37°C$, only two examples agglutinated cells suspended in saline, but 19 agglutinated cells suspended in albumin (Garratty *et al.* 1977). In some cases it is necessary to use an increased ratio of serum to cells to demonstrate clinically significant cold autoantibodies.

At any given temperature, enzyme-treated red cells take up more cold autoantibody than untreated cells and are agglutinated by potent anti-I up to about $38-40°C$ (Evans *et al.* 1965).

In studies with ^{131}I-labelled potent cold autoagglutinins maximally sensitized cells took up 8.9 mg of antibody/ml red cells, corresponding to rather more than 500 000 molecules per cell (Evans *et al.* 1965). The same authors found that the rate of association and dissociation of anti-I was unaffected by the presence of complement, suggesting that complement did not affect the binding of this antibody. On the other hand, Rosse and co-workers (1968), using the C1 transfer test, found that complement did affect the binding of some examples of anti-I. For example, in the presence of C1, fewer red cells were required to absorb the same amount of antibody (for further discussion see Chapter 3).

Complement binding

When normal red cells are sensitized *in vitro* with fresh serum containing anti-I some cells may be lysed (see below); unlysed cells react with anti-C3c and anti-C4c as well as with anti-C3g, anti-C3d and anti-C4d. On circulating red cells the only C3 and C4 components detectable are C3d and C3g (Lachmann *et al.* 1982; Voak *et al.* 1983), and C4d (and, possibly, C4g). Serum containing potent autoagglutinins is always capable of producing some lysis of normal red cells at $20°C$, although it may be necessary to adjust the pH of the serum to 6.8 to produce this effect (Dacie 1962, p. 468). Potent cold autoagglutinins that are readily lytic may be confused with biphasic haemolysin (Donath–Landsteiner antibody), but the latter antibody is non-agglutinating and almost always has anti-P specificity.

When the possibility of confusion between anti-I and biphasic haemolysin arises, the following comparison is useful in distinguishing between them (H Chaplin, personal communication): in one test, two samples of serum, one untreated and one acidified to pH 6.8, are incubated continuously (with red cells) at $20-25°C$ for 1 h and in the other, serum and red cells are first kept at $0°C$ for 30 min, then at $37°C$ for 30 min. Biphasic haemolysin gives maximal lysis under these latter conditions and is unaffected by acidification; on the other hand anti-I haemolysins are maximally lytic when incubated continuously at $20-25°C$, especially with acidified serum.

At low temperatures the agglutination caused by anti-I is very intense and when agglutination is dispersed some lysis may be observed due, apparently, to mechanical damage during dispersal of the agglutinates (Stats 1954). Although it has been claimed that potent cold autoagglutinins directly lyse red cells without the aid of complement (Salama *et al.* 1988), the effect may be a laboratory artefact.

Acquired resistance to complement-mediated lysis

When normal red cells are incubated at $20-30°C$ with anti-I serum and then warmed to $37°C$, anti-I is eluted but complement components remain bound to the red cell surface (Harboe 1964; Evans et al. 1965). As described in Chapter 3, bound C3b is very rapidly converted to iC3b, which is then cleaved relatively slowly, leaving only C3dg on the cell surface. Normal red cells exposed to anti-I and complement *in vitro* under conditions that are suboptimal for producing lysis become coated with α_{2D} (i.e. C3dg) and become resistant to lysis (Evans et al. 1968; De Wit and van Gastel 1970) and take up little or no β_{1A} (i.e. C3b) upon renewed exposure to anti-I and complement (Engelfriet et al. 1972; see also Jaffe et al. 1976).

Red cells made resistant to lysis by anti-I in the way just described are partially protected against lysis by anti-Le[b] (Engelfriet et al. 1972) and by anti-Le[a] (M Contreras and PL Mollison, unpublished observations). These findings are explained, presumably, by the fact that I and Lewis antigen sites are on molecules in close proximity and thus bring about the accumulation of C3dg molecules on closely similar areas of the red cell membrane. Cells coated with complement by exposure to serum at very low ionic strength are not protected against lysis by anti-I (De Wit and van Gastel 1970), possibly because the C3dg molecules are dispersed over the red cell surface and thus present in too low concentrations in the critical areas round I sites.

Circulating red cells of patients with CHAD are strongly coated with C3dg and are relatively resistant to red cell destruction. Thus, if a sample of red cells from a patient with CHAD is labelled with ^{51}Cr and re-injected into the circulation, the rate of red cell destruction is uniform and relatively slow. On the other hand, when red cells from a normal donor are injected, some 50% are destroyed in the first hour, although subsequently the rate of destruction is far slower (Evans et al. 1968; see below and also Chapter 10.

The question of transfusion in CHAD is discussed below.

Specificity of cold autoagglutinins associated with autoimmune haemolytic anaemia

Ii. In patients with CHAD the antibodies most commonly have I specificity, reacting with determinants on branched type 2 chains and occasionally have i specificity, reacting with determinants on linear type 2 chains (see Chapter 4). Antibodies (anti-j) reacting with both branched and linear type 2 chains have also

been described (Roelcke et al. 1994). I specificity can be verified by demonstrating that the serum reacts more strongly with adult than with cord red cells; several samples of cord cells should be tested, as some react relatively well with anti-I. The stronger reaction of anti-I with adult than with cord cells is sometimes more marked at 30°C than at lower temperatures (Burnie 1973). Occasionally, the antibody in CHAD has other specificities, as described below.

Pr and Sa. Unlike I, these antigens are expressed in equal strength on the red cells of adults and newborn infants. Most Pr antigens are destroyed by both proteases and sialidases. Anti-Pr and -Sa recognize the sialo-O-glycans of glycophorins. The reactivity of anti-Pr, as of some examples of anti-I, is greatly enhanced in low-ionic-strength solution (LISS), a fact that must be remembered when interpreting tests performed in this medium.

Anti-Pr has been found in patients, including newborn infants, with rubella (Geisen et al. 1975; König et al. 1992, 2001) and in patients with varicella (Northoff et al. 1987; Herron et al. 1993). Life-threatening autoimmune haemolytic anaemia occurring in a 6-week-old infant 5 days after receiving a diphtheria-pertussis-tetanus vaccination was attributed to an IgM cold-reactive autoantibody with probable anti-Pr specificity (Johnson et al. 2002). The infant survived after receiving transfusions from a donor who was homozygous for the extremely rare Mk phenotype and another individual who was homozygous for the vary rare MiVII phenotype.

Sialidase-susceptible antigens. Sia-11, Sia-b1 and Sia-lb1 (formerly Vo, F1 and Gd) are differentiation antigens (like I and i), created by sialylation of linear and branched type 2 chains (for a review of the biochemistry and serology of the above-mentioned specificities, see Roelcke 1989).

Other specificities

Rarely the specificity may be anti-A (Atichartakarn et al. 1985), anti-type 2 H (Uchikawa and Tokyama 1986), anti-P (von dem Borne et al. 1982), anti-M-like (Sangster et al. 1979; Chapman et al. 1982), anti-D (Longster and Johnson 1988), anti-Sd[x], later named anti-R[x] (Marsh et al. 1980; Bass et al. 1983) or anti-Ju (Göttsche et al. 1990a).

Anti-I and anti-i associated with acute infections

Following infection with *Mycoplasma pneumoniae* there is commonly a transient increase in the titre and thermal range of anti-I cold autoagglutinins. When the thermal range is high enough, the patient may develop an episode of haemolytic anaemia, which may be severe.

The fact that the titre of anti-I is increased following infection with *M. pneumoniae* suggests the possibility of the presence in that organism of I-like antigen. Although intact *M. pneumoniae* do not inhibit anti-I, lipopolysaccharide prepared from these organisms does. Furthermore, the cold agglutinins that develop in rabbits following the injection of *M. pneumoniae* are inhibited by these organisms (Costea *et al.* 1972). The erythrocyte receptors for mycoplasma are long-chain oligosaccharides of sialic acid joined by α (2–3) linkage to the terminal galactose residues of poly-N-acetyllactosamine sequences of Ii antigen type (Loomes *et al.* 1984).

Cold agglutinins with the specificity anti-Sia-b1 (or branched type 2 chains) frequently occur together with anti-I in the serum of patients with a *Mycoplasma pneumoniae* infection (König *et al.* 1988). However, the specificity of these antibodies is different from that of monoclonal anti-Sia-b1. Whereas the polyclonal antibodies recognize a determinant present on Oh cells, which is partially destroyed by endo-β-galactosidase, the epitope recognized by the monoclonal antibody is not present on Oh cells and is resistant to the enzyme. The antibodies may represent a post-infection autoimmune response against a sialo-type 2 structure common to Sia-b1 and I, which may be a receptor for *M. pneumoniae* (Roelcke *et al.* 1991).

Anti-I in very high titre has been found following infection with *Listeria monocytogenes*, which carries an I-like antigen: the patient had transient haemolytic anaemia (Korn *et al.* 1957). A transient increase in anti-I titre has also been described in a patient with systemic leishmaniasis associated with haemolytic anaemia (Kokkini *et al.* 1984) and following an acute cytomegalovirus infection not clearly associated with haemolytic anaemia (Pien *et al.* 1974).

In infectious mononucleosis, anti-i is frequently present as a transient phenomenon (Jenkins *et al.* 1965; Rosenfield *et al.* 1965). The antibodies rarely react *in vitro* above 24°C. Fewer than 1% of patients with mononucleosis develop a haemolytic syndrome (Worlledge and Dacie 1969).

In a few cases in which haemolytic anaemia complicated infectious mononucleosis and in which the patient's serum contained a potent cold agglutinin, the agglutinin was an IgG–IgM complex, the antibody being IgG and the IgM an anti-IgG antibody (Goldberg and Barnett 1967; Gronemeyer *et al.* 1981). In an exceptional case, the antibody although IgM, behaved serologically as a biphasic haemolysin: the agglutinin was active *in vitro* only up to 22°C, but exposure of red cells to the serum at 4°C, followed by warming of the mixture to 37°C, resulted in lysis (Burkart and Hsu 1979). In one, apparently unique, case anti-N was formed instead of the expected anti-i in a patient with infectious mononucleosis (Bowman *et al.* 1974).

Persistent anti-I and anti-i cold agglutinins not associated with haemolytic anaemia have also been found in the serum of patients with acquired immune deficiency syndrome (AIDS) or AIDS-related complex (Pruzanski *et al.* 1986). The thermal range of the antibodies was not established.

Is it necessary in clinical practice to determine the titre of cold agglutinins?

The serological diagnosis of CHAD is made by demonstrating the stronger reactivity at low temperatures and the wide thermal range of the antibody; activity can usually be demonstrated *in vitro* up to a temperature of 31°C. Determination of the titre is not worthwhile as a routine, although an association between a low titre and a response to corticosteroids has been observed (see below).

Red cell transfusion in patients with cold haemagglutinin disease

When red cells from a normal (I-positive) donor are transfused to a patient with CHAD due to anti-I, there is a phase of destruction that lasts until the cells have acquired resistance to complement-mediated destruction; during this phase, a proportion of the transfused population is destroyed within minutes; an identical phenomenon is observed with complement-activating alloantibodies (see Chapter 10). In CHAD, therefore, transfusion should be avoided if possible. If a transfusion is judged to be essential, the blood should be prewarmed, although a more important step is to nurse the patient in a warm room (see below). Red cells from ii adults have been shown to survive normally in patients with CHAD due to anti-I both in the chronic form (van Loghem *et al.* 1963) and in the transient form (Woll *et al.* 1974), but ii donors are seldom available. Unless the patient fails to respond to transfusion of red cells from random donors and it is known that ii donors are available, there is no point in determining the specificity of the cold agglutinins.

The presence of cold agglutinins complicates pre-transfusion testing (see Chapter 8).

Most patients with CHAD are not severely anaemic; if a haemolytic crisis does develop, red cell destruction can usually be arrested by putting the patient in a really warm environment (40°C). In cases in which the cold autoagglutinins have a low titre but a wide thermal range, treatment with corticosteroids has been successful (Lahav *et al.* 1989). Treatment with alpha-interferon resulted in a prompt clinical response and a considerable decrease of the titre of the cold agglutinins in two patients with severe CHAD (O'Connor *et al.* 1989; Fest *et al.* 1994). The successful use of rituximab, a monoclonal anti-CD20, in the treatment of CHAD is reported by Berentsen and co-workers (2004) who monitored 37 courses of rituximab given prospectively to 27 patients. Fourteen patients responded to their first course of treatment and 6 out of 10 responded to re-treatment. These authors conclude that rituximab is an effective and well-tolerated therapy for CHAD.

In a patient with scleroderma associated with severe haemolytic anaemia due to cold agglutinins, treatment with danazol (a gonadotrophin-release inhibitor) was followed by a rapid rise in Hb concentration (Lugassy *et al.* 1993).

Immunoglobulin structure of cold agglutinins

In chronic cold haemagglutin disease most examples of anti-I and anti-i are IgMκ, although a few IgMλ examples have been described (Pruzanski *et al.* 1974; Roelcke *et al.* 1974). All cold agglutinins with specificity for the I or i antigens are encoded by a single VH gene segment, VH4–34 (synonym: VH4–21; Silberstein *et al.* 1991; Pascual *et al.* 1992). The three-dimensional structure of the Fab of an anti-I (KAU) has been solved (Cauerhff *et al.* 2000). Potter and co-workers (2002) analysed this structure and proposed that I antigen interacts with antibody KAU via a hydrophobic patch in FR1 and the outside surface of CDRH3 rather than the conventional antigen binding site (Fig. 7.1). This raises the intriguing possibility that the conventional binding site of antibody KAU, and by inference of other cold agglutinins directed at I and i

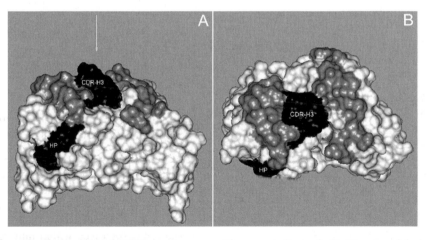

Fig 7.1 Crystal structure of cold agglutinin KAU, showing the hydrophobic patch in FR1 in relation to the conventional Ab combining site. (A) Space-filling representation of the surface of the V_H and V_L domains of KAU (Brookhaven Protein Data Bank code 1DN0). The hydrophobic patch (HP) and the CDR_H3 are depicted in black, the main body of the Ab is white, and the rest of the Ag binding site is grey. The arrow indicates the V_H:V_L axis and the location of the conventional Ag binding site. (B) View almost perpendicular to (A), looking down the axis of the V_H:V_L domain pair onto the conventional Ag binding site. Colour codes are as in (A). Figures were produced using INSIGHT II. From Potter *et al.* 2002 with permissions.

antigens, bind to additional as yet unidentified antigens. These authors draw an analogy between the binding of Ii carbohydrate structures to the hydrophobic patch on KAU and the way in which oligosaccharide chains of antibody molecules bind to a hydrophobic patch on the $C\gamma2$ domains of IgGFc. This alternative carbohydrate antigen-binding region also provides a possible explanation for the cold agglutinin activity of other V4–34 encoded antibodies including monoclonal anti-Ds (Thorpe *et al.* 1998).

Of the relatively few examples of anti-Pr, six were IgAκ and five of these had Pr_1 and one, Pr_a specificity (Angevine *et al.* 1966; Garratty *et al.* 1973; Roelcke 1973; Tonthat *et al.* 1976; Roelcke *et al.* 1993); one that was IgMκ was anti-Pr_2 and another (IgMλ), anti-Pr_3 (Roelcke *et al.* 1974, 1976). An IgAκ cold agglutinin had anti-Sa specificity (Roelcke *et al.* 1993).

IgM cold agglutinins with λ light chains are rarely directed against the I antigen. They are frequently cryoprecipitable and are often found in malignant conditions. Such agglutinins thus differ markedly from cold agglutinins with κ light chains.

Patients with chronic CHAD synthesize IgM at approximately 10 times the normal rate; treatment with alkylating agents results in a diminished rate of synthesis (Brown and Cooper 1970).

Occasionally, cold IgM anti-I is accompanied by a warm IgG autoantibody of the same or another specificity (see below). Examples of anti-I cold agglutinins that appeared to be solely IgG were described by Ambrus and Bajtai (1969) and Mygind and Ahrons (1973) and two cases in which the anti-Pr was IgG1κ have been described (Dellagi *et al.* 1981; Curtis *et al.* 1990). The latter case was unusual because the cold agglutinins failed to activate complement.

The possibility that IgM anti-I is always accompanied by at least traces of IgG and IgA autoantibodies is raised by the finding of Hsu and co-workers (1974). Using a PVP-augmented antiglobulin test in the autoanalyzer they found that, in patients with typical anti-I cold agglutinins, IgG and IgA could always be detected on the patient's red cells in addition to C3 and C4. Similarly, Ratkin and co-workers (1973) prepared eluates from 19 sera from patients with cold agglutinin disease and regularly found an excess of IgG and of IgA, both having agglutinating activity of relatively low titre. They interpreted their observations to mean that in patients in whom IgM autoantibodies predominated, autoantibodies of classes IgG and IgA were also regularly present, although in lower titre.

In mycoplasma infection, when a patient develops potent cold autoagglutinins of anti-I specificity as a transient phenomenon the antibody is made of heterogeneous IgM and contains both κ and λ light chains (Costea *et al.* 1966), although the heterogeneity is restricted (see Feizi 1977).

Production of cold autoagglutinins following repeated blood transfusions

Rous and Robertson (1918) observed that in rabbits transfused almost daily with the blood of other rabbits, cold autoagglutinins developed in about one-half of the animals. The animals with the most potent agglutinins developed a sudden anaemia, due perhaps to immune clearance of transfused cells. The agglutinins persisted in the animal's serum long after transfused cells had disappeared. Thus, in one case, 133 days after the last blood transfusion there was still gross autoagglutination on chilling the animal's blood.

Ovary and Spiegelman (1965) gave repeated injections of Hg^A-positive red cells to an Hg^A-negative rabbit: the animal produced not only the expected anti-Hg^A active at 37°C, but also a cold agglutinin.

The production of cold autoagglutinins in humans, following alloimmunization and in association with a delayed haemolytic transfusion reaction, has been observed only occasionally (see Chapter 11).

Cold (biphasic) autohaemolysins

In the syndrome of paroxysmal cold haemoglobinuria (PCH) the patient's serum contains a cold, complement-fixing antibody. This antibody, often referred to as the Donath–Landsteiner antibody after its discoverers, produces haemolysis both *in vitro* and *in vivo* when the blood is first cooled (to allow the binding of antibody) and then warmed (to provide optimal conditions for complement-mediated haemolysis). Because of this behaviour, the antibody is described as a 'biphasic haemolysin'.

Although biphasic haemolysin was originally described in a patient with tertiary syphilis, the majority of cases seen nowadays are associated with viral infections, particularly in children. In one series of 11 cases, only three were definitely syphilitic; of five which were definitely non-syphilitic, one followed measles and one mumps (Worlledge and Rousso 1965). Biphasic haemolysin may also occur transiently following chickenpox, influenza-like illness and prophylactic immunization with measles vaccine (Bird *et al.* 1976a).

Of 19 patients with biphasic haemolysin reported by Sokol and co-workers (1982, 1984), 17 were children. All patients were non-syphilitic. In 10 of the children the biphasic haemolysin developed after an upper respiratory tract infection. The other patients had infections with adenovirus type 2, influenza A virus or *Haemophilus influenzae*; one had chickenpox. The authors stressed the fact that in the acute form that typically occurs in children, the onset of the haemolytic anaemia is sudden, usually with haemoglobinuria, prostration and pallor. In the chronic form haemolysis is only mild; this form occurred in only two patients, one a child and the other an adult. Biphasic haemolysin in an adult patient with pneumonia due to *Klebsiella* was described by Lau and co-workers (1983).

In one series, all of 22 patients with biphasic haemolysins were children, who developed the antibodies after infection, usually of the upper respiratory tract (Göttsche *et al.* 1990b).

It has been suggested that for the prevalent non-syphilitic form of the syndrome the term Donath–Landsteiner haemolytic anaemia should be used rather than PCH, as the clinical manifestations are rarely paroxysmal, seldom precipitated by cold and not necessarily characterized by haemoglobinuria (Wolach *et al.* 1981).

Several estimates of the relative frequency of biphasic haemolysin in AIHA are available. In one series of 347 cases of AIHA, the antibody was found in six, i.e. fewer than 2% (Petz and Garratty 1980, p. 54). Similarly, of red cell autoantibodies from 2000 patients, 48 (2.4%) were biphasic haemolysins (Engelfriet *et al.* 1982). On the other hand, the antibody was present in four of 34 (12%) acute cases of AIHA in children in one series (Habibi *et al.* 1974) and in 17 out of 42 (40%) cases in another (Sokol *et al.* 1984). The 22 patients with biphasic haemolysins described by Göttsche and co-workers (1990b) were among 599 patients with AIHA, 68 of whom were children.

Although maximum haemolysis is observed when red cells are left with biphasic haemolysin and complement in the cold phase, the requirement for complement in the cold phase is not absolute. Thus when red cells are first left at 0°C with EDTA-treated serum containing fairly potent antibody then washed and incubated at 37°C with fresh normal serum, some haemolysis occurs (Polley *et al.* 1962). Similarly, Hinz and co-workers (1961a) found that if PNH red cells were used, haemolysis occurred quite readily when complement was supplied only in the warm phase of the reaction. An experiment described by Dacie (1962, p. 553) shows clearly that the reason why much more haemolysis is found when complement is present in the cold phase of the reaction is that, on warming, antibody very rapidly elutes from the red cells so that at higher temperatures there is usually too little antibody on the cells to activate complement. Hinz and co-workers (1961b) showed that optimal lysis occurred even when only C1 was present with antibody in the cold phase of the reaction; C4 could be present either in the cold or warm phases but C2 and C3 were essential in the warm phase.

False-negative results may be observed due to hypo-complementaemia and it may then be necessary to add fresh normal serum to demonstrate the presence of the biphasic haemolysin (Wolach *et al.* 1981).

In cases in which biphasic haemolysin is associated with syphilis (tertiary or congenital) the antibody is seldom active above 20°C; that is to say, red cells and serum must be cooled to a temperature below 20°C if there is to be haemolysis on subsequent warming. In cases in which the antibody appears transiently in children following infections, the thermal range is greater and the antibody may be active *in vitro* up to a temperature as high as 32°C (see Bird *et al.* 1976a). A monophasic haemolysin acting *in vitro* up to 32°C, in an adult, was described by Ries and co-workers (1971).

As mentioned above, potent cold autoagglutinins which are readily lytic may be confused with biphasic haemolysin, but the latter is usually non-agglutinating, produces substantially more lysis, is IgG rather than IgM and has anti-P rather than anti-I specificity. A test that helps to distinguish unusually lytic anti-I from biphasic haemolysin is described above.

Specificity. Classically, biphasic haemolysin has the specificity anti-P (Levine *et al.* 1963; Worlledge and Rousso 1965). Very occasionally, the specificity may be anti-'p' (see Chapter 4).

Biphasic haemolysins with anti-P specificity are inhibited by globoside: some are more strongly inhibited by the Forssman glycolipid, which contains the globoside structure with an additional terminal GalNAc residue, suggesting that the antibodies are probably evoked by Forssman antigens which are widespread in animal tissues and microorganisms (Schwarting *et al.* 1979). Chambers and Rauck (1996) described a case of childhood acute haemolytic anaemia following parvovirus infection. In this case the reticulocyte count was low (1.0%, attributed to parvovirus infection, see Chapter 4) despite profound anaemia (haematocrit 14.5%). As P antigen is both the receptor for parvovirus B19 and the target for most biphasic haemolysins the authors speculate that interaction of the virus with P antigen may have triggered an auto-anti-P response.

Occasionally, biphasic haemolysins have a specificity outside the P system: anti-IH (Weiner *et al.* 1964), anti-I (Engelfriet *et al.* 1968a; Bell *et al.* 1973a), anti-i, as described above, or anti-Pr like (Judd *et al.* 1986). In practice, determination of the specificity of biphasic haemolysins is not helpful in diagnosis. On the other hand, in children with antibodies of wide thermal range and severe red cell destruction, confirmation of anti-P specificity may be helpful in treatment, as transfusion of pp red cells is sometimes very successful (see below).

Immunoglobulin class. Biphasic haemolysin (of specificity anti-P) is composed of IgG (Adinolfi *et al.* 1962; Hinz 1963). If red cells are incubated at a temperature such as 15°C with fresh serum containing biphasic haemolysin and then washed at room temperature, they react weakly with anti-IgG but strongly with anti-C4 and anti-C3, as expected from the fact that the antibody elutes rapidly as the temperature is raised. During, and for some time after, an attack of haemoglobinuria, the red cells of patients with PCH give a positive direct antiglobulin test (DAT). Only complement components (presumably C3d and C4d) can be detected on the red cells.

Red cell transfusion in patients with biphasic haemolysins

Red cell transfusion is seldom required in PCH. When the thermal range of the antibody extends only to 20°C or so *in vitro*, the patient is not severely anaemic. In patients in whom the thermal range extends to 30°C or more, severe anaemia does occur occasionally but in these patients the disease is usually transient and recovery has usually begun before the question of transfusion has to be considered. The successful use of P-negative red cells (from a bank of frozen blood) has been reported (Rausen *et al.* 1975) but unwashed, unwarmed P-positive blood has also been used successfully in three affected children (Wolach *et al.*

1981). In a child with PCH and severe anaemia, who did not respond to transfusion of P-positive blood, the transfusion of P-negative blood resulted in a sustained rise in Hb level (I Franklin and M Contreras, personal observation). The use of plasmapheresis to remove the Donath–Landsteiner antibody and ameliorate severe autoimmune haemolytic anaemia in a child following gastroenteritis is described by Roy-Burman and Glader (2002). The authors consider that because production of the Donath–Landsteiner antibody is transient and relatively brief in post-viral illness, removal of the antibody by plasmapheresis is less likely to be followed by significant rebound antibody production.

Harmless warm autoantibodies

IgG subclass of harmless warm antibodies

The affinity of Fc receptors for IgG4 is very low and subjects with only IgG4 on their red cells are expected to have a positive DAT but no signs of red cell destruction. With IgG2, the situation is more complex because, as explained in Chapter 3, there are two alleles of the gene that encodes the FcRIIa receptor on macrophages. As a result, some subjects have a low-affinity receptor for IgG2 and, in the presence of an IgG2 autoantibody have a positive DAT without signs of red cell destruction; others have a high-affinity receptor and the potential to destroy IgG2-coated cells. Indeed, some patients with only IgG2 on their red cells have haemolytic anaemia (CP Engelfriet, unpublished observations). However, IgG2-mediated destruction depends upon antigen specificity; see pp. 227–228 and 426.

Although IgG1 and IgG3 readily adhere to Fc receptors and antibodies of these subclasses are expected to cause red cell destruction, in the case of IgG1, the number of molecules bound per cell must exceed a certain minimum number to bring about attachment to phagocytes and thus to cause red cell destruction (see below). Subjects with a relatively small number of IgG1 molecules per red cell are expected to have a positive DAT without signs of red cell destruction.

Positive direct antiglobulin test in apparently normal subjects

The fact that an apparently normal donor has a positive DAT is often first discovered when the donor's red cells are used in crossmatching. Sixty-five cases were found in this way in one region during a period in which one million donations were collected. Assuming that for every 10 donors detected one was missed, the frequency of donors with a positive DAT was estimated to be one in 14 000 (Gorst et al. 1980). In another prospective survey donors with a positive DAT were discovered either by antiglobulin testing or by noting autoagglutination of a blood sample in an automated or manual test and then doing an antiglobulin test. The frequency of donors with a positive DAT was one in 13 000 (Habibi et al. 1980). Although the results of these two surveys look very similar there were apparent differences between the two. In the first there was only C3d (and C4d) on the red cells of 28 of the 65 donors. All donors with a positive DAT were haematologically normal; of 32 of the donors followed for many years, 31 remained well and only one, with a strongly positive DAT with anti-IgG, developed AIHA (Gorst et al. 1980).

In the second series, immunoglobulin was detectable on the red cells in all of 69 cases (IgG in 67, IgM in 2). Ten per cent of the donors had subnormal Hb values; a further 29% had reticulocytosis, with or without hyperbilirubinaemia: 61% appeared to be normal haematologically but when Cr survival studies were carried out in a few of these subjects, results were below normal in about 50% of the cases (Habibi et al. 1980). It should be noted that 25% of the donors with a positive DAT were receiving methyldopa, a circumstance that might have debarred them from donation in many countries. In any case, it must be said that the evidence presented for a haemolytic state in many of the donors was rather slight. No donor had a reticulocyte count higher than about 4.5% or a bilirubin value higher than 2.2 mg/dl (37 μmol/l). Slightly reduced Cr survival in haematologically normal subjects is difficult to interpret. Finally, in many of the donors who were followed for a period of 1 year or more, haematological findings became normal.

A very much higher frequency of positive DATs in normal donors than that found in the two series mentioned above was reported by Allan and Garratty (1980), namely one in 1000, but the discrepancy may be more apparent than real, as over 90% of the reactions were only '1+' or less.

In 22 out of 23 normal donors with IgG on their red cells from the series of Gorst and co-workers (1980), the IgG subclass of the antibody was later investigated.

In 20 of the cases it was solely IgG1 and the number of IgG1 molecules per red cell varied from 110 to 950; in the remaining two subjects the red cells were coated only with IgG4 (Stratton et al. 1983). In another series of 10 subjects, five had only IgG1, three IgG4, one IgG2 and one both IgG1 and IgG3 (Allan and Garratty 1980).

In normal donors with a positive DAT, the specificity of the autoantibody, as in patients with AIHA, is often related to Rh (Issitt et al. 1976a; Habibi et al. 1980) but may be outside the Rh system, for example anti-Jk^a (Holmes et al. 1976) and anti-Xg^a (Yokohama and McCoy 1967).

In normal subjects with IgG on their red cells, the red cells may be agglutinated by anti-complement as well as anti-IgG, although the frequency with which both IgG and complement have been found has varied widely in different series, i.e. 15% (Gorst et al. 1980); 44% (Allan and Garratty 1980) and 70% (Issitt et al. 1976).

Positive direct antiglobulin test (IgG) in hypergammaglobulinaemia

An association has been observed between hypergammaglobulinaemia and a positive DAT. Of 50 patients with an increased concentration of IgG in their serum, 25 had a positive DAT without signs of increased red cell destruction. The eluates from the red cells were unreactive (Huh et al. 1988). In another study of 20 patients with an increased serum IgG and a positive DAT, there were no signs of increased red cell destruction. These eluates were also unreactive (Heddle et al. 1988). In a prospective study of 44 patients with increased serum IgG, the DAT was positive in the three patients with the highest IgG concentrations. The DAT became positive in two other patients who were treated with high-dose intravenous immunoglobulin and, again, the eluates were unreactive (Heddle et al. 1988). In patients with a positive DAT but with an unreactive eluate, a significant correlation has been observed between the strength of the DAT reaction and the serum IgG concentration (Clark et al. 1992).

C3d (and C4d) alone on red cells

In 40–47% of normal donors with a positive DAT, only complement is detected on the red cells (Allan and

Garratty 1980; Gorst *et al.* 1980). C3d can be demonstrated on all normal red cells by using a sufficiently potent anti-C3d serum (Graham *et al.* 1976) and both C3d and C4d can be demonstrated by using the sensitive PVP-augmented antiglobulin test (Rosenfield and Jagathambal 1978). The presence of these fragments on red cells is taken as evidence of continuing low-grade activation of complement (see Chapter 3). There is no reason to believe that autoantibodies of any kind are responsible for this activation and it is therefore not logical to discuss this subject under the general heading of 'harmless warm autoantibodies', but it is nevertheless convenient.

The amount of C3d on the red cells of normal adults has been estimated by using rabbit IgG anti-C3d and ^{125}I-labelled goat anti-rabbit IgG; in 174 normal adults there were estimated to be between 50 and 200 C3d molecules per red cell, i.e. too few to be detected in the ordinary DAT. There was no difference between males and females and no evidence of any change in the number of molecules per cell over the age range 20–65 years. There was also no evidence that the number was different in children (Chaplin *et al.* 1981). Other estimates of the number of C3d molecules per cell in normal adults are 207–427 (Freedman and Barefoot 1982) and 280–560 (Merry *et al.* 1983).

Weakly positive DATs due to increased amounts of C3d on the red cells appear to be relatively frequent in subjects who are ill. Dacie and Worlledge (1969) found that 40 out of 489 (8%) patients in hospital gave weakly positive antiglobulin reactions due to complement. Similarly, Freedman (1979) found that of 100 EDTA samples from hospital patients, taken at random, seven gave positive reactions with anti-C3d and anti-C4d; all seven patients were seriously ill. Again, in 8% of random hospital patients values greater than 230 C3d molecules per cell were found by Chaplin and co-workers (1981), who also noted that in random patients in hospital 33% had values for the numbers of C3d molecules per red cell that were above the range found in more than 90% of healthy adults.

In testing red cells with anti-C3d and anti-C4d, freshly taken EDTA blood should be used whenever possible, as the amounts of C3d and C4d on red cells in ACD blood may increase slightly during brief storage at 4°C (Engelfriet 1976); after 21 days of storage, the increase of C3d and C4d may be two-fold (H Chaplin, personal communication).

Positive direct antiglobulin test associated with various diseases, but without signs of increased red cell destruction

Malaria. A positive DAT has been found in 40–50% of West African children with falciparum malaria (Topley *et al.* 1973; Facer *et al.* 1979; Abdalla and Weatherall 1982). In most cases, only C3d is detected on the red cells but in some both C3d and IgG are present and, in a few, IgG alone. Although in one series there was a relationship between a positive DAT and anaemia (Facer *et al.* 1979), in the others there was not. It was suggested that a positive test might be associated with the development of immunity to malaria (Abdalla and Weatherall 1982).

On the other hand, some patients with falciparum malaria, with antibodies against triosephosphate, associated with a positive DAT, have a prolonged haemolytic anaemia (Ritter *et al.* 1993).

Kala azar. The presence of complement on the red cells of patients with this disorder was reported by Woodruff and co-workers (1972). Of 67 patients with kala azar, 33% tested prior to antimonial therapy had a positive DAT (Vilela *et al.* 2002).

Patients on α-methyldopa and other drugs. The development of a positive DAT without any evidence of a haemolytic process is very common in patients taking α-methyldopa and is found occasionally in patients taking a variety of other drugs. The subject is considered in more detail in the section on drug-induced haemolytic anaemia.

Patients with autoimmune haemolytic disease in spontaneous remission without signs of red cell destruction may have a positive DAT (Loutit and Mollison 1946). In a patient reported by Goldberg and Fudenberg (1968), the red cells were initially agglutinated by anti-IgG and anti-C3; the serum contained an IgM antibody reacting with IgG-coated red cells. After treatment with steroids, the patient went into complete haematological remission and the IgM antibody disappeared from the serum; however, the red cells were still strongly agglutinated by anti-IgG and anti-C3.

In a patient reported by von dem Borne and co-workers (1977), who initially suffered from severe AIHA, a long-lasting remission was induced with steroid therapy, and it was then found that the antibody on the patient's cells was predominantly IgG4; the coated red cells induced only weak rosetting with monocytes *in vitro* and it was postulated that there had been a switch in the subclass of the autoantibody, with production of a subclass IgG4, which was incapable of producing destruction *in vivo*.

Harmful warm autoantibodies

As mentioned above, antibodies reacting as well, or better, at 37°C than at lower temperatures are found in about 80% of all cases of AIHA. In the warm antibody type of AIHA, the DAT is almost always positive but the indirect test (for antibody in serum) is sometimes negative. Harmful warm autoantibodies are of two kinds: incomplete antibodies and haemolysins.

Incomplete warm autoantibodies

IgG alone has been found in 18.3% (Petz and Garratty 1975), 36% (Worlledge 1978) and 64% (Engelfriet *et al.* 1982) of cases.

IgG alone was found invariably in patients with a positive DAT associated with α-methyldopa in two series (Worlledge 1969; Issitt *et al.* 1976), although in a third, IgM and complement (Clq), in addition to IgG, were found on the red cells of all patients who developed α-methyldopa-induced haemolytic anaemia (Lalezari *et al.* 1982), results that could not be reproduced by one previous author (CP Engelfriet) or by Ben-Izhak and co-workers (1985). The detection of the IgM antibodies appears to depend on the anti-IgM serum used. It has been suggested that if the affinity of the anti-IgM for IgM is much greater than that of the IgM red cell antibodies for the red cell antigen, the IgM antibodies are removed from the red cell in the antiglobulin phase of the test (P Lalezari, personal communication).

IgG and complement have been found in 64.5% (Petz and Garratty 1980), 44.4% (Worlledge 1978) and about 34% (Engelfriet *et al.* 1982) of cases; in the latter series, IgG and complement were found on the red cells of all patients with a combination of IgG incomplete warm autoantibodies and warm haemolysins (see below).

When complement and IgG are found on the red cells of patients with incomplete warm autoantibodies, it does not follow that complement has been fixed by autoantibody. Some of the evidence for this assertion is as follows: (1) neither IgG incomplete warm autoantibodies present in the serum nor those detectable in an eluate from the red cells are capable of fixing complement *in vitro*; (2) in at least 50% of patients with IgA incomplete warm autoantibodies alone, complement is detectable on the red cells; and (3) the frequency with which both IgG and complement are found on the red cells is much higher in patients suffering from a typical immune complex disease such as systemic lupus erythematosus (SLE), than in other cases of the warm type of AIHA. Thus, in SLE, both IgG and complement were found on the red cells in all cases by Chaplin (1973) and Worlledge (1978), in virtually all cases by Petz and Garratty (1980) and in 81% of cases by Engelfriet and colleagues (1982).

IgG subclass of warm incomplete autoantibodies

IgG warm autoantibodies are IgG1 in the vast majority of patients (Engelfriet *et al.* 1982). IgG1 alone was found in 72% of patients and IgG1 with antibodies of another subclass in 25%. In only 23 out of 572 patients was no IgG1 detectable. IgG2 and IgG4 antibodies were found the least frequently. Table 7.2 shows the frequency with which IgG autoantibodies of only one subclass were detected, and the relation of the subclass of the autoantibodies to increased red cell destruction. Determination of the IgG subclass of autoantibodies in eluates can readily be achieved using commercially available gel tests (Fabijanska-Mitek *et al.* 1997).

As mentioned above, subjects whose red cells are coated with not more than 950 IgG1 molecules per cell show no signs of red cell destruction. On the other hand in patients with AIHA with only IgG1 on their red cells, the number of molecules per cell was found to be 1200 or more (Stratton *et al.* 1983). This finding agrees well with the observation that at least 1180 IgG1 anti-D molecules must be bound per cell for adherence to monocyte receptors to occur *in vitro* (Zupanska *et al.* 1986). There is a clear relationship between the number of IgG1 molecules per cell and the severity of haemolytic anaemia (van der Meulen *et al.* 1980). The role of IgG2 autoantibodies is uncertain; in subjects with high-affinity FcRIIa receptors, alloantibodies with A specificity are lytic but those with Rh specificity are not (Kumpel *et al.* 1996). IgG3 antibodies mediate lysis by monocytes even when present

265

Number of patients	IgG1	IgG2	IgG3	IgG4	Increased red cell destruction
416	+	–	–	–	75%
4	–	+	–	–	None
13	–	–	+	–	100%
5	–	–	–	+	None
438*					

Table 7.2 Presence or absence of increased red cell destruction in patients with IgG incomplete warm autoantibodies of only one subclass.

* 438 of 572 patients with IgG incomplete warm autoantibodies had antibody of only one subclass (CP Engelfriet, unpublished observations).

on red cells at too low a concentration to be detected in the normal DAT, which explains why the test is negative in some patients with AIHA. IgG4 autoantibodies do not cause red cell destruction.

The ability of different IgG subclasses to effect lysis of red cells is related to the nature of their interaction with Fc receptors and their ability to activate complement. The IgG Fc receptor family consists of several activating receptors and a single inhibitory receptor. Two activating receptors (FcγRI, FcγRIIIa) are common to humans and mice. Two additional receptors (FcγRIIa, FcγRIIIb) are found in humans but not in mice. The inhibitory receptor (FcγRIIb) is common to mice and man. Experiments carried out in mice lacking different Fc receptors have demonstrated that absence of activating receptors ablates tissue destruction in models of autoimmune disease, whereas inactivation of FcγRIIb exacerbates existing autoimmunity (reviewed in Hogarth 2002). Studies using transgenic mice expressing FcγRIIa show that crosslinking this receptor with antimouse platelet antibody results in a severe immune-mediated thrombocytopenia not found in transgene negative mice (McKenzie et al. 1999). Fossati-Jimack and colleagues (2000) injected different IgG subclass switch variants of a low-affinity auto-anti-red cell antibody (4C8) into mice to induce AIHA and compared the pathogenicity of the different antibodies. They found the highest pathogenicity with IgG2a (20- to 100-fold more potent than IgG1 or IgG2b) and IgG3 was not pathogenic at all. By comparing the results with wild-type mice and FcγR-deficient mice they could show that the differences in pathogenicity were related to the ability of the switch variants to react with the low-affinity FcγRIII. In a subsequent study, Azeredo da Silveira and co-workers (2002) compared subclass switch variants of a high-affinity anti-red cell autoantibody (34–3C) with those obtained with

the low-affinity antibody. They found that the high-affinity antibodies (IgG2a = IgG2b > IgG3) activated complement, whereas the low-affinity antibodies (and high-affinity IgG1) did not activate complement. The pathogenicity of high-affinity IgG2b and IgG3 isotypes was more than 200-fold higher than the corresponding low-affinity isotypes. This study in the mouse illustrates very clearly that a high density of cell-bound IgG is required for efficient binding and activation of C1, with complement activation being related to antibody affinity and the density and distribution of antigen.

Complement alone was found in about 10% of cases in two series (Worlledge 1978; Petz and Garratty 1980), although no cases of this kind were found in another series (Issitt *et al.* 1976). Only complement was found on the red cells of all patients with cold autoagglutinins, biphasic haemolysins or warm haemolysins without the simultaneous presence (see below) of incomplete warm autoantibodies (von dem Borne *et al.* 1969; Engelfriet *et al.* 1982).

As in all patients on whose red cells complement is bound *in vivo*, C3d (actually C3dg, see Chapter 3) is the subcomponent of C3 present on circulating red cells, and similarly C4d (possibly C4dg) is the only subcomponent of C4 present.

IgA. Incomplete warm autoantibodies may be solely IgA (Engelfriet *et al.* 1968b). IgA alone was found in 3 out of 291 cases in one series (Worlledge 1978), in 2 out of 102 cases in another series (Petz and Garratty 1980), and in 11 out of 1374 patients in a third series (Engelfriet *et al.* 1982). One example of an IgA incomplete autoantibody with Rh specificity (anti-e) has been described (Stratton *et al.* 1972). An IgA autoantibody with specificity for the third extracellular loop of band 3 has also been described (Janvier *et al.* 2002). For optimal conditions for detecting bound IgA in the antiglobulin test, see Chapter 8. In about 50% of patients with IgA autoantibodies, complement as well as IgA can be detected on the red cells.

The clinical course of patients with IgA incomplete warm autoantibodies is very similar to that of patients with IgG antibodies. Destruction of red cells by IgA antibodies is brought about by adherence to Fc receptors for IgA on monocytes and macrophages. It has been shown that adherence to this receptor leads to cytotoxic damage (Clark *et al.* 1984) or phagocytosis (Maliszewski *et al.* 1985). The FcR for IgA(FcαRI,CD89) belongs to the immunoglobulin superfamily and contains an extracellular region of 206 amino acids, a transmembrane domain of 19 amino acids and a cytoplasmic region of 41 amino acids. The extracellular region consists of two Ig-like domains, EC1 and EC2, and six potential sites for N-glycosylation. The receptor binds IgA1 and IgA2 with an equal affinity (Ding *et al.* 2003).

IgM incomplete warm autoantibodies occur with about the same frequency as IgA incomplete warm autoantibodies, i.e. in about 1% of patients with incomplete warm autoantibodies. For example, in one series of 1374 patients, 13 had only IgM autoantibody on their cells (always accompanied by complement), 13 had mixed IgG and IgM incomplete warm autoantibodies (and complement), and a single patient had a mixture of IgA and IgM incomplete warm autoantibodies together with complement (Engelfriet *et al.* 1982). The presence of autoantibodies of more than one immunoglobulin class on the red cells is associated with severe haemolytic anaemia (Ben-Izhak *et al.* 1985). Garratty and co-workers (1997) describe three severe cases (two fatal) of AIHA associated with warm IgM autoantibodies and point out that the specificities of each antibody (En[a], Wr[b] and Pr) are all associated with glycophorin A. The severity of AIHA caused by antibodies of these specificities may be related to the role of glycophorin A an inhibitor of red cell lysis by autologous complement (Okada and Tanaka 1983; Tomita *et al.* 1993, see Chapter 6).

Brain and co-workers (2002) obtained evidence that binding of lectins (*Maclura pomifera* and wheatgerm agglutinin) and antibodies to glycophorin A make the red cell membrane leaky to cations.

Warm autohaemolysins and agglutinins

Nearly all warm autohaemolysins react *in vitro* only with enzyme-treated red cells, although some examples weekly sensitize untreated red cells to agglutination by anti-complement serum. Most warm autohaemolysins react with antigens susceptible to destruction by phospholipase; the rest react with antigens that are hardly, if at all, susceptible; warm haemolysins show no specificity for Ii or Rh antigens (Wolf and Roelcke 1989).

Warm haemolysins, which are nearly always IgM, were the only autoantibodies found in 165 out of 2000 patients with red cell autoantibodies (Engelfriet *et al.* 1982). When only IgM warm haemolysins, reacting only with enzyme-treated cells *in vitro*, are demonstrable in a patient's serum, red cell survival is only slightly shortened (von dem Borne *et al.* 1969). IgM warm haemolysins also frequently occur together with incomplete warm autoantibodies, for example in 138 of the 2000 patients in one series (Engelfriet *et al.* 1982). Complement is found on the red cells of all patients with IgM warm autohaemolysins.

Rarely, warm autoantibodies are capable of agglutinating and haemolysing untreated normal red cells suspended in saline. Such autoantibodies were described by Chauffard and Vincent (1909), Dameshek and Schwartz (1938) and Dacie (1954), but are very rare. In one series they were found in only three of 2000 patients with red cell autoantibodies; their presence is associated with very severe intravascular haemolysis, which may be directly responsible for the death of the patient (Engelfriet *et al.* 1982).

Cold and warm autoantibodies occurring together

Patients with AIHA with both cold and warm autoantibodies in their serum are not as rare as was thought at one time: in one series the combination was recorded in 63 out of 865 patients (Sokol *et al.* 1981). In 25 of these patients studied in more detail, IgG and complement were detectable on the red cells in every case and anti-I or anti-i cold autoagglutinins, reactive at 30°C or above, were detectable in the serum. All the cases were severe; 56% were secondary, the commonest associated diseases being SLE and lymphoma (Sokol *et al.* 1983). In another series, a somewhat lower incidence of this kind of AIHA was reported, namely 12 out of 144 patients (Shulman *et al.* 1985); again, the haemolytic anaemia was severe in all cases and, again, many cases were secondary to SLE or lymphoma. Three of 46 patients with AIHA described by Kajii and colleagues (1991) had both IgGκ warm autoantibodies and IgMκ cold autoagglutinins. One patient had a lymphoma and the other two idiopathic AIHA. A few other cases have been described in which a patient with AIHA has had both IgG and IgM autoantibodies active at 37°C but in which the features have not been exactly the same as in the series described above. In one of these atypical cases both the IgM and the IgG autoantibodies reacted better in the cold but had a wide thermal range, the IgG antibody lysing enzyme-treated cells at 37°C (Moore and Chaplin 1973). In two other cases both IgM and IgG autoantibodies had anti-I specificity. There were many features that were quite atypical of CHAD; thus, the patients had a very severe haemolytic process unrelated to exposure to cold and responding well to steroids (Freedman and Newlands 1977). A case with many similarities was reported by Dacie (1967, p. 751).

Association of red cell autoantibodies, autoimmune haemolytic anaemia and carcinoma

Erythrocyte autoantibodies and carcinoma are found together 12–13 times more often than expected from their relative frequencies. In patients with carcinoma, warm autoantibodies were about twice as common as cold ones; about 50% of carcinoma patients with autoantibodies had AIHA (Sokol *et al.* 1994).

Negative direct antiglobulin test in autoimmune haemolytic anaemia

About 10% of patients with the clinical picture of AIHA have a negative conventional DAT (Garratty 1994). In many of these cases IgG, IgM or IgA auto-antibodies can be demonstrated by more sensitive methods (Petz and Branch 1983; Salama *et al.* 1985; Sokol *et al.* 1987). In five out of seven patients with a negative DAT on whose red cells an increased amount of IgG was detected with a more sensitive method, the anaemia was corrected by steroid therapy (Gutgsell *et al.* 1988).

Specificity of warm autoantibodies

Rh related

A few warm autoantibodies are specific for one particular Rh antigen such as e (Weiner *et al.* 1953) or D

(Holländer 1954); others react more strongly with e-positive than with e-negative samples (Dacie and Cutbush 1954) but the commonest pattern, found by Weiner and Vos (1963) in two-thirds of cases is to react well with all cells except for those of the type Rh_{null}.

Celano and Levine (1967) concluded that three specificities could be recognized: (1) anti-LW; (2) an antibody reacting with all samples except Rh_{null}; and (3) an antibody reacting with all samples including Rh_{null}.

Weiner and Vos (1963) classified their cases according to whether they reacted only with normal (nl) D-positive cells or also with 'partially deleted' (pdl) Rh-positive cells, for example D– –, or with both these types of cell and also with 'deleted' (dl) cells, i.e. Rh_{null}; of 50 cases tested by Marsh and co-workers (1972), three had specificity involving both Rh and U – about 40% of the antibodies in the series had no recognizable specificity. Anti-dl specificity, or 'no recognizable specificity' as some would call it, was found in 23 out of 33 cases associated with α-methyldopa and in 23 out of 30 normal subjects with a positive DAT by Issitt and co-workers (1976).

Subsequent biochemical studies have confirmed that many warm autoantibodies precipitate Rh polypeptides and RhAG from normal red cells, whereas others immunoprecipitate band 3, or band 3 and glycophorin A (Leddy *et al.* 1993). Iwamoto and co-workers (2001) expressed band 3, Rh polypeptides D, cE, ce, CE and chimeric antigens CE-D and D-CE in the eythroleukaemic line KU812 and tested the autoantibodies from 20 patients with AIHA for reactivity with the cloned transfected cell lines by flow cytometry. Fifteen of the autoantibody eluates reacted with at least one of the Rh expressing cell lines, and seven reacted with the band 3 expressing cell line.

Leddy and Bakemeier (1967) found a relationship between specificity and complement binding; with one exception, antibodies reacting weakly or not at all with Rh_{null} cells failed to bind complement, whereas 70% of antibodies reacting as well with Rh_{null} cells as with other cells did bind complement. A similar observation was made by Vos and co-workers (1970), namely that those eluates that fixed complement had broad specificities, as evidenced, for example, by the ability to react both with normal red cells and with Rh_{null} cells.

In patients who develop a positive DAT as a result of taking α-methyldopa, with or without haemolytic anaemia, the autoantibodies have the same Rh-like specificities as in idiopathic AIHA (Carstairs *et al.* 1966; Worlledge *et al.* 1966; Garratty and Petz 1975).

Often, mixtures of specific autoantibodies, for example auto-anti-e and autoantibodies with no recognizable specificity, occur together. In such cases the presence of the specific autoantibody may be suspected if the serum is titrated against red cells of different Rh phenotypes. Differential absorptions of the serum with R_1R_1, R_2R_2 and rr red cells confirm the presence of specific autoantibody or reveal a relative specificity (i.e. stronger reactions with red cells carrying certain antigens, e.g. E), when it has not previously been suspected. If the three red cells are properly selected, so as to cover between them the vast majority of important antigens, clinically significant alloantibodies can also be excluded (Wallhermfechtel *et al.* 1984). The additional use of polyethylene glycol (PEG) or LISS in the absorption procedure is reported to reduce markedly the number of absorptions required to identify alloantibodies in sera with autoantibodies and so decrease the time required for laboratory investigation (Cheng *et al.* 2001; Chiaroni *et al.* 2003).

When the autoantibody has a specificity resembling that of Rh alloantibodies, red cells that are compatible *in vitro* survive normally, or almost normally, in the recipient's circulation (Holländer 1954; Ley *et al.* 1958; Mollison 1959; Högman *et al.* 1960). In the example shown in Fig. 7.2, the patient was ccddee, with an autoantibody of apparent specificity anti-e. The mean lifespan of transfused e-positive (DCCee) red cells was about 8 days, which was similar to that of the patient's own red cells (see Dacie 1962, p. 450), whereas the survival of e-negative (DccEE) red cells was only slightly subnormal. For references to further similar cases in which red cell survival has been studied, see Petz and Swisher (1989, pp. 565–567).

Specificity mimicking that of alloantibodies with Rh specificity

A minority of warm autoantibodies at first sight appear to have the specificity of an Rh alloantibody, such as anti-E. For example, an eluate prepared from the red cells of a patient of phenotype DCCee may react more strongly with E-positive than with E-negative cells and thus appear to contain anti-E. However, in about 70% of such cases all antibody activity can be absorbed completely by red cells lacking the

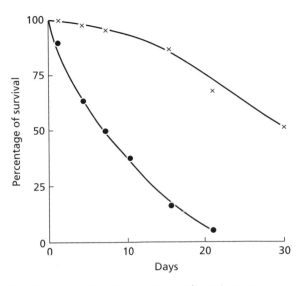

Fig 7.2 Survival, in a ddccee patient with autoimmune haemolytic anaemia, of e+ (DCCee) red cells (●), estimated by differential agglutination, and of e− (DccEE) cells (×), estimated by ^{51}Cr labelling and corrected for Cr elution. The patient's serum contained an autoantibody reacting preferentially with e+ cells. (The legend of this figure as published originally (Mollison 1959) stated incorrectly that the e+ cells were autologous and were labelled with ^{51}Cr.)

corresponding antigen, e.g. DCCee in the present example. The specificity of these autoantibodies seems in fact to be anti-Hr or anti-Hr$_0$ (Issitt and Pavone 1978).

The case reported by van't Veer and co-workers (1981) in which a negative DAT was found on the red cells of a patient with severe haemolytic anaemia, whereas strong autoantibodies of apparent anti-C and anti-e specificity were present in the serum demonstrates that such Rh specificities may be entirely illusory: not only (1) could the autoantibodies be absorbed with C-negative and e-negative cells, respectively, but also (2) during the episode in which the DAT was negative and the patient's red cells (DCcee) did not react *in vitro* with the patient's own autoantibodies, they reacted normally with auto-anti-C and allo-anti-e. The nature of the epitope with which such antibodies react is not known. Neither is it clear why the epitope should be so strongly associated with Rh alloantigens. The case reported by Rand and co-workers (1978) in which autoantibodies with anti-E

269

specificity were eluted from an E-negative patient's cells clearly demonstrates the mimicking nature of the specificity of the autoantibodies. Not only could the anti-E be absorbed to exhaustion by E-negative cells, but also the eluate from the E-negative cells used for absorption contained antibodies that again showed positive reactions only with E-positive cells. A possible explanation for this phenomenon is provided by observations on the specificity of anti-Is reported by Potter and co-workers (2002) who conclude that anti-I specificity is mediated through binding to a hydrophobic patch adjacent to the conventional antigen binding site (see p. 259). It is well established that many monoclonal anti-Ds are encoded by the same Ig gene (V4–34) as cold agglutinins and can exhibit cold agglutinin activity (Thorpe et al. 1998). The cold agglutinin activity itself could account for absorption of anti-D by D-negative red cells. Alternatively, the unusually high positive charge of anti-Ds and/or the considerable structural homology between D and CE polypeptides (discussed in Chapters 3 and 5; see also Thorpe et al. 1998) might predispose to absorption of these antibodies on all red cells irrespective of Rh phenotype. Some monoclonal anti-D recognized a ce polypeptide in which Arg145 was substituted by Thr, Thr 154 is not found in the D polypeptide. In this case, cold reactivity was ruled out as a possible explanation (Wagner et al. 2003).

Specificities outside the Rh system

The possible involvement of Wr^b in the specificity of autoantibodies was investigated by Issitt and co-workers (1976). Of 64 sera from patients with AIHA, two failed to react with Wr(a+ b–) cells and contained only anti-Wr^b; the remaining sera reacted with Wr(a+ b–) red cells but, after absorption with these cells to remove anti-dl, 32 could be shown to contain anti-Wr^b. The Wr^b antigen is formed by the association of band 3 with glycophorin A (see Chapter 6). Some, but not all, warm autoantibodies capable of co-precipitating band 3 and glycophorin A were shown to have anti-Wr^b specificity by Leddy et al. (1994). In patients with warm AIHA, autoantibodies with many other specificities are occasionally encountered, e.g. A (Szymanski et al. 1976); K, k and Kp^b in association with weakening of Kell antigens (see below); Kx (Sullivan et al. 1987); Jk^a (van Loghem and van der Hart 1954); Jk3 (O'Day 1987); N (Bowman et al.

1974); S (Johnson et al. 1978); U (Marsh et al. 1972); Vel (Szaloky and van der Hart 1971); I^T (Garratty et al. 1974); Ge (Reynolds et al. 1981); Sd^x (Denegri et al. 1983) and Sc1 (Owen et al. 1992). For others, see Garratty (1994).

Kell antibodies associated with autoimmune haemolytic anaemia

Several cases have been described in which a patient has developed a positive DAT, usually with overt haemolytic anaemia, and has been found to have autoantibodies of Kell specificity in the serum associated with weakening of Kell antigens. Seyfried and co-workers (1972) described a patient with potent anti-Kp^b in his serum; during the period of his acute illness his own red cells reacted with anti-Kp^b only after they had been treated with ficin. Sixteen weeks later, when the patient was better, Kell antigens were of normal strength. Beck and co-workers (1979) described a patient with similar serological findings but without AIHA. A patient has been described in whom, during consecutive relapses of autoimmune thrombocytopenia the Kell and Lutheran antigens became virtually undetectable. It was shown that this was due to transient absence of the Kell and Lutheran proteins during a relapse (Williamson et al. 1994). Other examples of weakening of red cell antigens in association with the appearance of alloantibodies or autoantibodies of the corresponding specificity are given in Chapter 3.

The frequency of autoantibodies with Kell specificity in patients with warm AIHA was estimated to be about 1 in 250 by Marsh and co-workers (1979).

Autoantibodies mimicking alloantibodies with specificity other than Rh

Autoantibodies may mimic the specificity of anti-K (Garratty et al. 1979; Viggiano et al. 1982); anti-Jk^b plus anti-Jk3 (Ellisor et al. 1983); anti-Kp^b (Manny et al. 1983; Puig et al. 1986), anti-Fy^b (Issitt et al. 1982; van't Veer et al. 1984), anti-Fy^a plus anti-Fy^b (Harris 1990) and anti-hr^B-like (Vengelen-Tyler and Mogck 1991). In all of these cases, the patient was negative for the corresponding antigen, the antibodies could be absorbed by red cells negative for the corresponding antigen, and eluates from such cells again showed the mimicking specificity.

Autoantibodies directed against non-polymorphic determinants

Some warm autoantibodies are directed against determinants that are clearly non-polymorphic. For example, anti-phospholipid antibodies, which occur in some patients with SLE and which may cause haemolytic anaemia (Arvieux et al. 1991) and antibodies against triosephosphate, found in some patients with falciparum malaria (see section on positive DAT in malaria, above).

Negative direct antiglobulin test despite warm autoantibodies in the serum

In a case reported by Seyfried and co-workers (1972), during an episode of severe haemolysis, the DAT on the patient's red cells was negative despite the presence of potent autoantibodies in the serum. The antibodies had anti-Kp^b specificity, and weak anti-Kp^b could be eluted from the patient's red cells. The antigens of the Kell system were severely depressed at the time when the DAT was negative, but were of normal strength after recovery. Cases of transient depression of LW, associated with appearance of anti-LW in the serum, and without haemolytic anaemia, are described in Chapter 5. Several further cases, similar to the case of Seyfried and co-workers, have been observed in which the autoantibodies have had the following specificities: anti-E (Rand et al. 1978); anti-Rh of undefined specificity (Issitt et al. 1982; Vengelen-Tyler et al. 1983); 'mimicking' anti-C + anti-e (see above) (van't Veer et al. 1981); anti-En^a (Garratty et al. 1983); anti-Kp^b (Brendel et al. 1985; Puig et al. 1986); specificity for a high-frequency antigen in the Kell system (Vengelen-Tyler et al. 1987); anti-Jk^a (Ganly et al. 1988); anti-Jk3 (Issitt et al. 1990) and anti-Fy^a + Fy^b (Harris 1990). In all the foregoing cases, there was total or severe depression of the antigens, against which the autoantibodies were directed (compare with Chapter 3). In some cases, although the DAT was negative, an eluate from the patient's red cells contained weak autoantibodies of the same specificity as those in the serum. In some cases the DAT had been positive before the episode of severe haemolysis. In other cases the patient presented with a negative DAT and the antibodies were first thought to be alloantibodies.

In a case reported by Herron and co-workers (1987) the autoantibodies were found to react much more strongly with old, i.e. relatively dense, red cells than with young cells and it was suggested that the DAT during an episode of severe haemolysis became negative because only young red cells remained in the circulation.

Role of CD47 in modulating the severity of autoimmune haemolytic anaemia in mice

CD47 is a glycoprotein present on all cells. In human red cells it is associated with the proteins of the band 3–Rh complex (see also Chapters 3 and 5). CD47 appears to inhibit phagocytosis of normal circulating red cells by ligating the macrophage inhibitory receptor signal regulator protein alpha (SIRPalpha; Oldenborg et al. 2000). Non-obese diabetic (NOD) mice spontaneously develop mild AIHA aged between 300 and 550 days, whereas CD47-deficient NOD mice develop a severe AIHA at age 180–280 days. In addition, CD47-deficient C57BL/6 mice are much more susceptible to experimental passive AIHA induced by anti-red cell monoclonal antibodies than their wild-type counterparts (Oldenborg et al. 2002). These results are consistent with a role for CD47 in antibody-mediated phagocytosis.

Transfusion as a stimulus for allo- and auto-antibody production

Young and co-workers (2004) carried out a retrospective analysis of blood bank records in order to determine the frequency of red cell autoimmunization associated with alloimmunization. They found 121 out of 2618 patients with a positive direct or indirect antiglobulin test (IAT) to have red cell autoantibodies. Forty-one of these patients also had alloantibodies and 12 of these developed their autoantibodies in temporal association with alloimmunization after recent blood transfusion. These authors conclude that auto-immunization and the development of AIHA should be recognized as a complication of allogeneic blood transfusion and recommend that once red cell auto-immunization is recognized, a strategy that minimizes exposure to allogeneic blood should be employed In total, 6 out of 16 D-negative patients who developed anti-D after transfusion with D-positive red cells also made IgG autoantibody and three of these patients suffered prolonged haemolysis (Frohn et al. 2003). Shirey and co-workers (2002) advocate prophylactic antigen-matched donor blood for patients with warm autoantibodies in order to minimize the risk of allo-antibody production.

Red cell transfusion and other therapy for patients with autoimmune haemolytic anaemia associated with warm autoantibodies

In severe AIHA, transfusion produces only a very transient increase in Hb concentration and carries an increased risk of: (1) inducing the formation of allo-antibodies; (2) increasing the potency of the auto-antibodies; and (3) inducing haemoglobinuria due to autoantibody-mediated red cell destruction (Chaplin 1979). Accordingly, even in severely anaemic patients, it is usually best to begin treatment with corticos-teroids, following which the Hb concentration usually starts to rise within 7 days (Petz and Garratty 1980, p. 392). If the effect of corticosteroids is not satis-factory, or if a quicker effect is needed, intravenous immunoglobulin (IVIG) can be given which, in very high doses (e.g. 0.4 g/kg per day) may have a very rapid effect (MacIntyre et al. 1985; Newland et al. 1986; Argiolu et al. 1990). However, in a study including 73 patients, IVIG had a rapid effect in only about 35% of cases, and particularly in patients with hepatomegaly and patients with a low pre-treatment haemoglobin. It is recommended that this treatment should be restricted to selected cases, for example to those in which the pre-treatment haemoglobin level is < 60–70 g/l or those with hepatomegaly (Flores et al. 1993).

Treatment with ciclosporin (4 mg/kg per day) can be tried and may result in a fairly rapid increase in Hb concentration (Hershko et al. 1990). Splenectomy is indicated only in patients who have failed to respond to steroids, IVIG and ciclosporin. In the patients with complete warm haemolysins IVIG may be valuable, as Ig has been found to inhibit complement-dependent lysis (Frank et al. 1992). Rituximab (monoclonal anti-CD20) has been used successfully in the treatment of AIHA in several studies. Shanafelt and co-workers (2003) consider that rituximab should be considered as salvage therapy for immune cytopenias that are refractory to both corticosteroid treatment and splenectomy. These authors report complete remission in 5 out of 12 patients with idiopathic thrombocytope-nia, and two out of five patients with AIHA. However, serious adverse effects have been reported (reviewed in Petz 2001). Jourdan and co-workers (2003) report

a case of severe AIHA that developed following rituximab therapy in a patient with a lymphopro-liferative disorder.

There have been several reports of a high incidence of alloantibodies in patients with the warm antibody type of autoimmune haemolytic anaemia (WAIHA) who have been transfused. In three series the frequency was 32–38% and was as high as 75% in patients who had received more than five transfusions (Branch and Petz 1982; Laine and Beattie 1985; James et al. 1988; reviewed by Garratty and Petz 1994). In these three series, the patient's serum was absorbed with auto-logous red cells before being tested for alloantibodies. In another series it was found that 44% of alloanti-bodies could not be detected before autoabsorption (Walhermfechtel et al. 1984). There has been one report indicating that red cell alloimmunization is rare in WAIHA (Salama et al. 1992) but the patients' sera were not absorbed with autologous red cells before being tested and alloantibodies may have been overlooked.

The risk of haemolysis after red cell transfusions in patients with AIHA with warm autoantibodies has been questioned. No instance of increased haemolysis was seen in 53 patients even in cases in which the trans-fused red cells were incompatible with autoantibodies detectable in the recipient's serum (Salama et al. 1992).

Transfusion is indicated only in special circum-stances, for example if the patient is severely anaemic and is going into cardiac failure, or has neurological signs, or has rapidly progressive anaemia, or is to undergo splenectomy. In most other circumstances it is better to use palliative measures, such as absolute bed rest, to counteract the decreased tolerance to exercise, while monitoring the Hb level.

If transfusions are given, it is important to group the patient's red cells for all clinically significant alloanti-gens, to facilitate the identification of any alloanti-bodies that may be produced. In patients who have previously been transfused or have been pregnant, it is also important to try to exclude the presence of allo-antibodies, which may be masked by the presence of autoantibodies. Either autoabsorption can be used or, if sufficient autologous red cells cannot be obtained, differential absorptions (see Chapter 8). It is helpful to obtain red cells from the patient before the first trans-fusion is given, and to store these at 4°C or frozen, so as to have cells for autoabsorptions if needed (Petz and Swisher 1989, p. 564).

When the presence of an alloantibody has been established, antigen-negative red cells must be selected for transfusion: the practice of transfusing 'least incompatible red cells' is not acceptable under these circumstances (see Laine and Beattie 1985).

In selecting red cells for transfusion, any blood group specificity of incomplete warm autoantibodies should when possible also be taken into account. In Rh D-negative females with auto-anti-e who have not yet reached the menopause, the red cells should, if possible, be e-negative as well as D-negative (i.e. ddccEE). In patients with auto-anti-e, e-negative (EE) red cells may survive better than e-positive cells (see Fig. 7.1) but may stimulate the production of anti-E (Habibi et al. 1974).

When transfusing patients with AIHA, packed red cells should be given in just sufficient quantities to raise the Hb concentration to a level that will make it possible for other therapy to be applied. In acute anaemia, oxygen may have to be given. A few patients need regular transfusions despite all other forms of therapy.

As mentioned above, the presence of warm auto-antibodies in the serum may make it difficult to detect alloantibodies (see also Chapter 8).

T-cell reactivity in AIHA

Peptides corresponding to sequences in the D and CE polypeptides stimulated proliferation of T cells from the peripheral blood and spleen of seven out of nine patients with AIHA. In total, four of the seven reactive patients had autoantibody to the Rh proteins. Multiple peptides were also stimulatory in two positive control donors who had been alloimmunized with D-positive red cells (Barker et al. 1997). Stimulation of peripheral blood mononuclear cells from patients with AIHA with D polypeptide resulted in either proliferation and secretion of γ-interferon or secretion of interleukin 10 (IL-10). Peptides derived from the D polypeptide that preferentially induced IL-10 secretion suppressed T-cell proliferation against D polypeptide, suggesting that it may be possible to ameliorate red cell autoantibody responses in man with inhibitory peptides (Hall et al. 2002). An important role for IL-10 in the function of peptide-induced regulatory T cells in vivo is apparent from successful peptide therapy, based on nasal administration of peptides corresponding to dominant T-cell epitopes, in mouse models of autoimmunity such as experimental allergic encephalomyelitis, which are associated with a devia-

tion from a Th1 to a regulatory IL-10 CD4+ T-cell response (Sundstedt et al. 2003).

Haemolytic anaemia in recipients of allografts

Alloantibodies produced by donor lymphocytes in grafted tissue may simulate autoantibodies in the recipient and cause haemolytic anaemia (see Chapter 11).

Positive direct antiglobulin tests due to anti-red cell antibodies in antilymphocyte globulin

Antilymphocyte globulin (ALG) is commonly prepared in horses and the serum contains antibodies against human red cells. Following the injection of ALG, the recipient's red cells acquire a positive DAT within 1–3 days (Lapinid et al. 1984; Swanson et al. 1984). The reaction between AHG reagent and the horse serum on the patient's red cells can be inhibited by adding diluted horse serum to the AHG reagent without interfering with the reaction between the AHG reagent and any human alloantibodies which may be bound to the patient's red cells (Swanson et al. 1984). In the serum of patients injected with ALG, autoantibodies can be detected, which usually show no obvious specificity but which occasionally have a Lu-related pattern (Anderson et al. 1985).

Occasionally, a positive DAT in a patient who has been injected with ALG is due to human red cell alloantibody; the alloantibody is derived from the plasma which has been added to the ALG to inhibit horse antibodies against human plasma proteins (Shirey et al. 1983).

Administration of ALG may occasionally produce immune red cell destruction; in the case described by Prchal and co-workers (1985) the DAT was negative with AHG reagent but positive with anti-horse immunoglobulin.

Antibodies against bound or induced antigens

Drug-induced immune haemolytic anaemia

Among cases of acquired immune haemolytic anaemia 18% were due to drugs in the series of Dacie and Worlledge (1969) and 12.4% in the series of Petz and Garratty (1980). The great majority of cases of drug-induced haemolytic anaemia were at one time due to α-methyldopa (Worlledge 1969) but this drug is now used much less frequently. Cases resulting from other drugs are very rare, penicillin-induced anaemia being the least uncommon (Petz and Garratty 1980). Recently, four cases of haemolytic anaemia (one fatal) have been described following piperacillin therapy (Arndt *et al.* 2002), one case attributed to tazobactum (Broadberry *et al.* 2004) and another to teicoplanin (Coluccio *et al.* 2004).

Most drug-induced immune haemolytic anaemias since the late 1980s have been caused by second- and third-generation cephalosporins, cefotetan and ceftriaxone respectively (Arndt and Garratty 2002; Petz and Garratty 2004). In total, 10 out of 35 cases of cefotetan-induced severe haemolytic anaemia studied by Garratty and co-workers (1999) were in patients who had received cefotetan prophylactically for obstetric and gynaecological procedures. Citak and co-workers (2002) report the development of haemolytic anaemia in a child with no underlying immune deficiency or haematological disease following treatment with ceftriaxone for a urinary tract infection. The patient had antibody against ceftriaxone and was successfully treated with high-dose corticosteroids.

Non-steroidal anti-inflammatory drugs (NSAIDs) can also induce very severe AIHA. Jurgensen and co-workers (2001) describe a case of fatal AIHA with multisystem organ failure and shock caused by diclofenac-dependent red cell autoantibodies.

The fluoroquinolones, ciprofloxacin and levofloxacin, have been associated with causing AIHA in single case reports (Lim and Alam 2003; Oh *et al.* 2003).

Most drug molecules are not large enough to induce an immune response but may become immunogenic when bound to a macromolecule, for example a protein at the surface of a cell, to form a hapten–carrier complex. Antibodies formed against such a complex may be specific for the hapten, the hapten–carrier combining site or the carrier alone (see Shulman and Reid 1993).

There are several ways in which drugs may be responsible for a positive DAT, often associated with immune haemolytic anaemia (reviewed in Issitt and Anstee 1998; Petz and Garratty 2004).

Drug adsorption mechanism

The drug may bind firmly to red cells; when an antibody is formed against the drug, the drug-coated cells may be destroyed. The drug antibodies can be detected *in vitro* with washed drug-coated cells. In these cases, the antibodies are directed against the drug alone (i.e. the hapten) and can be absorbed by the drug. This mechanism has been called 'the drug-adsorption mechanism' (Garratty and Petz 1975). Penicillin acts in this way and so, occasionally, do other drugs, particularly some of the cephalosporins (see Garratty 1994).

In about 3% of patients with bacterial endocarditis receiving massive doses of i.v. penicillin, a positive DAT develops but AIHA occurs only occasionally; the first case, associated with the prolonged administration of penicillin in high dosage (20 million units or more daily for weeks), was described by Petz and Fudenberg (1966): the patient's serum contained an IgG penicillin antibody of unusual potency. If it is necessary to continue giving penicillin to patients with AIHA due to penicillin antibodies, transfusions may be required. Normal red cells, uncoated with penicillin, will appear to be compatible on crossmatching but after transfusion will become coated *in vivo* and destroyed in the same way as the patient's cells.

Although penicillin antibodies are usually IgG they may be partly IgM (Fudenberg and German 1960) or solely IgM (Bird *et al.* 1975), in which case complement is bound and the red cells are agglutinated by anti-C3. In patients with immune haemolytic anaemia due to penicillin antibody, the antibody can invariably be demonstrated in high titre in the serum, using red cells coated *in vitro* with penicillin (Petz and Garratty 1980; Petz and Branch 1985).

IgM or IgG antibodies reactive with penicillin-coated red cells have been found in the serum of about 4% of haematologically normal subjects (Fudenberg and German 1960).

The benzyl-penicilloyl groups are the most immunogenic of the haptenic groups of penicillin (Garratty and Petz 1975).

Several cases of severe or even fatal haemolytic anaemia due to second- or third-generation cephalosporins have been described in which the drug adsorption mechanism was involved (see Garratty *et al.* 1992). In some of the cases the immune complex mechanism described below also seems to have been involved (Marani *et al.* 1994; Ogburn *et al.* 1994).

Trimolecular complex mechanism

The drug does not bind firmly to red cells so that drug-coated cells cannot be prepared. It has been suggested that in these cases, when antibodies are formed against the drug, immune complexes attach to the red cell. This immune complex theory has been criticized for the following reasons: (1) certain drugs cause haemolytic anaemia in some patients but immune thrombocytopenia in others implying that a specific membrane component is involved; (2) drug antibodies attach to the cell membrane by their Fab part suggesting specific binding rather than passive adsorption of immune complexes; (3) the drug antibodies cannot be absorbed by the drug alone and can only be detected by bringing red cells, free drug and antibodies together; and (4) the binding of the drug antibodies may depend on the presence of a particular red cell antigen, which implies that the drug binds to the cell surface, albeit loosely (Salama and Mueller-Eckhardt 1987a). It seems therefore more likely that a trimolecular complex of the drug, the drug antibody and a component on the red cell membrane is formed. (For a survey of the subject, see Shulman and Reid 1993 and Garratty 1994, who also gives a list of drugs acting in this way.) Drugs that produce red cell destruction by this mechanism can do so even when given in low doses. The haemolysis is arrested within 1–2 days of stopping the drug. The antibodies are often IgM and complement-activating and then only complement can be detected on the patient's red cells (Garratty and Petz 1975).

In some cases, the antibodies are directed against a metabolite rather then the drug itself (Salama and Mueller-Eckhardt 1985, 1987a,b; Kim et al. 2002). The antibodies can then be detected by using urine from subjects who have taken the drug. Bougie and co-workers (1997) describe a case of haemolytic anaemia and subsequent renal failure resulting from diclofenac in which the patient had an antibody specific for a glucuronide conjugate of a known metabolite of diclofenac (4'-OH hydroxydiclofenac). The antibody could be demonstrated in the patient's serum with red cells in the presence of urine taken from individuals who had ingested diclofenac. These authors point out that as glucuronidation is a common pathway of drug metabolism, studies on glucuronidation of other common medications associated with immune haemolytic anaemia should be considered.

Drug-induced autoantibody formation

The drug does not bind firmly to red cells, antibody against the drug is not formed, but IgG autoantibodies are induced. α-Methyldopa and levodopa are prime examples of drugs acting in this way. In 15–20% of patients receiving α-methyldopa, the DAT becomes positive after 3–6 months' treatment; the development of a positive DAT is dose dependent (Carstairs et al. 1966). Only about 1% of patients receiving the drug develop haemolytic anaemia.

It has been suggested that α-methyldopa induces red cell autoantibodies by inhibiting the activity of suppressor T lymphocytes (Kirtland et al. 1980). Although no effect on suppressor cells could be demonstrated in one investigation (Garratty et al. 1986), a drug, lobenzarit, which inhibits suppressor cell function, has been found to induce α-methyldopa type autoimmune haemolytic anaemia (Andou et al. 1994).

α-Interferon seems to be responsible for the development of autoantibodies to various structural proteins or receptors and for the exacerbation of autoimmune disease (Conlon et al. 1990). The development of warm red cell autoantibodies has been observed in a patient receiving α-interferon and IL-2 (Perez et al. 1991). These various effects are believed to be due to the inhibition of normal cellular immune suppressor mechanisms.

As stated above, some drugs that do not bind firmly to red cells induce both anti-drug antibodies and red cell autoantibodies, for example nomifensine (Martlew 1986; Salama and Mueller-Eckhardt 1987a), tolmetin and suprofen (van Dijk et al. 1989).

The inference has been drawn that even when drugs bind loosely to red cells, they can induce the formation of antibodies against a red cell antigen alone (Salama and Mueller-Eckhardt 1987a). Alternatively the drug could directly influence the immune response against autoantigens (Kirtland et al. 1980).

Non-specific adsorption of proteins

The drug may alter the red cell membrane in some way so that proteins are adsorbed non-specifically. Cephalosporin and cisplatin are believed to act in this way as a rule. This mechanism has not been shown to result in haemolytic anaemia unless antibodies against the drug are formed.

Effect of red cell antigens on the binding of drug–antibody complexes

In a case in which streptomycin was involved, the drug was apparently bound to the red cell membrane through chemical groups related to M and possibly D (Martinez-Letona *et al.* 1977). Several similar cases in which various drugs and different red cell antigens were involved have been reported (for a survey, see Garratty 1994).

Treatment of drug-induced haemolytic anaemia

In cases in which antibodies are involved against a drug that binds firmly to the red cell and in cases in which immune complexes are responsible for the destruction of the red cells, stopping the drug is sufficient to arrest the haemolytic process and treatment of the haemolytic anaemia is rarely necessary. In cases in which it is impossible to stop the drug and the patient is anaemic, red cell transfusions should be given. In AIHA induced by α-methyldopa, the drug must be stopped, but red cell destruction may continue for weeks or months. If treatment is required it is the same as for patients with drug-independent warm AIHA.

In occasional patients, autoantibodies disappear despite continued administration of the drug (Habibi 1983).

Antibodies against other bound antigens

Fatty acid-dependent agglutinin ('albumin agglutinin')

The serum of a small proportion of people agglutinates red cells suspended in albumin but not those suspended in saline (Weiner *et al.* 1956). Agglutination is found only with caprylate-treated albumin (Golde *et al.* 1969, 1973) and the antibody is in fact directed against sodium caprylate or other fatty acid salts and not against albumin at all (Beck *et al.* 1976). The term 'fatty acid-dependent agglutinin' is therefore preferable to the previously used 'albumin agglutinin'. Fatty acid-dependent agglutinins may cause false-positive reactions in slide tests in which blood grouping reagents containing albumin are used (Reid *et al.* 1975; Case 1976) and in the IAT test if albumin is used in the sensitizing phase of the reaction.

Antibiotics

Antibiotics are added to samples of red cells that are distributed commercially for the identification of alloantibodies. Such cells may give false-positive results if antibodies against the relevant antibiotic are present in a sample of serum. In a systematic search for such antibodies, Watson and Joubert (1960) found that 6 out of 1700 routine blood bank serum samples agglutinated chloramphenicol-treated cells. Three examples of an antibody of this kind were found to be IgM and two bound complement (Beattie *et al.* 1976). An IgA antibody agglutinating red cells suspended in 0.1 mg of neomycin/ml was described by Hysell and co-workers (1975). Antibodies vs. penicillin-treated red cells are described above.

Acriflavine

Some commercial anti-B-sera have acriflavine added to them as a colouring agent and this may be a cause of false-positive results if anti-acriflavine antibodies are present in a patient's serum, possibly as a result of previous exposure to acriflavine. The antibodies may cause agglutination of normal red cells in the presence of a 1 in 150 000 dilution of acriflavine (Beattie and Zuelzer 1968; Beattie *et al.* 1971).

Immune complexes adsorbed to red cells in vitro in ulcerative colitis

In occasional patients with ulcerative colitis, the DAT on clotted samples is positive but on anticoagulated samples is negative. Allogeneic red cells give a positive IAT with the patient's serum but a negative test with plasma. It is postulated that the patient's plasma contains an antibody against an activated coagulation factor and that, during clotting, immune complexes form and attach to the red cells (Garratty *et al.* 1980).

Lactose- or glucose-treated red cells

Antibodies have been described which agglutinated any red cells that had been incubated with lactose (Gray 1964) or glucose (Lewis *et al.* 1980). In the latter case, red cells from patients with diabetes reacted, although after incubation in saline, the cells were no longer agglutinated. Examples of anti-M and anti-N reacting only with lactose- or glucose-treated red cells are described in the preceding chapter.

Antibody against chemically altered red cells (the LOX antigen)

Red cells exposed to citrate–phosphate–dextrose

solution in particular batches of plastic blood packs may acquire a new red cell antigenic determinant 'LOX', reacting with an antibody present in normal serum. The development of this antigen is probably associated with sterilization of the packs with propylene oxide gas (Bruce and Mitchell 1981).

Polyagglutinability

Red cells are said to be polyagglutinable when they are agglutinated by almost all samples of normal human serum although not by the patient's own serum. The commonest forms of polyagglutinability are due to exposure, by the action of bacterial enzymes, of antigenic determinants (T, Tk, Th, Tx), which form part of the structure of the normal red cell membrane, but which are usually hidden. Another form of polyagglutinability is believed to be due to somatic mutation leading to the emergence of a line of red cells lacking an enzyme essential for the formation of normal red cell antigens; as a result, a normally hidden antigen, Tn, is exposed. In all the foregoing cases, the red cells are polyagglutinable because antibodies (anti-T, etc.) corresponding to the determinants are present in serum from all normal adults (although not in serum from newborn infants). Why these antibodies are in all normal sera is not known but, like anti-A and anti-B, this may be related to the widespread occurrence of the antigens in the environment. Chicks kept in germ-free conditions developed anti-T and anti-Tn when fed *Escherichia coli* O86 in their drinking water (Springer

and Tegtmeyer 1981). Tn has been found in several helminth parasites, including *Echinococcus granulosus*, *Taenia hydatigena* and *Fasciola hepatica* (Casaravilla *et al.* 2003) and in human skin mites (Kanitakis *et al.* 1997). Further forms of polyagglutinability may be due to the inheritance of an antigen (C3d, NOR or HEMPAS) for which a corresponding antibody is present in almost all normal human sera.

T activation

Exposure of T antigen in vitro

As Fig. 7.3 shows, the T determinant is normally covered by N-acetylneuraminic acid and can therefore be described as a cryptantigen. The antigen can be exposed by the action of bacterial or viral neuraminidases.

Anti-T and anti-Tn (see below), present in the serum of all subjects except infants, are presumably formed as a reaction to T and Tn present in many Gram-negative bacteria and vaccines (Springer *et al.* 1979; Springer and Tegtmeyer 1981).

Knowledge of T activation stems from the original observation that suspensions of red cells might become agglutinable by ABO-compatible serum after standing for many hours at room temperature, and that this agglutination was associated with infection of the suspension with certain enzyme-producing bacteria (Hübener 1925; Thomsen 1927; Friedenreich 1930). Very many organisms, including pneumococci, streptococci, staphylococci, clostridia, *E. coli*, *Vibrio*

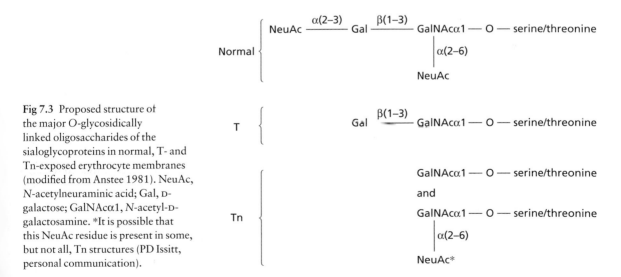

Fig 7.3 Proposed structure of the major O-glycosidically linked oligosaccharides of the sialoglycoproteins in normal, T- and Tn-exposed erythrocyte membranes (modified from Anstee 1981). NeuAc, N-acetylneuraminic acid; Gal, D-galactose; GalNAcα1, N-acetyl-D-galactosamine. *It is possible that this NeuAc residue is present in some, but not all, Tn structures (PD Issitt, personal communication).

cholerae and influenza viruses are capable of producing this effect *in vitro*.

Preparation of T-activated red cells. Add 11 mg of $CaCl_2$ to 100 ml of 0.85% NaCl to provide a solution containing approximately 10 mmol of $CaCl_2$/l. Add 0.2 ml of a solution containing 500 units of neuraminidase/ml to give an enzyme concentration of 1 unit/ml. This solution can be stored at 4°C for 1 year. Wash group O red cells four times in saline and make a 25% suspension of cells in the enzyme solution. Incubate at 37°C for 2–3 h. Remove the supernatant, wash the red cells in saline four times, make a 5% suspension in saline and check for T activation by testing with anti-T lectin (Howard 1979).

T-activated red cells can be kept for several weeks in Alsever's solution but must be washed thoroughly in saline before being used.

T sites on red cells

As there are 15 O-glycosidically linked oligosaccharides on each molecule of glycophorin A (α-SGP), and probably similar numbers on glycophorins C and B (β- and δ-SGPs), there are many potential T-antigen sites (around 20 million) on the red cell. There are also T-active structures on red cell membrane components other than SGPs, for example on gangliosides (Anstee 1980).

Activation of T receptor in vivo

T activation may occur *in vivo*. Usually, this polyagglutinability occurs as a transient phenomenon, disappearing within a few weeks or months of the time when it is first observed. The phenomenon is not very common; at a large Blood Transfusion Centre, only 10 cases were observed in 12 years (Stratton and Renton 1958).

In the past, T activation was almost always detected by finding discrepancies between the results of testing red cells and sera in the course of ABO grouping. Nowadays, monoclonal anti-A and -B are widely used and so T activation seldom causes trouble in blood grouping.

In many cases, the patient has an obvious bacterial infection, but the phenomenon has also been observed in apparently healthy subjects; for a review of some of the earlier reported cases, see Henningsen (1949). In a case reported by Reepmaker (1952), an organism that was shown to be capable of inducing T transformation was isolated from the patient's urine. Chorpenning and Hayes (1959) made the point that T transformation is not the only kind of polyagglutinability induced by bacterial infection, and that in many reported cases of polyagglutinability it was simply assumed that the change was T transformation.

Similarity of T activation to acquisition of 'B-like' antigen

Certain bacterial enzymes confer B-specificity on red cells as well as rendering them polyagglutinable (Marsh 1960; see also Chapter 4).

Reactions of T-activated cells

T-activated cells are agglutinated by all sera containing more than a trace of anti-T, that is to say, by sera from most adults. Anti-T is absent from cord serum but appears at or before the age of 2 months (F Stratton, personal communication). The agglutinin reacts best at room temperature and may be inactive at 37°C. Agglutinates due to anti-T may be large; there are many free cells present.

T-activated cells react most strongly with fresh serum and sometimes fail to react with serum that has been stored frozen (Stratton 1954). T-activated cells react better with sera containing anti-A than with those that do not (Race and Sanger 1975, p. 487).

T-activated cells fail to agglutinate in their own serum (the titre of anti-T being low presumably due to absorption by exposed T) and the cells give a negative DAT. At 37°C they are not sensitized to an antiglobulin serum by human sera that agglutinate them at room temperature.

An anti-T lectin can be extracted from the peanut, *Arachis hypogaea* (Bird 1964). Testing with peanut anti-T lectin is far more sensitive than testing with adult serum (Seger *et al.* 1980). Reactions of various types of polyagglutinable red cells with different lectins and with polybrene are shown in Table 7.3.

Use of polybrene in testing for T. Normal red cells (negatively charged) are agglutinated by polybrene (positively charged), but red cells, such as T-activated cells, which are deficient in sialic acid and thus have a reduced negative charge, are not. For a method of testing red cells with polybrene, see Issitt and Issitt (1975).

Table 7.3 Reactions of different kinds of polyagglutinable red cells (based on the publications of GWG Bird and co-workers).

	Arachis hypogaea	Dolichos biflorus*	Glycine soja†	GS II‡	Vicia cretica	Salvia sclarea	Leonurus cardiaca	Polybrene
T	+	−	+	−	+	−	+§	−
Tk	+	−	−	+	−	−	−	+
Th	+	−	−	−	+	−	−	+
Tx	+	−	−	−	−	−	−	+
Tn	−	+	+	−	−	+	−	−
Cad	−	+	+	−	−	−	+	+

* Tests with this lectin can be used only when the cells are group O or B.

† May not react with weaker examples of Cad.

‡ *Griffonia simplicifolia II.*

§ Weak reaction.

The deficiency of red cell sialic acid must exceed about 12% before cells fail to be agglutinated by 0.1 g/dl of polybrene in a test tube (EA Steane, personal communication, 1978), although with very dilute polybrene solutions (< 0.003 g/dl), red cells that have only a 10% reduction in sialic acid are agglutinated (Cartron *et al.* 1978). When polybrene in as high a concentration as 0.6 g/dl is used, prozones are observed, for example cells with 30% or more loss of sialic acid are not agglutinated (Cartron *et al.* 1978).

A typical case. In the recent past, when normal sera containing anti-T, in addition to polyclonal anti-A and -B, were used for ABO grouping, T-activated cells were recognized by finding discrepancies between the results of testing red cells and serum, as in the following case:

Mrs S was admitted to hospital with a septic abortion: mixed coliforms and non-haemolytic streptococci were grown from a vaginal swab. Her red cells were strongly agglutinated by anti-A serum and partially agglutinated by anti-B; her serum agglutinated and lysed B cells but failed to agglutinate A cells, suggesting that she really belonged to group A. On further testing, her red cells were found to be agglutinated by four adult AB sera, the reactions being strongest at 4°C and weakest at 37°C; the cells were not agglutinated by several samples of cord blood serum from group A infants.

The patient made a good recovery and 1 week after admission her cells were only very weakly polyagglutinable.

Polyagglutinability is frequent in newborn infants with necrotizing enterocolitis (Bird 1982) but will not be detected when monoclonal anti-A and -B are used for grouping. The diagnosis can be made with anti-T lectin.

Leucocytes and platelets also become T activated; platelet function is not impaired (Hysell *et al.* 1976).

Haemolytic syndromes due to T activation?

Most patients with T-activated cells do not have an associated haemolytic process. Although several cases have been reported in which such an association has been observed, it is difficult in some of the cases to be sure that T activation has been responsible. The difficulty of incriminating anti-T seems particularly great in infants, in whom anti-T, if present at all, is not strong. Moreover, in many of the cases described the patients have had an infection with *Clostridium perfringens*, an organism notorious for producing violent haemolytic syndromes.

In four cases described by van Loghem (1965), the Hb concentration was between 4.5 and 6.9 g/dl and serum haptoglobin was reduced. Two of the patients showed red cell autoagglutination. In the three cases in which organisms were isolated they were *C. perfringens*, *Staphylococcus aureus* and pneumococcus. In a patient reported by Moores and co-workers (1975), with a presumed lung infection following a stab wound, there was rapid improvement on treatment with antibiotics, but after 7 days there was a sudden deterioration and fall in Hb concentration to 3.4 g/dl and a reticulocytosis of 25%. T activation was demonstrated and anti-T eluted from the patient's red cells. F Stratton (personal communication) has seen four infants of 2 months old or less with T activation, associated with the development of severe anaemia. *E. coli* was implicated in one of the cases. In a child aged 14 months described by Rickard and co-workers (1969) the Hb concentration fell to 3.7 g/dl: the blood film showed spherocytes and Schumm's test was positive.

279

Further cases were described by Bird and Stephenson (1973) and by Tanaka and Okubo (1977).

In one case, the transfusion of normal plasma (containing anti-T) appeared to be the cause of a severe haemolytic transfusion reaction (HTR) (van Loghem *et al.* 1955). Among six further cases, there was severe haemolysis in one and mild haemolysis in three. It was recommended that patients with T activation should be transfused with washed red cells or platelets (William *et al.* 1989).

Scepticism about the haemolytic potential of anti-T was expressed by Heddle and co-workers (1977), who found no evidence of significant red cell destruction in three premature infants with T-activated red cells following the transfusion of blood components containing anti-T.

Haemolytic syndromes associated with polyagglutinability have been produced experimentally in guinea pigs following the injection of pneumococcal cultures (Ejby-Poulsen 1954a,b), and have been shown to occur spontaneously in rabbits in association with enteritis (Evans *et al.* 1963).

Other kinds of polyagglutinability due to bacterial enzymes or bacteria

Tk activation

This form of polyagglutinability of the red cells is similar to T activation in that it is a transient phenomenon associated with infection. The red cells are agglutinated by the Tk-specific lectin GS II, isolated from *Griffonia simplificifolia* seeds (Bird and Wingham 1972); they also react with peanut lectin, the reaction being greatly enhanced if the red cells are first treated with papain (Bird and Wingham 1972).

Tk cells have normal amounts of sialic acid, as indicated by the fact that they are agglutinated by polybrene (see Table 7.3). Further work indicates that Tk is exposed by the action of an endo-β-galactosidase produced by *Bacteroides fragilis* (Inglis *et al.* 1975a,b) or derived from *Escherichia freundii* (Doinel *et al.* 1980) or *Flavobacterium keratolyticus* (Liew *et al.* 1982). Endo-β-galactosidase exposes a terminal *N*-acetylglucosamine residue on carbohydrate chains of long-chain glycolipids and glycoproteins carrying highly branched *N*-glycans, notably band 3 (Doinel *et al.* 1980).

T and Tk activation associated with acquired B

In patients with acquired B the red cells often exhibit Tk polyagglutination with or without T activation. In reporting three patients it was pointed out that the changes in each were due to different bacterial enzymes and that, depending on the relative amounts of each of these enzymes, different phenotypes were produced, for example in one case T activation might predominate and in another, Tk (Judd *et al.* 1979 – see also Mullard *et al.* 1978; Janot *et al.* 1979).

In Tk polyagglutination H and A red cell antigens are weakened (Inglis *et al.* 1978), as are I and i (Andreu *et al.* 1979). These observations are consistent with the location of the majority of ABH and Ii antigens on complex *N*-glycans on the normal red cell (see Chapter 3).

VA polyagglutination

This condition is considered here for convenience although there is no evidence that it is caused by bacterial enzymes. The condition is characterized by persistent polyagglutination associated with haemolytic anaemia; the red cells are weakly agglutinated by almost all adult sera but only up to a temperature of 18°C. The abnormalities in the red cells include a slight reduction in sialic acid (3.7%) and a depression of H receptors (Graninger *et al.* 1977a,b). VA accompanied by Tk was reported by Beck *et al.* (1978). VA may represent one end of a Tk spectrum (Bird 1980).

Th activation

The Th antigen is exposed in infection with *Corynebacterium aquaticum* (Levene 1984). A neuraminidase that can be isolated from culture supernatant of *C. aquaticum* was shown to be responsible. The release of less than 20 μg of sialic acid per 10^{10} red cells appeared to lead to Th reactivity, whereas hydrolysis of greater amounts of sialic acid activates T (Sondag-Thull *et al.* 1989).

When Th is exposed (Bird *et al.* 1978), the red cells are agglutinated by peanut lectin, extracts from *Vieia eretica* (Bird and Wingham 1981), *Medicago disciformis* (Bird and Wingham 1983) and by polybrene, but not by lectins from *Glycine sofa*, GS II, *Salvia sclarea* or *Salvia horminin* (Bird *et al.* 1978); see Table 7.3.

In studying 200 paired samples of maternal and cord blood, the incidence of Th activation was found to be much higher in newborn infants (11% and their mothers 13%) than in blood donors (Wahl *et al.* 1989), in whom the incidence was 1.5% (Herman *et al.* 1987). In none of the cases were the red cells polyagglutinable, which shows that Th activation leads to polyagglutinability only in some cases.

Tx and Tr activation

The Tx antigen is exposed on red cells by pneumococcal enzymes (Bird *et al.* 1982). Tx cells are agglutinated by peanut lectin but not by other lectins. Transient Tx polyagglutination lasting 4–5.5 months was described in three siblings of one family by Wolach and co-workers (1987).

Reid and co-workers (1998) reported on an individual with an unusual form of polyagglutination, denoted Tr, the red cells giving a unique reaction pattern when tested with lectins.

Polyagglutinability due to adsorbed bacteria

Many bacteria or their thermostable products will adhere to red cells (Keogh *et al.* 1948; Jochem 1958a,b). The red cells will be polyagglutinable when the corresponding antibody is present in most samples of human serum. Antibodies to some bacteria, for example *Bacillus cereus*, do not agglutinate red cells coated with the bacteria but sensitize the cells to agglutination by antiglobulin serum (Weeden *et al.* 1960).

Tn red cells

Tn red cells, like T-activated cells, are deficient in sialic acid (Bird *et al.* 1971) and are polyagglutinable (Dausset *et al.* 1959), as anti-Tn, like anti-T, is present in all normal adult sera.

Apart from the fact that T and Tn are quite separate antigenic structures (see Fig. 7.2) Tn polyagglutination differs in three important respects from T polyagglutination or any other polyagglutination associated with infection: first, Tn agglutination is persistent; second, it is associated with haematological abnormalities; and third, affected subjects have two populations of red cells, one normal and one showing the Tn change. The condition (sometimes referred to as persistent mixed field polyagglutination) appears to be due to somatic mutation occurring in stem cells, leading to the emergence of a population of abnormal (Tn) red cells (as originally suggested by Bird *et al.* 1971, 1976b). Data supporting this concept are as follows: in subjects with Tn red cells there are also two populations of platelets, Tn positive and Tn negative (Cartron and Nurden 1979). Only Tn-positive platelets contain glycoprotein 1b with a modified oligosaccharide chain structure responsible for the expression of Tn antigen (Nurden *et al.* 1982). A similar abnormality is present on Tn-positive granulocytes (Cartron *et al.* 1981). It has also been found that a sizeable fraction of erythrocyte, granulocyte and megakaryocyte colonies grown from the bone marrow of a patient with the Tn syndrome appear to consist exclusively of either Tn-positive or Tn-negative cells, demonstrating the clonal origin of Tn cells (Vainchenker *et al.* 1982). Tn-positive B and T cells can also be demonstrated in patients with the Tn syndrome (Brouet *et al.* 1983) and, finally, expression of the Tn antigen has been demonstrated at a very early stage of differentiation, i.e. in colony-forming units (Vainchenker *et al.* 1985).

Initially, *N*-acetylgalactosamine bound glycosidically to serine and threonine of red cell glycoproteins (GalNAcα1-O-serine/threonine) was considered to be the only major antigen on Tn cells (Dahr *et al.* 1975). A deficiency in Tn cells of the GalNAc (β1,3)-D-galactosyl transferase, which normally generates the O-glycosidically linked oligosaccharides attached to the red cell sialoglycoproteins was described (Cartron *et al.* 1978). An explanation for the deficiency of this galactosyl transferase in Tn syndrome is provided by Ju and Cummings (2002). These authors show that expression of an active GalNAc(beta1,3)-D-galactosyl transferase requires the presence of a chaperone protein (Cosmc) encoded by a gene on the X chromosome at Xq23. In the Jurkat cell line that expresses Tn antigen, the galactosyl transferase gene is normal, but *Cosmc* has an inactivating mutation. Formal proof is required from analysis of *Cosmc* in DNA derived from patients with Tn syndrome but the analogy with paroxysmal nocturnal haemoglobinuria (PNH) is very compelling. Like Tn syndrome, PNH is an acquired clonal disorder affecting a subset of all blood cells. PNH results from inactivating mutations in a gene on the X chromosome (*PIG-A* on Xp22.1, reviewed in Young *et al.* 2000). Sialosyl-Tn (NeuAcα2–6GalNAcα1-o-serine/threonine) is also present in Tn cells (Kjeldsen *et al.* 1989). This disaccharide is absent in normal glycophorins and therefore the responsible transferase must be induced in Tn cells (Blumenfeld *et al.* 1992). The induction of this transferase is thus the second abnormality in Tn cells.

Although Tn polyagglutination usually persists for long periods, it has been known to disappear in four subjects; two of these disappearances were spontaneous, as neither patient was receiving cytotoxic therapy (Bird *et al.* 1976b). Although Tn polyagglutination is usually associated with neutropenia and thrombocytopenia (Gunson *et al.* 1970; Haynes *et al.* 1970) and may be associated with haemolytic anaemia (Bird *et al.* 1971), it is also found in normal subjects (Myllylä *et al.* 1971; Bird *et al.* 1976c). In a subject investigated by Myllylä and co-workers (1971) it was shown that the survival of the subject's red cells in his own circulation was normal and that no anti-Tn was demonstrable in the serum; when the red cells were injected into the circulation of a normal subject (i.e. with anti-Tn in the plasma) the cells were rapidly destroyed.

When normal red cells are transfused to a subject with Tn polyagglutination the transfused cells do not become Tn positive (Haynes *et al.* 1970).

Tn red cells are agglutinated by an extract of *Dolichos biflorus* (Gunson *et al.* 1970) and by snail anti-A but not by purified human anti-A (Bird 1978). They are also agglutinated by the lectins from *Salvia sclarea*, *Helix pomatia* and *Glycine sofa* (Bird 1978).

Tn red cells are best diagnosed by testing with an extract of *Salvia sclarea* (see Table 7.3). The lectin must be diluted to avoid non-specific activity but then reacts strongly with Tn cells and not at all with T-activated cells.

Exposure of T, Tn, sialylated Tn and Tk in malignant cells

Immunoreactive T antigen is present in the cytoplasm and on the outer cell membrane of about 90% of the major forms of carcinoma and T lymphoma, as determined by absorption of human anti-T antibodies and immunohistochemistry (Springer *et al.* 1974, 1983). In addition to T, carcinoma cells express Tn antigen. Tn antigen was detected by absorption of human anti-Tn antibody in 46 out of 50 primary breast carcinomas and in all six metastases originating from Tn-positive primary carcinomas. In total, 13 out of 25 (52%) anaplastic carcinomas, but only 2 out of 15 (13%) well-differentiated carcinomas had more Tn than T; one anaplastic carcinoma had neither antigen. Moreover, 18 out of 20 benign breast lesions had no Tn; the

two with Tn were premalignant. Tissue from 18 breast carcinomas reacted strongly with anti-Tn (Springer *et al.* 1985). Carcinoma-associated T antigen stimulates profound cellular and humoral immune responses in the patient, early in the disease and throughout its course (Springer *et al.* 1983). Monoclonal anti-T and anti-Tn, which reacted with T- and Tn-positive carcinoma cells, were prepared by Springer and co-workers (1983). Several monoclonal antibodies to T, Tn and sialylated Tn have been produced and used to explore the prognostic value of the respective antigens in cancer (O'Boyle *et al.* 1996; Rittenhouse-Diakun *et al.* 1998). Meichenin and co-workers (2000) used a monoclonal anti-Tk (LM389) to show that Tk is a colorectal carcinoma-associated antigen.

NOR, an inherited form of polyagglutinability

The red cells of a healthy young male were found to be agglutinable by 75 of 100 ABO-compatible sera; the red cell characteristic, NOR, associated with polyagglutinability was shown to be inherited in an apparently dominant manner by four other family members in two generations (Harris *et al.* 1982). The only other inherited characteristics associated with polyagglutinability are C3d and HEMPAS, described in the previous chapter. NOR can be distinguished from C3d by the failure of NOR red cells to react with an extract of *D. biflorus* and can be distinguished from the acquired forms of polyagglutinability, T, Tk, Th and Tn, by the failure of NOR red cells to react with an extract either of *Arachis hypogaea* or of *S. sclarea* (Harris *et al.* 1982). A second case was reported in a Polish family (Kusnierz-Alejska *et al.* 1999). Subsequent studies on the red cells of NOR+ individuals from this second family identified two neutral glycolipids unique to NOR+ cells reactive with anti-NOR and the lectin *Griffonia simplicifolia* IB4 (GSL-IB4). The structure of one of these glycolipids (NOR1) was determined to be Galα1–4GalNAcβ1–3Galα1–4Galβ1–4Glcβ1–CER(α-galactosyl-globoside; Duk *et al.* 2001). Duk and co-workers (2002) point out that GSL-IB4 can be used in a simple serological test with papain-treated red cells to detect NOR+ cells in individuals of group A and O but not of group B because the lectin also recognizes the Gal alpha1–3 structure. However, these authors found it necessary to absorb their GSL-IB4 preparation with normal group A1 cells to remove traces of other lectins found in GSL in order to render it useful for detection of NOR antigen.

Agglutinins for other normally hidden antigens

Antigens on enzyme-treated red cells

Agglutinins for red cells treated with various enzymes are found in all normal sera; for example, if trypsinized red cells are mixed with normal human serum and incubated for not more than 20 min and then centrifuged they will usually be found to be agglutinated, although if incubation is continued for 1 h only about 1% of samples will still be agglutinated (Rosenthal and Schwartz 1951; Rosenfield and Vogel 1951).

If normal serum is heated to 60°C for 2 h the agglutinin, which is IgM (Mellbye 1966), is inactivated; the heated serum can now be shown to contain a factor 'reversor', which renders cells non-agglutinable by normal serum (Spaet and Ostrom 1952). 'Reversor' is histidine (Mellbye 1967).

Although trypsin is adsorbed to red cells during enzyme treatment, the receptor with which the 'trypsin agglutinin' reacts is not trypsin itself but is probably a glycoprotein (Mellbye 1969a). Problems caused by such antibodies can be avoided by use of crystalline enzymes.

According to Mellbye (1969b), agglutinins specific for trypsin-, papain-, bromelin-, neuraminidase- and periodate-treated red cells can all be found in normal serum; each agglutinin can be removed only by absorption with the appropriate red cells. The agglutinin for trypsin-treated red cells is the only one found in cord serum and the only one whose reactions are reversed by the addition of histidine. In testing a very large series of normal samples, a warm haemolysin for papain-treated red cells was found in 0.1%. There was some crossreaction with trypsinized cells but none with bromelin-treated cells. The antibody did not affect the survival of red cells in vivo (Bell et al. 1973b). In one series in which the serum of normal donors was tested in the autoanalyzer, agglutinins reacting with bromelin-treated red cells were found in 2% of donors (Ranadazzo et al. 1973).

Autohaemolysin reacting with trypsinized red cells

Heistö and co-workers (1965) found that the serum of 94 out of 961 normal donors would haemolyse the subject's own trypsinized red cells; the haemolysin was twice as common in women as in men and was shown to be inherited; it was not inhibited by trypsin itself.

Antigens demonstrable on stored red cells and on freshly washed cells

A cold agglutinin reacting only with stored red cells

In the first example described, red cells became agglutinable after 4–7 days' storage at room temperature (Brendemoen 1952). Three further examples were found in women with severe haemolytic anaemia; the antibodies were active at 37°C as well as at lower temperatures. Fresh untreated red cells never reacted but they became agglutinable after brief enzyme treatment (Jenkins and Marsh 1961). A very thorough study of another case was published by Ozer and Chaplin (1963).

Evidence that the antigen on stored red cells might resemble low-density lipoprotein was found in one case (Beaumont et al. 1976) but a more recent study of two further cases indicates that during storage there is a gradual expression of galactose- or mannose-containing epitopes and that these are the determinants involved (Krugluger et al. 1994). Incidentally, these three patients did not have haemolytic anaemia.

An antibody reacting only with freshly washed red cells

This was described by Freiesleben and Jensen (1959). The donor's plasma would no longer agglutinate red cells after they had stood at room temperature for periods between 5 min and 4 h after washing (Allan et al. 1972). A later example not only agglutinated freshly washed red cells, but also bound complement to them; washed red cells were found to have a shortened ^{51}Cr survival time (Davey et al. 1979).

The changes in the red cell membrane induced by washing in sodium chloride, which renders the cells agglutinable, remain to be determined. It should be added that there is no reason to suppose that the phenomenon is related in any way to an enzyme, and that it is included in this section simply for lack of any more convenient place for it.

Red cell agglutination not due to antibodies

Rouleaux formation

If red cells are allowed to sediment in their own plasma,

they tend to adhere together in a characteristic way, 'like a pile of coins'. The rate of sedimentation of the red cells depends upon the degree of this tendency to aggregate so that rapid, intense rouleaux formation and a high erythrocyte sedimentation rate (ESR) go hand in hand.

The relation between the ESR and the plasma concentrations of 20 different proteins was determined by Scherer and co-workers (1975). The correlation coefficient was highest with fibrinogen, α-1-acid glycoprotein, α-2-macroglobulin, α-1-antitrypsin, caeruloplasmin and IgM. The best correlation between the concentration of various plasma proteins and ESR was obtained when the molar concentrations of fibrinogen, α-2-macroglobulin and IgM were summed.

Occasional samples of serum with high levels of immunoglobulin, as in myelomatosis, even when diluted with an equal volume of saline, may cause strong rouleaux formation. On the other hand, most samples of human serum, when diluted with an equal volume of saline, will not cause rouleaux formation – a fact that is of great value in distinguishing rouleaux formation from agglutination due to antibodies.

Dextran molecules produce rouleaux formation only when they exceed a certain size (Bull et al. 1949). It has been postulated that a monolayer of large dextran molecules serves to increase the distance between cells, so that there is weaker electrical repulsion, and at the same time provides a large absorption area on the cell surface, which provides a bridging force (Chien and Kung-Ming 1973).

It is often thought that rouleaux formation can be distinguished from true agglutination by simple microscopic examination, but in fact the distinction may be difficult to make. In large rouleaux, the cells do not all adhere together in neat piles but tend instead to form large clumps, which may easily be mistaken for agglutinates. Conversely, weak agglutination in colloid media can closely resemble rouleaux formation; this may be observed, for example, in the titration of partially neutralized immune anti-A sera against A cells in a medium of serum.

Other causes of non-specific agglutination of red cells

Colloidal silica

When solutions are autoclaved or stored in glass bottles, the solution may become contaminated by colloidal silica, particularly if the solution is alkaline. Colloidal silica is adsorbed by red cells and may be the cause of false-positive serological tests. Red cells suspended in a 1 in 200 dilution of plasma are completely protected against this effect (see previous editions of this book for references). The potential adverse effects of colloidal silica in serological tests have become of much less importance now that solutions are often stored in plastic rather than glass.

Chromic chloride, etc.

Many other substances cause red cells to agglutinate non-specifically, for example multivalent metallic ions such as Cr^{3+} or tannic acid. The antibiotic vancomycin, a polycation, also induces red cell aggregation (Williams and Domen 1989).

Wharton's jelly

Samples of blood contaminated with Wharton's jelly may agglutinate spontaneously (Wiener 1943, p. 49). Contamination of cord blood with a 1 in 1000 dilution of the jelly is enough to cause red cell clumping (Flanagan and Mitoma 1958). The clumping can be dispersed by adding hyaluronidase (Killpack 1950). The phenomenon is likely to cause trouble only when cord blood is collected by cutting the cord and allowing the blood to drain into the tube. For many reasons this is a very unsatisfactory way of obtaining a sample. A far better way is to take a blood sample with a syringe and needle from the umbilical vein.

References

Abdalla S, Weatherall DJ (1982) The direct antiglobulin test in *P. falciparum* malaria. Br J Haematol 51: 415–425

Adinolfi M (1965a) Anti-I in normal newborn infants. Immunology 9: 43

Adinolfi M (1965b) Some serological characteristics of the normal incomplete cold antibody. Immunology 9: 31

Adinolfi M, Polley MJ, Hunter DA et al. (1962) Classification of blood-group antibodies as β₂M or gamma globulin. Immunology 5: 566

Adinolfi M, Daniels C, Mollison PL et al. (1963) Evidence that 'normal incomplete cold antibody' is not a gamma globulin. Nature (Lond) 199: 389

Allan J, Garratty G (1980) Positive direct antiglobulin tests in normal blood donors. In: Abstracts, 16th Congress of the International Society of Blood Transfusion, Montreal

Allan CJ, Lawrence RD, Shih SC et al. (1972) Agglutination of erythrocytes freshly washed with saline solution. Four saline-auto-agglutinating sera. Transfusion 12: 306

Ambrus M, Bajtai G (1969) A case of an IgG-type cold agglutinin disease. Haematologia 3: 225

Anderson HJ, Aubuchon JP, Draper EK et al. (1985) Transfusion problems in renal allograft recipients. Anti-lymphocyte globulin showing Lutheran system specificity. Transfusion 25: 47–50

Andou S, Fujii S, Harada Y et al. (1994) α-Methyldopa type autoimmune haemolytic anemia caused by lobenzarit disodium of a nefenanine acid derivative and immunomodulator. Blood 83: 3097

Andreu C, Doinel C, Cartron JP et al. (1979) Induction of Tk polyagglutination by Bacteroides fragilis culture supernatants. Associated modifications of ABH and Ii antigens. Rev Fr Transfus Immunohématol 22: 551–561

Angevine CD, Andersen BR, Barnett EV (1966) A cold agglutinin of the IgA class. J Immunol 96: 578

Anstee DJ (1980) Blood group MNSs-active sialoglycoproteins of the human erythrocyte membrane. In: Immunobiology of the Erythrocyte. SG Sandler, J Nusbacher, MS Schanfield (eds). Progress in clinical and biological Research 43: 67–98. New York: Alan R Liss

Anstee DJ (1981) The blood group MNSs-active sialoglycoproteins. Semin Hematol 18: 13–31

Argiolu F, Diana G, Arnone M et al. (1990) High-dose intravenous immunoglobulin in the management of autoimmune hemolytic anemia complicating thalassemia major. Acta Haematol 83: 65–68

Arndt PA, Garratty G (2002) Cross-reactivity of cefotetan and ceftriaxone antibodies, association with hemolytic anemia, with other cephalosporions and penicillin. Am J Clin Pathol 118: 256–262

Arndt PA, Garratty G, Hill J et al. (2002) Two cases of immune hemolytic anemia, associated with anti-piperacillin, detected by the 'immune complex' method. Vox Sang 83: 273–278

Arvieux J, Schweizer B, Roussel B et al. (1991) Autoimmune haemolytic anaemia due to antiphospholipid antibodies. Vox Sang 61: 190–195

Atichartakarn V, Chiewsilp P, Ratanasirivanich P et al. (1985) Autoimmune haemolytic anaemia due to anti-B autoantibody. Vox Sang 49: 301–303

Azeredo da Silveira S, Kikuchi S, Fossati-Jimack L et al. (2002) Complement activation selectively potentiates the pathogenicity of the IgG2b and IgG3 isotypes of a high affinity anti-erythrocyte autoantibody. J Exp Med 195: 665–672

Barker RN, Hall AM, Standen GR et al. (1997) Identification of T-cell epitopes on the Rhesus polypeptides in autoimmune haemolytic anaemia. Blood 90: 2701–2715

Bass LS, Rao AH, Goldstein J et al. (1983) The Sd-antigen and antibody: biochemical studies on the inhibitory property of human urine. Vox Sang 44: 191–196

Beattie KM, Zuelzer WW (1968) A serum factor reacting with acriflavin causing an error in ABO cell grouping. Transfusion 8: 254

Beattie KM, Seymour DS, Scott A (1971) Two further examples of acriflavin antibody causing ABO cell typing errors. Transfusion 11: 107

Beattie KM, Ferguson SJ, Burnie KL et al. (1976) Chloramphenicol antibody causing interference in antibody detection and identification tests (Abstract). Transfusion 16: 174

Beaumont JL, Lorenzelli L, Delplanque B et al. (1976) A new serum liproprotein-associated erythrocyte antigen which reacts with a monoclonal IgM. The stored human red blood cell SHRBC antigen. Vox Sang 30: 36

Beck ML, Edwards RL, Pierce SR et al. (1976) Serologic activity of the fatty acid dependent antibodies in albumin-free systems. Transfusion 16: 434

Beck ML, Myers MA, Moulds J et al. (1978) Coexistent Tk and VA polyagglutinability. Transfusion 18: 680

Beck ML, Marsh WL, Pierce SR et al. (1979) Auto-anti-Kp^b associated with weakened antigenicity in the Kell blood group system: a second example. Transfusion 19: 197–202

Bell CA, Zwicker H, Rosenbaum DL (1973a) Paroxysmal cold hemoglobinuria (PCH) following mycoplasma infection: Anti-I specificity of the biphasic hemolysin. Transfusion 13: 138

Bell CA, Zwicker H, Nevius DB (1973b) Nonspecific warm hemolysins of papain-treated cells: Serologic characterization and transfusion risk. Transfusion 13: 207

Ben-Izhak C, Slechter Y, Tatorsky I (1985) Significance of multiple types of antibodies on red blood cells of patients with positive direct antiglobulin test: a study of monospecific antiglobulin reagents in 85 patients. Scand J Haematol 35: 102–108

Berentsen S, Ulvestad E, Gjertsen BT et al. (2004) Rituximab for primary chronic cold agglutinin disease: a prospective study of 37 courses of therapy in 27 patients. Blood 103: 2925–2928

Bird GWG (1964) Anti-T in peanuts. Vox Sang 9: 748

Bird GWG (1978) Significant advances in lectins and polyagglutinable red cells. 15th Congress of the International Society of Blood Transfusion, Paris

Bird GWG (1980) Lectins and red cell polyagglutinability: history, comments and recent developments. In: Polyagglutination, A Technical Workshop. Washington, DC: Am Assoc Blood Banks

Bird GWG (1982) Clinical aspects of red blood cell polyagglutinability of microbial origin. In: Blood Groups and other Red Cell Surface Markers in Health and Disease. C Salmon (ed.). New York: Masson Publishing

Bird T, Stephenson J (1973) Acute haemolytic anaemia associated with polyagglutinability of red cells. J Clin Pathol 26: 868

Bird GWG, Wingham J (1972) Tk: a new form of red cell polyagglutination. Br J Haematol 23: 759

Bird GWG, Wingham J (1981) *Vicia cretica*: a powerful lectin for T- and Th- but not Tk- or other polyagglutinable erythrocytes. J Clin Pathol 34: 69–70

Bird GWG, Wingham J (1983) 'New' lectins for the identification of erythrocyte cryptantigens and the classification of erythrocyte polyagglutinability: *Medicago disciformis* and *Medicago turbinata*. J Clin Pathol 36: 195–196

Bird GWG, Shinton NK, Wingham J et al. (1971) Persistent mixed-field polyagglutination. Br J Haematol 21: 443

Bird GWG, McEvoy MW, Wingham J (1975) Acute haemolytic anaemia due to IgM penicillin antibody in a 3-year-old child: a sequel to oral penicillin. J Clin Pathol 28: 321

Bird GWG, Wingham J, Martin AJ et al. (1976a) Idiopathic non-syphilitic paroxysmal cold haemoglobinuria in children. J Clin Pathol 29: 215

Bird GWG, Wingham J, Chester GH et al. (1976b) Erythrocyte membrane modification in malignant disease of myeloid and lymphoreticular tissues. II. Erythrocyte 'mosaicism' in acute erythroleukaemia. Br J Haematol 33: 295

Bird GWG, Wingham J, Pippard MJ et al. (1976c) Erythrocyte membrane modification in malignant disease of myeloid and lymphoreticular tissues. I. Tn-polyagglutination in acute myelocytic leukaemia. Br J Haematol 33: 289

Bird GWG, Wingham J, Beck ML et al. (1978) Th, a 'new' form of erythrocyte polyagglutination (Letter). Lancet i: 1215

Bird GWG, Wingham J, Seger R et al. (1982) Tx, a 'new' red cell cryptantigen exposed by pneumococcal enzymes. Rev Fr Transfus Immunohématol 25: 215–216

Blumenfeld OO, Lalezari P, Khorshidi M et al. (1992) O-linked oligosaccharides of glycophorins A and B in erythrocytes of two individuals with the Tn polyagglutinability syndrome. Blood 80: 2388–2395

Booth PB, Jenkins WJ, Marsh WL (1966) Anti-I^T: A new antibody of the I blood-group system occurring in certain Melanesian sera. Br J Haematol 12: 341

von dem Borne AEGKr, Engelfriet CP, Beckers D et al. (1969) Autoimmune haemolytic anaemias. II. Warm haemolysins: serological and immunochemical investigations and ^{51}Cr studies. Clin Exp Immunol 4: 333

von dem Borne AEGKr, Beckers D, van der Meulen FW et al. (1977) IgG4 autoantibodies against erythrocytes, without increased haemolysis. Br J Haematol 37: 137

von dem Borne AEGKr, Mol JJ, Joustra-Maas N et al. (1982) Autoimmune haemolytic anaemia with monoclonal

IgM (K) anti-P cold autohaemolysins. Br J Haematol 50: 345–350

Bougie D, Johnson ST, Weitekamp LA et al. (1997) Sensitivity to a metabolite of diclofenac as a cause of acute immune hemolytic anemia. Blood 90: 407–413

Bowman HS, Marsh WL, Schumacher HR et al. (1974) Auto anti-N immunohemolytic anemia in infectious mononucleosis. Am J Clin Pathol 61: 465

Brain MC, Prevost JM, Pihl CE et al. (2002) Glycophorin A-mediated haemolysis of normal human erythrocytes: evidence for antigen aggregation in the pathogenesis of immune haemolysis. Br J Haematol 119: 886

Branch DR, Petz LD (1982) A new reagent (ZZAP) having multiple applications in immunohematology. Am J Clin Pathol 78: 161–167

Brendel WL, Issitt PD, Moore RE et al. (1985) Temporary reduction of red cell Kell system antigen expression and transient production of anti-Kp^b in a surgical patient. Biotest Bull 2: 201–206

Brendemoen OJ (1952) A cold agglutinin specifically active against stored red cells. Acta Pathol Microbiol Scand 31: 574

Broadberry RE, Farren TW, Bevin SV et al. (2004) Tazobactum-induced haemolytic anaemia, possibly caused by non-immunological adsorption of IgG onto patient's red cells. Transfusion Med 14: 53–57

Brouet JC, Vainchenker W, Blanchard D et al. (1983) The origin of human B and T cells from multipotent stem cells: a study of the Tn syndrome. Eur J Immunol 13: 350–352

Brown DL, Cooper AG (1970) The *in vivo* metabolism of radioiodinated cold agglutinins of anti-I specificity. Clin Sci 38: 175

Bruce M, Mitchell R (1981) The LOX antigen: A new chemically-induced red cell antigen. Med Lab Sci 38: 177–186

Bull JP, Ricketts C, Squire JR et al. (1949) Dextran as a plasma substitute. Lancet i: 134

Burkart PT, Hsu TCS (1979) IgM cold-warm hemolysins in infectious mononucleosis. Transfusion 19: 535–538

Burnie K (1973) Ii antigens and antibodies. Can J Med Technol 35: 5

Carstairs KC, Breckenridge A, Dollery CT et al. (1966) Incidence of a positive direct Coombs test in patients on α-methyldopa. Lancet ii: 133

Cartron JF, Nurden AT (1979) Galactosyltransferase and membrane abnormality in human platelets from Tn-syndrome donors. Nature (Lond) 282: 621–623

Cartron JP, Andreu G, Cartron J et al. (1978) Demonstration of T-transferase deficiency in Tn-polyagglutinable blood samples. Eur J Biochem 92: 111

Cartron JP, Blanchard D, Nurden AT et al. (1981) Tn syndrome: a disorder affecting red cell, platelet and granulocyte cell surface components. In: Blood Groups and other Red Cell Surface Markers in Health and Disease. C Salmon (ed.). Paris: Masson Publishing

Casaravilla C, Freire T, Malgor R et al. (2003) Mucin-type O-glycosylation in helminth parasites from major taxonomic groups: evidence for widespread distribution of the T antigen (GalNAc-Ser/Thr) and identification of UDP-GalNAc: polypeptide N-acetylgalactosaminyltransferase activity. J Parasitol 89: 709–714

Case J (1976) Albumin autoagglutinating phenomenon as a factor contributing to false positive reactions when typing with rapid slide-test reagents. Vox Sang 30: 441

Cauerhff A, Braden BC, Carvalho JG et al. (2000) Three-dimensional structure of the Fab from a human IgM cold agglutinin. J Immunol 165: 6422–8

Celano MJ, Levine P (1967) Anti-LW specificity in autoimmune acquired hemolytic anemia. Transfusion 7: 265

Chambers LA, Rauck AM (1996) Acute transient hemolytic anemia with a positive Donath-Landsteiner test following parvovirus B19 infection. J Paediatr Hematol Oncol 18: 178–181

Chaplin H Jr (1973) Clinical usefulness of specific antiglobulin reagents in autoimmune hemolytic anemias. In: Progress in Hematology. EB Brown (ed.), vol. VIII. New York: Grune & Stratton

Chaplin H (1979) Special problems in transfusion management of patients with autoimmune hemolytic anemia. In: A Seminar on Laboratory Management of Hemolysis. Washington, DC: Am Assoc Blood Banks

Chaplin H, Nasongkla M, Monroe MC (1981) Quantitation of red blood cell-bound C3d in normal subjects and random hospitalized patients. Br J Haematol 48: 69–78

Chapman J, Murphy MF, Waters AH (1982) Chronic cold haemagglutinin disease due to an anti-M like auto antibody. Vox Sang 42: 272–277

Chauffard MA, Vincent C (1909) Anémie grave avec hemolysines dans le sérum; ictère hémolysinique. Ser Med (Paris) 28: 345

Cheng CK, Wong ML, Lee AW (2001) PEG adsorption of autoantibodies and detection of alloantibodies in warm autoimmune hemolytic anemia. Transfusion 41: 13–17

Chiaroni J, Touinssi M, Mazet M et al. (2003) Adsorption of autoantibodies in the presence of LISS to detect alloantibodies underlying warm autoantibodies. Transfusion 43: 651–655

Chien S, Kung-Ming J (1973) Ultrastructure basis of the mechanism of rouleaux formation. Microvasc Res 5: 155

Chorpenning FW, Hayes JC (1959) Occurence of the Thomsen-Friedenrich phenomenon in vivo. Vox Sang 4: 210

Citak A, Garratty G, Usel R et al. (2002) Ceftriaxone-induced haemolytic anaemia in a child with no immune deficiency or haematological disease. J Paediatr Child Health 38: 209–210

Clark DA, Dessypris EN, Jenkins DE et al. (1984) Acquired immune-hemolytic anemia associated with IgA erythrocyte coating: investigations of hemolytic mechanisms. Blood 64: 1000–1005

Clark JA, Tauley PC, Wallas CH (1992) Evaluation of patients with positive direct antiglobulin tests and non-reactive eluates discovered during pretransfusion testing. Immunohaematology 8: 9–12

Coluccio E, Villa MA, Villa E et al. (2004) Immune hemolytic anemia associated with teicoplanin. Transfusion 44: 73–78

Conlon KC, Urba WJ, Smith JW et al. (1990) Exacerbation of symptoms of autoimmune disease in patients receiving α-interferon therapy. Cancer 65: 2237–2242

Costea N, Yakulis V, Heller P (1966) Light chain heterogeneity of anti-I and anti-i antibodies. Fed Proc 25: 373

Costea N, Yakulis VJ, Heller P (1972) Inhibition of cold agglutinins (anti-I) by M. pneumoniae antigens. Proc Soc Exp Biol (NY) 139: 476

Crawford H, Cutbush M, Mollison PL (1953) Specificity of incomplete 'cold' antibody in human serum. Lancet i: 566

Curtis BR, Lamon J, Roelcke D et al. (1990) Life-threatening, antiglobulin test-negative, acute autoimmune hemolytic anemia due to a non-complement activating IgG1 κ cold antibody with Pr_a specificity. Transfusion 30: 838–843

Dacie JV (1950) Occurrences in normal human sera of 'incomplete' forms of 'cold' autoantibodies. Nature (Lond) 166: 36

Dacie JV (1954) The Haemolytic Anaemias, Congenital and Acquired, Part II. The Autoimmune Haemolytic Anaemias. London: Churchill

Dacie JV (1962) The Haemolytic Anaemias, Congenital and Acquired, Part II. The Auto-Immune Haemolytic Anaemias, 2nd edn. London: Churchill

Dacie JV (1967) The Haemolytic Anaemias, Congenital and Acquired, Part III. Secondary or Symptomatic Haemolytic Anaemias, 2nd edn. London: Churchill

Dacie JV, Cutbush M (1954) Specificity of auto-antibodies in acquired haemolytic anaemia. J Clin Pathol 7: 18

Dacie JV, Worlledge SM (1969) Auto-immune hemolytic anemias. In: Progress in Hematology, VI. EB Brown, CV Moore (eds), p. 82. New York: Grune & Stratton

Dacie JV, Crookston JH, Christenson WN (1957) 'Incomplete' cold antibodies: role of complement in sensitization to antiglobulin serum by potentially haemolytic antibodies. Br J Haematol 3: 77

Dahr W, Uhlenbruck G, Gunson HH et al. (1975) Molecular basis of Tn-polyagglutinability. Vox Sang 29: 36

Dameshek W, Schwartz SD (1938) The presence of hemolysins in acute hemolytic anemia; preliminary note. N Engl J Med 218: 75

Dausset J, Colombani J (1959) The serology and the prognosis of 128 cases of autoimmune hemolytic anaemia. Blood 14: 1280

Dausset J, Moullec J, Bernard J (1959) Acquired hemolytic anemia with polyagglutinability of red blood cells due to a new factor present in normal human serum (anti-Tn). Blood 14: 1079

Davey RJ, O'Gara C, McGinniss MH (1979) Incompatibility *in vitro* and *in vivo* demonstrated only with saline-suspended red cells. Vox Sang 36: 301–306

Dellagi K, Brouet JC, Schenmetzler *et al.* (1981) Chronic hemolytic anemia due to a monoclonal IgG cold agglutinin with anti-Pr specificity. Blood 57: 189–191

Denegri JF, Nangi AA, Sinclair M *et al.* (1983) Autoimmune haemolytic anaemia due to immunoglobulin G with anti-Sd^x specificity. Acta Haematol 69: 19–22

De Wit DC, van Gastel C (1970) Haemolysis in cold agglutinin disease: the role of C' and cell age in red cell destruction. Br J Haematol 18: 557

van Dijk BA, Barrera RP, Hoitsma A *et al.* (1989) Immune hemolytic anemia associated with tolmetin and suprofen. Transfusion 29: 638–641

Ding Y, Xu G, Yang M *et al.* (2003) Crystal structure of the ectodomain of human FcalphaRI. J Biol Chem 278: 27966–70

Doinel C, Andreu G, Cartron JP *et al.* (1980) Tk polyagglutination produced *in vitro* by an endo-beta-galactosidase. Vox Sang 38: 94–98

Duk M, Reinhold BB, Reinhold VN *et al.* (2001) Structure of a neutral glycosphingolipid recognised by human antibodies in polyagglutinable erythrocytes of the rare NOR phenotype. J Biol Chem 276: 40574–82

Duk M, Lisowska E, Kusnierz-Alejska G (2002) Serologic identification of NOR polyagglutination with *Griffonia simplificolia* IB4 lectin. Transfusion 42: 806

Ejby-Poulsen P (1954a) Experimentally produced polyagglutinability (T-transformation of erythrocytes *in vivo*) in guinea pigs infected with pneumococci. Nature (Lond) 173: 82

Ejby-Poulsen P (1954b) Haemolytic anaemia produced experimentally in the guinea pig by T-transformation of the erythrocytes *in vivo* with purified concentrated enzyme. Nature (Lond) 174: 929

Ellisor SS, Reid ME, Day TO *et al.* (1983) Autoantibodies mimicking anti-Jk^b plus anti-Jk3 associated with autoimmune haemolytic anaemia in a primipara who delivered an unaffected infant. Vox Sang 45: 53–59

Engelfriet CP (1976) C4 and C3 on red cells coated in *vivo* and in *vitro*. In: The Nature and Significance of Complement Activation. Raritan, NJ: Ortho Research Institute

Engelfriet CP, von dem Borne AEGKr, Moes M *et al.* (1968a) Serological studies in autoimmune haemolytic anaemia. Bibl Haematol 29: 473

Engelfriet CP, von dem Borne AEGKr, von dem Giessen M *et al.* (1968b) Autoimmune haemolytic anaemias. I. Serological studies with pure anti-immunoglobulin reagents. Clin Exp Immunol 3: 605

Engelfriet CP, von dem Borne AEGKr, Beckers ThAP *et al.* (1972) Autoimmune haemolytic anaemias. V. Studies on the resistance against complement haemolysis of red cells of patients with chronic cold agglutinin disease. Clin Exp Immunol 2: 255

Engelfriet CP, Beckers, ThAP, van't Veer MB *et al.* (1982) Recent advances in immune haemolytic anaemia. In: Recent Advances in Haematology. SR Hollan (ed.), pp. 235–251. Budapest: Akademia Kiado

Evans RS, Bingham M, Weiser RS (1963) A hemolytic system associated with enteritis in rabbits. II. Studies on the survival of transfused cells. J Lab Clin Med 62: 569

Evans RS, Turner E, Bingham M (1965) Studies with radio-iodinated cold agglutinins of ten patients. Am J Med 38: 378

Evans RS, Turner E, Bingham M *et al.* (1968) Chronic hemolytic anemia due to cold agglutinins. II. The role of C' in red cell destruction. J Clin Invest 47: 691

Fabijanska-Mitek J, Lopienska H, Zupanska B (1997) Gel test for IgG sublclass detection in auto-immune haemolytic anaemia. Vox Sang 72: 233–237

Facer CA, Bray RS, Brown J (1979) Direct Coombs antiglobulin reactions in Gambian children with *Plasmodium falciparum* malaria. I. Incidence and class specificity. Clin Exp Immunol 35: 119–127

Feizi T (1977) Immunochemistry of the Ii blood group antigens. In: Human Blood Groups. JF Mohn, RW Plunkett, RK Cunningham *et al.* (eds), pp. 164–171. Basel: S Karger

Fest T, deWazièzes B, Laney B *et al.* (1994) Successful response to alpha-interferon 2b in a refractory IgM auto-agglutinin-mediated hemolytic anemia. Am J Hematol 69: 147–149

Flanagan CJ, Mitoma TF (1958) Clumping (false agglutination) of blood from the umbilical cord. Am J Clin Pathol 29: 337

Flores G, Cunningham-Rundles C, Newland AC *et al.* (1993) Efficacy of intravenous immunoglobulin in the treatment of autoimmune haemolytic anaemia: results in 73 patients. Am J Hematol 44: 237–242

Fossati-Jimack L, Ioan-Facsinay A, Reininger L *et al.* (2000) Markedly different pathogenicity of four immunoglobulin G isotype-switch variants of a anti-erythrocyte autoantibody is based on their capacity to interact *in vivo* with the low-affinity Fcgamma receptor III. J Exp Med 191: 1293–1302

Frank M, Basta M, Fries LF (1992) The effects of intravenous immune globulin on complement-dependent immune damage of cells and tissues. Clin Immunol Immunopathol 62: 82–86

Freedman J (1979) False-positive antiglobulin tests in healthy subjects and in hospital patients. J Clin Pathol 32: 1014–1018

Freedman J, Barefoot C (1982) Red blood cell-bound C3d in normal subjects and in random hospital patients. Transfusion 22: 511–514

Freedman J, Newlands M (1977) Autoimmune haemolytic anaemia with the unusual combination of both IgM and IgG autoantibodies. Vox Sang 32: 61

Freedman J, Newlands M, Johnson CA (1977) Warm IgM anti-I^T causing autoimmune haemolytic anaemia. Vox Sang 32: 135

Freiesleben E, Jensen KG (1959) An antibody specific for washed red cells. Abstract 330, Commun 7th Congr Eur Soc Haematol, London

Friedenreich V (1930) The Thomsen Hemagglutination Phenomenon. Copenhagen: Levin and Munksgaard

Frohn C, Dumbgen L, Brand JM et al. (2003) Probability of anti-D development in D-patients receiving D+ RBCs. Transfusion 43: 893–8

Fudenberg HH, German JL (1960) Certain physical and biological characteristics of penicillin antibody. Blood 15: 683

Ganly PS, Laffan MA, Owen I et al. (1988) Auto-anti-Jk^a in Evans' syndrome with negative direct antiglobulin test. Br J Haematol 69: 537–539

Garratty G (1994) Review: immune hemolytic anemia and/or positive direct antiglobulin tests caused by drugs. Immunohaematology 10: 41–50

Garratty G, Petz LD (1975) Drug-induced immune hemolytic anemia. Am J Med 58: 398

Garratty G, Petz LD (1994) Transfusing patients with auto immune haemolytic anaemia (Letter). Lancet 341: 1220

Garratty G, Petz LD, Brodsky I et al. (1973) An IgA high-titer cold agglutinin with an unusual blood group specificity within the Pr complex. Vox Sang 25: 32

Garratty G, Petz LD, Wallerstein RO et al. (1974) Autoimmune hemolytic anemia in Hodgkin's disease associated with anti-I^T. Transfusion 14: 226

Garratty G, Petz LD, Hoops JK (1977) The correlation of cold agglutinin titrations in saline and albumin with haemolytic anaemia. Br J Haematol 35: 587

Garratty G, Gattler MS, Petz LD et al. (1979) Immune hemolytic anemia associated with anti-Kell and a carrier state for chronic granulomatous disease. Rev Fr Transfus Immunohématol 22: 529–549

Garratty G, Davis J, Myers M et al. (1980) IgG red cell sensitization associated with in vitro clotting in patients with ulcerative colitis (Abstract). Transfusion 20: 646

Garratty G, Brunt O, Greenfield B et al. (1983) An autoanti-En^a mimicking an alloanti-En^a associated with pure red cell aplasia (Abstract). Transfusion 23: 408

Garratty G, Prince H, Arndt P et al. (1986) In vitro IgG production following preincubation of lymphocytes with methyldopa and procainamide (Abstract). Blood 68(Suppl. 1): 108a

Garratty G, Nance S, Lloyd M et al. (1992) Fatal immune hemolytic anemia due to cefotetan. Transfusion 32: 269–271

Garratty G, Arndt P, Domen R et al. (1997) Severe autoimmune hemolytic anemia associated with IgM warm autoantibodies directed against determinants on or associated with glycophorin A. Vox Sang 72: 124–130

Garratty G, Leger RM, Arndt PA (1999) Severe immune hemolytic anemia associated with prophylactic cefotetan in obstetric and gynecologic procedures. Am J Obstet Gynecol 181: 103–104

Geisen HP, Roelcke D, Rehn K et al. (1975) Hochtitrige Kälteagglutinine der Spezifität Anti-Pr nach Rötelninfektion. Klin Wschr 53: 767–772

Goldberg LS, Barnett EV (1967) Mixed γG-γM cold agglutinin. J Immunol 99: 803

Goldberg LS, Fudenberg HH (1968) Warm antibody hemolytic anemia: prolonged remission despite persistent positive Coombs test. Vox Sang 15: 443

Golde DW, McGinniss MN, Holland PV (1969) Mechanism of the albumin agglutination phenomenon. Vox Sang 16: 465

Golde DW, Greipp PR, McGinniss MH (1973) Spectrum of albumin autoagglutinins. Transfusion 13: 1

Gorst DW, Rawlinson VI, Merry AH et al. (1980) Positive direct antiglobulin test in normal individuals. Vox Sang 38: 99–105

Göttsche B, Salama A, Mueller-Eckhardt C (1990a) Autoimmune hemolytic anemia caused by a cold agglutinin with a new specificity (anti-Ju). Transfusion 30: 261–262

Göttsche B, Salama A, Mueller-Eckhardt C (1990b) Donath-Landsteiner autoimmune hemolytic anemia in children. A study of 22 cases. Vox Sang 58: 281–286

Goverman J, Woods A, Larson L et al. (1993) Transgenic mice that express a myelin basic protein-specific T cell receptor develop spontaneous autoimmunity. Cell 72: 551–560

Graham HA, Davies DM Jr, Tigner JA et al. (1976) Evidence suggesting that trace amounts of C3d are bound to most human red cells. Transfusion 16: 530

Graninger W, Ramesis H, Fischer K et al. (1977a) 'VA', a new type of erythrocyte polyagglutination characterized by depressed H receptors and associated with hemolytic anemia. I. Serological and hematological observations. Vox Sang 32: 195

Graninger W, Poschmann A, Fischer K et al. (1977b) 'VA', a new type of erythrocyte polyagglutination characterized by depressed H receptors and associated with hemolytic anemia. II. Observations by immunofluorescence, electron microscopy, cell electrophoresis and biochemistry. Vox Sang 32: 201

Gray MP (1964) A human serum factor agglutinating human red cells exposed to lactose. Vox Sang 9: 608

Gronemeyer P, Chaplin H, Ghazarian V et al. (1981) Hemolytic anemia complicating infectious mononucleosis due to the interaction of an IgG cold anti-i and an IgM cold rheumatoid factor. Transfusion 21: 715–718

Gunson HH, Stratton F, Mullard GW (1970) An example of polyagglutinability due to the Tn antigen. Br J Haematol 18: 309

Gutgsell NS, Issitt PD, Tomasulo PA *et al.* (1988) Use of the direct enzyme-linked antiglobulin test (ELAT) in patients with unexplained anemia. Transfusion 28 (Suppl.): 36S

Habibi B (1983) Disappearance of alpha-methyldopa induced red cell autoantibodies despite continuation of the drug. Br J Haematol 54: 493–495

Habibi B, Homberg J-C, Schaison G *et al.* (1974) Autoimmune hemolytic anemia in children. A review of 80 cases. Am J Med 56: 61

Habibi B, Muller A, Lelong F *et al.* (1980) Autoimmunisation érythrocytaire dans la population 'normale'. 63 observations. Nouv Presse Méd 9: 3253–3257

Hall AM, Ward FJ, Vickers MA *et al.* (2002) Interleukin-10-mediated regulatory T-cell responses to epitopes on a human red cell autoantigen. Blood 100: 4529–4536

Harboe M (1964) Interactions between ^{131}I trace-labelled cold agglutinin, complement and red cells. Br J Haematol 10: 339

Harris T (1990) Two cases of autoantibodies that demonstrate mimicking specificity in the Duffy blood group system. Immunohematology 6: 87

Harris PA, Roman GK, Moulds JJ *et al.* (1982) An inherited rbc characteristic, NOR, resulting in erythrocyte polyagglutination. Vox Sang 42: 134–140

Haynes CR, Chaplin H Jr (1971) An enhancing effect of albumin on the determination of cold hemagglutinins. Vox Sang 20: 46

Haynes CR, Dorner I, Leonard GL *et al.* (1970) Persistent polyagglutinability *in vivo* unrelated to T-antigen activation. Transfusion 10: 43

Heddle NM, Blajchman MA, Bodner N *et al.* (1977) Absence of hemolysis of T-activated red cells following infusion of blood products. Atlanta, GA: Commun Am Assoc Blood Banks

Heddle NM, Kelton JG, Turchyn KL *et al.* (1988) Hypergammaglobulinemia can be associated with a positive direct antiglobulin test, a nonreactive eluate, and no evidence of hemolysis. Transfusion 28: 29–33

Heistö H, Harboe M, Godal HC (1965) Warm haemolysins active against trypsinized red cells: occurrence, inheritance, and clinical significance. Proc 10th Congr Int Soc Blood Transfus, Stockholm

Henningsen K (1949) A case of polyagglutinable human red cells. Acta Path Microbiol Scand 26: 339

Herman JH, Shirey RS, Smith B *et al.* (1987) Th activation in congenital hypoplastic anaemia. Transfusion 27: 253–256

Herron R, Clark M, Smith DS (1987) An autoantibody with activity dependent on red cell age in the serum of a patient with autoimmune haemolytic anaemia and a negative direct antiglobulin test. Vox Sang 52: 71–74

Herron B, Roelcke D, Orson C *et al.* (1993) Cold agglutinins with anti-Pr specificity associated with fresh varicella infection. Vox Sang 65: 239–242

Hershko C, Sonnenblick M, Ashkenazi J (1990) Control of steroid-resistant autoimmune haemolytic anaemia by cyclosporine. Br J Haematol 76: 436–437

Hinz CF (1963) Serologic and physiochemical characterization of Donath–Landsteiner antibodies from six patients. Blood 22: 600

Hinz CF Jr, Picken ME, Lepow IH (1961a) Studies on immune human hemolysis. I. The kinetics of the Donath–Landsteiner reaction and the requirements for complement in the reaction. J Exp Med 113: 177

Hinz CF Jr, Picken ME, Lepow IH (1961b) Studies on immune human hemolysis. II. The Donath–Landsteiner reaction as a model system for studying the mechanism of action of complement and the role of C'1 and C'1 esterase. J Exp Med 113: 193

Hogarth PM (2002) Fc receptors are major mediators of antibody based inflammation in autoimmunity. Curr Opin Immunol 14: 798–802

Högman C, Killander J, Sjölin S (1960) A case of idiopathic auto-immune haemolytic anaemia due to anti-e. Acta Paediatr 49: 270

Holländer L (1954) Study of the erythrocyte survival time in a case of acquired haemolytic anaemia. Vox Sang 4: 164

Holmes LD, Pierce SR, Beck M (1976) Autoanti-Jk[a] in a healthy donor (Abstract). Transfusion 16: 521

Howard DR (1979) Expression of T-antigen on polyagglutinable erythrocytes and carcinoma cells: preparation of T-activated erythrocytes, anti-T lectin, anti-T absorbed human serum and purified anti-T antibody. Vox Sang 37: 107–110

Hsu TCS, Rosenfield RE, Burkart P *et al.* (1974) Instrumented PVP-augmented antiglobulin tests. II. Evaluation of acquired hemolytic anemia. Vox Sang 26: 305

Hübener G (1925) Untersuchungen über Isoagglutination, mit besonderer Berücksichtigung scheinbarer Abweichungen vom Gruppenschema. Z Immun-Forsch 45: 223

Huh YO, Liu FJ, Rogge K *et al.* (1988) Positive direct antiglobulin test and high serum immunoglobulin G values. Am J Clin Pathol 90: 179–200

Hysell JK, Gray JM, Hysell JW *et al.* (1975) An anti-neomycin antibody interfering with ABO grouping and antibody screening. Transfusion 15: 16

Hysell JK, Hysell JW, Nichols ME *et al.* (1976) *In vivo* and *in vitro* activation of T-antigen receptors on leukocytes and platelets. Vox Sang 31: 9

Inglis G, Bird GWG, Mitchell AAB *et al.* (1975a) Erythrocyte polyagglutination showing properties of both T and Tk, probably induced by *Bacteroides fragilis* infection. Vox Sang 28: 314

Inglis G, Bird GWG, Mitchell AAB *et al.* (1975b) Effect of *Bacteroides fragilis* on the human erythrocyte membrane: pathogenesis of Tk polyagglutination. J Clin Pathol 28: 964

Inglis G, Bird GWG, Mitchell AAB *et al.* (1978) Tk poly-agglutination associated with reduced A and H activity. Vox Sang 35: 370

Issitt PD, Anstee DJ (1998) Applied Blood Group Serology, 4th edn. Durham, NC: Montgomery Scientific Publications

Issitt PD, Issitt CH (1975) Applied Blood Group Serology. Oxnard, CA: Spectra Biologicals

Issitt PD, Obarski G, Hartnett PL *et al.* (1990) Temporary suppression of Kidd system expression accompanied by transient production of anti-Jk3. Transfusion 30: 46–50

Issitt PD, Pavone BG (1978) Critical re-examination of the specificity of auto-anti-Rh antibodies in patients with a positive direct antiglobulin test. Br J Haematol 38: 63

Issitt PD, Pavone BG, Goldfinger D *et al.* (1976) Anti-Wr[b], and other autoantibodies responsible for positive direct antiglobulin tests in 150 individuals. Br J Haematol 34: 5

Issitt PD, Gruppo RA, Wilkinson SL *et al.* (1982) Atypical presentation of acute phase, antibody-induced haemolytic anaemia in an infant. Br J Haematol 52: 537–543

Iwamoto S, Kamesaki T, Oyamada T *et al.* (2001) Reactivity of autoantibodies of autoimmune hemolytic anemia with recombinant rhesus blood group antigens or anion trans-porter 3. Am J Haematol 68: 106–114

Jackson VA, Issitt PD, Francis BJ *et al.* (1968) The simultaneous presence of anti-I and anti-i in sera. Vox Sang 15: 133

Jaffe CF, Atkinson JP, Frank MM (1976) The role of complement in the clearance of cold agglutinin-sensitized erythrocytes in man. J Clin Invest 58: 942

James P, Rowe GP, Tozzo, GG (1988) Elucidation of alloantibodies in autoimmune haemolytic anaemia. Vox Sang 54: 167–171

Janot C, Andreu G, Schooneman F *et al.* (1979) Association des polyagglutinabilités de types T et B acquis. A propos d'une observation. Rev Fr Transfus Immunohématol 22: 375–385

Janvier D, Sellami F, Missud F *et al.* (2002) Severe autoimmune hemolytic anemia caused by a warm IgA autoantibody directed against the third loop of band 3 (RBC anion-exchange protein 1). Transfusion 42: 1547–1552

Jenkins WJ, Marsh WL (1961) Autoimmune haemolytic anaemia. Three cases with antibodies specifically active against stored red cells. Lancet ii: 16

Jenkins WJ, Koster HG, Marsh WL *et al.* (1965) Infectious mononucleosis: an unsuspected source of anti-i. Br J Haematol 11: 480

Jochem E-M (1958a) Rôle des streptocoques dans la panhé-magglutination et la polyagglutinabilité. Ann Inst Pasteur 95: 756

Jochem E-M (1958b) Rôle de *Bacillus anthracis* dans la panhémagglutination. Ann Inst Pasteur 95: 760

Johnson MH, Plett MJ, Conant CN *et al.* (1978) Auto-immune hemolytic anemia with anti-S specificity (Abstract). Transfusion 18: 389

Johnson ST, McFarland JG, Kelly KJ *et al.* (2002) Transfusion support with RBCs from an Mk homozygote in a case of autoimmune hemolytic anemia following diphtheria-pertussis-tetanus vaccination. Transfusion 42: 567–571

Jourdan E, Topart D, Richard B *et al.* (2003) Severe autoimmune hemolytic anemia following rituximab therapy in a patient with a lymphoproliferative disorder. Leuk Lymphoma 44: 889–890

Ju T, Cummings RD (2002) A unique molecular chaperone Cosmc required for activity of the mammalian core 1 beta 3-galactosyltransferase. Proc Natl Acad Sci USA 99: 16613–16618

Judd WJ, McGuire-Mallory D, Anderson KM *et al.* (1979) Concomitant T- and Tk-activation associated with acquired-B antigens. Transfusion 19: 293–298

Judd WJ, Wilkinson SL, Issitt PD *et al.* (1986) Donath–Landsteiner hemolytic anemia due to anti-Pr-like biphasic hemolysin. Transfusion 26: 423–425

Jurgensen JS, Seltsam A, Jorres A (2001) Fatal acute diclofenac-induced immune hemolytic anemia. Ann Hematol 80: 440–442

Kanitakis J, Al-Rifai I, Faure M *et al.* (1997) Demodex mites of human skin express Tn but not T (Thomsen Friedenreich) antigen immunoreactivity. J Cutan Pathol 24: 454–455

Keogh EV, North EA, Warburton MF (1948) Adsorption of bacterial polysaccharides to erythrocytes. Nature (Lond) 161: 687

Killpack WS (1950) Letter to the Editor Lancet ii: 827

Kim S, Song KS, Kim HO *et al.* (2002) Ceftriaxone induced immune hemolytic anemia: detection of drug dependent antibody by *ex vivo* antigen in urine. Yonsei Med J 43: 391–394

Kirtland HH, Mohler DN, Horwitz DA (1980) Methyldopa inhibition of suppressor-lymphocyte function. N Engl J Med 305: 825–832

Kjeldsen T, Hakomori S, Springer CF *et al.* (1989) Coexpression of sialosyl-Tn (NeuAcα(2–6)GalNAcα1-O-Ser/Thr) and Tn (GalNAcα1-O-Ser/Thr) blood group antigen on Tn erythrocytes. Vox Sang 57: 81–87

Kokkini G, Vrionis G, Liosis G *et al.* (1984) Cold agglutinin syndrome and haemophagocytosis in systemic leishmaniasis. Scand J Haematol 32: 441–445

König AL, Kreft H, Hengge U *et al.* (1988) Co-existing anti-I and anti-Fl/Gd cold agglutinins in infections by *Mycoplasma pneumoniae*. Vox Sang 55: 176–180

König AL, Keller HE, Braun RW *et al.* (1992) Cold agglutinins of anti-Pr specificity in rubella embryopathy. Ann Hematol 64: 277–280

König AL, Schabel A, Sugg U et al. (2001) Autoimmune hemolytic anemia caused by IgG lambda-monotypic cold agglutinins of anti-Pr specificity after rubella infection. Transfusion 41: 488–492

Korn RJ, Yakulis VJ, Lemke CE et al. (1957) Cold agglutinins in Listeria monocytogenes infections. Arch Intern Med 99: 573

Krugluger W, Köller M, Hopmeier P (1994) Development of a carbohydrate antigen during storage of red cells. Transfusion 34: 496–501

Kumpel BM, van de Winkel JGJ, Westerdaal NAC et al. (1996) Antigen topography is critical for interaction of IgG2 anti-red-cell antibodies with Fcγ receptors. Br J Haematol 94: 175–183

Kusnierz-Alejska G, Duk M, Storry JR et al. (1999) NOR polyagglutination and Sta glycophorin in one family: relation of NOR polyagglutination to terminal alpha-galactose residues and abnormal glycolipids. Transfusion 39: 32–38

Lachmann PJ, Pangburn MK, Oldroyd RG (1982) Breakdown of C3bi to C3c, C3d and a new fragment-C3g. J Exp Med 156: 205–216

Lahav M, Rosenberg I, Wysenbeek AJ (1989) Steroid-responsive idiopathic cold agglutinin disease: a case report. Acta Haematol 81: 166–168

Laine ML, Beattie KM (1985) Frequency of alloantibodies accompanying autoantibodies. Transfusion 25: 545–546

Lalezari P, Louie JE, Fadlallah N (1982) Serologic profile of alphamethyldopa-induced hemolytic anemia: correlation between cell-bound IgM and hemolysis. Blood 59: 61–68

Landsteiner K (1903) Über Beziehungen zwischen dem Blutserum und den Körperzellen. Münch Med Wschr 50: 1812

Landsteiner K, Levine P (1926) On the cold agglutinins in human serum. J Immunol 12: 441

Lapinid IM, Steib MD, Noto TA (1984) Positive direct antiglobulin tests with antilymphocyte globulin. Am J Clin Pathol 81: 514–17

Lau P, Sererat S, Moore V et al. (1983) Paroxysmal cold haemoglobinuria in a patient with klebsiella pneumonia. Vox Sang 44: 167–172

Leddy JP, Bakemeier RF (1967) A relationship of direct Coombs test pattern to autoantibody specificity in acquired hemolytic anemia. Proc Soc Exp Biol (NY) 125: 808

Leddy JP, Falany JL, Kissel GE et al. (1993) Erythrocyte membrane proteins reactive with human (warm-reacting) anti-red cell autoantibodies. J Clin Invest 91: 1672–1680

Leddy JP, Wilkinson SL, Kissel GE et al. (1994) Erythrocyte membrane proteins reactive with IgG (warm-reacting) anti-red blood cell autoantibodies; II. Antibodies coprecipitating band 3 and Glycophorin A. Blood 84: 650–656

Levene WA (1984) Polyagglutination in Israel. Thesis, Hebrew University, Hadassah Medical School, Jerusalem, pp. 1–68

Levine P, Gelano MJ, Falkowski F (1963) The specificity of the antibody in paroxysmal cold hemoglobinuria (PCH). Transfusion 3: 278

Lewis R, Reid M, Ellisor S et al. (1980) A glucose-dependent panhemagglutinin. Vox Sang 39: 205–211

Ley AB, Mayer K, Harris JP (1958) Observations on a 'specific autoantibody'. Proc 6th Congr Int Soc Blood Transfus, Boston, 1956

Liew YW, Bird GWG, King MJ (1982) The human erythrocyte cryptantigen Tk: exposure by an endo-beta galactosidase from Flavobacterium keratolyticus. Rev franç Transfus Immunohémat 25: 639–641

Lim S, Alam MG (2003) Ciprofloxacin-induced acute interstitial nephritis and autoimmune hemolytic anemia. Renal Failure 25: 647–651

van Loghem JJ (1965) Some comments on autoantibody induced red cell destruction. Ann NY Acad Sci 124: 465

van Loghem JJ, van der Hart M (1954) Varieties of specific auto-antibodies in acquired haemolytic anaemia. Vox Sang (OS) 4: 2

van Loghem JJ, van der Hart M, Land ME (1955) Polyagglutinability of red cells as a cause of severe haemolytic transfusion reaction. Vox Sang (OS) 5: 125

van Loghem JJ, Peetoom F, van der Hart M et al. (1963) Serological and immunochemical studies in haemolytic anaemia with high-titre cold agglutinins. Vox Sang 8: 33

Longster GH, Johnson E (1988) IgM anti-D as auto-antibody in a case of cold auto-immune haemolytic anaemia. Vox Sang 54: 174–176

Loomes LM, Uemura K, Childs RA et al. (1984) Erythrocyte receptors for Mycoplasma pneumoniae are sialylated oligosaccharides of Ii antigen type. Nature (Lond) 307: 560–562

Loutit JF, Mollison PL (1946) Haemolytic icterus (acholuric jaundice) congenital and acquired. J Pathol Bacteriol 58: 711

Lugassy G, Reitblatt T, Ducach A et al. (1993) Severe autoimmune hemolytic anemia with cold agglutinin and sclerodermic features: favorable response to danazol. Ann Hematol 67: 143–144

MacIntyre EA, Linch DC, Macey MG et al. (1985) Successful response to intravenous immunoglobulin in autoimmune haemolytic anaemia. Br J Haematol 60: 387–388

MacKenzie MR, Fudenberg HH (1972) Macroglobulinaemia: an analysis for forty patients. Blood 39: 874

Maliszewski CR, Shen L, Fanger MW (1985) The expression of receptors for IgA on human monocytes and calcitriol treated HL-60 cells. J Immunol 135: 3878–3881

Manny W, Levene C, Sela R et al. (1983) Autoimmunity and the Kell blood groups: autoanti-Kp^b in a Kp(a+ b−) patient. Vox Sang 45: 252–256

Marani T, Leatherbarrow MB, Armstrong KS et al. (1994) Carboplatin-induced immune hemolytic anemia (CIHA) due to an antibody reacting with features of both the immune complex (1C) and drug-adsorption (DA) mechanism (Abstract). Transfusion 34 (Suppl.): 20S

Marsh WL (1960) The pseudo B antigen. A study of its development. Vox Sang 5: 387

Marsh WL (1972) Scoring of hemagglutination reaction. Transfusion 12: 352

Marsh WL, Reid ME, Scott P et al. (1972) Autoantibodies of U blood group specificity in autoimmune haemolytic anaemia. Br J Haematol 22: 625

Marsh WL, Øyen R, Alicea E et al. (1979) Autoimmune hemolytic anemia and the Kell blood groups. Am J Hematol 7: 155–162

Marsh WL, Johnson CL, DiNapoli J et al. (1980) Immune hemolytic anemia caused by auto anti-Sd^x: a report on 6 cases (Abstract). Transfusion 20: 647

Martinez-Letona J, Barbolla L, Frieyro E et al. (1977) Immune haemolytic anaemia and renal failure induced by streptomycin. Br J Haematol 35: 561

Martlew VJ (1986) Immune haemolytic anaemia and nomifensine treatment in north-west England 1984–85: report of six cases. J Clin Pathol 39: 1147–1150

McKenzie SE, Taylor SM, Malladi P (1999) The role of the human Fc receptor Fc gamma RIIA in the immune clearance of platelets: a transgenic mouse model. J Immunol 162: 4311–4318

Meichenin M, Rocher J, Galanina O et al. (2000) Tk, a new colon tumor-associated antigen resulting from altered O-glycosylation. Cancer Res 60: 5499–5507

Mellbye OJ (1966) Reversible agglutination of trypsinised red cells by a γM globulin synthesized by the human foetus. Scand J Haematol 3: 310

Mellbye OJ (1967) Reversible agglutination of trypsinised red cells by normal human sera. Scand J Haematol 4: 135

Mellbye OJ (1969a) Properties of the trypsinised red cell receptor reacting in reversible agglutination by normal sera. Scand J Haematol 6: 139

Mellbye OJ (1969b) Specificity of natural human agglutinins against red cells modified by trypsin and other agents. Scand J Haematol 6: 166

Merry AH, Thomson EE, Rawlinson V et al. (1983) The quantification of C3 fragments on erythrocytes: estimation of C3 fragments on normal cells, acquired haemolytic anaemia cases and correlation with agglutination of sensitized cells. Clin Lab Haematol 5: 387–397

van der Meulen FW, de Bruin HG, Goosen PCM et al. (1980) Quantitative aspects of the destruction of red cells sensitized with IgG1 autoantibodies: an application of flow cytofluorometry. Br J Haematol 46: 47–56

Mollison PL (1956) Blood Transfusion in Clinical Medicine, 2nd edn. Oxford: Blackwell Scientific Publications

Mollison PL (1959) Measurement of survival and destruction of red cells in haemolytic syndromes. Br Med Bull 15: 59

Mollison PL (1983) Blood Transfusion in Clinical Medicine, 7th edn. Oxford: Blackwell Scientific Publications

Moore JA, Chaplin H Jr (1973) Autoimmune hemolytic anemia associated with an IgG cold incomplete anti-body. Vox Sang 24: 236

Moores P, Botha MC, Brink S (1970) Anti-N in the serum of a healthy type MN person: a further example. Am J Clin Pathol 54: 90

Moores P, Pudifin D, Patel PL (1975) Severe hemolytic anemia in an adult associated with anti-T. Transfusion 15: 329

Mullard GW, Haworth C, Le D (1978) A case of atypical polyagglutinability due to Tk transformation. Br J Haematol 40: 571

Murakami M, Nakajima K, Yamazaki K et al. (1997) Effects of breeding environments on generation and activation of autoreactive B-1 cells in anti-red blood cell autoantibody transgenic mice. J Exp Med 185: 791–794

Mygind K, Ahrons S (1973) IgG cold agglutinins and first trimester abortion. Vox Sang 23: 552

Myllylä G, Furuhjelm U, Nordling S et al. (1971) Persistent mixed field polyagglutinability. Electrokinetic and serological aspects. Vox Sang 20: 7

Newland AC, Macey AC, Macintyre EA et al. (1986) The role of intravenous IgG in autoimmune haemolytic anaemia. In: Abstracts, 21st Congr Int Soc Blood Transfus, Sydney

Northoff H, Martin A, Roelcke D (1987) An IgG κ monotypic anti-Pr$_{ih}$ associated with fresh varicella infection. Eur J Haematol 38: 85–88

Nurden AT, Dupuis D, Pidard D et al. (1982) Surface modifications in the platelets of a patient with alpha-N-acetyl-D-galactosamine residues, the Tn-syndrome. J Clin Invest 70: 1281–1291

O'Boyle KP, Markowitz AL, Khorshidi M et al. (1996) Specificity analysis of murine monoclonal antibodies reactive with Tn, sialylated Tn, T and monosialylated (2–6) T antigens. Hybridoma 15: 401–8

O'Connor B, Clifford JS, Lawrence WD et al. (1989) Alpha-interferon for severe cold agglutinin disease. Ann Intern Med 111: 255

O'Day T (1987) A second example of autoanti-Jk3. Transfusion 27: 442

Ogburn JR, Knauss MA, Thapar K et al. (1994) Cefotetan-induced immunohemolytic anemia (IHA) resulting from both drug adsorption and immune complex mechanisms (Abstract). Transfusion 34: 27S

Oh YR, Carr-Lopez SM, Probasco JM et al. (2003) Levofloxacin-induced autoimmune hemolytic anemia. Ann Pharmacother 37: 1010–1013

Okada H, Tanaka H (1983) Species-specific inhibition by glycophorins of complement activation via the alternative pathway. Mol Immunol 20: 1233–1236

Oldenborg PA, Zheleznyak A, Fang Y-F *et al.* (2000) Role of CD47 as a marker of self on red blood cells. Science 288: 2051–2054

Oldenborg PA, Gresham HD, Chen Y *et al.* (2002) Lethal autoimmune hemolytic anemia in CD47-deficient nonobese diabetic (NOD) mice. Blood 99: 3500–3504

Oldstone MBA (1998) Molecular mimicry and immune-mediated diseases. FASEB J 12: 1255–1265

Ovary Z, Spiegelman J (1965) The production of cold 'autohemagglutinins' in the rabbit as a consequence of immunization with isologous erythrocytes. Ann NY Acad Sci 124: 147

Owen I, Chowdhury V, Reid ME *et al.* (1992) Autoimmune hemolytic anemia associated with anti-Scl. Transfusion 32: 173–176

Ozer FL, Chaplin H (1963) Agglutination of stored erythrocytes by a human serum. Characterization of the serum factor and erythrocyte changes. J Clin Invest 42: 1735

Parish HJ, Macfarlane RG (1941) Effect of calcium in a case of autohaemagglutination. Lancet ii: 447

Pascual V, Victor K, Spellerberg M *et al.* (1992) VH restriction among human cold agglutinins. The VH4–21 gene segment is required to encode anti-I and anti-i specificities. J Immunol 149: 2337–2344

Perez R, Padavic K, Krigel R *et al.* (1991) Antierythrocyte autoantibody formation after therapy with interleukin-2 and gamma-interferon. Cancer 67: 2512–2517

Petz LD (2001) Treatment of autoimmune hemolytic anemia. Curr Opin Hematol 8: 411–416

Petz LD, Branch DR (1983) Serological tests for the diagnosis of immune haemolytic anaemias. In: Methods in Haematology: Immune Cytopenias. R McMillan (ed.), pp. 9–48. New York: Churchill Livingstone

Petz LD, Branch DR (1985) Drug-induced hemolytic anemia. In: Immune Hemolytic Anemias. H Chaplin (ed.), pp. 47–94. New York: Churchill Livingstone

Petz LD, Fudenberg HH (1966) Coombs-positive hemolytic anemia caused by penicillin administration. N Engl J Med 274: 171

Petz LD, Garratty G (1975) Laboratory correlations in immune hemolytic anemias. In: Laboratory Diagnosis of Immunologic Disorders. GN Vyas, DP Sites, G Brecher (eds). New York: Grune & Stratton

Petz LD, Garratty G (1980) Acquired Immune Hemolytic Anemias. New York: Churchill Livingstone

Petz LD, Garratty G (2004) Immune Hemolytic Anemias, 2nd edn. New York: Churchill Livingstone

Petz LD, Swisher SN (1989) Blood transfusion in acquired hemolytic anemias. In: Clinical Practice of Transfusion Medicine. LD Petz, SN Swisher (eds), pp. 549–582. New York: Churchill Livingstone

Pien FD, Smith TF, Taswell HF *et al.* (1974) Cold reactive antibodies in a case of congenital cytomegalo-virus infection. Am J Clin Pathol 61: 352

Polley MJ, Mollison PL, Soothill JF (1962) The role of 19S gamma globulin blood group antibodies in the antiglobulin reaction. Br J Haematol 8: 149

Potter K, Hobby P, Klijn S *et al.* (2002) Evidence for involvement of a hydrophobic patch on framework region 1 of human V4–34-encoded Igs in recognition of the red blood cell I antigen. J Immunol 169: 3777–3782

Prchal JT, Huang ST, Court WS *et al.* (1985) Immune hemolytic anemia following administration of antithymocyte globulin. Am J Haematol 19: 95–98

Pruzanski W, Cowan DH, Parr DM (1974) Clinical and immunochemical studies of IgM cold agglutinins with lambda type light chains. Clin Immunol Immunopathol 2: 234

Pruzanski W, Roelcke D, Donnelly E *et al.* (1986) Persistent cold agglutinins in AIDS and related disorders. Acta Haematol 75: 171–173

Puig N, Carbonell F, Marty ML (1986) Another example of mimicking Anti-Kp^b in a Kp(a+ b–) patient. Vox Sang 51: 57–59

Race RR, Sanger R (1975) Blood Groups in Man, 6th edn. Oxford: Blackwell Scientific Publications

Rand BP, Olson JD, Garratty G (1978) Coombs negative immune hemolytic anemia with anti-E occurring in the red blood cell eluate of an E-negative patient. Transfusion 18: 174

Randazzo P, Streeter B, Nusbacher J *et al.* (1973) A common agglutinin reactive only against bromelin-treated red cells (Abstract). Transfusion 13: 345

Ratkin GA, Osterland CK, Chaplin H Jr (1973) IgG, IgA and IgM cold-reactive immunoglobulin in 19 patients with elevated cold agglutinins. J Lab Clin Med 82: 67

Rausen AR, LeVine R, Hsu RCS *et al.* (1975) Compatible transfusion therapy for paroxysmal cold hemoglobinuria. Pediatrics 55: 275

Reepmaker J (1952) Relation between polyagglutinability of erythrocytes *in vivo* and the Hübener-Thomsen-Friedenreich phenomenon. J Clin Pathol 5: 266

Reid ME, Ellisor SS, Frank BA (1975) Another potential source of error in Rh-hr typing. Transfusion 15: 485

Reid ME, Halverson GR, Lee AH *et al.* (1998) Tr: a new bype of polyagglutination. Transfusion 38: 1005

Reviron M, Janvier D, Reviron J *et al.* (1984) An anti-I cold autoagglutinin enhanced in the presence of sodium azide. Vox Sang 46: 211–216

Reynolds MV, Vengelen-Tyler V, Morel PA (1981) Auto-immune haemolytic anaemia associated with autoanti-Ge. Vox Sang 41: 61–67

Rickard KA, Robinson RJ, Worlledge et al. (1969) Acute acquired haemolytic anaemia associated with polyagglutination. Arch Dis Childh 44: 102

Ries CA, Garratty G, Petz LD et al. (1971) Paroxysmal cold hemoglobinuria: report of a case with an exceptionally high thermal range Donath-Landsteiner antibody. Blood 38: 491

Rittenhouse-Diakun K, Xia Z, Pickhardt D et al. (1998) Development and characterisation of monoclonal antibody to T antigen: (gal beta 1–3GalNAc-alpha-O). Hybridoma 17: 165–173

Ritter K, Kuhlencord A, Thonssen R et al. (1993) Prolonged haemolytic anaemia in malaria and autoantibodies against triosephosphate isomerase. Lancet 342: 1333–1335

Roelcke D (1973) Specificity of IgA cold agglutinins: anti-Prl. Eur J Immunol 3: 206–212

Roelcke D (1989) Cold Agglutinins. Transfus Med Rev 3: 140–166

Roelcke D, Kreft H (1984) Characterisation of various anti Pr cold agglutinins. Transfusion 24: 210–213

Roelcke D, Ebert W, Feizi T (1974) Studies on the specificities of two IgM lambda cold agglutinins. Immunology 27: 879

Roelcke D, Ebert W, Geisen HP (1976) Anti-Pr3: serological and immunochemical identification of a new anti-Pr subspecificity. Vox Sang 30: 122

Roelcke D, Kreft H, Northoff H et al. (1991) Sia-b1 and I antigens recognized by Mycoplasma pneumoniae induced human cold agglutinins. Transfusion 31: 627–630

Roelcke D, Hack H, Kreft H et al. (1993) IgA cold agglutinins recognize Pr and Sa antigens expressed on glycophorins. Transfusion 33: 472–475

Roelcke D, Kreft H, Hack H et al. (1994) Anti-j: human cold agglutinins recognizing linear (i) and branched (I) type 2 chains. Vox Sang 67: 216–221

Rosenfield RE, Jagathambal (1978) Antigenic determinants of C3 and C4 complement components on washed erythrocytes from normal persons. Transfusion 18: 517

Rosenfield RE, Vogel P (1951) The identification of hemagglutinins with red cells altered with trypsin. Trans NY Acad Sci 13: 213

Rosenfield RE, Schmidt PJ, Calvo RC et al. (1965) Anti-i, a frequent cold agglutinin in infectious mononucleosis. Vox Sang 10: 631

Rosenthal MC, Schwartz L (1951) Reversible agglutination of trypsin-treated erythrocytes by normal human sera. Proc Soc Exp Biol (NY) 76: 635

Rosse WF (1968) Fixation of the first component of complement (C'la) by human antibodies. J Clin Invest 47: 2430

Rosse WF, Borsos T, Rapp HJ (1968) Cold-reacting antibodies: the enhancement of antibody fixation by the first component of complement (Cla). J Immunol 100: 259

Rous P, Robertson OH (1918) Free antigen and antibody circulating together in large amounts (hemagglutinin and agglutinogen in the blood of transfused rabbits). J Exp Med 27: 509

Rousey SR, Smith RE (1990) A fatal case of low titer anti-Pr cold agglutinin disease. Am J Hematol 35: 286–287

Roy-Burman A, Glader BE (2002) Resolution of severe Donath-Landsteiner autoimmune hemolytic anemia temporally associated with institution of plasmapheresis. Crit Care Med 30: 931–934

Rubin H, Solomon A (1967) Cold agglutinins of anti-i specificity in alcoholic cirrhosis. Vox Sang 12: 227

Sacher RA, Abbondanzo SL, Miller DK et al. (1989) Clinical and serologic findings of seven patients from one hospital and review of the literature. Am J Clin Pathol 91: 304–309

Salama A, Mueller-Eckhardt C (1985) The role of metabolite specific antibodies in nomifensine-dependent immune hemolytic anemia. N Engl J Med 313: 469–474

Salama A, Mueller-Eckhardt C (1987a) On the mechanisms of sensitization and attachment of antibodies to RBC in drug-induced immune hemolytic anemia. Blood 69: 1006–1010

Salama A, Mueller-Eckhardt C (1987b) Cianidanol and its metabolites bind tightly to red cells and are responsible for the production of auto- and/or drug-dependent antibodies against these cells. Br J Haematol 66: 263–266

Salama A, Mueller-Eckhardt C, Bhakdi S (1985) A two-stage immunoradiometric assay with 125I-staphylococcal protein A for the detection of antibodies and complement on human blood cells. Vox Sang 48: 239–245

Salama A, Gottsche B, Vaidya V et al. (1988) Complement-independent lysis of human red blood cells by cold hemagglutinins. Vox Sang 55: 21–25

Salama A, Berghöfer H, Mueller-Eckhardt C (1992) Red blood cell transfusion in warm-type autoimmune haemolytic anaemia. Lancet 340: 1515–1517

Sangster JM, Kenwright MG, Walker MP et al. (1979) Anti-blood group M autoantibodies with livedo reticularis, Raynaud's phenomenon and anaemia. J Clin Pathol 32: 154–157

Scherer R, Morarescu A, Ruhenstroth-Bauer G (1975) Die spezifische Wirkung der Plasmaproteine bei der Blutkörperchensenkung. Klin Wschr 53: 265

Schreiber AD, Herskovitz BS, Goldwein M (1977) Low-titer cold-hemagglutinin disease. Mechanism of hemolysis and response to corticosteroids. N Engl J Med 296: 1490

Schwarting GA, Kundu SK, Marcus DM (1979) Reaction of antibodies that cause paroxysmal cold hemoglobinuria (PCH) with globoside and Forssman glycosphingolipids. Blood 53: 186–192

Seger R, Joller P, Bird GWG et al. (1980) Necrotising enterocolitis and neuraminidase-producing bacteria. Helv Paediatr Acta 35: 121–128

Seyfried H, Corska B, Maj S *et al.* (1972) Apparent depression of antigens of the Kell blood group system associated with autoimmune acquired haemolytic anaemia. Vox Sang 23: 528

Shanafelt TD, Madueme HL, Wolf RC *et al.* (2003) Rituximab for immune cytopenia in adults: idiopathic thrombocytopenic purpura, autoimmune hemolytica anemia, and Evans syndrome. Mayo Clin Proc 78: 1340–1346

Shirey RS, Smith B, Sensenbrenner L *et al.* (1983) Red cell sensitization due to anti-D in an anti-lymphocyte globulin. Transfusion 23: 396–397

Shirey RS, Boyd JS, Parwani AV *et al.* (2002) Prophylactic antigen-matched donor blood for patients with warm autoantibodies: an algorithm for transfusion management. Transfusion 42: 1435–1441

Shulman WR, Reid PM (1993) Mechanisms of drug-induced immunologically mediated cytopenias. Transfus Med Rev 7: 215–229

Shulman IA, Branch DR, Nelson JM *et al.* (1985) Autoimmune hemolytic anemia with both cold and warm autoantibodies. JAMA 253: 1746–1748

Silberstein LE, Jefferies LC, Goldman J *et al.* (1991) Variable region gene analysis of pathologic human autoantibodies to the related i and I red blood cell antigens. Blood 78: 2372–2386

Sniecinski I, Margolin K, Shulman I *et al.* (1988) High-titer, high-thermal-amplitude cold agglutinin not associated with hemolytic anemia. Vox Sang 55: 26–29

Sokol RJ, Hewit S, Stamps BK (1981) Autoimmune haemolysis: an 18-year study of 865 cases referred to a regional transfusion centre. BMJ i: 2023–2027

Sokol RJ, Hewitt S, Stamps BK (1982) Autoimmune haemolysis associated with Donath–Landsteiner antibodies. Acta Haematol 68: 268–277

Sokol RJ, Hewitt S, Stamps BK (1983) Autoimmune haemolysis: mixed warm and cold type antibody. Acta Haematol 69: 266–274

Sokol RJ, Hewitt S, Stamps BK *et al.* (1984) Autoimmune haemolysis in childhood and adolescence. Acta Haematol 72: 245–257

Sokol RJ, Hewitt S, Booker DJ *et al.* (1987) Small quantities of erythrocyte bound immunoglobulins and autoimmune haemolysis. J Clin Pathol 40: 254–257

Sokol RJ, Booker OJ, Stamps R (1994) Erythrocyte antibodies, autoimmune haemolysis and cancer. J Clin Pathol 47: 340–343

Sondag-Thull P, Levene NA, Levene C *et al.* (1989) Characterisation of a neuraminidase from *Corynebacterium aquaticum* responsible for Th polyagglutination. Vox Sang 57: 193–199

Spaet TH, Ostrom BW (1952) Studies on the normal serum panagglutinin active against trypsinated human erythrocytes. I. The mechanism of agglutination reversal. J Clin Pathol 5: 332

Springer GF, Tegtmeyer H (1981) Origin of anti-Thomsen-Friedenreich (T) and Tn agglutinins in man and in white leghorn chicks. Br J Haematol 47: 453–460

Springer GF, Desai PR, Banatwala I (1974) Blood group MN specific substances and precursors in normal and malignant human breast tissue. Naturwissenschaften 61: 457

Springer GF, Desai PR, Murthy MS *et al.* (1979) Precursors of the blood group MN antigens as human carcinoma-associated antigens. Transfusion 19: 233–249

Springer GF, Desai PR, Fry WA *et al.* (1983) Patients immune response to CA-associated T antigen. In: Cellular Oncology, vol. 1. PJ Moloy, GL Nicolson (eds), pp. 99–130. New York: Praeger

Springer GF, Taylor CR, Howard DR *et al.* (1985) Tn, a carcinoma associated antigen, reacts with anti-Tn of normal human sera. Cancer 55: 561–569

Stats D (1954) Cold hemagglutination and cold hemolysis. The hemolysis produced by shaking cold agglutinated erythrocytes. J Clin Invest 24: 33

Strange CA, Cross J (1981) An anti-A agglutinin active only in the presence of borate. Vox Sang 41: 235–238

Stratton F (1954) Polyagglutinability of red cells. Vox Sang (OS) 4: 58

Stratton F, Renton PH (1958) Practical Blood Grouping, p. 87. Oxford: Blackwell Scientific Publications

Stratton F, Rawlinson VI, Chapman SA *et al.* (1972) Acquired hemolytic anemia associated with IgA anti-e. Transfusion 12: 157

Stratton F, Rawlinson VI, Merry AH *et al.* (1983) Positive direct antiglobulin test in normal individuals. II. Clin Lab Haematol 5: 17–21

Sullivan CM, Kline WE, Rabin BI *et al.* (1987) The first example of auto-anti-Kx. Transfusion 27: 322–324

Sundstedt A, O'Neil E, Nicolson KS *et al.* (2003) Role for IL-10 in suppression mediated by peptide-induced regulatory T cells *in vivo*. J Immunol 170: 1240–1248

Swanson JL, Issitt CH, Mann EW *et al.* (1984) Resolution of red cell compatibility testing problems in patients receiving anti-lymphoblast or anti-thymocyte globulin. Transfusion 24: 141–143

Szalóky A, van der Hart M (1971) An auto-antibody anti-Vel. Vox Sang 20: 376

Szymanski IO, Roberts PL, Rosenfield RE *et al.* (1976) Anti-A autoantibody with severe intravascular hemolysis. N Engl J Med 294: 995

Tanaka H, Okubo Y (1977) Acute acquired hemolytic anemia with T-polyagglutination. Ann Paediatr Jap 23: 49

Tegoli J, Harris JP, Nichols MF *et al.* (1970) Autologous anti-I and anti-M following liver transplant. Transfusion 10: 133

Terness P, Kirschfink M, Navolan D *et al.* (1995) Striking inverse correlation between IgG anti-F(ab')2 and autoantibody production in patients with cold agglutinin. Blood 85: 548–551

Thomsen O (1927) Ein vermehrungsfähiges Agens als Veränderer des isoagglutinatorischen Verhaltens der roten Blutkörperchen, eine bisher unbekannte Quelle der Fehlbestimmung. Z Immun-Forsch 52: 85

Thorpe SJ, Turner CE, Stevenson FK et al. (1998) Human monoclonal antibodies encoded by the V4–34 gene segment show cold agglutinin activity and variable multi-reactivity which correlates with the predicted charge of the heavy chain variable region. Immunology 93: 129–136

Tippett P, Noades J, Sanger R et al. (1960) Further studies of the I antigen and antibody. Vox Sang 5: 107

Tomita A, Radike EL, Parker CJ (1993) Isolation of erythrocyte membrane inhibitor of reactive lysis type II. Identification as glycophorin A. J Immunol 151: 3308–3323

Tonthat H, Rochant H, Henry A et al. (1976) A new case of monoclonal IgA kappa cold agglutinin with anti-Pr_1d specificity in a patient with persistent HB antigen cirrhosis. Vox Sang 30: 464

Topley E, Knight R, Woodruff AW (1973) The direct antiglobulin test and immunoconglutinin titres in patients with malaria. Trans R Soc Trop Med Hyg 67: 51

Tubbs RR, Hoffman GC, Deodhar SD et al. (1976) IgM monoclonal gammography. Histopathologic and clinical spectrum. Cleveland Clin Quart 43: 21

Uchikawa H, Tokyama H (1986) A potent cold autoagglutinin that recognizes type 2H determinant on red cells. Transfusion 26: 240–242

Vainchenker W, Testa U, Deschamps J et al. (1982) Clonal expression of the Tn antigen in erythroid and granulocyte colonies and its application to determination of the clonality of the human megakaryocyte colony assay. J Clin Invest 69: 1081–1091

Vainchenker W, Vinci G, Testa U et al. (1985) Presence of the Tn antigen on hematopoietic progenitors from patients with the Tn syndrome. J Clin Invest 75: 541–546

van't Veer MB, van Wieringen PMV, van Leeuwen I et al. (1981) A negative direct antiglobulin test with strong IgG red cell auto-antibodies present in the serum of a patient with autoimmune haemolytic anaemia. Br J Haematol 49: 393–386

van't Veer MB, van Leeuwen I, Haas FJLM et al. (1984) Red-cell autoantibodies mimicking anti-Fy^b specificity. Vox Sang 47: 88–91

Vengelen-Tyler V, Mogck N (1991) Two cases of 'hr^B-like' autoantibodies appearing as alloantibodies. Transfusion 31: 254–256

Vengelen-Tyler V, Goya K, Mogck W et al. (1983) Autoantibody-hr^B appearing as an alloantibody: report of two cases (Abstract). Transfusion 23: 408

Vengelen-Tyler V, Gonzalez B, Garratty G et al. (1987) Acquired loss of red cell Kell antigens. Br J Haematol 65: 231–234

Viggiano E, Clary NL, Ballas SK (1982) Autoanti-K antibody mimicking an alloantibody. Transfusion 22: 329–332

Vilela RB, Bordin JO, Chiba AK et al. (2002) RBC-associated IgG in patients with visceral leishmaniasis (kala-azar): a prospective analysis. Transfusion 42: 1442–1447

Voak D, Lachmann PJ, Downie DM et al. (1983) Monoclonal antibodies: C3 serology. Biotest Bull 4: 339–347

Vos GH, Petz LD, Fudenberg HH (1970) Specificity of acquired haemolytic anaemia autoantibodies and their serological characteristics. Br J Haematol 19: 57

Vroclans-Deiminas M, Boivin P (1980) Analyse des resultats observés au cours de la recherche d'une auto-sensibilisation anti-erythrocytaire chez 2400 malades. Rev Fr Transfus Immuno-hématol 23: 105–117

Wagner FF, Ladewig B, Flegel WA (2003) The RHCE allele ceRT: D epitope 6 expression does not require D-specific amino acids. Transfusion 43: 1248–54

Wahl CM, Herman JH, Shirey RS et al. (1989) The activation of maternal and cord blood. Transfusion 29: 635–637

Wallhermfechtel MA, Pohl B, Chaplin H (1984) Allo-immunization in patients with warm autoantibodies: a retrospective study employing 3 donor alloabsorptions to aid in antibody detection. Transfusion 24: 482–485

Watson KC, Joubert SM (1960) Haemagglutination of cells treated with antibiotics. Nature (Lond) 188: 505

Weeden AR, Datta N, Mollison PL (1960) Adsorption of bacteria on to red cells leading to positive antiglobulin reactions. Vox Sang 5: 523

Weiner W, Vos GH (1963) Serology of acquired hemolytic anemias. Blood 22: 606

Weiner W, Battey DA, Cleghorn TE et al. (1953) Serological findings in a case of haemolytic anaemia: with some general observations on the pathogenesis of the syndrome. BMJ ii: 125

Weiner W, Tovey GH, Gillespie EM et al. (1956) Albumin auto-agglutinating property in three sera. A pitfall for the unwary. Vox Sang 1: 279

Weiner W, Gordon EG, Rowe D (1964) A Donath-Landsteiner antibody (non-syphilitic type). Vox Sang 9: 684

Wiener AS (1943) Blood Groups and Transfusion, 3rd edn. Springfield, IL: CC Thomas

William RA, Brown EF, Hurst D et al. (1989) Transfusion of infants with activation of erythrocyte T antigen. J Pediatr 115: 949–953

Williams L, Domen RE (1989) Vancomycin-induced red cell aggregation. Transfusion 29: 23–26

Williamson LM, Poole J, Redman C et al. (1994) Transient loss of proteins carrying Kell and Lutheran red cell antigens during consecutive relapses of autoimmune thrombocytopenia. Brit J Haemat 87: 805–812

Wolach B, Heddle N, Barr RD et al. (1981) Transient Donath-Landsteiner haemolytic anaemia. Br J Haematol 48: 425–434

Wolach B, Sadan N, Bird GWG *et al.* (1987) Tx polyagglutination in three members of one family. Acta Haematol 78: 45–47

Wolf MW, Roelcke D (1989) Incomplete warm hemolysins. II. Corresponding antigens and pathogenetic mechanisms in autoimmune hemolytic anemias induced by incomplete warm hemolysins. Clin Immunol Immunopathol 51: 68–76

Woll JE, Smith CM, Nushbacher J (1974) Treatment of acute cold agglutinin hemolytic anemia with transfusion of adult i RBCs. JAMA 229: 1779

Woodruff AW, Topley E, Knight R *et al.* (1972) The anaemia of kala azar. Br J Haematol 22: 319

Worlledge SM (1969) Immune drug-induced haemolytic anaemias. Semin Haematol 6: 181

Worlledge S (1978) Results published in the 6th edition of this book, p. 397

Worlledge SM, Rousso C (1965) Studies on the serology of paroxysmal cold haemoglobinuria (PCH), with special reference to its relationship with the P blood group system. Vox Sang 10: 293

Worlledge SM, Carstairs KC, Dacie JV (1966) Autoimmune haemolytic anaemia associated with α-methyldopa therapy. Lancet ii: 135

Worlledge SM, Dacie JV (1969) Haemolytic and other anaemias in infectious mononucleosis, In Infectious Mononucleosis, eds RL Carter and HG Penman. Blackwell Scientific Publications, Oxford

Yasuda H, Ohto H, Motoki R *et al.* (1997) An EDTA-associated anti-B agglutinin: the role of ionised calcium. Transfusion 37: 1131–1136

Young NS, Abkowitz JL, Luzzatto L (2000) New insights into the pathophysiology of acquired cytopenias. Hematology (Am Soc Hematol Educ Program) 18–38

Young PP, Uzieblo A, Trulock E *et al.* (2004) Autoantibody formation after alloimmunisation: are blood transfusions a risk factor for autoimmune hemolytic anemia? Transfusion 44: 67–72

Zupanska B, Thomson EE, Merry AH (1986) Fc receptors for IgG1 and IgG3 on human mononuclear cells: an evaluation with known levels of erythrocyte-bound IgG. Vox Sang 50: 97–103

8 Blood grouping techniques

For the identification of red cell antibodies the reaction between red cell antigens and corresponding antibodies is usually detected by a method based on the agglutination test. In the traditional agglutination test, red cells suspended in a fluid medium are mixed with serum or plasma and incubated. The red cells are allowed to sediment or are centrifuged and then examined for agglutination. If no agglutinates are observed, the cells may be washed, mixed with antiglobulin reagent, centrifuged and re-examined for agglutination. Antiglobulin reagent is usually a mixture of antibody reactive with the Fc portion of IgG and antibody reactive with C3d, a complement component that becomes cell bound when activation of the complement system by antibody occurs (see Chapter 3). The sensitivity of agglutination tests is increased in various ways,

for example by using special media such as low-ionic-strength solutions (LISS), polyethylene glycol solutions (PEG) or by treating red cells with proteolytic enzymes.

Nowadays antibody detection is frequently carried out using the gel test (Fig. 8.1). In this case the antibody-containing serum is mixed with red cells, incubated on top of a dextran gel containing antiglobulin reagent and then centrifuged. Unagglutinated red cells pass through the gel whereas agglutinated cells are retained.

The most reliable results for the detection and identification of red cell antibodies are obtained by using a combination of tests. The particular combination of tests adopted in specialist blood group reference laboratories depends on such factors as the nature of the problems to be solved, including the urgency

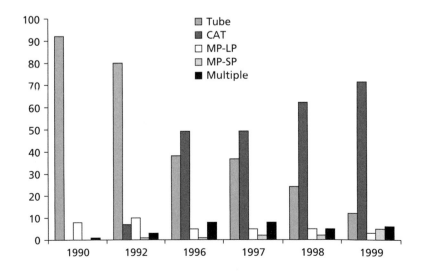

Fig 8.1 Trends in indirect antiglobulin test (IAT) technology used for antibody screening in the UK (y axis % participants). From Knowles *et al.* (2002). MP-LP, microplate (liquid phase); MP-SP microplate (solid phase); CAT (gel/column).

with which a result is needed, the technical expertise of the staff available and financial restraints.

In identifying red cell antigens, the test used depends on the characteristics of the antibodies available. The simplest technique is agglutination in saline, and this test can almost always be used when the relevant antibody is IgM. When the antibody is IgG it will usually be necessary to use some slightly more complicated procedure (commonly, addition of antiglobulin reagent or pre-treatment of red cells with proteolytic enzymes). A solid-phase system can also be used. In this case antibody is bound to a surface and the adherence of red cells (carrying the antigen) measured. The gel test can also be used for red cell antigen typing and involves incubating the antibody with red cells on top of a dextran gel and then distinguishing agglutinated red cells from unagglutinated cells by centrifugation.

Gel test and solid-phase methods are increasingly used in routine blood banking in preference to traditional agglutination methods because they are easier to perform and less dependent on the technical competence of the individuals performing the test. Monoclonal antibodies (see Chapter 3) have largely replaced polyclonal antibodies as reagents for routine blood grouping procedures based on agglutination.

The reaction between red cell antigens and antibodies may be detected in various other ways: for example, the antibody may be labelled with a radioisotope such as ^{125}I and the amount of ^{125}I bound to the cells measured. The antibody may be coupled to an enzyme and the binding of antibody to red cells measured by the amount of colour released from a suitable substrate, as in the enzyme-linked immunosorbent assay (ELISA). The antibody may be coupled to a fluorescent dye and the binding of antibody to red cells measured by its bound fluorescence using flow cytometry. When an antibody to a blood group antigen is labelled in one of these ways the test can be used to quantify the number of antigen sites per red cell in the sample examined or to compare the amount of antigen expression on red cells from different samples. However, it is more usual to label an anti-IgG preparation with radio-iodine, enzyme or fluorescein and to use this reagent for quantification of antigen sites or blood group antibody molecules bound, as in this case only one labelled antibody preparation is required to quantify the binding of many blood group antibodies.

The object of most blood grouping and antibody detection tests in clinical work is to provide completely compatible red cells for transfusion; the only question to be answered is: is a particular antigen or antibody absent or present? Quantitative tests are needed in assessing the significance of antibodies found in women in connection with pregnancy.

Blood typing can also be carried out using methods based on detection of the DNA sequence encoding blood group antigens rather than agglutination. These methods are particularly useful for determination of the blood group of a fetus at risk from haemolytic disease or neonatal anemia (see p. 503). Molecular methods can also be used to find antigen-matched donor red cells for patients with complex mixtures of antibodies when the typing reagents to the less common antigens, which are needed to screen for compatible blood by agglutination methods, are in short supply (see p. 336).

Quantitative differences between red cells from different donors

Homozygotes and heterozygotes

With respect to some red cell antigens, significant differences in reactivity are found between the cells of homozygotes and heterozygotes. Some examples are as follows: C, c, M, S K and Jk^a. This is an important consideration when selecting red cells for use in screening sera for the presence of blood group antibodies, as clinically significant antibodies may be missed when cells heterozygous for important antigens like K and Jk^a are used (Phillips and Voak 1996). In 1997, 95.5% of participants in the UK National External Quality Assessment Scheme were selecting screening cells that had homozygous expression of antigens (Knowles *et al.* 2002).

Differences between donors of the same phenotype

The reactivity of red cells from different individuals of the same phenotype is particularly variable with regard to the following antigens: P_1, I, i, Le^a, Le^b, Sd^a, Vel and Ch/Rg. This property is a useful aid to the identification of antibodies of these specificities.

Differences between newborn infants and adults

For details, see Chapter 3.

Effect of storage on red cell antigens

Storage above 0°C

When red cells were stored at 4°C either as whole blood mixed with CPDA-1 or -2, or with saline–adenine–glucose (SAG) additive for up to 35 or 42 days, respectively, very little loss of activity of red cell antigens other than M and P_1 was observed (Snyder et al. 1983; Myhre et al. 1984). Gradual loss of expression of the complement regulatory proteins DAF (Cromer blood group protein) and CD59 from stored packed red cells was observed over a period of 6 weeks by Long and co-workers (1993). Red cell microvesicles derived from outdated units of red cells have A, B, D, M, N, Ss and Fy^a activity as determined by adsorption studies (Oreskovic et al. 1992).

Red cells stored as clotted blood lose their antigenic activity more rapidly than when stored with citrate anticoagulant (Rosenfield et al. 1971). When blood is collected into plastic bags, if the donor line is not emptied immediately after collection and then refilled with blood mixed with anticoagulant, the clotted blood in the tubing is an unreliable source of red cells for compatibility tests (Jørgensen 1964). Furthermore, red cells stored as clotted blood may give false-positive reactions in the antiglobulin test owing to uptake of complement components during storage at 4°C.

Reagent red cells may be stored as whole blood with citrate–phosphate–dextrose (CPD) or acid–citrate–dextrose (ACD) but more usually they are stored as washed cells in a preservative solution. A modified Alsever's solution, with added inosine (with or without adenine) and with antibiotics is commonly used, permitting satisfactory storage for at least 35 days at 4°C.

Before being suspended in preservative solution, red cells should be freed, as far as possible, from leucocytes. Leucocytes contain proteolytic enzymes that, in the absence of plasma inhibitors, may cause lysis of red cells (Högman et al. 1978). In red cell suspensions stored in LISS in the presence of neomycin, proteolytic enzymes from leucocytes may damage red cell antigens. The damage occurs only when leucocytes are present in combination with LISS and neomycin (Malyska et al. 1983). The exact mechanism responsible for the damage is not known, but aminoglycoside antibiotics may promote the release of proteolytic enzymes from leucocytes. Damage to antigens was found to be much more serious with aminoglycoside antibiotics, such as neomycin, than with others (Allan et al. 1990). Red cells stored in LISS to which amphotericin B has been added are lysed rapidly, probably due to an increased susceptibility of red cells in LISS for sodium deoxycholate present in the amphotericin solution. However, frozen-thawed red cells can be stored safely for 21 days at 4°C in a LISS solution that does not contain either aminoglycoside antibiotics or amphotericin B (Allan et al. 1990). The following solution is recommended: glycine, 13.7 g; glucose, 8.5 g; NaCl, 1.9 g; Na_2HPO_4, 0.21 g; $NaH_2PO_4.2H_2O$, 0.23 g; adenine, 0.2 g; inosine, 0.4 g; chloramphenicol, 0.34 g and water to 1 l.

Frozen storage

When red cells were stored at −20°C in a citrate–phosphate–glycerol solution (see Appendix 12) for 1 year the only antigen found to react more weakly was P_1 (Crawford et al. 1954). After thawing the frozen cells, glycerol must be removed before the cells can be tested; removal is most conveniently carried out by washing; see Appendix 12.

Unfortunately, when red cells are stored at −20°C there may be extensive haemolysis, possibly dependent on the time for which the red cells were stored before freezing.

For storage for indefinite periods red cells must be kept at −80°C or lower. One very convenient method is known as 'glycigel'. Tubes containing a glycerol solution mixed with gelatin are kept available in the refrigerator. When red cells for storage are added to one of these tubes and the tube is warmed, the glycerol is released slowly as the gelatin melts and cell damage is minimized. The red cells are stored at −80°C or lower and, when wanted, are thawed and washed free from glycerol (Huggins et al. 1982; see also Appendix 11).

A very simple method for preparing red cells for frozen storage is to add dextrose or sucrose to them and then add the mixture dropwise from a syringe into liquid nitrogen (Meryman, 1956). Another method that has proved very satisfactory is the one described by Bronson and McGinniss (1962). Blood mixed with an equal volume of Alsever's solution is mixed with one-tenth of its volume of 50% glucose; a metal screen is dipped into the mixture, which is then frozen by immersion in liquid nitrogen. After storage in nitrogen vapour, the blood is thawed by placing the screen in a tube containing 5% glucose in saline at 40°C. The cells are then washed. In washing red cells that have been frozen in this way, better results are obtained if the thawed cells are first washed in a hypertonic solution (Burnie 1965). An alternative excellent method for reagent red cells utilizes polyvinyl pyrrolidone (PVP). PVP (molecular weight 44 000) is prepared as a 30% solution (w/v) in water, autoclaved, mixed well and stored in aliquots. Three volumes of PVP solution are added to 10 volumes of anticoagulated blood (or 45% suspension of red cells in PBS, pH7.4). The mixture is then added, dropwise, to liquid nitrogen. The frozen beads obtained are stored in a pre-chilled container in nitrogen vapour. To recover the cells, drop the beads into warm phosphate-buffered saline (PBS) pH 7.4 (approximately 2 ml of PBS per bead), centrifuge and wash three times with PBS (G Inglis, personal communication).

Freeze–thaw damage to red cells can be reduced using ice-binding proteins found in Antarctic sea ice diatoms (Kang and Raymond 2004).

Lyophilized red cells

The disaccharide trehalose functions to reduce dehydration in plants and animals living in desert habitats and can be used to reduce osmotic damage in stored red cells. Trehalose has been used for stabilization of dried red cell-coated microplates and may ultimately facilitate storage of red cells by lyophilization (Thorpe et al. 2002; Satpathy et al. 2004).

When whole units of blood are needed to provide cell panels, any method for the frozen storage of blood for transfusion is suitable (see Chapter 9).

Factors affecting red cell–antibody interactions

Serum vs. plasma

For antibody detection, plasma has the theoretical disadvantage, compared with serum, of containing anticoagulants that inhibit complement activation and therefore possibly interfere with the detection of some complement-activating antibodies. On the other hand, plasma is more convenient and is widely used in automated systems of grouping and antibody screening. A comparison of plasma and serum for antibody detection using the gel system has been reported (Scott et al. 1996).

Storage of sera

If there is no microbial contamination, at 4°C blood grouping sera retain their potency for 1–2 years; when stored at –20°C or less, they retain their potency for very many years.

The use of sodium azide is potentially hazardous. When solutions containing azide are discharged to waste via metal pipes, heavy metal azides, notably of copper or lead, are formed, which are readily detonated, explosive compounds. Copper azide is particularly sensitive to mechanical shock. Despite these potential hazards, sodium azide is still added to most commercial blood grouping reagents. Antibiotics such as those used in red cell suspensions may be used as a substitute for azide but corresponding antibodies are sometimes present in human sera (see Chapter 7) and then produce anomalous results.

Colouring agents

Dyes are frequently added to anti-A and anti-B reagents; usually blue is added to anti-A and yellow to anti-B; Patent blue V (E131) and Ariavit tartrazine (E102) in concentrations of 0.08 g/l are suitable. Although colour is convenient in identifying reagents, it must not be relied on, i.e. the reagent should be identified by reading the label, and the use of controls remains essential. A green dye is added to some polyspecific antiglobulin reagents.

Deterioration of complement on storage

When serum with an optimal concentration of complement is required it should be separated from red cells as soon as possible (Fischer et al. 1958). On storage of serum at 4°C there is just-detectable deterioration of complement after 24 h and readily detectable deterioration at 1 week (Polley and Mollison 1961).

Garratty (1970) found that over 60% of normal complement activity was required to avoid the risk of missing weak complement-binding antibodies. In a study of normal sera this level of activity was retained for less than 1 day at 37°C, for 1 day at room temperature, for 2 weeks at 4°C, for 2 months at –20°C and for at least 3 months at –55°C or below (see also Polley and Mollison 1961). Complement deteriorates far less rapidly in the plasma of ACD stored blood than in serum, possibly due to the diminished levels of Ca^{2+}

and Mg^{2+}; after three weeks at 4°C the average loss of haemolytic activity is only 9%. If ACD plasma is used as a source of complement, it must be recalcified (Reich *et al.* 1970).

Potentiators

The effect of colloids in potentiating agglutination is discussed in Chapter 3.

The colloid most widely used until recently in manual tests is bovine serum albumin (BSA), which is used in a concentration of 10–20% to enhance agglutination in reagents containing (IgG) antibodies and other potentiators, and in a concentration of 3–8% to enhance agglutination by reagents containing IgM antibodies or reduced and alkylated IgG antibodies. In 'normal' preparations of BSA, 5–10% of the protein is in the form of dimers or oligomers; the percentage may be increased to as high as 50% to produce 'polymerized albumin'. The potentiating effect is greatest with preparations containing the largest percentages of dimers and oligomers (Jones *et al.* 1969; Reckel and Harris 1978: ICSH 1982). With the advent of monoclonal antibodies as reagents, the use of albumin has diminished.

Polyethylene glycol (PEG) is used as a potentiator in the antiglobulin test (see below), but other substances, such as dextran and PVP, are no longer used in manual tests.

Proteolytic enzymes

As discussed in Chapter 3, treatment of red cells with certain enzymes renders them agglutinable by otherwise non-agglutinating antibodies.

The discovery that enzyme-treated RhD-positive red cells suspended in saline are agglutinated by otherwise non-agglutinating anti-Rh D was made by chance. In 1946, MM Pickles (personal communication) was trying to find out whether there was any connection between T-activated red cells and antibody-coated cells, such as those found in haemolytic disease of the newborn. D-positive and D-negative red cells were included with the various controls that were used. *Cholera vibrio*-treated D-positive red cells but not D-negative red cells were agglutinated by diluted incomplete anti-D (Pickles 1946). It was discovered soon afterwards that trypsin gave results similar to those with *C. vibrio* filtrate (Morton and Pickles 1947).

Several proteolytic enzymes are used in blood grouping tests: trypsin and chymotrypsin, which have a very restricted specificity, and bromelin, ficin and papain, which have a broad specificity for peptide bonds. Trypsin cleaves peptides that are C-terminal to lysine and arginine, whereas chymotrypsin catalyses cleavage primarily after the C-terminal of phenylalanine and tryptophan. Bromelin, ficin and papain are all thiol proteases with a cysteine residue at the active site, which must be in its reduced form for activation of the enzyme. Thiol proteases are readily inactivated under normal storage conditions as a result of oxidation of the thiol group of the cysteine or by binding of traces of heavy metal ions to the thiol group. Optimal activation of thiol proteases occurs on simultaneous addition of a thiol reducing agent, such as cysteine, and a heavy metal chelating agent such as EDTA (Kimmel and Smith 1954). Reducing agents have a greater effect on activity than do chelating agents (Scott *et al.* 1994).

Traditionally, in blood group serology, papain has been used in its activated form (for example Low's formulation containing cysteine and sometimes EDTA), whereas bromelin and ficin have been used inactivated. The activity of bromelin and ficin can be greatly increased by the addition of sulphydryl reducing agents (Scott *et al.* 1994).

Enzyme preparations should be standardized either by using azoalbumin as a substrate (Lambert *et al.* 1978; Scott and Whitton 1988), or by comparison with a standard enzyme preparation, using a standard blood grouping reagent. A lyophilized preparation of papain at 0.6 azoalbumin units and a lyophilized reference anti-D have been prepared by the International Society of Blood Transfusion (ISBT)/International Committee on Standardization in Haematology (ICSH) Working Party on Enzymes (Scott *et al.* 1994). In practice, enzyme preparations are frequently assessed for potency by subjective serological tests.

Effect of enzymes on particular red cell antigens

In the detection of Rh antibodies, tests with enzyme-treated red cells are extremely sensitive. Giles (1960) found that additional Rh antibodies were often revealed by tests with ficin-treated red cells: for example, 'pure' anti-D might be found to contain anti-C or anti-E, 'pure' anti-C to contain anti-e and 'pure' anti-E to contain anti-c.

The reactions of anti-P_1 and of Lewis and Kidd antibodies are stronger with enzyme-treated than with untreated red cells and Lewis and Kidd antibodies may lyse enzyme-treated red cells when they will not lyse untreated cells. Other antibodies that react more strongly with enzyme-treated than with untreated cells include anti-I and -i and the antibodies of the Colton and Dombrock systems.

Antigens inactivated or weakened by treatment with certain proteolytic enzymes include Fy^a, Fy^b, M, N, S, s, Yt^a, Xg^a, Ge, Ch, Rg, JMH, In^b, Knops system antigens, Cromer system antigens, Tn and Pr (Table 8.1). Crude preparations of bromelin, ficin and papain are mixtures of many proteolytic enzymes and these three enzyme preparations weaken most of the above antigens. On the other hand, crystalline trypsin and chymotrypsin have more selective effects: S, s and Fy^a are destroyed by chymotrypsin but not by trypsin, and K is only destroyed when both enzymes are used together; some antigens, for example M, N and Lu^a, are destroyed by either enzyme (Judson and Anstee 1977).

Lu^a and Lu^b were found to be unaffected by treatment with ficin or papain by G Garratty (personal communication), although variable effects were found by Poole and Giles (1982).

The low-frequency antigens of the MNSs system can be classified according to their sensitivity to trypsin treatment. The trypsin-sensitive determinants are located on glycophorin A, carrying MN determinants, whereas the trypsin-insensitive determinants are probably located on glycophorin B, carrying Ss determinants, although they may be located on glycophorin A close to the red cell membrane (Giles 1982).

The reactions of anti-Yt^a are not diminished by trypsin treatment of red cells but, in one series, six of six examples failed to react with cells treated with bromelin, chymotrypsin, ficin or papain (Rouger *et al.* 1982) and in another series, 8 out of 14 examples of anti-Yt^a failed to react with cells treated with ficin or papain (Vengelen-Tyler and Morel 1979).

The determinants Pr, Tn and T are weakened by treatment with proteolytic enzymes but are not inactivated. Some activity persists because the determinants occur not only on glycophorins A, C and D, which are split off the red cell membrane by most proteolytic enzymes, but are also carried on glycophorin B, which is not affected by treatment with most proteolytic enzymes (the exception being chymotrypsin).

In some cases, the antigens are damaged only by relatively high concentrations of enzyme. For example, in one investigation destruction of s was not observed until chymotrypsin levels of 132 units/ml were used and even at this level the receptor detected by one

example of anti-S was unaffected (Judson and Anstee 1977). Similarly, although T is not destroyed by concentrations of papain normally used in blood grouping tests (Bird *et al.* 1971) it is destroyed by 3–4% ficin or papain (Issitt *et al.* 1972).

Stability of enzymes on storage

Cysteine-activated papain stored at 4°C as a liquid at pH 5.4 loses about 50% of enzyme activity within 2 weeks; most of this loss is due to instability of the activator (ML Scott and PK Phillips, personal communication). Preparations that have not been cysteine activated are relatively stable during storage at 4°C (Stapleton and Moore 1959). Because of the instability of activated enzyme preparations, which may be the cause of false-positive or false-negative results (Holburn and Prior 1987), many users prepare their own enzyme solutions and store them at −20°C, at which temperature they may be kept for 6 months.

Liquid enzyme preparations can be stabilized in a form suitable for distribution by reversible inhibition of the enzyme by heavy metal ions; activated enzyme is recovered by the addition of a separately provided activator (ML Scott and PK Phillips, personal communication). As an activator, cysteine is unsuitable because of its instability; dithiothreitol (DTT) and glutathione are both stable on storage at 4°C but, as DTT added to activated papain destroys Kell antigens (Branch and Petz 1982), glutathione is preferred.

Low ionic strength

As described in Chapter 3, the rate of association of antibody with antigen is very greatly increased by lowering ionic strength. The advantages of using a low-ionic-strength medium are seen chiefly in tests with IgG antibodies (see section on antiglobulin tests, below). Nevertheless, it is a fairly common practice to use a low-ionic-strength medium instead of saline for the suspension of red cells. Most workers have found that with anti-A and anti-B results are similar with low-ionic-strength medium and with saline (Elliot *et al.* 1964; Löw and Messeter 1974; Moore and Mollison 1976). The reactivity of some cold alloagglutinins is enhanced in a low-ionic-strength medium so that their thermal range becomes wider, for example anti-A_1 and anti-P_1 (seventh edition, p. 519); others, for example two examples of anti-Pr_1 are detectable

Table 8.1 Effect of various proteases, sialidase and AET on high-frequency red cell antigens.

Antigen	Treatment							Antigen	Treatment						
	Tryp[1]	Chym[2]	T/C[3]	Pap[4]	Pro[5]	Sla[7]	AET[7]		Tryp	Chym	T/C	Pap	Pro	Sla	AET
MNS5 (U)	+*	+	+	+	+	+	+	H1 (H)	+	+	+	+	+	+	+
EnªTS	O†	+	O	O	O	+/O‡	+	XK1 (Kx)	+	+	+	+	+	+	+
EnªFS	+	+	+	O	O	+	+	GE2	O	w	O	O	O	+/O	+
EnªFR	+	+	+	+	+	+	+	GE3	O	+	O	+	O	+	+
RH17	+	+	+	+	+	+	+	GE4	O	+	O	O	O	O	+
RH29	+	+	+	+	+	+	+	CROMER1 (Crª)	+	O	O	+	+	+	w
LU2 (Luᵇ)	O	O	O	+	+	+	O	CROMER2 (Tcª)	+	O	O	+	+	+	w
LU3	O	O	O	+	+	+	O	CROMER5 (Drª)	+	O	O	+	+	+	w
LU4	O	O	O	+	+	+	O	CROMER6 (Esª)	+	O	O	+	+	+	w
LU5	O	O	O	+	+	+	O	CROMER7 (IFC)	+	O	O	+	+	+	w
LU6	O	O	O	I	+	+	O	CROMER9 (WESᵇ)	+	O	O	+	O	+	w
LU8	O	O	O	O	O	+	O	CROMER10 (UMC)	+	O	O	+	+	+	w
LU12	O	O	O	+	+	+	O	IN2 (Inᵇ)	O	O	O	O	O	+	O
LU13	O	O	O	+	+	+	O	COST1 (Csª)	+	+	+	+	+	+	+
LU17	O	O	O	+	+/O	+	O	COST3 (Ykª)	O	O	O	+	+	O	O
KEL2 (k)	+	w§	O	+	+	+	O	COST4 (Knª)	O	O	O	+	+	I	O
KEL4 (Kpᵇ)	+	w	O	+	+	+	O	COST6 (McCª)	O	O	O	+/O	w	+	O
KEL5 (Ku)	+	w	w	+	+	+	O	GY1 (Gyª)	w	+	w	+	w	+	w
KEL7 (Jsᵇ)	+	w	w	+	+	+	O	GY2 (IIy)	+	+	w	+	+	+	w
KEL11	+	w	O	+	+	+	O	I1 (I)	I	+	I	+	+	+	+
KEL12	+	w	w	+	+	+	O	I2 (I)	+	+	+	+	+	+	I
KEL13	+	w	w	+	+	+	O	ER1 (Erª)	+	+	+	+	+	+	+
KEL14	I	w	O	+	+	+	O	GLOBO1 (P)	+	+	+	+	+	+	+
KEL18	+	w	O	+	+	+	O	GLOBO3 (LKE)	+	+	+	+	+	+	+
KEL19	+	O	O	+	+	+	O	WR2 (Wrᵇ)	+	+	+	+	I	+	+
KEL22	+	w	O	+	+	+	O	Vel	+	+	+	+	+	+	+
FY3	+	+	+	+	+	+	+	Lan	+	+	+	I	+	+	+
FY6	+	O	O	O	O	+	+	Atª	+	+	+	+	+	+	+
JK3	+	+	+	+	+	+	+	Jrª	+	+	+	+	+	+	+
D12 (Diᵇ)	+	+	+	+	+	+	+	Oka	+	+	+	+	+	+	+
YT1 (Ytª)	+	O	O	O	O	+	O	JMH	O	O	O	O	+/O	+	O
SC1	+	+	+/O	+	+/O	+	+	Emm	+	+	+	+	+	+	+
CO1 (Coª)	+	+	+	+	+	+	+	AnWj	+	+	+	+	+	+	+
CO3	+	+	+	+	+	+	+	MB-2D10	+	w	w	+	O	+	+
LW5 (LWª)	+	w	+	+	O	+	O								
LW6 (Lwaᵇ)	+	w	w	+	O	+	O								
Ch	O	O	O	O	O	+	+								
Rg	O	O	O	O	O	+	+								

From Daniels G (1992) Immunohematology 9: 3.

* Antibodies positive with treated red cells.

† Antibodies negative with treated red cells.

‡ Antibodies with same specificity–different results.

§ Strong antibodies react; weaker antibodies do not.

[1] Trypsin.

[2] Chymotrypsin.

[3] Trypsin/chymotrypsin.

[4] Papain.

[5] Pronase.

[6] Sialidase.

[7] Aminoethylisothiouronium bromide.

only in a low-ionic-strength medium (O'Neill *et al.* 1986). The enhanced activity of cold alloagglutinins may complicate blood grouping and pre-transfusion testing if low-ionic-strength techniques are used in direct agglutination.

Confusion is caused by using the term 'low ionic strength' to describe a variety of solutions supplied with reagent kits. These may be used under the impression that their composition is identical with some of the earlier described solutions (e.g. Moore and Mollison 1976), although in fact, they may have a higher tonicity.

Polycations

Protamine and polybrene cause red cells to aggregate. The resulting very close contact allows crosslinking of red cells by IgG antibodies. Non-specific aggregation can be dispersed by the addition of a suitable agent and then only specific agglutinates remain. Manual tests in which a low-ionic-strength medium is used together with protamine have proved very sensitive in detecting alloantibodies. If no agglutination occurs the cells can be washed and antiglobulin serum added as a further step (Rosenfield *et al.* 1979; Lalezari and Jiang 1980). Details of a manual polybrene test (MPT) are given later.

Monoclonal vs. polyclonal antibodies

Monoclonal antibodies have several advantages over polyclonal antibodies: (1) they provide an unlimited supply of identical material; (2) they are free from unwanted contaminating antibodies, for example HLA antibodies or antibodies to low-frequency antigens, so that testing and quality control are far simpler; (3) they are free from naturally occurring antibodies such as anti-T so that they do not give false-positive results, for example with T-transformed red cells; (4) they are free from viruses of hepatitis and of HIV; and (5) their use avoids the need to immunize and plasmapherese human donors.

Murine monoclonal antibodies have at least two disadvantages: first, as their specificities may apparently vary at different concentrations, tests employing them must be very carefully standardized (MacDonald and Gerns 1986); second, they may give unexpected reactions, for example some potent monoclonal anti-A react weakly with some B cells and some potent anti-B react with A_1 cells (see Chapter 4). Other possible

disadvantages of monoclonal antibodies are mentioned in Chapter 3.

Antibodies of only certain specificities can be produced in mice. Some excellent human monoclonals have been produced (see Chapters 3, 4, 5 and 6). Monoclonal antibodies can be converted from IgG to IgM using recombinant DNA technology in order to make them more suitable for use as blood typing reagents. Lee and co-workers (2004) describe the production and use of humanized chimeric IgM monoclonal anti-Fy^a and anti-Js^b. Dimeric Fab of anti-N and anti-M specificities have been produced using recombinant techniques and expression in *Escherichia coli*. These dimeric Fabs had similar agglutinating properties to the corresponding bivalent IgG antibodies (Czerwinski *et al.* 2002). (Polyclonal anti-M and anti-N are usually of the IgG class and are direct agglutinins because the M, N antigens are located at the amino terminus of glycophorin A, some distance from the lipid bilayer, enabling IgG to bridge two red cells in suspension; see Chapter 3.)

Reduced and alkylated IgG antibodies

As described in Chapter 3, after mild chemical reduction and alkylation IgG3 incomplete antibodies will agglutinate red cells suspended in saline. Agglutination is greatly enhanced by adding polymerized BSA to a final concentration of 6–8%. Reagents containing reduced anti-D have been superseded by monoclonal IgM anti-D.

Agglutination tests

In the agglutination reaction two separate processes may be recognized: first, the uptake of antibody onto the red cells and second, the adherence to one another of the antibody-coated cells. In agglutination tests, the red cells may be allowed to come into contact with one another by sedimentation or the process may be accelerated by the use of centrifugation.

Tests with untreated red cells in saline

Need to wash red cells

For traditional serological tests, red cells should be washed free of their own plasma. If this is not done, clots will form when the red cells (contaminated with fibrinogen) are mixed with serum, which contains residual thrombin. Other reasons for washing red cells are as follows: (1) plasma tends to cause rouleaux formation, which interferes with the interpretation of agglutination tests; (2) plasma contains anticoagulants that are anti-complementary and may thus interfere with the detection of complement-binding antibodies; (3) various substances added to red cell suspensions, for example lactose or neomycin, are occasionally responsible for agglutination when corresponding antibodies are present in the patient's plasma (see Chapter 7); most of the antibodies concerned do not react with red cells washed in saline; (4) ABO, Lewis, Chido/Rodgers and Ii antigens are present in the plasma and may inhibit the corresponding antibody in the test serum; and (5) plasma may contain so-called albumin autoagglutinins which used to cause false-positive reactions when whole blood was added to a serum albumin mixture (see p. 272).

Optimal period of incubation

The optimal period is determined first by the rate of combination of antibody with red cells and, second, by the time taken for antibody-coated cells to come into contact with one another. Factors affecting the uptake of antibody, namely the ratio of serum to cells, the period of incubation, temperature and the tonicity of the medium, are discussed in Chapter 3. Contact between antibody-coated cells occurs relatively slowly if the red cells are simply left to sediment in a column, for example in a test tube. Alternatively, the cell suspension can be centrifuged.

Tests in tubes

Tubes in racks can easily be placed in a waterbath (at 37°C), incubator or heat block. The period of incubation is usually 45 min. The red cells can be allowed to sediment or the tubes can be centrifuged. The tube is then tapped and rolled to resuspend the cells. If no agglutinates are seen with the naked eye the tube can be examined with a hand lens, over a magnifying mirror or under a low-power microscope.

Microplates (microtitre plates)

Microplates are clear plastic plates containing, as a rule, 96 wells (8 × 12). With V-shaped wells, very weak cell suspensions (0.03%) can be used, but with U-shaped wells, 1–2% suspensions are optimal. One small volume (e.g. 20 µl) of serum is added to an equal volume of red cell suspension. The plates are centrifuged. As a rule, U wells are agitated and read in a conventional way. V wells are tilted at 75°C to the horizontal for 10 min. Unagglutinated cells stream down the side of the well as a smooth thin line; agglutinated cells remain as a button. The use of microplates has several advantages: the method is very much more sensitive than that of other agglutination systems, primarily because very weak cell suspensions can be used; very small amounts of reagents are needed; titrations are easier with multi-channel pipettes and grades of reactions can be compared. A problem with microplates is that some antibody reagents cannot be used undiluted because their high viscosity causes red cells to adhere to the side of the wells. This problem arises particularly when potentiated anti-D reagents and, to a lesser extent, when anti-A and anti-B reagents are used. The problem can be overcome by diluting the reagents with saline. Some monoclonal antibodies adhere to the plastic solid phase and a positive reaction is seen as a monolayer of cells, whereas a negative reaction is seen as a button or stream. A semi-automated system is mentioned in a later section. For a review of the use of microplates, see Blood Transfusion Task Force (1991).

Slide tests

Slide tests should be used only if equipment for other tests is not available. As water evaporates rapidly from the large surface area, slide tests must be read within 5 min or so; in practice, reagents that produce strong agglutination within 1–2 min are normally used and the tests are employed simply for rapid determination of ABO and RhD groups. As the results are read macroscopically, strong cell suspensions (20% or more) should be used to facilitate the detection of agglutination.

Tests in capillary tubes

A method of Rh grouping in capillary tubes was described by Chown (1944) and Chown and Lewis (1946; 1951). Two important advantages of the method are that each test required only 5 µl of serum and that results can be read in 15 min. For a review of the many applications of capillary tube tests, see Crawford (1987).

Methods using proteolytic enzymes

One- vs. two-stage methods

One-stage methods. In a method described by Löw (1955), enzyme (cysteine-activated papain), serum and cells are mixed together, thus allowing enzyme treatment of the cells and the reaction of antigen and antibody to occur simultaneously. Evidently, in such a method an opportunity is provided for the cleavage of Ig molecules by the enzyme. The proteolytic effect of the enzyme is diminished by protease inhibitors in serum (Travis and Salvesen 1983) but such inhibitors also reduce the effect of enzyme on the red cells. *Although one-stage methods are sufficiently sensitive to give reliable results with potent blood grouping reagents, they are unsuitable for antibody detection or determination of specificity with manual techniques.*

Two-stage method. In this method, washed red cells are first treated with an enzyme, then washed again and incubated with serum. The method has two substantial advantages over a one-stage method: first, no opportunity is provided for degradation of Ig by enzyme; second, enzyme treatment and red cell–antibody interaction can each be carried out at its optimal pH. For papain and bromelin treatment of red cells, the optimal pH is 5.4–5.8, as determined by serological results in a two-stage technique (Scott *et al.* 1987). The optimal pH for binding of anti-D to red cells is 6.5–8.0 (Hughes-Jones *et al.* 1964a), although the optimum for antibodies of other specificities may be different.

A two-stage papain technique in which washing of the cells after papain treatment is replaced by the addition of a specific papain inhibitor, E-64, has been described by Scott and Phillips (1987). This technique permits optimal enzyme treatment of the red cells while avoiding digestion of immunoglobulins following the addition of serum. It thus combines the sensitivity of two-stage tests with the convenience of one-stage tests. The inhibitor E-64 can also be used for bromelin (Ogasawara and Mazda 1989).

In automated blood grouping machines, red cells are suspended in enzyme solution and incubated briefly before being mixed with the sera.

A comparison of one- and two-stage methods

In a study by the ISBT/ICSH Working Party on Enzymes, the sensitivities of a two-stage method and of various one-stage methods, namely one-stage mixing (Löw 1955), one-stage layering (Dodd and Eeles 1961), a one-stage phase technique (Odell *et al.* 1983) and the phased inhibitor technique (Scott and Phillips 1987) were compared. Only the two-stage technique was found to be sensitive enough to be used for the detection of antibodies. When papain or bromelin was used at 0.6 azoalbumin units, the two-stage technique was slightly more sensitive than the standard LISS spin-tube IAT (Scott *et al.* 1994). A disadvantage of the two-stage technique is that false-positive reactions occur when the enzyme activity is too great. Use of the ISBT/ICSH reference preparation should allow the standardization of enzyme preparations and techniques in individual laboratories and thus avoid false-positive results.

The clinical significance of antibodies detectable only with enzyme-treated red cells ('enzyme-only antibodies') has been much discussed. As described in Chapter 10, such antibodies are sometimes capable of causing accelerated destruction of small volumes of incompatible red cells, but they seem hardly ever to cause clinically significant haemolysis. In a retrospective study on serum samples from 10 000 recently transfused patients, 35 were found to contain enzyme-only antibodies. In total, 19 out of the 35 patients had been transfused with incompatible red cells and only one had developed a DHTR. However, in 17 of these 19 cases the antibody was anti-E and, in most cases at least, may well have been naturally occurring. In the remaining two cases, the specificities were anti-c and anti-e and in the first of these a DHTR developed (Issitt *et al.* 1993).

As tests with enzyme-treated cells detect many clinically insignificant antibodies, they should not be used in pre-transfusion testing. On the other hand, enzyme-only antibodies may be found in the early stages of primary immunization, for example in pregnancy and in patients (e.g. those with thalassaemia) receiving regular transfusion.

Role of ionic strength

The effects of low ionic strength and of enzyme treatment of cells are not additive (Atchley *et al.* 1964; Elliot *et al.* 1964). In external quality assessment surveys the use of low ionic strength was found to have no influence on results obtained with enzyme techniques (Holburn and Prior 1987).

The manual polybrene test

As discussed in a later section, protamine and poly-brene are used in certain automated techniques for antibody detection; they are also used in manual tests. In the low-ionic polycation test, protamine is used and in the manual polybrene test (MPT), polybrene. Of these two tests, the most satisfactory appears to be the MPT, as it requires fewer manipulations and only a very brief incubation period at room temperature.

One millilitre of a low-ionic-strength medium (dextrose-EDTA) is added to two drops of a 10% cell suspension and two drops of serum; after 1 min at room temperature, two drops of 0.05% polybrene are added, the tubes are spun, and the supernatant is decanted. Two drops of a citrate–dextrose solution are added to disperse polybrene-induced aggregation and the contents of the tube are mixed by gentle rolling. After examining the tube for agglutinates, the red cells can be washed and the antiglobulin test carried out. As C3 and C4 may bind non-specifically at low ionic strength, the antiglobulin reagent should not contain anticomplement (Lalezari and Jiang 1980).

A modified test in which two drops of serum are mixed with one drop of a 3% suspension of red cells and 0.6 ml of low-ionic-strength medium was used by Ferrer and co-workers (1985). This test was found to be more sensitive than the original test described by Lalezari and Jiang (1980).

For the detection of most antibodies, the MPT was found to be more sensitive than either the standard two-stage enzyme method or the IAT (Fisher 1983). However, anti-K and anti-Fy[a] (particularly the former) are often missed, and may be missed even when the MPT test is followed by a test with antiglobulin serum (Fisher 1983; Ferrer et al. 1985; Malde et al. 1986). Using a commercial kit for the MPT, 31 of 47 anti-Ks were not detected and this MPT test was therefore considered to be unsuitable as a primary technique for the detection of alloantibodies (Letendre et al. 1987).

For large-scale red cell typing the MPT was found to be as good as routine microplate testing but twice as quick. Antiglobulin serum was needed only for Kell grouping (Etges et al. 1982). Satisfactory results were observed in another series, although antiglobulin serum was used for testing with anti-Jk[a], -S and -s as well as with -K (Anderson and Patel 1984). The MPT has also been recommended for red cell antibody screening, provided that appropriate positive and negative controls are used (Ferrer et al. 1985); the test carried out in microplates was found to be as sensitive as the tube test (Lown and Ivy 1988).

False-positive results in agglutination tests

The commonest cause is rouleaux formation. Dilution of serum with an equal volume of saline greatly diminishes or completely abolishes rouleaux. Dextran is a potential source of trouble but only high-molecular-weight preparations (no longer used as plasma substitutes) cause rouleaux formation of untreated red cells. Enzyme-treated red cells may be intensely aggregated even by Dextran 40 (Selwyn et al. 1968).

The next commonest cause of false-positive results is the presence of cold autoagglutinins. These antibodies (usually anti-I) produce strong agglutination up to a temperature of about 25°C, or even sometimes up to 32°C, but are very seldom active at a temperature of 37°C. If red cells and serum are not pre-warmed to 37°C before being mixed, subsequent warming to 37°C may fail to disperse agglutination completely.

When there is difficulty in distinguishing between rouleaux formation and autoagglutination it is helpful to prepare dilutions of the serum in saline (1 in 2 and 1 in 4) and to incubate these with the subject's own red cells, first at 4°C and then at 37°C. Potent autoagglutinins should react very strongly at 4°C and weakly or not at all at 37°C; furthermore, diluting the serum 1 in 4 should have little or no effect on the degree of agglutination. By contrast, rouleaux formation should be more pronounced at 37°C than at 4°C; it should be very much weaker in a 1:2 dilution than in undiluted serum and should be completely absent in the 1:4 dilution.

Spontaneous agglutination of antibody-coated cells in albumin

A problem that arises when albumin is used as a potentiator of agglutination is that red cells sensitized with an autoantibody in vitro or in vivo may agglutinate spontaneously in concentrations of albumin as low as 6% (Garratty et al. 1984). It is therefore essential, as a routine, to carry out a control test in which the red cells are mixed with potentiating agent alone. The term potentiating agent is used because some reagents which contain albumin may contain other potentiating agents so that the control used must be one supplied by the manufacturer of the reagent containing everything except the reagent antibody (White *et al.* 1974; Garratty *et al.* 1984).

Mixed field agglutination

This term is used to describe the presence of agglutinated and unagglutinated cells in a red cell suspension treated with an agglutinin. The term is often used to imply that two phenotypically distinct populations of red cells are present, as in mosaics, chimeras, subjects who have been transfused, women whose circulation contains fetal red cells, and subjects some of whose red cells have undergone T or Tn transformation. On the other hand, a similar appearance may be seen in red cell suspensions of a single phenotype, either when the red cells have relatively few antigen sites (e.g. 'weak' varieties of A) or when the agglutinin is of low titre. Lutheran antibodies characteristically produce a mixed field appearance of large agglutinates with many free cells and anti-Sd^a produces small agglutinates in a sea of free cells.

Although mixed field agglutination is included in the present section under the general heading of 'agglutination of red cells suspended in saline', it may be observed in any agglutination reaction, for example between antibody-coated red cells and antiglobulin serum. For example, when the direct antiglobulin test (DAT) is performed in a patient who is having a DHTR, a mixed field may be observed, for (as a rule) only the donor cells are agglutinated.

Again, if an IAT with anti-D is performed on red cells from a D-negative mother whose circulation contains a substantial number of D-positive red cells, owing to a transplacental haemorrhage (TPH) from her fetus, a mixed field will be observed and may be misinterpreted as meaning that the mother has a weak D antigen. When a mixed field due to the presence of two phenotypically distinct populations is suspected, there are many tests that can be done to confirm or refute the suspicion. For example, tests may be made with sera containing alloantibodies of various specificities, which may reveal that there are two populations of red cells present, differing with respect to many antigens. Alternatively, the agglutinated cells may be separated from the agglutinated cells by differential sedimentation and the agglutinated cells may then be disagglutinated and tested.

In detecting the presence of two different populations of red cells, the gel test (see p. 313) is excellent. In both techniques, one population of cells will remain at the top of the gel (agglutinated) and the other will go to the bottom of the tube or column (unagglutinated). The gel test has been successfully used to detect mixed red cell populations in patients who had received a bone marrow transplant (ZagoNovaretti *et al.* 1993).

Tests for lysis of red cells

Tests for alloantibodies that lyse red cells (haemolysins) are no longer used in blood grouping: first, because, apart from some examples of anti-A and anti-B, most blood group antibodies will not readily lyse red cells and, second, because the lytic property of serum deteriorates rapidly on storage due to the decay of complement. Nevertheless, in some circumstances, it is valuable to know whether or not a serum sample is lytic: (1) if a serum causes specific lysis, it establishes the fact that it contains a complement-binding antibody; (2) if a serum is readily lytic *in vitro* at 37°C, the antibody is likely to cause intravascular lysis of incompatible red cells (although this information would usually be of interest only in a retrospective investigation); (3) in circumstances in which group O blood has to be used for transfusion to group A or B subjects, a screening test for lytic anti-A and anti-B may be the best for detecting really 'dangerous' group O donors (see p. 323); and (4) if an infant is suspected of having ABO haemolytic disease, the diagnosis is virtually excluded by showing that the mother's serum will not lyse the infant's red cells (Crawford *et al.* 1953).

Apart from anti-A and anti-B, the commonest lytic antibody encountered is anti-Le^a. Other strongly lytic alloantibodies are all rare, i.e. anti-H (in *hh*– subjects), anti-P, anti-PP$_1$P^k and anti-Vel. Autohaemolysins are described in Chapter 7.

In crossmatching tests, lytic antibodies may be a cause of false-negative results; most of the cells may be lysed and the remainder may be unagglutinated. It is therefore essential to examine the supernatant for lysis before examining the cell button for agglutination, and before washing the cells in the antiglobulin test.

Use of human serum as a source of complement

In testing for haemolysins, it is preferable to use very fresh serum, i.e. serum taken within the previous

2 h (see Chapter 4). When stored serum is tested for haemolysins, fresh serum should be added as a source of complement.

In testing for anti-A or anti-B lysins, group O serum from which anti-A and anti-B have been absorbed may be used. In detecting lytic anti-Le[a] or anti-Le[b], serum from Le(a– b–) subjects, free from Lewis antibodies, may be used. Alternatively in detecting lysis by Lewis antibodies, a two-stage test may be used and then the Lewis group of the serum used as a source of complement in the second stage is of no importance (Polley and Mollison 1961).

Use of animal serum as a source of complement

For details, see Chapter 3.

Importance of ratio of serum to cells

For details, see Chapter 4.

Enzyme treatment of cells

Some examples of anti-Le[a], anti-Le[b] and anti-Jk[a] will lyse untreated red cells; other examples will lyse only enzyme-treated cells.

^{51}Cr release method

The technique of estimating the release of ^{51}Cr from ^{51}Cr-labelled group A_1 red cells incubated with anti-A is referred to in Chapter 9. In addition to being convenient for demonstrating very weak haemolysins this method is useful for demonstrating the presence of a very small proportion of A_1 red cells in a mixture of A_1 and O cells, for example in measuring the proportion of A_1 cells in blood group chimeras (Booth et al. 1957). The method can also be used to estimate the survival of transfused A cells in an O subject (see Chapter 11 and Appendix 7).

The antiglobulin test (Coombs' test)

By definition, non-agglutinating (incomplete) antibodies are those that fail to agglutinate red cells suspended in saline. In the antiglobulin reaction, red cells coated with incomplete antibodies, for example IgG anti-Rh, are agglutinated by anti-IgG, which links the IgG molecules on neighbouring red cells. The principle of the test was described by Moreschi (1908) who showed that if rabbit red cells were incubated with a dose of goat anti-rabbit red cell serum too small to produce agglutination, and then washed, they were strongly agglutinated by rabbit anti-goat serum.

The antiglobulin test was rediscovered and introduced into clinical medicine by Coombs and co-workers (1945) who showed that it could be used either to detect incomplete blood group antibodies in serum – the IAT – or to detect the sensitization of red cells in vivo, as in haemolytic disease of the newborn (Coombs et al. 1946) – the DAT.

Most non-agglutinating blood group antibodies are IgG and are detected by an anti-IgG serum. A few IgM antibodies are incomplete, for example Lewis antibodies, which, at 37°C, usually fail to agglutinate red cells but may be detectable by the IAT using anti-IgM (Polley et al. 1962), although they are best detected with anti-complement.

The fact that an anti-human globulin (AHG) reagent might react with complement components on red cells was first described by Dacie and co-workers (1957) and it was subsequently shown that the main complement components detected were C4 (Jenkins et al. 1960; Pondman et al. 1960) and C3 (Harboe et al. 1963).

Antibodies required in antiglobulin reagents

As described above, AHG reagents may be used to detect IgM and IgA, as well as IgG antibodies on red cells and may also be used to detect various components of complement.

In considering which antibodies are required in AHG reagents, a distinction must be made between reagents used in detecting alloantibodies by the IAT and those used in diagnosing sensitization in vivo by the DAT.

Antiglobulins for indirect tests

In the detection of alloantibodies, using the routine spin-antiglobulin test, anti-IgG is clearly essential but anti-IgM is not required. All incomplete IgM antibodies described so far bind complement and can be detected more readily with anti-complement than with anti-IgM, because each bound IgM molecule leads to the binding of many complement molecules. Some blood group antibodies (e.g. anti-A, anti-B, anti-D) may be partly IgA (Adinolfi et al. 1966) but are then always also partly IgG so that anti-IgG can be used for their detection. A single weak example of anti-K was wholly IgA (Pereira *et al.* 1989).

In detecting alloantibodies by conventional antiglobulin techniques the presence of anti-complement in the AHG reagent often leads to stronger reactions and very occasionally leads to the detection of antibodies, which would otherwise be missed (for references, see the eighth and earlier editions of this book). When using the conventional spin-antiglobulin test for the detection of alloantibodies the reagent must contain anti-complement. On the other hand, reagents lacking anti-complement are often used in the PEG–IAT, and in the MPT followed by an IAT. Reagents containing anti-complement as well as anti-IgG can be used in these tests but particular care must then be taken to avoid false-positive results.

In deciding which anti-complement components to include in AHG reagents, there are good grounds for preferring anti-C3 to anti-C4: in the activation of complement by the classical pathway, more C3b than C4b is bound, and during storage at 4°C, more C4d than C3d is bound to red cells non-specifically (Engelfriet 1976; Garratty and Petz 1976). The choice of the particular anti-C3 component is more difficult. When C3b is bound to red cells it is converted rapidly to iC3b, which reacts with anti-C3c, -C3d and -C3g. iC3b is then further cleaved; C3c is split off, leaving only C3d and C3g on the cell surface (see Chapter 3). The advantage of using anti-C3c is that C3c is found on cells only as a consequence of antibody binding, although the use of too high a concentration of anti-C3c may give false-positive results (Voak *et al.* 1986a). The disadvantage of using anti-C3c is that the period of incubation in the IAT must be limited to about 30 min, after which the amount of C3c remaining on the cells may be suboptimal. As some laboratories use longer periods of incubation, it has been recommended that either anti-C3d (Giles and Engelfriet 1980) or anti-C3g (Voak *et al.* 1986a) should be included in AHG reagents. In both cases, the concentration must be too low to detect the small amount of C3dg present in small amounts on normal red cells and in larger amounts on stored cells and on cells incubated in fresh normal serum (see Stratton and Rawlinson 1976). When using polyclonal anti-C3d, false-positive results are not due solely to the detection of C3d but may be due to the synergistic effect of various antibodies against complement components,

each present on the red cells in too low a concentration to be detected separately. Unwanted positive results are less of a problem when using monoclonal anti-C3d, although even then there may be trouble (Voak *et al.* 1986a).

One of the two polyspecific antiglobulin reference reagents, made available by the ISBT and the ICSH, reagent RIIIM, is a blend of polyclonal anti-IgG and monoclonal anti-C3c and anti-C3d. The other reference reagent (R3P) is entirely polyclonal (see Engelfriet and Voak 1987). Antiglobulin reagents that are blends of murine monoclonal anti-IgG and either monoclonal anti-C3d or monoclonal anti-C3d and C3c have been described and found to be as satisfactory as reagents containing polyclonal anti-IgG (Betremieux *et al.* 1994; Moulds *et al.* 1994). In 1999 the ISBT/ISCH working party on international reference reagents produced a third reference reagent for antihuman globulin to replace those made available in 1987 (Case *et al.* 1999).

AHG reagents for direct tests

In the detection of autoimmune haemolytic anaemia (AIHA) and drug-induced haemolytic anaemia, using the DAT, anti-IgM is not needed in addition to anti-IgG because IgM autoantibodies are always complement binding and can be detected better with anti-complement. Anti-IgA is needed very rarely because it is very rare for IgA alone to be detectable on the red cells (see Chapter 7). It is simpler to use monospecific anti-IgA to test cells that are negative with a polyspecific reagent than to include anti-IgA in the polyspecific reagent.

The main components of complement found on red cells from patients with AIHA are C3dg and C4d (see Chapter 7). So far, no case of AIHA has been described in which one of these components has been present without the other. Because polyspecific reagents for the IAT contain anti-C3d or anti-C3g, which, although present in restricted amount, will readily detect the large amounts of C3dg found on red cells of patients with AIHA, the same polyspecific reagent can be used for the DAT and the IAT.

Production of antiglobulin reagents

In most laboratories, commercially available AHG reagents are used. For those who wish to produce their own reagents, a survey of methods of production is available (Engelfriet *et al.* 1984).

Heteroagglutinins in antiglobulin reagents

When AHG reagents produced in animals are used, heteroagglutinins are a potential source of trouble; methods of dealing with this problem have been described previously (seventh edition, pp. 507–508). If AHG reagents are to be used with enzyme-treated cells, residual heteroagglutinins must be removed by absorption with enzyme-treated cells.

The reaction with bound immunoglobulin

In the IAT, red cells are first incubated with serum to allow the uptake of antibody (and, in some cases, the binding of complement) and are then washed and tested with an AHG reagent.

Reaction between anti-IgG and IgG-coated red cells

Using radioiodine-labelled antiglobulin serum, the maximum number of anti-IgG molecules that can combine with an anti D (IgG) molecule on a red cell surface was estimated to be six to nine by Costea and co-workers (1962) and Rochna and Hughes-Jones (1965). Near-saturation of the antigen sites of an IgG (anti-D) molecule is obtained by having a free equilibrium concentration of 10–15 µg of anti-IgG per ml; that is to say, after the uptake by anti-D of the maximum number of anti-IgG molecules, 10–15 µg of anti-IgG per ml should remain in solution. With an initial IgG concentration of 15 µg/ml the amount of antibody taken up by sensitized red cells after 4 min is 95% of the final equilibrium value (Rochna and Hughes-Jones 1965).

Prozones

If an excess of anti-IgG serum is added to a sample of IgG-sensitized red cells, agglutination is inhibited. This prozone phenomenon was investigated by van Loghem and co-workers (1950) and considered to be due to the fact that, with antiglobulin in excess, all the IgG molecules attached to the red cells are coated with anti-IgG so that no 'bridges' can be formed by particular anti-IgG molecules reacting with unsaturated IgG molecules on different red cells. An example of a prozone is shown in Table 8.2.

This type of prozone can be eliminated by washing the cells after incubation with AHG; presumably removal of excess unbound AHG facilitates lattice formation by removing competition between bound and unbound AHG molecules (Salama and Muller-Eckhardt 1982).

Optimal concentration of anti-IgG

Surprisingly, there is no apparent correlation between the anti-Ig concentration and the serological activity of anti-IgG reagents (Gardner et al. 1983). Accordingly, such reagents must be assessed serologically; see Engelfriet and Voak (1987).

A single dilution of a particular AHG reagent is usually optimal for detecting almost all examples of anti-D. On the other hand, a lower dilution may be optimal for detecting occasional alloantibodies of other specificities. There is some evidence that aberrant behaviour with anti-IgG sera is related to the specificity of the alloantibody concerned. Specificities which are suspect in this regard are anti-Jk[a] (see Table 8.2), anti-Fy[a] (Pollack et al. 1962) and anti-S, -s, -Xg[a], -Yt[a] and -Vel (Issitt 1977). It should be emphasized that many alloantibodies of these specificities are best detected with the dilution of AHG reagent that is optimal for detecting anti D but it may be necessary to compromise by selection of a somewhat lower dilution for routine use.

Because of the heterogeneity of Ig molecules the use of many donors to provide pooled IgG, and the pooling of anti-IgG from many immunized animals, is desirable in producing reagents for routine use.

Diluent for antiglobulin reagents

AHG reagents are usually provided at their optimal dilution and for storage at 4°C. Various diluents are employed; the following one is convenient: 0.1 mol/l of NaCl, 0.05 mol/l of phosphate pH 7.2, 1 g/l of Na_4 EDTA $2H_2O$, 10 g/l BSA and 1 g/l of sodium azide. Use of a low-ionic-strength diluent does not appear to enhance reactions of AHG reagents, perhaps because bound IgG antibodies extend beyond the 'ionic cloud' surrounding red cells (Leikola and Perkins 1980a). However, the use of low-ionic-strength antiglobulin serum in the LISS–IAT has been found to increase the sensitivity of the test (Ahn et al. 1987).

Dyes may be added to AHG reagents to provide a means of checking that the reagent has been added to tubes. Green is the colour most frequently used

Table 8.2 Comparison of optimal dilutions of a particular anti-human globulin serum (Goat, H39), for cells sensitized with an example of anti-Rh (Avg.) and one of anti-Jk^a (Cro.).

Red cells sensitized with the following dilutions of antiserum (as reciprocals)		Dilutions of anti-IgG from Goat (H39) (as reciprocals)						
		50	100	500	1000	5000	10 000	50 000
Anti-Rh (Avg.)	256	++	+++	+++	++	+	(+)	–
	512	++	++	+++	++	+	–	–
	1024	+	++	++	+	–	–	–
	2048	+	++	++	+	–	–	–
	4096	–	+	+	+	–	–	–
	8192	–	–	(+)	Wk	–	–	–
Anti-Jk^a (Cro.)	2	+	+	(+)	–	–	–	–
	4	+	+	(+)	–	–	–	–
	8	–	(+)	–	–	–	–	–

for commercial polyspecific reagents and a suitable depth of colour is provided by mixing 0.08 g/l of Ariavit tartrazine (E102) with 0.02 g/l of Patent blue V(E131).

Relationship between number of bound IgG molecules and reactions with anti-IgG

Using the spin-antiglobulin test, the minimum number of IgG anti-D molecules per cell detectable with anti-IgG is between 100 and 150 (Romano *et al.* 1973; Burkart *et al.* 1974; Stratton *et al.* 1983). The minimum detectable number of IgG anti-A and anti-B molecules per red cell bound to the red cells of either adults or newborn infants is also about 150 (Romano *et al.* 1973). In normal subjects with a negative DAT the number of IgG molecules per red cell was found to be in the range of 5–90 (Merry *et al.* 1982). The findings of Jeje and co-workers (1984) were almost identical. In both series the average number of IgG molecules per red cell was between 30 and 40.

A correlation exists between agglutination strength and the number of IgG molecules bound per cell in both the DAT and the IAT (Merry *et al.* 1984); in the IAT anti-K bound under low-ionic-strength conditions required a greater number of bound molecules for a given agglutination strength than antibodies of other specificities. The number of molecules per cell required for maximal agglutination with anti-IgG is in the range of 500–2000 (Petz and Garratty 1980; Schmitz *et al.* 1981; Merry *et al.* 1984). As the number of IgG molecules bound per red cell in AIHA frequently exceeds 2000, the strength of agglutination in the DAT is of limited value as an indicator of the degree of antibody sensitization.

Inhibition of anti-IgG by IgG in solution

When using an AHG reagent containing about 10 μg of anti-IgG per millilitre, obvious weakening of the reaction between anti-IgG and IgG-coated cells is not likely to occur unless the level of IgG in the suspending medium reaches about 10 μg/ml. As normal serum contains about 10 μg of IgG per millilitre it must be diluted at least 1000 times during washing of antibody-coated red cells to avoid false-negative results. A better safety margin is a dilution of about 5000.

Suppose that one incubates 0.08 ml (two drops) of test serum with 0.04 ml of cell suspension, that 4 ml of saline is used for each wash and that 0.1 ml of supernatant is left with the cells after each wash: a single wash then dilutes the serum only 18-fold; three washes will dilute the original serum almost 6000-fold and will therefore be adequate. Nevertheless, as many commercial AHG reagents appear to contain much less than 10 μg of IgG/ml, it is advisable to wash the red cells four times. The danger of false-negative reactions owing to inadequate washing is reduced when two volumes of AHG reagent are used to one volume of washed cell suspension. When cell-washing centrifuges are used, correct maintenance of the machines is essential (Voak *et al.* 1986b).

Reactions of anti-IgM

Many IgM antibodies are agglutinins active at 37°C and the reactions of these antibodies are not enhanced by the addition of anti-IgM. However, certain IgM antibodies act as agglutinins only at temperatures up to about 25°C or 30°C, and at 37°C may act as incomplete antibodies and then be demonstrable by the antiglobulin test using anti-IgM. Polley and co-workers (1962) found that the following antibodies behaved in this way: anti-Le^a (eight out of eight examples), anti-HI and anti-P$_1$ (single, selected potent examples) and allo-anti-I (from an i donor). In addition to these cold antibodies, a few examples of warm incomplete IgM antibodies were found that were capable of sensitizing red cells to agglutination by anti-IgM, namely one out of three examples of anti-K and 3 out of 15 examples of anti-Jk^a (Polley et al. 1962).

The agglutination produced by anti-IgM is weak compared with that produced by anti-IgG, perhaps because of the small number of IgM molecules attached to the red cells. Therefore, when the antibody concerned binds complement it is always easier to detect it by incubating red cells with antibody and complement and then testing the cells with an anti-complement reagent.

Red cells coated only with IgM can be prepared by sensitizing Le(a+) cells with serial dilutions of EDTA-treated serum containing potent anti-Le^a. At some dilution the anti-Le^a fails to agglutinate the cells but sensitizes them to agglutination by anti-IgM. Another method which has been used successfully is to prepare purified IgM anti-D and treat it with 2-mercaptoethanol (2-ME). The treated preparation will fail to agglutinate D-positive red cells but will sensitize them to agglutination by anti-IgM. Anti-Le^a treated with 2-ME will not sensitize Le(a+) red cells to agglutination by anti-IgM because the IgM subunits have a very low affinity (Holburn 1973).

Reactions of anti-IgA

Anti-A and anti-B are quite commonly partly IgA, as are potent examples of anti-D; Lutheran antibodies may also be partly IgA. Relatively few tests have been made to see whether antibodies of other specificities, for example anti-K, are also partly IgA.

Red cell antibodies are seldom made solely of IgA; although a few autoantibodies of this kind have been reported, only a single such alloantibody has been described (see p. 307).

A convenient way of preparing red cells coated with IgA (and also IgG) is simply to take a number of anti-D sera (e.g. 10) from hyperimmunized subjects and use them to sensitize D-positive red cells. Several samples in the batch are likely to sensitize red cells to anti-IgA. The fact that the reactions are not due to contaminating anti-IgG can be confirmed by adding IgG (0.1 g/l) to the anti-IgA serum. An alternative method is to use chromic chloride to couple IgA myeloma protein to red cells (see Chapter 13).

Anti-IgA sera, like anti-IgG, exhibit prozones and usually react optimally at a considerable dilution, such as 1 in 500 (seventh edition, p. 514).

The reaction with bound complement

Unlike anti-IgG reagents, anti-complement reagents produced in animals do not exhibit obvious prozones. On the other hand, monoclonal anti-C3d reagents, because of their high antibody concentrations, exhibit prominent prozones so that, unless the reagents are adequately diluted, negative reactions may be observed (D Brazier, personal communication, 1985).

When testing red cells coated with complement components, less washing of the coated cells is required after incubation with serum because of the relatively low concentrations of C3 and C4 in serum (see seventh edition, p. 514). Anti-C3g is not neutralized by serum at all because C3g is not expressed on native C3.

Preparation of complement-coated red cells

For methods, see Engelfriet et al. (1987).

Quantification of anti-complement components

The optimal concentrations of anti-C3b and anti-C3c are 1–2 µg/ml, i.e. similar to those of anti-IgG (Gardner et al. 1983). In the ISBT/ICSH reference antiglobulin reagents, the titre of anti-C3c with red cells coated with iC3b is 32–64; that of anti-C3d with C3d-coated cells is 2–4 and should not be higher if false-positive results are to be avoided.

Technique of antiglobulin tests

In the IAT, red cells are first incubated with serum to

allow the uptake of antibody and, in some cases, complement, and are then washed and tested with an AHG reagent. In the DAT the cells are simply washed and tested. The uptake of antibody and complement in the indirect test will be discussed first.

The uptake of antibody

The sensitivity of antibody detection is affected by several variables which determine the rate and extent of antibody uptake.

Effect of the ratio of serum to red cells. The amount of antibody taken up per red cell is at a maximum when the ratio of serum to cells is about 1000:1 (Hughes-Jones *et al.* 1964b). Under normal conditions the ratio is much lower. For example, when one volume of serum is incubated with one volume of a 3% suspension of red cells, the ratio of serum to cells is 33:1. The effect of lowering the cell concentration *from 2.5% to 0.5% is* shown in Table 8.3.

Dropper pipettes used for dispensing serum and commercially supplied red cell suspensions were found to deliver between 17 and 43 drops/ml. Moreover, the PCV of the red cell suspensions varied by a factor of 2. When two drops of serum were added to one drop of cell suspension, the ratio of serum to cells varied from 19:1 to 70:1 (Beattie, 1980).

The titre in the normal-ionic-strength solution (NISS) IAT of most Rh antibodies and of some Kell antibodies was four times higher when four volumes of serum were used instead of one volume with 3% cell suspen-

sion, i.e. a serum–cells ratio of about 130:1. Similar results were obtained in tests with ficin-treated cells and in low-ionic polycation tests (Ahn *et al.* 1987).

Effect of period of incubation. The time taken for the maximum uptake of antibody depends on the concentrations of antigen and antibody and also on the binding constant of the reaction. Typical figures for incubation at 37°C, with a final concentration of DCcee cells of 2% in 'NISS' and of anti-D, with a binding constant of 10^8 l/mol, of 1 µg/ml are: maximum uptake after 4 h; 40% of this amount after 15 min, 87% after 1 h and 99% after 2 h (NC Hughes-Jones, personal communication; see also Hughes-Jones *et al.* 1962). Evidently, the period for which cells and serum are incubated in serological tests is somewhat arbitrary; 30 min is adequate to detect most antibodies, although some weak antibodies need longer incubation (see AABB, 1993); in cases of urgency, shorter periods may be used.

Effect of temperature. In detecting Rh antibodies, incubation at 37°C is optimal (see Chapter 3). In IATs, scores were never higher at 30°C than at 37°C, not only with Rh antibodies but also with those of the Kell, Duffy and Kidd systems. On the other hand, although incubation at 22°C gave lower scores with about 50% of Rh antibodies, it gave the same scores with Kidd antibodies and with 80–90% of Duffy and Kell antibodies. At 10°C scores were as high as at 37°C with 60% of SsU antibodies (Arndt and Garratty 1988). Many monoclonal Rh antibodies react optimally at room temperature.

Effect of low ionic strength. As discussed above, the uptake of antibody is much more rapid at low ionic strength. With many alloantibodies, the titre was found to be increased when red cells were suspended in low-ionic-strength medium but the effect on undiluted serum was not tested (Elliot *et al.* 1964; Hughes-Jones *et al.* 1964b). In view of the observation that red cells exposed to serum at low ionic strength take up complement non-specifically, there was, for a time, reluctance to use a low-ionic-strength medium for routine tests. However, Löw and Messeter (1974) showed that when red cells were suspended in a solution of sodium glycinate containing 0.03 mol/l NaCl, false-positive results were not a problem, and this finding was confirmed (Moore and Mollison 1976). The latter authors gave details of a more convenient method of preparing

Table 8.3 Effect of: (1) red cell concentration (2.5% vs. 0.5%) and (2) saline vs. LISS as a suspending medium, on the reactions of Fy (a +) cells with anti-Fy^a in the indirect antiglobulin test.

Serum dilutions	Cells in saline		Cells in LISS	
	2.5%	0.5%	2.5%	0.5%
1 in 2	$^1/_2$	$1^1/_2$	3	4
1 in 8	0	1	2	3

One volume of diluted serum incubated with one volume of cell suspension for 10 min at 37°C, cells washed and tested with anti-IgG by the spin-antiglobulin technique; strength of agglutination on an arbitrary scale of 0–4.

LISS; incidentally, LISS is prone to growth of bacteria and is best sterilized by filtration. A method of performing IATs using LISS-suspended red cells is as follows.

Red cells are washed twice in saline and then once in LISS; a 3% suspension of red cells in LISS is then prepared. One volume of this suspension is added to an equal volume of serum (drops may be used except with plastic test tubes, for which it is better to use some form of automatic pipette to ensure that the drops of cell suspension and serum are equal in volume). The mixture is incubated at 37°C for 10 min and the red cells are then washed three times; use of LISS for cell washing leads to only slightly stronger reactions than when the cells are washed in saline. Finally, the washed cells are tested with antiglobulin serum in the usual way.

In the technique of Löw and Messeter (1974), ionic strength is reduced by about 20%. In the polybrene technique described by Lalezari and Jiang (1980), ionic strength is reduced by about 80% and the period of incubation, at room temperature, is reduced to 1 min (see p. 304); there is a similar reduction in ionic strength and incubation period in the test of Szymanski and Gandhi (1983).

The chief advantage of suspending red cells in LISS rather than in saline lies in the increased rate of uptake of antibody. Although maximum antibody coating may be observed after a period of incubation as short as 5 min, it has been recommended that 10 min of incubation should be used as a routine because results are sometimes stronger at 10 min than at 5 min (Moore and Mollison 1976).

The only clinically significant antibody that tends to react less well in a low-ionic-strength medium is anti-K. In one investigation, 3 out of 16 samples failed to react, and one of these was associated with an HTR (Molthan and Strohm 1981). In another investigation, 2 out of 195 examples were detected with LISS but not with saline, and the remainder was detected with both (Dankbar et al. 1986). The problem of failing to detect anti-K at low ionic strength can be overcome by using a serum–cell ratio of at least 40:1 (Voak et al. 1982).

Using ^{125}I-labelled anti-IgG, Merry and co-workers (1984) observed an accelerated rate of uptake in LISS of antibodies of several specificities but anti-K antibodies were the exception, less antibody being bound in LISS than in saline.

A disadvantage of the use of LISS is that occasional serum samples give a positive IAT with all red cells, including the subject's own cells (see, for example,

Morel and Vengelen-Tyler 1979). Red cells suspended in LISS give enhanced reactions with common cold alloantibodies such as anti-A_1 and anti-P_1, but this potential disadvantage can be almost completely overcome by eliminating a room temperature incubation phase and by warming red cells and serum to 37°C before mixing them.

The use of a low-ionic-strength antiglobulin serum in the LISS–IAT was found to increase the sensitivity of the test and, particularly with stored sera, to result in fewer non-specific reactions than with the conventional LISS–IAT (Ahn et al. 1987).

Use of albumin (BSA–IAT)

Although albumin enhances the uptake of some alloantibodies, its use adds to the complexity and cost of testing. As emphasized above, the simplest and most effective way of increasing sensitivity is to increase the ratio of serum to cells.

'Spin-tube' antiglobulin test

In this test, a weak (3%) suspension of washed sensitized red cells is mixed with antiglobulin serum in a tube, which is then briefly centrifuged, so as to produce a cell button without packing the cells too firmly. The cells are gently resuspended and examined for agglutination either with a hand lens or under the low power of a microscope.

Use of an inverted microscope provides a convenient means of examining the cells microscopically within the tube and avoids the need to transfer the cells to a microscope slide.

Although an immediate spin after adding red cells to antiglobulin serum seems to be optimal for detecting IgG-coated red cells, red cells coated with IgA may be better detected after cells and antiglobulin serum have been in contact for a longer period, for example 5–10 min (Sturgeon et al. 1979). When the results after an immediate spin are negative, therefore, the tube may be respun after 10 min and read again. C3d reactions may be stronger when cells and antiglobulin serum are incubated before being centrifuged (G Garratty, personal communication).

Use of enzyme-treated cells. Some antibodies that fail to sensitize untreated red cells to agglutination by antiglobulin serum may be detected if enzymetreated red cells are used (Unger 1951). The enzyme–antiglobulin method is particularly suitable for detecting anti-Jk^a (van der Hart and van Loghem 1953). It will also reveal the presence of the antigen Le^a on red cells, which, by other methods, appear to be O Le(a– b+) (Cutbush et al. 1956).

As described above, false-positive results obtained with enzyme-treated cells are sometimes due to the presence of heteroagglutinins in antiglobulin sera. Another potential source of false positives is overtreatment with the enzyme.

Polyethylene glycol indirect antiglobulin test (PEG–IAT)

PEG, a water-soluble polymer, potentiates red cell–antibody interactions in the antiglobulin test (Nance and Garratty 1987). A 20% solution of PEG of molecular weight 4000 was found to be optimal. Of 25 weak antibodies tested, 64% reacted more strongly in the PEG–IAT than in LISS–IAT or in the MPT, 28% reacted equally well in all three techniques and 8% reacted more weakly in the PEG–IAT test. It was found that many false-positive reactions occurred if the antiglobulin serum used contained anti-complement.

Several studies have confirmed the superiority of the PEG–IAT over the LISS–IAT and the BSA–IAT. Reactions tend to be stronger in the PEG–IAT than in the other two tests and a few clinically significant antibodies are detected only in the PEG–IAT and not in the BSA–IAT or the LISS–IAT (Slater et al. 1989; De Man and Overbeeke 1990; Wenz et al. 1990; Shirey et al. 1994; Barrett et al. 1995).

In detecting most warm antibodies, the PEG–IAT, in which anti-IgG or -Ig is used, is more sensitive than the BSA–IAT, although in this latter test a polyspecific reagent containing anti-complement is used. On the other hand, a few antibodies were detected in the BSA–IAT or the LISS–IAT but not in the PEG–IAT: an anti-Jk^a (Slater et al. 1989); two anti-Vel and one anti-P, ascribed to low affinity of the antibodies (MAM Overbeeke, personal communication); and Lutheran antibodies, whose reactivity seems to be reduced by PEG (Fisher 1990).

As mentioned above, the MPT, particularly if it is followed by a test with antiglobulin serum (MPT–IAT), is also more sensitive than the conventional antiglobulin test. In fact it is as sensitive as the PEG–IAT (R Knight, personal communication). For the antiglobulin test

following the MPT, an antiglobulin reagent without anti-complement is used. If either the MPT–IAT or the PEG–IAT replaces the conventional antiglobulin test for the detection of alloantibodies, anti-complement will no longer be required in the antiglobulin reagent.

The gel test

In this test, special microtubes filled with Sephadex gel are used (Lapierre et al. 1990). For the detection of saline agglutinins a neutral gel is applied, and for the antiglobulin test, a gel containing antiglobulin reagent. Gels containing red cell antiserum can also be used. The red cells are centrifuged through the gel. In a negative reaction, all cells collect at the bottom of the tube, whereas in a positive reaction the cells are trapped in the gel. The test is easy, sensitive and reproducible. Advantages are that the antiglobulin test can be performed without washing the cells, that small quantities of reagents are used and that after the reaction has occurred the gels can be kept for at least 24 h, allowing second opinions to be sought and photocopies of the tubes to be made.

With the commercial version of the test (DiaMed-ID Micro Typing System) contradictory results were at first reported. Some found it to be more sensitive than other tests, such as the MPT, a microplate IAT, the LISS–IAT and a two-stage papain test (Bromilow et al. 1991). Others found it less sensitive than a semi-solid-phase microplate IAT (Voak et al. 1991) or the LISS–IAT (Phillips 1992) and even slightly less sensitive than the saline-IAT (Pinkerton et al. 1993a,b). However, in most subsequent studies the gel test has been found to be more sensitive than the traditional antiglobulin test (Bromilow et al. 1993; Phillips and Whitton 1993; Lillevang et al. 1994, Titlestad et al. 1997). At the same time, the DiaMed-ID test has been found to be less reliable than the immediate spin-tube technique in detecting ABO incompatibility between serum from B donors and A$_2$B cells (Cummins and Downham 1994). Phillips and co-workers (1997) proposed that the failure of the gel test to detect weak ABO incompatibilities results from shear forces applying during centrifugation through the gel, which do not occur in the spin-tube method. They further note that this failure of the gel method is unlikely to have any clinical significance because the weak ABO antibodies missed react poorly, if at all, at 37°C. Performing the DAT with the gel test is easier and more sensitive than spin-tube and has the added advantage of minimizing exposure of blood bank personnel to risk from infectious samples, particularly in areas of the world where blood-borne diseases are prevalent (Nathalang *et al.* 1997). A variation of the gel test in which glass beads are placed in a microcolumn together with a diluent has also been developed (Reis et at. 1993).

Tests in microplates

An antiglobulin test in microplates was first described by Wegmann and Smithies (1966) and found to be suitable for routine use (Crawford *et al.* 1970). The reliability of the antiglobulin test in microplates for the detection of red cell alloantibodies was confirmed in three large studies (Crawford *et al.* 1988). Because of the small volume in which the reaction is carried out, the cells should be washed four times (Crawford *et al.* 1988). Several variations of this technique are used (Gordon and Ross 1987). Both V- and U-shaped wells can be used and to reduce stickiness the use of saline containing 0.1% BSA and/or 0.02% Tween 20 for washing the cells is recommended. The advantages of the test are sensitivity and the need for only very small quantities of reagents and cells.

Antiglobulin reagents standardized for spin-tube tests may produce a prozone in liquid-phase microplate tests. Accordingly, the optimal dilution of each batch of antiglobulin reagent must be determined (Voak *et al.* 1990). Dilution may compromise anti-complement activity and make anti-IgG more prone to neutralization. Washing procedures, particularly when automated, must be strictly controlled.

The detection of bound complement

When fresh serum is available and it is not anti-complementary, optimal results are obtained by carrying out the test in exactly the same way as for detecting bound IgG. When testing stored serum in which the complement components may have decayed, fresh normal serum should be added. For example, one volume of fresh normal serum may be added to three volumes of the antibody-containing serum, and the IAT then carried out on the mixture.

Lewis antibodies in the test serum may inadvertently be neutralized by the addition of Lewis substances to the serum, unless Le(a– b–) serum is used as a source of complement. On the other hand when a two-stage test

is used, the red cells being incubated first with antibody and then with complement, fresh serum of any Lewis group may be used as a source of complement (Polley and Mollison 1961).

Two-stage test. Stored sera may become strongly anti-complementary. It may then become difficult to detect the presence of antibodies that are best detected (such as anti-Le[a]) by a technique based on complement binding. The difficulty can be overcome by first incubating the red cells with EDTA-treated serum, washing them and then incubating them with fresh serum. The presence of EDTA in the first stage prevents the binding of altered complement (once described as 'complementoid'), which may otherwise block the binding of normal complement in the second stage of the test (Polley and Mollison 1961).

False-negative results in antiglobulin tests

The most important cause of false-negative results is failure to wash the red cells adequately. To demonstrate that a negative result is not due to neutralization of antiglobulin by residual serum, a drop of D-sensitized red cells should be added. In tube tests, the mixture is spun before being read. An inverted microscope is particularly convenient for this procedure, as the antiglobulin is all retained within the tube. It is particularly important that the D-sensitized red cells are not too strongly sensitized, because strongly sensitized cells may be agglutinated by partially neutralized AHG reagent. The cells should not give stronger reactions than 1+ to 2+ in the IAT (Voak *et al.* 1986b).

Another important cause of false-negative reactions is excessive agitation in reading the test (Voak *et al.* 1986b). The 'tip and roll' procedure, combined with reading under an inverted microscope, or careful transfer of the cell button to a slide with reading under a standard microscope are advised.

Wash solutions should be buffered to pH 7.0–7.4. Failure to detect clinically significant antibodies may be due to the use of wash solutions with pH values below pH 5 or of solutions that have been autoclaved and stored in plastic containers (Bruce *et al.* 1986).

False-positive results in antiglobulin tests

One may distinguish between genuine false-positive results, due to unwanted antibodies such as heteroagglutinins in the antiglobulin serum (see p. 307), and those positive results that are 'true' in that they indicate the presence of globulin on the red cells, but are unwanted, in that they have no obvious clinical significance.

Heteroagglutinins were a source of false-positive results when polyclonal reagents were used but are, of course, absent from monoclonal reagents.

Agglutinins against enzyme-treated red cells. Three out of nine AHG reagents tested by Beck and co-workers (1976) reacted with enzyme-treated normal red cells, due to residual antispecies antibodies. This observation underlines the need to use suitable controls when testing enzyme-treated red cells with AHG reagents, for example when testing C3d cells produced by enzyme treatment of C3b cells. Under these circumstances, the positive reaction may be due to agglutinins for enzyme-treated red cells rather than to anti-C3d (Beck *et al.* 1976).

Automation of serological tests

The inducement to use mechanized methods of blood grouping (McNeil *et al.* 1963) came from the hope of introducing greater reliability and of avoiding drudgery. These hopes were largely realized with the development of machines such as the Technicon Autogrouper and the Kontron Groupamatic. The Autogrouper used a continuous flow system and comprised a dozen or more channels simultaneously, each with a different antiserum or reagent red cell. The Groupamatic used individual wells for each reaction between red cells and antibody. These machines have now largely been superseded by the Olympus PK 7200, which, like the Groupamatic, uses individual wells for each reaction between red cells and antibody. All the foregoing machines are controlled by a computer; manual intervention is not required, greatly reducing the chance of transcription errors. The machines are designed to deal with large numbers of blood samples and are not suitable for the average hospital blood bank. Most UK hospital blood banks with full automation use gel methods for both grouping and antibody screening. A minority use solid-phase microplate systems (R Knight, personal communication).

Continuous flow systems

In these systems, antisera and red cells are pumped continuously through coils, where agglutination is recog-

nized and the result recorded as positive or negative. Individual samples are automatically sampled and kept separate with air bubbles. Using bar-coded samples, the computer matches the result to the corresponding sample.

Two main methods have been used, either with the large Autogroupers or with single-channel autoanalyzers: in the first the red cells are treated with a protease, e.g. 0.1% bromelin, and a polymer is added to the reaction medium, 0.25% PVP, K-9 (Rosenfield *et al.* 1964) or methylcellulose (Marsh *et al.* 1968); in the second, a low-ionic-strength medium is used, together with polybrene (Lalezari 1968). A disadvantage of the low-ionic-strength method is that it fails to detect some examples of anti-K. The autoanalyzer is still used for antibody quantification (see below).

Systems using individual reaction wells

The Kontron Groupamatic machines are fully automated instruments that identify bar-coded samples, perform ABO and Rh grouping, detect antibodies and print out results automatically. Once enzyme-treated red cells and plasma have been dispensed into each of a series of wells on a disc, the disc is agitated to mix the contents of the wells, centrifuged and remixed. Reactions are read automatically by a simple photometric system (Matté 1971).

In the Olympus machines (PK7100 and PK7200), which are also fully automatic, the reactions take place in special microplates, each containing 120 wells with a stepped profile: agglutinates adhere to the sides of the well but unagglutinated cells fall to the bottom and form a button. The reactions are interpreted by a simple photometric system (PK7100) or by image analysis (PK7200). These systems have several advantages: <25 μl of reactants are needed. Using monoclonal reagents, tests for many red cell antigens can be made successfully, weak antigens being well detected.

Gel systems and semi-automated microplate systems

Semi-automated systems designed to handle and read both microplates for grouping and microtubes for antibody screening are available, as is an automated system for the DiaMed-ID (Parker *et al.* 1995). A semi-automated PEG–IAT microplate method was found to be comparable with conventional tube and gel tests for K, Fy^a and Jk^a typing (Diedrich *et al.* 2001).

A semi-automated fluorescence cytometric method is described by Roback and co-workers (2004).

Solid-phase systems

In the first-described solid-phase technique, red cells were attached to the inner surface of plastic tubes to form a monolayer. The cells were incubated with antibody-containing serum, washed and then lysed to release Hb and produce a colourless background. After incubation with anti-IgG, a 0.2% suspension of IgG- or complement-coated cells was added. In a positive reaction, the coated cells were bound to the monolayer (Rosenfield *et al.* 1976).

Various semi-automated solid-phase assays for ABO and Rh D grouping, antibody detection and crossmatching have been described. For red cell grouping, monoclonal anti-A, -B and -D are absorbed to microplate wells; enzyme-treated cells are added and the plates centrifuged. In positive reactions, the cells adhere to the face of the well, whereas in negative reactions the cells form a button in the centre of the well. For serum grouping, the solid phase is prepared by coating the wells with rabbit anti-human red cell antibody, which then binds enzyme treated A and B cells. The cells are lysed and the Hb washed out. Test serum is now added and anti-A or -B, if present, binds to the red cell ghosts. Binding is demonstrated by adding indicator A or B cells, centrifuging and reading. Automated reading is performed at 405 nm using a spectrophotometer (ELISA reader), with the light beam offset to pass 1.5 mm from the centre of the well in order to avoid the cell button in negative reactions. In tests on over 2000 donors there were very few discrepancies compared with conventional agglutination techniques, and these could be resolved by the use of computer-aided image analysis (Sinor *et al.* 1985).

In an alternative approach, the detection of haemoglobin peroxidase in adherent cells is used as an indicator system for ABO and D grouping (Moore 1984). Using this method with wells optimally coated with IgM monoclonal anti-A, anti-B or anti-D, it is possible to group cells without the need for enzyme pretreatment (Scott 1991).

The solid-phase assay with red cell adherence is also applicable to antibody screening and compatibility testing (Rachel *et al.* 1985). Red cells are incubated with the patient's serum, washed and then suspended in antiglobulin serum. The suspension is transferred to IgG-coated wells, centrifuged and read visually or photometrically. A disadvantage of this test is that only IgG antibodies are detected and that there is no reaction with anti-complement to facilitate the detection of complement-binding IgG antibodies. This disadvantage can be overcome by coating the plates with AB serum in which complement has been activated with heat-aggregated immunoglobulin to ensure that the AB serum contains a sufficient amount of C3d (Guigner *et al.* 1988). Alternatively (as in the Biotest Solid Screen System) the plate is coated with antibodies against the anti-IgG (e.g. anti-rabbit). In a positive reaction, sensitized red cells that have been incubated with anti-IgG adhere to the solid phase. In a development of this test (Solidscreen II), an activated plate with a high affinity for the AHG reagent, detecting both IgG and C3-coated red cells, is used (Uthemann and Poschmann 1990). In comparing two solid-phase techniques, the Capture-R (CR) and the Capture-R Reading Screen (RS) it was found that not all antibodies detected in a saline-IAT were detected by these methods. On the other hand, some clinically significant antibodies, such as anti-K, anti-Fy^a, anti-Jk^a and Mc^a were only detected in the CR and some (anti-Jk^a, anti-E) only in the RS (Haslam *et al.* 1995).

The problem of having to centrifuge the microplates between each of the required five to six washes can be overcome by fixing the red cells or ghosts to the wells, after which ELISA washes can be used. Suitable methods include fixation of cells by using anti-human red cell antibodies, as described above, or treating plates with poly-L-lysine or glutaraldehyde so that red cells will adhere. Systems of this kind can easily be introduced into a routine blood bank. A fully automated system using microplates to determine ABO and D types and solid-phase red cell adherence assays for antibody detection and IgG crossmatching was found to have an accuracy comparable with standard manual methods (Sandler *et al.* 2000).

In a very thorough investigation of factors governing the results of solid-phase blood grouping tests, it was found that the amount of antibody bound to the solid phase was correlated with sensitivity. The optimal pH for binding was about pH 7 for monoclonal anti-A and -B but was pH 9.0–10.5 for monoclonal anti-D. When concentrations of monoclonal antibodies were too high, less antibody was bound. Selection of antibodies for solid-phase techniques was shown to be essential. For further details, see Scott (1991).

A solid-phase system for testing individual samples outside the laboratory has been devised (Plapp *et al.* 1986). Anti-A or anti-B is bound covalently to individual nylon squares that are then attached to plastic strips to form 'dipsticks'. A drop of blood is added to the dipstick; after 1 min the stick is rinsed with saline; a positive result is indicated by the red colour of adhering cells. From a technical point of view, this method seems likely to be more reliable than determining ABO groups on cards on which anti-A and anti-B have previously been dried (Eldon 1955). Nevertheless, objections to both systems are the same, namely that it is difficult to devise controls that are as reliable as those available when liquid blood group reagents are used, and that serum cannot be tested to confirm ABO groups.

Quantification of red cell antibodies

Antibody titres

The classical method of determining antibody 'strength' is to determine the titre of a serum, expressed as the reciprocal of the highest dilution of the serum that will produce a detectable reaction with selected red cells. There are several reasons why this method gives only a very approximate indication of antibody concentration. First, the method is unsound in principle as it estimates only the amount of antibody bound to red cells, not the amount of antibody in the serum. At the endpoint of the titration, agglutination is caused by the relatively small number of antibody molecules in the serum with the highest affinity, and therefore the proportion of such molecules in the serum has a considerable influence on its titre. As an example, if two sera each contain the same concentration of an antibody but one example has a binding constant 10 times higher than the other then the antibody with the higher binding constant will have a titre approximately 10 times greater than the other (Hughes-Jones 1967). Second, as usually carried out, dilution of the serum is performed in a series of double-dilution steps. This method is inaccurate and, unless special precautions are taken, traces of serum are carried over from one dilution to another. In practice, the titres of anti-D sera determined by a manual method have been found to be poorly correlated with the antibody concentrations of the same sera determined by an isotope method (Hughes-Jones 1967).

A score is a better estimate of antibody concentration than a titre. To determine a score all positive reactions obtained with serial, doubling dilutions of an antiserum are given a value based on the strength of the reaction, e.g. $++++=10, +++=8$, etc. The sum of these values is the score (see Marsh 1972).

For routine determinations of antibody concentration, the autoanalyzer gives far more reliable results than those given by titration.

Use of the autoanalyzer

A single-channel autoanalyzer, using the bromelin–methylcellulose method, provides a simple method of quantifying anti-D with fair reproducibility, for example with a coefficient of variation of 17%. Reproducibility is substantially better than that of manual titration (Judd and Jenkins 1970). Nevertheless, interlaboratory reproducibility is not very good, having a coefficient of variation of about 20% (Fleetwood and McNeill 1990).

In a comparison with the ^{125}I antiglobulin method, two-thirds of estimates of anti-D made in the autoanalyzer agreed to within 24% (Moore and Hughes-Jones 1970).

Despite the considerable inherent assay variability the autoanalyzer is still widely used for the quantification of anti-D (Bowell *et al.* 1982) and anti-c (Kozlowski *et al.* 1995) in pregnancy and for the quantification of anti-D immunoglobulin preparations.

[125]I-labelled antiglobulin

Direct labelling of antibody with radio-iodine

When whole serum is labelled with radio-iodine, lipids are labelled in addition to serum proteins. When the labelled serum is incubated with the red cells the lipids exchange rapidly between the serum and cells and mask the specific uptake of antibody (Hughes-Jones and Gardner 1962). Methods exist for greatly reducing non-specific uptake but are too tedious for routine use. Purified IgG is now used for labelling.

Use of radio-iodine-labelled anti-IgG

In this technique, ^{125}I-labelled anti-IgG is used to estimate the number of IgG molecules on washed sensitized red cells. An advantage is that a given batch of labelled anti-IgG can be used to estimate the amount of antibody in many different sera. The technique has been used particularly in estimating the amount of anti-D in preparations intended for immunoprophylaxis, although concentrations of anti-D as low as 1 µg of anti-D/ml can be measured (Hughes-Jones and Stevenson 1968).

An assay based on the consumption of anti-IgG by sensitized red cells, the remaining anti-IgG being measured by precipitation with ^{125}I-labelled IgG in the presence of PEG, has been described (van de Winkel et al. 1988). The reproducibility of this technique was found to be excellent.

Enzyme-linked immunosorbent assay

The ELISA technique was adapted by Leikola and Perkins (1980b) for the quantification of IgG antibody on red cells. Anti-IgG was conjugated to alkaline phosphatase using glutaraldehyde and was calibrated by adding doubling dilutions to tubes containing fixed quantities of IgG; p-nitrophenyl phosphate was added as substrate; the reaction was stopped after 30 min with NaOH and the yellow colour measured at 405 nm. Similarly, the anti-IgG conjugate was added to antibody-coated red cells followed by substrate and the colour measured. It was found that the test was two to three doubling dilution steps more sensitive than a conventional antiglobulin test and that as little as 5 ng/ml of anti-D could be detected.

In a further paper, the authors described the use of the enzyme-linked antiglobulin test (ELAT) to study the uptake of antibodies on to red cells suspended in LISS (Leikola and Perkins 1980a). ELAT has been used to detect fetal D-positive cells in the circulation of D-negative women; the lowest concentration of D-positive cells that could be detected reliably corresponded to a transplacental haemorrhage of about 6 ml of red cells (Riley et al. 1982).

ELATs have also been used to quantify IgG, IgM, IgA or C3 on the red cells of patients with AIHA (Kiruba and Han 1988; Sokol et al. 1988).

A method for quantification of anti-D in alloimmunized patients and in anti-D immunoglobulin preparations using ELISA is described (Lambin et al. 1998; Ahaded et al. 1999). Red cells (10% suspension) are sensitized with anti-D (<1.2 µg/ml) at 37°C for 2 h, the antibody-D polypeptide immune complexes solubilized

in the non-ionic detergent Triton X-100 (20–24°C for 30 min) and recovered from the supernatant after centrifugation. The immune complexes are then captured in microplates coated with rabbit anti-mouse IgG Fc and monoclonal mouse anti-human IgG Fc. Binding of human anti-D is measured using alkaline phosphatase-labelled rabbit anti-human IgG. The method can be modified for quantification of IgG subclasses by substitution of mouse anti-human IgG subclass-specific monoclonal antibodies for the mouse anti-human IgG Fc. These authors report an excellent correlation between their ELISA and autoanalyser measurements and consider the method to be more sensitive than flow cytometric methods.

A competitive enzyme-linked immunoassay (EIA) for the quantification of monoclonal anti-D for prophylaxis has also been described (Thorpe et al. 2003a). Fifty monoclonal anti-D were quantified by inhibition of red cell binding of biotinylated monoclonal anti-D (BRAD-5) and their potencies estimated against the international reference preparation (IRP) for anti-D Ig. Two antibodies were insufficiently inhibitory and so could not be quantified and 11 showed dose responses not parallel to those of the other monoclonal antibodies and the IRP. These authors conclude that competitive EIA is suitable for quantifying most monoclonal anti-D.

Flow cytometry

A flow cytometer provides delivery of a single file of cells or other particles in suspension through a focused laser beam. Signals due to light scattering and/or emission of fluorescence are available for analysis or may be used as a basis for cell sorting.

Flow cytometry has been used to measure the amount of antibody bound to red cells (DeBruin et al. 1983), to estimate the amount of antibody of different samples of coated red cells giving maximum agglutination in the antiglobulin test (Nance and Garratty 1984), to estimate the density of antigen sites on red cells (Langlois et al. 1985; Bockstaele et al. 1986; McHugh et al. 1987), to analyse the distribution of c, D and E epitopes; to measure the relative density of D sites on selected samples of red cells and to quantify the relative numbers of cell-bound IgG1 and IgG3 anti-D molecules (see Chapter 5); to study the relative numbers of IgG1 and IgG3 anti-D molecules in anti-D preparations used for immunoprophylaxis and to assess the degree of red cell sensitization by IgG1 and IgG3 anti-D monoclonals in experimental studies (see Chapter 5) and in studies relating IgG1 and IgG3 anti-D concentrations to the severity of HDN (see Chapter 12). Flow cytometry has also been used to measure the survival of compatible and incompatible red cells (see Chapters 9 and 10) and to detect fetal D-positive red cells in the circulation of D-negative women (see Chapter 12).

Austin and McIntosh (2000) compared five methods for quantification of 10 serum samples containing anti-D by flow cytometry. Plotting the mean anti-D value for each sample as a percentage of the value determined by autoanalyzer revealed wide variability between the methods. These authors concluded that further validation of the flow cytometric method was required before routine application. In a subsequent study, a flow cytometric assay was compared with autoanalyzer quantification with more favourable results (flow cytometry gave values ranging from 87% to 129% of the value obtained by autoanalyzer). It was concluded that flow cytometry is a suitable method for quantifying polyclonal anti-D immunoglobulins (Schaffner *et al.* 2003).

Relative sensitivity of different methods of antibody detection

The indirect antiglobulin test

The lowest concentration of IgG anti-D detectable by the standard IAT is about 10 ng/ml; using this test in external quality assessment surveys 98% of unselected participants were able to detect 11 ng/ml (Pinkerton *et al.* 1984).

ELAT was found to be distinctly more sensitive than the IAT, the lowest concentrations detectable being 4 and 10 ng/ml respectively (Postoway *et al.* 1985). In one recent survey, 100% of participants detected anti-D at a concentration of 0.1 IU/ml, i.e. 0.02 µg/ml (UK NEQUAS for blood group serology).

Other manual methods

Two-stage tests with enzyme-treated cells are generally believed to be more sensitive than the IAT in detecting IgG anti-D, although no evidence in support of this view was obtained in proficiency testing described by Pinkerton and co-workers (1984).

The manual low-ionic-strength polybrene test is capable of detecting about 1 ng of anti-D/ml without an antiglobulin stage (M Contreras, unpublished observations). Although no quantitative studies have been done, it seems that the PEG antiglobulin test is even more sensitive. The titre of 10 out of 11 alloantibodies was found to be higher in the PEG test than in the polybrene test (Nance and Garratty 1987).

The autoanalyzer

Using the low-ionic-strength polybrene method, or the bromelin–methyl cellulose method, the lowest concentration of IgG anti-D detectable is approximately 2 ng/ml.

Reference preparations

Anti-A, anti-B, anti-A,B and incomplete anti-D and anti-c as well as complete anti-c and anti-E are available as reference preparations from the World Health Organization and can be used for determining minimal acceptable levels of potency of reagents. The first anti-D immunoglobulin reference preparation (68/419) contains 60 µg of anti-D; 1 µg is equivalent to 5 IU (Gunson *et al.* 1980). Comparative studies of this preparation, a national standard, two commercial and two national preparations for clinical use showed that the isotope method, manual haemagglutination and the autoanalyzer all gave similar values (Bangham *et al.* 1978). A lyophilized anti-D immunoglobulin preparation (01/572) was adopted by WHO as the second international standard for anti-D immunoglobulin with an assigned potency of 285 IU/ampoule (Thorpe *et al.* 2003b). The new standard was calibrated against 68/419 and two other preparations in a collaborative international study involving 25 laboratories in 15 countries. Most laboratories (20 out of 25) assayed the preparations using an autoanalyzer, competitive enzyme-linked immunoassay (see above) or flow cytometry. The new standard was designated the standard for anti-D immunoglobulin, Lot 4 by the United States Food and Drug Administration Center for Biologics Evaluation and Research and as the first Biological Reference Preparation for anti-D immunoglobulin by the European Directorate for the Quality of Medicines. In view of limited supplies of reference preparations, individual countries and laboratories should set up their own working standards after determining the relation of such standards to the international reference preparation. For up-to-date information about the availability of WHO standards see http://www.nibsc.ac.uk/biological.html.

As mentioned above, a lyophilized anti-D reference preparation for standardizing enzyme activity has been developed by the ISBT/ICSH. A lyophilized anti-D preparation for monitoring the performance of routine antibody detection tests and of test operators is also available (Phillips et al.1998).

An anti-c reference preparation suitable for use as a standard in quantifying anti-c in the autoanalyzer is available (Phillips 1987). Polyspecific reference antiglobulin reagents available from the ISBT and ICSH have been mentioned above.

Some countries (e.g. the USA and the UK) have established their own reference preparations, which are supplied to manufacturers, whose reagents must match or exceed the potency of the reference preparations.

The potencies of the international standards and reference preparations are expressed in units. The use of units rather than mass is undoubtedly appropriate when dealing with impure substances or compounds of varying potency but seems far less appropriate when describing the amount of IgG anti-D, which is of known molecular weight. Clearly, it is no more accurate to use units than micrograms; both are subject to the same errors of measurement. The use of micrograms has two advantages: first it conveys more information, as, for example, it is possible to calculate the number of molecules of antibody attached to red cells under various conditions. Second, whereas when units are used a stable reference preparation is essential, when micrograms are used the amount of antibody present can be redetermined at any time by a new estimation.

The selection of compatible red cells

The serological crossmatch

In selecting compatible blood, the traditional practice is first to determine the patient's ABO and Rh D groups, second to 'screen' the patient's serum for red cell antibodies other than anti-A and anti-B and, third, having selected blood of the same ABO and Rh D group, to crossmatch the donor's red cells against the recipient's serum. These three steps will be considered in turn.

Determination of the recipient's ABO and RhD groups

The determination of the ABO groups differs from the determination of other blood groups in two ways. First, the ABO system is by far the most important blood group system in transfusion practice; second, the ABO system is the only one in which the antigens present on the red cells can usually be predicted from a knowledge of the antibodies present in the serum.

The standard method of determining the ABO group of a sample is therefore to test the red cells against monoclonal anti-A and anti-B and to test the serum against group A and group B red cells. Traditional practice includes testing the red cells against anti-A,B to detect weak group A samples that are not agglutinated by anti-A from a group B donor but this is not necessary when monoclonal anti-A selected to react with weak A is used. Monoclonal anti-B used for ABO grouping should not react with acquired B antigen. In grouping recipients, it is not necessary to recognize weak groups of A; recipients with weak group A may be safely transfused with group O blood.

It is usual to test the serum against A_1 rather than A_2 cells, as A_1 cells have more A antigen and thus serve better to detect anti-A. In some subjects of subgroups A_2 and A_2B, the serum contains anti-A_1; in that case, the serum has to be retested to demonstrate that it will not react with A_2 cells. Testing for ABO antibodies in the serum can be omitted for neonates or if a secure automation system is used. In the latter case, there must be at least one historic record where the results of testing for serum antibodies is recorded and the current cell group must be identical with all historical records (Chapman et al. 2004).

When speed is essential and when a tube test is used, the mixtures can be centrifuged immediately. For rapid RhD grouping, IgM monoclonal anti-D reagents are available for tube or slide tests. When tests have to be done in a hurry it is more convenient to use blood mixed with an anticoagulant than clotted blood because with the clotted samples there may be delay in separating the clot and obtaining the red cells from the bottom of the tube.

In the absence of a secure automation system two IgM monoclonal anti-D reagents not reactive with DVI cells (see Chapter 5) should be used to determine the D phenotype (Chapman et al. 2004). Most monoclonals fail to react with one or more of the D variants so it is advisable to use a combination of two monoclonals, which together recognize all common variants in the population being tested.

In determining the patient's D group, the risk of failing to detect weak or partial D should be ignored. If a recipient with a weak D antigen is misclassified as D-negative and transfused with D-negative blood, no harm will be done. The IAT should *not* be used to detect weak D samples, as there is a substantial chance of a false-positive result (see later). Such an error might lead to the subject being transfused with D-positive blood, or, if pregnant or recently delivered, not receiving anti-D immunoglobulin.

In view of the known frequency of errors in ABO and D grouping, due mainly to clerical mistakes, it is important to minimize the risk of error by separating the procedure into distinct tasks and using different members of staff to perform each task (e.g. separating the documentation of reaction patterns from the final interpretation; Chapman *et al.* 2004).

Whenever a patient's blood groups are determined, the results should be recorded so that if further samples from the same patient are tested the results can be compared.

Positive and negative controls should be used on a regular basis.

Error rates in blood grouping

Proficiency testing schemes have shown how difficult it is to eliminate errors in ABO and RhD grouping. Results on samples sent to some 2000 laboratories indicated that the average error rate was 0.64% (Myhre *et al.* 1977). In trials carried out in Canada over a 4-year period, the frequency of major errors in ABO grouping was between 0.13% and 0.14%; errors in RhD typing fell from 0.66% to 0.23% over the period (Pinkerton *et al.* 1979, 1981).

In a review of the UK National External Quality Assessment Scheme over the period 1985–2000 it was found that error rates for ABO grouping fell from 0.19% in 1984/1985 to 0.05% in 1998/2000. This improvement was attributed to the elimination of technical errors in misgrouping A_2B samples as group B, with the residual errors being due to transcription, transposition or misinterpretation. In contrast, error rates for RhD grouping did not change significantly over the same period (0.25% in 1984/85 and 0.21% in

1998/2000), at least 70% of the errors in 1998/2000 were the result of transcription or transposition (Knowles *et al.* 2002). These findings emphasize the importance of involving two members of staff in the overall process of documentation and interpretation of grouping results.

Screening tests on the serum of potential recipients

The advantages of screening the serum of potential recipients for the presence of alloantibodies are as follows. First, when the screening test can be carried out well in advance of transfusion and when alloantibodies are detected there will be time to identify the antibody and select compatible units. Second, special red cells can be used for the screening test, which have been obtained from donors homozygous for alleles such as c, E, Jk^a and Fy^a; such red cells react far more strongly than cells from heterozygotes and their use is essential for the detection of some weak alloantibodies. It is virtually impossible to find a single donor who is homozygous for all the relevant alleles and the usual practice is to select two to three donors who between them are homozygous for the most important alleles such as c and Jk^a. In screening sera for alloantibodies, different samples of red cells should not be pooled, as this may lead to failure to detect antibodies (De Silva and Contreras 1985; Knowles *et al.* 2002).

In screening, the LISS antiglobulin test is considered the most suitable method (Knowles *et al.* 2002; Chapman *et al.* 2004). The PEG–IAT and the IAT in microplates are also considered to be as sensitive. However + or ++ reactions may easily be missed in spin-tube IATs due to inappropriate reading, particularly in large-scale screening (see Engelfriet and Reesink 1995). Great advantages of gel/column agglutination techniques are that reading is much easier and that results can be checked by others.

For pregnant women and patients who have been transfused recently, who could be developing an immune response, a second test, such as the MPT, should be used in addition.

In patients who are to undergo operations involving induced hypothermia there is no need to screen the serum at a temperature below 37°C. No convincing account has ever been published of red cell destruction caused, during hypothermia, by a red cell alloantibody active *in vitro* only at a temperature below 37°C.

Antibodies passively transferred by injections of immunoglobulin. D-negative patients receiving injections of anti-D immunoglobulin may, of course, have detectable amounts of anti-D in their plasma for considerable periods after injection. They may also have detectable amounts of antibodies of other specificities if these are present in sufficient concentration in the immunoglobulin. In one such case, passively transferred anti-E, anti-Le^b and anti-HI, all IgG, were detected in a patient who had received 900 μg of anti-D immunoglobulin (Wright *et al.* 1979).

Errors in antibody detection

Two kinds of error may be distinguished: those due to technical errors and those inherent in the techniques used. As an example of the first kind, one may take the results of quality control exercises in which participants used various techniques.

In a comparative study carried out in Canada and the UK about 17% of participants failed to detect anti-D at 0.1 IU (0.02 μg) per millilitre and about 1.5% failed to detect anti-D at 0.25 IU (0.05 μg) per ml (Pinkerton *et al.* 1985). In the UK between 1991 and 1998 a progressive improvement in the performance of the IAT was noted such that by 1998 100% of participants detected anti-D at a concentration of 0.1 IU (Knowles *et al.* 2002).

In the UK, error rates for false-negative antibody screens have fallen from 3.2% in 1984/1985 to 0.5% in 1998/2000. In contrast with ABO and D typing the majority of these errors result from technical problems relating to test sensitivity and have been lower with the antiglobulin method than with other methods. Thus, in detecting anti-D at a concentration of 0.05 μg/ml error rates were as follows: antiglobulin test, 2–3%; with an albumin method, 14–21%; and using enzyme-treated cells 27–49% (Holburn and Prior 1986). Although most laboratories used a one-stage enzyme technique, even two-stage enzyme techniques proved to be less reliable than antiglobulin techniques. Nevertheless, the incidence of false-positive results was significantly higher in the antiglobulin test than in any other technique (Holburn and Prior 1984, 1986). By 1999 most laboratories in the UK had abandoned the use of enzyme-treated cells and direct saline agglutination tests relying solely on the indirect antiglobulin method. In the same period, traditional tube technology was largely replaced by the use of gel/column

methods (see Fig. 8.1). When cells heterozygous for Jk^a are used for antibody screening using gel/column technology anti-Jk^a may be missed (Knowles *et al.* 2002).

Selection of donor blood (red cells)

In countries where blood is collected at transfusion centres, most hospitals rely entirely on the description on the label of the unit of blood and make no further tests on it. In the UK, for example, it is not considered necessary to verify the ABO and D groups of units received from a Blood Transfusion Centre. In the USA, the ABO group of all units and the D group of all D-negative units must be verified.

Limitation of the supply of D-negative blood very occasionally makes it necessary to consider giving D-positive blood to D-negative recipients. If the recipient is a male who has not been transfused before, and particularly if the recipient is elderly, the transfusion of D-positive blood is not likely to lead to trouble. Anti-D is not likely to be formed for several weeks after the transfusion, so that if further transfusions are needed within a few days of the first transfusion more D-positive blood can be given (provided that cross-matching is carried out with a sample obtained on the day of transfusion). Although it may be defensible to give D-positive blood to D-negative males, it must be an absolute rule that D-positive blood is never transfused to a D-negative female who is still capable of childbearing.

In a D-negative woman who has reached the menopause, the transfusion of D-positive blood is much less safe than in a D-negative man because the woman may have been sensitized by pregnancy. Such a case, in which a woman developed a severe DHTR after her first transfusion, is described in Chapter 11. Donations for D-negative patients immunized to D must be C negative and E negative as well as D negative, because subjects who make anti-D often make anti-C(G) or anti-E as well. However, for D-negative patients who have not made anti-D it is sufficient to give blood that is D negative and the donor red cells need not also be C negative and E negative (compare with Chapter 5).

When alloantibodies active at 37°C, other than anti-A, -B and -D are present, or have been present in the past but are no longer detectable, for example anti-Jk^a, red cells lacking the corresponding antigens must be selected for transfusion.

Is it practicable to try to prevent immunization to antigens other than D?

In females who have not yet reached the menopause. It seems worth giving serious consideration to the possibility of trying to prevent the formation of anti-K and anti-c. It is relatively easy to avoid using K-positive blood for K-negative recipients, but finding c-negative blood for c-negative recipients involves a substantial extra amount of work. Nevertheless, as haemolytic disease of the newborn due to anti-D becomes less common, the possibility of preventing immunization of women by c may seem worth pursuing.

In patients who receive multiple transfusions. It is very likely that antibodies will be made to the more immunogenic of the red cell alloantigens that the patients themselves lack. For patients with sickle cell disease or thalassaemia, a strong case has been made for using red cells matched for Rh antigens (C, c, E, e) and K in addition to ABO and D. A retrospective analysis of 137 alloimmunized patients with sickle cell disease in the USA demonstrated that production of all alloantibodies would have been prevented for more than one-half of these patients if matching for these antigens had been undertaken (Castro *et al.* 2002). As approximately 13.6% of random white blood donors would be expected to match for these antigens, these authors concluded that such an approach is feasible. They also noted that extending the matching further to include S, Fy^a and Jk^b would have prevented alloimmunization in 70% of patients, but as only 0.6% of white donors in the USA would match such a protocol this approach did not represent a realistic strategy. In a different study, where extended antigen matching was not performed it was concluded that delayed serological and/or haemolytic transfusion reactions occurring in alloimmunized sickle cell patients (29% of paediatric patients and 47% of adults) did not result in severe clinical outcome 'in most instances' (Aygun *et al.* 2002). A survey of 37 academic medical centres in the USA and Canada revealed that 73% routinely provide antigen-matched blood for sickle cell patients. Of these, 89% match for C, E and K (Afenyi-Annan *et al.* 2004). Much of the difficulty in providing extensive antigen-matching blood for patients with sickle cell disease in Europe and the USA stems from the relatively small number of black donors in these countries. A comparison of the frequency of alloanti-bodies in 190 sickle cell patients in Jamaica compared with 37 patients in the UK revealed a striking difference. Only 2.6% of Jamaicans transfused had alloantibodies in comparison with 76% of those transfused in the UK. Multiple anti-bodies occurred in 63% of UK residents but in no Jamaicans (Olujohungbe *et al.* 2001).

Screening of the donor's plasma

When group O whole blood is transfused to recipients of groups A, B or AB and when the donor's plasma contains potent anti-A,B, a haemolytic reaction may be produced (see Chapters 10 and 11). The risk is diminished when plasma-reduced blood is used and further diminished by the use of red cell concentrates or red cells suspended in additive solutions.

In some hospitals it is the custom to give group O blood (O, D-negative blood for female recipients or for previously transfused males) in grave emergencies without any compatibility tests. When this is done, the risk of producing a haemolytic reaction from anti-A or anti-B in the donor's plasma can be greatly reduced by selecting group O donors with low-titre antibodies. A commonly used test is to screen for high-titre anti-A,B using A_1B cells suspended in saline containing AB substance. Donors whose serum gives a positive reaction in this test are considered to be dangerous if their blood is transfused to patients of groups other than O. This test can be performed in parallel with automated ABO and D grouping. Many transfusion services put a special label on group O units with high-titre anti-A or anti-B, to indicate that these units should be used only for group O recipients.

There is some evidence that a test for anti-A and anti-B lysins might be better than a test for high-titre agglutinins in excluding 'dangerous' group O donors (Grove-Rasmussen *et al.* 1953; fifth edition, p. 530).

Very few haemolytic reactions due to the presence in the donor's plasma of antibodies other than anti-A and anti-B have been described (see Chapter 11). The increasing use of red cells suspended in additive solutions is likely to make such accidents even rarer in the future. In screening the plasma of donors, a relatively simple test, capable of detecting potent antibodies to the most clinically important antigens, is needed. In large donor centres, screening is undertaken on automated machines. Pools of six donor sera can be safely used in the solid-phase Immunocor-Capture ™-R system (Beck *et al.* 1991).

The results of screening the serum of more than 84 000 blood donors during 1975 were described by Giblett (1977). The overall frequency of antibodies was relatively low, i.e. 0.32%, due partly to the fact that the average age of the donors was only about 30 years. Of the antibodies, 68% were anti-D. In the donors with no history of transfusion or pregnancy the frequency of antibodies was 0.04%. It was pointed out that by testing the serum of donors giving a history of previous transfusion or pregnancy, and by also testing the serum of all D-negative donors, only about 1 in 10 000 sensitized donors would be undetected. In view of the fact that the undetected antibodies would virtually always be of low titre it seems quite unjustified to devote much effort to their detection. Certainly, the use of the antiglobulin test in these circumstances seems very wasteful of time and money (Giblett 1977).

Crossmatching tests

Ottenberg (1908) was the first to apply Landsteiner's discovery of the blood groups to transfusion practice by testing for lysis and agglutination of donor's red cells by the recipient's serum as a preliminary to transfusion. During the following few years it was found that in over 100 cases in which the patient's serum did not lyse the donor's red cells no haemoglobinuria developed. By contrast, when there was lysis *in vitro* in the 'cross' test (as it was then called – see Ottenberg 1937), there was always some intravascular lysis in the recipient (Ottenberg and Kaliski 1913). Crossmatching tests capable of detecting incomplete antibodies became widely used only in the mid-1940s, after the discovery of the effects of suspending red cells in albumin and of using antiglobulin serum. However, a test in which whole citrated blood from donor and recipient was mixed in various proportions was introduced much earlier by Weil (1915). As pointed out by Rosenfield (1977), the use of this test may have first revealed RhD antibodies in human sera, as the test was positive in five cases of serious reactions following ABO-compatible transfusions described by Unger (1921).

As described above, it is standard practice to screen the serum of potential recipients for red cell alloantibodies. When this has been done, an abbreviated crossmatch procedure can be used, of which the main purpose is to detect ABO incompatibility due, for example, to misidentification of the patient (see below).

When preliminary screening has not been done, the test used for crossmatching must be capable of detecting virtually all clinically significant antibodies. In the detection of red cell alloantibodies the IAT is undoubtedly the best single test available. As discussed earlier, the ratio of serum to cells is very important in determining sensitivity; if possible, not less than four volumes of serum should be mixed with one volume of a 2–5% suspension of red cells in isotonic saline. After 3 min at room temperature, the tube is centrifuged; the supernatant is examined for lysis and the cells are then resuspended and examined for agglutination. If the test is negative at this stage the tube is incubated at 37°C for at least 30 min; the cells are then washed four times, antiglobulin serum is added, the tube centrifuged once more and the cells examined for agglutination. When the test is carried out at low ionic strength the incubation time can be reduced to 10 min (for further details, see earlier section on the anti-globulin test).

In patients who are to undergo surgery involving hypothermia, crossmatching tests (like screening tests) should be carried out, as usual, at 37°C.

Type and screen

In many blood transfusion laboratories a great many units of blood (or red cell concentrates) are crossmatched each day for patients who are most unlikely to require transfusion, for example patients who are to undergo a surgical procedure in which it is unusual for blood to be transfused. To avoid units of blood being reserved unnecessarily the policy was adopted in such cases of simply grouping the patient's red cells and screening the serum for abnormal antibodies, i.e. type and screen (Henry *et al.* 1977). The fact that the patient's serum has been screened for unexpected antibodies should ensure almost complete transfusion safety (Boral and Henry 1977). To exclude ABO incompatibility either an abbreviated crossmatch is done or the ABO groups of donors and patient are checked before transfusion (see below). The type and screen procedure is now not only used for patients who are to undergo an elective surgical procedure but, in many hospitals, for all patients except (1) patients in whose blood abnormal red cell antibodies are or have been detectable, (2) patients who have received multiple blood transfusions and (3) newborn infants. For these patients a full crossmatch including an indirect antiglobulin test should always be carried out.

The concept of a maximum surgical blood order schedule (MSBOS) has proved extremely valuable. MSBOS is a list of elective surgical procedures, together with the number of blood units required, based on a retrospective analysis of actual usage in each hospital. A satisfactory order meets the requirements of 90% of patients (Friedman 1979). For a detailed discussion, see Standard Haematology Practice (1991).

Abbreviated crossmatching (immediate-spin vs. computer issue)

As mentioned above, when typing and screening is not followed by a crossmatch including an IAT, in order to exclude ABO incompatibility, either an abbreviated crossmatch must be done or the donor's and patient's ABO groups must be checked with anti-A and anti-B reagents.

An abbreviated crossmatch can comprise the so-called immediate-spin or non-serological methods such as electronic issue. The UK BCSH recommend computer issue without a serological crossmatch as the method of choice when a laboratory wishes to replace the IAT crossmatch with an alternative method. This is because of concerns about lack of standardization of the immediate-spin method (O'Hagan et al. 1999).

The immediate-spin method is simply to mix a saline suspension of donor red cells with recipient's serum in a tube, centrifuge immediately and examine for agglutination. The justification for using only an abbreviated crossmatch when the patient's serum has already been screened for antibodies lies in the observation that very few antibodies are detected by rigorous crossmatching that have not been detected by screening. For example, Heistø (1979) reported the results of screening more than 20 000 patients by rather an elaborate technique, involving an IAT with two different cells containing most of the red cell alloantigens and a papain technique against R_1R_2 cells, which revealed alloantibodies in approximately 0.75% of the patients. Only 5030 of the patients became recipients and, in these, compatibility tests revealed previously undetected antibodies in only three cases (0.06%); all three antibodies were very weak. Results reported by Oberman and co-workers (1978) were similar and led the authors to conclude that if blood that had been carefully screened by the antiglobulin test was subsequently released, after a crossmatch consisting only of an immediate spin, there would have been only about

a 0.06% chance that an extremely weak antibody of potential clinical significance would have gone undetected.

The conclusions of Walker (1982) were almost identical. He calculated that the risk that an antibody to a low-frequency antigen, missed on screening, might be the cause of incompatibility because it was missed on subsequent abbreviated crossmatching was approximately 0.06% and that such an event would very seldom be of clinical significance because most of the antibodies concerned cause little or no red cell destruction. Although these calculations led Walker (1982) to conclude that there was no need to do an antiglobulin crossmatching test for patients about to undergo surgery who were unlikely to require a blood transfusion, he stated that he would like to retain the antiglobulin test in routine crossmatching procedures for patients who actually needed blood.

In a later study, some 47 000 crossmatches were performed for about 17 500 patients, whose serum was also screened for alloantibodies. Of 284 clinically significant antibodies, 30 were detected only during crossmatching, using the IAT. Of the 30 antibodies, 24 were directed to low-frequency antigens but were otherwise unidentified; the remaining six had the following specificities: anti-C^W (two cases), -Kp^a, -M, -Mi^a and -Jk^a. In view of the relatively high incidence of antibodies to low-frequency antigens detected only by crossmatching, together with the relatively low cost of retaining the antiglobulin test, the authors concluded that the antiglobulin test should be retained for crossmatching (Motschman et al. 1985).

To replace the immediate-spin crossmatch a computer crossmatch can be used. The computer crossmatch is performed only for patients without unexpected antibodies in the past or present and with a record of two (or more) concordant results of ABO and Rh D typing (Butch et al. 1994). Furthermore, it requires software that does not permit the issue of ABO-incompatible blood (Judd 1998; Chapman et al. 2000). Computer crossmatching can result in a considerable reduction in blood wastage and significant savings in laboratory workload (Cox et al. 1997; Miyata et al. 2004).

Errors in abbreviated crossmatching

Problems in detecting ABO incompatibility by the immediate spin have been reported. When an immediate spin was used, or a spin after a very short period of incubation, the reaction between A_2B cells and B serum was missed in about 40% of cases although other ABO-incompatible combinations were detected reliably (Berry-Dortch et al. 1985).

Using an immediate spin in 1000 combinations of patients with blood group B and donors with blood group A_2B, incompatibility was detected in only 40% of the cases using a test in saline and in 64.4% using LISS. Incompatibility was also missed sometimes with other combinations (Shulman et al. 1987). These findings do not seem to be very worrying because misgrouping of A_2B donor units as B is rare.

When the centrifugation step in the immediate-spin crossmatch was delayed for 2 min, no agglutination and only weak to moderate lysis was seen in 5 out of 200 crossmatches between group O serum and group A_1 red cells. The absence of agglutination was presumed to be due to steric hindrance by C1 fixed on the red cells. In all five cases, agglutination occurred when the red cells were suspended in saline containing EDTA (Shulman and Calderon 1991). Failure to detect ABO incompatibility when centrifugation is not delayed may be due to a prozone effect if the antibodies in the patient's serum are exceptionally strong, probably because C1 is immediately fixed on the red cells (Judd et al. 1988).

Using a polybrene method, incompatibility between A_2 and anti-A, and B and anti-B, was missed in a substantial number of cases (Mintz and Anderson 1985), presumably because IgM antibodies are less reactive in polybrene. In contrast to these findings, when red cells suspended in LISS were incubated with serum at 37°C for 10 min before being spun, only one example of anti-A (and none of anti-B) was missed in the course of testing nearly 3000 sera (Trudeau et al. 1981).

It seems that the most reliable method of all, in looking for ABO incompatibility, is to follow a test for agglutination by the antiglobulin test; the increased sensitivity may be due partly to the longer period for which the red cells are incubated and partly to the potential for detecting bound complement.

Another reason for retaining the antiglobulin test in crossmatching is simply that because in practice there are so many potential sources of error, some redundancy seems desirable. At the same time, it is clear that if the IAT is omitted from crossmatching, in patients in whom no antibodies have been found on screening, the risk of giving incompatible blood will be extremely small.

Crossmatching in patients having repeated transfusions

In patients who are having blood transfusions every day or two there is a temptation to obtain a large sample of serum and use this for crossmatching for several successive transfusions. One must remember that any one of a series of transfusions may stimulate a secondary response in a previously immunized subject and that the antibody may rapidly increase in titre once it has appeared. In order to minimize the risk of failing to detect newly formed alloantibodies, one should insist on having serum taken not more than 24 h before the next proposed transfusion.

On the other hand, if incompatible red cells are transfused to a patient whose serum contains a weak antibody, all the antibody may be temporarily absorbed so that if the patient requires a further transfusion, serum taken before the first transfusion may be best for crossmatching. Most cases of this kind can be diagnosed by carrying out a DAT on the patient's red cells at the time of the second or later transfusions provided that enough sensitized donor cells are still present.

If a previously identified antibody has been temporarily absorbed or is no longer detectable, donors who are negative for the corresponding antigen must be selected. For example, if a patient is known to have had anti-c but the antibody is no longer detectable, the patient should receive blood from donors known to be c negative.

A suggested routine for patients receiving a series of transfusions is to screen the pre-transfusion serum and all subsequent serum samples against red cells containing the common red cell antigens (see above). The pre-transfusion samples of red cells should be taken into a suitable preservative solution and stored at 4°C in case further blood grouping tests are needed; in identifying any antibodies that the patient may form, it is extremely helpful to know the patient's red cell phenotype and it is evidently far easier to determine this on a pre-transfusion sample than on one taken after the patient has received many units of blood. Molecular methods may be useful for blood typing the patient post transfusion (see p. 336).

Compatibility tests in newborn infants

At birth the only alloantibodies present in the sera of

most infants are those that have been transferred across the placenta from the mother's circulation. In the occasional cases in which alloagglutinins formed by the infant are present, they are found in only trace amounts. It can be assumed that a sample of red cells compatible with the mother's serum will not cause any immediate untoward effects if transfused to the infant. For example, if the mother is group B and the infant group O, group B red cells transfused at the time of birth will usually be compatible with the infant's serum and are expected to have a normal survival (see cases reported by Jervell 1924; Wiener 1943, p. 74; Pickles 1949; first edition, p. 241).

Although the mother's red cells are almost always compatible with her infant's serum at the time of birth, they should not be used when she is RhD positive and her infant is D negative. For infants of less than 4 months old, the following procedures have been recommended. Both the infant's and the mother's ABO and RhD groups should be determined; the mother's serum should be screened for irregular antibodies and a DAT should be done on the infant's red cells. If the mother's screening test and the infants DAT are both negative, blood of the same ABO and D groups as the infant may be issued without crossmatching (but see below for exceptions), even after repeated transfusions, provided that the ABO and D groups of the donor unit are checked before transfusion (Standard Haematology Practice 1991).

Haemolytic transfusion reactions may occur in infants with undiagnosed haemolytic disease of the newborn. For example, increased jaundice may follow the transfusion of D-positive blood to an infant with RhD haemolytic disease. There are special risks in group A or B infants born to group O mothers. In mature infants with ABO haemolytic disease, transfused adult A_1 red cells are destroyed more rapidly than the infant's own red cells and severe jaundice or even haemoglobinuria may result (see Chapter 12). In premature A or B infants born to O mothers, ABO haemolytic disease is believed not to occur because the A and B antigens are so poorly developed. On the other hand, the transfusion of group A or B red cells may be followed by hyperbilirubinaemia and haemoglobinuria, due to destruction of the donor's red cells by passively acquired IgG anti-A or anti-B (see Chapter 12). Because of this risk, it has been recommended that in infants of group O mothers, group O red cells should be transfused unless it has been shown that the mother's

IgG anti-A or -B titre is less than 32 (Standard Haematology Practice 1991).

Cases in which all donors seem incompatible

In some circumstances it may be very difficult to find a donor whose red cells do not react with the patient's serum *in vitro*.

1 The commonest cause of apparent incompatibility is potent rouleaux formation. If the presence of rouleaux can be confirmed, for example by showing that serum diluted with an equal volume of saline does not produce clumping and that the IAT is negative, the red cells can safely be transfused.

2 The next commonest cause of difficulty in finding compatible blood is in patients whose serum contains potent cold autoagglutinins. If the agglutinin is active at a temperature of about 30°C or higher, the patient will probably have a positive DAT (owing to complement components on the red cells) and transfused red cells will have a subnormal survival. However, in these circumstances transfusion is not dangerous if the patient is warmed and kept in a warm room. The problem, then, is mainly to avoid overlooking an alloantibody. In performing compatibility tests, the suspension of donor's red cells and the sample of the recipient's serum should be warmed separately to 37°C before being mixed and tests should be read (microscopically) on warm slides. In carrying out the IAT, the cells should be washed in warm saline. If tests are carried out in this way, it should be possible to detect an alloantibody, as the cold autoantibody is unlikely to interfere. If the cold autoantibody is anti-I, it can sometimes be removed from the patient's serum by absorption at 4°C with the patient's own enzyme-treated red cells or with rabbit red cell stroma.

3 Patients whose serum contains potent warm autoantibodies present more of a problem, as when the IAT is carried out all samples of red cells may be incompatible. Occasionally, by titrating the serum with a selected panel, some definite specificity such as anti-e may be recognized and compatible cells can then be selected. More often, the serum reacts to some extent with all samples of red cells. Under those circumstances there is some possibility that an alloantibody will be overlooked, particularly when the patient has received many previous transfusions.

Some useful advice on the detection of alloantibodies in patients with AIHA was given by Petz and Garratty

(1980, pp. 366–372). Among the points made by the authors were the following:

• It is useful to determine the patient's red cell phenotype before embarking on blood transfusion.

• If the patient's serum reacts with all normal red cells, it may be possible to identify the presence of an alloantibody by noting that the serum reacts more strongly with some panel cells than it does with the patient's cells.

• An attempt may be made to remove autoantibody from the patient's serum, by absorption with the patient's own red cells, after eluting autoantibody from them.

• A single absorption at 37°C may be enough to remove a low-titred autoantibody, and four absorptions should suffice for the removal of a potent antibody.

• Autoantibody can be eluted from the patient's red cells by the use of either chloroquine or 'ZZAP', which is a mixture of papain and DTT (Branch and Petz 1982).

• After absorption the serum is retested. If it no longer reacts with the patient's own cells (from which autoantibody has been eluted) one can conclude that the autoantibody has been removed and tests may be made for alloantibodies in the ordinary way.

• If the serum still reacts with all red cells it may need further absorptions or, of course, it may contain an alloantibody reacting with a high-frequency antigen.

• When insufficient red cells are available from the patient, donor red cells of known phenotypes can be used for differential absorption (Petz and Garratty 1980).

The risk that an alloantibody will be present in the serum of a patient with AIHA is of course much greater in patients who have received repeated transfusions. In a series in which alloantibodies were unmasked by a differential absorption procedure, using donor red cells, alloantibodies were found in 6 out of 19 patients who had received more than five previous transfusions; 42% of the alloantibodies were undetectable before absorption (Wallhermfechtel et al. 1984). Using a similar procedure, clinically significant alloantibodies were found in 41 out of 109 patients (38%) with warm autoantibodies (Laine and Beattie 1985), although this very high figure suggests that some of the 'alloantibodies' may really have been autoantibodies with mimicking specificities (see Chapter 7).

When the patient's serum contains an alloantibody reacting with a high-frequency antigen, a national or international panel of donors of rare groups or a bank of frozen red cells such as the Bank of Frozen Blood of the Council of Europe may be able to supply compatible blood. Alternatively, the patient's close relatives can be tested, as they have a greatly increased chance of being suitable donors.

It should be realized that the importance of antibodies of certain specificities such as anti-K is very different in different populations.

Should an autocontrol be included in crossmatching tests?

In the past, when a test at room temperature was included in the crossmatch procedure, testing of the patient's red cells against his or her own serum (autocontrol) was desirable to avoid confusing autoantibodies with alloantibodies. When, as at present, crossmatching is carried out only at 37°C, an IAT carried out as an autocontrol on the patient's own red cells is only dubiously worthwhile. Such a test very seldom detects AIHA (Kaplan and Garratty 1985) and very seldom detects an alloantibody bound to transfused red cells: in a series of almost 800 patients with a positive DAT following transfusion within the preceding 14 days, only six were due to alloantibodies bound to transfused red cells and not detectable in the patient's serum (Judd et al. 1986).

Errors in identifying the donor or recipient

It is well known that most incompatible transfusions result not from failure to detect antibodies but rather from mistakes in identification of samples or patients. There are four stages at which errors can occur: (1) labelling of the sample taken from the patient; (2) laboratory errors such as transposing tubes during serological tests; (3) releasing the wrong unit from the blood bank; and (4) failure to identify the recipient correctly. Any one of these errors can result in giving the 'wrong' blood. Methods of estimating the frequency with which the wrong red cells are given are discussed in Chapter 11.

In a very thorough analysis from the Mayo Clinic, it was found that the overall error rate for blood bank procedures was almost 0.3% between 1990 and 1992. An error was defined as any deviation from standard operating procedures and included such minor errors as mis-spelling names. It was emphasized that, in reducing errors, attention should be given to the introduction of better systems, rather than trying to reduce human error (Taswell *et al.* 1994).

Identification of patients and units of blood

Many systems have been described for minimizing the risk of misidentification. The essentials are for patients to be identified in some second way in addition to their name, for example by number or date of birth; for the laboratory to enter the details on a label that is securely attached to units of blood found to be compatible for the patient; and for some responsible person to check these details at the bedside against those of the patient who is to receive the blood. It is important that tubes should not be labelled before samples are taken from patients. In practice, pre-labelled tubes are not infrequently filled with blood from the wrong patient.

Wristbands carrying details of identification are an important means of avoiding misidentification. It is very important that they should not be removed from patients before surgery as may happen if they are found to be in the way of putting up i.v. lines. A survey by the American College of Pathologists showed that identification based on wristbands was subject to a disturbingly high rate of errors, although these could be greatly reduced by appropriate monitoring (Renner *et al.* 1993).

The use of bar codes, for marking of wristbands and for the identification of units of blood can further reduce hazards. The bar codes can be read at the bedside and the information then checked against data entered in the hospital's computer (Taswell *et al.* 1994; Murphy and Kay 2004).

Donor–recipient compatibility can be verified by feeding appropriate data (including bar codes) into a computer and eliminating the abbreviated crossmatch (see above, Miyata *et al.* 2004). A method of making it physically impossible to transfuse a unit unmatched against the patient's serum has been described. A three-letter code is issued to the patient and the same code is attached to a sample from the patient and to units crossmatched against the patient's serum. Units issued by the blood bank are enclosed in containers that cannot be opened without feeding in the patient's code (Mercuriali *et al.* 1996).

Another method in use in some countries is to confirm the ABO group of the recipient and of donor units at the bedside. This practice is a legal requirement in France and a recommended practice in Germany but is not completely satisfactory, perhaps because the people carrying out the bedside tests are often relatively inexperienced. Genetet and Mannoni (1978) commented that in their experience the practice had failed to detect gross errors of ABO mismatching either because of faulty technique or because of the 'climat d'urgence'.

Omission of compatibility tests in desperate cases

These are cases in which the clinician decides that blood must be given at once if the patient's life is to be saved. It must be emphasized that few cases fall into this category, as all but the most severe cases of blood loss can be temporarily treated with infusions of saline or a plasma substitute while compatibility tests are being performed.

If blood must be given without any preliminary tests, group O blood must be used; in addition, if it is to be transfused to a woman who is not known to be D positive, the blood must be D negative.

Tovey (1974) pointed out that if group O, D-negative, K-negative blood is given to recipients who are known to be D negative (or have not been D grouped) and group O, c-negative, K-negative blood is used for patients known to be D positive, the risk of giving incompatible red cells is extremely small.

Identification of antibodies

When an antibody is found on screening, its specificity must be determined, using a suitable panel of red cells, and then blood of a theoretically compatible group selected for crossmatching. If the antibody is first identified there will be a double check on each donor. For example, if the antibody is found to be anti-c, c-negative blood can be obtained either from a transfusion centre or by testing any available units with known anti-c serum. This blood can then be matched directly against the patient's serum. Use of the patient's serum alone for donor selection is inadvisable, because if the anti-c is relatively weak it may fail to detect the antigen on the cells of cC donors.

Use of a panel of red cells

When a single antibody specificity is present, most red cell alloantibodies can readily be identified by testing them against a suitable panel of red cells. Detailed recommendations for preparing reagent red cells have been published (Guidelines for the Blood Transfusion Service 1993). The selection of blood group phenotypes for inclusion in a panel should take account of the frequency of blood group antigens and antibodies in the local population. For example, anti-Di[a] is extremely unusual in Caucasians but relatively common in Far Eastern and South American populations. Consequently, it is essential to include at least one Di[a]+ cell in red cell panels used in areas with a Far Eastern or South American population but this would not necessarily be the case in certain parts of Europe. Likewise, the inclusion of a K+ panel cell would be essential in Europe and the USA, but not necessarily in the Far East (Table 3.3). When tests against panel cells do not immediately reveal the specificity or specificities of antibodies in a patient's serum, there are a number of additional steps that can be taken. Weak antibodies of certain specificities may react only with the red cells of donors with homozygous expression of the antigen and so inspection of the panel with this in mind can be helpful. Anti-c, anti-Jk[a] and anti-M are examples of antibodies that react more strongly with homozygous cells.

Some antibodies (anti-P$_1$, -Sd[a], -Ch, -Kn[a] and -Cs[a]) show a wide spectrum of reactions with red cells from donors whose red cells carry the corresponding antigens in various degrees of strength. Often the behaviour of an antibody in vitro provides valuable clues to its identity. Antibodies which agglutinate saline-suspended red cells are likely to belong to the ABO, Ii, Lewis, P or MN systems or to be anti-Sd[a]. The Sd[a], Le[a] Le[b], P$_1$, Ch/Rg, Cs[a], Yk[a] and Kn[a] antigens are much stronger in some samples of cells than in others. Agglutination by anti-Sd[a] and anti-Lu[a] gives a 'mixed field' appearance with discrete clusters of red cells in a field of completely unagglutinated cells. Agglutination by Lewis antibodies gives a peculiar 'stringy' appearance.

Antibodies that can be demonstrated by the IAT but not by agglutination in saline are more likely to belong to the Rh, Kell, Duffy and Kidd systems. If reactions are obtained with anti-complement the antibody is virtually certain not to belong to the Rh system. Conversely, if no reactions are obtained with anti-complement the antibody cannot belong to the Lewis system, provided that the red cells have been incubated with serum containing complement.

Antibodies that can be demonstrated by the IAT but fail to react with enzyme-treated red cells are most likely to be anti-Fy[a], -Ch/Rg, -JMH, -S or -Lu[b].

When an antibody has been identified, it must be remembered that it may not be the only one present. For example, if anti-D is identified the serum should be tested against a small panel of D-negative cells carrying the main other red cell antigens.

When a mixture of antibodies is present it is often useful to test the reactivity of the serum with the panel cells using several different techniques (saline room temperature, enzyme-treated panel cells) in addition to the antiglobulin test. The use of enzyme-treated cells is particularly valuable because the enzyme sensitivity of most blood group antigens is known (see Table 8.1). An example of the use of this approach to investigate a serum with a mixture of antibodies is given in Fig. 8.2.

Another important aid is knowledge of the ethnic origin of the patient. For example, anti-In[b] is not infrequent in India and Pakistan but is rare elsewhere. The In[b] antigen is papain sensitive so an antibody reacting with all panel cells by saline and IAT but negative with papain-treated cells in a patient originating from these countries has a reasonable probability of being anti-In[b].

Specific inhibition

In identifying antibodies it is sometimes helpful to demonstrate that they are specifically inhibited. Some group-specific substances can be obtained from human milk (I), saliva (e.g. A, B, H, Le[a]) or urine (e.g. Sd[a]); P$_1$ substance can be obtained from human or sheep hydatid cyst fluid or pigeon egg white. Alternatively, synthetic oligosaccharides or peptides can be used, for example group B trisaccharide to inhibit anti-B or glycophorin A peptides to inhibit antibodies to MNS system antigens (Johe et al. 1991). Recombinant DNA technology can be used to produce soluble blood group-active proteins for use as inhibitors. Soluble CR1 and soluble DAF have been used to inhibit Knops system antibodies and Cromer system antibodies respectively (Moulds and Rowe 1996; Daniels et al. 1998). Another approach is to use recombinant DNA technology to express a particular blood group antigen on cells other than red cells and to use these cells to identify the presence of a particular blood group antibody within a mixture of antibodies (Reid et al. 2000a).

	Patient's serum		
	IAT	IAT	18°C (RT)
Cells	Untreated	Papain	
1	4	4	1
2	4	4	2
3	2	4	3
4	4	0	0
5	4	4	2
6	3	0	1
7	2	4	0
8	4	0	3
9	3	0	2
Patient	0		0
	e.g. anti-S+Jk^a+Fy^a+P1		

Cell 1 → Papain resistant
Cell 3 → Papain enhanced
Cells 4–8 → Variable strength reactions
Cell 9 → Papain sensitive

Fig 8.2 Investigation of a broadly reacting serum.

Use of AET reagents

Treatment of red cells with thiol reagents such as 2-aminoethylthiouronium bromide (AET) results in the weakening or loss of some blood group antigens that are carried on red cell surface proteins where the tertiary structure is maintained by intrachain disulphide bonding. AET treatment of red cells was first reported to inactivate Kell system antigens (Advani *et al.* 1982). It is now clear that antigens of several other systems (including Lutheran, Cromer, Knops, Indian, Yt, LW, JMH) are also inactivated (Table 8.1). AET-treated red cells provide another very useful tool for the identification of blood group antibodies in complex mixtures, particularly when used in parallel with protease-treated red cells.

Value of knowing the subject's full red cell phenotype

The identification of antibodies is greatly simplified by knowing the full blood groups of the patient. With this information one can deduce what antibodies the patient can make and devise a strategy for investigating the serum, for example by absorbing the patient's serum with a red cell that expresses only one of the antigens against which the patient could make antibody and eluting antibody from those cells to see if the antibody is present. A variety of absorption methods have been used to recover antibody from red cells (see below and also tenth edition, pp. 274–276). The heat

method of elution is useful because of its simplicity; the acid elution method is more effective in terms of yield of antibody (see below).

Isolation of antibodies by absorption and elution from red cells

Often a serum contains several alloantibodies and it may then be desirable to absorb out or neutralize the unwanted ones or to extract the wanted ones.

Absorption

If only a limited amount of the appropriate red cells is available, more antibody will be removed by two absorptions with one-half of the quantity of red cells than with a single absorption with the whole amount. When the antibody to be removed is haemolytic, the serum should first be heated to 56°C for 30 min to inactivate complement. Alternatively, absorption may be carried out strictly at 0°C, or EDTA added, in which case a two-stage IAT (see p. 314) must be used in testing the absorbed serum.

Absorption of anti-A and anti-B should in any case be carried out at 0–4°C because absorption at 37°C may fail to remove agglutinins active at a lower temperature. Absorption is performed by first washing the red cells three times in saline and then adding an equal volume (or some lesser volume) of packed red cells to the serum and leaving the mixture at 0–4°C for 30 min. The serum is now tested to see if it is capable of agglutinating A$_1$

red cells and, if so, further absorptions are performed until the serum will no longer react at all. It is desirable to use the least number of absorptions that will suffice, as there is a tendency for the activity of the serum to be slightly reduced by each absorption, due to dilution by saline mixed with packed cells.

Anti-A and anti-B are removed more efficiently if the red cells are enzyme treated. Papain-treated cells are commonly used. It may be possible to take advantage of the fact that some antigens are destroyed by enzymes. For example, Eaton and co-workers (1956) used enzyme-treated AB, Yt(a+) cells to remove anti-A and anti-B, but not anti-Yt^a, from a serum containing all three antibodies.

Elution

Antibodies that have been bound specifically to antigens on red cells (or other cells) can be dissociated by heat, changes in pH or treatment with organic solvents. Organic solvents are no longer widely used and will not be described here (for details, see tenth edition).

Heat. In the first method to be described, washed red cells and a small volume of saline are heated to 56°C for 5 min; after centrifugation, antibody is recovered in the pink supernatant (Landsteiner and Miller 1925). This method has the great advantages of speed and simplicity. It is satisfactory for eluting anti-A and anti-B from red cells, as in the diagnosis of ABO haemolytic disease of the newborn or for eluting other antibodies that bind more strongly at low temperatures. However, the yield of warm antibodies compares unfavourably with that of other methods. In one study, using ^{131}I-labelled IgG anti-D, only one-third of the amount of antibody originally bound to the red cells was obtained in active form in the eluate (Hughes-Jones *et al.* 1963).

Low pH. As discussed in Chapter 3, breaking of the bonds between antibody and antigen can be accomplished by lowering pH. The acid–digitonin method (Kochwa and Rosenfield 1964) involves red cell lysis but methods in which pH is lowered to 3.0 or less without lysing the red cells have been described (Rekvig and Hannestad 1977; Louie *et al.* 1986; see also Byrne 1991).

Maximizing the yield of antibody in eluates

The most strongly binding antibody is obtained from red cells with relatively weak antigens. For example, elution of anti-D from weak D red cells yields antibody that binds very strongly; in contrast, elution from D– – cells yields a very weakly binding antibody, detectable only with enzyme-treated D– – cells (Goodman and Masaitis 1964). A weak antibody in an eluate can be concentrated by addition of commercially available beads to which the protein A, protein G or anti-Ig has been coupled, centrifugation to recover the beads and elution of the bound antibody under acidic conditions (pH 2.5–4).

Identification of autoantibodies

In investigations on cold autoagglutinins, blood should be collected into a warm screw-capped container and put into a Thermos flask containing water at 37°C and transferred from there directly into a heated centrifuge. By following this procedure it should be possible to separate serum from a sample that has never been cooled to more than a degree or two below body temperature. If it is necessary to harvest serum from a clotted sample that has been allowed to cool, the sample should be warmed to 37°C for at least 1 h before the serum is separated (Issitt and Jackson 1968).

As the specificity of most cold autoagglutinins is anti-I or anti-i, sera should initially be tested against red cells from a normal adult and from a sample of cord blood. The specificity of anti-I and anti-i is often masked unless dilutions of the serum are tested at 20°C or higher with adult and cord cells. When examining cold autoagglutinins, the possibility of other specificities should not be overlooked (e.g. very rarely the specificity of a cold autoagglutinin may be anti-M).

In absorbing cold agglutinins from serum, centrifugation of the sample following absorption at 0°C should preferably be carried out at a similar temperature; if it is necessary to centrifuge the sample at room temperature, efficiency of absorption can be improved by returning the tubes to 0°C for a period before separating the serum (Issitt and Jackson 1968).

As described in Chapter 3, treatment of serum with sulphydryl compounds under suitable conditions inactivates IgM but not IgG antibodies. This can sometimes be useful when testing the serum of a patient with cold haemagglutinin disease for the presence of IgG alloantibodies. The method may also be helpful in forecasting the possibility of haemolytic disease of the newborn (see Chapter 12). A solution of 20 mmol DTT in saline (15.48 g/l) is commonly used; the solution remains stable for many months at −20°C. One volume of the solution is mixed with one volume of undiluted serum and left at room temperature for 15 min. Treatment with iodacetamide (IAA) to prevent reassociation of 7S units is unnecessary with whole serum but is indicated with eluates. IAA should be added to a final concentration of 25 mmol/l and the mixture left for 1 h at room temperature before being dialysed against saline overnight at 4°C.

Warm autoantibodies may exhibit clear-cut specificity within the Rh system although as a rule specificity is not very pronounced (see Chapter 7); an eluate prepared from the patient's red cells should be tested against a panel of red cells of known Rh phenotypes including e-negative cells (R_2R_2).

Treatment of red cells with 'ZZAP' (cysteine-activated papain and DTT) results in complete dissociation of autoantibodies, but MNSs, Duffy and Kell antigens are destroyed (Branch and Petz 1982).

Treatment of red cells with chloroquine is useful as a preliminary step in determining the phenotype of red cells with a positive DAT. In one study, after treatment for 2 h with chloroquine, 83% of samples that initially had a positive DAT were no longer agglutinated by anti-IgG (Edwards et al. 1982).

Elution of antibodies by chloroquine was found to be much more efficient at 30°C and 37°C than at 18°C or 25°C. The DAT was virtually negative or very weak after 2 h treatment at 30°C and 30 min at 37°C. Red cell antigens (D, C, E, Kell, Duffy and Kidd antigens) were well preserved after 2 h at 30°C but began to deteriorate after treatment for more than 30 min at 37°C (Beaumont et al. 1994).

A technique in which microwave irradiation was used to dissociate IgG from red cells proved to give better results than treatment with chloroquine, particularly when the DAT was strongly positive (McCullough et al. 1993).

Methods of antibody identification utilized in the specialist blood group reference laboratory

Use of null phenotypes

For most blood group systems, rare individuals have been described whose red cells lack all of the known antigens within the system, e.g. Rh_{null}, Ko, Co(a− b−), Lu(a− b−), Fy(a− b−), Jk(a− b−). These cells can be particularly useful for identifying antibodies against high-frequency antigens reacting with all panel cells. Frequently, it will be necessary to prepare eluates containing the antibody of interest before testing with null cells in order to avoid problems with ABO group incompatibility. Alternatively, anti-A and/or anti-B can be removed from a serum by passing it through a column to which an appropriate oligosaccharide has been attached. For example, anti-B can be removed by passage through a column to which group B oligosaccharide has been bound. Very satisfactory results have been obtained using purified human A and B substances instead of oligosaccharides (A Lubenko and S Gee, personal communication).

Monoclonal antibody-specific immobilization of erythrocyte antigens (MAIEA) has proved to be very valuable in localizing various red cell antigens to specific membrane proteins. This method is particularly useful for identifying antibodies in the Knops system (Petty et al. 1997). Knops system antibodies are not uncommon but, as they are not clinically significant, it is useful to be able to identify them when they are the cause of incompatible crossmatch and so avoid unnecessary delays to transfusion. The red cells are incubated with a red cell alloantibody, washed, incubated with a murine monoclonal antibody against a particular membrane protein (CR1 in the case of Knops antigens) and then washed again. A lysate is prepared and incubated in wells coated with anti-mouse IgG, to which the monoclonal antibody binds. In order to discover whether the alloantibody has also been bound to the complex, a suitably labelled (e.g. fluorescein labelled) anti-human IgG is added. If binding occurs, it can be concluded that the relevant human antigen is situated on the particular membrane protein. This principle was first applied to the detection of platelet-specific antibodies and the localization of platelet antigens to a particular membrane glycoprotein (MAIPA test; see Chapter 13) and has also been used for the detection and localization of granulocyte antigens (MAIGA). Note that false-negative results may be obtained if the alloantigen and protein-specific antigen are in close proximity so that one antibody blocks binding of the other.

Western blotting and/or immune precipitation can be useful in assisting the identification of the specificity of an antibody, as these methods determine the molecular size of the protein with which the antibody reacts.

A particularly useful application of Western blotting is in the analysis of MNS system variants involving the Miltenberger antigens. As many of the MNS variants have characteristic mobilities upon SDS-polyacrylamide gel electrophoresis, it is possible to determine the zygosity of cells expressing different Miltenberger antigens using this method (King *et al.* 1989).

Matuhasi–Ogata phenomenon

This phenomenon consists of the absorption of compatible antibody together with incompatible antibody on to red cells. For example, when group B, D-negative red cells were incubated with anti-B and anti-D, an eluate prepared from the cells was found to contain anti-D as well as anti-B (Matuhasi 1959). The phenomenon occurs with mixtures of sera each containing a single antibody as well as with a serum containing more than one antibody (Ogata and Matuhasi 1964). Confirmatory observations have been published (Allen *et al.* 1969). From an investigation in which labelled non-specific IgG was used it was concluded that the finding of unexpected antibodies in eluates might be due to non-specific uptake of IgG rather than to the adherence of antibodies to antigen–antibody complexes (Bove *et al.* 1973). This phenomenon is usually recognized without difficulty because the amount of unexpected antibody in the eluate is usually small and gives only weak reactions (Issitt and Anstee 1998, pp. 1132–1133).

Investigations to determine the serological cause of a haemolytic transfusion reaction

Methods of investigating transfusion reactions are discussed in Chapter 11, and this section deals only with tests to be used in obtaining evidence of serological incompatibility.

The first step should be to repeat the ABO and Rh D grouping of donor and recipient, using both pre- and post-transfusion samples from the latter. The sample alleged to have been taken from the patient before transfusion may in fact have come from another individual. A remote possibility is that the donor blood has been wrongly labelled. The next step is to repeat crossmatching.

When pre-transfusion serum is scarce, as it often is, it is best to use post-transfusion serum first and to keep the pre-transfusion serum in reserve.

When repeat crossmatching provides no evidence of incompatibility, despite the fact that the recipient has suffered a severe haemolytic transfusion reaction, the possibility of an interchange of samples must be considered.

In one case, serum alleged to have been taken from a certain group O patient was found to contain anti-B (titre of 64) but no anti-A. The serum contained A substance and had evidently come from a group A patient. Group A blood had been crossmatched with this serum and had been transfused to the group O patient whose name was on the label of the serum specimen (fourth edition, p. 464).

If it becomes clear that incompatible blood has been transfused due to a 'mix-up' of samples, it should be remembered that a second patient may be at risk and immediate steps should be taken to see what is happening to the second patient involved in the mix-up.

The DAT should also be carried out on pre- and post-transfusion samples. If an antibody is found in the recipient's serum but cannot readily be identified, a pre-transfusion sample of the recipient's red cells should be grouped as fully as possible to give some clue to the specificity of the antibody.

The blood group antibodies most frequently involved in haemolytic transfusion reactions, after anti-A, anti-B and anti-D, are anti-c, anti-E, anti-K, anti Fy^a and anti-Jk^a in approximately that order and, accordingly, tests to discover whether the patient's red cells carry the corresponding antigens will be very helpful.

If group O blood has been transfused to A, B or AB recipients, it may be helpful to determine the haemolysin and indirect antiglobulin titres of anti-A and anti-B in the donor's plasma. The patient's own red cells are expected to give a positive DAT for at least a day or two after the transfusion of incompatible plasma. Other findings are summarized in Chapter 10. Another possibility to consider is that the red cells of one transfused unit have been destroyed by antibody passively transferred from another (see Chapter 11).

When no pre-transfusion sample is available and the patient has been transfused with blood from many donors, it may be difficult to decide which red cells belong to the patient and which are the transfused ones. To resolve this problem, use can be made of the fact that the youngest cells in the patient's circulation (i.e. the least dense) will be predominantly his of her own. To separate these cells from the others, high-speed centrifugation of blood samples in test tubes

(Renton and Hancock 1964) or in capillary tubes, with or without phthalate esters has been employed (Wallas *et al.* 1980; Reid and Toy 1983). It may be difficult to obtain good separation within 72 h of transfusion because stored red cells initially have a relatively low density and the reticulocyte count may not reach a peak for some days after transfusion (Branch and Petz 1982; Reid and Toy 1983). Another approach to distinguishing between donor and recipient red cells is to use flow cytometry, identifying reticulocytes by staining with fluorescent Thiazole orange and using fluorescence-labelled antibodies to determine the antigen content of donor and recipient red cells (Griffin *et al.* 1994). Yet another approach is to use molecular methods to determine the blood group phenotype of the patient (see below).

Molecular methods of red cell grouping

Once the blood group genes had been cloned it was a comparatively simple matter to compare the DNA sequences from individuals with different blood group phenotypes and so deduce the genetic mechanisms responsible for different blood group antigen structures (see Chapters 4–6). In most cases the genetic mechanism giving rise to blood group antigens is a single nucleotide substitution, which changes a codon so that a different amino acid is incorporated into the polypeptide of the blood group-active protein when the mRNA is translated (known as a single nucleotide polymorphism or SNP). The genetic basis of the antigens K (K1) and k (K2) is given in Fig. 8.3 to illustrate this point. Provided that this is the only mechanism whereby K and k can be created at the surface of the red cell, determination of the nature of the base (C or T) in the middle of codon 193 will determine which antigen is present. The two most commonly used methods are restriction fragment length polymorphism (RFLP) and allele-specific primers (ASPs). Both methods employ the polymerase chain reaction (PCR) (described in Plate 16.1). RFLP analysis requires the use of a restriction enzyme that will cleave the DNA sequence when one of the bases defining the SNP is present but not when the other is found. For the Kk SNP, the restriction enzyme BsmI specifically cleaves the nucleotide sequence GAATGC found when K is expressed but not when k is expressed (see Fig 8.3). This means that DNA containing the SNP when amplified by PCR and then exposed to BsmI will con-

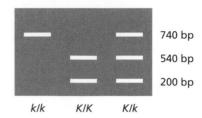

Restriction enzyme BsmI specificity GAATGC

K   AACC**GAATGC**TG

k   AACCGAA**C**GCTG

740 bp
540 bp
200 bp

k/k   K/K   K/k

Fig 8.3 *K/k* genotyping by restriction fragment length polymorphism (RFLP).

tain DNA fragments of different sizes, depending on whether or not K or k is encoded. If the DNA is from someone homozygous for the k SNP one large DNA fragment will be present. If the K SNP is homozygously expressed two smaller DNA fragments will be produced. If the DNA sample is from an individual of type Kk then three fragments will be found when the DNA samples are separated on agarose gels (Fig 8.3; Lee *et al.* 1995a; Murphy *et al.* 1996).

ASP uses a different approach. In this case one of the oligonucleotides used to prime the PCR has its 3' base specific for the sequence corresponding to the allele to be detected. The other oligonucleotide primer anneals to a sequence common to both polymorphic sequences. The result is that DNA is amplified by the PCR when one allele is present but not when the other is found. It is necessary to include primers for the amplification of a suitable control (housekeeping) gene in this type of assay to provide a positive control for the presence of DNA in the PCR (Fig 8.4; Avent and Martin 1996; Hessner *et al.* 1996; Lee *et al.* 1996).

An accurate method that generates simultaneous typing for both alleles is DNA sequencing. In this method an initial PCR produces a product of 400 base-pairs encompassing the region of the polymorphism. The PCR product is excised from an agarose gel and a second PCR is carried out to generate products for DNA sequencing. Two PCRs are performed with each sample, one using the forward primer and the other the reverse primer. Alignment of the two derived sequences against a reference sequence ensures accurate geno-typing (Fig 8.5).

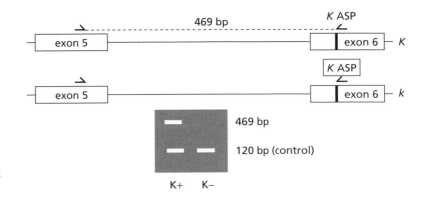

Fig 8.4 Predicting K phenotype using allele-specific primer.

Another method uses real-time PCR. In this allelic discrimination assay, two probes each labelled with a different reporter dye are used. Each probe is specific for one allele. As the PCR progresses, a reporter dye is released from the probe and detected by laser. Samples are assigned to the correct genotype from analysis of the endpoint fluorescence signal of each reporter dye in comparison with signals from control DNA samples analysed on the same 96-well plate.

These relatively straightforward methods for detection of SNPs are not applicable to the detection of D antigen, where different approaches must be used because of the complexity of the antigen itself and the very different molecular bases for the D-negative phenotype found in different ethnic groups (see Chapters 5 and 12 for details).

There are a number of situations where it is valuable to type red cell antigens by molecular methods.

Clinical management of fetuses at risk of haemolytic disease of the newborn

Molecular methods for determination of blood group from fetal DNA and for the determination of *RhD* zygosity are discussed in Chapter 12.

Determining the red cell phenotype of chronically transfused patients

Several groups have reported successful determination of the blood group phenotype of patients who had received multiple transfusions using molecular methods (Wenk and Chiafari 1997; Legler *et al.* 1999; Reid *et al.* 2000b; Rozman *et al.* 2000). It is clear from these studies that residual DNA from donor blood is not a barrier to the use of SNP detection assays. Consistent with this, Lee and co-workers (1995b) report >99.9% clearance of allogenic leucocytes within hours of transfusion of non-leucodepleted red cells. Such a strategy can be particularly useful in establishing the patient's phenotype if this has not been determined prior to the production of multiple alloantibodies. The allele discrimination assay is the preferred method for typing multi-transfused patients because DNA can be extracted and the assay set up and run on the same day with the results available as soon as the assay has been

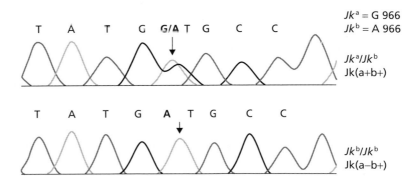

Fig 8.5 Kidd typing by DNA sequencing.

run. A further benefit results from the assay being run in a closed system, which avoids the potential risk of contamination with other PCR products during processing. Use of a microplate format allows simultaneous typing for all desired alleles (P Martin, personal communication).

Determining the red cell phenotype of donors

Molecular methods are useful when donors are required who express a red cell phenotype for which antisera are not readily available, such as a particular Dombrock phenotype (Rios *et al.* 2001; Wu *et al.* 2001).

Automated molecular typing

Technologies for rapid simultaneous screening of large numbers of SNPs have been developed and applied to blood group typing (Denomme and van Oene 2005; Hashmi *et al.* 2005).

Quality assurance for molecular blood grouping

An international workshop on molecular blood group typing involving 30 laboratories found error rates from 0% to 11% for different polymorphisms (Daniels *et al.* 2005).

References

AABB (1993) Technical Manual, 11th edn. Bethesda, MD: Am Assoc Blood Banks

Adinolfi A, Mollison PL, Polley MJ *et al.* (1966) γA blood group antibodies. J Exp Med 123: 951

Advani H, Zamor J, Judd WJ *et al.* (1982) Inactivation of Kell blood group antigens by 2-amino-ethylisothiouronium bromide. Br J Haematol 51: 107–115

Afenyi-Annan A, Wood Johnson R, Brecher ME (2004) Pretransfusion phenotype matching for sickle disease patients. Transfusion 44: 619

Ahaded A, Debbia M, Beolet M *et al.* (1999) Evaluation by enzyme-linked immunosorbent assay of IgG anti-D and IgG subclass concentrations in immunoglobulin preparations. Transfusion 39: 515–521

Ahn JH, Rosenfield RE, Kochwa S (1987) Low ionic antiglobulin tests. Transfusion 27: 125–133

Allan JC, Bruce M, Mitchell R (1990) The preservation of red cell antigens at low ionic strength. Transfusion 30: 423–426

Allen FH Jr, Issitt P, Degnan T *et al.* (1969) Further observations on the Matuhasi-Ogata phenomenon. Vox Sang 16: 47

Anderson HJ, Patel S (1984) Red cell phenotyping using hexadi-methrine bromide (Polybrene) in a microplate system. Transfusion 24: 353–356

Arndt P, Garratty G (1988) Evaluation of the optimal incubation temperature for detecting certain IgG antibodies with potential clinical significance. Transfusion 28: 210–213

Atchley WA, Bhagavan NV, Masouredis SP (1964) Influence of ionic strength on the reaction between anti-D and D positive red cells. J Immunol 93: 701

Austin EB, McIntosh Y (2000) Anti-D quantification by flow cytometry: a comparison of five methods. Transfusion 40: 6–9

Avent ND, Martin PG (1996) Kell typing by allele-specific PCR (ASP). Br J Haematol. 93: 728–30

Aygun B, Padmanabhan S, Paley C *et al.* (2002) Clinical significance of RBC alloantibodies and autoantibodies in sickle cell patients who received transfusions. Transfusion 42: 37–43

Bangham DR, Kirkwood TBL, Whybrow G *et al.* (1978) International collaborative study of assay of anti-D (anti-Rho) immunoglobulin. Br J Haematol 38: 407

Barrett VJ, Stubbs JR, Stuardi K *et al.* (1995) Analysis of the routine use of polyethylene glycol (PEG) as an enhancement medium. Immunohaematology 11: 11–13

Beattie KM (1980) Control of the antigen-antibody ratio in antibody detection/compatibility tests. Transfusion 20: 277–284

Beaumont AE, Stamps R, Booker DJ *et al.* (1994) An improved method for removal of red cell-bound immunoglobulin using chloroquine solution. Immunohematology 10: 22–24

Beck ML, Hicklin B, Pierce SR (1976) Unexpected limitations in the use of commercial antiglobulin reagents. Transfusion 16: 71

Beck ML, Hardman JT, Briseno AM (1991) Antibody detection using pooled sera and a solid phase system. Immunohaematology 7: 73–75

Berry-Dortch S, Woodside CH, Boral LI (1985) Limitations of the immediate spin crossmatch when used for detecting ABO incompatibility. Transfusion 25: 176–178

Betremieux C, Verschelde M, Keyser L *et al.* (1994) Serological and immunochemical evaluation of a new polyspecific monoclonal anti-human globulin blend of anti-IgG and anti-C3d monoclonal antibodies. Vox Sang 67 (Suppl. 2): 122

Bird GWG, Shinton NK, Wingham J *et al.* (1971) Persistent mixed-field polyagglutination. Br J Haematol 21: 443

Blood Transfusion Task Force (1991) Microplate techniques in liquid phase blood grouping and antibody screening. In: Standard Haematology Practice. BE Roberts (ed.), pp. 164–188. Oxford: Blackwell Scientific Publications

Bockstaele DR, Berneman ZN, Muylle L *et al.* (1986) Flow cytometric analysis of erythrocytic D antigen density profile. Vox Sang 51: 40–46

Booth PB, Plant G, James JD *et al.* (1957) Blood chimerism in a pair of twins. BMJ i: 1456

Boral LI, Henry JB (1977) The type and screen: a safe alternative and supplement in selected surgical procedures. Transfusion 17: 163

Bove JR, Holburn AM, Mollison PL (1973) Non-specific binding of IgG to antibody-coated red cells (the 'Matuhasi-Ogata phenomenon'). Immunology 25: 793

Bowell PJ, Wainscot JS, Peto TEA *et al.* (1982) Maternal anti-D concentrations and outcome in rhesus haemolytic disease of the newborn. BMJ 285: 327–329

Branch DR, Petz LD (1982) A new reagent (ZZAP) having multiple applications in immunohematology. Am J Clin Pathol 78: 161–167

Bromilow IM, Adams KE, Hope J *et al.* (1991) Evaluation of the ID-gel test for antibody screening and identification. Transfus Med 1: 159–161

Bromilow IM, Eggington JA, Owen GA *et al.* (1993) Red cell antibody screening and identification. A comparison of two column technology methods. Br J BioMed Sci 50: 329–333

Bronson WR, McGinniss MH (1962) The preservation of human red blood cell agglutinogens in liquid nitrogen: study of a technique suitable for routine blood banking. Blood 20: 478

Bruce M, Watt AH, Hare W *et al.* (1986) A serious source of error in antiglobulin testing. Transfusion 26: 177–181

Burkart P, Rosenfield RE, Hsu TCs *et al.* (1974) Instrumented PVP-augmented antiglobulin tests. I. Detection of allogeneic antibodies coating otherwise normal erythrocytes. Vox Sang 26: 289

Burnie KL (1965) The recovery of red cells from blood samples stored in liquid nitrogen. Can J Med Technol 27: 179

Butch SH, Judd WJ, Stenes EA *et al.* (1994) Electronic verification of donor-recipient compatibility: the computer crossmatch. Transfusion 34: 105–109

Byrne PC (1991) Use of modified acid/EDTA elution technique. Immunohematology 7: 46–47

Case J, Ford DS, Chung A *et al.* (1999) International reference reagents: antihuman globulin. An ISBT/ICSH joint working party report. International Society of Blood Transfusion. International Committee for Standardisation in Haematology. Vox Sang 77: 121–7

Castro O, Sandler SG, Houston-Yu P *et al.* (2002) Predicting the effect of transfusing only phenotype-matched RBCs to patients with sickle cell disease: theoretical and practical implications. Transfusion 42: 684–90

Chapman JF, Milkins C, Voak D (2000) The computer crossmatch: a safe alternative to the serological crossmatch. Transfus Med 10: 251–6

Chapman JF, Elliott C, Knowles SM *et al.* (2004) Guidelines for compatibility procedures in blood transfusion laboratories. Transfus Med 14: 59–73

Chown B (1944) A rapid, simple and economical method for Rh agglutination. Am J Clin Pathol 14: 144

Chown B, Lewis M (1946) Further experiences with the slanted capillary method for the Rh typing of red cells. Can Med Assoc J 55: 66

Chown B, Lewis M (1951) The slanted capillary method of rhesus blood-grouping. J Clin Pathol 4: 464

Coombs RRA, Mourant AE, Race RR (1945) A new test for the detection of weak and 'incomplete' Rh agglutinins. Br J Exp Pathol 26: 255

Coombs RRA, Mourant AE, Pace RR (1946) *In vivo* isosensitization of red cells in babies with haemolytic disease. Lancet i: 264

Costea N, Schwartz R, Constantoulakis M *et al.* (1962) The use of radioactive antiglobulin for the detection of erythrocyte sensitization. Blood 20: 214

Cox C, Enno A, Deveridge S *et al.* (1997) Remote electronic blood release system. Transfusion 37: 960–964

Crawford H, Cutbush M, Mollison PL (1953) Hemolytic disease of the newborn due to anti-A. Blood 8: 620

Crawford H, Cutbush M, Mollison PL (1954) Preservation of red cells for blood-grouping tests. Vox Sang (OS) 4: 149

Crawford MN, Gottman FE, Gottman CA (1970) Micro plate system for routine use in blood bank laboratories. Transfusion 10: 258–263

Crawford MN, Wolford FE, Pilkington PM *et al.* (1988) Identification of antibodies on microplates. Immunohematology 4: 11–12

Crawford RJ, Mitchell R, Burneti AK *et al.* (1987) Who may give blood? BMJ 294: 572

Cummins D, Downham B (1994) Failure of DiaMed-ID microtyping system to detect major ABO incompatibility. Lancet 343: 1649

Cutbush M, Giblett ER, Mollison PL (1956) Demonstration of the phenotype Le(a+b+) in infants and in adults, Br J Haematol 2: 210

Czerwinski M, Krop-Watorek A, Lisowska E *et al.* (2002). Construction of dimeric F(ab) useful in blood group serology.Transfusion 42: 257–64.

Dacie JV, Crookston JH, Christenson WN (1957) 'Incomplete' cold antibodies: role of complement in sensitization to antiglobulin serum by potentially haemolytic antibodies. Br J Haematol 3: 77

Daniels G (1992) Effect of enzymes on and chemical modification of high frequency red cell antigens. Immunohematology 8: 53–57

Daniels GL (1992) Blood group antigens on treated red cells. Immunohematology 8: 55

Daniels GL, Green CA, Powell RM *et al.* (1998) Haemagglutination inhibition of Cromer blood group antibodies with soluble recombinant decay-accelerating factor. Transfusion 38: 332–336

Daniels GL, van der Schoot CE, Olsson ML (2005) Report of the First International Workshop on molecular blood group genotyping. Vox Sang 88: 136–142

Dankbar DT, Blake BE, Pierce SR et al. (1986) Comparison of anti-K reactivity using saline and LISS tests (Abstract). Transfusion 26: 549

DeBruin HG, De Leur-Ebeling I, Aaij C (1983) Quantitative determination of the number of FITC molecules bound per cell in immuno-fluorescence flow cytometry. Vox Sang 45: 373–377

De Man AJM, Overbeeke MAM (1990) Evaluation of the polyethylene glycol antiglobulin test for detection of red blood cell antibodies. Vox Sang 58: 207–211

Denomme GA, van Oene M (2005) High-throughput multiplex single-nucleotide polymorphism analysis for red cell and platelet antigen genotypes. Transfusion 45: 660–666

De Silva M, Contreras M (1985) Pooled cells versus individual screening cells in pre-transfusion testing. Clin Lab Haematol 7: 369–373

Diedrich B, Andersson J, Sallander S et al. (2001) K, Fy(a), and Jk(a) phenotyping of donor RBCs on microplates. Transfusion 41: 1263–7

Dodd BE, Eeles DA (1961) Rh antibodies detectable only by enzyme technique. Immunology 4: 337

Eaton BR, Morton JA, Pickles MM et al. (1956) A new antibody, anti- Yt^a, characterizing a blood group of high incidence. Br J Haematol 2: 333

Edwards JM, Moulds JJ, Judd WJ (1982) Chloroquine dissociation of antigen-antibody complexes. A new technique for typing red blood cells with a positive direct antiglobulin test. Transfusion 22: 59–61

Eldon K (1955) Simultaneous ABO and Rh groupings on cards in the laboratory or at the bedside. Dan Med Bull 2: 33

Elliot M, Bossom E, Dupny ME et al. (1964) Effect of ionic strength on the serologic behaviour of red cell isoantibodies. Vox Sang 9: 396

Engelfriet CP (1976) C4 and C3 on red cells coated in vivo and in vitro. In: The Nature and Significance of Complement Activation. Raritan, NJ: Ortho Research Institute

Engelfriet CP, Holburn AM, Leikola J et al. (1984b) The production of anti-human globulin reagent for use in immuno-haematology. WHO, League of Red Cross Societies, Lab/84.8

Engelfriet CP, Reesink HW (1995) What is the best technique for the detection of red cell alloantibodies? Int Forum Vox Sang 69: 292–300

Engelfriet CP, Voak D (1987) International reference polyspecific anti-human globulin reagents. Vox Sang 43: 241–247

Engelfriet CP, Overbeeke, MAM, Voak D et al. (1987) The anti-globulin test (Coombs test) and the red cell. In:

Progress in Transfusion Medicine, vol. 2. JD Cash (ed.). Edinburgh: Churchill Livingstone

Etges CC, Callicoat PA, Smith DM Jr (1982) A polybrene microplate technique for large-scale red cell typing (Abstract). Transfusion 22: 429

Ferrer Z, Wright J, Moore BPL et al. (1985) Comparison of a modified manual hexadimethrine bromide (Polybrene) and a low-ionic-strength solution antibody detection technique. Transfusion 25: 145–148

Fischer H, Fritsche W, Argenton H (1958) Die Bedeutung des Properdinsystems für den normalen und gesteigerten Blutzellabbau. Klin Wschr 36: 411

Fisher ES (1990) Reduction of Lutheran antibody reactions with polyethylene glycol. Abstracts ISBT and AABB Joint Congress, Los Angeles, Scientific Section, 611

Fisher GA (1983) Use of the manual polybrene test in the routine hospital laboratory. Transfusion 23: 151–154

Fleetwood P, McNeill O (1990) Quality assurance of anti-D quantitation. Transfusion Med (Suppl.) 1: 44

Friedman BA (1979) Analysis of surgical blood use in United States hospitals with application to the maximum surgical blood order schedule. Transfusion 19: 268–278

Gardner B, Ghosh S, Brazier DM et al. (1983) Quantitative quality control of antiglobulin reagents. Clin Lab Haematol 5: 215–229

Garratty G (1970) The effect of storage and heparin on serum complement activity with particular reference to the detection of blood group antibodies. Am J Clin Pathol 54: 531

Garratty G, Petz LD (1976) The significance of red cell bound complement components in development of standards and quality assurance for the anti-complement components of antiglobulin sera. Transfusion 16: 297

Garratty G, Postoway N, Nance SJ et al. (1984) Spontaneous agglutination of red cells with a positive direct antiglobulin test in various media. Transfusion 24: 214–217

Genetet B, Mannoni P (1978) La Transfusion. Paris: Flammarion

Giblett ER (1977) Blood group alloantibodies: an assessment of some laboratory practices. Transfusion 17: 229

Giles CM (1960) Survey of uses for ficin in blood group serology. Vox Sang 5: 467

Giles CM (1982) Serological activity of low frequency antigens of the MNSs system and reappraisal of the Miltenberger complex. Vox Sang 42: 256–261

Giles CM, Engelfriet CP (1980) Working Party on the Standardization of Antiglobulin Reagents of the ISBT/ICSH Expert Panel on Serology. Vox Sang 38: 178–179

Goodman HS, Masaitis L (1964) Binding characteristics of RH antibodies and their serologic properties. Vox Sang 9: 6

Gordon I, Ross D (1987) Large-scale blood grouping and antibody screening using microplates and an automated reader for ABO and Rh determination. In: The Use of Microplates in Blood Group Serology. R Knight, G Poole (eds), pp. 20–25. Manchester: British Blood Transfusion Society

Griffin GD, Lippert LE, Pow NS *et al.* (1994) A flow cytometric method for phenotyping recipient red cells following transfusion. Transfusion 34: 233–237

Grove-Rasmussen M, Shaw RS, Marceau E (1953) Hemolytic transfusion reaction in group-A patient receiving group-O blood containing immune anti-A antibodies in high titer. Am J Clin Pathol 23: 828

Guidelines for the Blood Transfusion Service (1993) 2nd edn. London: HMSO

Guigner F, Domy M, Angue M *et al.* (1988) Comparison between a solid-phase low-ionic-strength antiglobulin test and conventional low-ionic-strength antiglobulin test: assessment for the screening of antierythrocyte antibodies. Vox Sang 55: 30–34

Gunson HH, Bowell PJ, Kirkwood TBL (1980) Collaborative study to recalibrate the international reference preparation of anti-D immunoglobulin. J Clin Pathol 33: 249–253

Harboe M, Müller-Eberhard HJ, Fudenberg HH *et al.* (1963) Identification of the components of complement participating in the antiglobulin reaction. Immunology 6: 412

van der Hart M, van Loghem JJ (1953) A further example of anti-Jk[a]. Vox Sang (OS) 3: 72

Hashmi G, Shariff T, Seul M *et al.* (2005) A flexible array format for large scale, rapid blood group DNA typing. Transfusion 45: 680–688

Haslam GM, Sajur J, Fournier J (1995) A comparison of two solid phase systems for antibody detection. Immunohematology 11: 8–10

Heistø H (1979) Pretransfusion blood group serology: limited value of the antiglobulin phase of the cross-match when a careful screening test for unexpected antibodies is performed. Transfusion 19: 761–763

Henry JB, Mintz P, Webb M (1977) Optimal blood ordering for elective surgery. JAMA 237: 451

Hessner MJ, McFarland JG, Endean DJ. (1996) Genotyping of KEL1 and KEL2 of the human Kell blood group system by the polymerase chain reaction with sequence specific primers. Transfusion 36: 495–9

HMSO (1993) Guidelines for the Blood Transfusion Service, 2nd edn, London: HMSO

Högman CF, Hedlund K, Åkerblom O *et al.* (1978) Red blood cell preservation in protein-poor media. I. Leukocyte enzymes as a cause of hemolysis. Transfusion 18: 233

Holburn AM (1973) Quantitative studies with [125I] IgM anti-Le[a]. Immunology 24: 1019

Holburn AM, Prior D (1984) The UK National Quality Assessment Scheme in blood group serology. Compatibility testing 1981–1982: performance and practice. Clin Lab Haematol 6: 325–340

Holburn AM, Prior D (1986) The UK National External Quality Assessment Scheme in blood group serology. ABO and D groupings, and antibody screening 1982–1983. Clin Lab Haematol 8: 243–256

Holburn AM, Prior D (1987) The UK National External Quality Assessment Scheme in blood group serology. Compatibility testing 1983–1984: the influence of variables in test procedures on detection of incomplete antibodies. Clin Lab Haematol 9: 33–48

Huggins CE, Parker BH, Milbury CS *et al.* (1982) 'Glycigel': a practical technique for preservation of small aliquots of red cells (Abstract). Transfusion 22: 408

Hughes-Jones NC (1967) The estimation of the concentration and the equilibrium constant of anti-D. Immunology 12: 565

Hughes-Jones NC, Gardner B (1962) The exchange of ^{131}I-labelled lipid and ^{131}I-labelled protein between red cells and serum. Biochem J 83: 404

Hughes-Jones NC, Stevenson M (1968) The anti-D content of IgG preparations for use in the prevention of Rh haemolytic disease. Vox Sang 14: 401

Hughes-Jones NC, Gardner B, Telford R (1962) The kinetics of the reaction between the blood-group antibody anti-c and erythrocytes. Biochem J 85: 466

Hughes-Jones NC, Gardner B, Telford R (1963) Comparison of various methods of dissociation of anti-D, using ^{131}I-labelled antibody. Vox Sang 8: 531

Hughes-Jones NC, Gardner B, Telford R (1964a) The effect of pH and ionic strength on the reaction between anti-D and erythrocytes. Immunology 7: 72

Hughes-Jones NC, Polley MJ, Telford R *et al.* (1964b) Optimal conditions for detecting blood group antibodies by the antiglobulin test. Vox Sang 9: 385

ICSH (1982) Working party on the standardization of albumin reagents. Unpublished report

Issitt PD (1977) The antiglobulin test and the evaluation of antiglobulin reagents. II. The IgG-anti-IgG and IgA-anti-IgA reactions and the evaluation of anti-IgG. Advances in Immunohematology 4, no. 5. Oxnard, CA: Spectra Biologicals

Issitt PD, Anstee DJ. (1998) Applied Blood Group Serology, 4th edn. Durham, NC: Montgomery Scientific Publications

Issitt PD, Jackson VA (1968) Useful modifications and variations of techniques in work on I system antibodies. Vox Sang 15: 152

Issitt PD, Issitt CH, Moulds J *et al.* (1972) Some observations on the T, Tn and Sd[a] antigens and the antibodies that define them. Transfusion 12: 217

Issitt PD, Combs MR, Bredehoeft SJ *et al.* (1993) Lack of clinical significance of 'enzyme-only' red cell alloantibodies. Transfusion 33: 284–293

Jeje MO, Blajchmann MA, Steeves K *et al.* (1984) Quantitation of red cell-associated IgG using an immunoradiometric assay. Transfusion 24: 473–176

Jenkins GC, Polley MJ, Mollison PL (1960) Role of C′4 in the antiglobulin reaction. Nature (Lond) 186: 482

Jervell F (1924) Untersuchungen über die Lebensdauer des transfundierten roten Blutkörperchen beim Menschen. Acta Pathol Microbiol Scand 1: 20

Johe KK, Vengelen-Tyler V, Leger R et al. (1991) Synthetic peptides homologous to human glycophorins of the Miltenberger complex of variants of MNSs blood group system specify the epitopes for Hil, SJL, Hop and Mur antisera. Blood 78: 2456–2461

Jones JM, Kekwick RA, Coldsmith KLG (1969) Influence of polymer on the efficacy of serum albumin as a potentiator of 'incomplete' Rh agglutinins. Nature (Lond) 224: 510

Jørgensen JR (1964) Delayed haemolytic transfusion reaction caused by anti-c and anti-E. Dan Med Bull 11: 1

Judd WJ (1998) Requirements for the electronic crossmatch. Vox Sang 74 (Suppl.) 2: 409–417

Judd WJ, Jenkins WJ (1970) Assay of anti-D using the Technicon AutoAnalyzer and the international standard anti-D typing serum. J Clin Pathol 23: 801

Judd WJ, Barnes BA, Steiner EA et al. (1986) The evaluation of a positive direct antiglobulin test (auto-control) in pre-transfusion testing revisited. Transfusion 26: 220–224

Judd WJ, Steiner, EA, O'Donnell DB et al. (1988) Discrepancies in reverse ABO typing due to prozone. How safe is the immediate-spin crossmatch? Transfusion 28: 334–338

Judson PA, Anstee DJ (1977) Comparative effect of trypsin and chymotrypsin on blood group antigens. Med Lab Sci 34: 1

Kang JS, Raymond JA (2004) Reduction of freeze-thaw-induced hemolysis of red blood cells by an algal ice-binding protein. Cryo Lett 25: 307–10

Kaplan HS, Garratty G (1985) Predictive value of direct antiglobulin test results. Diagnostic Med 8: 29–33

Kimmel JR, Smith EL (1954) Crystalline papain. I. Preparation, specificity and activation. J Biol Chem 207: 515

King MJ, Poole J, Anstee DJ (1989) An application of immunoblotting in the classification of the Miltenberger series of blood group antigens. Transfusion 29: 106–112

Kiruba R, Han P (1988) Quantitation of red cell-bound immunoglobulin and complement using enzyme-linked antiglobulin consumption assay. Transfusion 28: 519–542

Knowles SM, Milkins CE, Chapman JF et al. (2002) The United Kingdom National External Quality Assessment Scheme (Blood Transfusion Laboratory Practice): trends in proficiency and practice between 1985 and 2000. Transfus Med 12: 11–23

Kochwa S, Rosenfield RE (1964) Immunochemical studies of the Rh system. I. Isolation and characterization of antibodies. J Immunol 92: 682

Kozlowski CL, Lie D, Shwe KH et al. (1995) Quantification of anti-c in haemolytic case of the newborn. Transfus Med 5: 37–42

Lalezari P (1968) A new method for detection of red blood cell antibodies. Transfusion 8: 372

Lalezari P, Jiang AF (1980) The manual polybrene test: a simple and rapid procedure for detection of red cell antibodies. Transfusion 20: 206–211

Laine ML, Beattie KM (1985) Frequency of alloantibodies accompanying autoantibodies. Transfusion 25: 545–546

Lambert R, Edwards J, Anstee DJ (1978) A simple method for the standardization of proteolytic enzymes used in blood group serology. Med Lab Sci 35: 233

Lambin P, Ahaded A, Debbia M et al. (1998) An enzyme-linked immunosorbent assay for the quantitation of IgG anti-D and IgG subclasses in the sera of alloimmunized patients. Transfusion 38: 252–261

Landsteiner K, Miller CP (1925) Serological studies on the blood of the primates. II. The blood groups in anthropoid apes. J Exp Med 42: 853

Langlois RG, Bigbee WL, Jensen RH (1985) Flow cytometric characterization of normal and variant cells with monoclonal antibodies specific for glycophorin A. J Immunol 134: 4009–4017

Lapierre Y, Rigal D, Adam J et al. (1990) The gel test: a new way to detect red cell antigen-antibody reactions. Transfusion 30: 109–113

Lee E, Burgess G, Halverson GR et al. (2004) Applications of murine and humanized chimaeric monoclonal antibodies for red cell phenotyping. Br J Haematol 126: 277–281

Lee S, Wu X, Reid M et al. (1995a) Molecular basis of the Kell (K1) phenotype. Blood 85: 912–916

Lee S, Bennett PR, Overton T et al. (1996) Prenatal diagnosis of Kell blood group genotypes: KEL1 and KEL2. Am J Obstet Gynecol 175: 455–459

Lee TH, Donegan EA, Slichter S, Busch MP (1995b) Transient increase in circulating donor leukocytes after allogeneic transfusions in immunocompetent recipients compatible with donor cell proliferation. Blood 85: 1207–1214

Legler TJ, Eber SW, Lakomek M et al. (1999) Application of RHD and RHCE genotyping for correct blood group determination in chronically transfused patients. Transfusion 39: 852–855

Leikola J, Perkins HA (1980a) Red cell antibodies and low ionic strength: a study with enzyme-linked antiglobulin test. Transfusion 20: 224–228

Leikola J, Perkins HA (1980b) Enzyme-linked antiglobulin test: an accurate and simple method to quantify red cell antibodies. Transfusion 20: 138–144

Letendre PL, Williams MA, Ferguson DJ (1987) Comparison of a commercial hexadimethrine bromide method and low-ionic-strength solution for antibody detection with special reference to anti-K. Transfusion 27: 138–141

Lillevang ST, Georgsen J, Kristensen T (1994) An antibody screening test based on the antiglobulin gel technique, pooled test cells and plasma. Vox Sang 66: 210–215 van Loghem JJ, Kresner M, Coombs RRA *et al.* (1950) Observations on a prozone phenomenon encountered in using the anti-globulin sensitization test. Lancet ii: 729

Long KE, Yomtovian R, Kida M *et al.* (1993) Time-dependent loss of surface complement regulatory activity during storage of donor blood. Transfusion 33: 294–300

Louie *et al.* (1986) Preparation of intact antibody from red cells in autoimmune haemolytic anaemia (Abstract). Transfusion 26 (Suppl.): 550

Löw B (1955) A practical method using papain and incomplete Rh-antibodies in routine Rh blood-grouping. Vox Sang (OS) 5: 94

Löw B, Messeter L (1974) Antiglobulin test in low-ionic strength salt solution for rapid antibody screening and cross-matching. Vox Sang 26: 53

Lown JAG, Ivy JG (1988) Laboratory techniques. Polybrene technique for red cell antibody screening using microplates. J Clin Pathol 41: 556–557

McCullough JS, Torloni AS, Brecker ME *et al.* (1993) Microwave dissociation of anti-antibody complexes: a new elution technique to permit phenotyping of antibody-coated red cells. Transfusion 33: 725–729

MacDonald EB, Gerns LM (1986) The use of murine monoclonal antibodies in blood grouping. Abstracts, 19th Congr Int Soc Blood Transfus, Sydney

McHugh TM, Reid ME, Stites DP *et al.* (1987) Detection of the human erythrocyte surface antigen Gerbich by flow cytometry using human antibodies and phycoerythrin for extreme immunofluorescence sensitivity. Vox Sang 53: 231–234

McNeil G, Helmick WM, Ferrari A (1963) A preliminary investigation into automatic blood grouping. Vox Sang 8: 235

Malde R, Kelsall G, Knight RC *et al.* (1986) The manual low-ionic strength polybrene technique for the detection of red cell antibodies. Med Lab Sci 43: 360–363

Malyska H, Kleeman JE, Masouredis SP *et al.* (1983) Effects on blood group antigens from storage at low ionic strength in the presence of neomycin. Vox Sang 44: 375–384

Marsh WL (1972) Scoring of hemagglutination reaction. Transfusion 12: 352

Marsh WL, Nichols ME, Jenkins WJ (1968) Automated detection of blood group antibodies. J Med Lab Technol 25: 335

Matté C (1971) Le Groupamatic, appareil pour la détermination automatique des groupes sanguins. Proc 12th Congr Int Soc Blood Transfus, Moscow

Matuhasi T (1959) Plasma protein and antibody fractions observed from the serological point of view. Proc 15th Gen Assembly Jap Med Congr, Tokyo 4: 80

Mercuriali F, Inghilleri G, Colotti MT *et al.* (1996) Bedside transfusion errors: analysis of 2 years use of a system to monitor and prevent transfusion errors. Vox Sang 70: 16–21

Merry AH, Thomson EE, Rawlinson V *et al.* (1982) A quantitative antiglobulin test for IgG for use in blood transfusion serology. Clin Lab Haematol 4: 393–402

Merry AH, Thomson EE, Rawlinson VI *et al.* (1984) Quantitation of IgG on erythrocytes: correlation of number of IgG molecules per cell with the strength of the direct and indirect antiglobulin tests. Vox Sang 47: 73–81

Meryman HT (1956) Mechanics of freezing in living cells and tissues. Science 124: 515

Mintz PD, Anderson G (1985) Limitations of polybrene to detect ABO incompatibility (Abstract). Transfusion 25: 451

Miyata S, Kawai T, Yamamoto S *et al.* (2004) Network computer-assisted transfusion management system for accurate blood component-recipient identification at the bedside. Transfusion 44: 364–372

Mollison PL (1951) Blood Transfusion in Clinical Medicine. Oxford: Blackwell Scientific Publications

Mollison PL (1967) Blood Transfusion in Clinical Medicine, 4th edn. Oxford: Blackwell Scientific Publications

Mollison PL (1972) Blood Transfusion in Clinical Medicine, 5th edn. Oxford: Blackwell Scientific Publications

Mollison PL (1983) Blood Transfusion in Clinical Medicine, 7th edn. Oxford: Blackwell Scientific Publications

Molthan L, Strohm PL (1981) Hemolytic transfusion reaction due to anti-Kell undetectable in low-ionic-strength solution. Am J Clin Pathol 75: 629–631

Moore BPL, Hughes-Jones NC (1970) Automated assay of anti-D concentration in plasmapheresis donors. In: Advances in Automated Analysis. Technicon Int Congr, Chicago

Moore HC, Mollison PL (1976) Use of a low-ionic-strength medium in manual tests for antibody detection. Transfusion 16: 291

Moore HH (1984) Automated reading of red cell antibody identification tests by a solid phase antiglobulin technique. Transfusion 24: 218–221

Morel P, Vengelen-Tyler V (1979) LISS autoagglutinins of no apparent clinical significance (Abstract). Transfusion 19: 647

Moreschi C (1908) Neue Tatsachen über die Blutkörperchen Agglutinationen. Zbl Bakt 46: 49 and 456

Morton JA, Pickles MM (1947) Use of trypsin in the detection of incomplete anti-Rh antibodies. Nature (Lond) 159: 779

Motschman TL, Reisner RK, Taswell HF (1985) Evaluation of the antibody screen and crossmatch (Abstract). Transfusion 25: 451

Moulds JM, Rowe KE (1996) Neutralisation of Knops system antibodies using soluble complement receptor 1. Transfusion 36: 517–520

Moulds MM, Spruell P, Lomas C. *et al.* (1994) Experience in the use of a monoclonal polyspecific anti-human globulin reagent for antibody investigation. Vox Sang 67 (Suppl. 2): 121

347

Murphy MF, Kay JD (2004) Barcode identification for transfusion safety. Curr Opin Hematol 11: 334–338

Murphy MT, Fraser RH, Goddard JP (1996) Development of a PCR-based diagnostic assay for the determination of KEL genotype in donor blood samples. Transfus Med 6: 133–7

Myhre BA, Koepke JA, Polesky HF et al. (1977) The CAP blood bank comprehensive survey program: 1975. Am J Clin Pathol 68 (Suppl.) 175

Myhre BA, Demaniew S, Nelson EJ (1984) Preservation of red cell antigens during storage of blood with different anticoagulants. Transfusion 24: 499–501

Nance S, Garratty G (1984) Correlates between in vivo hemolysis and the amount of rbc bound IgG measured by flow cytometry (Abstract). Blood 64 (Suppl. 1): 88a

Nance SJ, Garratty G (1987) A new potentiator of red blood antigen-antibody reactions. Am J Clin Pathol 87: 633–635

Nathalang O, Chuansumrit A, Prayoonwiwat W et al. (1997) Comparison between conventional tube technique and the gel technique in direct antiglobulin tests. Vox Sang 72: 169–171

Oberman HA, Barnes BA, Friedman BA (1978) The risk of abbreviating the major crossmatch in urgent or massive transfusion. Transfusion 18: 137

Odell WR, Roxby DR, Ryall RG (1983) A LISS spin enzyme method for the detection of red cell antibodies and use in routine antibody screen procedures. Transfusion 23: 373–376

Ogasawara K, Mazda T (1989) Differences in substrate specificities for cysteine proteinases used in blood group serology, and the use of bromelain in a two-phase inhibitor technique. Vox Sang 57: 72–76

Ogata T, Matuhasi T (1964) Further observations on the problems of specific and cross reactivity of blood group antibodies. Proc 9th Congr Int Soc Blood Transfus, Mexico, 1962, p. 528

O'Hagan J, White J, Milkins CE et al. (1999) Direct agglutination crossmatch at room temperature (DRT): the results of a NEQAS (BTLP) Questionnaire. Transfus Med 6 (Suppl. 1): 42

Olujohungbe A, Hambleton I, Stephens L et al. (2001) Red cell antibodies in patients with homozygous sickle cell disease: a comparison of patients in Jamaica and the United Kingdom. Br J Haematol 113: 661–665

O'Neill P, Shulman IA, Simpson RB et al. (1986) Two examples of low ionic strength-dependent autoagglutinins with anti-Pr_a specificity. Vox Sang 50: 107–111

Oreskovic RT, Dumaswala UJ, Greenwalt TJ (1992) Expression of blood group antigens on red cell microvesicles. Transfusion 32: 848–849

Ottenberg R (1908) Transfusion and arterial anastomosis. Some experiments in arterial anastomosis and a study of transfusion with presentation of two clinical cases. Ann Surg 47: 486

Ottenberg R (1937) Reminiscences of the history of blood transfusion. J Mt Sinai Hosp 4: 264

Ottenberg R, Kaliski DJ (1913) Accidents in transfusion. Their prevention by preliminary blood examination: based on experience of one hundred and twenty-eight transfusions. JAMA 61: 2138

Parker PI, Scott Y, McArdle B et al. (1995) Automated blood grouping by gel technology. Br J Biomed Sci 52: 266–70

Pereira A, Monteagudo J, Rovira M et al. (1989) Anti-K1 of the IgA class associated with Morganella morganii infection. Transfusion 29: 549–551

Petty AC, Green CA, Poole J et al. (1997) Analysis of Knops blood group antigens on CR1(CD35) by the MAIEA test and by immunoblotting. Transfus Med 7: 55–62

Petz LD, Garratty G (1980) Acquired Immune Hemolytic Anemias. New York: Churchill Livingstone

Phillips P, Voak D (1996) Can pooled red cells be used for antibody screening of patients' specimens? Transfus Med 6: 320–323

Phillips P, Voak D, Knowles S et al. (1997) An explanation and the clinical significance of the failure of microcolumn tests to detect weak ABO and other antibodies. Transfus Med 7: 47–53

Phillips P, Voak D, Downie M et al. (1998) New reference reagent for the quality assurance of anti-D antibody detection. Transfus Med 8: 225–230

Phillips PK (1987) A preparation for calibrating the assay of the blood group antibody anti-c. Br J Haematol 65: 57–59

Phillips PK (1992) External quality assessment of blood grouping, antibody screening and crossmatch procedures within the United Kingdom. In: Quality Assurance in Transfusion Medicine. G Rock, MJ Seghatchian (eds), vol. 1. Boca Raton, FL: CRC Press

Phillips PK, Whitton CM (1993) Detection of anti-Fy^a, anti-D and anti-Jk^a in relation to the genotypes of the panel red cells. Report of a UK NEQAS survey. Transfus Med 3: 123–127

Pickles MM (1946) Effect of cholera filtrate on red cells as demonstrated by incomplete Rh antibodies. Nature (Lond) 158: 880

Pickles MM (1949) Haemolytic Disease of the Newborn. Oxford: Blackwell Scientific Publications

Pinkerton PH, Wood DE, Burnie KL et al. (1979) Proficiency testing in immunohematology in Ontario, Canada, 1975–1977. Am J Clin Pathol 72: 559–563

Pinkerton PH, Wood DE, Burnie KL et al. (1981) Proficiency testing in immunohaematology in Ontario, Canada 1977–1979. Clin Lab Haematol 3: 155–164

Pinkerton PH, Zuber ED, Barr RM et al. (1984) Sensitivity of routine blood bank methods for the detection of anti-D as determined during proficiency testing. Am J Clin Pathol 82: 326–329

Pinkerton PH, Zuber ED, Wood DE *et al.* (1985) Proficiency testing in immunohaematology in Ontario, Canada, and in the United Kingdom: a comparative study. J Clin Pathol 38: 570–574

Pinkerton PH, Chan R, Ward J *et al.* (1993a) Sensitivity of column agglutination technology in detecting unexpected red cell antibodies. Transfus Med 3: 275–279

Pinkerton PH, Ward J, Chan R *et al.* (1993b) An evaluation of a gel technique for antibody screening compared with a conventional table method. Transfus Med 3: 201–205

Plapp FV, Rachel JM, Simor CT (1986) Dipsticks for determining ABO blood groups. Lancet i: 1465–1466

Pollack W, Hager HJ, Hollenberger LL Jr (1962) The specificity of anti-human gamma globulin reagents. Transfusion 2: 17

Polley MJ, Mollison PL (1961) The role of complement in the detection of blood group antibodies. Special reference to the antiglobulin test. Transfusion 1: 9

Polley MJ, Mollison PL, Soothill JF (1962) The role of 19S gamma globulin blood group antibodies in the antiglobulin reaction. Br J Haematol 8: 149

Pondman KW, Rosenfield RE, Tallal L *et al.* (1960) The specificity of the complement antiglobulin test. Vox Sang 5: 297

Poole J, Giles CM (1982) Observations on the Anton antigen and antibody. Vox Sang 43: 220–222

Postoway N, Nance S, O'Neill P *et al.* (1985) Comparison of a practical differential agglutination procedure to flow cytometry in following the survival of transfused red cells (Abstract). Transfusion 25: 453

Rachel JM, Sinor LT, Beck ML *et al.* (1985) A solid-phase antiglobulin test. Transfusion 25: 24–26

Reckel RP, Harris J (1978) The unique characteristics of covalently polymerized bovine serum albumin solutions when used as antibody detection media. Transfusion 18: 397

Reich ML, Heilweil L, Fischel EE (1970) Complement preservation in citrated human blood. Transfusion 10: 14

Reid ME, Rios M, Powell VI *et al.* (2000a) DNA from blood samples can be used to genotype patients who have recently received a transfusion. Transfusion 40: 48–53

Reid ME, Rios M, Yazdanbakhsh K (2000b) Applications of molecular biology techniques to transfusion medicine. Semin Hematol 37: 166–176

Reid ME, Toy PT (1983) Simplified method for recovery of autologous red cells from transfused patients. Amer J Clin Path 79: 364–366

Reis KJ, Chachowski R, Cupido A *et al.* (1993) Column agglutination technology: the antiglobulin test. Transfusion 33: 639–643

Rekvig OP, Hannestad K (1977) Acid elution of blood group antibodies from intact erythrocytes. Vox Sang 33: 280

Renner SW, Horvanitz PH, Bachner P (1993) Wristband identification error reporting in 712 hospitals. Arch Pathol Lab Med 117: 573–577

Renton PH, Hancock JA (1964) A simple method of separating erythrocytes of different ages. Vox Sang 9: 183

Riley JZ, Ness PM, Taddie SJ *et al.* (1982) Detection and quantitation of fetal maternal hemorrhage utilizing an enzyme-linked antiglobulin test. Transfusion 22: 472–474

Rios M, Hue-Roye K, Storry JR *et al.* (2001) Molecular basis of the Dombrock null phenotype. Transfusion 41: 1405–1407

Roback JD, Barclay S, Hillyer CD (2004) Improved method for fluorescence cytometric immunohematology testing. Transfusion 44: 187–196

Roberts B (ed.) (1991) Standard Haematology Practice, vol. 1, on behalf of the British Committee for Standardisation in Haematology. Oxford: Blackwell Scientific Publications

Rochna E, Hughes-Jones NC (1965) The use of purified ^{125}I-labelled anti-γglobulin in the determination of the number of D antigen sites on red cells of different phenotypes. Vox Sang 10: 675

Romano EL, Hughes-Jones NC, Mollison PL (1973) Direct antiglobulin reaction in ABO-haemolytic disease of the newborn. BMJ i: 524

Rosenfield RE (1977) In memoriam Alexander S Wiener. Haematologia 11: 5

Rosenfield RE, Szymanski IO, Kochwa S (1964) Immunochemical studies of the Rh system: III. Quantitative hemagglutination that is relatively independent of source of Rh antigens and antibodies. Cold Spring Harb Symp Quant Biol 29: 427

Rosenfield RE, Berkman EM, Nusbacher J *et al.* (1971) Specific agglutinability of erythrocytes from whole blood stored at 4°C. Transfusion 11: 177

Rosenfield RE, Kochwa S, Kaczera Z (1976) Solid-phase serology for the study of human erythrocytic antigen-antibody reactions. Abstracts, 15th Congr Int Soc Blood Transfus, Paris, pp. 27–33

Rosenfield RE, Shaikh SH, Innella F *et al.* (1979) Augmentation of hemagglutination by low ionic conditions. Transfusion 19: 499–510

Rouger PH, Dosda F, Girard M *et al.* (1982) Étude de la sensibilité de l'antigène Yt^a aux enzymes protéolytiques. Rev Transfus Immunohématol 25: 45–47

Rozman P, Dovc T, Gassner C. (2000) Differentiation of autologous ABO, RHD, RHCE, KEL, JK, and FY blood group genotypes by analysis of peripheral blood samples of patients who have recently received multiple transfusions. Transfusion 40: 936–942

Salama A, Mueller-Eckhardt C (1982) Elimination of the prozone effect in the antiglobulin reaction by a simple modification. Vox Sang 42: 157–160

Sandler SG, Langeberg A, Avery N *et al.* (2000) A fully automated blood typing system for hospital transfusion services. ABS2000 Study group. Transfusion 40: 201–207

Satpathy GR, Torok Z, Bali R *et al.* (2004) Loading red blood cells with trehalose: a step towards biostabilization. Cryobiology 49: 123–136

Schaffner G, Kayser T, Tonjes A *et al.* (2003) Validation of flow cytometry to quantify the potency of anti-D immunoglobulin preparations. Vox Sang 84: 129–136

Schmitz N, Djibey I, Kretschmer V *et al.* (1981) Assessment of red cell autoantibodies in autoimmune haemolytic anaemia of warm type by a radioactive anti-IgG test. Vox Sang 41: 224–230

Scott ML (1991) The principles and applications of solid-phase blood group serology. Tranfus Med Rev 5: 60–72

Scott ML, Phillips PK (1987) Sensitive two-stage papain technique without cell washing. Vox Sang 52: 67–70

Scott ML, Whitton CM (1988) Standardization of papain reagents by measurement of active sites using a synthetic inhibitor, E-64. Transfusion 28: 24–28

Scott ML, Johnson CA, Phillips PK (1987) The pH optima for papain and bromelin treatment of red cells. Vox Sang 52: 223–227

Scott ML, Voak D, Phillips PK *et al.* (1994) Review of the problems involved in using enzymes in blood group serology: provision of freeze-dried ICSH/ISBT protease enzyme and anti-D reference standards. Vox Sang 67: 89–99

Scott Y, Parker P, McArdle B *et al.* (1996) Comparison of plasma and serum for antibody detection using DiaMed tubes. Transfus Med 6: 65–67

Selwyn JG, Seright W, Donald J *et al.* (1968) Matching blood for recipients of dextrans. Lancet ii: 1032

Shirey RG, Boyd JS, Ness PM (1994) Polyethylene glycol versus low-ionic-strength solution in pretransfusion testing: a blinded comparison study. Transfusion 34: 368–370

Shulman, IA, Calderon C (1991) Effect of delayed centrifugation or reading on the detection of ABO incompatibility by the immediate-spin crossmatch. Transfusion 31: 197–200

Shulman IA, Meyer EA, Lam HT *et al.* (1987) Additional limitations of the immediate spin crossmatch to detect ABO incompatibility (Letter). Am J Clin Pathol 87: 667

Sinor LT, Rachel JM, Beck ML *et al.* (1985) Solid-phase ABO grouping and Rh typing. Transfusion 25: 21–23

Slater JL, Griswold DJ, Wojtyniak LS *et al.* (1989) Evaluation of the polyethylene glycol-indirect antiglobulin test for routine compatibility testing. Transfusion 29: 686–688

Snyder EL, Hezzey A, Joyner R *et al.* (1983) Stability of red cell antigens during prolonged storage in citrate-phosphate-dextrose and a new preservative solution. Transfusion 23: 165–166

Sokol RJ, Hewitt S, Booker DJ *et al.* (1988) An enzyme-linked direct antiglobulin test for assessing erythrocyte bound immunoglobulins. J Immunol Methods 106: 31–35

Standard Haematology Practice (1991) Volume 1. B Roberts (ed.) on behalf of the British Committee for Standardisation in Haematology. Oxford: Blackwell Scientific Publications

Stapleton RR, Moore BPL (1959) A tube test for Rh typing using papain and incomplete anti-D. J Lab Clin Med 64: 640

Stratton F, Rawlinson VI (1976) C3 components on red cells under various conditions. In: The Nature and Significance of Complement Activation. Raritan, NJ: Ortho Research Institute

Stratton F, Rawlinson VI, Merry AH *et al.* (1983) Positive direct antiglobulin test in normal individuals. II. Clin Lab Haematol 5: 17–21

Sturgeon P, Smith LE, Chun HMT *et al.* (1979) Autoimmune hemolytic anemia associated exclusively with IgA of Rh specificity. Transfusion 19: 324–328

Taswell HF, Galbreath JL, Harmsen WS (1994) Errors in transfusion: detection, analysis, frequency and prevention. Arch Pathol Lab Med 118: 405–410

Thorpe SJ, Fox B, Sands D (2002) A stable lyophilised reagent for use in a potential reference assay for quantification of anti-D in immunoglobulin products. Biology 30: 315–321

Thorpe SJ, Fox B, Turner C *et al.* (2003a) Competitive enzyme-linked immunoassay of monoclonal immunoglobulin G anti-D preparations. Transfus Med 13: 153–159

Thorpe SJ, Sands D, Fox B *et al.* (2003b) A global standard for anti-D immunoglobulin. i. International collaborative study to evaluate a candidate preparation. Vox Sang 85: 313–321

Titlestad K, Georgsen J, Andersen H *et al.* (1997) Detection of irregular red cell antibodies: more than 3 years experience with a gel technique and pooled screening cells. Vox Sang 73: 246–251

Tovey GH (1974) Preventing the incompatible blood transfusion. Haematologia 8: 389

Travis GH, Salvesen GS (1983) Human plasma proteinase inhibitors. Annu Rev Biochem 52: 655–709

Trudeau LR, Judd WJ, Oberman HA *et al.* (1981) Is a room temperature crossmatch necessary for the detection of ABO errors? (Abstract). Transfusion 21: 625

Unger LJ (1921) Precautions necessary in selection of a donor for blood transfusion. JAMA 76: 9

Unger LJ (1951) A method for detecting Rh_0 antibodies in extremely low titer. J Lab Clin Med 37: 825

Utheman H, Poschmann A (1990) Solid-phase antiglobulin test for screening and identification of red cell antibodies. Transfusion 30: 114–116

Vengelen-Tyler V, Morel P (1979) Serological and IgG subclass characterization of multiple examples of Cartwright[a] (Yt[a]) and Gerbich antibodies (Abstract). Transfusion 19: 650

Voak D, Downie DM, Haigh T *et al.* (1982) Improved antiglobulin tests to detect difficult antibodies: detection of anti-Kell by LISS. Med Lab Sci 39: 363–370

Voak D, Downie DM, Moore BPL *et al.* (1986a) Anti-human globulin reagent specification. The European and ISBT/ICSH view. Biotest Bull 1: 7–22

Voak D, Downie DM, Moore BPL *et al.* (1986b) Quality control of anti-human globulin tests: use of replicate tests to improve performance. Biotest Bull 1: 41–52

Voak P, Dapier JAF, Boulton FE *et al.* (1990) Guidelines for microplate techniques in liquid-phase blood grouping and antibody screening. Clin Lab Haematol 12: 437–460

Voak P, Downie PM, Campbell G *et al.* (1991) Optimal specification of AHG and microplate IAM for antibody detection with greater sensitivity than the Diamed gel test (Abstract). Transfus Med (Suppl. 2), Abstract 37

Walker RH (1982) Is a crossmatch using the indirect antiglobulin test necessary for patients with a negative antibody screen. In: Safety in Transfusion Practices. HF Polesky, RH Walker (eds). Skokie, IL: College of American Pathologists

Wallas CH, Tanley PC, Gorrell LP (1980) Recovery of autologous erythrocytes in transfused patients. Transfusion 20: 332–336

Wallhermfechtel MA, Pohl B, Chaplin H (1984) Alloimmunization in patients with warm autoantibodies: a retrospective study employing 3 donor alloabsorptions to aid in antibody detection. Transfusion 24: 482–485

Wegmann TG, Smithies O (1966) A simple hemagglutination system requiring small amounts of red cells and antibodies. Transfusion 6: 67

Weil R (1915) Sodium citrate in the transfusion of blood. JAMA 64: 425

Wenk RE, Chiafari PA (1997) DNA typing of recipient blood after massive transfusion. Transfusion 37: 1108–1110

Wenz B, Apuzzo J, Shah DP (1990) Evaluation of the polyethylene glycol-potentiated indirect antiglobulin test. Transfusion 30: 318–321

White WD, Issitt CH. McGuire D (1974) Evaluation of the use of albumin controls in Rh phenotyping. Transfusion 14: 67

Wiener AS (1943) Blood Groups and Transfusion, 3rd edn. Springfield, IL: CC Thomas

van de Winkel JGJ, Tax WJM, Groeneveld A *et al.* (1988) A new radiometric assay for the quantitation of surface-bound IgG on sensitized erythrocytes. J Immunol Methods 108: 95–103

Wright J, Freedman J, Lim FC *et al.* (1979) Crossmatch difficulties following the prophylactic use of Rh immune globulin. Can Med Assoc J 120: 1235–1238

Wu GG, Jin SZ, Deng ZH *et al.* (2001) Polymerase chain reaction with sequence-specific primer-based genotyping of the human Dombrock blood group DO1 and DO2 alleles and the DO gene frequencies in Chinese blood donors. Vox Sang 81: 49–51

Zago-Novaretti MC, Pulley FL, Dorlhiac-Lacer PE *et al.* (1993) Use of the gel test to detect mixed red blood cell populations in bone marrow transplantation patients. Vox Sang 65: 161–162

The transfusion of red cells

The survival of transfused red cells

A human red cell, newborn and released into the circulation, has a lifespan of about 120 days. Transfused red cells also survive for long periods in the recipient's circulation. However, cells of different ages co-exist in the collection bag, so survival and lifespan are not interchangeable terms. Less than 1% of the red cells transfused are destroyed each day, which explains why red cell transfusion is so effective. Most cells are removed from circulation by the natural course of ageing; others meet a premature end as the result of chance destruction, disease-related debility or, in the case of transfusion, attack by alloantibodies.

Estimates of red cell survival are not often needed in clinical practice. However, they can be helpful when a compatibility problem arises, for example when serologically compatible red cells have been involved in a haemolytic transfusion reaction. In contrast, red cell recovery and survival studies continue to be essential in establishing the value of new methods of red cell preservation and modification.

Studies of red cell survival depend upon techniques for 'labelling' cells, either by injecting some isotopic precursor that will be taken up by a cohort of developing cells or more often by withdrawing an aliquot of cells of mixed age and applying some traceable marker. An ideal marker would label only the red cell, adhere tightly and unchanged for the duration of the study, prove non-toxic to the cell and the recipient, lack immunogenicity after repeated injections and, if radioactive, provide sufficient energy for detection and imaging without measurable risk to the patient. The labelling method should be easy and inexpensive. No

such label has been found. Instead, a variety of labels are available depending upon the requirements of the study. For most purposes, ^{51}Cr, an isotope with relatively low emission energy and a long half-life (27.7 days), has become the preferred red cell label. Nevertheless, because much of our present knowledge about the survival time of transfused red cells, compatible and incompatible, fresh and stored, was obtained by applying the method of differential agglutination (see Appendix 7), this method will be described, together with results observed when fresh normal compatible red cells are transfused to normal subjects.

Estimation of survival by antigenic differentiation

In 1911, a method for investigating the fate of red cells transfused from one animal to another was first described by Todd and White (1911). This technique consisted of preparing a serum that would haemolyse the red cells of one bull (Y), but not those of another bull (Z) *in vitro*. After transfusing blood from bull Z to bull Y, the mixture of cells in a sample from bull Y could be analysed by adding anti-Y serum; the recipient's (Y) cells were haemolysed and the intact cells of the donor (Z) were then counted.

Ashby (1919) applied this principle to the investigation of red cell survival in humans. After transfusing group O blood to group A recipients, she took blood samples and incubated them with anti-A serum; the A cells were agglutinated and the group O cells could be counted. Subsequently, differences within other blood group systems were used for the same purpose, including MN (Landsteiner *et al.* 1928) and Rh (Mollison and Young 1942; Wiener 1943).Differential agglutination can be used in two ways. Either the recipient's red cells can be agglutinated and the donor's red cells recognized by their failure to agglutinate ('indirect' differential agglutination) or the donor's red cells can be agglutinated using a serum that does not react with the recipient's red cells ('direct' differential agglutination) (Dekkers 1939).

'Indirect' differential agglutination (or haemolysis)

'Indirect' differential agglutination enables the number of surviving red cells to be counted. Provided that highly potent and specific antisera are used and that a sufficient number of red cells are counted, reliable quantitative estimates can be obtained. Visual counting with a cell chamber is accurate ($\pm$ 5%) if tedious, but the method can be automated with an impedance counter (Valeri *et al.* 1985).

Todd and White (1911) used haemolysis rather than agglutination to 'remove' the recipient's red cells. A useful modification, applicable to human blood when the recipient is group A and the donor O, was introduced by Mayer and D'Amaro (1964): the recipient's group A cells are lysed with the immune reagent and the remaining group O cells are then washed and lysed so that their number can be assessed spectrophotometrically. An improvement on this method, in which the mixture of red cells is labelled with ^{51}Cr before lysis, so that quantitative estimates can be obtained by radioactive counting, has been described (see seventh edition and Appendix 7).

Direct method of differential agglutination

Recognition of the survival of foreign red cells by directly agglutinating them with a serum that does not react with the recipient's own red cells is valuable chiefly in the retrospective investigation of suspected incompatibility (see Chapter 11). The method provides only semi-quantitative estimates of survival. The major weaknesses of differential agglutination are the inability to measure the survival of the subject's native cells, and the risk of inadvertent sensitization to antigens other than those of interest, which might lead to a spurious diagnosis of haemolysis (Adner *et al.* 1963).

Rosetting tests

These tests, most commonly used for detecting a small number of D-positive red cells in the circulation of a D-negative subject, are described in Chapter 12.

Use of flow cytometry

Using a suitable alloantibody and fluorescein-labelled anti-immunoglobulin G (IgG), red cell populations in a transfused subject can be identified directly or, indirectly, on the basis of antigenic differences.

As an example of direct identification, after transfusing C-positive red cells to a C-negative patient, blood samples from the recipient were treated with anti-C and then with fluorescein-conjugated anti-IgG; the C-positive cells were then quantified by passage through a flow cytometer (Garratty 1990). As an example of indirect identification, after injecting 10-ml of D-negative red cells to a D-positive patient, and treating samples as above but using anti-D, the non-fluorescent (D-negative) cells were counted (Issitt *et al.* 1990).

Survival of transfused red cells in normal subjects

When compatible red cells are transfused in therapeutic amounts, the number of surviving cells in the recipient's circulation diminishes steadily over a period of 110–120 days (Wiener 1934; Mollison and Young 1942; Callender *et al.* 1945), indicating that all red cells have the same lifespan. Transfused blood is then presumed to contain cells of all ages, in equal numbers: approximately one-hundredth of the total number is 1 day old, another hundredth 2 days old, and so on. Thus, on each day after transfusion, one-hundredth of the number reaches the end of its lifespan and disappears from the circulation.

In males, the survival curve was found to be linear, from which it may be deduced that normally little or no random destruction of red cells occurs. In females, survival was curvilinear, indicating some random loss. Although menstruation seems the most likely cause of this loss, the complicated mathematical treatment of the data suggests that additional factors may be involved (Callender *et al.* 1947).

As there is normally little or no random loss in males, the survival time is determined by donor rather than by recipient factors. In one careful study, red cells from two donors were transfused, in each case to three recipients, and found to have 'potential lifespans' (after correction for any random loss detected) of 114 (± 8) and 129 (± 5) days respectively (Eadie and Brown 1955). For other estimates, see below. Derivation of mean red cell lifespan from red cell survival curves is described in Appendix 6.

The hypothesis that red cells have a more or less constant lifespan implies that after a certain period in the circulation the red cells become susceptible to some physiological removal mechanism. The nature of such a mechanism is discussed below.

Methods of separating red cells according to age

Separation by density. As a unit of blood contains cells of all ages, separation of a cohort of young cells ('neocytes') that circulate longer than average could extend the interval between transfusions and decrease total transfusions and transfusional iron overload (Propper 1982). Although this concept has not yet resulted in successful therapy, efforts to separate young cells by density gradient methods continue (Simon *et al.* 1989; Spanos *et al.* 1996). The densest red cells in normal human blood have an MCV of 86.7 fl, compared with 91.7 fl for unselected cells and 99.3 fl for the lightest cells (Vincenzi and Hinds 1988). Red cell density increases throughout the lifespan of red cells. When ^{59}Fe was administered to normal human subjects and blood samples were taken at intervals and centrifuged, the ^{59}Fe was found in increased amounts in the lightest cells for about the first 20 days; the ratio of ^{59}Fe in the top:bottom layers equalized between days 20 and 50, and fell below unity between 50 and 90 days. After 90 days, ^{59}Fe began to reappear in the top layer as a result of label re-utilization (Borun *et al.* 1957). Similarly, when cohorts of red cells were labelled in rabbits, using glycine-2–^{14}C, and fractions were separated in a discontinuous gradient of bovine serum albumin (BSA), the glycine was found in progressively denser fractions. By day 60, all was in the lowest 50% and most was in the lowest 10% (Piomelli *et al.* 1967).

In rabbits, the survival of red cells *in vivo* diminishes with increasing cell density. For example, the time after injection of labelled cells for ^{51}Cr survival to fall to 10% varied as follows: top 10% of centrifuged cells, 56 days; unfractionated cells, 42 days; bottom 10%, 28 days (Piomelli 1978). Red cells were separated on an arabino-galactose gradient. In another study in which red cells were separated by simple centrifugation, ^{51}Cr survival was also longer (T_{50}Cr 11.2 days) for cells from the top fraction than for unselected cells (T_{50}Cr 9.6 days), and was very much shorter (3.6 days) for cells from the bottom fraction (Gattegno *et al.* 1975).

In human red cells separated on a self-forming Percoll gradient, a relationship has also been demonstrated between increasing red cell density and (1) an increase in the band 4.1a:4.1b ratio and (2) loss of maximum deformability, both of which have previously been shown to be related to red cell age (for 4.1a:4.1b, see below). The content of the complement receptor CR1 and cell membrane complement regulator, decay-accelerating factor (DAF), diminished linearly with increasing density, and both were about 50% lower in dense compared with light cells (Lutz *et al.* 1992).

Despite the foregoing evidence, many investigators contend that, apart from the low density of very young red cells, no clear relationship exists between red cell density and age, as measured by ^{59}Fe (Luthra *et al.* 1979) or both ^{59}Fe and HbA$_{1c}$ (van der Vegt *et al.* 1985a) as age markers. Similarly, using biotin to tag circulating red cells in rabbits and using avidin to separate cells labelled 50 days previously, the densest fraction was only two to three times enriched in old cells (Dale and Norenberg 1990). The most likely explanation for the discrepant views seems to be that the precise method used to separate red cells by density makes a big difference to the results obtained. Although the results of Gattegno and co-workers cited above indicate that red cells can be separated by age by simple centrifugation, the results of others suggest that for such separation density gradient separation is essential (Piomelli *et al.* 1967).

Separation by volume. Red cells can be separated by volume using countercurrent centrifugation. Using ^{59}Fe and HbA$_{1c}$ as markers, this method achieves a linear separation by age. With elutriation, mean cell volume (MCV) is found to fall linearly with age, whereas mean corpuscular Hb concentration (MCHC) remains constant, indicating that red cells lose Hb during ageing; the loss of Hb has been estimated to be as high as 25% during the lifetime of the red cell (van der Vegt *et al.* 1985a). Shedding of Hb-containing vesicles is likely to be responsible for Hb loss (Lutz 1978; Dumaswala and Greenwalt 1984). Cell size can also be determined by flow cytometric analysis of the forward light scatter (Mullaney et al. 1969). Using this method, red cells have been shown to lose A and B antigens with ageing (Fibach and Sharon 1994).

Although red cell surface area decreases with ageing, cell volume decreases even more. Thus, the ratio of surface area to volume increases and osmotic fragility decreases (van der Vegt et al. 1985b).

Obtaining old red cells by suppressing erythropoiesis

In animal experiments, populations of old red cells have been obtained by giving fortnightly transfusions of red cells from donors of the same inbred strain of rats. Every 2 weeks, some of the hypertransfused animals were sacrificed to obtain blood for transfusion to others. By keeping the recipients polycythaemic, haematopoiesis was suppressed and contamination with reticulocytes was minimized. As cell ageing progressed, there was a steady reduction in MCV and some loss of Hb from the cells (Ganzoni et al. 1971).

In other experiments in which this method was used, although in mice rather than rats, after 8 weeks the $t_{1/2}$ of the red cells had fallen from the normal 15 days to < 1 day. The most obvious alteration in membrane proteins was an increase in the 4.1a:4.1b ratio, a change postulated to be due to the conversion of 4.1b to 4.1a as cells age. In the mouse, cell density did not increase significantly with age (Mueller et al. 1987).

Some differences between young and old red cells

Using all of the three methods of separation described above, MCV has been found to diminish steadily with ageing.

The content of some red cell enzymes, hexokinase for example, is much higher in reticulocytes than in mature red cells and falls rapidly as the reticulum is lost, although some activity persists throughout the red cell lifespan (Zimran et al. 1990). With other enzymes, for example pyruvate kinase, the loss is slow and progressive throughout the red cell lifespan. These kinetics make pyruvate kinase a reliable marker for red cell age.

The densest red cells, with a specific gravity of more than 1.110, display autologous IgG on their surface that can be eluted by heating to 47°C. The IgG is an autoantibody to terminal galactosyl residues that are normally hidden by membrane sialic acid. These residues are exposed on the densest red cells and can be exposed on lighter cells by treating the cells with a suitable proteolytic enzyme (Alderman et al. 1980, 1981). Only 4% of the circulating red cells have a specific gravity of more than 1.110 and only these cells give a positive direct antiglobulin test (DAT) (Khansari 1983). These observations have been interpreted to mean that red cell ageing is associated with progressive loss of cell membrane, leading to exposure of normally hidden structural components ('cryptantigens') for which there are naturally occurring antibodies in the serum. The autoantibody-coated red cells become bound to, and subsequently engulfed by, tissue macrophages.

There is also a correlation between increasing red cell density and loss of DAF (see above) and C8-binding protein, both of which are deficient in red cells from patients with paroxysmal nocturnal haemoglobinuria, leading to the speculation that aged red cells may disintegrate through complement-mediated lysis (Ueda et al. 1990). On the other hand, even the densest red cells are far from a pure sample of the oldest cells and evidence from methods other than density separation is needed before the mechanism by which senescent red cells are removed from the circulation can be established (Beutler 1988).

Variation in lifespan within a population of red cells

The hypothesis that in healthy subjects all red cells live for about 110–120 days is doubtless an oversimplification. For one thing, existing data are insufficiently precise to distinguish between a strictly linear disappearance slope and one that is slightly curvilinear, although data obtained both with differential agglutination and with di-isopropyl-^{32}P-phosphofluoridate (DF^{32}P) labelling suggest that the slope may be very close to linear in most males.

When survival curves are approximately linear, a small variation in red cell lifespan will be revealed by a 'tail' at the end of the curve (see Fig. 9.1 for an example). If the linear portion of the slope, i.e. up to about 80 days, is extrapolated to the time axis the standard deviation of red cell lifespan can be deduced by the proportion of red cells surviving at this time (Dornhorst 1951). Estimates made in this

355

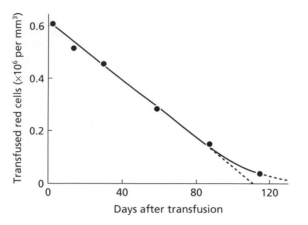

Fig 9.1 Survival of transfused red cells in a male adult. Until elimination of the cells is almost complete, the points fall on a slope that is linear or slightly curvilinear. If the slope is assumed to be linear, mean cell life, estimated by extrapolation of the line to the time axis, is 114 days. The persistence of a few transfused cells beyond 114 days is due to variation in red cell lifespan (see text).

way suggest that the standard deviation of lifespan may be as short as 6 days in normal subjects (first edition, p. 104). Obvious 'tails' can be seen in some published curves (Eadie and Brown 1955; Szymanski *et al.* 1968).

The effect of splenectomy

Following splenectomy, red cell survival has been found to be normal in humans and rabbits (Miescher 1956a; McFadzean *et al.* 1958), although slightly prolonged in rats (Belcher and Harris 1959). Splenectomy prolongs the survival of red cells with disordered membrane proteins; however, red cell survival differs depending on the specific hereditary defect (Reliene *et al.* 2002).

The effect of plethora

Although it is sometimes tacitly assumed that subjects rendered plethoric by transfusion suffer increased destruction of red cells, in fact no evidence of this exists. In newborn infants with a packed cell volume (PCV) as high as 0.64 after transfusion the survival of transfused red cells is normal (Mollison 1943, 1951, p. 111).

Estimation of survival using ^{51}Cr

Red cells can be labelled with ^{51}Cr by incubating them with radioactive sodium chromate (Gray and Sterling 1950). Radioactive chromate diffuses through the membrane via the band 3 anion channel and binds predominantly to the β-chains of Hb (Pearson and Vertrees 1961).

The method of ^{51}Cr labelling has two great advantages over that of differential agglutination: (1) the subject's own red cells can be labelled; and (2) the survival of very small volumes (0.1 ml or less) of red cells can be studied. Furthermore, sites of red cell sequestration can be identified using surface counting, the degree of intravascular haemolysis can be estimated in short-term tests (see Chapter 10), and blood loss in the stools can be estimated. ^{51}Cr liberated from red cells, destroyed either within the bloodstream or within the mononuclear phagocyte system, is not re-utilized. Unfortunately, the ^{51}Cr method suffers from several serious disadvantages: survival curves have to be corrected for leakage (elution) of ^{51}Cr from intact cells to obtain estimates of true red cell survival. Furthermore, the high doses required for detection and the long half-life all place limitations on serial survival studies and scanning for sites of sequestration. Serial recovery studies are possible if the first is performed with a low dose (5 uCi); successively higher doses are used with the subsequent re-infusions, and adjustment for background is made in the analysis.

^{51}Cr elutes from red cells at the rate of approximately 1% per day (Ebaugh *et al.* 1953). In addition, during the first 2 or 3 days (mainly during the first 24 h) there is additional, so-called 'early loss' (Mollison and Veall 1955) so that normal ^{51}Cr survival at 24 h is only about 96% (instead of about 98%) of the 10-min value (see below). The rate at which ^{51}Cr elutes from red cells is affected by the technique of labelling (Mollison 1961a; Szymanski and Valeri 1970). With studies of stored red cells, 24-h survival data are expressed without correcting for elution (Moroff *et al.* 1999).

Two methods of labelling have been shown to give similar results, namely the 'citrate wash' method (Mollison 1961b; Garby and Mollison 1971) and an acid–citrate–dextrose (ACD) method in which packed red cells are labelled (Bentley *et al.* 1974). Both of these methods have been recommended by ICSH (1971, 1980), but the ACD method is more convenient and

Table 9.1 Mean Cr survival in normal subjects and correction factors which convert the Cr survival into 'true' red cell survival (mean red cell lifespan 115 days) when the 'citrate wash' method is used (Garby and Mollison 1971)*.

Day	Cr survival	Correction factor	Day	Cr survival	Correction factor
0	100.0		16	70.7	1.22
1	96.2	1.03	17	69.3	1.23
2	94.0	1.05	18	67.8	1.25
3	92.0	1.06	19	66.3	1.26
4	90.1	1.07	20	64.9	1.27
5	88.2	1.08	21	63.4	1.29
6	86.5	1.10	22	62.0	1.31
7	84.7	1.11	23	60.5	1.32
8	83.1	1.12	24	59.1	1.34
9	81.4	1.13	25	57.6	1.36
10	79.9	1.14	26	56.2	1.38
11	78.3	1.16	27	54.7	1.40
12	76.7	1.17	28	53.3	1.42
13	75.2	1.18	29	51.9	1.45
14	73.7	1.19	30	50.4	1.47
15	72.2	1.20			

* Note that although the T_{50}Cr with this method of labelling is on the average just over 30 days, with some other methods it may be shorter.

The values in the table were reproduced in ICSH (1971). Almost identical values were obtained by Bentley *et al.* (1974) using the method of labelling described in Appendix 2.

has therefore been selected as the reference method (see Appendix 2 for details). Table 9.1 gives values for ^{51}Cr survival obtained using the citrate wash method. The table also gives factors that convert observed ^{51}Cr values on any particular day to true red cell survival, assuming that the normal mean lifespan is 115 days. The results thus corrected for ^{51}Cr elution are then analysed as described in Appendix 6.

Using the ACD method recommended by ICSH, similar correction factors were derived. This finding is reassuring, because the factors were derived from a comparison between the results of ^{51}Cr and di isopropyl phosphofluoridate (DFP) labelling, whereas the factors given in Table 9.1 were obtained by comparing ^{51}Cr results with those expected from normal survival. Furthermore, the figures in Table 9.1 were derived from the survival of allogeneic red cells, whereas those of Bentley and co-workers were based on autologous red cell survival.

In another recommended method, after incubating ACD or CPD blood with $Na_2{}^{51}CrO_4$, ascorbic acid is added to reduce hexavalent ^{51}Cr to the trivalent form and thus stop any further uptake, and the whole

mixture is then injected. However, after 15 min of incubation of red cells with $Na_2{}^{51}CrO_4$ at 37°C, uptake of ^{51}Cr is virtually arrested, even when ascorbic acid is not added, so that the value of adding ascorbic acid is doubtful. The disadvantage of the method compared with methods in which washed red cells are injected is that accurate estimates of red cell volume require that the amount of ^{51}Cr in the supernatant of the injection suspension be measured and allowed for. Also, even when only red cell survival is being measured, the amount of ^{51}Cr in the plasma of samples drawn within the first 24 h must be estimated. Finally, ascorbate may damage red cells with certain metabolic abnormalities, particularly those with glucose-6-phosphate dehydrogenase deficiency (Beutler 1957).

Half-life ($T_{1/2}$) is not an accurate term to describe red cell survival kinetics. The curvilinear slope of ^{51}Cr survival in normal subjects cannot be fitted by a simple exponential and the time taken for survival to fall to 50% of its original value should be expressed as the T_{50} ('half-survival'), not the $T_{1/2}$.

The mean normal T_{50}Cr is about 31 days and in 95% of healthy subjects falls within the range 25–37 days

357

Table 9.2 Relation between $T_{50}Cr$, derived red cell lifespan and relative rate of Cr elution is normal, i.e. about 1% per day) (from Mollison 1981).

$T_{50}Cr$ (days)	Mean red cell life span (days)	Rate of red cell destruction
31	115	×1
23	54*	×2
18	38*	×3
14	27*	×4

* Destruction assumed to be random.

(Mollison 1981). When $T_{50}{}^{51}Cr$ is less than 25 days it is best to correct results for ^{51}Cr elution and deduce mean red cell lifespan (ICSH 1971, 1980) using the method of analysis described in Appendix 6. As Table 9.2 shows, the $T_{50}{}^{51}Cr$ is not a satisfactory index of red cell destruction as it bears no simple relation to mean red cell lifespan.

Note that when ^{51}Cr survival is within normal limits, correction factors should not be applied in the hope of securing a good estimate of true red cell survival. When survival is within normal limits, the daily loss of ^{51}Cr by elution is approximately equal to the daily loss of red cells and variations in the rate of ^{51}Cr elution therefore have a relatively large effect on the estimate of true survival.

The rate of ^{51}Cr elution in healthy subjects was found to vary from 0.70% to 1.55% per day (mean 1.0, SD 0.07) by Bentley and co-workers (1974). In patients with haematological diseases, values of between 0.6% and 2.3% per day were found by Cline and Berlin, and between 0.6% and 2.0% by Garby and Mollison (Cline and Berlin 1962; Garby and Mollison 1971). These figures for the variability of elution must somewhat overestimate the true variability, as they are derived from a comparison of estimates of ^{51}Cr and DFP survival and are thus affected by the error of both estimates.

In a wide variety of diseases, estimation of red cell lifespan based on ^{51}Cr measurements corrected for elution agrees well with DFP measurements (Eernisse and van Rood 1961; Finke *et al.* 1965; Garby and Mollison 1971). As expected, though, the ^{51}Cr method is insensitive in detecting slight increases in red cell destruction (Cline and Berlin 1963b; Finke *et al.* 1965).

Early loss. There is a great deal of evidence that 'early loss' of ^{51}Cr is not due to damage to red cells during labelling or washing; the extent of the loss is not related to the dose of ^{51}Cr used, nor to the number of times the cells have been washed. Moreover, the same early loss is observed when red cells are labelled *in vivo* by injecting a small dose of $Na_2{}^{51}CrO_4$ intravenously (Hughes-Jones and Mollison 1956). Further evidence was supplied by Kleine and Heimpel (1965) in experiments in which red cells were labelled with $DF^{32}P$ in a donor from whom a sample was taken 48 h later. The cells were now also labelled with ^{51}Cr. After cell injection into a recipient, the loss of ^{51}Cr exceeded that of $DF^{32}P$ by about 5% in 24 h. Presumably, 'early loss' is due to the relatively loose binding of a small fraction of ^{51}Cr.

Toxic effect of chromate on red cells

$Na_2{}^{51}CrO_4$ is available with a specific activity of 7×10^9 Bq (20 mCi)/mg. Even when 2 mBq of ^{51}Cr is used to label as little as 0.2 ml of red cells, the dosage of chromate, expressed as the dose of ^{51}Cr, will only be about 5 µg/ml of red cells. No effect on red cell survival has been noted at doses up to 20 µg ^{51}Cr/ml cells, although abnormal survival curves have been found when 35 µg ^{51}Cr/ml cells or more are used (Donohue *et al.* 1955; Hughes-Jones and Mollison 1956).

^{51}Cr survival in the very young and the very old

Red cells of newborn infants. The following values for the $T_{50}{}^{51}Cr$ have been recorded: 20 days (Hollingsworth 1955); 22.8 days compared with 27.5 for adults (Foconi and Sjölin 1959); 24 days compared with 30 days for adults (Gilardi and Miescher 1957); 17.5 days compared with 25 days for adults (E Giblett, unpublished observations, 1955). The $T_{50}{}^{51}Cr$ of red cells from premature infants injected into adults was found to be 15.8 days by Foconi and Sjölin (Foconi and Sjölin 1959) and to be 16 days by Gilardi and Miescher (1957).

In children aged 2.5 years or more. ^{51}Cr survival is the same as in adults (Remenchik *et al.* 1958).

^{51}Cr red cell survival in elderly subjects. ^{51}Cr red cell survival was found to be normal in five patients aged 70–90 years by Miescher and co-workers (1958),

in 10 men and 12 women aged 80–94 years by Woodfield-Williams and co-workers (Woodfield *et al.* 1986), and in 11 subjects aged 70–90 years by Hurdle and Rosin (1962).

Use of non-radioactive chromium (^{52}C). Human red cells contain about 0.8 µg ^{51}Cr/l cells. Following incubation with $Na_2{}^{52}CrO_4$, i.e. ordinary non-radioactive sodium chromate, they readily take up large amounts of ^{51}Cr. Although glutathione reductase is slightly inhibited at ^{51}Cr levels as low as 2 µg/ml of red cells, no effect on red cell survival has been noted at levels up to 20 µg/ml of cells (see above). Following the injection of about 20 ml of packed red cells labelled with a total of about 40 µg of ^{51}Cr (2 µg/ml of red cells), in a subject with a total circulating red cell volume of 2 l, the concentration of Cr is expected to be 20 µg/l of cells, i.e. 20 times the normal level. Using Zeeman electrothermal adsorption spectrophotometry, with a graphite furnace attachment, Cr concentrations between 1 and 7 µg/l can be estimated with a coefficient of variation of 4.7% (Heaton *et al.* 1989a). When red cell volume was estimated using ^{52}Cr, results were similar to those observed with ^{51}Cr-labelled red cells or with estimates deduced from plasma volume. Similarly, estimates of the 24-h survival of stored red cells agree with those based on ^{51}Cr labelling (Heaton *et al.* 1989a,b). In another study, in which red cells in 130 ml of blood was labelled with a total of 250 µg of ^{52}Cr, and results compared with those obtained with ^{51}Cr in the same subjects, the $T_{50}Cr$ values by the two methods were almost identical (Sioufi *et al.* 1990). Although the idea of using non-radioactive Cr is attractive, the need to use relatively large volumes of red cells, the somewhat elaborate technology and the relative inaccuracy make the method in its present form less attractive than the use of ^{51}Cr.

Other methods of random labelling of red cells

Use of di-isopropyl phosphofluoridate

Di-isopropyl phosphofluoridate (DFP) binds to a serine residue of membrane cholinesterase in red cells and other cells such as platelets, and also binds to plasma cholinesterase. DFP has been used to label red cells *in vitro*, using ^3H-DFP (Cline and Berlin 1963a) or $DF^{32}P$ (Bratteby and Wadman 1968). With the latter, as the maximum amount of DFP that binds

irreversibly to red cells is about 0.15 µg/ml cells and as the maximum available specific activity of $DF^{32}P$ is about 400 µCi/mg (14.8 MBq/mg), at least 50 ml of red cells must be labelled if not less than 2 µCi (74 kBq) are to be injected. In most experiments, $DF^{32}P$ has been injected intravenously, thus labelling the whole red cell mass. Some 4% of the label is lost in the first 24 h, probably as a result of the labelling process, but thereafter no loss is detectable. Some of the loss in the first 24 h may be due to labelling of leucocytes and platelets, but almost all the injected $DF^{32}P$ is bound by red cells. Using a linear fit, estimates of mean red cell lifespan have been close to 120 days (Cohen and Warringa 1954; Bove and Ebaugh 1958; Garby 1962; Heimpel *et al.* 1964; Bentley *et al.* 1974).

Biotinylation

Biotin is a water-soluble member of the vitamin B complex and is found predominantly within the cell. Biotin has a very high binding affinity for avidin, a protein found in egg white and in bacteria. The binding between biotin and avidin is rapid and sufficiently tight as to be irreversible for weeks. The unusually high binding constant between biotin and avidin allows red cells that have been labelled with biotin to be diluted after injection *in vivo* and subsequently quantified accurately with avidin tagged with either a radioactive isotope or a fluorochrome such as fluorescein. When rabbit red cells were treated in this way, estimates of red cell survival were similar to those obtained with ^{14}C-cyanate (Suzuki and Dale 1987). The method has been applied to the selective extraction of aged red cells from the circulation of rabbits whose red cells were labelled 50 days beforehand to investigate the relationship between red cell age and density (Dale and Norenberg 1990).

In a study in which human red cells were labelled with biotin *in vitro* and then used to estimate total circulating red cell volume, estimates agreed well, in most cases, with simultaneous estimates made with ^{51}Cr. Cavill and co-workers (1988) found biotin labelling unsuitable for estimating red cell survival: in some cases all of the label disappeared within 1 week, a result that was associated with the subject's recent consumption of eggs, which are rich in avidin. On the other hand, biotin has been used to label murine red cells both *in vitro* and *in vivo*, giving similar values for red cell lifespan (Hoffman-Fezer *et al.* 1993). Mock

359

and co-workers (1999) found biotin labelling to be an accurate method to measure red cell survival in humans. A major advantage of the method is absence of exposure to radiation, which makes it particularly suitable for infants and for gravid women. However, biotin labelling does alter red cell antigens (Cowley *et al.* 1999). Furthermore, 3 out of 20 subjects who had labelling studies performed developed transient IgG antibodies directed against biotin-coated red cells (Cordle *et al.* 1999). As yet the clinical significance of these antibodies is unknown, as is the chance that they will limit the use of this method for serial survival studies.

^{99m}Tc and ^{111}In

Technetium (^{99m}Tc) is a useful label for red cell volume determinations (see below), but its short half-life and elution characteristics make it unsuitable for recovery studies, let alone determination of red cell survival. Indium (^{111}In) has been used as a red cell label, but it elutes more readily and less predictably than does ^{51}Cr which makes it somewhat less accurate (AuBuchon and Brightman 1989). However, its higher emission energy permits imaging of the site of cell sequestration when that is desired with a lower dose than that of ^{51}Cr.

Use of Hb differences between donor and recipient

The survival of normal red cells transfused to patients with haemoglobinopathies, particularly sickle cell and HbC disease, can be studied by preparing haemolysates, separating normal from abnormal Hb by electrophoresis and estimating the amount of each type. Like the method of differential agglutination, this method is particularly useful when the decision to estimate red cell survival is made after transfusion. It can also be used when, because of serological similarities between donor and recipient, differential agglutination is impracticable. The method has the added advantage of not involving exposure to radio-activity (Restrepo and Chaplin 1962). Automated analysis can now distinguish Hb variants and detect small differences extremely accurately (Mario *et al.* 1997).

Methods of labelling a 'cohort' of red cells

By a 'cohort' is meant a population produced over a limited period of time. Cohort labelling is primarily an investigative tool for determining normal red cell lifespan and reduction of survival in hereditary red cell disorders. A cohort of cells can be labelled by pulse injection of the iron isotope ^{59}Fe to normal subjects and withdrawal of a blood sample about 5 days later. However, an unacceptably large amount of radioactivity has to be used and extensive re-utilization of iron occurs with this method (Ricketts *et al.* 1977).

Reticulocytes will take up iron *in vitro* (Walsh *et al.* 1949) and cells labelled in this way have been used successfully to demonstrate the destruction of red cells by alloantibodies and to investigate the subsequent fate of the labelled Hb (Jandl *et al.* 1957).

Use of ^{15}N-labelled glycine and of ^{14}C-labelled compounds

A subject's own red cells can be labelled by administering oral ^{15}N-glycine, the glycine being incorporated into the haem of newly synthesized Hb. The concentration of labelled nitrogen per unit mass of red cells does not reach its peak for about 25 days, begins to fall on about the eightieth day and then declines steeply. The interval between the mid-point of the rise and the declining portion of the graph was determined to be 127 days, and this value was defined as the average lifetime of the cells (Shemin 1946).

Although it was originally believed that Hb, and thus ^{15}N, could not be lost from intact red cells, the decrease in labelled haem which began about 60 days after peak values had been reached suggests that label is, in fact, lost (Mollison 1961a, p. 173). There is now direct evidence that red cells lose Hb during their lifespan (van der Vegt *et al.* 1985b). Because of the relatively slow incorporation of labelled haem, the loss of label from intact red cells and the re-utilization of the label, measurements with ^{15}N-glycine, although providing valuable information about Hb metabolism, do not add anything important to knowledge of the lifespan of human red cells. Measurements with glycine-2–^{14}C in human subjects (Berlin *et al.* 1954) indicate that the method is open to the same criticisms that apply to the ^{15}N method.

Use of DF^{32}P

Cohort labelling with DF^{32}P was achieved by first injecting a large dose of unlabelled DFP to produce a temporary block of further uptake, and 6–9 days later,

Table 9.3 Survival of allogeneic and autologous red cells labelled with ^{51}Cr (Mollison 1981).

Donors[†]		Recipients		Cr survival at 28 days (%)	
Sex (initials)	No.	No. of studies		Mean	SD
*Allogeneic red cells**					
F (M.S.)	18	18		53.4	5.1
F (M.L.)	8	11		58.4	4.4
F (K.B.)	9	18		51.4	4.1
M (H.S.)	14	14		55.2	4.5
Autologous red cells[†]	13	13		52.5	

* All recipients of allogeneic cells were D-negative 'non-responder' males; for sources of data see text.
[†] Cr survival at 28 days deduced from the data of Bentley *et al.* (1974).

when new (unblocked) red cells had been produced, injecting DF^{32}P. Using this method, red cells produced in response to acute blood loss were shown to have a survival time which was distinctly shorter than that of normal red cells (Neuberger and Niven 1951; Cline and Berlin 1962).

Summary of normal survival of red cells

There are several reasons why generally acceptable values for the mean and range of true red cell survival in normal subjects have not yet been established: the number of studies is not large, many different techniques have been used and, perhaps above all, the data have been interpreted in many different ways. The main difficulty is that the disappearance curve of the red cells is not, as a rule, defined with sufficient precision so that it is usually not possible to determine whether the points should be fitted by a straight line or a curvilinear slope. Even a minor degree of curvilinearity implies a substantially lower mean survival time (Mills 1946). Accordingly, if a straight line is fitted to points that really fall on a slightly curvilinear slope, mean cell life is overestimated.

The survival of transfused (allogeneic) red cells differs little if at all from that of autologous red cells, as shown by the close similarity of results obtained with differential agglutination and (using autologous red cells) with DF^{32}P. The same point is made in Table 9.3, which compares the survival of ^{51}Cr-labelled allogeneic and autologous red cells. All the estimates for allogeneic cells are of the survival of D-positive red cells from one of four donors in selected D-negative

recipients who failed to make anti-D after at least two injections of D-positive red cells given at an interval of 5–6 months and were judged to be non-responders (Mollison 1981). The figure for the survival of autologous red cells is deduced from the data of Bentley and co-workers (1974).

Rapid destruction of transfused red cells in certain haemolytic anaemias

The shorter the red cell survival, the less important are the technical inaccuracies of the labelling method. In all of those conditions in which a haemolytic anaemia is due to some extrinsic mechanism rather than to any intrinsic red cell defect, transfused normal red cells are expected to undergo accelerated destruction. Nevertheless, if the donor's red cells are compatible with the autoantibody in the recipient's circulation, their survival may be almost normal (see Chapter 7). In haemolytic anaemia associated with potent cold autoagglutinins, when normal (I-positive) red cells are transfused, they undergo rapid destruction until the C3 bound to them by anti-I has been cleaved, leaving only C3d,g on their surface (see Chapter 10).

Diminished survival of transfused red cells in aplastic anaemia

In aplastic anaemia, the survival of the patient's own red cells is usually moderately reduced and this reduction is not due to haemorrhage (Lewis 1962). In a case reported by Loeb and co-workers (1953), the survival of transfused red cells was moderately reduced, as it was in the case illustrated later in the text (see Fig. 9.7). The reduced survival of the patient's own red cells is presumably due to dyserythropoiesis (Cavill *et al.* 1977), but the reduced survival of transfused red cells has not been explained.

Increased red cell destruction in fever

Fever, resulting from the intravenous injection of pyrogen, the intramuscular injection of heated milk or from external heating results in an increase in red cell destruction, affecting old red cells more than young ones (Karle 1969).

Diminished survival of red cells due to haemorrhage

Loss of blood in the stools. In patients with a low platelet count, poor survival of transfused red cells may be due not to haemolysis but to chronic bleeding into the gastrointestinal tract. If ^{51}Cr-labelled red cells are injected into the circulation, the amount of blood lost in the stools can be measured by estimating faecal ^{51}Cr content. Correction for blood loss can then be applied so as to discover whether the survival curve, corrected in this way, is normal. According to Hughes-Jones (1958a), the normal daily loss of blood in the stools is about 0.5 ml (or 0.2 ml of red cells); this figure is a little lower than that obtained by Ebaugh and Beekin (1959) who, using a quantitative benzidine method, estimated the daily loss as 2 ml of whole blood.

Loss of blood by venous sampling. Corrections are also needed if substantial amounts of blood are withdrawn during the course of estimating red cell survival. When the amount of blood lost from the circulation is $x\%$ of the blood volume, the corrected survival is calculated by:

$$\text{Observed survival} \times \frac{100}{100 - x} \qquad (9.1)$$

This is the appropriate correction whatever the percentage of surviving cells at the time the sample is taken (Mollison 1961a, p. 208).

Suppose ^{51}Cr-labelled cells are injected into a subject whose blood volume is 4500 ml. By the 20th day after injection, 10 samples each of 15 ml (i.e. total 150 ml or 3.33% of the blood volume) have been withdrawn. The observed ^{51}Cr survival is 55%; corrected survival is:

$$55 \times \frac{100}{100 - 3.33} \quad \text{or } 57\% \qquad (9.2)$$

Hypersplenism

In nine patients with chronic lymphocytic leukaemia with splenomegaly (average splenic weight approximately 2000 g), the mean T_{50}Cr was 21 days, but increased to 27 days by 1 year after splenectomy (Christensen 1971). Similarly, in three patients with cryptogenic splenomegaly, the T_{50}Cr was found to be 15–25 days, but became normal after splenectomy (McFadzean *et al.* 1958). Red cell survival diminishes in animals when splenomegaly is induced by implanting percorten (Miescher 1956b).

Radionuclide scanning after injection of ^{51}Cr-labelled red cells may provide evidence of splenic sequestration and help to predict the effectiveness of splenectomy for patients with shortened red cell survival (McCurdy and Rath 1958). Monitoring radioactivity over the spleen compared with the liver with reference to a precordium measurement as the neutral 'blood pool' may foretell remission after splenectomy in patients with severe autoimmune haemolytic anaemia. However, accurate measurement, analysis and interpretation require experienced hands. Sequestration studies are far less predictive for other causes of shortened red cell survival and for mild, chronic autoimmune haemolysis (Parker *et al.* 1977).

Survival of transfused red cells in haemolytic anaemia due to an intrinsic red cell defect

In haemolytic anaemia caused by an inherited red cell defect (e.g. hereditary spherocytosis, haemoglobinopathies and red cell enzyme deficiencies), compatible red cells are expected to survive normally. For example, the survival of transfused red cells from qualified allogeneic donors is entirely normal in hereditary spherocytosis (Dacie and Mollison 1943) and in sickle cell anaemia (Callender *et al.* 1949).

Although normal survival of transfused red cells has also been described in many patients with thalassaemia major (Evans and Duane 1949; Hamilton *et al.* 1950), diminished survival has been reported in patients who have been repeatedly transfused. Among

20 children with thalassaemia major who received regular transfusions, many appeared to require transfusion unduly frequently. In six out of seven selected cases, 50% of transfused red cells were eliminated in 5–9 days and, although no blood group antibodies could be detected, low-grade alloimmunization is one likely explanation. After splenectomy, the transfusion requirements were reduced to between one-fifth and one-third (Lichtman *et al.* 1953). The possible induction of immunological tolerance in children with thalassaemia in whom transfusion is begun early in life is discussed in Chapter 3.

Transfused red cells from healthy donors survive normally in patients with paroxysmal nocturnal haemoglobinuria (Dacie and Firth 1943; Mollison 1947). Erythrocyte microvesicles from stored transfused blood transfer glycophosphatidyl inositol (GPI)-linked proteins *in vivo* to deficient cells, which may improve survival of the native cells as well (Sloand *et al.* 2004).

Estimation of mean red cell lifespan in haemolytic anaemia. See Appendix 6.

Storage of red cells in the liquid state

History

The first account of the storage of red cells was published by Fleig (1910); 80 ml of blood was drawn from rabbits and defibrinated. The red cells were washed in isotonic spa water and kept in an icebox for up to 7 days before being returned to the donor animal. A rise in the red cell count following transfusion suggested that some of the red cells were viable.

A spoonful of sugar

In 1915, Well (1915) also showed that citrated blood stored in an icebox for several days could be transfused safely to animals. The work of Rous and Turner (1916) established a milestone. As red cells were believed to be impermeable to sugars, different sugars were tested in the hope that their colloid properties might prevent haemolysis. Blood taken from one rabbit, stored for up to 12 days in a citrate–sucrose solution and then transfused to another rabbit that had just been bled, prevented the development of anaemia. When human blood was stored, dextrose was found to be marginally better than sucrose in diminishing lysis.

Accordingly, a solution containing dextrose was recommended for the storage of human blood and was soon afterwards used for transfusion (see below). This recommendation proved to be fortunate, because at the time dextrose was not recognized to have the strikingly favourable effect on the metabolism of stored red cells, which sucrose lacks. More than 20 years later, the addition of dextrose to citrated blood was found to decrease the rate of hydrolysis of ester phosphorus during storage (Aylward *et al.* 1940), and the suggestion was made that dextrose exerted its favourable effects by providing energy for the synthesis of phosphate compounds, particularly DPG and ATP (Maizels 1941).

Blood stocks and banks

The discoveries of Rous and Turner were put to practical use in the First World War by Robertson (1918). Working with the Allied Expeditionary Forces in Belgium, and during a relatively quiet period, Robertson bled donors into Rous–Turner solution (500 ml of blood added to 350 ml of 3.8% trisodium citrate and 850 ml of 5.4% dextrose). After gravity sedimentation had been allowed to occur in an icebox for 4–5 days, the red cells had settled to a volume of 800 or 900 ml and, after 2 weeks or so, to 500 ml. After removing the supernatant solution, the volume was reconstituted to 1000 ml with 2.5% gelatine in saline. Twenty-two transfusions of this mixture were given to 20 recipients, mainly soldiers suffering from severe haemorrhage. The results were apparently as good as those observed with fresh blood. The usual storage time was from 10 to 14 days, but some units of red cells stored for up to 26 days were transfused. Robertson pointed out that the chief advantage of this system was the great convenience of having a stock of blood at hand for busy times, an advantage which remains to this day.

After the end of the First World War, interest in the storage of blood seems to have evaporated and revived only in the 1930s, first in the Soviet Union. Filatov (1937) reported that by the end of 1936 many thousands of transfusions of stored blood had been given in Leningrad and elsewhere (Filatov 1937). According to Riddell (1939), by about 1937 all large hospitals in Russia were using stored blood almost to the exclusion of fresh blood. Donors attended their local 'Central

Institute', where blood was taken and stored and distributed to hospitals as required.

The concept of a blood bank ('it is obvious that one cannot obtain blood unless one has deposited blood') was formulated by Fantus (1937), who set up the first such bank at Cook County Hospital in Chicago in 1937, although the practice of refrigerated storage probably antedated this by at least 2 years (Lundy *et al.* 1936). The analogy, appropriate at the time, has proved to be both resilient and regrettable, as on the one hand it links blood with money, whereas on the other, it fails to stress the constant daily need for replenishment. A more accurate comparison might be made with a pipeline or a supply chain (Jones 2003).

The first attempt to supply the transfusion needs of an army in the field seems to have been made during the Spanish Civil War when between August 1936 and January 1939 stored blood was supplied from a centre in Barcelona; 9000 l of blood was obtained from donors during a period of 2.5 years (Jorda 1939). Only group O donors were used. Blood was drawn into a citrate–glucose solution and six donations, each of about 300 ml, were pooled in a special robust container and stored under a pressure of two atmospheres of air.

The outbreak of the Second World War led to the rapid organization of transfusion services equipped to collect and store whole blood on a large scale. At first, citrate alone was used in many services before the value of adding dextrose was rediscovered. A great deal of further work was then done in an attempt to find better preservative solutions. The main advance that resulted from all this work was the discovery of the value of acidifying the citrate–dextrose solution.

The acid test: a tart cell is a happy cell

Between 1938 and 1942 several publications confirmed that the rates of efflux of potassium from red cells and of lysis were diminished when blood was stored with an acid diluent (Cotter and McNeal 1938; Jeanneney and Servantie 1939; Maizels 1941; Maizels and Paterson 1940; Wurmser *et al.* 1942). Nevertheless, no attempt was made to use acidified solutions in clinical practice, mainly because some feared that they might be harmful. The incentive to test acidified solutions for clinical use arose from a major inconvenience in preparing solutions of trisodium citrate and dextrose: when they were autoclaved together, substantial

caramelization occurred. When acidified citrate–dextrose solutions were autoclaved, little or no caramelization developed. As it would be simpler and easier to autoclave the entire preservative solution in the blood container rather than to add autoclaved dextrose separately, a systematic study of ACD solutions was carried out by Loutit and co-workers (1943). Blood stored in these solutions produced minimal effects on the recipient's acid–base balance – in fact it produced a slight alkalosis due to the catabolism of citrate. Additionally and unexpectedly, red cell survival after storage was much improved. These findings led to the immediate introduction of an ACD solution as the standard preservative in the UK (Loutit and Mollison 1943), although ACD came into wider use only after the end of the Second World War.

The work of Rapoport (1947) showed an association between the ATP content of stored red cells and their viability (1947). Later, Gabrio and co-workers (1955a,b) found that the ATP content of stored red cells could be restored almost completely by incubation with adenosine and that restoration of the ATP content was accompanied by an increased post-transfusion survival. Adenosine was never used in routine transfusion practice because of its toxicity, but a few years later adenine, a far less toxic substance, was discovered to be capable, together with inosine, of 'rejuvenating' stored red cells (Nakao *et al.* 1960). Furthermore, adenine alone, when added at the beginning of storage, retarded the rate of loss of red cell viability (Simon 1962; Simon *et al.* 1962).

Until about 1960, the primary criterion for satisfactory preservation of red cells was maintenance of viability. However, following the discovery of the role of 2,3 DPG in releasing oxygen from HbO_2 and the realization that red cell DPG was not well maintained with current methods of preservation, attention switched to the quality of stored red cells. Relevant measures of quality and function of stored red cells remain a major challenge.

Collection of blood to provide components

At one time, all blood was collected as whole blood. Increasingly, whether by manual, semi-automated or automated techniques, blood is collected primarily for separation into components. Using special plastic collection bags with one to three satellites, it is possible, by centrifugation, to process each donation into red cells, plasma and platelets. The procedure can be carried out with some semi-automation, as in the 'bottom and top' Optipress system of Baxter or in the Compomat system of NPBI (Chapter 14). Alternatively, plasma alone can be collected by plasmapheresis or red cells, plasma, platelets and other cells can be collected, with or without plasma, using blood cell separators (Chapter 17).

Although citrate remains the anticoagulant in all of these methods, the composition of the solution into which the blood is drawn, and in which individual components are stored, will vary according to need and preference. Whenever the plasma obtained is to be fractionated, a relatively low concentration of citrate, such as 4% citrate or as in the solution called half-strength CPF (0.5CPD) is desirable, although not appropriate if the red cells or platelets are to be stored (see Appendix 9). Special solutions for red cell storage are described below.

A unit of whole blood contains a volume of 450–500 ml. No standard for Hb content has been agreed upon, although the lowest acceptable Hb concentration for blood donors assures that each unit of allogeneic whole blood will contain at least 50 g of Hb. Red cells are prepared by centrifugation to remove plasma or by haemapheresis. The Council of Europe (2003) standard defines this unit as Hb of 45 g and a haematocrit between 65% and 75%; the United States Pharmacopoeia (USP) has proposed a Hb content of 50 g in a volume of 180–325 ml. A unit of red cells that has been leucocyte depleted is required to contain 42.5 g or more (CoE = 43 g), whereas a frozen, deglycerolized unit must have a minimum of 40 g (CoE = 36 g). These definitions are arbitrary and an effort to harmonize these and other 'product specifications' would be welcomed.

The optimum temperature at which whole blood and the different components should be held prior to processing and storage is dictated by several considerations. If whole blood is kept at ambient temperature (20–25°C) for some hours, the granulocytes will ingest some contaminating bacteria. On the other hand, keeping CPD blood at ambient temperature for as little as 8 h results in a loss of 50% of the 2,3-DPG content of the red cells (Högman 1994). Although refrigeration is best for preserving red cells, including the maintenance of DPG levels, cooling results in the loss of platelet viability. This chapter will address red

cell transfusion; transfusion of other components is addressed in Chapter 14.

As demand for plasma and platelets increased, methods of separating blood at the time of collection into red cells and platelet-rich plasma (PRP) were developed. Nowadays, in many blood collection centres, red cells are separated and stored at 4°C in a special 'additive' solution; platelets are harvested from PRP or buffy coats and stored at about 22°C; the plasma is frozen for fresh-frozen plasma (FFP), for the production of cryoprecipitate or further fractionated to obtain immunoglobulin (IVIg) and other valuable derivatives. Thus, the emphasis in blood collection and storage is no longer solely on red cells, but rather on the optimal harvesting and storage of several blood constituents. In this chapter, only the storage of red cells is considered.

Deleterious changes occurring during storage

When blood is mixed with an anticoagulant solution and stored at 4°C, the red cells change shape from discs to echinocytes and finally to spheres, become more rigid, shed lipid, exhibit various biochemical changes, particularly a fall in ATP and DPG content, and progressively lose the ability to survive in the circulation after transfusion. As is the case with people, some red cells age more gracefully than others; there is great donor-to-donor variability. When studies of storage conditions are undertaken, paired studies of the same donor yield the most accurate comparisons.

Loss of viability

Unlike wine and fine violins, red cells do not improve with age. From a practical point of view the most important change that occurs in red cells during storage is loss of viability, their capacity to survive in the recipient's circulation after transfusion. Figure 9.2 shows results with ACD, the standard preservative solution from the mid-1940s to the mid-1960s. As described later, with solutions now in use red cell viability declines more slowly. Nevertheless, the same pattern is observed. After relatively short periods of storage (up to about 14 days for ACD), a small proportion of the cells is removed from the circulation within the first 24 h of transfusion, but the rest survive normally. After longer storage (28 days for ACD) about one-quarter of the cells is removed within 24 h

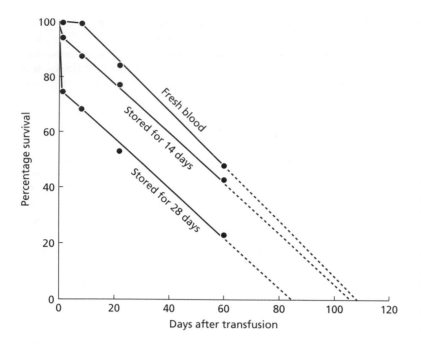

Fig 9.2 Post-transfusion survival of red cells of fresh blood compared with that of red cells stored in acid–citrate–dextrose at 4°C for 14–28 days. When stored red cells are transfused, some leave the circulation in the first 24 h after transfusion but the rest survive well (results obtained by the method of differential agglutination, revised from Mollison 1951, p. 13).

and, although the survival of the remainder is prolonged, it is not quite as long as that of unstored cells. The viability of a sample of stored red cells cannot be accurately predicted from any measurement made *in vitro*, so that measurements of post-transfusion survival remain essential in developing improved methods of preservation.

The fact that some red cells stored for a period at 4°C survive as well as fresh red cells indicates that red cells do not age during storage in the same way as they do in the circulation.

Changes in red cell metabolism

Normal red cell metabolism. Breakdown of glucose is the only source of energy for red cells. Glucose readily penetrates the red cell membrane and is phosphorylated and metabolized, with lactate as the end product. The first part of this process involves some energy-consuming steps in which the adenosine triphosphate (ATP) loses one inorganic phosphate radical and is transformed to adenosine diphosphate (ADP). Later in the metabolic pathway, ATP is regenerated with a net gain of 2 ATP molecules per molecule of glucose. In the circulating red cell, most of the total adenine nucleotides are present in the form of ATP; the other nucleotides, ADP and adenosine monophosphate (AMP), are present in much lower concentrations. The mean values (as mmol/l) are: ATP, 1.552; ADP, 0.160; AMP, 0.014 (Ericson *et al.* 1983). The mean ATP value corresponds to 4.56 µmol/g Hb. Other published estimates are somewhat lower, i.e. approximately 3.5 µmol/g Hb (Bensinger *et al.* 1977; Heaton *et al.* 1984).

Metabolism in stored red cells. During prolonged storage at 4°C, the normal high energy level is not sustained, resulting in a decrease in ATP and an increase in ADP and AMP. AMP is deaminated and dephosphorylated to hypoxanthine, which cannot be used by the red cell for resynthesis of adenine nucleotides. However, when adenine is added to the storage medium it combines with phosphoribosyl pyrophosphate to form AMP. In this way, the total concentration of adenine nucleotides can be maintained for several weeks, even if the ATP concentration decreases.

Phosphorylation of glucose is the source of energy for stored red cells and cannot continue when ATP is depleted. Although red cell ATP and viability are often associated, they are not well correlated. For example, when red cells are stored in a solution of bicarbonate, adenine, glucose, phosphate and mannitol, which results in the maintenance of high DPG levels but in a fall in ATP levels to about 10% of normal, as many as 87% of the cells may be viable (Wood and Beutler 1967). The content of total adenylates, AMP, diphosphate (ADP and triphosphate (ATP)), is more closely associated with survival than is ATP content alone (Högman *et al.* 1985). When red cells are supplied with glucose and adenine and stored at 4°C, the ATP content is maintained at the initial level or increases slightly for 1–4 weeks but then falls progressively.

DPG (2,3-diphosphoglycerate or -biphosphoglycerate), whose role in regulating the oxygen affinity of Hb has been mentioned briefly above, is present in red cells in a higher concentration than that of ATP, namely 13–15 µmol/g Hb (Bensinger *et al.* 1977), corresponding to about 5 µmol/l of red cells. The cellular concentration of DPG is regulated by a mutase (synthesis from 1,3DPG) and a phosphatase (dephosphorylation to 3-phosphoglycerate). When the intracellular pH drops below 7.2, the phosphatase is activated and the concentration of DPG decreases (Duhm 1974). In ACD blood, the fall starts as early as the third to fifth days of storage and starts not much later in CPD blood. Red cells stored in the commonly used additive solutions [saline–adenine–glucose–mannitol (SAGM), Adsol, AS-3, etc.] lose most of their DPG within 14 days (Högman *et al.* 1983; Heaton *et al.* 1984; Simon *et al.* 1987). The observation that the oxygen dissociation curve of stored blood is 'shifted to the left', indicating that stored red cells release oxygen to the tissues less readily than do fresh red cells was made before the role of DPG had been recognized (Valtis and Kennedy 1954). After transfusion, the DPG level is restored, although relatively slowly (Beutler and Wood 1969).

An important factor in the maintenance of a normal DPG concentration is the intracellular pH (pHi). The pH of blood is strongly temperature dependent. In freshly collected blood, the pHi is about 7.2 at 22°C but 7.6 at 4°C (Minakami 1975). Even after rapid cooling of whole CPD blood to room temperature, storage for 24 h results in a rapid fall in DPG (Pietersz *et al.* 1989), owing to metabolic acidification to a pH below 7.2, a level at which the breakdown of DPG is accelerated. At 4°C the decrease is slower, owing to the lower rate of metabolism. Collection in ACD results in a lower initial pH than collection in CPD (a less acid solution, see Appendix 9). Methods of raising intracellular pH to permit better maintenance of DPG are discussed below. The temporary shift in the oxygen dissociation curve of transfused stored red cells is of little clinical significance in only moderately stressed patients but may be important in critical clinical situations (Collins 1980; Apstein *et al.* 1985; Marik and Sibbald 1993).

Changes in shape and rigidity

During storage red cells change from discs to echinocytes and then to spheres. After 8 weeks' storage with ACD, this change is virtually complete, but if the cells are stored with adenine and inosine most of the cells retain their original discoid shape and viability is greatly increased (Nakao *et al.* 1960). Furthermore, if red cells are stored with ACD alone for 8 weeks and then incubated with adenine and inosine, many of the red cells change from spheres to discs and viability is partially restored (Nakao *et al.* 1962). A study of the relation between shape and viability indicated that the two are highly correlated in rejuvenated, but not in non-rejuvenated, samples. A possible explanation is that time is needed for the rejuvenation process. Time for shape change is available when cells are rejuvenated *in vitro* but may not be available when non-rejuvenated cells are transfused, so that discoid cells are trapped in the spleen before the storage changes can be reversed (Högman *et al.* 1987a).

On storage, metabolic depletion leads to dephosphorylation of spectrin and loss of red cell deformability (Mohandas 1978). Whereas 100% of fresh red cells can pass through a pipette of minimal dimensions 2.85 µm (thought to be similar to that of the microcirculation in the spleen), after 3 weeks' storage in ACD, only about 80% of cells can pass (Weed and LaCelle 1969).

Increase in plasma Hb and loss of membrane lipid

During storage, spontaneous lysis of a small fraction of red cells takes place and vesicles containing both lipid and Hb from intact red cells are shed. In plasma from stored blood, microvesicles contribute more than free Hb to total plasma Hb. In a study of the effect of the plasticizer DEHP, after storage for 21 days in CPD, figures were as follows: in plastic without DEHP, total plasma Hb was 149 mg/dl and free Hb 44.6 mg/dl. Corresponding figures for storage in plastic with DEHP were 81.3 and 7.6 (Greenwalt *et al.* 1991). In suspensions of red cells in SAGM (see below), stored at 4°C for 42 days (without mixing), spontaneous lysis, expressed as total plasma Hb divided by total Hb, amounts to 0.60% (Högman *et al.* 1987b). Standards for maximum percentage of haemolysis at outdate have been established to validate the storage period (< 1%) (Moroff *et al.* 1999).

Although an increased rate of spontaneous lysis with any preservative solution indicates that viability will be poor, absence of lysis does not indicate that viability will be good. For example, red cells stored for 14 days in a trisodium citrate–sucrose solution show less than 1% haemolysis, even although almost all of the cells are non-viable (Mollison and Young 1941, 1942). Similarly, certain phenothiazine compounds inhibit red cell haemolysis on storage (Halpern *et al.* 1950), but do not increase the post-transfusion survival (Chaplin *et al.* 1952).

Increase in red cell sodium and plasma potassium

The Na^+–K^+ ATPase is highly sensitive to decreases in temperature. As a consequence, when blood is cooled to 4°C, sodium diffuses into the cells and potassium leaks out until electrochemical equilibrium across the red cell membrane is reached. The increased potassium content of the plasma of stored blood presents a potential hazard to neonates, although under almost all other circumstances it can be ignored (see Chapter 15).

Changes in osmotic fragility

The composition of the preservative is a factor affecting the osmotic fragility of stored red cells. For example, red cells stored with sucrose, which does not penetrate the red cell membrane, have an increased osmotic resistance, although they have a very poor survival. In contrast, red cells stored with a relatively large volume of 5% dextrose have an increased osmotic fragility but survive well (Mollison and Young 1942).

In stored cells, a major component of the increase in osmotic fragility results from the accumulation of lactate and, to a lesser extent, from the substitution of chloride ion for a diminished cell content of 2,3-DPG. However, in addition to the overall increase in osmotic fragility produced by the increased intracellular osmotically active material, there is a fragile tail of red cells. These cells are the first to be lost following

re-injection into the circulation and are presumably a subpopulation that has lost the most membrane (and thus surface area) during storage (Beutler *et al.* 1982).

Effect of storage medium

The rate at which the above-described changes occur can be slowed by adjusting pH to a level at which some of the important red cell enzymes can continue to function, and by providing metabolic precursors such as dextrose and adenine.

Effect of pH

For the preservation of red cell viability, an initial extracellular pH (pHe) of about 7.0 appears to be optimal. Acidified preservative solutions, such as ACD, prevent the rise in pH which would otherwise occur on cooling blood from 37°C to 4°C and help to maintain normal metabolism, including the maintenance of ATP levels. Even after 3 weeks' storage, about 70% of the red cells remain viable.

As Fig. 9.2 shows, when red cells stored with ACD are transfused after about 2 weeks' storage, approximately 10% are removed from the circulation in the first 24 h and the rest survive normally. In contrast, when red cells are stored with trisodium citrate glucose, a solution that has a pH about 0.8 units higher than ACD, 24-h survival falls to about 50% after 1 week (second edition, p. 11).

During storage, pH falls due to the production of lactic and pyruvic acids from glycolysis. As a result, pHi falls to a level (< 7.2) at which glycolysis is inhibited and DPG phosphatase is activated. After about 2 weeks' storage, red cell DPG falls almost to zero. At a pH above 7.2, a high concentration of DPG is maintained (Duhm 1974) due to ready availability of the substrate of DPG mutase and a low activity of DPG phosphatase.

The fall in pHi can be prevented by washing the red cells in citrate before storage, which results in a loss of chloride ions and a gain in OH^- ions (Meryman *et al.* 1991). Red cells washed in a Cl^--free medium and stored in a citrate–phosphate–glucose–adenine solution had a pHi of 7.6. Red cell DPG rose to double the initial value and fell below normal only after 8 weeks (Matthes *et al.* 1994). Washing of red cells before storage is impracticable, but a method derived from it that is suitable for routine use is described below.

Prolonged red cell storage has been reported by increasing the volume and buffering capacity of the additive solution (Hess *et al.* 2003). Longer storage can be achieved by alkalinizing the additive solution so that ATP is generated in excess of utilization. However, above pH 7.2, glycolysis is diverted to DPG production and ATP production is inhibited. The addition of 30 mEq per litre of sodium bicarbonate led to the buffering of 9 mmol of protons, in addition to the eight buffered by Hb, allowing the pH to be maintained above 6.6 and the red blood cell ATP concentration above 3 mol per gram of Hb for 12 weeks. Moreover, *in vivo* recovery was 78% at 24 h (Hess *et al.* 2003).

Addition of glucose

In glycolysis, dextrose is phosphorylated by ATP and the phosphorylated dextrose is catabolized to pyruvic or lactic acid. In the process of glycolysis, ATP is generated from ADP. Although glycolysis is substantially slowed at 4°C, red cell preservation is greatly enhanced by adding dextrose to the storage medium and the optimum amount to add depends on the length of storage. For example, in red cells from whole blood mixed with standard citrate–phosphate–dextrose–adenine solution, there is enough dextrose for maintenance of ATP levels for 35 days, but after 42 days the amount is suboptimal (Dawson *et al.* 1976).

Addition of adenine

Red cell preservation is greatly improved by adding adenine and inosine (Nakao *et al.* 1962) or adenine alone (Simon 1962) to the storage medium. The addition of adenine in a final concentration of 0.5 mmol/l to ACD blood increased 24-h survival after 42 days' storage from 49% to 74% (Simon 1962). Later work showed that an initial concentration of 0.25 mmol/l was sufficient for this length of storage (Åkerblom and Kreuger 1975).

Toxicity of adenine. No adverse clinical reactions attributable to adenine were noted in a series of more than 5000 transfusions of blood to which 35 mg (approximately 0.26 mmol) adenine per unit had been added (de Verdier 1966). The only potential hazard seems to be the formation of the metabolite 2,8-dioxyadenine (DOA), which is poorly soluble and may

be deposited in renal tubules (Åkerblom *et al.* 1967). In practice, the only patients at risk are those who have massive transfusions and, even then, risk appears to be minimal. In one study, no impairment of renal function was found in patients who had received approximately 17 units of ACD-adenine blood (Westman 1972). In another study, of six patients who had died in the immediate postoperative period, DOA crystals were found in the kidneys in three of the patients, who had received, respectively, 17, 46 and 95 mg of adenine per kilogram of body weight (Falk *et al.* 1972; Westman 1974). CPD-adenine blood (final concentration of adenine 0.25 mmol/l or approximately 34 mg/l) appears to be safe for exchange transfusion in newborn infants, even when repeated exchange transfusions have to be given (Kreuger 1976). The safety of adenine (and other additives) has not been proven for extremely ill premature infants, particularly those with hepatic and renal insufficiency. However, several decades of extensive use of blood preserved in additive solutions has shown no reason for concern.

Effect of mixing red cells during storage

Mixing whole blood or red cells at various intervals during storage has clear-cut beneficial effects: in blood stored with CPD or ACD-adenine, red cells in units mixed daily had a significantly better 24-h survival, a higher ATP content and less spontaneous lysis than did unmixed units (Dern *et al.* 1970). Red cells stored in SAGM solution (see above) showed less spontaneous lysis and shed fewer microvesicles if the suspension was mixed weekly (Högman *et al.* 1987a). Red cells stored in an additive solution such as Adsol and mixed daily were as well preserved after 8 weeks, as judged by morphological index, ATP and lysis, as unmixed cells stored for 6 weeks (Meryman *et al.* 1994). The beneficial effect of mixing is presumed to be due to dissipation of acid metabolites, which otherwise collect in the bottom layer of stored red cells, and to ensuring the even supply of nutrients.

Reversibility of storage changes *in vivo*

Changes observed in stored red cells are at least partly reversible *in vivo*: after relatively brief periods of storage the majority of the cells show shape changes and increased rigidity, although after transfusion most cells are viable.

Changes in the composition of stored red cells following transfusion can be studied after separating donor red cells from samples of the recipient's blood, using the technique of differential agglutination (Crawford and Mollison 1955). This method has been used to study the rate at which changes in 2,3-DPG and electrolytes are reversed *in vivo*.

Rate of restoration of red cell 2,3-diphosphoglycerate in vivo

In two studies of red cells stored as whole blood mixed with ACD and transfused to patients, results were as follows: in the first, in three subjects, at least 25% of the DPG content was restored within 3 h and more than 50% within 24 h; in the second, also in three subjects, about 45% was restored in 4 h and about 66% at 25 h (Beutler and Wood 1969; Valeri and Hirsch 1969). In studies of normal volunteers whose red cells had been stored for 35 days with AS-1 or AS-3 (Appendix 8), results were not very different: DPG levels returned to 50% of normal in 7 h and almost to 95% at 72 h. The rate of regeneration was slower with red cells stored as CPDA-1 blood, owing possibly to lower intracellular levels of glucose and adenine (Heaton *et al.* 1989c).

Reversal of electrolyte changes

The concentration of potassium in stored red cells is restored to normal very slowly after transfusion. Red cells previously stored in ACD for 15–16 days did not regain a normal content for more than 6 days after transfusion, although their sodium content became normal within 24 days (Valeri and Hirsch 1969). Similarly, red cells previously stored for 1–3 months at –20°C in a citrate–glycerol mixture did not regain normal potassium values until 4 days after transfusion (Crawford and Mollison 1955).

Best methods of storing red cells

Storage as whole blood

The best solution devised so far for addition to whole blood is citrate–phosphate–dextrose–adenine, version CPDA-1 (Appendix 9). When 14 ml of this solution are added per 100 ml of blood, the final concentration of adenine is 33.8 mg/l or 0.25 mmol/l.

This concentration is suitable for maintaining red cell ATP in stored whole blood and is better than 0.5 mmol/l in maintaining DPG levels (Kreuger and Åkerblom 1980). In a collaborative trial from six laboratories, the mean 24-h survival for 50 studies in which red cells were stored as whole blood with CPDA-1 for 35 days was 79%, SD ± 10% (Moore *et al.* 1981).

Effect of excess anticoagulant. During the course of an ordinary donation, the first red cells to be collected are necessarily mixed with an excess of anticoagulant solution. Red cells from the first 100 ml of blood to be collected into ACD and stored for 28 days were found to have a 24-h survival of 20–32% compared with 44–61% for the whole unit (Gibson *et al.* 1956). Similarly, when blood was incubated at 37°C for 30 min with one-half of its volume or more of ACD the 24-h survival of the red cells was 50% or less at 24 h (Mayer *et al.* 1966, 1970). A recent suggestion that part of this discrepancy relates to a technical artefact involving increased ^{51}Cr elution from cells labelled in a low pH medium has merit, at least for baboon red cells, but needs to be confirmed by studies of human red cells (Valeri *et al.* 2003a).

When a full unit of blood cannot be collected from a donor, damage to the red cells may occur as a result of the relatively high ratio of anticoagulant solution to blood in the collection container. A study in which varying volumes of blood were collected into a fixed amount of ACD or CPD intended for 350 ml of blood, and were then stored for 21 days, indicated that, with ACD only collections of 400 g or more should be accepted, although with CPD those of 300 g were satisfactory. With storage periods as long as 35 days, red cells of units 'undercollected' into CPDA-1 are actually at an advantage, presumably due to the higher ratio of nutrients to cells. In a carefully controlled study, donations of 275 ml had a mean 24-h survival of 87.7% compared with 78.8% for standard donations of 450 ml (Davey *et al.* 1984).

In one type of cell separator (MCS-3P, Haemonetics Corp.), anticoagulant is added to whole blood at a constant ratio during collection, which may account for the improved *in vitro* characteristics of red cells collected with this instrument, namely higher ATP and 2,3-DPG, and better red cell deformability (Matthes *et al.* 1994). On the other hand, in a crossover study viability of red cells collected with the MCS-3P did not differ significantly from manual collection after 35 days' storage (Regan *et al.* 1997).

Storage as red cells

If most of the supernatant plasma preservative solution is removed and loosely packed red cells are stored, viability is as well maintained as in whole blood. For example, in a comparison with blood taken into CPD-adenine, after 5 weeks the mean 24-h survival was 78.7% for storage as whole blood and 76.5% for storage as red cells (Kreuger *et al.* 1975).

When tightly packed red cells are stored, there is less residual preservative solution, and extra nutrients must be supplied for optimum preservation (Beutler and West 1979). In trials of a solution of CPDA-2 containing increased dextrose and adenine (Appendix 9), red cells stored for 42 days as concentrates with a PCV of 0.75 had a mean 24-h survival of 76.7% and those with a PCV of 0.85 had a mean survival of 70.6%. Although CPDA-2 appears superior to CPDA-1 when red cells are to be stored as concentrates (Sohmer *et al.* 1981), the preservative has not been commercialized because of the development of the additive solution approach to red cell concentrate preservation (see below).

Storage as resuspended red cells ('additive solutions')

The idea of storing separated red cells with a nutrient solution containing adenine and glucose was proposed in 1964 (Fischer 1965) and has since been widely adopted. In one system, platelets, buffy coats and plasma are separately harvested from units of whole blood and the red cells are stored in a saline–adenine–glucose–mannitol solution (SAGM, Appendix 10). In one trial, after 42 days the mean survival was 77.4%, SD 4.7% (Högman *et al.* 1983). In trials of a solution containing 60% more adenine and nearly 2.5 times as much glucose (Adsol, Appendix 10), mean 24-h survival after 35 days was 86% and after 49 days was 76% (Heaton *et al.* 1984). Results with other additive solutions containing glucose and adenine (e.g. AS-3, see Appendix 10) have been similar (Simon *et al.* 1987).

Although viability is well maintained with the solutions described in the preceding paragraph, DPG levels are depleted within 2 weeks (Hogman *et al.* 1983).

As mentioned earlier, better maintenance of DPG depends on raising pHi. A practical method of achieving this without impairing maintenance of viability has been described. Blood is collected into a solution containing only one-half of the usual amount of citrate (0.5 CPD, Appendix 9). The purpose of this is twofold: first, the red cells can subsequently be suspended in a citrate-containing solution without increasing the total amount of citrate to be transfused to undesirable limits; and second, the yield of factor VIII from plasma is greater when the citrate concentration is reduced. Red cells are separated and stored with an investigational red cell additive solution, RAS2 (Erythrosol), containing citrate, phosphate, adenine and mannitol; glucose is contained in a separate length of plastic tubing attached to the end of the cell pack and added separately (see Appendix 10). This is necessary because RAS2 has a pH of 7.3 and glucose caramelizes if autoclaved at this pH. Under these conditions, DPG fell to 67% after an initial holding period of 8 h at room temperature but was still at this level after 28 days; 24-h survival after 49 days was $78.9 \pm 7.1\%$ (Högman *et al.* 1993).

Rejuvenation of stored red cells *in vitro*

Even after prolonged storage, the ATP content and post-transfusion survival of stored red cells can be restored to near pre-collection values by incubation of the red cells *in vitro* with adenosine (Gabrio *et al.* 1955b). Striking effects are observed on incubation with inosine and adenine. For example, red cells stored for 8 weeks as blood mixed with ACD have the appearance of smooth spheres and their ATP content is very low. After incubation at 37°C for 1 h with inosine and adenine, they regain their original discoid shape, their ATP level rises to near-normal values and their survival *in vivo* is greatly improved (Nakao *et al.* 1962).

DPG levels of stored red cells can be restored, and even increased to supranormal levels, by incubation with inosine, phosphate and pyruvate (McManus and Borgese 1961). Pyruvate greatly increases the amount of DPG produced, probably by oxidizing NADH to NAD and thus preventing the inhibition of glyceraldehyde phosphate dehydrogenase caused by NADH (Duhm *et al.* 1971). As an example of what can be achieved, stored red cells in which the DPG content had fallen from an initial 4.2 mmol/l red cells to

0.35 mmol/l were incubated at 37°C for 4 h with final concentrations of 10 mmol/l of inosine, 4 mmol/l of phosphate and 4 mmol/l of pyruvate; the DPG level rose to almost 6 mmol/l of red cells (Oski *et al.* 1971).

Estimation of viability of stored red cells

Although the factors causing loss of red cell viability are now much better understood, no *in vitro* method can predict with great accuracy how a given sample of stored red cells will survive in the circulation. As noted above, the same holds true for *in vitro* assays of red cell function. Direct measurement of post-transfusion survival therefore continues to play an essential role in the development of improved methods of red cell preservation.

When red cells that have been stored for a relatively short period are injected into the circulation, some cells are cleared within a few hours but the rest survive normally. With longer storage, the percentage cleared within the first few hours increases progressively and after prolonged storage all the cells are cleared rapidly. In practice, knowledge of the percentage survival at 24 h makes it possible to predict how the whole population will survive and there is therefore little reason to continue assays beyond this time.

In view of the fact that, in a population of stored red cells, some are cleared within the mixing time (Fig. 9.3), percentage survival cannot be estimated accurately unless a labelled population of fresh red cells is also injected. True survival can then be determined from estimation of total circulating red cell volume (RCV) or as a ratio of stored–fresh red blood cell survival. On the other hand, when the proportion of non-viable red cells is relatively small, satisfactory estimates can be made by an extrapolation method (see below), without injecting a second labelled population.

Methods that have been used for estimating the percentage survival of stored red cells have been reviewed elsewhere (Mollison 1984). Here, only two methods will be described.

In the *double-label method*, the sample of stored (autologous) cells is labelled with one isotope (^{51}Cr) and a sample of fresh (autologous) red cells is labelled with a second isotope (e.g. [99m]Tc). The two lots of labelled red cells are injected as a mixed suspension. RCV is estimated from the ^{99m}Tc values in samples taken at 5–10 min and the percentage survival of the ^{51}Cr-labelled stored cells is calculated from a sample

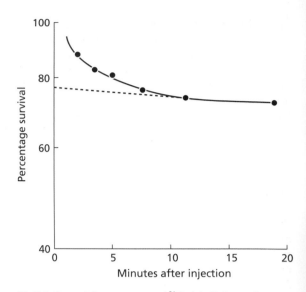

Fig 9.3 Rate of disappearance of ^{51}Cr-labelled stored red cells from the circulation during the 20 min following injection. The red cells were from blood that had been stored for 42 days at 4°C with acid–citrate–dextrose and inosine. The true percentage survival 24 h after injection was about 50%. Each observation is based on a comparison with the survival of fresh red cells labelled with ^{32}P and injected at the same time. If survival had been based on the ^{51}Cr estimates alone, taking samples from 10 min onwards and extrapolating the estimates to zero time (– – –) to obtain a figure for apparent 100% survival, 24-h survival would have been estimated as 65% (50/77), instead of 50%.

taken at 24 h. This method is the most accurate available. When RCV is estimated simultaneously with two lots of fresh red cells, each labelled with a different isotope, the results agree closely, as expected from the fact that the two lots of cells are injected in the same suspension and that common standards are prepared. Using ^{51}Cr and ^{32}P, the mean value for RCV estimates with the two isotopes differed by less than 0.1% with an SD of 0.9% (Mollison *et al.* 1958). Using ^{51}Cr and ^{99m}Tc, in two series the mean value of estimates with ^{99m}Tc was about 1.2% higher in one small series (Jones and Mollison 1978) and 0.9% higher in another (Beutler and West 1984).

As an alternative to using a second red cell label to estimate RCV, ^{125}I has been used to estimate plasma volume and RCV has then been deduced. This method is far less satisfactory; it has a substantially larger error as: (1) the volumes of labelled plasma and of red cell suspension that are injected are different; (2) different standards are prepared from plasma and from the red cell suspension; and (3) in deducing RCV from plasma volume, a factor has to be assigned for the H_B/H_V ratio (see Appendix 4). Apart from the greater error involved in estimating RCV in this indirect way, ^{125}I has a substantially greater radiotoxicity than ^{99m}Tc.

In the *single-label method*, which is simpler but less accurate than the double red cell label method, a sample of stored red cells is labelled with ^{51}Cr and injected; a series of samples is taken and the values are extrapolated to zero time to obtain an estimate of the 100% survival value. In using this second method it is evident that the first sample must not be taken before mixing is virtually complete, and sampling must be confined to a period during which the rate of cell destruction is more or less constant. Mixing is usually not complete for 3–5 min after injection (Strumia *et al.* 1968). In a series in which samples were taken at 2.5-min intervals, the points between 5 and 15 min after injection were well fitted by a single exponential but the 20-min value was above the line, indicating that destruction had slowed by this time. When RCV was estimated by extrapolating a line through the 5- to 15-min values to zero time, the estimates of RCV were within ± 5% of the true value (obtained from the ^{99m}Tc estimate), provided that the 24-h survival was above 70%. When survival was below this value, RCV was overestimated by about 25%. For example, in one case the true survival, estimated from a ^{99m}Tc estimate of RCV, was 13.3%, but if calculated from the RCV determined by extrapolation was 16.9%. This overestimate can either be expressed as: 3.6/13.3 × 100 (27%) or as 16.9 – 13.3, (3.6%). The latter figure is the one that is important in practice and the error of the extrapolation method is not large enough to be important (Beutler and West 1984). Using this second method of interpreting results, in a series in which the survival rate was always greater than 60% and usually greater than 70%, the single-isotope method overestimated survival by only 1–4.3% (Beutler and West 1985). In another study, in which the 24-h survival rate by a double red cell labelling method averaged 78.2%, survival by the extrapolation method was overestimated by about 3%. When true survival was less than 75%, the overestimate was about 5% (Heaton *et al.* 1989d).

Because of its low and stable rate of elution, ^{51}Cr has become the standard label for red cell viability studies. ^{99m}Tc and ^{111}In have been proposed but have not proved popular for red cell storage studies (Marcus *et al.* 1987).

Survival of stored red cells taken from different subjects

In estimating the post-transfusion survival of stored red cells, allowance must be made for the significant differences between donors. Dern and co-workers (1966) carried out at least two tests on each of 28 subjects whose blood was stored in ACD for 21 days and found consistent differences between subjects. Whereas the inherent experimental error, including the error of the method, biological variation between tests on the same subject, etc., had an SD of 6.4, the SD of differences between subjects was 6.6. Similar observations have been made by others; for example, Finch (CA Finch, personal communication, 1955) found that whereas the red cells of most normal donors, after storage in ACD for 3 weeks, had a 24-h survival of 70–85%, those taken from one particular donor regularly had a survival of only 60–65%. Another example is provided by Table 9.4, which shows that the 24- and 48-h survival of subjects 2 and 3 was consistently better than that of subjects 1 and 4. In another series in which red cells from six donors were stored in two different ACD solutions, after 28 days the ranking order of the donors with regard to survival was almost identical. It was particularly striking that one donor had the best survival on both occasions, and one by far the worst; in this latter subject (RP) the 24-h survival was 41% and 33% on the two occasions, compared with mean values of 74% and 75% in the other five subjects (Mishler *et al.* 1979). Further investigations on the red cells of RP showed that during storage their rate of loss of deformability was substantially greater than in other subjects (Card *et al.* 1983).

In another investigation, donors were selected according to the results of previous measurements of autologous red cell survival after storage. From these previous measurements, nine were predicted to have better than average survival and four worse than average. Further measurements of the survival of autologous red cells after storage showed that observed survival correlated reasonably well ($r = 0.648$) with predicted survival (Myhre *et al.* 1990).

In the above paragraph, autologous rather than allogeneic red cells were used in all series (with the possible exception of that of CA Finch) but, as described

	(A) No preliminary incubation*			(B) Preliminary incubation*		
	Survival (%)† at			Survival (%)† at		
Subject	10 min	24 h	48 h	10 min	24 h	48 h
1	94	65	67	92	54	53
2	82	79	76	91	74	74
3	94	82	82	87	75	71
4	80	66	66	78	58	59
Mean	87.5	73.0	72.8	87.0	65.3	64.3

Table 9.4 Effect of a preliminary 2-h incubation at 37°C before 28 days' storage at 4°C on the subsequent post-transfusion survival of autologous red cells (Mollison 1961b).

For the 24-h figures (A vs. B), $t = 3.68$, $P < 0.05 > 0.01$.

* In order to avoid systematic bias, the red cells of subjects 1 and 2 were stored first by method A, then by method B, and those of subjects 3 and 4 first by method B, and then by method A.

† Survival determined by a double labelling method. Fresh red cells labelled with ^{32}P to determine RCV; stored cells labelled with ^{51}Cr; results corrected for Cr elution.

in the series in the paragraph below, the point is not an important one.

In comparing two methods of red cell preservation, it is essential either to use a relatively large number of subjects or, if only a few subjects are used, to compare both methods in the same subject. An example is given in Table 9.4. Note that if method B had been used to store the red cells of subjects 2 and 3 and method A for subjects 1 and 4, the conclusion would have been reached that method B gives a better 24-h survival rate (mean 74.5%) than method A (mean 65.5%) – the reverse of the truth.

In the absence of alloimmunization, recipient characteristics exert a relatively minor effect on the survival of donor red cells. In two different studies, the survival of stored red cells from any particular subject appeared to be the same in the subject's own circulation as in the circulation of a recipient injected with part of the same sample (Dern 1968; Shields 1969b; Dern *et al.* 1970).

Differences between young and old red cells

The effect of increasing periods of storage on the post-transfusion survival of red cells calls for some comment. For red cells in storage, getting older is not getting better. As already mentioned, the survival curve of red cells stored for relatively short periods (under 2 weeks) in a suitable preservative solution is characterized by destruction of up to 10% of the cells within the first 24 h with normal survival of the

remainder, removal of about 1% a day. This finding suggests that the cells rendered non-viable are a random sample of the population and that the remainder are still capable of normal survival. The idea that young and old red cells are equally susceptible to damage by storage receives support from an observation of Ozer and Chaplin (1963) using an antiserum that agglutinated stored red cells but not fresh red cells; young cells became agglutinable on storage to the same extent as old red cells.

Red cells stored for 28 days or more in ACD show a different survival pattern (see Fig. 9.2). About one-quarter is removed in 24 h and the remainder disappear at a rate distinctly faster than 1% a day. This finding suggests that after relatively long periods of storage, young red cells suffer more than old red cells, or alternatively that post-transfusion survival of all the red cells is adversely affected. In experiments in dogs, after storage for 20 days young red cells were far more severely damaged than old red cells (Gabrio and Finch 1954).

Effect of storage temperature on maintenance of red cell viability

The refrigeration of blood is expected to slow metabolism and, thus, to enhance preservation, and to slow the growth of possible bacterial contaminants. Blood is commonly stored at a temperature of between 2°C and 6°C, but the reasons for the choice of this temperature are not obvious. Presumably, the intention has always been simply to keep blood as cold as possible without allowing it to freeze. In fact, blood mixed with ACD solution freezes at about −0.5°C and may be supercooled to −3°C and maintained indefinitely at that temperature without freezing (Strumia 1954). It might, therefore, appear that a temperature in the region of, say, 0°C to 2°C ought to be used, rather than 2–6°C. It is rather surprising that so few attempts have been made to discover the optimal temperature for red cell preservation.

Only one study has been published of the effect on red cell viability of varying the storage temperature in the range −10°C to +10°C, but it provides valuable information. The red cells of four subjects were stored on successive occasions at −10°C, −2°C, +4°C and +10°C for 34 days before being labelled with ^{51}Cr and re-injected into the subject's circulation. It was thus possible to compare the survival of each subject's red cells at the four temperatures. The same solution, containing glycerol as well as citrate, phosphate and dextrose was used throughout. The mean post-transfusion (24-h) survival after 34 days' storage was: −10°C, 80%, −2°C, 78%, +4°C, 63%, +10°C, 52% (Hughes-Jones 1958b). The trend is interesting even if the differences are within the margin of error for the assay.

Blood can be kept at 20–24°C for many hours before being stored at 4°C with very little adverse effect, provided that it is cooled rapidly to 22°C after collection. Holding at 20–24°C for up to 24 h, followed by storage at 4°C (with Adsol) for up to 42 days had scarcely any effect on survival: comparing a holding period at 20–24°C of 24 h with 8 h, survival after 35 days was 79.4% vs. 79.0% and after 42 days was 73.0% vs. 76.2% (Moroff et al. 1990).

Warming blood to 22°C for 24 h after storage at 4°C (in ACD) for various periods was found to have a slightly adverse effect compared with storage at 4°C throughout: the survival figures were as follows (unwarmed results first): after 7 days, 92% vs. 87%; after 21 days, 84% vs. 78%; and after 28 days, 75% vs. 62% (Shields 1970).

Red cells deteriorate rapidly at 37°C in ACD. The DPG level falls to 20% in 5 h. After 24 h, only 30% of the cells are viable and after 48 h, virtually none (Jandl and Tomlinson 1958). Even if blood is incubated at 37°C for only 2 h immediately after withdrawing it from the donor and is then stored for 28 days, red cell survival diminishes significantly compared with the survival of red cells from the same donor stored for the same period but without 2-h incubation (Table 9.4).

In experiments on rabbit red cells, incubation at 41.5°C for 8 h was shown to produce substantial damage, with survival at 4.5 h only 60% (Karle 1969).

Effect of delayed cooling on 2,3-diphosphoglycerate in red cells

Extended storage of whole blood at 22°C decreases the concentration of red cell DPG, whether or not the units have been rapidly cooled to this temperature (Pietersz et al. 1989). Estimates of the fall in 2,3-DPG in CPD or CPD-Adsol blood kept at ambient temperature for 6–8 h are: after 6 h, 13% (Avoy et al. 1978) and 27% (Moroff et al. 1990), and after 8 h, 43% (Moroff et al. 1990). Prompt cooling to below 15°C prevents the loss of DPG from red cells. Blood taken freshly (into bottles) has a temperature of 30°C, but within 2 h of putting single bottles (or bags) into a ventilated cold room, the temperature of the blood has fallen below 15°C (Prins 1970).

Effect of plasticizers on stored red cells

Di (2-ethylhexyl) phthalate

As described in Chapter 15, the plasticizer phthalate leaches into blood during storage. The plasticizer is taken up by the red cell membrane and has the effect of diminishing the rate of progressive lysis of the red cells and of enhancing resistance to hypotonic lysis (Rock et al. 1983; Estep et al. 1984; Horowitz et al. 1984). In a convincing experiment, addition of phthalate to stored blood had the effect of substantially slowing the rate of loss of viability of the red cells, whether they are stored in plastic or glass containers (AuBuchon et al. 1988). For a brief discussion of the toxicity of phthalates, see Chapter 15.

Butyryl-n-trihexyl citrate

Because of the potential toxicity of phthalates, a new type of plastic, PL-2209, incorporating butyryl-n-trihexyl citrate (BTHC), a plasticizer that is less toxic than di (2-ethylhexyl) phthalate (DEHP), has been tested. Like DEHP, BTHC reduces red cell lysis during storage, although to a lesser extent. Red cell viability is as well maintained with either plastic (Buchholz et al.

375

1989; Högman *et al.* 1991). Few countries have eliminated blood bags containing DEHP, in part because of the odour of BTHC, but primarily because of the increased cost.

Effect of irradiation of red cells, stored either beforehand or subsequently

A dose of 25 Gy is required for complete T-cell inactivation in stored red cells as measured by a limiting dilution assay of proliferation (Pelszynski *et al.* 1994). Doses of this order applied to red cell suspensions that are then stored, affect red cell viability adversely. In a paired study in eight normal subjects, blood was drawn into AS-1, irradiated with 30 Gy and then stored for 42 days; compared with non-irradiated blood from the same subjects, 24-h red cell survival was lower (68.5% vs. 78.4%), as was ATP (Davey *et al.* 1992). A more detailed study of red cells stored in AS-1 suggested that red cell viability is maintained for 28 days from collection, regardless of when the cells are irradiated, but that irradiation of cells at day 14 after collection impairs viability to an unacceptable degree if the cells are stored for a full 42 days (Moroff *et al.* 1999). In the USA, the FDA and the AABB recommend that red cells may be irradiated throughout their shelf-life but may be subsequently stored for only 28 days (or up to the end of the storage period for the non-irradiated product if this is less). This recommendation is not supported by the data above, although a reduction in 24-h red cell survival (< 75%) may be a reasonable trade-off for avoiding GvHD. The current data support a standard that permits storage up to 28 days after collection regardless of the day of irradiation. The CoE has adopted a standard that meets this requirement (Council of Europe 2003).

When red cells are irradiated and then stored, supernatant potassium increases substantially. With 30 Gy, an approximate doubling within 48 h has been noted (Ramirez *et al.* 1987) and, after 42 days, an increase to a mean of 78 mEq/l compared with 43 mEq/l in non-irradiated control samples (Davey *et al.* 1992). The increased amount of potassium in the red cell supernatant following irradiation and storage is of no clinical significance except in exchange transfusions or when massive transfusions are given to infants.

Effect of irradiation before freezing. In a controlled study, red cells were exposed to 15 Gy before being stored at 4°C for 6 days, then frozen in glycerol and stored for 8 weeks. After 6-day storage at 4°C, supernatant potassium was about twice as high with the irradiated cells but, after freezing and deglycerolization, there were no differences between irradiated and control groups with respect to ATP, DPG and survival *in vivo* (Suda *et al.* 1993).

Storage of red cells in the frozen state

Satisfactory storage of red cells in the frozen state became possible when it was discovered that red cells, mixed with glycerol, could be frozen and thawed without damage (Smith 1950). Rabbit red cells, after being dialysed free of glycerol and transfused, were capable of circulating *in vivo* (Sloviter 1951) and human red cells, previously frozen to −79°C in glycerol, survived well in humans (Mollison and Sloviter 1951).

Red cells must be rendered glycerol free before being transfused and, unfortunately, rapid, simple, inexpensive closed-system methods for doing so have proved elusive. For these reasons, small use has been made of frozen red cell depots. Nevertheless, prolonged storage is invaluable in some circumstances and evolving technology may alter the use of frozen red cell reserves (Bandarenko *et al.* 2004).

Effects of freezing

The damaging effects of freezing are related to the rate of cooling: at slow rates, there is time for water to leave the cell in response to the osmotic gradient created when extracellular water freezes. Many of the tissue-damaging effects of freezing are those expected from exposure of the tissues to a hypertonic solution followed (on thawing) by exposure to an isotonic solution. This observation suggests that the salt concentration is responsible for cell injury caused by freezing and thawing (Lovelock 1953a). However, later work suggests that, at slow rates of freezing, the loss of intracellular water and the associated reduction in cell volume, rather than the absolute concentration of solutes, is responsible for injury (Meryman 1971). The mechanism of damage seems to be either intracellular dehydration or stress to the cell membrane (Meryman 1989).

With rapid freezing, there is time for only part of the freezable water to leave the cell so that there is less dehydration and the cells may largely escape injury (Meryman 1989). Frog cells subjected to ultra-rapid cooling and thawing can be recovered intact (Luyet and Gehenio 1940). On the other hand, cooling at even faster rates leaves too little time for water to leave the cell and damage occurs due to formation of intracellular ice rather than to the effects of hypertonicity (Mazur *et al.* 1972).

Substances that protect against damage by freezing

Substances that do not penetrate cells

Damage to cells during freezing can be reduced by adding a substance that does not penetrate the cell membrane but increases solution viscosity and reduces the optimum cooling velocity (Meryman 1989). Substances that have been shown to be effective include various sugars and colloids, including dextrose, lactose, sucrose, albumin, hydroxyethyl starch (HES), polyvinyl pyrrolidone (PVP) and dextran. With all of these substances the rates of freezing and thawing must be very rapid if lysis is to be avoided.

The addition of glucose to blood has been used to reduce damage during very rapid freezing and thus preserve red cells for serological tests. If a small volume of citrated blood is mixed with an equal volume of 20% glucose and immediately frozen, only 2–3% lyses on thaw (Florio *et al.* 1943). Similarly, red cells can be mixed with glucose and then sprayed into liquid nitrogen; the resulting droplets are kept at the temperature of liquid nitrogen (–196°C) and subsequently thawed by being dropped into warm saline (Meryman 1956).

Substances that penetrate red cells

Several cell-penetrating substances have been shown to prevent damage during the slow freezing and thawing of red cells, but of these, glycerol stands out because of its low toxicity. Glycerol limits ice formation and provides a liquid phase in which salts are distributed as cooling proceeds so that excessive hypertonicity is avoided (Lovelock 1953b). Glycerol is most effective in protecting those cells that it permeates fairly rapidly; human red cells are ideal in this regard.

Use of glycerol

In 1949 Polge (1949) discovered by fortunate accident that glycerol protects spermatozoa against the otherwise lethal effects of freezing, and soon afterwards Smith (1950) found that red cells could also be protected. The following description of the way in which the protective effect of glycerol was discovered is based on published accounts (Sloviter 1976; Parkes 1985), supplemented by a personal communication from C Polge.

In 1948 a group under AS Parkes was attempting to preserve spermatozoa in the frozen state; fructose was added because it is the principal metabolic substrate for sperm and is present in moderately high concentration in seminal fluid – but it did not work. C Polge joined the group and decided to try again. He obtained from a cold room a bottle labelled 'laevulose' (another name for fructose) which contained a solution that had been made some weeks earlier. Spermatozoa were suspended in this solution and, after freezing and thawing, were found to be actively motile. In a freshly prepared solution of laevulose, after freezing and thawing, all sperm were non-motile. It was suggested that the solution might need to be aged but, after being aged, a new batch did not work. Meanwhile, almost the entire original bottle of 'laevulose' had been used up.

The remaining amount of 'laevulose' was then given to an organic chemist who soon found that no reducing sugar was present but that there was a lot of protein; the presence of glycerol was discovered when some of the solution was passed through a Bunsen burner flame and gave off the characteristic odour of acrolein. In the cold room a bottle of laevulose labelled 'albumin-glycerol' (a solution used for histological preparations) was found. It was presumed that labels had become detached in the cold room and had been re-attached to the wrong bottles.

Rate of freezing and optimal glycerol concentration

When red cells are frozen slowly, for example over a period of 30–60 min, they must be mixed with sufficient glycerol to yield a final concentration of 4.5 mol/l (approximately 10% w/v) if haemolysis is to be avoided (Hughes-Jones *et al.* 1957). On the other hand, when freezing is relatively rapid, as when the blood–glycerol mixture in a thin-walled metal container is plunged into liquid nitrogen, the final concentration of glycerol need be only 20% w/v (Pert *et al.* 1963). In the process developed by Krijnen *et al.* using the same concentration of glycerol, the blood reaches 0°C only after about 8 min, but cooling is then very rapid (about 2°C/s) (Krijnen *et al.* 1964).

When red cells are to be frozen only to $-20°C$, a final glycerol concentration of 3.0 mol/l is sufficient to prevent lysis. If the dextrose concentration is raised to about 220 mmol/l, the glycerol concentration can be reduced to about 1.4 mol/l (see below).

Addition of glycerol to red cells and storage at low temperature

If solutions containing more than about 50% (w/v) glycerol are added to blood, some haemolysis results. The addition of 50% (w/v) glycerol in citrate to an equal volume of blood yields a final concentration of approximately 30% (w/v) in the fluid phase of the mixture, because the glycerol mixes not only with the plasma, but also with the water space in the red cells that accounts for about 65% of their volume. If a final concentration exceeding 30% (w/v) glycerol is to be attained, it is best to add the glycerol in stages (Hughes-Jones et al. 1957).

Storage temperature and maintenance of viability – blowing hot and cold

Red cells mixed with a glycerol–citrate–phosphate solution and stored at $-20°C$ deteriorate very slowly. After 3 months' storage, the post-transfusion survival is only slightly less than that of fresh cells (Chaplin et al. 1954). Even after 18 months' storage, more than 50% of the red cells are still viable (Hughes-Jones et al. 1957). With a glyceroldextrose–adenine–phosphate solution, 24-h survival after 10 months' storage was found to be more than 85% (Meryman and Hornblower 1978).

At lower storage temperatures, deterioration slows further. At temperatures in the range of $-40°C$ to $-50°C$ there does not seem to be any definite deterioration in red cell survival over a period of up to 1 year or more (Chaplin et al. 1957; Hughes-Jones et al. 1957), although Chaplin and co-workers (1957) deduced that after 5 years' storage at this temperature, post-transfusion survival would have fallen to 70%.

Storage at $-79°C$ (achieved by adding solid CO_2 to a bath of alcohol) was used in some of the earlier experiments with glycerol-treated red cells and shown to give satisfactory preservation (Mollison et al. 1952; Brown and Hardin 1953). After a period of storage as long as 21 months at this temperature, post-transfusion survival may be as good as after storage for only a few weeks (Chaplin et al. 1956).

Haynes and co-workers (1960) stored glycerolized red cells at $-80°C$ to $-120°C$ and found no evidence of deterioration with time; the two samples stored for the longest periods (36 and 44 months) had a post-transfusion survival of about 95%. Similarly, 90% of cells stored for up to 7 years at $-80°C$ and then stored at $4°C$ for 48 h survived at 24 h (Valeri et al. 1970). Storage for up to 21 years at $-80°C$ was reported by Valeri and co-workers (1989). Mean 24-h survival with various methods was 80–85%. Red cells have now been frozen for as long as 37 years and after freeze–thaw–wash have mean recovery values of 75%, less than 1% haemolysis, and normal ATP, 2,3-DPG and P50, and 60% of normal red cell K(+) levels (Valeri et al. 2000).

Methods suitable for routine use

Storage at $-20°C$

If the concentration of dextrose is increased to about 0.2 mol/l in a mixture of red cells, dextrose and glycerol, the glycerol concentration can be reduced to about 1.4 mol/l in the final mixture and still permit freezing to $-20°C$ and subsequent thawing without lysis. After a single wash in a solution containing mannitol and a relatively high concentration of dextrose, the red cells can be resuspended in a buffered, glycerol-free solution containing dextrose and adenine and stored at $4-6°C$ for up to 35 days. The whole process is carried out in a closed system, using special interconnected bags. In tests in 10 subjects, red cells stored at $-20°C$ for 56 days, followed by storage at $4-6°C$ for 14–21 days, mean 24-h survival was 75.5%. Recovery in vitro was 96% (Lovric and Klarkowski 1989).

Storage at $-80°C$

The advantage of using a high glycerol concentration (4.0 mol/l or more) is that not only can freezing be slow, but subsequent storage can be at a temperature as high as $-65°C$ ($-80°C$ is usually preferred), so that mechanical refrigeration can be used. Moreover, the frozen red cells can be transported in solid carbon dioxide ('dry ice', temperature $-79°C$).

Glycerol can be added to red cells in their original plastic bags (Valeri et al. 1981); a minor modification of this method is described in Appendix 12. Although plastic blood containers of standard design can be used with this process, polyolefin is preferred to polyvinylchloride because there is less haemolysis during freezing and the containers are less brittle at −80°C. The standard method of deglycerolization after thawing is to dilute the thawed glycerolized blood with 12% sodium chloride and, after allowing the mixture to equilibrate for 5 min, to wash the red cells with 3 l of saline. The cells are finally resuspended in 0.9% saline with 0.2% dextrose.

Storage at −120°C or −196°C – as cold as any stone

The advantage of this method is that the final glycerol concentration can be as low as 2.25 mol/l (Krijnen 1970). However, the disadvantages are that special containers must be used for freezing and storage and, because the temperature must not be allowed to rise above −120°C, the containers must be stored in and transported in liquid nitrogen (−196°C).

Removal of glycerol from red cells – reducing osmotic stress

If red cells that have been stored with glycerol are to be transfused, their glycerol content must be reduced to about 1–2% or they will swell and haemolyse on contact with plasma as water enters the cells more rapidly than glycerol can exit them. The number of washes needed can be substantially reduced by first exposing the red cells to a hypertonic solution of a non-penetrating substance, such as citrate, which causes the cells to shrink and lose much of the glycerol so that they can subsequently be washed in saline with little haemolysis (Lovelock 1952).

In the method of Meryman and Hornblower (1972), 12% NaCl is added to a red cell glycerol mixture, followed after 3 min by a relatively large volume of 1.6% NaCl. Thereafter, the cells can be washed in a suitable automated blood processor. Wash solutions suitable for use with all of these machines were described by Valeri (1975). Although the process is a major improvement over manual processing, thawed and washed cells must be used within 24 h of thaw.

A functionally closed blood processor (Haemonetics ACP 215) for glycerolization and deglycerolization of red cells, originally developed for military use, is now licensed for preservatives used in the civilian sector.

Red cells can now be stored post thaw for up to 15 days with adequate recovery and survival (Valeri et al. 2001; Bandarenko et al. 2004).

Red cells containing sickle Hb

A particular problem arises when U-negative or Fy(a−b−) red cells are required. Many donors with these phenotypes have HbS (AS or SS) and special care is needed when deglycerolizing such red cells. Sickle (SS) red cells, prepared for autologous use on rare occasions, can be washed successfully if 4 l, rather than 2 l, of washing solution is introduced into the red cell washer, together with the thawed red cells, before carrying out the usual deglycerolization procedure (see above). The same presumably applies to AS cells. If no extra washing solution is used and the red cells are introduced too rapidly into the cell washer, the cells tend to pack into a semi-solid dark gel. After storage of sickle cells in glycerol at −85°C, losses during thawing and processing are higher than with normal red cells, but results after about 3 years are much the same as after shorter periods of storage (Castro et al. 1981).

Red cell losses during processing

One disadvantage of freezing processes involves small losses of red cells at various stages which, when added together, may become substantial. Valeri (1974) estimated these losses after varying periods of storage before and after freezing. When red cells were frozen at −80°C in 40% w/v glycerol, then thawed, processed and transfused within 4 h, 86–92% of the original number of red cells was available for transfusion.

The concept of 'therapeutic effectiveness' was introduced by Valeri and Runck (1969) to take account of losses in vitro and in vivo. The index of therapeutic effectiveness (ITE) is simply the recovery in vitro, i.e. the number of red cells available for transfusion as a percentage of the number in the original unit, multiplied by the percentage survival in vivo at 24 h. Calculation of this index emphasizes that figures for post-transfusion survival alone give too optimistic a picture of the value of freezing as a means of pre-servation. For example, in the work of Valeri and co-workers (1989) survival in vivo after storage for up to 21 years was 80–85% but the ITE was 70–75.

379

Storage of red cells before freezing

Red cells that are to be frozen in glycerol can be stored as ACD blood for up to 7 days without any adverse effect on their ultimate survival (Valeri 1965). Red cells stored at 4°C for as long as 42 days in a nutrient-additive solution 'AS-3', then frozen in glycerol and stored for 8 weeks, had an *in vitro* recovery of 81% and a 24-h survival of 78%, giving an ITE of 63% (Rathbun *et al.* 1989).

Rejuvenation of stored red cells followed by freezing

Red cells that had been stored as packed cells for 23 days were incubated at 37°C for 1 h with a solution containing pyruvate, inosine, glucose, phosphate and adenine. The cells were then mixed with glycerol and stored at −80°C for up to 12 months. After thawing and washing, they were transfused to anaemic patients. Such red cells had a 24-h survival of approximately 82% compared with 71% for cells that had not been incubated with the 'rejuvenation' solution before being frozen. The rejuvenated red cells had a normal 2,3-DPG content, whereas the non-rejuvenated cells had almost no 2,3-DPG (Valeri and Zaroulis 1972). In a controlled study of red cells stored for 42 days in AS-3 and rejuvenated before cryopreservation, the frozen cells, after deglycerolization, had a mean ATP level of 146% and mean 2,3-DPG of 115%. The mean 24-h red cell survival exceeded 75% (Lockwood *et al.* 2003).

Storage of red cells at 4°C after freezing

Red cells that have been frozen and stored for up to 18 months can be satisfactorily preserved for up to three weeks at 4°C after thawing. However, some solutions, such as Adsol, that are suitable for the refrigerated storage of red cells have proven unsatisfactory for the preservation of previously frozen cells. One solution that gives satisfactory preservation is AS-3 (see Appendix 10). After 2 weeks at 4°C, mean 24-h survival was 85% and ITE 80%; after 3 weeks, the figures were 77% and 72% respectively (Moore *et al.* 1993).

Use of substances other than glycerol

Dimethylsulphoxide is as effective as glycerol in protecting cells against damage by freezing but has no clear advantage (eighth edition 1987, p. 156).

PVP is potentially advantageous because it does not permeate red cells and therefore allows the cells to be transfused after thawing without first having to be washed. Unfortunately, the method results in substantial haemolysis, and post-transfusion red cell survival is only about 70% (Morrison *et al.* 1968). The toxicity profile may render PVP unsuitable for human use.

Results with HES are similar to those observed with PVP. A mean 24-h survival of 83.4%, in a small number of subjects, has been reported (Thomas *et al.* 1996). As is the case with 20% w/v glycerol, red cells frozen with HES in a 14% solution must be frozen in liquid nitrogen at −197°C and stored at −150°C.

Compared with sugars, colloids such as HES, PVP and dextran decrease the amount of Hb liberated from the individual cell without appreciably decreasing the number of damaged cells. The extent to which dextran decreases the lysis of red cells during freezing and thawing thus underestimates the real extent of damage (Zade-Oppen 1968). Similarly, with PVP, post-transfusion haemoglobinuria after the transfusion of frozen red cells is a problem. PVP is thought to seal defects in red cell membranes that become apparent when the PVP is washed away in the circulation (Williams 1976).

Indications for the use of frozen red cells

The main advantage of storing blood in the frozen state is that the red cells can be kept for an indefinite period so that it becomes possible to accumulate units of blood of rare red cell phenotypes. Accordingly, when a patient has developed alloantibodies that make it difficult to find compatible blood, it may be possible to find sufficient compatible units in the frozen red cell bank to supply the patient's needs. The alternative of trying to find suitable donors willing to be bled at short notice is likely to be far more difficult. Units of autologous blood for patients with particularly difficult transfusion problems have been stored in frozen blood repositories; however, such units are often left unused, either because patients do not subsequently require transfusion, move away from the storage site or even forget that such units are in storage (Depalma *et al.* 1990).

When autologous red cells have been collected but, for one reason or another have to be stored for more than a few weeks, freezing is the only appropriate method of preservation (Goldfinger *et al.* 1993). Frozen red cells may be useful in paediatric practice, for example when a premature infant requires a series of transfusions.

Frozen (and washed) red cells have the advantage of being virtually free from plasma, leucocytes and platelets.

Strategic red cell reserves

If cryopreservation of red cells and subsequent processing could be made simple and inexpensive enough, blood collectors might consider accumulating stocks of red cells of common groups (particularly group O) to avoid the periodic shortages of supply that occur when blood is stored in the liquid state. So far, cost and logistics have discouraged collection centres from using frozen red cells in this way. One estimate is that the cost of units stored in the frozen state is three times that of units stored in the liquid state (Chaplin 1984). However, this estimate refers to storage at −80°C in a high glycerol concentration. Storage at −20°C in a low glycerol concentration would be more practical.

Frozen red cell reserves have also been proposed as a strategy to address emergency blood needs during disasters and as protection against an acute loss of qualified donors as might occur following an epidemic or an act of bioterrorism. At one point the USA military blood programme stored more than 60 000 units of group O cells in frozen depots around the world. Several issues need to be addressed before embarking upon such a strategy. First, even major disasters require relatively little immediate transfusion support, and whatever is needed is available from liquid inventory (Klein 2001). Second, blood from frozen stores cannot be readily mobilized; the thaw–wash procedure takes approximately 1 h per unit and requires large numbers of instruments and trained staff to produce 30 units a day. In contrast, 1000 liquid units can be mobilized in 2 h. Third, substantial breakage with component loss occurs when cells are shipped in the frozen state (Valeri *et al.* 2003b). Finally, long-term frozen reserves must be designed to meet future donor eligibility requirements. This involves a separate inventory of frozen specimens suitable for testing should new screening tests be introduced, a mechanism of updating donor history for new qualification requirements, and data to support new processing

procedures, such as pathogen reduction technology, that are introduced years after the cells have been frozen. However, the availability of functionally closed systems for freezing and post-thaw washing with a 14-day post-thaw liquid shelf-life makes a frozen reserve as a back-up to liquid reserves more practical. Periodic rotation of inventory, such that turnover is complete in 3 or 4 years, will minimize the risk of unnecessary discard while allowing a method to 'backfill' the use of liquid reserves for emergencies. Such a programme has been used to help manage blood shortages and outdating (R Gilcher, personal communication).

The transfusion of red cells in anaemia

The treatment of acute haemorrhage has been considered in Chapter 2. The present chapter deals only with patients who have a more or less normal blood volume.

Physiological compensations for anaemia

Tissues cannot 'bank' oxygen. Blood can be thought of as a pipeline that delivers oxygen continuously from pulmonary alveoli to capillary beds. In healthy subjects, the oxygen delivery system exceeds resting oxygen needs by several fold. In chronic anaemia, the reduced capacity of the blood to carry oxygen is compensated for by (1) an increase in cardiac output, (2) redistribution of blood flow and (3) increase in the 2,3-DPG content of the red cells, which causes a shift to the right in the oxygen dissociation curve, so that at a given degree of oxygen saturation of Hb, oxygen is more readily given up to the tissues (Duke and Abelmann 1969; Finch and Lenfant 1972). As an example, assuming that the oxygenation in the lungs is normal and that a capillary Po_2 of 30 mmHg has to be maintained, an equal amount of oxygen can be released from 8 4 g of Hb when the oxygen dissociation curve is shifted to the right (P_{50} 32 mmHg) as from 14.0 g of Hb when the oxygen dissociation curve is normal, i.e. P_{50} 27 mmHg (Högman 1971).

Despite the compensatory change in the oxygen dissociation curve, the amount of oxygen delivered to the tissues = cardiac output × arterial oxygen content. As the oxygen content is diminished in anaemia, the anaemic patient can maintain the overall supply of oxygen to the tissues only by increasing cardiac output and thus reducing the cardiac reserve. The inverse relationship between Hb concentration and cardiac output has been well documented (Chapler and Cain 1986). Accordingly, if transfusion is considered for a chronically anaemic patient, the advantage of raising the arterial oxygen content has to be weighed against the hazards of overloading an already hyperkinetic circulation.

Signs and symptoms of chronic anaemia

Anaemia is a general sign of disease, not a diagnosis. In all categories of anaemia, the physiological changes and symptoms, apart from those of acute volume loss in the rapidly bleeding patient, differ primarily in severity and are related to the degree of anaemia and the rapidity of its development. Cardiac output responds relatively quickly to hypoxia, so that elevated heart rate (and stroke volume, should one be in a position to measure it), especially with modest exertion, is an early sign. Pallor, emphasized to generations of medical students, is appreciated only with moderate to extreme reductions in Hb concentration as blood is redistributed from the skin to internal organs. Pale conjunctivae, tongue, mucous membranes and nail beds evidence the altered perfusion. Pale optic fundi may be accompanied by retinal haemorrhages. As cardiac output increases, patients may experience tinnitus and palpitations. Rapid respiration and shortness of breath at rest should be considered as disturbing evidence of oxygen deficit and evidence of cardiac decompensation. Dizziness and fainting are common as anaemia progresses, but apprehension, changes in mentation and leg cramps are indications of severe oxygen deprivation and presage coma and death.

Effect of transfusion on the circulation

Normovolaemic subjects

In subjects with a previously stable blood volume, rapid transfusion produces a transient rise in venous pressure, but venous pressure falls to normal as soon as the transfusion is stopped, even although blood volume may remain above normal for many hours afterwards. For example, in one normal subject the transfusion of 1600 ml of serum in 14 min produced a considerable increase in plasma volume, as shown by a fall in Hb concentration of 23.5%. Venous pressure rose from 0 to 10.5 cm H_2O during the transfusion; 14 min after the end of the transfusion, venous pressure (measured in an antecubital vein) was only 1 cm H_2O, although the Hb concentration was still 20% below the pre-transfusion level (Sharpey-Schafer and Wallace 1942a).

After large rapid transfusions of serum or blood, vital capacity is diminished, an indication that part of the added fluid is accommodated in the blood vessels of the lungs. However, the degree of reduction in vital capacity accounts for only a part of the additional volume and doubtless the larger veins and subcapillary venous plexus also accommodate extra fluid (Loutit et al. 1942; Sharpey-Schafer and Wallace 1942a).

Rate of extrusion of plasma from the circulation. When cats were transfused with an amount of plasma equal to their initial plasma volume in less than 1 h, plasma volume returned to its original value within 24 h (Florey 1941). Similarly, in human subjects with a stable blood volume transfused with 700–2100 ml of serum in 7–27 min, in most instances plasma volume was only slightly above its initial value at 1 h, although readjustment took more than 24 h in a few subjects (Sharpey-Schafer and Wallace 1942b).

Rate of readjustment of blood volume after transfusion

Relatively few observations have been made on the rate of readjustment of blood volume after transfusions of red cell suspensions or whole blood. In four patients transfused with approximately 500 ml of concentrated red cell suspensions in 20–40 min, Hb concentration, PCV and donor red cell concentration were all about 10% greater in the 24- and 48-h samples than in the sample taken 5 min after transfusion. These observations indicate that blood volume was temporarily increased by an amount approximately equal to the volume transfused. In eight further cases, an average of 1010 ml of citrated blood was transfused in periods varying from 20 to 85 min, and samples were taken in the same way. Again, the estimates at 24 and 48 h all showed a rise in values of about 10% compared with the immediate post-transfusion sample (Mollison 1947). These figures do not refer to the total change in values produced by transfusion, but to the shift in values following the end of transfusion.

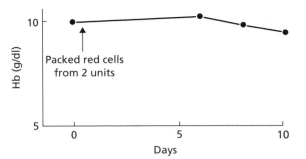

Fig 9.4 Failure of the haemoglobin (Hb) concentration to rise materially following transfusion in a patient with chronic renal insufficiency. Transfused red cells were shown to survive normally (see Fig. 9.5), and the failure of the Hb concentration to rise was evidently due to very slow readjustment of blood volume.

Because some subjects take as long as 24 h to readjust blood volume, the effects of the transfusion of large amounts of blood must always be carefully monitored, particularly in those patients whose venous pressure is elevated prior to transfusion.

Rate of readjustment of blood volume in newborn infants

A 3.5-kg infant has at birth a blood volume of about 270 ml and another 120 ml or so in the placental circulation. Provided that the cord is not tied until about 5 min after birth most of the blood in the placenta is transferred to the infant. The circulating red cell mass cannot be measured accurately from the indirect measurement of haematocrit or estimated by mathematical calculations of red cell volume (Strauss et al. 2003). During the following 3–4 h, the amount of plasma lost from the circulation is greater than the amount transferred from the placenta, so that plasma volume actually shrinks slightly (Mollison et al. 1950; Usher et al. 1963). More than 70 ml of plasma may leave the circulation in the first 30 min after birth (Usher et al. 1963).

In a previous edition of this book, an example was given of the rapid readjustment of blood volume in a 5-week-old infant transfused in 20 min with 75 ml of citrated blood. Readjustment of blood volume was virtually complete by the time a sample was taken 5 min after transfusion (Mollison 1961a, p. 129).

Diminished control of blood volume in renal insufficiency

If patients with diminished renal function are transfused, the resulting increase in blood volume is far more prolonged than in normal subjects. Because of this prolonged expansion of blood volume the Hb concentration may fail to rise during the day or two following a transfusion, and this may lead to a suspicion that the transfused red cells have been eliminated. Figures 9.4 and 9.5 demonstrate a case of this kind (Mollison 1961a, p. 52). As Fig. 9.4 shows, the patient's Hb concentration failed to rise following transfusion of red cells from 2 units of blood (1 unit = 420 ml of blood with 120 ml of ACD). Four weeks later, a further transfusion of red cells from 1 unit of blood was given and at the same time 10 ml of the red cells was labelled with ^{51}Cr and injected. The red cells were eliminated at the normal rate (Fig. 9.5), although the individual estimates of survival did not fall on a smooth curve, presumably due to fluctuations in blood volume produced by further transfusions during the observation period.

The failure of subjects with impaired renal function to correct blood volume promptly after transfusion was demonstrated by Hillman (1964). Two subjects with renal failure, one of whom was anuric, received 525 ml of stored, pooled plasma. Two hours later, the increase in blood volume still amounted to 90% of the volume of plasma transfused, whereas in normal subjects the figure was approximately 60%. The increase in plasma volume persisted for at least 5 h.

Post-transfusion rise in Hb concentration in patients with splenomegaly

In patients with massive splenomegaly, transfusion of a given quantity of blood produces a relatively small increase in Hb concentration; for example, in patients without a major degree of splenomegaly (spleen palpable no more than 5 cm below the costal margin or not palpable at all), transfusion of 1 unit of whole blood (approximately 180 ml of red cells) increased Hb concentration by 0.9 ± 0.12 g/dl; in subjects with splenomegaly the increase was 0.6 ± 0.16 g/dl (Huber et al. 1964). A spleen that weighs more than 750 g contains 13–66% of the total red cell mass (Motulsky et al. 1958; Strumia et al. 1962).

383

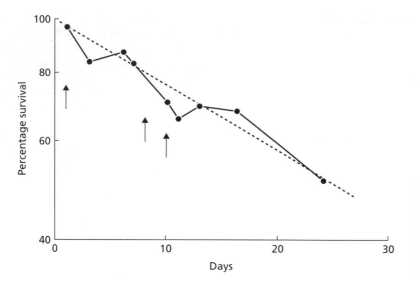

Fig 9.5 Red cell survival (^{51}Cr) in a patient with chronic renal insufficiency (see Fig. 9.4). Following each transfusion (↑), the concentration of labelled red cells was depressed for several days due to slow readjustment of blood volume.

Rate of transfusion in subjects with a normal circulation

Subjects without any circulatory impairment are not harmed by a temporary increase in blood volume. Transfusion of one unit of red cells per hour is perfectly safe. Rigorous control of infusion rate is not routinely required. However, for infants and patients at risk of volume overload, infusion pumps approved for blood administration provide accurate volume control. If infusion pumps are not available, a convenient way of checking the rate of transfusion is to hang the bag of red cells on a spring balance; the weight is noted at the time when transfusion is started and at any subsequent time the amount of red cells given can be readily determined.

The risk of overloading the circulation

Transfusion-related circulatory overload is under-appreciated and under-reported. Over a 7-year period, 1 in 3168 patients transfused with red blood cells at the Mayo Clinic developed evidence of circulatory overload; after a bedside consultation service was introduced, the frequency rose to 1 in 708 patients, the increase undoubtedly related to improved awareness (Popovsky and Taswell 1985). A separate retrospective analysis of 385 elderly orthopaedic surgery patients detected a volume overload rate of approximately 1%, even although the intraoperative blood loss was small and the transfusion volume only 1–2 units (Audet *et al.* 1998).

Patients with any degree of congestive cardiac failure must be transfused with caution. The risk of overloading the circulation can be minimized by (1) using red cells instead of whole blood and (2) administering a diuretic. Urinary output should be monitored. The risk of volume overload is greatly increased in patients with renal failure, who may not respond at all to the administration of diuretics.

Signs and symptoms of circulatory overloading

Volume overloading produces a rise in central venous pressure, an increase in the amount of blood in the pulmonary blood vessels and a diminution in lung compliance. These changes may elicit symptoms of headache, chest tightness and hyperpnoea; a dry cough is common. If these warning signs are neglected, pulmonary oedema soon develops and crepitations can be heard over the dependent parts of the lungs. One need not await dyspnoea and elevated jugular venous pressure to halt transfusion and initiate management for circulatory overload (upright positioning, oxygen, diuretics and positive pressure ventilation as indicated).

Hypertensive encephalopathy has been reported as an occasional consequence of transfusion in patients with nephritis. However, this syndrome is multifactorial

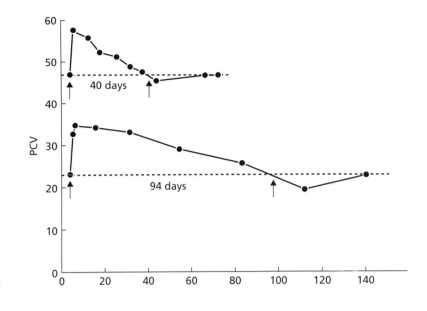

Fig 9.6 Changes in packed cell volume (PCV) following transfusion. Upper curve: a group of normal subjects (data from Pace *et al.* 1947). Lower curve: a single subject with chronic nephritis. In both curves the arrows mark the departure from, and return to, a baseline (Mollison 1954).

and may be initiated solely by an acute elevation of blood pressure (Hinchey *et al.* 1996). There is no evidence that transfusion per se presents some specific risk.

Hypertension, convulsions, severe headache and cerebral haemorrhage have been reported in patients with sickle cell disease or thalassaemia, following successive transfusions over a short period of time (Royal and Seeler 1978; Wasi *et al.* 1978).

Effect of transfusion on red cell production

When transfusions are administered to normal animals, red cell production diminishes. In a series of normal human subjects transfused with 1000 ml of red cells, PCV rose on average from 0.465 to 0.585 and remained above the pre-transfusion level for 40 days (Pace *et al.* 1947) (Fig. 9.6, upper curve). Had red cell production remained normal, the PCV should have remained above the pre-transfusion level for 110–120 days. Transfusion-induced plethora inhibits production of erythropoietin and results in low (but not absent) circulating levels (Spivak 1993). Further evidence of suppression of red cell production was provided by a fall in the reticulocyte count following transfusion. In children with severe thalassaemia, regular transfusions suppress marrow activity and permit normal bone growth.

Deductions about survival of transfused red cells based on changes in packed cell volume following transfusion

It was once thought that the survival time of red cells could be deduced by producing plethora, either by transfusion or by transient exposure to low oxygen tension, and then noting the time taken for Hb concentration to return to its normal level. However, this method gives a correct result only if red cell production remains approximately constant, as it may when already depressed (see Fig. 9.6, lower curve). If production diminishes, the time for which the Hb concentration remains elevated is much less than the mean lifespan of the red cells (see Fig. 9.6, upper curve). If red cell production were to cease altogether after transfusion, the population of red cells would diminish in a linear fashion, reaching zero at about 115 days. Reference to the upper curve in Fig. 9.6 shows that if the initial slope of the curve immediately after transfusion is extended to the time axis, it does in fact intersect it at about 120 days, suggesting that production was temporarily arrested following transfusion.

Figure 9.7 shows some observations in a patient with aplastic anaemia. The slope of fall of the PCV, if extrapolated, would have reached zero 50 days after transfusion; thus it could have been concluded that the average red cell lifespan was 50 days or less. Estimates

385

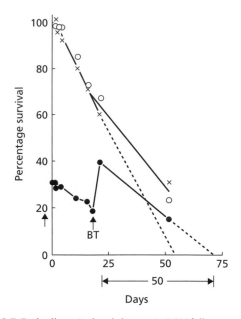

Fig 9.7 Red cell survival and changes in PCV following transfusion in a patient with aplastic anaemia. X, survival of patient's own red cells; O, survival of transfused red cells. The survival results are similar and extrapolation of the initial slope of the curve gives an estimate of mean lifespan of approximately 50 days. ●, PCV. After each blood transfusion (BT), PCV fell steadily: if the slope is extrapolated it intersects the baseline after about 50 days.

of survival of the patient's own red cells and of transfused red cells showed that the lifespan was in fact about 50 days.

As a rough guide, if the changes in PCV or Hb concentration following transfusion are plotted, and the initial slope, when extrapolated, intersects the time axis at 115 days or more, it does not prove that survival is normal; but if the time axis is intersected at some earlier time, such as 50 days, it can safely be concluded that the survival of the transfused red cells is reduced.

The transfusion trigger

The decision to transfuse red cells balances the potential benefits, decreased morbidity and mortality and increased functional recovery, and the potential risks, the side-effects of transfusion. Friedman and co-workers (1980) introduced the term 'transfusion trigger' to describe the factors that motivate physicians to order blood transfusion. In their study of 535 031 male and female surgical patients, they determined the importance of PCV as a component of this transfusion trigger as well its arbitrary use.

As mentioned (Chapter 2), a Consensus Conference in 1988 emphasized the folly of relying on a single Hb value as an indication for transfusion (Consensus Conference 1988). Nevertheless, physicians still rely heavily on Hb level to guide the transfusion decision; transfusions are infrequently ordered when Hb exceeds 100 g/l and commonly prescribed when Hb falls below 60 g/l; between these values is where most controversy arises. No combination of assays has yet proved superior to careful observation and good clinical judgement in determining the best regimen for patients with chronic anaemia.

Experiments in baboons (Wilkerson et al. 1988), pigs (Rasanen 1992) and dogs (Van der Linden et al. 1998) indicate that the critical Hb concentration lies between 30 and 40 g/l. Trials of acute normovolaemic haemodilution in healthy volunteers and surgical patients found the limit of critical oxygen delivery in humans at about 50 g/l (Weiskopf et al. 1998; Leung et al. 2000). Almost all of the clinical data regarding the transfusion trigger derive from studies of surgical patients or patients in the intensive care setting, rather than from patients with chronic anaemia. The major exception is the well-documented complications of severe anaemia in patients with thalassaemia major (see below).

The retrospective cohort of patients who refused transfusion for religious reasons has been cited previously (see Chapter 2). In the largest consecutive series of such patients, mortality rose as preoperative Hb fell, and postoperative Hb of 50–60 g/l was associated with a strikingly high mortality (Carson et al. 2002). Both animal and human data suggest that patients with cardiovascular disease (CVD) tolerate anaemia less well than do patients without CVD (Spahn et al. 1994; Hogue et al. 1998; Carson et al. 2002).

Several observational studies address the issue of transfusion trigger in the perioperative setting. In the largest, a review of 8787 consecutive patients age 60 or older who were hospitalized between the years 1983 and 1993 with hip fracture, perioperative transfusion at Hb of 80 g/l or above did not appear to influence 30- or 90-day mortality (Carson et al. 1998). Other studies have reported increased myocardial infarction and mortality with increased PCV in patients undergoing coronary artery bypass graft (CABG) and an association between transfusion and organ dysfunction and mortality in ICU patients, suggesting that arbitrary transfusion in these settings is unwarranted (Spiess *et al.* 1998; Vincent *et al.* 2002). Somewhat in contrast, observational studies of patients with vascular surgery and prostate surgery documented increased cardiovascular events in patients with PCV of less than 28% (Nelson *et al.* 1993; Hogue *et al.* 1998). In the largest retrospective review of medical patients, a cohort study of 78 974 Medicare patients who suffered myocardial infarction stratified by presenting PCV and adjusted for comorbidity, mortality was lower in those patients who were transfused when Hb fell below 110 g/l than in patients who were not (Wu *et al.* 2001). A large retrospective cohort study of 5793 elderly patients who underwent hip fracture repair suggested that a higher Hb level is associated with better early functional recovery (Lawrence *et al.* 2003). Although these studies are not strictly comparable and the results seem at best inconsistent, and at worst contradictory, several conclusions may be drawn: (1) there is no obvious transfusion trigger; (2) patients with CVD seem to fare better at higher PCV; and (3) the best available data suggest a transfusion trigger in the range of 70 g/l with a higher level (90–100) for patients with CVD.

The only adequately powered prospective controlled trial enrolled 838 consecutive intensive care unit patients with HB < 90 g/l and randomized 418 of them to either a restrictive (Hb < 70 g/l, maintain 70–90) or a liberal (Hb < 100 g/l, maintain 100–120) transfusion regimen (Hebert *et al.* 1999). Interpretation of the results remains controversial. Overall, 30-day mortality was similar in the two groups (18.7% vs. 23.%, *P* = 0.11). However, mortality rates were significantly lower with the restrictive transfusion strategy among patients who were less acutely ill and among patients who were less than 55 years of age, but not among patients with clinically significant cardiac disease. The mortality rate during hospitalization was significantly lower in the restrictive strategy group. Although the study suffers several weaknesses (the large number of patients excluded after enrolment, the failure to continue the randomization regimens after patients left the ICU setting, the failure to stratify randomization according to disease severity such as APACHE score and absence of a current practice control arm), it does suggest that younger patients are receiving too much red cell transfusion (average

5.6 units) during intensive care management when the Hb is as high as 100 g/l.

Transfusion with intermittent blood loss

Anaemia due to recurrent haemorrhage

Patients who have become anaemic as a result of recurrent haemorrhage should be transfused unless it is reasonably certain that risk of further haemorrhage has abated. For example, patients with recent haematemesis and whose Hb concentration falls as low as about 70 g/l are at risk lest a further fall in Hb from rebleeding precipitates circulatory failure and makes transfusion particularly hazardous. The frequency of rebleeding from oesophageal varices is about 30%. Bleeding recurs in 30–50% of peptic ulcers with non-bleeding visible vessels and adherent clots that are not treated with endoscopy and in 1–12% of patients treated with invasive inpatient therapy (Sung *et al.* 2003). Overall mortality rate for bleeding peptic ulcers remains about 6–7%. However, invasive therapies clearly improve prognosis (Barkun *et al.* 2003). Early transfusion in these settings seems prudent lest rebleeding prove fatal before endoscopic or surgical interventions can be undertaken.

Anaemia due to repeated blood sampling

The amount of blood lost due to sampling for diagnostic tests may be substantial.

In *premature infants* in intensive care units, the amount of blood removed for tests of various kinds is such that the infants must be transfused regularly if severe anaemia is to be avoided (see below).

In *adults* whose entire hospital stay was in general wards, the total blood loss in sampling averaged 175 ml in one study. In the same study, patients who spent all or part of their time in ICUs average a sampling loss of 762 ml; the loss in patients with arterial lines was 944 ml (four samples a day). In about 50% of patients transfused during their hospital stay, losses from phlebotomy (the equivalent of more than 1 unit of red cells) contributed to the transfusion requirement (Smoller and Kruskall 1986, 1989). Phlebotomy is still a significant source of blood loss. A multicentre study of critically ill patients found that the daily volume of blood lost through blood sampling averaged 41 ml (Vincent *et al.* 2002).

Red cell transfusion in premature infants

In newborn infants, erythropoiesis is suppressed for many weeks following birth, as the relatively high Hb values of the fetus are not needed in extrauterine life. In full-term infants, the Hb concentration levels off at about 100–110 g/l at the age of 2–3 months but in premature infants, lower Hb values are reached. One important reason for this difference is that in premature infants, compared with full-term infants, the erythropoietin output in response to anaemia is reduced (Strauss 1994). Administration of recombinant erythropoietin (and iron) significantly increases erythropoiesis, but marginally enough to decrease the average number of transfusions or donor exposures per infant in hospitalized infants of 1000-g birth weight (Ohls *et al.* 2001). In any case, the amounts of red cells lost by premature infants as a result of blood sampling demand replacement (Madsen *et al.* 2000). As an example of the quantities involved, in 59 premature infants with birthweights of less than 1500 g, a mean of 22.9 ml of packed red cells was lost during the first 6 weeks of life; 26% of the infants had a cumulative loss that exceeded their red cell mass at birth (Nexo *et al.* 1981). Even with microsampling practices, the average premature infant receives one transfusion of 35–39 ml (Ohls *et al.* 2001). The usual practice is to give cell transfusions when 5–10% of the estimated total blood volume has been removed (Strauss *et al.* 1990).

Other presently accepted indications for red cell transfusions in newborn infants are to maintain PCV above 0.40 during respiratory distress or in symptomatic congenital heart disease, and to treat congestive cardiac failure and episodes of severe apnoea (Strauss *et al.* 1990). Transfusing otherwise well premature infants simply to maintain Hb levels above 100 g/l was found to confer no benefit (Blank *et al.* 1984).

It is usual to transfuse red cells (PCV 0.65) in relatively small amounts, for example 10 ml/kg, over 3–4 h. In providing blood for transfusion to infants, the use of 'paedipacks' has several advantages. Paedipacks consist of a main pack containing enough anticoagulant for 250 ml of blood and three attached, initially empty, packs into which convenient amounts of anticoagulated blood from the main pack can be transferred. When an infant needs several transfusions over a relatively short period of time, blood from the same donor can be used. When the period is not more than about 4 weeks, the packs can be stored at 4°C; if transfusions are to be given over a longer period, the donor can be recalled after 2–3 weeks for a further donation of 250 ml into a paedipak. Alternatively, aliquots of blood from the same donor can be frozen and thawed, one at a time, as needed, or drawn into separate containers using sterile docking technique. The infant is exposed to blood of only a single donor, thus minimizing the chance of the formation of alloantibodies to blood cells and the chance of acquiring an infectious agent such as CMV. At the same time, special testing of donors, for example for anti-CMV, is minimized. Blood is used efficiently, as a single donation suffices for several transfusions. When relatively small amounts of blood are required, donors weighing less than 50 kg, who might otherwise qualify, can be bled. The practice of using 'walking donors,' donors whose blood can be drawn freshly on any number of occasions, for transfusion to one or more infants, has been generally condemned. Testing is often inadequate, records tend to be unsatisfactory and practical difficulties complicate taking of blood by syringe (Oberman 1974).

For premature infants, the practice until recently has been to transfuse blood stored for not more than 1 week. It is now generally agreed that this restriction is unnecessary.

Although blood components given to mature infants are not irradiated routinely, irradiation is advised for all components to be transfused either to infants *in utero* or to newborn infants of birthweight less than 1200 g (Strauss *et al.* 1990). A dose of 25–30 Gy is commonly used. As described earlier, when red cells are stored after irradiation, the rate of potassium loss increases. However, the increased amount of potassium in the plasma does not pose any threat in most transfusions. For example, when 10 ml of packed red cells per kilogram, stored for as long as 14 days after irradiation, are transfused over 3 h into a peripheral vein, the amount of potassium transfused per hour is substantially less than the normal requirement of about 0.08 mmol/h. There is therefore no need to wash the red cells. The situation is different when large volumes of irradiated stored blood are given during an exchange transfusion or during extracorporeal circulation or when there is pre-existing hyperkalaemia or pronounced renal failure, or when relatively large volumes of blood are being given by intracardiac transfusion (Strauss 1990).

Death attributed to increased potassium in transfused red cell concentrate has been described.

A 3-week-old full-term infant that had just undergone cardiac bypass surgery developed widening of the QRS complex accompanied by a fall in blood pressure and death following transfusion of 60 ml (2×30 ml) of 32-day-old red cells (PCV 0.75) in 10–15 min via a central venous line. The potassium level in the plasma infused was approximately 60 mmol/l and the total amount of potassium in the transfused cells therefore $0.06 \times 0.2 \times 60$ mmol = 0.90 mmol. Serum potassium after transfusion and before death was 8.9 mmol/l (Hall *et al.* 1993).

For infants in general, red blood cells collected in anticoagulant-additive solutions and administered in small aliquots over the shelf-life of the component to decrease donor exposure has supplanted the use of fresh red blood cells. The safety of several anticoagulant-preservative and red cell additive solutions has been documented (Luban 2002). Less well established are the indications for transfusing infants of all maturities. Haemoglobin or haematocrit alone remains a common but insensitive guide unless clinical findings such as oxygen desaturation, apnoea and bradycardia are part of the algorithm that is used to define transfusion need. Non-invasive assays that reflect the pathophysiology of oxygen delivery are needed in this patient population even more than in the adult.

The administration of erythropoietin (epoietin alpha or beta) to infants of very low birthweights (750–1500 g) during the first 6 weeks of life reportedly reduces the need for transfusion; a PCV of at least 0.32 without transfusion was maintained by 27.5% of treated infants but by only 4.1% of control subjects (Maier *et al.* 1994, 2002). However, although recombinant erythropoietin (and iron) clearly increases erythropoiesis in premature infants, the impact on transfusion requirement is at best marginal (Ohls *et al.* 2001). In practice, erythropoietin should probably be given only to infants of 800–1300 g without severe illness (Strauss 2001).

Transfusion in chronic anaemia

When there is continuous severe underproduction of red cells, as in aplastic anaemia, or production of red cells with a greatly diminished lifespan, as in thalassaemia major, regular transfusion may be essential.

Transfusion requirements when red cell production is negligible: aplastic and hypoplastic anaemia

If normal adult mean red cell lifespan is 115 days and mean red cell volume (male) is 30 ml/kg, normal daily red cell production is 30/115 ml red cells/kg per day or approximately 0.26 ml red cells/kg per day. Thus in a male weighing 70 kg, mean red cell production is approximately 18 ml of red cells per day. To maintain an Hb concentration of two-thirds of the normal (100 g/l) would require only 12 ml of red cells per day.

In considering the transfusion requirements of a patient with complete failure of red cell production, the above calculations refer to red cells that have a mean life expectancy of 115 days. By contrast, red cells taken from the circulation are of mixed ages and have an average life expectancy of 115/2 or 57.7 days. Thus the daily requirement of transfused red cells to maintain an Hb concentration of 100 g/l in a 70-kg adult male who is making no red cells at all is approximately 12×2 or 24 ml/day. If a unit of stored blood contains 200 ml of red cells and, allowing for some loss of red cells rendered non-viable by storage and from red cells left in the blood container and tubing, an average of almost 1 unit per week will have to be transfused. Even more will be needed when the survival of transfused red cells is reduced.

The goal of transfusion therapy in anaemia of minimal production is to maintain acceptable function and quality of life at an Hb level that will not suppress residual erythroid production. For patients with acquired aplastic anaemia, this is rarely an issue. However, for those with congenital red cell hypoplasia, such as Diamond–Blackfan anaemia, maintaining an Hb concentration of between 70 and 80 g/l may allow sufficient innate marrow activity to reduce transfusional iron accumulation.

Thalassaemia: a paradigm of maximal ineffective erythropoiesis

Most patients with the classic homozygous form of β-thalassaemia major who do not undergo stem cell transplantation require transfusions from the first 6 months of life if they are to survive. Haemoglobin concentration ranges from 20 to 70 g/l; patients with Hb as low as 50 g/l can survive and live productively well into adulthood. However, if a regular transfusion regimen is not established early, the classic picture of severe untreated β-thalassaemia develops: profound anaemia, hepatosplenomegaly, endocrine dysfunction and progressive bone deformities caused by expansion of blood-forming cells in the marrow cavities. Bone abnormalities result in the characteristic appearance (thalassaemic 'chipmunk' facies, frontal bossing, short stature), radiological features (cortical thinning, 'hair-on-end' skull, compressed vertebrae) and pathological fractures, primarily of long bones and vertebrae. Most of these changes are irreversible.

The guiding principle in managing β-thalassaemia major is to provide the minimum transfusion needed to ensure normal growth, development and quality of life. Modest transfusion will prevent the symptoms and signs of anaemia, heart failure and growth retardation; transfusion to a peak Hb of 60–70 g/l will not suppress ineffective erythropoiesis. Currently, the common practice in treating children with thalassaemia major is to maintain a baseline Hb at 90–100 g/l, a level sufficient to suppress overactivity of the bone marrow (Piomelli 1995; Cazzola et al. 1997). Determination of the serum transferrin receptor has been used to document adequate suppression of endogenous ineffective erythropoiesis at these levels of Hb (Cazzola et al. 1995).

The moderate transfusion recommendation is not without controversy. An early study compared a regimen of 'hypertransfusion' in which washed, frozen red cells were transfused every 4–5 weeks to maintain the PCV above 0.27, with a regimen of 'supertransfusion' in which the PCV was maintained at a level above 0.35 (Hb 120 g/l). The introduction of supertransfusion was accompanied by an initial increase in the red cell requirement, but after 1–4 months all patients maintained a PCV of over 0.35 on a transfusion schedule that was identical to that of hypertransfusion. This development was attributed to a mean decrease in blood volume ('marrow contraction') of about 20% following supertransfusion. In turn, erythropoiesis decreased significantly (Propper et al. 1980). Many clinicians now believe that the same result can be attained with less transfusion, thus avoiding accelerated transfusional haemosiderosis with its associated life-threatening consequences (Chapter 15).

Encouraging results with induction of fetal Hb using erythropoietin, hydroxyurea and other agents nourish the hope that at least some of these patients will be able to avoid lifelong transfusion maintenance (Rachmilewitz et al. 1995; Bradai et al. 2003).

Before recombinant human erythropoietin became available, some 25% of patients on dialysis for end-stage renal disease needed red cell transfusions. Treatment with erythropoietin avoids the need for transfusion in at least 97% of patients (Mohini 1989). To avoid various circulatory complications, the PCV should not be allowed to rise too rapidly and blood pressure should be monitored carefully (Groopman et al. 1989).

Transfusion of younger-than-average red cells ('neocytes'): the rose of youth

Using a cell separator it is possible to collect a selected population of red cells that is younger than average ('neocytes'). The $T_{50}Cr$ of such cells is appreciably longer than that of unfractionated cells, in one study 43.8 days compared with 27.8 days (Propper et al. 1980), and in another 47.4 days with an estimated mean cell age of 30 days compared with 29.5 days for unfractionated red cells (Corash et al. 1981). Similarly, using fractions obtained with an IBM-2991 cell washer, the red cell half-life, after correction for ^{51}Cr elution, was found to be 43.9 days for the younger fractions and 34.7 days for the older fractions (Bracey et al. 1983). In another study, also using the IBM-2991 cell washer, the top 50% of the cells had a $t_{50}Cr$ of 40 and 42 days in two patients compared with 29 days for unselected cells (Graziano et al. 1982). In one patient who received the top 30% of the cells, the $T_{50}Cr$ was 56 days, a very high value considering that if all the cells had had an age of only 1 day the $T_{50}Cr$ would not have been expected to be longer than 70 days (the $T_{1/2}$ of ^{51}Cr elution). In measurements made with DFP, and thus giving estimates of true lifespan, red cells were taken from the upper and lower halves of red cells in a unit of blood, after spinning for an additional 30 min. ^{14}C-DFP and ^{3}H-DFP were used to label the cells in vitro. Linear slopes of disappearance were observed and mean lifespans were approximately 120 days for cells from the upper half and just over 80 days for cells from the lower half (Sharon 1991).

When neocytes were used for transfusion to selected children with thalassaemia, the intervals between transfusions could be increased. On the other hand, although the use of neocytes allows transfusion of smaller amounts of red cells or less frequent transfusion while maintaining the same PCV, the method has not proved effective in practice. In a prospective double-blind trial, the results of using younger-than-average red cells were compared with those using unselected red cells in the treatment of transfusion-dependent patients with thalassaemia major. The younger-than-average red cells were obtained by centrifuging blood at 3000 rev/min for 15 min in an IBM-2991 cell washer and collecting the least dense 50% of the cells. The reticulocyte counts of these 'young' red cells were on the average 2.5 times higher than those in the original units. The patients receiving 'young red cells' experienced a slight reduction in blood consumption, but no reduction in the fall of Hb between transfusions or any increase in the interval between transfusions. The marginal reduction in the rate of iron loading brought about by using young red cells prepared in this particular way did not justify the expense, time and effort involved and the increased donor exposures (Marcus et al. 1985). This conclusion seems unlikely to be reversed by the contention that neocyte-enriched blood can be prepared more cheaply by simple centrifugation, as two to three times as many donors are needed to produce neocyte-enriched units as to produce ordinary units (Hogan et al. 1986; Simon et al. 1989).

Exchange transfusion in treating anaemia

Indications for exchange transfusion are discussed briefly in Chapters 12 and 18. Here only the problem of exchange transfusion in sickle cell disease will be discussed.

Exchange transfusion in sickle cell disease

Exchange transfusion is used in HbSC and SD diseases and in sickle β-thalassaemia as well as in SS disease. The objects are to increase the concentration of red cells containing HbA and to decrease the concentration of abnormal sickle cells and thus to diminish blood viscosity and improve the microcirculation. Recently, work on the possible contribution of red cell adhesion to vaso-occlusion in sickle cell disease has led to other hypotheses regarding the mechanism of the transfusion effect. Erythrocytes that express predominantly Hb S (SS RBC) adhere to both endothelial cells as well as to extracellular matrix proteins to a degree far greater than do normal red cells. Multiple lines of evidence have shown that the Lutheran protein can undergo activation that increases its ability to mediate

adhesion to laminin, and the LW protein, a known receptor for leucocyte integrins, has also been described as being expressed more strongly by SS RBC. The vaso-occlusive process in patients with sickle cell disease is likely to involve interactions between Hb S red blood cells, vascular endothelium and leucocytes (Parise and Telen 2003).

No clinical data support a single ideal level of HbA-containing cells. However, as few as 30% of transfused cells decrease blood viscosity and at mixtures of > 50%, resistance to membrane filterability approaches normal (Kurantsin-Mills et al. 1988). In non-emergent circumstances, high concentrations of HbA can be achieved by simple transfusion because of the differential survival of sickle and transfused cells. Simple transfusion has been shown to improve renal concentrating ability and splenic function in young sickle cell patients (Keitel et al. 1956; Pearson et al. 1970).

In order to reduce the proportion of sickle-prone cells in a short time without increasing the PCV to unacceptable levels, automated exchange transfusion must be performed (Klein et al. 1980). If the pre-transfusion PCV is very low, it is advisable to increase it only moderately, because a high PCV increases the risk of microcirculatory occlusion, particularly in SC disease (Milner 1982). The progress of the exchange can be monitored by measuring the proportions of HbA and S and the patient's total Hb concentration. Red cell exchange has been shown to improve exercise tolerance in an experimental setting and to reduce the periodic oscillations in cutaneous blood flow thought to reflect improved microcirculation in this disorder (Miller et al. 1980; Rodgers et al. 1984). Exchange transfusion has advantages over simple transfusion: the patient's short-lived sickle cells are removed with a consequent decrease in iron load; blood viscosity is more effectively lowered; risks of circulatory overload are diminished; and PCV is not raised to an unacceptably high level. Transfusion prophylaxis is now clearly indicated for children at high risk for stroke. A randomized controlled study demonstrated a risk reduction of 90% in the patients who were maintained at levels of HbS < 30% by simple or exchange transfusion (Adams et al. 1998). This result confirms earlier experience and indicates that in this group of children with sickle cell anaemia, transfusion therapy should begin before the first event and continue indefinitely. A long-term exchange programme may be preferable for patients at high risk for stroke who have developed iron overload to levels associated with organ damage (Kim *et al.* 1994).

Exchanges are also used to treat priapism, recurrent severe vaso-occlusive crises unresponsive to conventional therapy, refractory ankle ulcers, severe pneumonia, meningitis, aplastic crises, severe episodes of red cell destruction and splenic sequestration crises (Milner 1982).

The current view remains that in the management of sickle cell disease, chronic transfusion therapy, with the sole object of correcting low Hb levels or of preventing painful crises, is not indicated, mainly because of the risk of red cell alloimmunization that may hinder future transfusions. Other risks are those of hyperhaemolysis, thrombosis of peripheral veins and of venous access (Charache 1982). Delayed haemolytic transfusion reactions seem to be particularly common in patients with sickle cell disease (see Chapter 11).

Exchange transfusion prior to surgery. If a general anaesthetic needs to be administered to a patient with SS disease, avoidance of very low arterial oxygen tension during the procedure is critical. The risk of sickling may be reduced by performing preoperative transfusion (Morrison *et al.* 1978; Fullerton *et al.* 1981). Nevertheless, one review concluded that the advantages of partial exchange transfusion before surgery did not outweigh the risks (Searle 1973). Moreover, the risks of severe sickling crises are evidently small in experienced hands. Homi and co-workers (1979) studied 284 anaesthetic procedures in patients with sickle cell disease and reported that two-thirds of the patients underwent surgery without any transfusion; the complication rate was lower in the untransfused patients (13%) than in those receiving perioperative transfusions (28%). In an observational study, simple transfusion has reduced the rate of post-operative complications for 717 sickle cell patients undergoing low-risk procedures, although transfusion did not reduce the risk of moderate-risk procedures such as cholecystectomy and hip replacement (Koshy *et al.* 1995). Except for unusual circumstances, partial exchange transfusion does not seem necessary. In a randomized study of 551 sickle cell disease patients undergoing 604 surgical procedures, a conservative simple transfusion regimen to increase the Hb level to 10 g/dl was as effective as an aggressive regimen to lower the HbS level to < 30% with respect to perioperative non-transfusion-related complications. The

patients in the aggressive regimen group received twice as many units of blood, had a proportionally increased red blood cell alloimmunization rate and had more haemolytic transfusion reactions (Koshy *et al.* 1995). The results of this and other studies suggest that if prophylactic preoperative exchange transfusion is used, it should be limited to patients undergoing high-risk procedures in whom simple transfusion could not effectively raise the HbA level to > 70%.

Red cell exchange transfusion has proved to be beneficial in patients with proliferative SC retinopathy undergoing surgery for retinal detachment (Brazier *et al.* 1986). The exchange decreases the risk of vaso-occlusive sickling and improves the blood flow in the anterior segment.

Exchange transfusion in pregnancy. There is no general agreement regarding the prophylaxis of complications of pregnancy by transfusing women with Hb SS or SC disease. Some recommend routine exchange transfusion to maintain the HbA level above 20% (Morrison *et al.* 1980), whereas others recommend exchange only for patients with severe anaemia or acute complications (Milner 1982). The only randomized trial of transfusion during pregnancy has shown that prophylactic transfusion sufficient to reduce the incidence of painful crises did not reduce other maternal morbidity or perinatal mortality (Koshy *et al.* 1988).

Many clinicians prefer to use leucocyte-reduced red cells to reduce the risk of febrile reactions that are common in recurrently transfused patients and may exacerbate sickling crises.

Transfusion other than intravenously

Uptake of red cells injected intraperitoneally

John Hunter (1984) gave large intraperitoneal transfusions of rabbit blood to other rabbits, and showed that the recipient's red cell count was raised for approximately 21 days.

Hahn (1944) gave intraperitoneal injections of red cells tagged with radio-iron to a dog. The red cells moved promptly into the circulation via the lymphatics. Nevertheless, uptake was not complete 1 week after the injections.

In humans, quantitative estimates have been made using ^{51}Cr-labelled red cells. Pritchard and Weisman (1957) found that labelled cells appeared in the

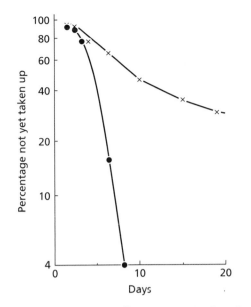

Fig 9.8 Rate of appearance of ^{51}Cr-labelled red cells in the circulating blood after injecting the cells intraperitoneally into an infant. For convenience, the 'percentage not yet taken up' has been plotted. For example, when 20% of the injected red cells have appeared in the circulating blood, the point is plotted as 80% 'not yet taken up'. ×, uptake after injecting 1 ml of labelled red cells; ●, uptake after injecting 20 ml of labelled red cells.

circulation within 24 h and reached a maximum at 3–11 days. In two patients reported previously, about 24 h passed before any appreciable number of cells appeared in the circulation. In the first patient, a child aged 1 week with severe spina bifida, an injection of 1 ml of red cells was taken up very slowly, but when 20 ml of red cells were injected, 50% of the cells were taken up in 5 days. Uptake was almost complete in 8 days (Fig. 9.8) In a second case, a child with thalassaemia major weighing 18 kg, more than 50% of the cells were taken up into the circulation by the fourth day after intraperitoneal transfusion of 350 ml of citrated blood (Mollison 1961a, p. 119).

Intramuscular injection

When red cells are injected intramuscularly, only very small amounts reach the circulation. In experiments in rabbits, 5 ml of a 40% suspension of ^{51}Cr-labelled red cells was injected into three or four different sites, and samples were taken over the following 2 weeks. The maximum radioactivity in samples of washed red cells never exceeded 0.5% of the injected dose in one case and 0.2% in the other (Mollison 1961a, p. 123).

Transfusion of red cell suspensions in anaemia

Transfusions of washed red cells were given as early as 1902 by Hédon. At that time transfusion of defibrinated blood was considered dangerous and Hédon decided to try the effect of washing the red cells and giving them as a suspension. Using both rabbits and dogs, he showed that when an animal was bled to the point of exsanguination, it could be rescued rapidly with transfusions of red cells in saline. He also tried the effect of packed red cells. In a rabbit bled of 145 ml over a period of 2 h to the point of potentially terminal convulsions, the rapid injection of red cells from 100 ml of blood from another rabbit, suspended to a total volume of 66 ml in saline, produced immediate improvement with complete recovery at 48 h.

Red cell concentrates

Castellanos (1937) was the first to use concentrated suspensions of red cells rather than whole blood for transfusion in humans. The use of such suspensions is logical whenever it is important to introduce red cells into a patient's circulation with the least possible disturbance of blood volume. In fact, other considerations led to the widespread use of red cells. During the Second World War, plasma was collected on a large scale. The hope of salvaging red cells that would otherwise be discarded led to clinical trials of the red cell residues (MacQuaide and Mollison 1940). An incidental advantage of using red cells rather than whole blood was a reduction in the rate of reactions. In an early series, severe febrile reactions were noted to be three times less common with packed red cells (MacQuaide and Mollison 1940). In retrospect, this reduction was probably due to the practice of removing as much of the buffy coat as possible in preparing the packed red cells (see Chapter 15).

Red cell concentrates are preferable to whole blood in transfusing patients with severe anaemia. The PCV of concentrates varies widely according to the method of preparation: sedimented cells usually have a PCV of 0.65–0.70, 30% of the original plasma and all the original leucocytes and platelets. Centrifuged cells have a PCV of 0.80 and 15% of the original plasma.

Centrifuged cells with the buffy coat squeezed off have a PCV of more than 0.90, 5–10% of the plasma, less than 30% of the platelets and less than 10% of the leucocytes. Addition of about one-third of the volume of saline to centrifuged red cells lowers the PCV to 0.70 and reduces the viscosity from about 5 times to only 1.3 times that of whole blood (Prins 1970).

Washed suspensions of red cells are not needed very often. Patients for whom they may be indicated are as follows:

1 Infants or fetuses requiring intrauterine transfusion, given either via the fetal peritoneal cavity or directly into umbilical cord vessels.

2 Patients who have had, or are likely to have, reactions to the transfusion of plasma proteins, e.g. patients with class-specific anti-IgA (where donors lacking IgA are not available) or patients with subclass-specific anti-IgA. In patients with anti-IgA, very thorough washing (six times) is needed (see Chapter 15).

3 Patients who have had severe allergic transfusion reactions for which no cause can be found.

4 Patients with T-activated red cells who require transfusion; see Chapter 7.

5 Very occasional patients with severe autoimmune haemolytic anaemia due to haemolysins in whom the supply of complement in transfused plasma may exacerbate red cell destruction.

6 Patients with paroxysmal nocturnal haemoglobinuria (PNH). PNH red cells are very susceptible to lysis by complement and are lysed *in vitro* by the interaction of leucocyte antigens and antibodies (Sirchia *et al.* 1970). Some authorities recommend the use of washed red cells for transfusion (Rosse 1990), although the overall frequency of reactions is apparently no lower than when ABO-identical unwashed cells are used. Avoidance of ABO isoagglutinins rather than removal of plasma proteins seems to be the crucial factor (Brecher and Taswell 1989).

For details of *frozen and thawed red cells*, see Chapter 14.

References

Adams RJ, McKie VC, Brambilla D *et al.* (1998) Stroke prevention trial in sickle cell anemia. Control Clin Trials 19: 110–129

Adner PL, Foconi S, Sjölin S (1963) Immunization after intravenous injection of small amounts of 51Cr-labelled red cells. Br J Haematol 9: 288

Åkerblom O, Kreuger A (1975) Studies on citrate-phosphate-dextrose (CPD) blood supplemented with adenine. Vox Sang 29: 90

Åkerblom O, de Verdier C-H, Finnson M (1967) Further studies on the effect of adenine in blood preservation. Transfusion 7: 1

Alderman EM, Fudenberg HH, Lovins RE (1980) Binding of immunoglobulin classes to subpopulations of red blood cells separated by density-gradient centrifugation. Blood 55: 817–822

Alderman EM, Fudenberg HH, Lovins RE (1981) Isolation and characterization of an age-related antigen present on senescent human red blood cells. Blood 58: 341–349

Apstein CS, Dennis RC, Briggs L *et al.* (1985) Effect of erythrocyte storage and oxyhemoglobin affinity changes on cardiac function. Am J Physiol 248: H508–H515

Ashby W (1919) The determination of the length of life of transfused blood corpuscles in man. J Exp Med 29: 267

AuBuchon JP, Brightman A (1989) Use of indium-111 as a red cell label. Transfusion 29: 143–147

AuBuchon JP, Estep TN, Davey RJ (1988) The effect of the plasticizer di-2-ethylhexyl phthalate on the survival of stored RBCs. Blood 71: 448–452

Audet AM, Andrzejewski C, Popovsky MA (1998) Red blood cell transfusion practices in patients undergoing orthopedic surgery: a multi-institutional analysis. Orthopedics 21: 851–858

Avoy DR, Ellisor SS, Nolan NJ (1978) The effect of delayed refrigeration on red cells, platelet concentrates and cryoprecipitable AHF. Transfusion 18: 160

Aylward FX, Mainwaring BR, Wilkinson JF (1940) Effects of some preservatives on stored blood. Lancet i: 685

Bandarenko N, Hay SN, Holmberg J *et al.* (2004) Extended storage of AS-1 and AS-3 leukoreduced red blood cells for 15 days after deglycerolization and resuspension in AS-3 using an automated closed system. Transfusion 44: 1656–1662

Barkun A, Bardou M, Marshall JK (2003) Consensus recommendations for managing patients with nonvariceal upper gastrointestinal bleeding. Ann Intern Med 139: 843–857

Belcher EH, Harriss E (1959) Studies of red cell lifespan in the rat. J Physiol (Lond) 146: 127

Bensinger TA, Chillar RK, Beutler E (1977) Prolonged maintenance of 2, 3-DPG in liquid blood storage: use of an internal CO_2 trap to stabilize pH. J Lab Clin Med 89: 498

Bentley SA, Glass HI, Lewis SM (1974) Elution correction in 51Cr red cell survival studies. Br J Haematol 26: 179

Berlin NI, Lawrence JH, Lee HC (1954) The pathogenesis of the anemia of chronic leukemia: measurement of the life-span of the red blood cell with glycine-2-C14. J Lab Clin Med 44: 860

Beutler E (1957) The glutathione instability of drug-sensitive red cells. A new method for the *in vitro* detection of drug sensitivity. J Lab Clin Med 39: 84

Beutler E (1988) Isolation of the aged. Blood Cells 14: 1–5

Beutler E, West C (1979) The storage of hard-packed red blood cells in citrate-phosphate-dextrose (CPD) and CPD-adenine (CPDA-1). Blood 54: 280–284

Beutler E, West C (1984) Measurement of the viability of stored red cells by the single-isotope technique using ^{51}Cr. Transfusion 24: 100–104

Beutler E, West C (1985) Measurement of the viable Adsol-preserved human red cells (Letter). N Engl J Med 312: 1392

Beutler E, Wood L (1969) The *in vivo* regeneration of red cell 2,3-diphosphoglyceric acid (DPG) after transfusion of stored blood. J Lab Clin Med 74: 300

Beutler E, Kuhl W, West C (1982) The osmotic fragility of erythrocytes after prolonged liquid storage and after reinfusion. Blood 59: 1141–1147

Blank JP, Sheagren TG, Vajaria J (1984) The role of rbc transfusion in the premature neonate. Am J Dis Child 138: 831–833

Borun ER, Figueroa WG, Perry SM (1957) The distribution of Fe59 tagged human erythrocytes in centrifuged specimens as a function of cell age. J Clin Invest 36: 676

Bove JR, Ebaugh FG Jr (1958) The use of diisopropyl fluorophosphate32 for the determination of *in vivo* red cell survival and plasma cholinesterase turnover ratio. J Lab Clin Med 51: 916

Bracey AW, Klein HG, Chambers S et al. (1983) *Ex vivo* selective isolation of young red blood cells using the IBM-2991 cell washer. Blood 61: 1068–1071

Bradai M, Abad MT, Pissard S et al. (2003) Hydroxyurea can eliminate transfusion requirements in children with severe beta-thalassemia. Blood 102: 1529–1530

Bratteby L-E, Wadman B (1968) Labelling of red blood cells *in vitro* with small amounts of di-iso-propyl-fluorophosphonate (DF32P). Scand J Clin Lab Invest 21: 197

Brazier DJ, Gregor ZJ, Blach RK (1986) Retinal detachment in patients with proliferative sickle cell retinopathy. Transact Ophthalmol Soc UK 105: 100–105

Brecher ME, Taswell HF (1989) Paroxysmal nocturnal hemoglobinuria and the transfusion of washed red cells. A myth revisited. Transfusion 29: 681–685

Brown IJ, Hardin HF (1953) Recovery and *in vivo* survival of human red cells. Arch Surg 66: 267

Buchholz D, Aster R, Menitove J (1989) Red blood cell storage studies in a citrate-plasticized polyvinyl chloride container. Transfusion 29 (Suppl.): 8S

Callender STE, Powell EO, Witts LJ (1945) The life-span of the red cell in man. J Pathol Bact 57: 129

Callender STE, Powell EO, Witts LJ (1947) Normal red cell survival in men and women. J Pathol Bact 59: 519

Callender STE, Nickel JF, Moore CV (1949) Sickle-cell disease: studied by measuring the survival of transfused red blood cells. J Lab Clin Med 34: 90

Card RT, Mohandas N, Mollison PL (1983) Relationship of post-transfusion viability to deformability of stored red cells. Br J Haematol 53: 237–240

Carson JL, Duff A, Berlin JA et al. (1998) Perioperative blood transfusion and postoperative mortality. JAMA 279: 199–205

Carson JL, Noveck H, Berlin JA et al. (2002) Mortality and morbidity in patients with very low postoperative Hb levels who decline blood transfusion. Transfusion 42: 812–818

Castellanos A (1937) La transfusion de globules. Arch Med Infant 6: 319

Castro O, Hardy KP, Winter WP et al. (1981) Freeze preservation of sickle erythrocytes. Am J Hematol 10: 297–304

Cavill I, Ricketts C, Napier JA et al. (1977) Ferrokinetics and erythropoiesis in man: red-cell production and destruction in normal and anaemic subjects. Br J Haematol 35: 33–40

Cavill I, Trevett D, Fisher J (1988) The measurement of the total volume of red cells in man: a non-radioactive approach using biotin. Br J Haematol 70: 491–493

Cazzola M, De Stefano P, Ponchio L et al. (1995) Relationship between transfusion regimen and suppression of erythropoiesis in beta-thalassaemia major. Br J Haematol 89: 473–478

Cazzola M, Borgna-Pignatti C, Locatelli F et al. (1997) A moderate transfusion regimen may reduce iron loading in beta-thalassemia major without producing excessive expansion of erythropoiesis. Transfusion 37: 135–140

Chapler CK, Cain SM (1986) The physiologic reserve in oxygen carrying capacity: studies in experimental hemodilution. Can J Physiol Pharmacol 64: 7–12

Chaplin H Jr (1984) Editorial retrospective. Frozen red cells revisited. N Engl J Med 311: 1696–1698

Chaplin H Jr, Crawford H, Cutbush M (1952) The effects of a phenothiazine derivative (RP3300) on red cell preservation. J Clin Pathol 5: 9

Chaplin H Jr, Crawford H, Cutbush M (1954) Post-transfusion survival of red cells stored at −20°C. Lancet i: 852

Chaplin HJ, Crawford H, Cutbush M (1956) The preservation of red cells at −79°C. Clin Sci 15: 27

Chaplin HJ, Schmidt PJ, Steinfeld JL (1957) Storage of red cells at sub-zero temperatures, further studies. Clin Sci 16: 651

Charache S Moyer MA (1982) Treatment of patients with sickle cell anemia – another view. In: Advances in the Pathophysiology, Diagnosis and Treatment of Sickle Cell Disease. Progress in Clinical and Biological Research. Scott RB (ed.). New York: Alan R Liss, pp. 73–81.

Christensen BE (1971) Effects of an enlarged splenic erythrocyte pool in chronic lymphocytic leukaemia. Scand J Haematol 8: 92

Cline MI, Berlin NI (1962) Red blood-cell life span using DFP32 as a cohort label. Blood 19: 715

Cline MJ, Berlin NI (1963a) An evaluation of DF32P and 51Cr as methods of measuring red cell life span in man. Blood 22: 459

Cline MJ, Berlin NI (1963b) The red cell chromium elution rate in patients with some hematologic disease. Blood 21: 63

Cohen JA, Warringa MGPJ (1954) The fate of P32 labelled di-isopropylfluorophosphonate in the human body and its use as a labelling agent in the study of the turnover of blood plasma and red cells. J Clin Invest 33: 459

Collins JA (1980) Abnormal hemoglobin-oxygen affinity and surgical hemotherapy. In: Surgical Hemotherapy. Collins JA and Lundsgard-Hangen P (eds). Basel: S Karger

Consensus Conference (1988) Perioperative red blood cell transfusion. JAMA 260: 2700–2703

Corash L, Klein H, Deisseroth A (1981) Selective isolation of young erythrocytes for transfusion support of thalassemia major patients. Blood 57: 599–606

Cordle DG, Strauss RG, Lankford G et al. (1999) Antibodies provoked by the transfusion of biotin-labeled red cells. Transfusion 39: 1065–1069

Cotter J, McNeal WJ (1938) Citrate solution for preservation of fluid blood. Proc Soc Exp Biol (NY) 38: 751

Council of Europe (2003) Guide to the Preparation, Use and Quality Assurance of Blood Components. Strasbourg: Council of Europe Press, p. 17

Cowley H, Wojda U, Cipolone KM et al. (1999) Biotinylation modifies red cell antigens. Transfusion 39: 163–168

Crawford H, Mollison PL (1955) Reversal of electrolyte changes in stored red cells after transfusion. J Physiol (Lond) 129: 639

Dacie JV, Firth D (1943) Blood transfusion in nocturnal haemoglobinuria. BMJ i: 626

Dacie JV, Mollison PL (1943) Survival of normal erythrocytes after transfusion to patients with familial haemolytic anaemia (acholuric jaundice). Lancet i: 550

Dale GL, Norenberg SL (1990) Density fractionation of erythrocytes by Percoll-hypaque results in only a slight enrichment for aged cells. Biochim Biophys Acta 1036: 183–187

Davey RJ, Lenes BL, Casper AJ (1984) Adequate survival of red cells from units 'undercollected' in citrate-phosphate-dextrose-adenine-one. Transfusion 24: 319–322

Davey RJ, McCoy NC, Yu M (1992) The effect of prestorage irradiation on posttransfusion red cell survival. Transfusion 32: 525–528

Dawson RB, Ellis TJ, Hershey RT (1976) Blood preservation. XVI. Packed red cell storage in CPD-adenine. Transfusion 16: 179

Dekkers HJN (1939) The fate of the transfused red blood cells. Acta Med Scand 99: 587

Depalma L, Palmer R, Leitman SF et al. (1990) Utilization patterns of frozen autologous red blood cells. Experience in a referral center and a community hospital. Arch Pathol Lab Med 114: 516–518

Dern RJ (1968) Studies on the preservation of human blood. III. The posttransfusion survival of stored and damaged erythrocytes in healthy donors and patients with severe trauma. J Lab Clin Med 71: 254

Dern RJ, Gwinn RP, Wiorkowski JJ (1966) Studies on the preservation of human blood. Variability in erythrocyte storage characteristics among healthy donors. J Lab Clin Med 67: 955

Dern RJ, Wiorkowski JJ, Matsuda T (1970) Studies on the preservation of human blood. V. The effect of mixing anticoagulated blood during storage on the poststorage erythrocyte survival. J Lab Clin Med 75: 37

Donohue DM, Motulsky AG, Giblett ER (1955) The use of chromium as a red cell tag. Br J Haematol 1: 249

Dornhorst AC (1951) The interpretation of red cell survival curves. Blood 6: 1284

Duhm J (1974) Metabolism and function of 2,3-diphosphoglycerate in red blood cells. In: The Human Red Cell in vitro. TJ Greenwalt, GA Jamieson (eds). New York: Grune and Stratton, pp. 111–148

Duhm J, Deuticke B, Gerlach E (1971) Complete restoration of oxygen transport function and 2,3-diphosphoglycerate concentration in stored blood. Transfusion 11: 147

Duke M, Abelmann WH (1969) The hemodynamic response to chronic anemia. Circulation 39: 503–515

Dumaswala U, Greenwalt TJ (1984) Human erythrocytes shed exocytic vesicles in vivo. Transfusion 24: 490–497

Eadie GS, Brown W Jr (1955) The potential life-span and ultimate survival of fresh red blood cells in normal healthy recipients as studied by simultaneous 51Cr tagging and differential hemolysis. J Clin Invest 34: 629

Ebaugh FJ, Beekin WL (1959) Quantitative measurement of gastro-intestinal blood loss. II. Determination of 24-hour fecal blood loss by a chemical photospectrometric technique. J Lab Clin Med 53: 777

Eernisse JG, van Rood JJ (1961) Erythrocyte survival time determinations with the aid of DF32P. Br J Haematol 7: 382

Ericson A, Niklasson F, de Verdier C-H (1983) A systematic study of nucleotide analysis of human erythrocytes using an anionic exchanger and HPLC. Clin Chim Acta 127: 47–59

Estep TN, Pedersen RA, Miller T (1984) Characterization of erythrocyte quality during the refrigerated storage of whole blood containing di-(2-ethylhexyl) phthalate. Blood 64: 1270–1276

Evans RS, Duane R (1949) Hemolytic anemias; recent advances in diagnosis and treatment. Calif Med 70: 1

Falk JS, Lindblad GTO, Westman BTM (1972) Histopathological studies on kidneys from patients treated with large amounts of blood preserved with ACD-adenine. Transfusion 12: 376

Fantus B (1937) The therapy of the Cook County Hospital. JAMA 108: 128

Fibach E, Sharon R (1994) Changes in ABH antigen expression on red cells during *in vivo* aging: a flow cytometric analysis. Transfusion 34: 328–332

Filatov AN (1937) (Abstract). Int Abstracts Surg 66: 500

Finch CA, Lenfant C (1972) Oxygen transport in man. N Engl J Med 286: 407–415

Finke J, Heimpel H, Hoffman G (1965) Vergleichende Untersuchungen zur Bestimmung der Erythrozytenlebenszeit mit Cr51 und DFP32 beim Menschen. Nucl Med (Amst) 4: 349

Fischer H (1965) Preservation of human blood in the liquid state: the practical importance of some new media. Proc 10th Congr Int Soc Blood Transfus, Stockholm. Bibl Haematol 23(3): 616.

Fleig C (1910) Les eaux minérales. Mileux vitaux. Serothérapie artificielle et balnéothérapie tissulaire par leur injection dans l'organisme. Academie des Sciences et Lettres de Montpellier. Mémoires de la Section de Médecine. 2ᴱ série, 3:1

Florey JW, Jennings JM (1941). The effects of massive injections of blood, plasma and serum into normal cats. Unpublished Report to the Medical Research Council, London, UK

Florio PHL, Stewart M, Mugrage ER (1943) The effect of freezing on erythrocytes. J Lab Clin Med 28: 1486

Foconi S, Sjölin S (1959) Survival of Cr51 labelled-red cells from newborn infants. Acta Paediat (Uppsala) 48 (Suppl.) 117: 18

Friedman BA, Burns TL, Schork MA (1980) An analysis of blood transfusion of surgical patients by sex: a question for the transfusion trigger. Transfusion 20: 179–188

Fullerton MW, Philippart AI, Sarnaik S (1981) Preoperative exchange transfusion in sickle cell anemia. J Pediatr Surg 16: 297–300

Gabrio B, Finch CA (1954) Erythrocyte preservation. I. The relation of the storage lesion to *in vivo* erythrocyte senescence. J Clin Invest 33: 242

Gabrio BW, Donohue DM, Finch CA (1955a) Erythrocyte preservation. V. Relationship between chemical changes and viability of stored blood treated with adenosine. J Clin Invest 34: 1509

Gabrio BW, Hennessey M, Thomasson JEA (1955b) Erythrocyte preservation. IV. The *in vitro* reversibility of the storage lesion. J Biol Chem 215: 357

Ganzoni AM, Oakes R, Hillman RS (1971) Red cell ageing *in vivo*. J Clin Invest 50: 1373

Garby L (1962) Analysis of red-cell survival curves in clinical practice and the use of di-isopropylfluoro phosphonate (DF32P) as a label for red cells in man. Br J Haematol 8: 15

Garby L, Mollison PL (1971) Deduction of mean red cell life-span from 51Cr survival curves. Br J Haematol 20: 527

Garratty G (1990) Flow cytometry; its applications to immunohaematology. In: Blood Transfusion: the Impact of New Technologies. C Marcela (ed.) Baillière's Clinical Haematology, pp. 267–287

Gattegno L, Bladier D, Cornillat P (1975) Ageing *in vivo* and neuraminidase treatment of rabbit erythrocytes: influence on half-life assessed by 51Cr labelling. Hoppe-Zeyler's Z Physiol Chem 356: 391

Gibson JG, Murphy WJ, Scheitlin WA (1956) The influence of extra-cellular factors involved in the collection of blood in ACD on maintenance of red cell viability during refrigerated storage. Am J Clin Pathol 26: 855

Gilardi VA, Miescher P (1957) Die Lebensdauer von autologen und homologen Erythrocyten bei Frühgeborenen und Elteren Kindern. Schweiz Med Wschr 87: 1456

Goldfinger D, Capon S, Czer L *et al.* (1993) Safety and efficacy of preoperative donation of blood for autologous use by patients with end-stage heart or lung disease who are awaiting organ transplantation. Transfusion 33: 336–340

Gray SJ, Sterling K (1950) The tagging of red cells and plasma proteins with radioactive chromium. J Clin Invest 29: 1604

Graziano JH, Piomelli S, Seaman C (1982) A simple technique for preparation of young red cells for transfusion from ordinary blood units. Blood 59: 865–868

Greenwalt TJ, McGuinness CG, Dumaswala UJ (1991) Studies in red blood cell preservation: 4. Plasma vesicle hemoglobin exceeds free hemoglobin. Vox Sang 61: 14–17

Groopman JE, Molina J-E, Scadden DT (1989) Hematopoietic growth factors. Biology and clinical applications. N Engl J Med 321: 1449–1457

Hahn PF, Miller LL, Rosbscheit-Robbins FS (1944) Peritoneal absorption. Red cells labeled by radio-iron hemoglobin move promptly from the peritoneal cavity into the circulation. J Exp Med 80: 77

Hall TL, Barnes A, Miller JR (1993) Neonatal mortality following transfusion of red cells with high plasma potassium levels. Transfusion 33: 606–609

Halpern BN, Dreyfus B, Bourdon G (1950) Influence favorable sur la conservation du sang des dérivés de la phénothiazine. Presse Med 58: 1151

Hamilton HE, Sheets RF, De Gowin EL (1950) Studies with inagglutinable erythrocyte counts. II. Analysis of mechanism of Cooley's anemia. J Clin Invest 29: 714

Haynes LL, Tullis JL, Pyle HM (1960) Clinical use of glycerolized frozen blood. JAMA 173: 1657

Heaton A, Miripol J, Aster R (1984) Use of Adsol preservation solution for prolonged storage of low viscosity AS-1 red blood cells. Br J Haematol 57: 467–478

Heaton WAL, Hanbury CM, Keegan TE (1989a) Studies with nonradioisotopic sodium chromate I. Development of a technique for measuring red cell volume. Transfusion 29: 696–702

Heaton WAL, Keegan T, Hanbury CM (1989b) Studies with nonradioisotopic sodium chromate II. Single and double-label 52Cr/51Cr post-transfusion recovery estimations. Transfusion 29: 703–707

Heaton A, Keegan T, Holmes S (1989c) In vivo regeneration of red cell 2,3-diphosphoglycerate following transfusion of DPG-depleted AS-1, AS-3 and CPDA-1 red cells. Transfusion 71: 131–136

Heaton WAL, Keegan T, Holme S (1989d) Evaluation of 99m Technetium/51 Chromium post-transfusion recovery of red cells stored in saline, adenine, glucose, mannitol for 42 days. Vox Sang 57: 37–42

Hebert PC, Wells G, Blajchman MA et al. (1999) A multi-center, randomized, controlled clinical trial of transfusion requirements in critical care. Transfusion Requirements in Critical Care Investigators, Canadian Critical Care Trials Group. N Engl J Med 340: 409–417

Heimpel H, Erdmann H, Hoffman G (1964) Tierexperimentelle Untersuchungen zur Markierung von Erythrozyten mit radioaktivem Diisopropylfluorphosphat (DFP32). Nucl Med (Amst) 4: 32

Hess JR, Hill HR, Oliver CK et al. (2003) Twelve-week RBC storage. Transfusion 43: 867–872

Hillman RS (1964) Pooled human plasma as a volume expander. N Engl J Med 271: 1027

Hinchey J, Chaves C, Appignani B et al. (1996) A reversible posterior leukoencephalopathy syndrome. N Engl J Med 334: 494–500

Hoffman-Fezer G, Mysliwietz J, Mortlbauer W (1993) Biotin labeling as an alternative nonradioactive approach to determination of red cell survival. Ann Hematol 67: 81–87

Hogan VA, Blanchette VS, Rock G (1986) A simple method for preparing neocyte-enriched leukocyte-poor blood for transfusion-dependent patients. Transfusion 26: 253–257

Högman CF (1971) Oxygen affinity of stored blood. Acta Anaesthesiol Scand 45 (Suppl.): 53–61

Högman CF (1994) Recent advances in the preparation and storage of red cells. Vox Sang 67 (Suppl. 3): 243–246

Högman CF, Åkerblom O, Hedlund K et al. (1983) Red cell suspensions in SAGM medium. Further experience of in vivo survival of red cells, clinical usefulness and plasma-saving effects. Vox Sang 45: 217–223

Högman CF, de Verdier CH, Ericson A et al. (1985) Studies on the mechanism of human red cell loss of viability during storage at +4 degrees C in vitro. I. Cell shape and total adenylate concentration as determinant factors for post-transfusion survival. Vox Sang 48: 257–268

Högman CF, de Verdier CH, Borgstrom L (1987a) Studies on the mechanism of human red cell loss of viability during storage at +4 degrees C. II. Relation between cellular morphology and viability. Vox Sang 52: 20–23

Högman CF, de Verdier CH, Ericson A et al. (1987b) Studies on the mechanism of human red cell loss of viability during storage at +4 degrees C in vitro. III. Effects of mixing during storage. Vox Sang 53: 84–88

Högman CF, Eriksson L, Ericson A et al. (1991) Storage of saline-adenine-glucose-mannitol-suspended red cells in a new plastic container: polyvinylchloride plasticized with butyryl-n-trihexyl-citrate. Transfusion 31: 26–29

Högman CF, Eriksson L, Gong J et al. (1993) Half-strength citrate CPD combined with a new additive solution for improved storage of red blood cells suitable for clinical use. Vox Sang 65: 271–278

Hogue CW Jr, Goodnough LT, Monk TG (1998) Perioperative myocardial ischemic episodes are related to hematocrit level in patients undergoing radical prostatectomy. Transfusion 38: 924–931

Hollingsworth JW (1955) Life-span of fetal erythrocytes. J Lab Clin Med 45: 469

Homi J, Reynolds J, Skinner A (1979) General anaesthesia in sickle-cell disease. BMJ i: 1599–1601

Horowitz B, Stryker MH, Wardman AA (1984) Stabilization of red blood cells by the plasticizer, diethylhexylphthalate. Vox Sang 48: 150–155

Huber H, Lewis SM, Szur L (1964) The influence of anaemia, polycythaemia and splenomegaly on the relationship between venous haematocrit and red-cell volume. Br J Haematol 10: 567

Hughes-Jones NC (1958a) Measurement of red-cell loss from gastro-intestinal tract, using radioactive chromium. BMJ i: 493

Hughes-Jones NC (1958b) Storage of red cells at temperatures between +10°C and –20°C. Br J Haematol 4: 249

Hughes-Jones NC, Mollison PL (1956) Interpretation of 51Cr survival curves. Clin Sci 15: 207

Hughes-Jones NC, Mollison PL, Robinson MA (1957) Factors affecting the viability of erythrocytes stored in the frozen state. Proc Roy Soc Lond B 147: 476

Hunter W (1884) The demonstration of the life of red blood corpuscles as ascertainable by transfusion. Proc Roy Soc Edinb 13: 849

Hurdle ADF, Rosin AJ (1962) Red cell volume and red cell survival in normal aged people. J Clin Pathol 15: 343

ICSH (1971) Recommended methods for radioisotope red-cell survival studies. Br J Haematol 21: 241

ICSH (1980) Recommended methods for radioisotope red-cell survival studies. Br J Haematol 45: 659–666

Issitt PD, Valinsky JE, Marsh WL (1990) In vivo red cell destruction by anti-Lu6. Transfusion 30: 258–260

Jandl JH, Tomlinson AS (1958) The destruction of red cells by antibodies in man. II. Pyrogenic, leukocytic and dermal responses to immune hemolysis. J Clin Invest 37: 1202

Jandl JH, Jones AR, Castle WB (1957) The destruction of red cells by antibodies in man. I. Observations on the sequestration and lysis of red cells altered by immune mechanisms. J Clin Invest 36: 1428

Jeanneney G, Servantie L (1939) Influence du pH et de la nature du citrate de soude employé, sur le rapport sodium/potassium du plasma sanguin citraté. Soc Biol Bordeaux 130: 473

Jones J, Mollison PL (1978) A simple and efficient method of labelling red cells with 99mTc for determination of red cell volume. Br J Haematol 38: 141

Jones RL (2003) The blood supply chain, from donor to patient: a call for greater understanding leading to more effective strategies for managing the blood supply. Transfusion 43: 132–134

Jorda FD (1939) The Barcelona Blood-Transfusion Service. Lancet i: 773

Karle H (1969) Destruction of erythrocytes during experimental fever. Quantitative aspects. Br J Haematol 16: 409

Keitel H, Thompson D, Itano H (1956) Hyposthenuria in sickle cell anemia: a reversible defect. J Clin Invest 35, 998–1001.

Khansari N (1983) Mechanisms for the Removal of Senescent Human Erythrocytes from Circulation: Specificity of the Membrane-bound Immunoglobulin G. Ireland: Elsevier Scientific Publishers, pp. 49–58

Kim HC, Dugan NP, Silber JH et al. (1994) Erythrocytapheresis therapy to reduce iron overload in chronically transfused patients with sickle cell disease. Blood 83: 1136–1142

Klein HG (2001) Earthquake in America. Transfusion 41: 1179–1180

Klein HG, Garner RJ, Miller DM et al. (1980) Automated partial exchange transfusion in sickle cell anemia. Transfusion 20: 578–584

Kleine N, Heimpel H (1965) The early loss of radioactivity in 51Cr survival curves: destruction of cells or loss of the label? Blood 26: 819

Koshy M, Burd L, Wallace D et al. J (1988) Prophylactic red-cell transfusions in pregnant patients with sickle cell disease. A randomized cooperative study. N Engl J Med 319: 1447–1452

Koshy M, Weiner SJ, Miller ST et al. (1995) Surgery and anesthesia in sickle cell disease. Cooperative Study of Sickle Cell Diseases. Blood 86: 3676–3684

Kreuger A (1976) Adenine metabolism during and after exchange transfusions in newborn infants with CPD-adenine blood. Transfusion 16: 249

Kreuger A, Åkerblom O (1980) Adenine consumption in stored citrate-phosphate-dextrose-adenine blood. Vox Sang 38: 156–160

Kreuger A, Åkerblom O, Hogman CF (1975) A clinical evaluation of citrate-phosphate-dextrose-adenine blood. Vox Sang 29: 81

Krijnen HW, de Wit JJF, Kuivenhoven ACJ (1964) Glycerol treated human red cells frozen with liquid nitrogen. Vox Sang 9: 559

Krijnen HW Kuivenhoven ACJ, De Wit JJFM (1970) The preservation of blood cells in the frozen state. In: Modern Problems of Blood Preservation. W Speilmann, S Seidl (eds). Stuttgart: Gustav Fischer

Kurantsin-Mills J, Klug PP, Lessin LS (1988) Vaso-occlusion in sickle cell disease: pathophysiology of the microvascular circulation. Am J Pediatr Hematol Oncol 10: 357–372

Landsteiner K, Levine P, Janes ML (1928) On the development of isoagglutinins following transfusions. Proc Soc Exp Biol (NY) 25: 672

Lawrence VA, Silverstein JH, Cornell JE et al. (2003) Higher Hb level is associated with better early functional recovery after hip fracture repair. Transfusion 43: 1717–1722

Leung JM, Weiskopf RB, Feiner J et al. (2000) Electrocardiographic ST-segment changes during acute, severe isovolemic hemodilution in humans. Anesthesiology 93: 1004–1010

Lewis SM (1962) Red-cell abnormalities and haemolysis in aplastic anaemia. Br J Haematol 8: 322

Lichtman HC, Watson RJ, Feldman F (1953) Studies on thalassemia. Part I. An extracorpuscular defect in thalassemia major. Part II. The effects of splenectomy in thalassemia major with an associated acquired hemolytic anemia. J Clin Invest 32: 1229

Lockwood WB, Hudgens RW, Szymanski IO et al. (2003) Effects of rejuvenation and frozen storage on 42-day-old AS-3 RBCs. Transfusion 43: 1527–1532

Loeb V Jr, Moore CV, Dubach R (1953) The physiological evaluation and management of chronic bone marrow failure. Am J Med 15: 499

Loutit JF, Mollison PL (1943) Advantages of a disodium-citrate-glucose mixture as a blood preservative. BMJ ii: 744

Loutit JF, Mollison MD, van der Walt ED (1942) Venous pressure during venesection and blood transfusion. BMJ ii: 658

Loutit JF, Mollison PL, Young IM (1943) Citric acid-sodium-citrate-glucose mixtures for blood storage. Quart J Exp Physiol 32: 183

Lovelock JE (1952) Resuspension in plasma of human red blood cells frozen in glycerol. Lancet i: 1238

Lovelock JE (1953a) The haemolysis of human red blood cells by freezing and thawing. Biochim Biophys Acta 10: 414

Lovelock JE (1953b) The mechanism of the protective action of glycerol against haemolysis by freezing and thawing. Biochim Biophys Acta 11: 28

Lovric VA, Klarkowski DB (1989) Donor blood frozen and stored between −20°C and −25°C with 35-day post-thaw shelf life. Lancet i: 71–73

Luban NL (2002) Neonatal red blood cell transfusions. Curr Opin Hematol 9: 533–536

Lundy JS, Tovell RM, Tuohy EB (1936) Annual report for 1935 of the section of anesthesia: Including data of blood transfusion. Proc Staff Meet Mayo Clin 11: 921–932

Luthra MG, Friedman JM, Sears DA (1979) Studies of density fractions of normal human erythrocytes labelled with iron-59 *in vivo*. J Lab Clin Med 94: 879–896

Lutz HU (1978) Vesicles isolated from ATP-depleted erythrocytes and out of thrombocyte-rich plasma. J Supramol Struct 8: 375–389

Lutz HU, Stammler P, Fasler S (1992) Density separation of human red blood cells on self forming Percoll gradients: correlation with cell age. Biochim Biophys Acta 1116: 1–10

Luyet BJ, Gehenio PM (1940) Life and Death at Low Temperature. Normandy, MO: Biodynamica

MacQuaide DHG, Mollison PL (1940) Treatment of anaemia with concentrated red cell suspensions. BMJ ii: 555

Madsen LP, Rasmussen MK, Bjerregaard LL et al. (2000) Impact of blood sampling in very preterm infants. Scand J Clin Lab Invest 60: 125–132

Maier RF, Obladen M, Scigalla P (1994) The effect of epoietin beta (recombinant human erythropoietin) on the need for transfusion in very-low-birth-weight infants. N Engl J Med 330: 1173–1178

Maier RF, Obladen M, Muller-Hansen I et al. (2002) Early treatment with erythropoietin beta ameliorates anemia and reduces transfusion requirements in infants with birth weights below 1000 g. J Pediatr 141: 8–15

Maizels M (1941) Preservation of organic phosphorous compounds in stored blood by glucose. Lancet i: 722

Maizels M, Paterson JH (1940) Survival of stored blood after transfusion. Lancet ii: 417

Marcus CS, Myhre BA, Angulo MC (1987) Radiolabelled red cell viability. I. Comparison of 51Cr, 99mTc, and 111In for measuring the viability of autologous stored red cells. Transfusion 27: 415–419

Marcus RE, Wonke B, Bantock HM (1985) A prospective trial of young red cells in 48 patients with transfusion-dependent thalassaemia. Br J Haematol 60: 153–159

Marik PE, Sibbald WJ (1993) Effect of stored-blood transfusion on oxygen delivery in patients with sepsis. JAMA 269: 3024–3029

Mario N, Baudin B, Aussel C et al. (1997) Capillary iso-electric focusing and high-performance cation-exchange chromatography compared for qualitative and quantitative analysis of hemoglobin variants. Clin Chem 43: 2137–2142

Matthes G, Tofote U, Krause K-P (1994) Improved red cell quality after erythroplasmapheresis with MCS-3P. J Clin Apheresis 9: 183–188

Mayer K , D'Amaro J (1964) Improvement of methods of differential haemolysis by haemoglobinometry. Scand J Haematol 1: 331

Mayer K, Ley AB, D'Amaro J (1966) Impairment of red cell viability by exposure to 'excess' acid-citrate dextrose. Blood 28: 513

Mayer K, Dwyer A, Laughlin JS (1970) Spleen scanning using ACD-damaged red cells tagged with 51Cr. J Nucl Med 11: 455

Mazur P, Leibo SP, Chu EHY (1972) A two-factor hypothesis of freezing. Exp Cell Res 71: 345

McCurdy PR, Rath CE (1958) Splenectomy in hemolytic anemia; results predicted by body scanning after injection of Cr51-tagged red cells. N Engl J Med 259: 459–463

McFadzean AJS, Todd D, Tsang KC (1958) Observations on the anemia of cryptogenetic splenomegaly. I. Hemolysis. Blood 13: 513

McManus TF, Borgese TA (1961) Effect of pyruvate on metabolism of inosine by erythrocytes. Fed Proc 20: 65

Meryman HT (1956) Mechanics of freezing in living cells and tissues. Science 124: 515

Meryman HT (1971) Osmotic stress as a mechanism of freezing injury. Cryobiology 8: 489–500

Meryman HT (1989) Cryopreservation of blood cells and tissues. In: Clinical Practice of Transfusion Medicine. LD Petz, SN Swisher (eds). Edinburgh: Churchill Livingstone, pp. 297–314

Meryman HT, Hornblower M (1972) A method for freezing and washing red blood cells using a high glycerol concentration. Transfusion 12: 145

Meryman HT, Hornblower M (1978) Advances in red cell freezing (Abstract). Transfusion 18: 632

Meryman HT, Hornblower M, Keegan T (1991) Refrigerated storage of washed red cells. Vox Sang 60: 88–98

Meryman HT, Hornblower M, Syring R et al. (1994) Extending the storage of red cells at 4°C. Transfus Sci 15: 105–115

Miescher P (1956a) Le mécanisme de l'erythroclasie a l'état normal. Rev Hematol 11: 248

Miescher P (1956b) Hypersplenie. Helv Med Acta 23: 457

Miescher P, Burger H, Gilardi A (1958) Die Lebensdauer von 51Cr-markierten Erythrocyten in verschiedenen Lebensaltern. Strahlentherapie 38 (Suppl. 3): 236

Miller DM, Winslow RM, Klein HG et al. (1980) Improved exercise performance after exchange transfusion in subjects with sickle cell anemia. Blood 56: 1127–1131

Mills JN (1946) The life-span of the erythrocyte. J Physiol (Lond) 105: 16

Milner PF (1982) Chronic transfusion regimens for sickle cell disease. In: Advances in the Pathophysiology, Diagnosis and Treatment of Sickle Cell Disease, Progress in Clinical and Biological Research. RB Scott (ed.). New York: Alan R Liss, pp. 97–107

Minakami ST (1975) Effect of intracellular pH (pHi) change on red cell glycolysis. In: The Human Red Cell *in vitro*. GJ Brewer (ed.). New York: Alan Liss, pp. 111–148

Mishler JM, Darley JH, Haworth C (1979) Viability of red cells stored in diminished concentration of citrate. Br J Haematol 43: 63–67

Mock DM, Lankford GL, Widness JA et al. (1999) Measurement of red cell survival using biotin-labeled red cells: validation against 51Cr-labeled red cells. Transfusion 39: 156–162

Mohandas N (1978) Effects of heat and metabolic depletion on erythrocyte deformability, spectrin extractability and phosphorylation. In: The Red Cell. GI Brewer (ed.). New York: Alan R Liss

Mohini R (1989) Clinical efficacy of recombinant human erythropoietin in hemodialysis patients. Semin Nephrol 9 (Suppl. 1): 16–21

Mollison PL (1943) The survival of transfused red cells in haemolytic disease of the newborn. Arch Dis Child 18: 161

Mollison PL (1947) The survival of transfused erythrocytes, with special reference to cases of acquired haemolytic anaemia. Clin Sci 6: 137

Mollison PL (1951) Blood Transfusion in Clinical Medicine. Oxford: Blackwell Scientific Publications

Mollison PL (1956) Blood Transfusion in Clinical Medicine, 2nd edn. Oxford: Blackwell Scientific Publications

Mollison PL (1961a) Blood Transfusion in Clinical Medicine, 3rd edn. Oxford: Blackwell Scientific Publications

Mollison PL (1961b) Further observations on the normal survival curve of 51Cr-labelled red cells. Clin Sci 21: 21

Mollison PL (1981) Determination of red cell survival using 51Cr. In: A Seminar on Immune-Mediated Cell Destruction. Chicago, IL: Am Assoc Blood Banks

Mollison PL (1983) Blood Transfusion in Clinical Medicine, 7th edn. Oxford: Blackwell Scientific Publications

Mollison PL (1984) Methods of determining the posttransfusion survival of stored red cells. Transfusion 24: 93–96

Mollison PL (1987) Blood Transfusion in Clinical Medicine, 8th edn. Oxford: Blackwell Scientific Publications

Mollison PL, Young IM (1941) Failure of in vitro tests as a guide to the value of stored blood. BMJ ii: 797

Mollison PL, Young IM (1942) In vivo survival in the human subject of transfused erythrocytes after storage in various preservative solutions. Quart J Exp Physiol 31: 359

Mollison PL, Sloviter HA (1951) Successful transfusion of previously frozen human red cells. Lancet ii: 862

Mollison PL, Veall N (1955) The use of the isotope 51Cr as label for red cell. Br J Haematol 1: 62

Mollison PL, Veall N, Cutbush M (1950) Red cell volume and plasma volume in newborn infants. Arch Dis Child 25: 242

Mollison PL, Sloviter HA, Chaplin H, Jr (1952) Survival of transfused red cells previously stored for long periods in the frozen state. Lancet ii: 501

Mollison PL, Robinson MA, Hunter DA (1958) Improved method of labelling red cells with radioactive phosphorus. Lancet i: 766

Moore GL, Peck CC, Sohmer PR (1981) Some properties of blood stored in anticoagulant CPDA-1 solution. A brief summary. Transfusion 21: 135–137

Moore GL, Hess JR, Ledford ME (1993) In vivo viability studies of two additive solutions in the post thaw preservation of red cells held for three weeks at 4°C. Transfusion 33: 709–712

Moroff G, Holme S, Heaton WAL (1990) Effect of an 8-hour holding period on in vivo and in vitro properties of red cells and Factor VIII content of plasma after collection in a red cell additive system. Transfusion 30: 828–830

Moroff G, Holme S, AuBuchon JP et al. (1999) Viability and in vitro properties of AS-1 red cells after gamma irradiation. Transfusion 39: 128–134

Morrison FS, Mollison PL, Robson DC (1968) Posttransfusion survival of red cells stored in liquid nitrogen. Br J Haematol 14: 215

Morrison JC, Whybrew WD, Bucovaz ET (1978) Use of partial exchange transfusion preoperatively in patients with sickle cell hemoglobinopathies. Am J Obstet Gynecol 132: 59–63

Morrison JC, Schneider JM, Whybrew WD (1980) Prophylactic transfusions in pregnant patients with sickle hemoglobinopathies: benefit versus risk. Obstet Gynecol 56: 274–280

Motulsky AG, Casserd F, Giblett ER (1958) Anemia and the spleen. N Engl J Med 259: 1164

Mueller TJ, Jackson CW, Dockter ME (1987) Membrane skeletal alterations during in vivo mouse red cell aging. J Clin Invest 79: 492–499

Mullaney PF, Vanvilla MA, Coulter JR et al. (1969) Cell sizing: a light scattering photometer for rapid volume determination. Rev Sci Instrum 40: 1029–1032

Myhre BA, Marcus CS, Wheeler NC (1990) The prediction of autologous red cell survival. Ann Clin Lab Sci 20: 258–262

Nakao K, Wada T, Kamiyama T (1962) A direct relationship between adenosine triphosphate-level and in vivo viability of erythrocytes. Nature (Lond) 194: 877

Nakao M, Nakao T, Arimatsu Y (1960) A new preservative medium maintaining the level of adenosine triphosphate and the osmotic resistance of erythrocytes. Proc Jap Acad 36: 43

Nelson AH, Fleisher LA, Rosenbaum SH (1993) Relationship between postoperative anemia and cardiac morbidity in high-risk vascular patients in the intensive care unit. Crit Care Med 21: 860–866

Neuberger A, Niven JSE (1951) Haemoglobin formation in rabbits. J Physiol 112: 292

Nexo E, Christensen NC, Olesen H (1981) Volume of blood removed for analytical purposes during hospitalization of low-birthweight infants. Clin Chem 27: 759–761

Oberman HA (1974) Transfusion of the neonatal patient. Transfusion 14: 183–184

401

Ohls RK, Ehrenkranz RA, Wright LL et al. (2001) Effects of early erythropoietin therapy on the transfusion requirements of preterm infants below 1250 grams birth weight: a multicenter, randomized, controlled trial. Pediatrics 108: 934–942

Oski FA, Travis SF, Miller LD (1971) The in vitro restoration of red cell 2,3-diphosphoglycerate levels in banked blood. Blood 37: 52

Ozer FL, Chaplin H (1963) Agglutination of stored erythrocytes by a human serum. Characterization of the serum factor and erythrocyte changes. J Clin Invest 42: 1735

Pace N, Lozaer EL, Consolazio WV (1947) The increase in hypoxia tolerance of normal men accompanying the polycythemia induced by transfusion of erythrocytes. Am J Physiol 148: 152

Parise LV, Telen MJ (2003) Erythrocyte adhesion in sickle cell disease. Curr Hematol Rep 2: 102–108

Parker AC, MacPherson AI, Richmond J (1977) Value of radiochromium investigation in autoimmune haemolytic anaemia. BMJ 1: 208–209

Parkes AS (1985) Off-beat Biologist; the Autobiography of AS Parkes. Cambridge: The Galton Foundation

Pearson HA, Vertrees KM (1961) Site of binding of chromium 51 to haemoglobin. Nature (Lond) 189: 1019

Pearson HA, Cornelius EA, Schwartz AD et al. (1970) Transfusion-reversible functional asplenia in young children with sickle-cell anemia. N Engl J Med 283: 334–337

Pelszynski MM, Moroff G, Luban NL et al. (1994) Effect of gamma irradiation of red blood cell units on T-cell inactivation as assessed by limiting dilution analysis: implications for preventing transfusion-associated graft-versus-host disease. Blood 83: 1683–1689

Pert JH, Schork PK, Moore R (1963) A new method of low-temperature blood preservation using liquid nitrogen and a glycerol sucrose additive. Clin Res 11: 197

Pietersz RNI, de Korte D, Reesink HW (1989) Storage of whole blood for up to 24 hours at ambient temperature prior to component preparation. Vox Sang 56: 145–150

Piomelli S (1995) The management of patients with Cooley's anemia: transfusions and splenectomy. Semin Hematol 32: 262–268

Piomelli S, Lurinsky G, Wasserman LR (1967) The mechanism of red cell aging. 1. Relationship between cell age and specific gravity evaluated by ultracentrifugation in a discontinuous density gradient. J Lab Clin Med 69: 659

Piomelli S, Seaman C, Reibman J et al. (1978). Separation of younger red cells with improved survival in vivo, an approach to chronic transfusion therapy. Proc Natl Acad Sci USA 75, 3474

Polge C, Smith AU, Parkes AS (1949) Revival of spermatozoa after vitrification and dehydration at low temperatures. Nature (Lond) 164: 666

Popovsky MA, Taswell HF. Circulatory overload: An underdiagnosed consequence of transfusion (Abstract). Transfusion 25, 469. 1985

Prins HK, Loos JA (1970) Studies on biochemical properties and viability of stored packed cells. In: Modern Problems of Blood Preservation. EW Spielmann, S Seidl (eds). Stuttgart: Gustav Fischer

Pritchard JA, Weisman R Jr (1957) The absorption of labeled erythrocytes from the peritoneal cavity of humans. J Lab Clin Med 49: 756–761

Propper RD (1982) Neocytes and neocyte-gerocyte exchange. Prog Clin Biol Res 88: 227–233

Propper RD, Button LN, Nathan DG (1980) New approaches to the transfusion management of thalassaemia. Blood 55: 55–60

Rachmilewitz EA, Aker M, Perry D et al. (1995) Sustained increase in haemoglobin and RBC following long-term administration of recombinant human erythropoietin to patients with homozygous beta-thalassaemia. Br J Haematol 90: 341–345

Ramirez AM, Woodfield DG, Scott R (1987) High potassium levels in stored irradiated blood (Letter). Transfusion 27: 444–445

Rapoport S (1947) Dimensional, osmotic and chemical changes of erythrocytes in stored blood. I. Blood preserved in sodium citrate, neutral and acid citrateglucose (ACD) mixtures. J Clin Invest 26: 591

Rasanen J (1992) Supply-dependent oxygen consumption and mixed venous oxyhemoglobin saturation during isovolemic hemodilution in pigs. Chest 101: 1121–1124

Rathbun EJ, Nelson EJ, Davey EJ (1989) Posttransfusion survival of red cells frozen for 8 weeks after 42-day liquid storage in AS-3. Transfusion 29: 213–217

Regan F, Teesdale P, Garner S et al. (1997) Comparison of in vivo red cell survival of donations collected by Haemonetics MCS versus conventional collection. Transfusion Med 7: 25–28

Reliene R, Mariani M, Zanella A et al. (2002) Splenectomy prolongs in vivo survival of erythrocytes differently in spectrin/ankyrin- and band 3-deficient hereditary spherocytosis. Blood 100: 2208–2215

Remenchik AP, Schuckmell N, Dyniewicz IM (1958) The survival of Cr51-labelled autogenous erythrocytes in children. J Lab Clin Med 51: 753

Restrepo FA, Chaplin H (1962) Measurement of in vivo survival of red blood cells by means of starch block hemoglobin electrophoresis. Am J Clin Pathol 6: 557

Ricketts C, Cavill I, Napier JA (1977) The measurement of red cell lifespan using 59Fe. Br J Haematol 37: 403–408

Riddell V (1939) Blood Transfusion. Oxford: Oxford University Press

Robertson OH (1918) Transfusion with preserved red blood cells. BMJ i: 691

Rock G, Tocch M, Tackaberry E (1983) Plasticized red blood cells: good or bad? (Abstract). Transfusion 23: 426

Rodgers GP, Schechter AN, Noguchi CT *et al.* (1984) Periodic microcirculatory flow in patients with sickle-cell disease. N Engl J Med 311: 1534–1538

Rosse WF (1990) Clinical Immunohematology: Basic Concepts and Clinical Applications. Oxford: Blackwell Scientific Publications

Rous P, Turner JR (1916) Preservation of living red blood corpuscles *in vitro*. II. The transfusion of kept cells. J Exp Med 23: 219

Royal JE, Seeler RA (1978) Hypertension, convulsions, and cerebral haemorrhage in sickle-cell anaemia patients after blood-transfusion. Lancet ii: 1207

Searle JF (1973) Anaesthesia in sickle cell states. A review. Anaesthesia 28: 48

Sharon BI, Honig G (1991) Management of congenital hemolytic anemias. In: Principles of Transfusion Medicine. EC Rossi, TL Simon, GS Moss (eds). Baltimore, MA: Williams and Wilkins, pp. 131–149

Sharpey-Schafer EP, Wallace J (1942a) Circulatory overloading following rapid intravenous injections. Lancet ii: 304

Sharpey-Schafer EP, Wallace J (1942b) Retention of injected serum in the circulation. Lancet i: 699

Shemin DR (1946) The life-span of the human red blood cell. J Biol Chem 166: 627

Shields CE (1969) Effect of adenine on stored erythrocytes evaluated by autologous and homologous transfusion. Transfusion 9: 115

Shields CE (1970) Studies on stored whole blood: IV. Effects of temperature and mechanical agitation on blood with and without plasma. Transfusion 10: 155

Simon ER (1962) Red cell preservation: further studies with adenine. Blood 20: 485

Simon ER, Chapman RG, Finch CA (1962) Adenine in red cell preservation. J Clin Invest 41: 351

Simon TL, Marcus CS, Myhre BA (1987) Effects of AS-3 nutrient additive solution on 42 and 49 days of storage of red cells. Transfusion 27: 178–182

Simon TL, Sohmer P, Nelson EJ (1989) Extended survival of neocytes produced by a new system. Transfusion 29: 221–225

Sioufi HA, Button LN, Jacobson MS (1990) Nonradioactive chromium technique for red cell labeling. Vox Sang 58: 204–206

Sirchia G, Ferrone S, Mercuriali F (1970) Leukocyte antigen-antibody reaction and lysis of paroxysmal nocturnal hemoglobinuria erythrocytes. Blood 36: 334–336

Sloand EM, Mainwaring L, Keyvanfar K *et al.* (2004) Transfer of glycosylphosphatidylinositol-anchored proteins to deficient cells after erythrocyte transfusion in paroxysmal nocturnal hemoglobinuria. Blood 104: 3782–3788

Sloviter HA (1951) *In vivo* survival of rabbit's red cells recovered after freezing. Lancet i: 1350

Sloviter HA (1976) Physiological and metabolic aspects of freezing erythrocytes with historical notes. In: Clinical Uses of Frozen-thawed Red Blood Cells. New York: Alan R Liss

Smith AU (1950) Prevention of haemolysis during freezing and thawing of red blood-cells. Lancet ii: 910

Smoller BR, Kruskall MS (1986) Phlebotomy for diagnostic laboratory tests in adults. Pattern of use and effect on transfusion requirements. N Engl J Med 314: 1233–1235

Smoller BR, Kruskall MS, Horowitz GL (1989) Reducing adult phlebotomy blood loss with the use of pediatric-sized blood collection tubes. Am J Clin Pathol 9: 701–703

Sohmer PR, Beutler E, Moore GL (1981) Clinical trials with CPD-A2 (Abstract). Transfusion 21: 600

Spahn DR, Smith LR, Schell RM *et al.* (1994) Importance of severity of coronary artery disease for the tolerance to normovolemic hemodilution. Comparison of single-vessel versus multivessel stenoses in a canine model. J Thorac Cardiovasc Surg 108: 231–239

Spanos T, Ladis V, Palamidou F *et al.* (1996) The impact of neocyte transfusion in the management of thalassaemia. Vox Sang 70: 217–223

Spiess BD, Ley C, Body SC *et al.* (1998) Hematocrit value on intensive care unit entry influences the frequency of Q-wave myocardial infarction after coronary artery bypass grafting. The Institutions of the Multicenter Study of Perioperative Ischemia (McSPI) Research Group. J Thorac Cardiovasc Surg 116: 460–467

Spivak JL (1993) The clinical physiology of erythropoietin. Semin Hematol 30: 2–11

Strauss RG (1990) Routinely washing irradiated red cells seems unwarranted (Editorial). Transfusion 30: 675–677

Strauss RG (1994) Erythropoietin and neonatal anemia (Editorial). N Engl J Med 330: 1227–1228

Strauss RG (2001) Managing the anemia of prematurity: red blood cell transfusions versus recombinant erythropoietin. Transfusion Med Rev 15: 213–223

Strauss RG, Sacher RA, Blazina JF (1990) Commentary on small-volume red cell transfusions for neonates. Transfusion 30: 565–570

Strauss RG, Mock DM, Johnson K *et al.* (2003) Circulating RBC volume, measured with biotinylated RBCs, is superior to the Hct to document the hematologic effects of delayed versus immediate umbilical cord clamping in preterm neonates. Transfusion 43: 1168–1172

Strumia MM (1954) Analytical review: the preservation of blood for transfusion. Blood 9: 1105

Strumia MM, Dugan A, Taylor L (1962) Splenectomy in leukemia and myelofibrosis: changes in the erythrocytic values. Am J Clin Pathol 37: 491

Strumia MM, Strumia PV, Dugan A (1968) Significance of measurement of plasma volume and of indirect estimation of red cell volume. Transfusion 8: 197

Suda BA, Leitman SF, Davey RJ (1993) Characteristics of red cells irradiated and subsequently frozen for longterm storage. Transfusion, 33: 389–392

Sung JJ, Chan FK, Lau JY et al. (2003) The effect of endoscopic therapy in patients receiving omeprazole for bleeding ulcers with nonbleeding visible vessels or adherent clots: a randomized comparison. Ann Intern Med 139: 237–243

Suzuki T, Dale GL (1987) Biotinylated erythrocytes: in vivo survival and in vitro recovery. Blood 70: 791–795

Szymanski IO, Valeri CR (1970) Factors influencing chromium elution from tagged red cells in vivo and the effect of elution on red cell survival measurements. Br J Haematol 19: 397

Szymanski IO, Valeri CR, McCallum LE (1968) Automated differential agglutination technic to measure red cell survival. I. Methodology. Transfusion 8: 65

Thomas MJG, Parry ES, Nash SG (1996) A method for the cryopreservation of red blood cells using hydroxyethyl starch as a cryoprotectant. Transfusion Sci 17: 385–396

Todd C, White RG (1911) On the fate of red blood corpuscles when injected into the circulation of an animal of the same species: with a new method for the determination of the total volume of blood. Proc Roy Soc Lond B 84: 255

Ueda E, Kinoshita T, Terasawa T (1990) Acetylcholinesterase and lymphocyte function-associated antigen 3 found on decay-accelerating factor-negative erythrocytes from some patients with paroxysmal nocturnal haemoglobinuria are lost during erythrocyte ageing. Blood 75: 762–769

Usher R, Shepard M, Lind J (1963) The blood volume of the newborn infant and placental transfusion. Acta Paediatr (Uppsala) 52: 497

Valeri CR (1965) The in vivo survival, mode of removal of the non-viable cells, the total amount of supernatant hemoglobin in deglycerolized, resuspended erythrocytes. I. The effect of the period of storage in ACD at 4°C prior to glycerolization. II. The effect of washing deglycerolized, resuspended erythrocytes after a period of storage at 4°C. Transfusion 5: 273

Valeri CR (1974) Factors influencing the 24-hour post-transfusion survival and the oxygen transport function of previously frozen red cells preserved with 40 per cent w/v glycerol and frozen at −80°C. Transfusion 14: 1

Valeri CR (1975) Simplification of the methods for adding and removing glycerol during freeze-preservation of human red blood cells with the high or low glycerol methods: biochemical modification prior to freezing. Transfusion 15: 195

Valeri CR, Hirsch NM (1969) Restoration in vivo of erythrocyte adenosine triphosphate, 2,3-diphosphoglycerate, potassium ion, and sodium ion concentrations following the transfusion of acidcitrate-dextrose-stored human red blood cells. J Lab Clin Med 73: 722

Valeri CR, Runck AH (1969) Long term frozen storage of human red blood cells: studies in vivo and in vitro of autologous red blood cells preserved up to six years with high concentrations of glycerol. Transfusion 9: 5

Valeri CR, Zaroulis CG (1972) Rejuvenation and freezing of outdated stored human red cells. N Engl J Med 287: 1307

Valeri CR, Szymanski IO, Runck AH (1970) Therapeutic effectiveness of homologous erythrocyte transfusions following frozen storage at −80°C for up to seven years. Transfusion 10: 102

Valeri CR, Valeri DA, Anastasi J et al. (1981) Freezing in the polyvinylchloride plastic collection bag: a new system for preparing and freezing non-rejuvenated and rejuvenated red blood cells. Transfusion 21: 138–149

Valeri CR, Landrock RD, Pivacek LE et al. (1985) Quantitative differential agglutination method using the Coulter Counter to measure survival of compatible but identifiable red blood cells. Vox Sang 49: 195–205

Valeri CR, Pivack LE, Gray AD (1989) The safety and therapeutic effectiveness of human red cells stored at −80°C for as long as 21 years. Transfusion 29: 429–437

Valeri CR, Ragno G, Piracek LE et al. (2000) An experiment with glycerol frozen red blood cells stored at −80°C for up to 37 years. Vox Sang 79: 168–174

Valeri CR, Ragno G, Pivacek LE et al. (2001) A multi-center study of in vitro and in vivo values in human RBCs frozen with 40-percent (wt/vol) glycerol and stored after deglycerolization for 15 days at 4 degrees C in AS-3: assessment of RBC processing in the ACP 215. Transfusion 41: 933–939

Valeri CR, MacGregor H, Giorgio A et al. (2003a) Comparison of radioisotope methods and a nonradioisotope method to measure the RBC volume and RBC survival in the baboon. Transfusion 43: 1366–1373

Valeri CR, Lane JP, Srey R et al. (2003b) Incidence of breakage of human RBCs frozen with 40-percent wt/vol glycerol using two different methods for storage at −80 degrees C. Transfusion 43: 411–414

Valtis DJ, Kennedy AC (1954) Defective gas-transport function of stored red blood cells. Lancet i: 119

Van der Linden P, Schmartz D, De Groote F et al. (1998) Critical haemoglobin concentration in anaesthetized dogs: comparison of two plasma substitutes. Br J Anaesth 81: 556–562

de Verdier C-H, Finson M, Garby L et al. (1966) Experience of blood preservation in ACD adenine solution. Proc 10th Congr Europ Soc Haematol, Strasbourg 1965

van der Vegt SGL, Ruben AMT, Werre JM (1985a) Counterflow centrifugation of red cell populations: a cell age related separation technique. Br J Haematol 61: 393–403 van der Vegt SGL, Ruben AMT, Werre JM (1985b) Membrane characteristics and osmotic fragility of red cells, fractionated with anglehead centrifugation and counter flow centrifugation. Br J Haematol 61: 405–413

Vincent JL, Baron JF, Reinhart K et al. (2002) Anemia and blood transfusion in critically ill patients. JAMA 288: 1499–1507

Vincenzi FF, Hinds TR (1988) Decreased Ca pump ATPase activity associated with increased density in human red blood cells. Blood Cells 14: 139–148

Walsh RJ, Thomas ED, Chow SK (1949) Iron metabolism. Heme synthesis in vitro by immature erythrocytes. Science 110: 396

Wasi P, Na-Nakorn S, Pootrakul P (1978) A syndrome of hypertension, convulsion, cerebral haemorrhage in thalassaemic patients after multiple blood-transfusions. Lancet ii: 602

Weed RI, LaCelle PL (1969) ATP dependence of erythrocyte membrane deformability. In: Red Cell Membrane Structure and Function. GA Jamieson, TJ Greenwalt (eds). Philadelphia, PA: Lippincott

Weiskopf RB, Viele MK, Feiner J et al. (1998) Human cardiovascular and metabolic response to acute, severe isovolemic anemia. JAMA 279: 217–221

Well R (1915) Sodium citrate in the transfusion of blood. JAMA 64: 425

Westman BJM (1972) Serum creatinine and creatinine clearance after transfusion and ACD-adenine blood and ACD blood. Transfusion 12: 371

Westman M (1974) Studies for evaluation of blood preservation procedures with special regard to the oxygen release function and the toxicity of adenine. PhD Thesis, University of Uppsala, Sweden

Wiener AS (1934) Longevity of the erythrocyte (Letter to the Editor). JAMA 102: 1779

Wiener AS (1943) Blood Groups and Transfusion. Springfield, IL: CC Thomas

Wilkerson DK, Rosen AL, Sehgal LR et al. (1988) Limits of cardiac compensation in anemic baboons. Surgery 103: 665–670

Williams RJ (1976) A proposed mechanism for PVP cryoprotection (Abstract). Cryobiology 13: 653

Wood L, Beutler E (1967) The viability of human blood stored in phosphate adenine media. Transfusion 7: 401

Woodfield G, Giles C, Poole J (1986) A further null phenotype (Sc-1–2) in Papua New Guinea. Proceedings of the 19th Congress of the International Society of Blood Transfusion, Sydney, p. 651

Woodford-Williams E, Webster D, Dixon MP (1962) Red cell longevity in old age. Geront Clin (Basel) 4: 183

Wu WC, Rathore SS, Wang Y et al. (2001) Blood transfusion in elderly patients with acute myocardial infarction. N Engl J Med 345: 1230–1236

Wurmser R, Filitti-Wurmser S, Briault R (1942) Sur la conservation du sang. Rev Can Biol 1: 372

Zade-Oppen AMM (1968) The effect of mannitol, sucrose, raffinose and dextran on posthypertonic hemolysis. Acta Physiol Scand 74: 195

Zimran A, Forman L, Suzuki T et al. (1990) In vivo aging of red cell enzymes: study of biotinylated red blood cells in rabbits. Am J Hematol 33: 249–254

10 Red cell incompatibility *in vivo*

Transfused cells are regarded as incompatible if their survival in the recipient's circulation is curtailed by antibodies. The realization that transfusions are inevitably incompatible if donor and recipient belong to different species was made only by degrees.

Transfusion of animal red cells to humans: keeping the sheep from the door

The first person transfuse to a human being was Professor J Denis who, with the help of a surgeon Mr C Emmerez, gave transfusions of lamb's blood or calf's blood to five different patients. His most famous, and last, recipient was a man (Mauroy) with an 'inveterate phrensy, occasioned by a disgrace he had received in some Amours'. Denis hoped that 'the calf's blood by its mildness and freshness might possibly allay the heat and ebulition of his blood'. The first two transfusions given to him apparently relieved his mania, although following the second his arm became hot, his pulse rose, sweat burst out over his forehead, he complained of pain in his kidneys, became sick to the stomach and passed black urine the next day. After this transfusion the patient became so much better that plans for a further transfusion were temporarily abandoned (Denis 1667–68). However, at the insistence of the patient's wife a third transfusion was attempted early in 1668. There were technical difficulties and only a few drops of blood were extracted from the patient and probably no blood at all transfused. Nevertheless, the patient died the same night. The case came before the Court at Châtelet on 27 April 1668 and the cause of death was examined; it was concluded that the patient's wife had been putting arsenic in his broth (for further details see Jeanneney and Ringenbach 1940; Hall and Boas Hall 1967; Keynes 1949, 1967). Although the transfusion probably had nothing to do with the patient's death, the episode was seized on by the opponents of transfusion who succeeded in having the procedure banned.

Work by Blundell (1824) indicating the need to use a donor of the same species has been referred to in an earlier chapter. Blundell's work was fully confirmed by Ponfick (1875), who showed that if the red cells of a donor of another species were transfused, they underwent rapid intravascular lysis. Ponfick also showed that when the red cells of a donor of one species were mixed *in vitro* with the serum of another, haemolysis occurred.

Despite Blundell's earlier work, an enthusiasm for transfusion and difficulty in recruiting human donors led to a considerable vogue for giving transfusions of lamb's blood during the last quarter of the nineteenth century (Gesellius 1874; Hasse 1874). Not all physicians were impressed, particularly as lamb's blood, except when used in very small quantities, invariably escaped via the kidneys (Fagge 1891). A witticism of the time ran that for a transfusion three sheep were needed: the donor, the recipient and the doctor (Zimmerman and Howell 1932).

Transfusions between members of the same species

The first studies of red cell survival following transfusion between members of the same species (bulls) were described by Todd and White (1911) in animals that had not previously been transfused. In fact, all the donor red cells were eliminated within a few days, presumably through the action of naturally occurring antibodies. Ashby (1919), who used a similar

406

technique to study red cell survival following transfusions between humans, found prolonged survival, due no doubt to the selection of ABO-compatible red cells.

Scope of this chapter

The present chapter is concerned mainly with experimental studies of the survival *in vivo* of small amounts of incompatible red cells and with theoretical deductions from the results. Chapter 11 deals with the clinical effects of the accidental transfusion of relatively large amounts of incompatible blood.

Some of the factors that affect the rate and site of destruction include: (1) the characteristics of the antibody, namely binding constant, Ig class and IgG subclass, ability to activate complement, thermal range and plasma concentration; (2) the characteristics of the antigen, namely abundance of sites on the cell surface and association with complement activation (both related to antigen specificity); (3) the number of red cells transfused; (4) the presence of the relevant antigen in the plasma; and (5) the phagocytic activity of the mononuclear phagocyte system (RES). In analysing the effects of these variables, tests with volumes of red cells as small as 1 ml or less have proved very helpful. The injection of such amounts almost never produces untoward symptoms in the recipient, causes virtually no immediate change in the concentration of antibody and does not tax the capacity of the RES. Accordingly, the main factors determining the rate of red cell destruction are the various characteristics of the antibody, including its concentration. The characteristics of the antigen also affect the result but this source of variability can be eliminated by using red cells from a single donor or can be minimized by using red cells of a particular phenotype or 'grade' of antigen.

In the present chapter, the results of tests with small volumes of red cells will be considered first from a qualitative point of view, that is to say from the patterns of red cell destruction observed, and second from the quantitative point of view, using evidence derived from investigations in which the amounts of antibody and antigen involved have been determined. The situation encountered in clinical practice, in which relatively large numbers of incompatible red cells are transfused, will then be discussed.

Estimation of survival of incompatible red cells

When incompatible red cells are transfused by accident, as a rule the only way to study their survival is with a serological method. For example, if the donor red cells are group N and the recipient is group M, differential agglutination with anti-M will provide estimates of the survival of the unagglutinated group N donor red cells. If the donor is Rh D positive and the recipient D negative, the donor red cells can be recognized by direct agglutination with anti-D or, if the recipient has formed anti-D, the surviving red cells can be recognized by the direct antiglobulin test (DAT) (Wiener and Peters 1940; Dacie and Mollison 1943). If a flow cytometer is available, quantitative estimates can be made whenever an antigenic difference between the red cells of the donor and the recipient exists, and suitable antisera are available (Garratty and Arndt 1999).

Ordinarily, the transfusion service does not perform an extended phenotype on the patient's red cells. As a result, no serological target for differential agglutination may be obvious after transfusion has taken place. However, if even modest erythropoiesis continues, the youngest circulating cells should belong to the recipient. The serologist can make use of this finding to separate the young from the old cells with a capillary gradient method and phenotype the separated (autologous) cells to identify the best serological target (Wallas *et al.* 1980). Here too, flow cytometry has become a method of choice (Griffin *et al.* 1994; Garratty and Arndt 1999). An elegant non-serological technique can be used should the transfused patient be one with a sickling disease. Red cells from patients with SS or SC haemoglobin (Hb) resist lysis with hypotonic saline. When a specimen from such a transfused patient is exposed to hypotonic saline (0.3%), the transfused cells are lysed and the native cells can then be resuspended in isotonic solution and phenotyped (Brown 1988). Semi-quantitative estimates of the Hb variant can be determined by electrophoretic techniques.

In experiments in which incompatible red cells are deliberately transfused, various labels can be used. For example, in studying the response of D-negative recipients to D-positive red cells, cord red cells can be transfused and their survival determined by making counts by the acid-elution method. However, the method of most general application and greatest precision is that of labelling with ^{51}Cr (see Chapter 9).

The following pages describe experiments to determine the relation between the serological characteristics of antibodies and the effects that they produce *in vivo*. The scope of tests with small volumes of incompatible red cells in ordinary transfusion practice has been discussed briefly elsewhere (Mollison 1981) and a method of carrying out such tests is described on p. 435. In clinical practice, tests are indicated only when it is uncertain whether the injected red cells will survive normally. When increased destruction is expected and the studies are being performed with the sole intention of increasing knowledge, the investigator must use an approved research protocol, secure prior authorization from the appropriate ethical committee and obtain the subject's informed consent.

Labelling of incompatible red cells: the chrome standard

Labelling with radionuclides remains the best method, as the survival of amounts less than 1 ml can be estimated accurately. Although flow cytometry offers certain advantages, the opportunity to store serial samples for example, the need to inject about 10 ml of red cells (Garratty and Nance 1990; Issitt *et al.* 1990) is a disadvantage. Kumpel and co-workers (2000) performed clearance studies using 4 ml of autologous D+ cells coated with anti-D at two concentrations (5 or 10 µg anti-D/ml of red cells) transfused to two subjects at separate times and survival studies using 5 ml of frozen-thawed D+ cells transfused to five D–subjects with no detectable anti-D. Flow cytometry is now the best method for typing reticulocytes in mixed cell populations (Griffin *et al.* 1994). None of the flow cytometric assays exhibited the necessary sensitivity or accuracy in quantification of the rare events to provide reliable data for the calculation of the initial clearance rate, the red cell half-life or the mean cell lifespan of transfused red cells. The inability to enumerate rare fluorescence-labelled cells was due mainly to the presence of 'background' events, which were a considerable problem when the coating level of anti-D was less than 3000 molecules of IgG per cell. If these techniques can be made more sensitive, they may become the method of choice.

Almost all of the results discussed in the present chapter were obtained using ^{51}Cr, which, when survival is to be followed for more than a few hours, remains the best label. For labelling with other radionuclides and with biotin, see Chapter 9. With ^{51}Cr, loss of label from red cells is slow, about 3% in the first 24 h with only about 1% per day thereafter (see Chapter 9). The $T_{1/2}$ of radioactive decay is 27.7 days, which allows studies over a period of weeks if necessary. In contrast, when red cells are labelled with ^{99m}Tc, about 4% of the label is lost from the red cells during the first hour. The rate of loss over the next 2 or 3 h is similar, but thereafter the rate slows and the loss in the first 24 h is about 30%. The rate of loss of indium (^{111}In or ^{113}In) appears to be 3–5% during the first 15 min after injection and approximately 15% in the first 24 h. ^{99m}Tc and ^{111}In appear to be suitable for detecting substantial destruction occurring in the first few hours after injection, but ^{51}Cr must be used if small amounts of destruction are to be detected reliably or if survival is to be followed for longer periods. For further details and references, see Appendix 2.

Use of ^{51}Cr

A dose of 0.2–0.5 µCi (7–18 kBq)/kg may be used, for example 12–30 µCi in a 60-kg adult. Using ^{51}Cr with a specific activity of 100 µCi/µg, a maximum of 0.3 µg of Cr will be added. Thus, even when the amount of red cells injected is as small as 0.3 ml, the amount of ^{51}Cr (1 µg/ml of red cells) will be well below the level that is likely to produce any interference whatever with the survival of the red cells.

The common indication for injecting small numbers of donor red cells is to determine whether survival will be normal. A 1-ml aliquot usually suffices for this use. In a few other circumstances, injection of smaller aliquots may be advisable. For patients whose serum contains potent incomplete antibodies (those detected only with antiglobulin reagents), a dose of 0.5 ml of red cells is recommended, as infusions as small as 1 ml have been known to provoke shivering and fever. For subjects whose serum contains haemolytic antibodies, tests should be performed with caution and no more than 0.1–0.2 ml of red cells should be injected.

When early rapid destruction of donor red cells appears unlikely, a sample drawn from the recipient 3 min after the injection of the cells may be used as the 100% survival value. In most normal subjects, mixing is at least 98% complete by 3 min (Strumia *et al.* 1958; Mollison 1959a) (Fig. 10.1) and appreciable destruction of injected red cells within the mixing period occurs only with relatively potent antibodies; an

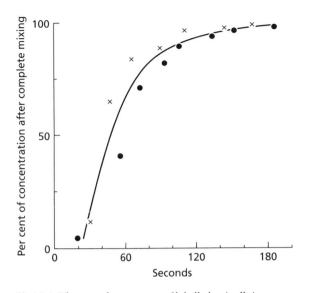

Fig 10.1 The rate of appearance of labelled red cells in samples taken from one superficial arm vein after injecting the cells into a vein in the other arm. Two different samples of the subject's own red cells were injected, labelled with ^{51}Cr (●) and ^{32}P (×) respectively. One sample was injected about 30 s after the other, but in each case the times are expressed as seconds from the mid-point of injection to the mid-point of the sample. '100%', the concentration attained after complete mixing, based on samples taken 10–20 min after injection (Mollison 1959a).

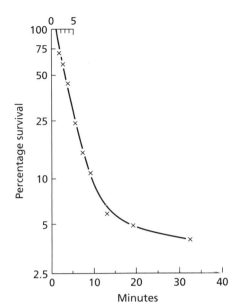

Fig 10.2 Survival *in vivo* of a sample of red cells from an Fy(a+) donor; the cells were labelled with ^{51}Cr, incubated with purified IgG anti-Fy^a and with complement, and reinjected into the donor. Red cell volume was determined by simultaneous injection of another sample of the donor's red cells labelled with ^{32}P but otherwise untreated. Mixing was probably incomplete at 2 min; a line drawn through estimates of survival at 2.8, 3.7 and 5.6 min intersects the time axis at about 1 min after the mid-point of injection. The initial rate of destruction has a $T_{1/2}$ of 2 min; the rate of destruction starts to slow 5–10 min after injection of the cells (Mollison 1962, case 3b).

example is given in Fig. 10.2. If such early destruction is suspected, an estimate of the patient's red cell volume will be required, and is best obtained by labelling a sample of the patient's own red cells with either ^{99m}Tc or ^{111}In and injecting these labelled red cells and the ^{51}Cr-labelled donor red cells as a single suspension ('double label' technique).

Qualitative aspects of red cell destruction by alloantibodies

As described in Chapter 3, red cells are not directly damaged by antibodies. The attachment of antibodies leads to destruction in one of two ways: either complement is activated leading to damage to the red cell surface by C8–9 followed by lysis; or the red cells, coated with antibody or complement (C3b, iC3b), or with both antibody and iC3b, become attached to a phagocyte, leading to loss of membrane, lysis or engulfment.

Predominantly intravascular destruction

With rare exceptions, the only antibodies that produce intravascular lysis of the majority of the red cells transfused are those that are readily lytic *in vitro* and the mechanisms are probably identical. The commonest antibodies of this kind are anti-A, anti-B and anti-A,B. As Fig. 10.3 shows, within 2 min of injecting ABO-incompatible red cells, the plasma may contain Hb equivalent to 90% of the amount contained in the injected intact red cells (Jandl *et al.* 1957; Cutbush and Mollison 1958). For antibodies other than those in the ABO system (e.g. anti-Vel and anti-Le^a), *in vitro* haemolysis and intravascular haemolysis may not correlate as well.

When ABO-incompatible red cells that are lysed incompletely by the recipient's serum *in vitro*, because

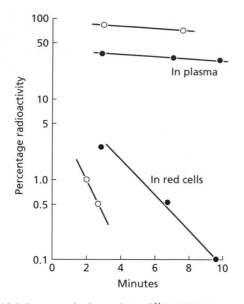

Fig 10.3 Intravascular haemolysis of ^{51}Cr-labelled ABO-incompatible red cells. ○, B cells injected into a group A recipient. ●, A_2 cells injected into a group O recipient (Cutbush and Mollison 1958).

either the antibody or the antigen is relatively weak, are transfused, fewer than one-half of the injected red cells may be lysed intravascularly. Figure 10.3 shows an example in which, following the transfusion of a small volume of A_2 red cells to a group O recipient, only 40% of the Hb was found in the plasma immediately after injection.

When the anti-A or anti-B in the recipient's plasma is weakly lytic so that lysis is observed *in vitro* only when the ratio of serum to cells exceeds about 500:1, destruction of the transfused cells may take place predominantly in extravascular sites with only 10% of the injected radioactivity being found in the plasma (Jandl *et al.* 1957).

When destruction by anti-A and anti-B is very rapid, 99.9% of the cells may be lysed within 10 min (see Fig. 10.3). When destruction is slower, some cells may survive for relatively long periods having, presumably, acquired resistance to complement-mediated destruction.

Certain other antibodies, particularly anti-PP$_1$P^k and anti-Vel, which are readily haemolytic *in vitro*, seem capable of causing predominantly intravascular

lysis of incompatible red cells, but no quantitative data have been published.

Many examples of anti-Le^a and rare examples of anti-Le^b lyse red cells *in vitro*, but as a rule the lysis is relatively slow. Accordingly, when small amounts of incompatible red cells are injected, the cells may be cleared by the RES before there has been time for haemolysis to occur. If relatively large amounts of incompatible red cells are transfused, some intravascular haemolysis may be observed. Exceptionally potent Lewis antibodies may produce some intravascular haemolysis even when small amounts of incompatible red cells are injected.

In the case reported by Mollison and co-workers (1963), 0.5 ml of ^{51}Cr-labelled Le(b+) red cells were injected at a time when the titre of anti-Le^b in the patient's serum was approximately 100. A sample taken 4 min later contained 60% of surviving cells with 13% of the injected radioactivity in the plasma: the sample at 13 min contained 16% of surviving cells and 7% of the injected radioactivity in the plasma. The discrepancy between the amounts of Hb in the two plasma samples suggested that some degree of haemolysis might have occurred after the samples had been withdrawn; this possibility emphasizes the need to separate cells from plasma promptly when making observations of this kind.

Erythrophagocytosis accompanying lysis by anti-A and anti-B

As mentioned above, not all ABO-incompatible red cells are lysed in the plasma. Presumably, most of the remainder are engulfed by cells of the RES but some are engulfed by neutrophils, so that erythrophagocytosis is observed in films of peripheral blood (Hopkins 1910; Ottenberg 1911). Gross neutropenia may be produced by the injection of as little as 10 ml of ABO-incompatible red cells.

Predominantly extravascular destruction

All antibodies except those that are readily haemolytic *in vitro* bring about extravascular destruction of red cells, chiefly in sinusoids of the liver and spleen. The maximum rate of disappearance of red cells from the bloodstream corresponds to the clearance of rather more than one-third of the blood per minute (Mollison 1962); that is, k, the fractional rate of red cell clearance = approximately 0.35/min.

As $k = \dfrac{\log_e 2}{T_{1/2}} \text{min}, \quad T_{1/2} = \dfrac{0.693}{0.35} = 1.9 \text{ min}$ (10.1)

When clearance occurs with a $T_{1/2}$ of the order of 2 min, surface counting shows that approximately 75% of the cells have been sequestered in the liver and approximately 10% in the spleen (Mollison and Hughes-Jones 1958).

Antibodies that fail to activate complement, of which anti-Rh D is exemplary, bring about destruction predominantly in the spleen (Jandl 1955; Mollison *et al.* 1955; Jandl and Greenberg 1957). In predominantly splenic destruction, the maximum rate of clearance observed corresponds to a $T_{1/2}$ of approximately 20 min ($k =$ approximately 0.035/min); more than 90% of the cells are removed in the spleen (Hughes-Jones *et al.* 1957). Under these circumstances, the rate of clearance of red cells is limited by the rate of blood flow through the spleen.

As the blood flow through the liver is approximately 10 times greater than that through the spleen, antibodies such as anti-D must not achieve efficient red cell destruction in the liver. In fact in splenectomized subjects, red cells heavily coated with anti-D are cleared with a $T_{1/2}$ of the order of 3–5 h, indicating that, on a weight basis, the liver is about 100 times less efficient than the spleen at removing D-sensitized red cells from the circulation (Crome and Mollison 1964).

It has been proposed that in the spleen, because the packed cell volume (PCV) of the blood is higher, plasma IgG competes with bound IgG antibodies for Fc receptors on macrophages far less successfully than it does in the liver (Engelfriet *et al.* 1981). By contrast, the adherence of complement-coated cells is not inhibited by plasma and therefore the cells bind to macrophages just as well in the liver as they do in the spleen.

'Lag' before the onset of extravascular destruction: delayed but not denied

When the percentage survival of incompatible red cells is plotted against the time after their injection into the circulation there is an apparent 'lag' before destruction begins. The most obvious explanation is that accelerated destruction cannot begin until the cells have taken up sufficient antibody but, like many obvious explanations, this one is probably incomplete or incorrect. Even if cells are previously sensitized by antibodies

in vitro or rendered non-viable by storage, the lag before the onset of destruction persists. In a series of measurements with such 'altered' red cells this delay was found to be 1.35 min, SD 0.45 (Mollison 1962). The most likely explanation for this 'lag' is an anatomic one. The circulation time through the portal circuit is slower than circulation through the rest of the body so that the time required for cells to pass from the point of injection to the sampling point (arm vein) may be of the order of 1–2 min. Accordingly, a blood sample taken from an arm vein less than 1 min after the injection of incompatible cells will not include any cells that have transited the portal circulation and thus it will appear that no cells have been cleared from the circulation (Mollison 1962).

After the injection of incompatible red cells, which must take up antibody before becoming susceptible to rapid clearance by the RES, a somewhat longer lag is observed. In 10 cases in which the antibody concerned was capable of agglutinating red cells suspended in saline, the mean apparent delay was 2.20 min, SD 0.75; and in 12 cases involving incomplete, complement-binding antibody, the mean delay was 4.0 min, SD 1.5 (Mollison 1962). Obvious examples of lags are provided by several figures in this chapter (see Figs 10.5, 10.6 and 10.7).

When the concentration of antibodies in the serum is very low, long delays may be observed. For example, in a D-negative subject injected with 1 µg of intramuscular anti-D and infused 24 h later with 0.3 ml of D-positive red cells, the maximum rate of red cell destruction began about 5 days afterward (Mollison and Hughes-Jones 1967). A similarly long delay was observed by Schneider and Preisler (1966) after injecting small amounts of low titre anti-D and D-positive red cells into D-negative subjects. The delay is due partly to the time taken for the uptake of IgG into the circulation and partly to the time taken for antigen and antibody to come into equilibrium at very low concentrations (Mollison and Hughes-Jones 1967).

Release of some Hb into the circulation in predominantly extravascular destruction: a touch of pink

Jandl and co-workers (1957) found that when D-positive red cells were injected into subjects whose plasma contained anti-D, or when D-positive red cells were incubated with anti-D *in vitro* and then re-injected,

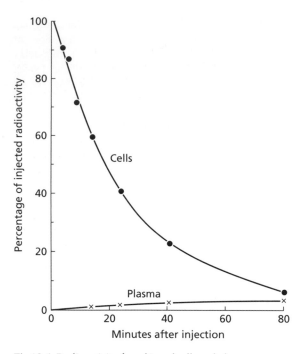

Fig 10.4 Radioactivity found in red cells and plasma following the injection of ^{51}Cr-labelled D-sensitized red cells. A small amount of radioactivity appears in the plasma about 10 min after the injection and reaches a maximum after about 1 h. This radioactivity in the plasma represents Hb liberated into the circulation (Mollison 1959a).

haemoglobinaemia developed within a few minutes of the injection and increased steadily to reach a peak 2 or 3 h after the injection.

In a previous edition, it was shown that when amounts of ^{51}Cr-labelled, anti-D-coated red cells of less than 1 ml are injected and the rate of clearance of the cells is approximately 0.035/min, the maximum amount of radioactivity in the plasma is usually 2–5%, reached about 1–2 h after injection (10th edition, p. 321; see also Fig. 10.4). Allowing for the fact that ^{51}Cr and Hb are being cleared steadily throughout this period, the amount released probably corresponds to about 10% of the number of red cells injected.

Jandl and co-workers (1957) found that in subjects injected with approximately 10 ml of red cells, the maximum plasma Hb concentration did not as a rule exceed 6% of the amount injected in the red cells, although in one subject injected with a larger volume of red cells (about 20 ml) the plasma Hb concentration reached the equivalent of 12% of the amount

injected in the red cells. Presumably when amounts of this order are injected the capacity of the RES to clear the Hb–haptoglobin complex is taxed, clearance is slowed and Hb tends to build up in the plasma. Alternatively, it is possible that intravascular haemolysis takes place in the absence of complement fixation and activation.

Haemoglobinaemia associated with predominantly extravascular destruction is thought to occur when red cells are lysed by the lysosomal enzymes released by macrophages following contact of the antibody-coated cell with the macrophage (Fleer *et al.* 1978; Kurlander *et al.* 1978). Thus, the process is postulated to be the same as that observed in antibody-dependent cell-mediated cytotoxicity tests *in vitro*.

Relation between antibody characteristics and patterns of red cell destruction

Those antibodies, whether IgM or IgG, that activate complement but cause either no lysis *in vitro* or only slow lysis characteristically bring about destruction of red cells in the liver. Initially, destruction is rapid with a $T_{1/2}$ of a few min, but after 5–20 min, and usually between 5 and 10 min, destruction slows abruptly. With IgM, antibody destruction is all but arrested, but with IgG antibody, destruction continues, although at a reduced rate (Mollison 1989). These patterns do not point to two populations of red cells, one susceptible and one resistant to rapid destruction. Rather, the whole population is susceptible to rapid destruction initially, but destruction slows as iC3b on the red cells is inactivated. Accordingly, the initial rate of destruction is obtained by extrapolating the tangent to the initial slope to the time axis, rather than by subtracting the 'slow component' (see Fig. 10.6b).

Those IgG antibodies that do not activate complement, for example anti-D, some examples of anti-K and -Fy^a, characteristically bring about red cell destruction in the spleen, often with no measurable destruction in the liver. Destruction produced by immune non-complement-binding IgG antibodies is typically described by a single exponential, even when the rate of destruction is very slow. On the other hand, some naturally occurring, non-complement-binding IgG antibodies (anti-D, anti-E) exhibit removal kinetics described by at least two components.

Although evidence reviewed in previous editions of this book appeared to indicate that non-complement-binding IgM antibodies could cause red cell destruction, a re-appraisal of the data suggests that they do not. As macrophage receptors specific for IgM have not been confirmed, if haemolysis can be effected through IgM binding alone, some other mechanism must be postulated.

The following sections contain examples of destruction by the various kinds of antibody described above.

Complement-binding IgM antibodies

Complement-binding IgM alloantibodies, the commonest of which are anti-A, -B, -A1, -HI, -P1, -Le^a and -Le^b, almost all occur naturally. Of this list, only anti-A and anti-B are often strongly lytic *in vitro* and *in vivo*. Lewis antibodies may cause slow lysis *in vitro* but only rarely cause intravascular haemolysis. Anti-A$_1$, -HI and -P$_1$ are almost never lytic *in vitro*; rare examples activate complement to the C3 stage and, when active at 37°C, may be capable of destroying small volumes of incompatible red cells *in vivo*.

Some examples of the patterns of destruction produced by complement-binding IgM antibodies are as follows.

Anti-A and anti-B

As described above, anti-A and anti-B commonly bring about the intravascular destruction of a proportion of injected incompatible red cells (see Fig. 10.3).

In subjects with hypogammaglobulinaemia, who often have very low levels of circulating anti-A and anti-B, destruction may be almost entirely extravascular. Destruction may be relatively rapid with an initial rate corresponding to a $T_{1/2}$ of a few minutes, with some slowing apparent after 10–20 min (Chaplin 1959); or 50% may be removed with a $T_{1/2}$ of a few minutes with much slower removal ($T_{1/2}$ 1.5 days) of the remainder (van Loghem 1965). In some cases there is no evidence of initial hepatic destruction, as in a case in which destruction was predominantly splenic with a $T_{1/2}$ of 12 h (van Loghem 1965); complement activation may be too weak to influence the mode of destruction in such cases. In still other cases, survival is only slightly subnormal with a $T_{50}Cr$ of 9–15 days. Similarly, in three healthy group A subjects without serologically detectable anti-B, the $T_{50}Cr$ was 10–21 days (van Loghem 1965). In these various cases,

destruction was probably influenced by an IgG component of antibody.

The effect of low concentrations of anti-B has also been investigated by injecting small volumes of B cells and of anti-B serum into a patient of group A with hypogammaglobulinaemia in whom group B cells had previously been found to have a $T_{50}Cr$ of 9–15 days; with varying amounts of anti-B the rate of destruction ranged from 1% to 14% per minute (Jandl and Kaplan 1960). It can be inferred from the data that slowing of destruction occurred after 6–21 min when 20–90% of the cells had been destroyed.

Experiments in which cells have been sensitized *in vitro* with anti-A or anti-B and then injected into the circulation of either healthy subjects or subjects with complement deficiency are described below in the section on sequestration and release of injected red cells.

Anti-Le^a and anti-Le^b

Most examples of anti-Le^a give a positive indirect antiglobulin test (IAT) with anti complement at 37°C and cause some destruction *in vivo* of a small dose of Le(a+) red cells. With potent anti-Le^a the initial rate of clearance may have a $T_{1/2}$ as short as 1.9 min, but the rate is slower than this with less potent antibodies (Mollison *et al.* 1955; Cutbush *et al.* 1956).

When group O, Le(b+) red cells were injected into the circulation of a group A subject, whose plasma contained potent anti-Le^a, 20–50% of the transfused red cells were destroyed owing to the small amount of Le^a substance carried on group O, Le(b+) red cells (Cutbush *et al.* 1956; Fig. 10.5).

A few examples of anti-Le^b react at 37°C with cells of the same ABO group as the recipient. With those that do, the pattern of destruction is the same as with anti-Le^a. For example, in one case in which a patient's plasma contained unusually potent anti-Le^b reactive at 37°C *in vitro*, the initial rate of destruction of group O, Le(a– b+) red cells had a $T_{1/2}$ of 4.5 min; destruction slowed abruptly after about 10 min and 44% of the cells were still present in the circulation at 6 h (Mollison 1959c).

In five cases in which anti-Le^b was active only at 30°C or less, survival of a small volume of Le(b+) red cells was normal at 24 h; in three others in which anti-Le^b was active at 37°C, 24-h survival ranged from 6% to 58%; in each of the three cases a two-component survival curve was observed (Davey 1982).

413

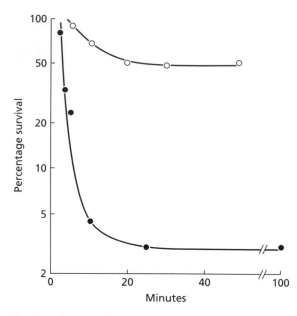

Fig 10.5 Clearance due to complement-binding IgM antibody (anti-Le^a) (Mollison 1986). ○, 1 ml of Le(a+ b+) red cells injected into a subject whose plasma contained anti-Le^a. After a delay of 3 min, 50% of the cells are cleared rapidly, the initial rate of destruction having a $T_{1/2}$ of about 9 min. The rate of clearance starts to diminish within 10 min of injection and percentage survival is the same at 20 and 50 min (Cutbush *et al.* 1956). ●, 1 ml of Le(a+ b–) red cells injected into the same subject; after a delay of about 2.3 min, 95% of the cells are cleared with a $T_{1/2}$ of 2 min. The rate of clearance starts to diminish within 10 min of injection and percentage survival is the same at 100 as at 24 min (observations during first 10 min only published by Mollison and Cutbush 1955).

Anti-A$_1$-HI and -P$_1$

Most examples of these antibodies are not active *in vitro* above a temperature of about 25°C and are incapable of causing destruction of injected red cells. In cases in which the antibody has reacted *in vitro* at 37°C, or has given definite reactions only up to 30–34°C, with dubious reactivity at 37°C, there has been some hepatic destruction initially with slowing after 10 min and with only slightly subnormal survival thereafter. For anti-A$_1$, see Cutbush and Mollison (1958) and Mollison and co-workers (Mollison *et al.* 1978); for anti-HI, see Mollison (1959a) and for anti-P$_1$ see Mollison and co-workers (Mollison *et al.* 1955) and Fig. 10.6.

A close relationship has been observed between thermal range *in vitro* and destruction of a 1-ml dose *in vivo*. For example, in one case in which anti-HI was weakly active at 31°C *in vitro*, no destruction whatever occurred in the 40 min following injections of 1 ml of red cells and in another, in which, at 37°C, the antibody only doubtfully agglutinated red cells but weakly sensitized them to agglutination by an anti-complement reagent, 20% destruction occurred in the first 20 min with virtually normal survival thereafter (PL Mollison, unpublished observations). In a further case in which weak agglutination and a positive reaction with anti-complement was observed at 37°C with anti-P$_1$, 50% of the cells were destroyed in 20 min (see Fig. 10.6).

Anti-H

In three O$_{HM}^{B}$ subjects with weak or undetectable anti-B and anti-H (or -HI), 4-ml amounts of group B and O cells underwent 40–70% destruction; in a fourth subject, following the injection of 58 ml of group B cells, there was little or no destruction (Lin-Chu and Broadberry 1990), possibly because the number of antibody molecules bound per cell was too small.

In contrast, the anti-H present in subjects with the Oh (Bombay) phenotype is strongly lytic *in vivo*. When a small sample of ^{51}Cr-labelled group O donor red blood cells was infused into one such individual, the $T_{1/2}$ of the infused cells was 6 min, with 2% of the cells surviving at 24 h. A similar study using the patient's own labelled red blood cells demonstrated 100% survival at 24 h. Anti-H was active in saline at 4°C, 22°C and 37°C and by the IAT. The antibody(ies) showed both IgM and IgG components. The anti-H titre at 37°C rose from 4 prior to the infusion of the O cells to 32 at 1 week post infusion, and a partial haemolysin appeared. Saliva inhibition studies demonstrated that the antibody was neutralizable prior to the group O exposure but was not neutralizable 1 week post exposure (Davey *et al.* 1978).

Auto-anti-I

This antibody is considered here because the pattern of destruction of injected I-positive red cells follows the same two-component kinetics as seen with the foregoing alloantibodies. In three patients with cold haemagglutinin disease (CHAD) with potent auto-anti-I, following the injection of a small dose of ^{51}Cr-labelled

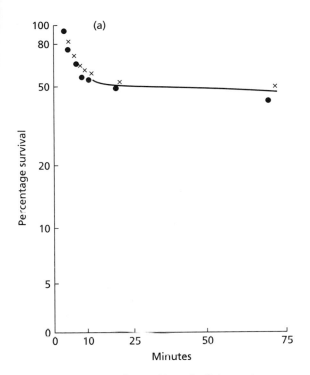

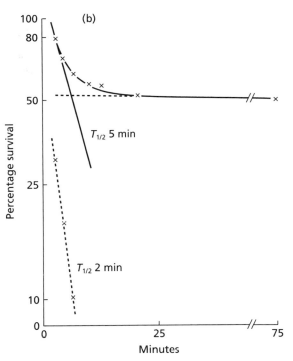

Fig 10.6 Destruction of P_1-positive red cells in a patient whose serum contained anti-P_1, weakly active at 37°C. (a) P_1-positive red cells labelled with ^{32}P were injected as an ice-cold suspension (•) and red cells from the same donor labelled with ^{51}Cr were injected as a warm (39°C) suspension (×) immediately afterwards. The temperature of the suspension at the time of injection did not appear to influence the survival (Mollison *et al.* 1955). (b) Deduction of the initial rate of destruction of the warm suspension from (a).

If it is (incorrectly) assumed that there are two subpopulations of red cells, one susceptible to rapid destruction and one resistant, the half-time of clearance of the susceptible population, plotted as the difference between the observed points and the extrapolated 'slow' component, is estimated to be 2 min. If it is (correctly) assumed that all cells are initially susceptible, the initial rate of destruction is estimated to have a half-time of 5 min (Mollison 1989).

I-positive red cells a two-component curve was observed: 30–60% of the cells were removed in 40–120 min with much slower removal of the remaining cells, i.e. $T_{1/2}$ 5–10 days (Evans *et al.* 1968). In a case in which detailed observations were made over the first 35 min, destruction started to slow 5–10 min after injection of the red cells and was very slow after 20 min, by which time about one-third of the cells had been destroyed (Mollison 1985).

Anti-M

This antibody almost never binds complement. In one exceptional case (Cutbush and Mollison 1958), the serum, containing only IgM anti-M, weakly sensitized M+N–, but not M+N+, red cells to agglutination by anti-complement. Following the injection of test doses of red cells, 65% of M+N– cells were removed with a half-time of 4 min; the rate of destruction slowed after 10 min. M+N+ cells were removed with a half-time of 4.5 days.

Effect of temperature of injected red cells

In a subject with anti-P_1 weakly reactive *in vitro* at 37°C (see Fig. 10.6) and in another with anti-M reactive *in vitro* at 34°C, although not at 37°C (Mollison 1959b), one sample of labelled incompatible red cells was warmed to 37°C and one, labelled with a different isotope, was cooled in ice water, following injection. Survival curves of the injected cells were superimposable.

415

Effect of hypothermia on cold alloantibodies

As most cold alloantibodies are IgM and complement binding, the issue of clinical significance in patients subjected to artificial hypothermia recurs frequently. Most transfusion services have long ago abandoned antibody screening at temperatures below 30°C, and virtually all hospitals crossmatch blood at a temperature of 37°C, even for patients undergoing procedures that involve deep hypothermia. Given the dearth of adverse events reported, it is likely that cold alloantibodies inactive at 37°C but active at some lower temperature such as 25°C or 30°C rarely, if ever, cause clinically significant red cell destruction when the patient is cooled. Although some shortening of red cell lifespan may result from the cold alloantibody, accurate assessment of red cell survival is confounded by changes in blood volume induced by haemorrhage and transfusion. One approach to this problem is to inject two labelled suspensions of red cells, one susceptible and one resistant to destruction, and note whether the ratio of the two populations changes during hypothermia. In a case investigated in this way, no evidence of destruction by anti-P was observed when the patient was cooled, but some destruction had occurred before cooling so that the cells had presumably become resistant to complement-mediated destruction.

Clinical data concerning cold agglutinins, hypothermia and haemolysis are limited. An oft-cited case report involves a patient with *Mycoplasma pneumoniae*, cold agglutinins and a haemolytic anaemia that may have resulted from vigorous treatment of hyperpyrexia with a cooling mattress (Niejadlik and Lozner 1974). Other anecdotes involve cold agglutinins in extracorporeal circuits and agglutination in the plastic tubing during plasmapheresis. None is particularly convincing. Perhaps the most reassuring data involve *in vivo* survival of M (M+N–) red cells in two patients with anti-M studied during hypothermia. The low-titre, IgM antibodies did not react at 30°C. ^{51}Cr survival studies performed with 2 ml of labelled blood documented normal circulation of M (M+N–) cells at 37°C, and no accelerated loss of these cells at blood temperatures between 16° and 28°C. One patient received 187 ml of MN (M+N+) red cells when the blood temperature was 25°C without evidence of a clinical transfusion reaction and without development of a positive DAT (Kurtz *et al.* 1983).

Complement-binding IgG antibodies

As described in Chapter 6, IgG antibodies of certain specificities, for example anti-A and anti-B, anti-K, -Fy^a and -Yt^a, occasionally bind complement. Sera containing Kidd antibodies usually bind complement, but recent data challenge the belief that IgG is implicated (Yates *et al.* 1996).

Anti-K

In one subject, Kk cells had a curvilinear slope of destruction. The initial rate had a $T_{1/2}$ of less than 20 min, but by 1–2 h the $T_{1/2}$ was more than 1 h. Surface counting showed that in the initial phase, destruction occurred mainly in the liver, and in the later phase mainly in the spleen (Hughes-Jones *et al.* 1957). When KK cells were injected the initial rate of clearance had a $T_{1/2}$ of 6 min and destruction slowed about 20 min after injection (Fig. 10.7). In a further case, about 80% of the cells were removed with an initial $T_{1/2}$ of 6 min. After about 30 min, the $T_{1/2}$ had lengthened to about 30 min (Cutbush and Mollison 1958).

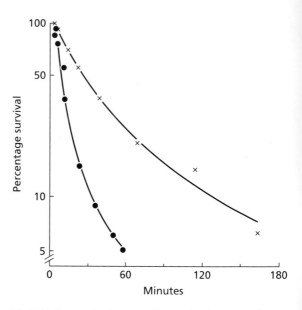

Fig 10.7 Destruction by a complement-binding example of anti-K of 1-ml doses of K-positive red cells. ●, KK cells (10th edition, p. 325); ×, Kk cells (Hughes-Jones *et al.* 1957).

Anti-Fy^a

One example was studied extensively: in the subject (RD) in whom anti-Fy^a was first identified, Fy (a+) cells showed a two-component curve of destruction. The initial rate of destruction had a $T_{1/2}$ of 4 min but, after 15 min, by which time 90% of the cells had been cleared, destruction became very much slower (Cutbush and Mollison 1958). In tests in which Fy (a+) cells were sensitized *in vitro* with purified anti-Fy^a from RD, up to 90% of the cells were cleared with a $T_{1/2}$ that could be as short as 2.5 min (Cutbush and Mollison 1958). Destruction slowed abruptly about 10 min after injection of the red cells (Fig. 10.8; see also Fig. 10.2). The results of quantitative tests are described in a later section.

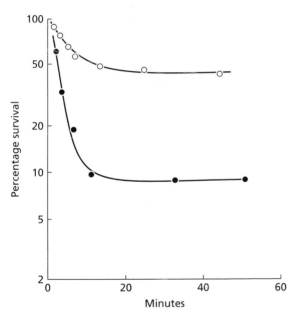

Fig 10.8 Clearance due to complement-binding IgG antibody (anti-Fy^a). Red cells (ml) of two Fy (a+) donors were coated *in vitro* with different amounts of anti-Fy^a and returned to each donor's circulation. The anti-Fy^a was a purified IgG fraction from a donor, RD (Mollison 1986). ○, After a delay of about 1 min, clearance begins with an initial $T_{1/2}$ of 8 min, but slows abruptly after about 10 min (Mollison 1962, case 6a; rate of clearance recalculated). ●, After a delay of about 1.2 min, clearance begins with an initial $T_{1/2}$ of 2 min, but slows abruptly after about 10 min (Mollison 1962, case 5; rate of clearance recalculated).

Anti-Jk^a and anti-Jk^b

In one case, Jk^{a}Jk^a cells were cleared with a $T_{1/2}$ of 4 min, 99% of cells being removed within 30 min of injection. In the same subject Jk^{a}Jk^b cells were cleared with a $T_{1/2}$ of about 80 min and no slowing was observed during the 60 min after injection for which survival was followed (Cutbush and Mollison 1958). In two other cases, substantially slower destruction was observed: for an example of anti-Jk^a, cells were cleared with a $T_{1/2}$ of 75 min (Fudenberg and Allen 1957), and for an example of anti-Jk^b, destruction also appeared to be described by a single exponential, with 90% of the cells being cleared in a period of 24 h (Howard *et al.* 1982). The exponential slopes sometimes associated with destruction by anti-Jk^a may be explained by the recent observation that, apparently, only IgM (and not IgG) Kidd antibodies bind complement (Yates *et al.* 1996).

In one unusual case, in which anti-Jk^a could be detected only by the manual polybrene test, destruction was rapid and more than 50% of the ^{51}Cr was found in the plasma within 1 h (Maynard *et al.* 1988).

Anti-Yt^a

In a patient with a complement-binding IgG example of this antibody, approximately 85% of Yt (a+) cells were cleared within 12 min, the remainder being cleared much more slowly (Bettigole *et al.* 1968).

Acquired resistance to complement-mediated destruction

In almost all the curves of destruction described above, owing to complement-binding antibodies, whether IgM or IgG, a common pattern emerges: destruction is initially rapid, with a $T_{1/2}$ of a few minutes indicating hepatic destruction, but after an interval which may be as short as 5 min or as long as 60 min (most commonly about 10 min) destruction slows abruptly. The slowing of destruction appears to result from cleavage of C3b, leaving on the red cell surface C3d,g which does not mediate red cell destruction through receptor-mediated macrophage uptake.

Acquired resistance of red cells to destruction by alloantibodies was described by Möller in mice (Möller 1964). The effect could be produced both *in vitro* and *in vivo* and depended on specific antibody and on some host factor, subsequently identified as complement. A similar effect was demonstrated in CHAD by Evans and co-workers (1967, 1968), who described the mechanism of resistance to complement-mediated lysis by cold agglutinins. Transfused red cells underwent rapid destruction initially but, within an hour, destruction slowed and the remaining cells were destroyed far more slowly. Donor red cells could be rendered relatively resistant to destruction by exposure to CHAD serum *in vitro*. Resistance to destruction was associated with the accumulation of complement on the red cell membrane. Similar observations were reported by Engelfriet and co-workers (1972) who discussed the possibility that the accumulation of α_{2D} (C3dg) on the red cell membrane might block the attachment of further C3 molecules (Jaffe *et al.* 1976).

Further work confirmed that the presence of functionally active C3 on the red cells was essential for hepatic sequestration and that cells coated with C3d (or C3dg) alone were not cleared from the circulation. The active forms of C3, C3b and iC3b have specific receptors on phagocytic cells (Nicholson-Weller *et al.* 1982). The inactive product, found on the red cells of patients with CHAD, is C3dg (Lachmann *et al.* 1982). Acquired resistance of transfused ABO-incompatible red cells to destruction was strongly suggested by observations published by Akeroyd and O'Brien (1958). After the transfusion of group AB cells to a group A patient, some surviving cells could be demonstrated after 6 weeks, even although the recipient's serum contained an anti-B lysin. When a new sample of AB cells was injected, 90% of the cells were removed from the circulation within 45 min.

Acquired resistance to destruction suggests the presence on the red cells of C3dg around the sites of antibody attachment. Chaplin and co-workers (1983) have shown that 85–95% of bound C3d disappears from circulating red cells in 5–8 days. Red cell destruction that depends on complement activation should be able to continue, although at a greatly reduced rate. The slowing of the rate of destruction, observed some 10 min after injection of red cells into the circulation, should be much less with IgG than with IgM antibodies, as IgG alone can mediate erythrophagocytosis, whereas IgM antibodies depend on complement activation. The difference between the effects produced by IgG and IgM complement-binding antibodies has been illustrated above. For example, with IgG anti-K, after

the initial rapid phase of destruction, the subsequent phase (with KK cells) continued with a $T_{1/2}$ of 30 min. In contrast, in destruction by IgM anti-P_1, after the initial phase of rapid destruction the rate became too small to measure. For further examples, see Mollison (1989).

Sequestration and release of complement-coated red cells

When red cells are sensitized *in vitro* with a complement-binding IgM antibody, or with complement alone, a proportion of the injected population is cleared rapidly but some or all of the red cells slowly return to the circulation. The initial disappearance is presumably mediated by attachment of the C3b- or iC3b-coated red cell to a macrophage. When iC3b is cleaved, leaving only C3dg on the red cell, the cell is released back into the circulation. This temporary trapping followed by the release of complement-coated red cells has been demonstrated in various experiments:

1 When a sample of red cells from a group B subject was incubated with anti-B and then re-injected into the circulation, 26% of the cells were removed almost immediately but returned to the circulation during the next 2 h (Jandl and Simmons 1957).

2 When the red cells of a patient with CHAD were exposed to their own serum at 4°C *in vitro* and then re-injected, about 40% were removed in 15 min. More than one-half of the cells returned to the circulation within 60 min and most within 24 h (Lewis *et al.* 1960).

3 In experiments in which red cells were coated with complement alone by exposure to their own serum at low ionic strength, 25–40% were sequestered following re-injection into the circulation; some cells returned within 60 min and almost all within 24 h (Mollison *et al.* 1965).

4 In C6-deficient rabbits, when red cells were coated *in vitro* with human anti-I and then re-injected, so that they bound C4, C3 (and C5), 45–95% were sequestered but most of the cells returned to the circulation in 2–3 h (Brown *et al.* 1970). For further observations, see Schreiber and Frank (1972) and Atkinson and Frank (1974a).

5 When group A or B cells were coated *in vitro* with relatively small amounts of purified anti-A or anti-B (20 IgM molecules per coated cell), about 30% disappeared within the first 12 min after re-injection into

the circulation, but almost all reappeared within the next 3 h. As the density of molecules per cell was increased, the proportion of cells that reappeared in the circulation after initial sequestration diminished. In two subjects with low levels of C2 and C4, cells coated with moderate amounts of IgM antibody survived normally. Thus IgM molecules alone appear incapable of effecting accelerated red cell destruction and that removal depends upon complement fixation (Atkinson and Frank 1974b).

Rate of cleavage of C3b *in vitro and in vivo*

Conversion of C3b to iC3b takes about 1 min *in vitro*. In blood, where cells express a cofactor, further cleavage of the molecule splits off C3c and leaves only C3dg on the cell surface with a $T_{1/2}$ of about 20 min (see Chapter 3). This rate of cleavage is consistent with the observation that destruction of complement-coated red cells may slow within 5–10 min of their injection into the circulation (Mollison 1986). On the other hand, it does not agree well with the observation that the release of temporarily sequestered complement-coated red cells takes about 2–3 h. The reason for the discrepancy is unknown. Possibly, iC3b is less accessible when it is attached to CR3.

Role of IgM *and of complement in producing irreversible sequestration*

When incompatible red cells are injected into a subject with a complement-binding antibody that appears to be solely IgM, a portion of the red cells is rapidly cleared and these cells do not return to the circulation. On the other hand, when red cells are sensitized *in vitro* with an IgM complement-binding antibody, many of the cells that are initially sequestered later return to the circulation. Neither IgM antibody nor complement alone causes red cell destruction. Although C3b seems to be involved primarily in bringing about attachment to macrophages rather than in promoting ingestion, macrophages activated by a lymphokine show complement-dependent phagocytosis (Griffin and Mullinax 1985). The enhanced activity of macrophages in infection is mentioned in Chapter 3. The effect of IgM in phagocytosis seems to be either to enhance in some unspecified way complement-mediated cell removal or to bring about the binding of critical numbers of complement molecules.

Non-complement-binding IgM antibodies

In previous editions of this book, several examples of destruction by IgM antibodies that seemed to be non-complement binding were described. Re-examination of the evidence has cast doubt on the interpretation of the data. However, the example of anti-M which produced rapid destruction of MM red cells should not have been described as non-complement binding, nor should the IgM fraction of the rabbit alloantibody anti-Hg[A] (Mollison 1986). The examples of IgM Rh antibodies that were reported to effect red cell destruction were probably contaminated with an amount of IgG that was too small to be detected by immunoelectrophoresis, but sufficient when given intravenously to have caused the clearance of D-positive cells that was observed. In summary, no evidence is available that non-complement-binding IgM antibodies play a role in accelerated red cell destruction.

Non-complement-binding IgG antibodies

Virtually all examples of IgG anti-D and most examples of IgG anti-K, anti-S and anti-Fy[a] fail to bind complement. Antibodies of this kind bring about red cell destruction predominantly in the spleen (Jandl 1955; Mollison *et al.* 1955; Hughes-Jones *et al.* 1957; Jandl and Greenberg 1957; Cutbush and Mollison 1958; Crome and Mollison 1964); Fig. 10.9.

As discussed in a later section, with most of the antibodies mentioned above, the small numbers of corresponding antigen sites limit the number of molecules of IgG bound per cell to about 25 000 or fewer. On the other hand, with anti-c, owing to the greater number of c sites, a theoretical maximum of about 80 000 molecules of anti-c per red cell can be bound. In retrospect, this fact probably explains the relatively rapid clearance of c-positive red cells in a subject whose serum contained both IgM and IgG anti-c. In this subject, cc red cells were cleared with a $T_{1/2}$ of 2.8 min, indicating clearance of 70% of the blood at a single passage through the liver (Fig. 10.10), a finding originally believed to indicate clearance by IgM anti-c (Cutbush and Mollison 1958). The subsequent recognition that the serum also contained relatively potent IgG anti-c, and the finding that c sites were more abundant than D sites, led to the re-interpretation of the data (Mollison 1989). The number of anti-c molecules bound per cell has been

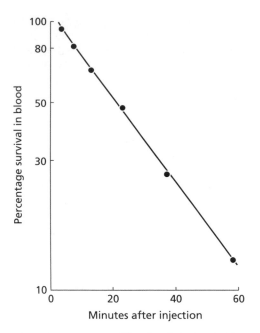

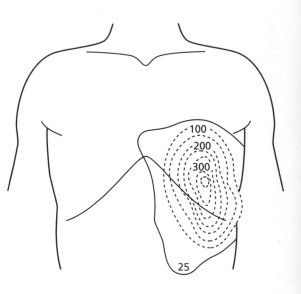

Fig 10.9 Destruction of ^{51}Cr-labelled Kk red cells in a subject with non-complement-binding anti-K. The points are fitted by a single exponential with a $T_{1/2}$ of 19 min. After the cells had been cleared from the circulation, surface counting showed that virtually all the ^{51}Cr was localized in the area of the spleen (Hughes-Jones *et al.* 1957, case 3).

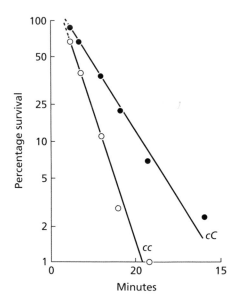

Fig 10.10 Clearance of c-positive red cells in a subject whose serum contained both IgG and IgM anti-c. cc cells (○) were cleared with a $T_{1/2}$ of 2.8 min, and cC cells (●) with a $T_{1/2}$ of 5.6 min (Cutbush and Mollison 1958).

estimated as approximately 57 000 (NC Hughes-Jones, personal communication). The degree of coating with IgG needed to produce complete clearance of coated red cells at a single passage through the spleen and the degree needed to produce some clearance by the liver are discussed below.

The fact that red cells coated with anti-D are removed from the circulation predominantly in the spleen can be turned to advantage. Clearance of antibody-coated red cells has been used as a functional diagnostic assay in several circumstances. First, scanning with a gamma camera following the injection of radiolabelled D-sensitized red cells can be used to locate aberrant splenic tissue. Second, the presence of a splenunculus (accessory spleen), as in a patient with hereditary spherocytosis who relapses following splenectomy, can be demonstrated (MacKenzie *et al.* 1962).

Third, estimation of the rate of clearance of D-positive red cells coated with an amount of anti-D that would normally be cleared in a single passage through the spleen can be used to determine whether splenic size or splenic blood flow are abnormal. For example, in a patient with hereditary spherocytosis with a spleen later shown at operation to weigh 395 g, D-sensitized red cells were cleared with a $T_{1/2}$ of just over 8 min compared with the normal $T_{1/2}$ of about 18–22 min (Mollison 1970). In a second example, a subject with a normal-sized spleen that was suspected to have been damaged at a previous operation cleared D-sensitized red cells with a $T_{1/2}$ of 60 min, strongly suggesting that the spleen was infarcted and had a much reduced blood flow. This finding was confirmed at operation (Mollison 1979, p. 504). Finally, in subjects in whom the RES is partially blocked by immune complexes, as in lupus erythematosus, clearance of D-sensitized red cells is much slower than in normal subjects (Frank *et al.* 1979). Similarly, in adults with AITP injected with 1–1.5 g of IgG/kg body weight, the rate of clearance of D-sensitized red cells was slowed (Fehr *et al.* 1982).

In splenectomized subjects, D-positive red cells coated with an amount of anti-D sufficient to bring about maximal clearance in a subject with a spleen are cleared with a $T_{1/2}$ of about 5 h (Jandl and Greenberg 1957; Crome and Mollison 1964; Brown 1983). When red cells are more heavily coated with anti-D, removal with a $T_{1/2}$ as short as 90–160 min may reflect a component of hepatic sequestration (Crome and Mollison 1964; Brown 1983). Hepatic destruction of red cells carrying only moderate amounts of IgG is partially inhibited by plasma IgG blockage of Fc receptors on the macrophages. On the other hand, when the number of IgG molecules bound to red cells exceeds a certain value, which differs for IgG1 and IgG3, plasma IgG becomes a much less efficient blocker of receptor sites (Engelfriet *et al.* 1981).

Naturally occurring Rh antibodies

The survival of small volumes of incompatible red cells has been studied in a few subjects with naturally occurring anti-E or anti-D; although, in the past, naturally occurring Rh antibodies have been assumed to be solely IgM, recent investigations using more sensitive tests indicate that most if not all antibodies are partly IgG.

Anti-E. Anti-E is the most common naturally occurring Rh antibody, but its effect on the survival of E-positive red cells has been studied in very few cases. In the subject described by Vogt and co-workers (1958) the survival curve had an interesting shape, about one-quarter of the cells being cleared with a $T_{1/2}$

of 20 min and the rest with a $T_{1/2}$ of several hours. This example of anti-E may well be alloimmune, rather than 'naturally occurring', as the subject had received transfusions of E-positive blood 52 and 41 days before the test was carried out. On the other hand, in the series described by Jensen and co-workers (1965), one subject who had not been transfused previously exhibited survival of E-positive red cells that was only slightly subnormal (T_{50}Cr 19.5 days).

In a small series studied by Contreras and co-workers (1987), survival was normal in one case but was reduced in two others. In one of these cases, approximately two-thirds of the cells were removed with a $T_{1/2}$ of a few hours and the rest with a $T_{1/2}$ of almost 5 days. In the other, 25% of cells were cleared in 24 h. The antibodies were at least partly IgG.

Anti-D. As described in Chapter 5, the kind of naturally occurring anti-D found on screening in the autoanalyzer and by no other method is IgG and cold reacting. In one subject with an antibody of this kind, T_{50}Cr was 19 days, only slightly reduced (Perrault and Högman 1972). Strictly normal survival was found in one case by Lee and co-workers (1984). In another series of three examples of naturally occurring anti-D in males, survival was virtually normal in one but greatly reduced in the remaining two. In one of these, about 75% of the cells were removed with a $T_{1/2}$ of a few hours, the remainder with a $T_{1/2}$ of approximately 6 days. In the remaining case, all the cells were removed with a $T_{1/2}$ of 2 h (Contreras *et al.* 1987). In summary, normal or almost normal red cell survival has been found in some subjects with naturally occurring anti-E or anti-D, but definitely reduced survival has been found in others. A puzzling feature of these latter cases has been the two component curves of survival, with slowing occurring as a rule some hours after injection of red cells into the circulation (Fig. 10.11).

Destruction by non-complement-binding IgG antibodies of other specificities

Observations on the rate of clearance of test doses of incompatible red cells, produced by alloantibodies of many other specificities, have been published. The following list is far from complete: At[a], Jr[a], Ok[a] (Chapter 6); Co[b] (Dzik and Blank 1986); Cr[a], IFC (Chapter 6); Do[a] (Polesky and Swanson 1966); Do[b] (Shirey *et al.* 1998); HLA (van der Hart *et al.* 1974; Nordhagen and

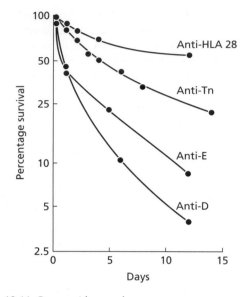

Fig 10.11 Curves with more than one component, associated with destruction by antibodies believed to be non-complement activating. Anti-HLA-28, survival of red cells on which HLA-28 was very strongly expressed, in a patient whose serum contained anti-HLA-28 (Nordhagen and Aas 1978). Anti-Tn, survival of red cells from a patient with Tn transformation in a normal subject, i.e. with anti-Tn (Myllyla *et al.* 1971). Anti-E and anti-D, survival of E-positive and D-positive red cells, respectively, in subjects whose serum contained naturally occurring anti-E and anti-D (Contreras *et al.* 1987).

Aas 1978; Panzer *et al.* 1984); Hy (see Chapter 6); In^a (Badakere *et al.* 1980); In^b (Ferguson and Gaal 1988; Lan (Clancey *et al.* 1972; Lampe *et al.* 1979); Lu^b (Cutbush and Mollison 1958; Peters *et al.* 1978); Lu6 (Issitt *et al.* 1990); LW^b (Sistonen *et al.* 1981); M, Mi^a (Cutbush and Mollison 1958); N (Ballas *et al.* 1985); S,s (Fudenberg and Allen 1957); Sc3 (see Chapter 6); Wr^a (Cutbush and Mollison 1958); Yt^a (Gobel *et al.* 1974; Ballas and Sherwood 1977; Silvergleid *et al.* 1978; Davey and Simpkins 1981).

Non-destructive IgG antibodies

Antibodies not expected to cause red cell destruction are: (1) those that are active only at temperatures below 37°C; (2) those that are active at 37°C, but are solely IgM and do not bind complement; and (3) those that are IgG, but are confined to subclasses IgG4 or IgG2 (but see Chapter 12) or are IgG1 often, but not

always, present in low concentration (Garratty and Nance 1990). As in most cases, IgG subclass has not been determined, and often cannot be determined because of the low antibody concentration; this characteristic is rarely helpful in determining whether a particular IgG antibody will, or will not, cause red cell destruction.

Examples of antibodies of the following specificities, although active *in vitro* at 37°C, and although shown to be, or presumed to be, IgG, have failed to bring about the destruction of small doses of incompatible red cells: Ch (Moore *et al.* 1975; Tilley *et al.* 1977; Silvergleid *et al.* 1978); Cs^a (Shore and Steane 1977); JMH (Sabo *et al.* 1978); K11 (Kelley *et al.* 1998); Kn^a, McC^a (Silvergleid *et al.* 1978; Baldwin *et al.* 1985); Lu^a (Greendyke and Chorpenning 1962); LW (Tregellas 1978; Cummings *et al.* 1984; Chaplin *et al.* 1985); Xg^a (Sausais *et al.* 1964); Yk^a (Tilley *et al.* 1977; Lau *et al.* 1994); Yt^a (Dobbs *et al.* 1968; Mollison 1983, p. 428). However, as these reports are often of single examples, these antibodies should still be respected when selecting blood for transfusion unless rare antigen-negative red cells are not available.

Relation between results of cellular bioassays and destruction *in vivo*

On the whole, good correlation has been found between the results of monocyte or macrophage monolayer tests and evidence of destruction *in vivo*. In the first series to be described, 25 antibodies (anti-Yt^a, -Jr^d, -Ch, -JMH, etc.) that had failed to cause haemolytic transfusion reactions or haemolytic disease of the newborn resulted in low values in the assay, whereas two that had caused either a haemolytic transfusion reaction or had rapidly destroyed ^51Cr-labelled red cells yielded high values (Schanfield *et al.* 1981). In another series, six antibodies (all anti-Yt^a, -Ge or -Lan) that had not caused haemolytic reactions after the transfusion of incompatible red cells or (in two cases) had not rapidly destroyed ^51Cr-labelled red cells gave a negative monocyte monolayer assay, whereas five antibodies (anti-Yt^a, -Ge or -Lan) that had rapidly destroyed labelled red cells gave positive results. Two of these five were anti-Lan, and these yielded positive results only when fresh serum was used for the assay (Nance *et al.* 1987).

In one series, four patients with anti-McC^a, -JMH or -Hy^a had negative macrophage assays but destroyed incompatible red cells at an accelerated rate in a short-term survival assay. The survival rate of labelled cells was 89–95% at 1 h, but the authors argued that the $T_{50}Cr$ of 12–15 days indicated that the risk of haemolysis was best estimated by this longer study (Baldwin *et al.* 1985). However, these long-term cell survival data are unreliable as evidence of antibody-mediated destruction, as some patients had chronic bleeding and others were transfused during the study period.

In patients with anti-Yt[a] in whom the antibody had first been detected less than 6 weeks previously, the MMA was positive (more than 3% reactive monocytes) in 24 out of 30; of eight who were transfused with Yt (a+) blood, three with a negative MMA had no adverse events; of five with a positive MMA, two had a mild delayed haemolytic transfusion reaction (DHTR). A positive MMA was significantly less common (6 out of 33) in patients in whom anti-Yt[a] had been detected more than 6 weeks previously. Of 10 of these who were transfused with Yt(a+) blood, the only patient with a positive MMA had a mild DHTR (Eckrich *et al.* 1995).

In addition to these relatively extensive studies, numerous single cases have been reported: an example of anti-Cr[a] that brought about more than 40% destruction of a small volume of incompatible red cells in 4 h gave a clearly positive result in a monocyte monolayer test (McSwain and Robins 1988); on the other hand, an example of anti-Lu12, which destroyed 50% of a small dose of incompatible red cells *in vivo*, did not react in a mononuclear assay (Shirey *et al.* 1988). In a patient who had formed an antibody against the Cromer-related antigen Tc[a], the survival at 24 h of a test dose of incompatible red cells was within normal limits and an MMA was normal at a time when the antibody was a mixture of IgG2 and IgG4. Some years previously, the antibody had also been partly IgG1, and an MMA had been well above normal limits (Anderson *et al.* 1991).

Using a test for monocyte phagocytosis (see Chapter 3), a negative result was obtained with an example of an IgG1 monoclonal anti-D that failed to destroy D-positive red cells *in vivo* (Crawford *et al.* 1988); and using a test for adherence to, and phagocytosis by, monocytes and an ADCC(M) assay (see Chapter 3), positive results were obtained with two monoclonal anti-Ds, one IgG1 and one IgG3 (Wiener *et al.* 1988) that were subsequently shown to produce accelerated clearance of D-positive red cells *in vivo* (Thomson *et al.* 1990). The same two monoclonal antibodies yielded moderately strong results when tested 'blind' in a number of bioassays with monocytes, although they gave only weak reactions in an ADCC(M) assay (Report from 9 Collaborating Laboratories 1991).

Limited data with a chemiluminescence assay suggest that results are similar to those with MMA (Hadley *et al.* 1999). Although bioassays have not yet been demonstrated to predict the speed and extent of red cell destruction produced by particular antibodies, they do seem to be able to distinguish between those antibodies that produce accelerated destruction of red cells and those that do not. As adhesion is only one of several functions of the monocyte involved in red cell destruction, it should come as no surprise that MMA results do not correlate perfectly with clinical findings. Although they are not often used in this way, bioassays should prove valuable adjuncts to crossmatching when the recipient has an antibody of questionable clinical significance. Like serological tests, bioassays cannot be expected to predict delayed haemolytic reactions in patients who have sustained primary immunization to a red cell antigen, but have no evidence of circulating alloantibody.

Effect of antigen content of red cells

Earlier sections have provided several examples of differences in the rate of destruction of two samples of red cells, depending on their membrane antigen content. The purpose of this section is to bring these observations together and to add a few additional ones.

Subgroups of A

The injection of 30–40 ml of A_1 blood to group O recipients produced haemoglobinaemia, and in 3 out of 5 cases, clinical reactions, whereas the same amount of A_2 blood produced neither haemoglobinaemia nor reactions (Wiener *et al.* 1953). Further evidence of the relative resistance of A_2 cells is provided by cases in which an A_2 or A_2B recipient is transfused with A_1 or A_1B blood and then with group O blood containing potent anti-A. The A_1 or A_1B red cells are destroyed preferentially.

Although red cells with a weak A antigen are relatively resistant to damage by anti-A, a haemolytic reaction following the transfusion of A_X blood has been reported in a patient whose serum contained potent anti-A. The pre-transfusion titre was 1000 vs. A_1 cells and 8 vs. A_X cells (Schmidt *et al.* 1959).

B red cells in newborn infants

Although the A and B antigens are considerably weaker in newborn infants than in adults, in experiments in which 1 ml of group B cord red cells was injected into group A mothers whose anti-B titre never exceeded 32, all of the red cells were destroyed within 20 min and usually within 5 min, mainly via intravascular lysis (Sieg *et al.* 1970).

Differences in the P_1 and Lewis antigens

Differences in the serological 'strength' of P_1 antigen in different P_1-positive blood samples correlate with the degree of red cell destruction *in vivo*. For example, in a patient whose serum contained a strong anti-P_1, 49% and 51% of the red cells of one P_1-positive donor were destroyed on two different occasions. In between these two tests, the red cells of another P_1-positive donor, whose red cells reacted more strongly *in vitro*, were injected and 60% were destroyed rapidly *in vivo* (PL Mollison, personal communication). Similarly, in a patient whose serum contained anti-Le^a, the red cells of adult donors of the phenotype Le(a+ b–) were removed with a $T_{1/2}$ of approximately 2 min, whereas those of infant donors of the phenotype Le(a+ b+) were removed with a $T_{1/2}$ of 3–5 min (Cutbush *et al.* 1956).

Differences between red cells from homozygotes and heterozygotes

An example of the slightly more rapid destruction of cc red cells compared with Cc by anti-c is shown in Fig. 10.8 and a similar difference between the rate of destruction of KK and Kk cells by anti-K is shown in Fig. 10.7. Considerably more rapid destruction of Jk^{a}Jk^a red cells than of Jk^{a}Jk^b cells by anti-Jk^a and a large difference between the rate of destruction of MM and MN cells has also been described (Cutbush and Mollison 1958).

Survival curves with more than one component

As discussed above, acquired resistance to complement-mediated destruction seems to be the commonest cause of survival curves with two components. There are only a few examples of two-component survival curves that seem not to be due to acquired resistance to complement-mediated destruction:

1 *Destruction by anti-Tn.* When red cells from a patient with 'mixed field polyagglutinability', only 50% of whose red cells were agglutinated by anti-Tn, were injected into a normal subject, almost one-half of the cells disappeared within a few days. The remaining cells had a longer, although still subnormal, survival (Myllyla *et al.* 1971); see Fig. 10.11.

2 *Destruction by anti-B* of a selected population of 'unagglutinable group B red cells'. A large volume of group B red cells was treated with group O serum containing potent anti-B. The unagglutinated cells were separated and treated with a fresh lot of the same group O serum. The process was repeated until a suspension of cells was obtained which was free from agglutinates and was inagglutinable by the anti-B serum. The selected cells were now injected into the group O donor of the potent anti-B and were destroyed far more slowly than an unselected population of group B cells injected into the same donor. After injection of the selected cells, the usual slowing in the rate of destruction occurred 10–20 min after injection; some 13% of the red cells continued to circulate at 24 h and the subsequent survival of these could not be described by a single exponential (Winkelstein and Mollison 1965).

3 *Destruction by anti-Hy.* Fewer than 50% of the cells had a $T_{1/2}$ of 2–3.5 days and the rest had a $T_{1/2}$ of 15 days. The antibody was IgG and apparently non-complement binding (Hsu *et al.* 1975).

4 *Destruction by anti-HLA.* As mentioned above, destruction has been observed in a few cases and, in these, two-component curves have been observed, often with slowing of the rate of destruction after only 1 day. For an example see Fig. 10.11.

5 *Destruction by anti-Lu^b.* In one case, destruction of Lu (a– b+) red cells was associated with a multicomponent clearance curve (Cutbush and Mollison 1958), although in two other cases destruction could be described by single exponentials (Tilley *et al.* 1977; Peters *et al.* 1978).

6 *Destruction by anti-Yt^a.* In a case described by Davey and Simpkins (1981), 20% of the cells were removed in the first 30 min. The remaining cells had a $T_{1/2}$ of about 4 days.

7 *Destruction by naturally occurring Rh antibodies (IgG).* As described above, two-component survival

curves associated with naturally occurring anti-E and anti-D have been observed. In some cases some cells were cleared with a $T_{1/2}$ of several hours and the remainder with a $T_{1/2}$ of several days; for examples, see Fig. 10.11.

In considering the above results, heterogeneity of antigen seems a likely explanation for examples 1, 2, 3 and 4; complement activation may have been overlooked for examples 5 (case 1) and 6. No explanation can be offered for no. 7.

Quantitative aspects of the destruction of transfused red cells by alloantibodies

When small amounts of red cells are transfused, the rate of red cell destruction by any particular antibody is determined by the number of antibody molecules combined with each cell. This number is affected by many factors: the concentration of antigen, which depends both on the number of red cells transfused and on the number of antigen sites per cell; the concentration of antibody in the plasma; and the equilibrium constant of the reaction between antigen and antibody and its degree of heterogeneity.

When a large volume of incompatible red cells is transfused, the cells are destroyed more slowly than when a small volume is transfused. Two independent factors determine this difference; first, as the amount of antibody in the recipient's plasma is limited, the amount taken up by each incompatible red cell diminishes as the number of transfused cells increases (in principle, antibody-mediated red cell destruction may be limited by complement availability, but there are few circumstances in which this limitation appears to be of practical importance); second, the number of red cells that can be removed by the RES in unit time is limited. In some circumstances the amount of antibody bound by various amounts of red cells can be calculated or even directly measured. On the other hand, there is little information about the functional capacity of the RES and the way in which it is affected by the 'load' of antibody-coated red cells.

This rather complicated situation will be dealt with by first reviewing experiments in which the destruction of small numbers of red cells by known amounts of antibody has been studied. Then the limited capacity of the RES will be considered, and finally the situation encountered in clinical practice will be described, in which both the limited amount of antibody and the limited capacity of the RES decrease the rate of red cell destruction.

Relation between number of antibody molecules per cell and rate of clearance

The relation between the average number of antibody molecules on each red cell and the rate of red cell clearance can be determined, or estimated, in three types of experiment. First, red cells can be sensitized with antibody *in vitro* before being re-injected into the circulation. Second, an antibody compatible with the recipient's red cells can be injected, followed (or preceded) by an injection of red cells incompatible with the injected antibody; for example, anti-D and D-positive red cells can be injected into a D-negative volunteer. Third, incompatible red cells can be injected into the circulation of a subject whose plasma contains the corresponding antibody.

When red cells are sensitized with antibody *in vitro*, the amount of antibody on the cells can be determined either by using a labelled antibody or by using a labelled antiglobulin serum. When antigen and antibody reach equilibrium only *in vivo*, the amount of antibody on the cells can be estimated by a flow cytometric method; alternatively, it can be calculated if the concentration and equilibrium constant of the antibody are known, together with the number of incompatible red cells taking part in the reaction and the volume within which the reaction is taking place. Further details are given below.

Injections of red cells coated in vitro *with antibody*

Red cells coated in vitro *with non-complement-binding antibody.* In studying the relation between the degree of antibody coating and the rate of red cell destruction, there are two advantages in using red cells sensitized *in vitro*: first, the subject's own red cells can be sensitized, and second, the amount of antibody on the red cells at the time of injection can be measured directly. The main disadvantage of using red cells sensitized *in vitro* is that after injection of the red cells into the circulation, the antibody dissociates progressively from the cells, so that the initial rate of destruction, obtained by drawing a tangent to the initial slope, has to be determined for comparison with the degree of antibody coating. In practice, it is easy to find antibodies with a

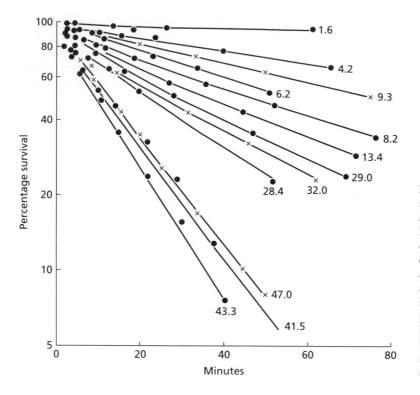

Fig 10.12 Clearance of D-positive red cells coated *in vitro* with various amounts of a particular anti-D. Purified IgG, prepared from this donor's serum, was used to coat the cells. The figures against each slope are the estimates of the amount of antibody on the red cells at the time of injection as micrograms of antibody per millilitre of red cells. In three cases (×) the estimates were made with labelled antiglobulin serum and in the remainder were made using labelled anti-D (Mollison *et al.* 1965).

relatively slow rate of dissociation so that for periods up to about 1 h the rate of red cell destruction approximates a single exponential (Cutbush and Mollison 1958; Mollison 1959c; Crome and Mollison 1964; Mollison *et al.* 1965).

Figure 10.12 shows experiments carried out with a single example of anti-D. There is a close relation between the degree of antibody coating and the rate of clearance.

In Figure 10.13, results in three of the cases shown in Fig. 10.12 have been replotted to show tangents to the initial slopes, which give the initial rates of red cell destruction. Coating with 28.4 μg of anti-D/ml red cells (10 400 antibody molecules per cell) gives an initial rate of 0.04/min, i.e. at the upper limit for clearance solely in the spleen. If approximately 10 000 molecules of anti-D per red cell are needed to produce clearance at a single passage through the spleen, anti-K must be more efficient in producing clearance. The maximum number of anti-K molecules bound cannot exceed about 5000 per red cell (as the number of

K sites per cell does not exceed about 6000) and yet anti-K can bring about clearance with a $T_{1/2}$ of 20 min (see Fig. 10.9).

Coating with 47.0 μg of anti-D/ml (17 000 antibody molecules per cell) gives clearance with an initial rate of 0.07/min (see Fig. 10.13), indicating substantial clearance in the liver as well as in the spleen. As the maximum number of D sites on red cells of common phenotypes is about 25 000, the maximum number of anti-D molecules with which red cells can be coated is approximately 20 000. In one experiment in which red cells were thought to have been maximally coated with anti-D, the initial rate of clearance had a $T_{1/2}$ of 5.6 min, corresponding to clearance of about 35% of the blood at each passage through the liver (Mollison 1989).

Because c sites are approximately three times as numerous as D sites it is possible for red cells to bind about 60 000 molecules of IgG anti-c per cell, and then as many as 70% of the cells are cleared at a single passage through the liver.

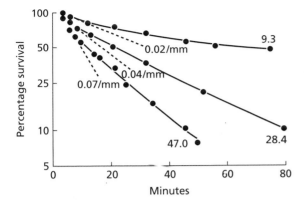

Fig 10.13 Clearance of D-positive red cells coated with different amounts of anti-D; the figures against each curve indicate the amount of anti-D on the cells, as µg/ml red cells, at the time of injection. Three of the cases from Fig. 10.12 have been replotted to show the slight curvilinearity of the slopes (due to elution of about 25% of the antibody during the first hour after injection). The initial rates of destruction are estimated by drawing tangents (– – –) to the initial slopes (modified from Mollison 1989).

Effect of IgG subclass of anti-D on rate of clearance

The experiments illustrated in Figs 10.12 and 10.13 were carried out with antibody derived from a single donor. With an assay using monoclonal anti-IgG1 and anti-IgG3, about one-quarter of the IgG molecules on D-positive red cells incubated with this polyclonal antibody are IgG3, and the rest are IgG1. Tests on other polyclonal anti-D sera have shown that in about three of four sera, fewer than 20% of the molecules bound to red cells are IgG3. With preparations of pooled IgG anti-D used for immunoprophylaxis, a smaller proportion of the anti-D molecules bound are IgG3 (Gorick and Hughes-Jones 1991).

In ADCC assays, the mean activity of IgG3 anti-D is clearly greater than that of IgG1 anti-D, but evidence concerning the relative effectiveness of the two subclasses *in vivo* is conflicting. In one comparison of two monoclonal anti-D, the IgG1 monoclonal (FOG-1) was definitely less effective than the IgG3 monoclonal (BRAD-3) in producing clearance of D-positive red cells (Thomson *et al.* 1990). However, in other experiments, the same IgG3 monoclonal was less effective

than a different IgG1 monoclonal (BRAD-5). The ability of the antibodies to react with FcγRI and FcγRIII appeared to correlate with their ability to bring about clearance (Kumpel and Judson 1995). Studies by Kumpel (1997) demonstrated a functional dichotomy between these two subclasses of anti-D: IgG3-coated red cells were lysed preferentially by monocytes mediated predominantly through FcγR1 interactions, whereas haemolysis of IgG1-sensitized cells was mediated mainly by FcγRIII on NK cells (Kumpel 1997). It is interesting that the presence of the FcγRIIIa-V158 allele polymorphism compromises the efficiency of removal of red cells coated with monoclonal IgG3 anti-D, although no delay in clearance is appreciated with polyclonal anti-D (Kumpel *et al.* 2003). In the experiments of Thomson (1990), the IgG3 monoclonal was slightly more effective than a polyclonal anti-D from a single donor, but the same monoclonal was slightly less effective than a pooled polyclonal preparation.

Rate of clearance affected by recipient differences and by red cell differences

Autologous red cells of different subjects, coated with a certain number of molecules of a particular anti-D, may be cleared at very different rates (Williams *et al.* 1985; Thomson *et al.* 1990). Furthermore, the red cells of a single donor, coated with approximately the same amount of antibody (2500 molecules per red cell), were cleared with half-times ranging from 26 to 81 min in different subjects (Williams *et al.* 1985). In the studies just referred to, HLA groups were not determined but it has been shown that defective Fc receptor function is associated with HLA-B8/Drw3. In patients with dermatitis herpetiformis, who are positive for these antigens and in normal subjects with the same HLA antigens, the clearance of anti-D-coated red cells is slower than normal in about 50% of cases (Lawley *et al.* 1981).

Red cells sensitized in vitro *with a complement-binding IgG antibody.* Some quantitative experiments with an immunoglobulin preparation containing complement-binding anti-Fy^a have been reported. The amount of antibody required for a maximal rate of clearance ($T_{1/2}$ of the order of 2 min) was found to be 5–9 µg/ml red cells; an example is shown in Fig. 10.14.

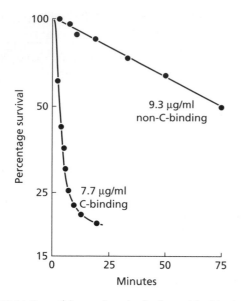

Fig 10.14 Rate of destruction of red cells sensitized *in vitro* with similar amounts of a C-binding antibody (an example of anti-Fy[a]) and of a non-C-binding antibody (anti-D) (Mollison *et al.* 1965).

Injections of anti-D and D-positive red cells given to D-negative subjects

The advantage of this type of experiment is that, provided the antibody is injected about 48 h before the red cells, a steady plasma level is reached and at some interval after injecting the red cells, antigen and antibody come into equilibrium and a constant rate of destruction ensues.

In experiments in which monoclonal IgG antibody (usually 300 µg) was injected intramuscularly followed in 48 h by 3 ml of D-positive red cells intravenously, the amount of anti-D bound was estimated by a flow cytometric method involving enzyme-linked immunosorbent assay (ELISA). The number of D-positive red cells present, when only a small amount of IgG anti-D was bound, was determined using IgM anti-D, biotin-conjugated anti-IgM and streptavidin (Kumpel and Judson 1995). At 3 h after injecting the red cells, the amount of anti-D bound correlated well with the rate of clearance of the cells as judged by the time taken for the initial red cell concentration to fall to 50%. In effecting clearance, an IgG1 monoclonal (BRAD-5) was almost as efficient as polyclonal anti-D and better than an IgG3 monoclonal (BRAD-3). In

seven subjects injected with 300 µg of BRAD-5 the mean number of anti-D molecules bound per red cell was about 6000 and the mean time for clearance of one-half of the red cells was about 6 h. The amount of antibody found on the red cells was close to the amount calculated from the affinity of the antibodies and the plasma anti-D levels achieved in the subjects (Kumpel and Judson 1995). The rates of red cell destruction observed, in relation to the amounts of bound antibody, for both monoclonal and polyclonal anti-D, were much slower than those found in the experiments illustrated in Figs 10.10 and 10.11.

In another series of experiments, the amount of anti-D injected varied from 1 to 1000 µg; the anti-D was polyclonal and obtained from a single donor and was often injected (intramuscularly) immediately after injecting the red cells (intravenously). The amount of anti-D bound to the red cells at equilibrium was calculated from the amount of red cells and antibody injected, the predicted plasma volume and extravascular space, the known equilibrium constant of the antibody, etc. When 250–1000 µg of anti-D was injected at the same time as the red cells there was a delay of 2–5 h before the onset of red cell destruction but then clearance was rapid ($T_{1/2}$ 2.5 h or less). Under these circumstances the amount of antibody on the cells cannot be calculated. On the other hand, when 1 µg of anti-D was injected intramuscularly 24 h before injecting 0.3 ml of red cells intravenously a maximum rate of red cell destruction was reached at 5–7 days and could thereafter be described by a single exponential with a $T_{1/2}$ of 2.7 days. Assuming that equilibrium between antigen and antibody was reached 1 week after injection, and using the method of calculation described below, about 1% of the antibody was bound, corresponding to about 10 molecules per cell. There was no detectable destruction of the injected red cells at 48 h (72 h after injecting the antibody), and the delay in the onset of destruction was likely to result from the time required for antigen and antibody to come into equilibrium at these very low concentrations (Mollison and Hughes-Jones 1967).

In other experiments in which 1 µg of IgG anti-D was injected intramuscularly and 0.8 ml of D-positive red cells intravenously, widely varying rates of destruction were observed; in the example shown in Fig. 10.15, the rate of destruction (after correcting the observations for elution of ^{51}Cr) has a $T_{1/2}$ of about 5 days. As the figure shows, the rate of destruction

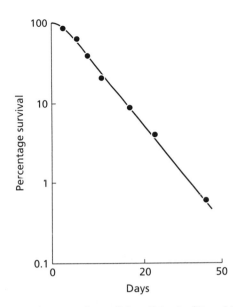

Fig 10.15 Clearance of a small dose (0.8 ml) of D-positive red cells, in an non-immunized D-negative subject, by passively administered IgG anti-D (1 μg) injected intramuscularly. After an initial delay (see text), the rate of clearance becomes constant and remains so for at least 42 days (Contreras and Mollison 1983).

Table 10.1 Plasma levels of anti-D expected after i.m. and i.v. injection of 100 μg of antibody.

Time	Plasma anti-D concentration (μg/ml)	
	i.m.	i.v.
5 min	0	0.033
3 h	0.002	0.032
9 h	0.005	0.029
1 days	0.010	0.024
3 days	0.015	0.015
5 days	0.014	0.012

From Smith *et al.* (1972).

appears to remain constant over the 6-week period of observation. This finding is hard to explain in view of the fact that IgG has a half-life of approximately 3 weeks.

Difference between intramuscular and intravenous injection. As Table 10.1 shows, when a given dose of anti-D is injected, the maximum plasma concentration when the i.v. route is used is about 2.5 times greater than when the i.m. route is used and, following i.m. injection, the maximum plasma concentration is reached only after about 48 h. It is not surprising that when D-positive red cells are injected at the same time as anti-D, clearance is much more rapid when the i.v. route is used. In a comparison made by Jouvenceaux and co-workers (1969) in which 300 μg of anti-D were injected together with 0.5 ml of red cells, the cells were cleared in 6 h when anti-D was given intravenously but only after 48 h when anti-D was injected intramuscularly. Some comparisons made by Huchet and co-workers (1970) with larger amounts of red cells are described below.

Injection of incompatible red cells

As the number of antigen sites on red cells has been determined in many blood group systems, it may be possible to estimate the maximum number of antibody molecules that can be bound and to draw relevant inferences. For example, the number of K sites has been estimated at not more than about 5000 per red cell (see Chapter 6). As anti-K has been shown to bring about clearance at a single passage through the spleen (Hughes-Jones *et al.* 1957), it seems that only 5000 molecules of IgG per cell are needed for maximal splenic clearance.

As another example, the fact that c sites are about three times as numerous as D sites explains the fact that anti-c can bring about far more rapid destruction than anti-D (see p. 426 and Fig. 10.10).

Estimation of amount of antibody combined with red cells at equilibrium *in vivo*. The following data are needed:
1 The molar concentration of antigen:
– The number of red cells transfused;
– The number of antigen sites per red cell;
– The number of molecules in 1 mole (Avogadro's number);
– The space within which red cells and antibody equilibrate;
2 The molar concentration of antibody:
– The plasma antibody concentration;
– The molecular weight of the antibody;
3 The equilibrium constant of the antibody (K_0) and its heterogeneity index (a).

429

The fraction of antibody bound to the red cells at equilibrium is given by the equation:

$$\frac{(Kc)^a}{1 + (Kc)^a} \qquad (10.2)$$

where c is the concentration of free antigen at equilibrium, K is the equilibrium constant, and a is the heterogeneity index.

For an example of the application of this method, see the eighth edition of this book (Mollison 1987, pp. 553–554), where it was applied to the case described by Chaplin (1959). It was pointed out that A and B red cells, because of the large number of antigen sites per cell, can bind very large amounts of antibody so that antibody concentration can be detectably diminished by the transfusion of as little as 4 ml of red cells. On the other hand, because Rh D sites are some 40 times less numerous than A and B, D-positive red cells can absorb relatively small amounts of anti-D.

Differences between IgG antibodies (non-complement-binding) in producing clearance

As IgG antibodies are composed of different subclasses that vary in their ability to bring about red cell destruction, it is not surprising that the relation between antibody concentration and the rate of clearance is variable. For example, in three cases in which the survival of 1 ml of incompatible red cells was measured, the relation between indirect antiglobulin titre and the rate of clearance (as a $T_{1/2}$) was as follows: anti-D, titre 2, $T_{1/2}$ 1.5 h; anti-E, titre 2, $T_{1/2}$ 3.5 days; anti-c, titre 8, $T_{1/2}$ 6 days (Mollison 1972, p. 499).

Another example of large differences in biological effectiveness between antibodies of similar concentration was as follows: in two cases in which anti-D could barely be detected using a sensitive version of the IAT capable of detecting as little as 2 ng of antibody per millilitre, 1 ml of D-positive red cells was cleared in less than 24 h in one instance but in about 30 days in the other (Mollison et al. 1970). In another series of experiments, using anti-D from a single donor, the injection of 12.5 µg (expected to produce a plasma concentration at 48 h of about 2 ng/ml) brought about clearance of a 0.3-ml dose of red cells with a $T_{1/2}$ of 24 h (Mollison and Hughes-Jones 1967).

Other evidence of the relative effectiveness of one specific polyclonal anti-D is as follows: when a very small dose (less than 1 ml) of D-positive red cells was injected intramuscularly, together with 1 µg of anti-D intramuscularly into a D-negative subject, the red cells were cleared with a half-time of 53 h (Mollison and Hughes-Jones 1967), but with a similar dose of D-positive red cells and pooled anti-D from many donors, the mean red cell survival time in 13 recipients was 24 days (Contreras and Mollison 1983). As described above, on D-positive red cells incubated with the first serum, about one-third of the antibody molecules are IgG3, although whether this finding explains the relative effectiveness of this anti-D in bringing about red cell destruction is uncertain.

Experiments with passively administered antibody incompatible with the recipient's red cells

See end of chapter.

The destruction of relatively large volumes of incompatible red cells

In the present section some examples are given of the rates of red cell destruction observed after incompatible transfusions. When destruction is predominantly intravascular, its rate and extent are limited only by the supply of antibody and complement.

As anti-A and anti-B are often partly IgG as well as partly IgM, the relation between the anti-A and anti-B antibody concentration and the amount of haemolysis produced is expected to be variable.

When destruction is due to anti-D, the rate of destruction is affected by the number of antibody molecules bound per cell, by the subclass of the antibody and by the capacity of the RES.

The capacity of the mononuclear phagocyte system

When red cell destruction depends on phagocytes, the rate of destruction must be limited by the number and activity of the relevant phagocytic cells. This limitation must apply to the destruction of both non-viable stored red cells and antibody-coated cells, even although the mechanism of destruction in the two cases is believed to be different.

Experiments with non-viable stored red cells in rabbits show that whereas 100% of a 0.1-ml dose was

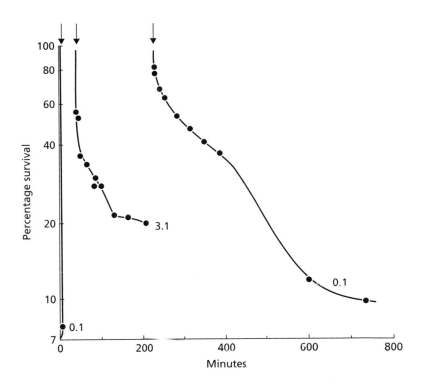

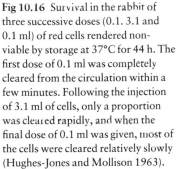

Fig 10.16 Survival in the rabbit of three successive doses (0.1. 3.1 and 0.1 ml) of red cells rendered non-viable by storage at 37°C for 44 h. The first dose of 0.1 ml was completely cleared from the circulation within a few minutes. Following the injection of 3.1 ml of cells, only a proportion was cleared rapidly, and when the final dose of 0.1 ml was given, most of the cells were cleared relatively slowly (Hughes-Jones and Mollison 1963).

cleared very rapidly (Fig. 10.16), only 60% of a 3.1-ml dose was cleared within the first few minutes after injection. From these and other experiments it was concluded that in rabbits injected with non-viable stored red cells up to about 2 ml of red cells per kilogram could be removed within 8 min (Hughes-Jones and Mollison 1963).

Partial blockage of the capacity for 'immediate removal' is also shown by Figure 10.16. The second 0.1-ml dose given after an intervening injection of 3.1 ml of non-viable red cells is cleared much more slowly than the first dose of 0.1 ml.

In humans, the rate of clearance of non-viable stored red cells varies inversely with the dose: when the dose of cells was approximately 0.25 ml/kg, half of the cells were removed in 30 min, but when the dose was approximately 1.5 ml/kg, clearance of one-half of the cells took more than 3 h (Noyes *et al.* 1960).

Estimation of the maximum capacity of the RES is complicated by the fact that destruction sometimes occurs predominantly in the spleen, which contains only a small part of the whole RES. Thus, the rate at which large numbers of D-positive red cells are destroyed is likely to be determined chiefly by the

capacity of the spleen, whereas the rate at which large numbers of stored red cells are destroyed may be determined by the capacity of the whole RES. This distinction is not absolute, as red cells heavily coated with anti-D are destroyed partly in the liver and, conversely, when stored red cells are injected, part of the non-viable population may be removed only in the spleen.

Table 10.2 contrasts the rate of clearance of large and small amounts of red cells calculated to have been coated with similar amounts of anti-D. As the table shows, when cells were coated with approximately 8 µg/ml, 160 ml red cells were cleared with a $T_{1/2}$ of 14 h and 1 ml with a $T_{1/2}$ of 1 h. When cells were coated with 1.6–2.0 µg/ml, 400 ml of red cells were cleared with a $T_{1/2}$ of the order of 72 h and 5.1 ml with a $T_{1/2}$ of 3.7 h.

In the examples given above, when anti-D was injected intravenously it was assumed that the reaction took place within a space equal to the plasma volume, estimated at 3000 ml.

When anti-D was injected intramuscularly 48 h before the red cells were injected, and when the red cells were subsequently cleared with a $T_{1/2}$ of 12 h or less, the amount of anti-D in the plasma was deduced

431

Reference	Red cells		Clearance $T_{1/2}$ (h)
	ml	µg anti-D per ml	
Eklund and			
Nevanlinna (1971)	160	8.1	14
Mollison *et al.* (1965)*	1	8.0	1
Hughes-Jones and			
Mollison (1968)	400	1.6	72
Huchet *et al.* (1970)	5.1	2.0	3.7

Table 10.2 Clearance of large and small amounts of D-positive red cells coated with similar amounts of anti-D.

* Value given by Mollison *et al.* (1965) determined directly; other values calculated as described in text.

from the figures given in Table 10.1 and the reaction was again estimated to take place within a volume of 3000 ml. However, when the anti-D was injected intramuscularly and destruction took place with a half-time measured in days, it was assumed that red cells and anti-D came into equilibrium within a space equal to twice the plasma volume.

An estimate of the maximum capacity to remove D-incompatible red cells is provided by an experiment reported by Mohn and co-workers (1961). After the injection of a large volume of very potent anti-D into a D-positive volunteer, the average rate of red cell destruction may be calculated at approximately 0.15 ml/kg/h, although the maximum rate was probably about 0.25 ml/kg/h (420 ml red cells destroyed in 24 h).

In experiments in rabbits with phenylhydrazine-damaged red cells, the maximum rate of removal of the cells from the circulation was approximately 0.5 ml/kg/h (Hughes-Jones and Mollison 1963).

Destruction of relatively large volumes of ABO-incompatible red cells

When the recipient's plasma contains potent anti-A and anti-B, the red cells (approximately 200 ml) of a unit of blood may be destroyed by intravascular lysis within 1 hour or, perhaps, within minutes (see Chapter 11).

When the titre of anti-A, or anti-B, is low, all detectable antibody may be removed by the transfusion of an amount of red cells as small as 4 ml (Chaplin 1959). Even when the antibody titre is considerably greater, the titre may be appreciably reduced by the

transfusion of relatively small amounts of blood. For example, in one series of observations the transfusion of 25 ml of A_1 blood reduced the titre against A_1 cells from 32 to 2; in another case in the same series the transfusion of 40 ml of A_2 blood reduced the titre against A_2 from 8 to 1 (Wiener *et al.* 1953).

After the transfusion of therapeutic quantities of blood, alloagglutinins may become temporarily undetectable and the transfused red cells survive normally until there has been an anamnestic response and sufficient antibody has been produced to bring about accelerated red cell destruction. In previous editions of this book, an example was given of a case in which, following the transfusion of 1000 ml of citrated group B blood to a group A patient with an anti-B titre of 32, group B red cells survived normally for about 4 days after transfusion but were then all eliminated within a few days as the anti-B reappeared (Mollison 1972, p. 504). A case in which 7.5 units of group A blood were transfused to a group O recipient and eliminated over a period of about 6 days with minimal signs of red cell destruction is described in Chapter 11. A similar case in which 3 units of group A blood were transfused to a group O patient and cleared progressively over about 4 days without any clinical signs of red cell destruction was described by Bucholz and Bove (1975).

Following the transfusion of ABO-incompatible blood, particularly when the recipient's pre-transfusion plasma contains only low-titre anti-A or anti-B, surviving incompatible red cells may be found for days or even weeks after the transfusion. Presumably, such cells are coated with C3dg and are thus resistant to complement-mediated destruction.

An elderly group O woman with carcinoma of the lung was inadvertently transfused with 600 ml of B blood. Haemoglobinuria was noted but there were no other untoward signs. Examination of a saline suspension of red cells taken from the patient on the following day showed the presence of small agglutinates that were identified as surviving B red cells (Mollison 1943).

The case of Akeroyd and O'Brien (1958), in which some group AB surviving cells were found for 6 weeks after transfusion despite a haemolysin titre of 4 in the recipient's serum, has been described above. A very similar case was observed (M Metaxas, personal communication, 1964): a group O patient was transfused with 8 units of A blood on the day after an operation. Some jaundice was noted clinically, but there were no other abnormal signs. Four days after blood transfusion, the anti-A titre was 4; by the eighth day it was 128 and the antibody was now capable of causing some lysis of A cells *in vitro*. During this period, and subsequently, the serum haptoglobin concentration remained normal. Group A cells could easily be detected in the circulation for up to 25 days after transfusion. Similar results have been observed in dogs, particularly when the transfused red cells contain a 'weak' antigen (Swisher and Young 1954).

Complement as a limiting factor in red cell destruction

If fresh human serum is absorbed with an equal volume of red cells sensitized with a complement-binding antibody, about five successive absorptions are required to remove all complement activity from the fresh serum (10th edition, p. 342). Although the amount of complement removed by different antibodies doubtless varies widely, in most situations antibody rather than complement is likely to be the limiting factor determining the destruction of incompatible red cells. Two possible exceptions are patients whose serum complement level is already low before transfusion and infants with haemolytic disease of the newborn due to ABO incompatibility (see Chapter 12).

In haemolytic anaemia due to auto-anti-I, the level of serum complement may in fact be diminished and complement may become a limiting factor in red cell destruction. Evans and co-workers (1968) observed that the transfusion of washed red cells regularly reduced the complement titre. They found that when two transfusions of red cells were given within a day or two of one another, the second unit survived better than the first and they considered that this might be due to a reduction in serum complement levels. Evans and co-workers (1965) had observed previously that in some patients the transfusion of fresh normal plasma apparently increased the rate of destruction of the patient's own red cells, possibly by supplying complement. Experimental work in dogs indicating that the rapid destruction of red cells occurs only as long as both antibody and complement are available in the recipient's plasma was reported by Christian (1951).

Destruction of relatively large volumes of Rh D-positive red cells

Information on the rate of destruction of relatively large amounts of D-positive red cells by anti-D is available from several different sources. First, accidental transfusions of D-positive blood to subjects who are already immunized to Rh D; second, inadvertent transfusions of D-positive blood to D-negative subjects who are not already immunized to Rh D, but who are given a dose of anti-D in the hope of suppressing primary immunization; third, experimental transfusions of large amounts of D-positive red cells together with large doses of anti-D to D-negative subjects to determine the conditions under which Rh D immunization is suppressed; fourth, the administration of large doses of anti-D to D-negative women who are found to have relatively large amounts of D-positive fetal red cells in their circulation after delivery; and finally, the experimental administration of potent anti-D to D-positive volunteers. This last category is considered in a later section, but the others will be considered here.

Transfusions of D-positive blood to D-immunized subjects. Figure 10.17 shows the survival of therapeutic quantities of D-positive red cells in three cases.

In case A, the plasma contained potent anti-D and the rate of destruction of red cells following the transfusion of 4 units of D-positive blood was of the order of 200–300 ml of red cells a day, almost maximal for destruction by anti-D (see above).

Following the transfusion of relatively large amounts of D-positive red cells to subjects whose serum contains potent anti-D, a considerable number of surviving D-positive red cells are usually found for at least 24 h after the transfusion. It is also usual to find

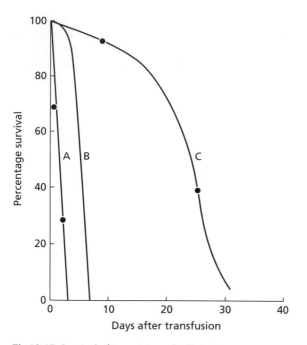

Fig 10.17 Survival of D-positive red cells in D-negative recipients (estimates by differential agglutination). Case A, potent anti-D present at time of transfusion: 4 units transfused. Case B, very weak anti-D present at time of transfusion; delayed haemolytic transfusion reaction (curve diagrammatic). Case C, no anti-D present at time of transfusion but present by day 39.

free anti-D, as expected from the rather poor absorbing capacity of D-positive red cells for anti-D due to the relatively small number of D antigen sites.

Suppose that a patient's serum has an anti-D concentration of 10 μg/ml, corresponding approximately to an indirect antiglobulin titre of 500. If plasma volume is assumed to be 3000 ml, there will be 3×10^4 μg of anti-D in the plasma. If 2 units of D-positive red cells are transfused containing 400 ml of red cells, and 30 μg of anti-D are taken up by each millilitre of red cells to yield maximal saturation, the total amount of anti-D absorbed would be 1.2×10^4 μg or only about one-half of the total amount in the plasma.

'Case B' shown in Fig. 10.17 is hypothetical in the sense that it is based on a number of cases (7th edition, p. 604). When the patient's serum contains only a trace of anti-D at the time of transfusion, the antibody titre usually increases very rapidly so that signs of increased red cell destruction become apparent on about the fourth or fifth day after transfusion, and the circulation may be completely cleared of incompatible cells by the seventh day. Further details of this kind of case are given in the following chapter.

Finally, Fig. 10.17 shows an example of a case (C) in which primary Rh D immunization developed following transfusion. As the figure shows, survival was subnormal at 28 days and some time between 28 and 39 days had fallen to zero, by which time anti-D was detectable in the serum. The transfusion was given 20 days before the patient delivered her first infant, so that it is possible, though unlikely, in this case that primary immunization had already been induced by fetal red cells.

Inadvertent transfusion of D-positive blood to D-negative subjects followed by injections of anti-D. In a D-negative woman who had been inadvertently transfused with 2 units of D-positive blood (approximately 400 ml of red cells), following an i.m. injection of 1000 μg of anti-D the red cells were cleared with a $T_{1/2}$ of approximately 3 days (Hughes-Jones and Mollison 1968). Assuming that the red cells equilibrated with the antibody available in the whole IgG space, approximately two-thirds of the amount of injected antibody was bound to the red cells, corresponding to occupancy of about 5% of the antigen sites, equivalent to 1.6 μg of anti-D per millilitre of red cells (Table 10.2).

In another case, following the inadvertent transfusion of 400 ml of D-positive blood (160 ml of red cells) to a D-negative woman, plasma containing about 2500 μg of anti-D was transfused over the course of 2 h. The transfusion was then stopped because the patient developed rigors and fever. The rate of clearance was estimated to have a $T_{1/2}$ of approximately 14 h (Eklund and Nevanlinna 1971). At equilibrium, an estimated 7.3 μg of anti-D was bound per millilitre of red cells (see Table 10.2).

In Chapter 5, details of four cases are presented in which between 1 and 3 units of D-positive blood were transfused, following which between 3000 and 7750 μg of anti-D were infused in divided doses. All red cells were cleared within 2–8 days; see Table 5.6 on p. 196.

Injections of anti-D following massive transplacental haemorrhage. Massive transplacental haemorrhage (TPH) is arbitrarily defined as the presence in the mother's circulation of more than about 10 ml of fetal red cells, as found in about two per 1000 recently delivered women (Chapter 12). In this section, a few examples are given of the rates of clearance of D-positive red cells that have been observed after giving various amounts of anti-D.

Intramuscular injections of anti-D. In a case in which a mother's circulation was estimated to contain 60 ml of fetal red cells, an injection of 500 µg of anti-D brought about clearance with a $T_{1/2}$ of 5–6 days (Hughes-Jones and Mollison 1968). A similar rate of clearance was observed in a case in which a TPH of an estimated 175 ml of red cells was treated with a dose of 500 µg of anti-D (de Wit and Borst-Eilers 1972). Distinctly more rapid clearance, with removal of all D-positive cells within 5 days, was observed in one case in which a TPH of 75 ml of red cells was treated with 1500 µg of anti-D (CD de Wit and E Borst-Eilers, personal communication) and in another in which a TPH of about 85 ml of red cells was treated with 1000 µg of anti-D (Woodrow *et al.* 1968).

In two cases in which the size of TPH was estimated to be equivalent to 28 and 43 ml of red cells, respectively, two successive intramuscular injections each of 600 µg were given at an interval of 1–3 days; the cells were not completely cleared for 5–7 days (Huchet *et al.* 1970). As pointed out in Chapter 14, some injections that are intended to be intramuscular are in fact deposited into subcutaneous fatty tissue. When this occurs, appearance of IgG in the plasma will be delayed.

Intravenous injections of anti-D. The much more rapid clearance of D-positive red cells following infusion of anti-D is emphasized by contrasting the two cases just described, in which the anti-D was injected into muscle with two other cases in which the volume of TPH was greater, equivalent to 60 and 88 ml of red cells respectively. In these cases, a single infusion of 600 µg of anti-D resulted in clearance with a $T_{1/2}$ of the order of 85 min (Huchet *et al.* 1970).

Interpretation of tests made with small numbers of incompatible red cells

When the results of serological tests are difficult to interpret, estimating the survival of small volumes of ^{51}Cr-labelled red cells from potential donors may be useful. The following procedure is suggested.

Method

One millilitre of red cells will be labelled with ^{51}Cr. If the recipients are likely to require at least 2 units of red cells, one should consider the merit of pooling 1 ml of citrated blood from each of two potential donor units and labelling red cells in the pool. Most of these tests will be in circumstances in which early rapid destruction of injected red cells is not expected. The first sample is taken at 3 min and the concentration of donor red cells in this sample is assumed to represent 100% survival. A minimum two further samples are drawn at 10 and 60 min after injection. The plasma of these two samples must be counted as well as samples of whole blood in order to detect any substantial degree of intravascular destruction. When survival is normal, and when the samples are counted to a statistical accuracy of ± 1%, the 60-min value should be at least 97%. Destruction must be at least 5% before there is a 95% chance that the 60-min value will be less than 97% (Mollison 1981). The chance of detecting a slight increase in the rate of red cell destruction is greatly improved by sampling over a longer period. When 5% destruction is the lower limit of detection, a 5-h sample may detect a rate of destruction of 1% per hour. When early rapid destruction of injected red cells is suspected, a double red cell labelling method must be used.

The shape of the survival curve during the first 60 min provides some indication of the likelihood of a secondary immune response. When a two-component curve is observed, with much slower destruction between 10 and 60 min than between 3 and 10 min, the antibody probably binds complement and the surviving cells have probably acquired resistance to complement-mediated destruction. Some IgM, cold-reacting complement-binding antibodies have not been associated with a secondary immune response. Other complement-binding antibodies, either IgM or IgG, are warm reacting; with these, an immune response is usually observed. Similarly, when the curve of red cell destruction is a single exponential, the antibody concerned will probably be a non-complement-binding IgG and the injection of incompatible red cells is almost certain to be followed by an immune response. If survival of the small volume of incompatible red cells is adequate and supports the safety of transfusing full units of incompatible red cells, the chance of a delayed haemolytic transfusion reaction will depend on whether the cells provoke a secondary immune response.

A note of the recommendations of ICSH for determining red cell survival using ^{51}Cr

The document published by a panel of the International Committee on Standardization in Haematology (ICSH 1980) was concerned chiefly with the conduct of autologous red cell survival tests in patients suspected of having a haemolytic process. The recommendations included methods of labelling with ^{51}Cr, timing of blood samples, corrections for ^{51}Cr elution and analysis of the resulting corrected red cell survival curves. These methods were not intended to be applied to investigating the survival of red cells from a potentially incompatible donor, and separate recommendations were provided for the use of ^{51}Cr-labelled red cells as a test for compatibility. For this purpose, the document recommends that 0.5 ml of red cells should be labelled and that blood samples should be taken 3, 10 and 60 min after injection. These recommendations have been widely ignored by authors claiming to have followed the technique proposed by ICSH. For example, in testing for compatibility *in vivo*, some authors have used the methods devised for estimating the survival of autologous red cells. These methods are wholly inappropriate when the survival curve has more than one component. Others have injected 10 ml or so of red cells instead of 0.5 ml. Although from a practical point of view, the precise amount of cells injected is not particularly important, from a scientific standpoint, and for comparison purposes, it is desirable to use the standard procedure. Another common practice is to draw the first sample from the recipient 10 or even 30 min after injecting the incompatible cells. The recommendation to take the first sample at 3 min was based on the observation of the lag of about 2.5 min before destruction begins, except when destruction is extremely rapid (see Fig. 10.2). As in most cases mixing is almost complete by 3 min, a sample taken at this time can be used as the 100% survival value with relatively little error (Mollison 1989). If the first sample is not taken for 10 min or more after injection, the major component of destruction may be missed. With destruction by complement-activating antibodies, the rate of destruction may be rapid for the first 10 min and then slow abruptly.

Difference between the survival of large and small volumes of incompatible red cells: size matters

In rabbits, the difference between the rate of clearance of small and large amounts of incompatible red cells is relatively small at high antibody concentrations, but substantial at low antibody concentrations. For example, when sufficient IgG anti-Hg^A was injected into an Hg (A–) rabbit to give an indirect antiglobulin titre of 256, the time taken for the destruction of 50% of a dose of Hg (A+) red cells was 18 min for a 1.0-ml/kg dose of red cells and 7 min for a 0.01-ml/kg dose. However, when the titre was only 16, the times were 102 h and 18 min respectively. With IgM antibodies, the largest amount of antibody injected resulted in a titre of only 2, and this titre was associated with a clearance $T_{1/2}$ of 2.5 min when a 0.01-ml/kg dose of Hg (A+) red cells was injected. With a 1-ml/kg dose, only one-third of the cells were cleared within the first hour after injection and one-third of the cells were still present in the circulation at 72 h (Burton and Mollison 1968).

Few observations have been made in man. In a patient with a very low concentration of anti-B, 4 ml of group B cells were destroyed within minutes, whereas the survival of a unit of red cells was almost normal (Chaplin 1959). Because of the large number of B antigen sites on red cells, 4 ml of cells were enough to absorb virtually all the plasma antibody. In a patient with anti-A$_1$ weakly active at 37°C, after the injection of about 0.55 ml of A$_1$ red cells (two different tests on two successive days), about 65% of the cells were destroyed within 30 min. Two days later, after the injection of 18.9 ml of cells, only about 45% of the cells were destroyed in the first 30 min (Mollison *et al.* 1978). When incompatibility is due to some other antigens, the amount of available antibody may not be the only factor involved; the capacity of the RES may play some part as well.

Attempts to inhibit the destruction of incompatible red cells

Several approaches can be envisaged: (1) specific inhibition of particular antibodies by injecting blood group-specific substances; (2) inhibition of complement activity; (3) interference with the activity of the RES; (4) red cell exchange; and (5) plasmapheresis.

All have been tried, but unequivocal success has been achieved only with the first.

Injections of soluble group-specific substances

The only blood group substances available in a purified form are A, B, Le^a and Le^b. The injection of a sufficient amount of these substances would be expected to neutralize all circulating antibody so that temporarily, red cells of a theoretically incompatible group would survive normally in the circulation. In the case of anti-A and anti-B, the effect would not be expected to be long lived, as an immune response would usually follow; complete suppression of antibody might then be impossible and the incompatible red cells would undergo accelerated destruction.

In the case of anti-Le^a and anti-Le^b, the situation is more promising for two reasons: first, Lewis antibodies are mainly IgM and, such as IgM anti-A and anti-B, are readily inhibited. In fact, Lewis antibodies are much easier to inhibit because they are usually far weaker than most examples of anti-A and anti-B. The IgG component of anti-A and anti-B is much more difficult to inhibit than is the IgM component. Second, after trans-

fusion to a Le(a– b–) subject, Le(a+) and Le(b+) red cells lose their Lewis antigens and become Le(a– b–). As this transformation occurs within a few days of transfusion, the red cells are likely to have become Le(a– b–) by the time that Lewis antibodies have appeared in high concentration in the recipient's plasma if a secondary immune response has been induced.

The suggestion that Le^a substance in transfused plasma might play a decisive role in preventing haemolytic transfusion reactions from anti-Le^a was first proposed by Brendemoen and Aas (1952), who had observed a haemolytic reaction in a subject transfused with packed red cells from O, Le(a+) blood.

In a case described by Mollison and co-workers (1963), anti-Le^a and anti-Le^b were neutralized by the injection of Lewis substances to allow the successful transfusion of Le(b+) blood (see Figs 10.18 and 10.19). Although in this case potent purified Lewis substances were used for suppression, preliminary observations with the transfusion of relatively small amounts of Le(a+ b–) plasma had shown that plasma alone could not only suppress all detectable antibody but allow the subsequent normal survival of Le(a+ b–) red cells (see Fig. 10.18). The subject was group B, Le(a– b–), and his serum contained anti-Le^a and anti-Le^b. He was scheduled to

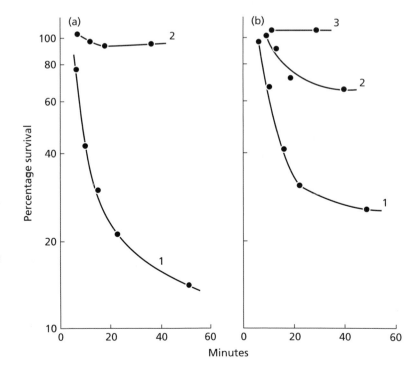

Fig 10.18 Survival of 0.5-ml amounts of group O, Le(a+ b–) red cells (a) and of group O, Le(b+) red cells (b), before (1) and after (2) the transfusion of 200 ml of Le(a+ b–) plasma. After the second test, 0.4 ml of a 1% solution of purified Le^b substance was infused and the survival of group O, Le(b+) red cells was estimated once more (3) (Mollison *et al.* 1963).

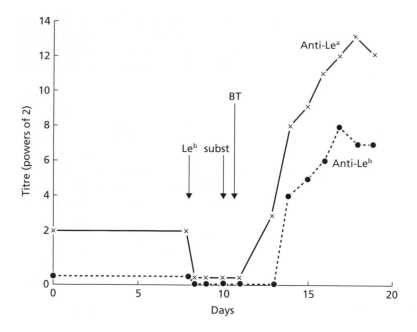

Fig 10.19 Changes in the titre of Lewis antibodies in a group B, Le(a– b–) subject before and after the transfusion of large amounts of group B, Le(b+) blood. The transfusion was preceded by the injection of two doses of Le^b substance, one given immediately before transfusion and one given 48 h beforehand (from Mollison *et al.* 1963).

undergo an operation, involving cardiac bypass, for which the blood of large numbers of donors was expected to be needed. In order to avoid the difficulty of finding sufficient group B, Le(a– b–) donors, suppression of the Lewis antibodies and use of Le(b+) donors was planned. Preoperative tests of the survival of Le(a+) and Le(b+) red cells before and after the transfusion of Le(a+) plasma and injection of purified Le^b substance are shown in Fig. 10.18.

Immediately before operation, a further injection of purified Le^b substance was given. During the operation and the following 36 h, the patient lost a considerable amount of blood and a total of 34 units of Le(a– b+) blood and 13 units of Le(a– b–) blood was transfused. There was no evidence that the haemorrhage was related to incompatibility.

As Fig. 10.19 shows, within 48 h after the end of the blood transfusion, anti-Le^a and anti-Le^b had reappeared in the patient's circulation. There were still no signs of a haemolytic reaction and the transfused red cells reacted very weakly with anti-Le^b. Within a few days the cells were phenotypically Le(a– b–).

In a second case, of an A$_1$, Le(a– b–) woman whose serum contained a relatively strong anti-Le^b and a weak anti-Le^a, a preliminary test showed that within 30 min of infusion approximately 60% of A$_2$, Le(b+) cells and 10% of A$_1$, Le(b+) red cells were destroyed. Following a transfusion of 250 ml of EDTA-plasma

from the A$_2$, Le(b+) donor, a second aliquot of A$_2$, Le(b+) red cells was infused and the red cells showed no evidence of destruction within the following 30 min. Le(b+) blood was transfused without incident (10th edition, p. 346).

Other cases in which Lewis antibodies were neutralized by the transfusion of plasma alone and in which several units of Le(a+) or Le(b+) blood were subsequently transfused without a clinical reaction were described by Hossaini (1972), Pelosi and co-workers (1974), Andorka and co-workers (1974) and Athkambhira and Chiewsilp (1978). In one case, a relatively potent anti-Le^b was not completely inhibited by the transfusion of about 800 ml of group A, Le(b+) plasma (Morel *et al.* 1978) (supplemented by personal communication).

In summary, the relative lack of difficulty caused by Lewis antibodies in blood transfusion seems to be due partly to the effect of Lewis substances in the donor's plasma in neutralizing corresponding antibodies in the recipient's plasma and partly to the chameleon-like behaviour of red cells that within a few days of transfusion assume the phenotype of the recipient.

The addition of soluble A and B substances to group O plasma to produce partial inhibition of anti-A and anti-B is described below.

Inhibition of complement activity

The effect of heparin. As described in Chapter 3, heparin prevents the activation of complement *in vitro* only at concentrations of the order of 100 IU/ml, but lower concentrations than this may have some inhibitory effect on red cell destruction *in vivo*. A concentration of 69 IU/ml was effective in inhibiting relatively slow destruction by anti-I in rabbits although 28 IU/ml was ineffective (Cooper and Brown 1971). Rosenfield and co-workers (1967) reported that concentrations as low as 20 IU/ml might prevent the destruction of antibody-coated red cells in rats.

C1-esterase inhibitor. The use of C1-esterase inhibitor has been considered as a therapeutic measure in autoimmune haemolytic anaemia (AIHA) with warm haemolysins (see Chapter 7) and has potential value in preventing destruction by complement-binding alloantibodies, particularly those that are IgM.

Intravenous immunoglobulin. Intravenous immunoglobulin (IVIG) inhibits the uptake of complement by target cells: (1) in guinea pigs treated with 600 mg of IVIG/kg per day for 2 days, clearance of IgM-sensitized guinea pig red cells, which is wholly complement dependent, was reduced, although the effect was relatively small, for example at 90 min, survival of injected red cells was about 60% compared with about 45% in control animals (Basta *et al.* 1989a); (2) in guinea pigs given a single slow infusion of 1800 mg of IVIG/kg, 3 h before being subjected to Forssman shock, survival was prolonged and/or death prevented, an effect believed to have been due to suppression of C3 fragment uptake on target cells (Basta *et al.* 1989b) Further work indicated that IVIG is an effective inhibitor of the deposition of C4b and C3b on target cells (Basta *et al.* 1991).

Interference with the activity of the mononuclear phagocyte system

Two methods have been tried, the injection of corticosteroids to reduce monocyte activity and the injection of IgG to compete with bound antibody for Fc receptor sites.

The effect of corticosteroids. In AIHA, the administration of corticosteroids results in a slowing of red cell destruction within a few days. The most important effect of corticosteroids is to decrease the amount of lysosomal enzymes released following contact between antibody-coated cells and phagocytes (Fleer *et al.* 1978).

In animal experiments, administration of large doses of corticosteroids has been shown to interfere with the sequestration of antibody-coated red cells in rats and guinea pigs (Kaplan and Jandl 1961; Atkinson and Frank 1974a). Only a few observations have been made in humans: in eight subjects who were given 1–3 ml of ^{51}Cr-labelled ABO-incompatible cells, the administration of 90 mg of prednisolone 30 min before and at the same time as the injection of incompatible cells failed to prevent the rapid intravascular destruction of the cells (Hewitt *et al.* 1961). This result is not surprising, as the destruction of ABO-incompatible cells by potent antibodies is predominantly intravascular and macrophages are not involved. On the other hand, suggestive evidence of a small diminution of the rate of clearance of D-sensitized red cells was observed in six patients with rheumatoid arthritis after 5 days of corticosteroid therapy (Mollison 1962).

Intravenous IgG. IVIG has been used with apparent success in a case in which anti-Kp^b was involved (Kohan *et al.* 1994).

A man, aged 50 years, with rectal cancer, who had been transfused during surgery with 2 units of blood, was found to have an unexpectedly low PCV (0.10). Following the transfusion of 50 ml of red cells he developed a severe febrile reaction accompanied by intense lumbar pain. His serum was found to contain anti-Kp^b. He was started on a regimen of 400 mg of IVIG/kg per day together with 500 mg of hydrocortisone. After 24 h he was transfused uneventfully with 2 units of Kp (b+) blood and the PCV rose to 0.18.

The authors have subsequently reported success using this regimen in five additional patients who required transfusion of non-ABO incompatible units (Kohan *et al.* 1994).

Destruction of transfused red cells without serologically demonstrable antibodies

The cases to be considered fall into two classes: (1) those in which at some stage of the investigation the antibody is in fact detected so that its specificity and characteristics are known, and (2) those in which no antibody can be demonstrated *in vitro* so that its presence is simply inferred.

Antibody demonstrable at some stage: now you see it

In delayed haemolytic transfusion reactions, antibody may be detected for the first time after the onset of red cell destruction, as described in the following chapter. In the past, cases have also been described in which antibodies have previously been found but have since become undetectable and in which small amounts of theoretically incompatible red cells have been rapidly destroyed (Fudenberg and Allen 1957; Chaplin and Cassell 1962). In one case, after the transfusion of a unit, an immediate haemolytic reaction occurred (Fudenberg and Allen 1957). Now that more sensitive tests for antibody detection have been introduced, cases of this kind are rarely observed.

Accelerated destruction of transfused red cells during primary immunization

In primary Rh D immunization, accelerated clearance of D-positive red cells can often be observed before anti-D can be detected.

The survival of a first injection of 1 ml of D-positive red cells in previously non-immunized D-negative subjects has been studied in two series. In the first, R_1R_2 red cells were injected and in the second, R_2R_2 cells. In both series, the red cells were labelled with ^{51}Cr and samples were obtained weekly after injection. Subjects who failed to form anti-D within 6 months of a first injection were given a second injection of labelled cells (Samson and Mollison 1975; Contreras and Mollison 1981). Taking the two series together, nine subjects formed anti-D after the first injection and six more after a second injection. Among these 15 responders were four subjects with normal survival at 28 days but who nevertheless made anti-D within 6 months. Conversely, five subjects eliminated virtually all the injected red cells within 28 days of a first injection but formed serologically detectable anti-D only after a second injection.

Further information about the time of onset of accelerated destruction during primary immunization can be obtained from the paper by Woodrow and co-workers (1969). Repeated injections of ^{51}Cr-labelled D-positive red cells from 5–10 ml of blood were given

to 11 D-negative subjects and followed for 7 days in each instance. The intervals between injections varied, but were most often 4–9 weeks. Seven subjects formed anti-D, and in three of these, subnormal survival was noted 10–23 weeks before anti-D could be detected.

Accelerated destruction during secondary immunization

In the two series referred to above, in which two injections of ^{51}Cr-labelled D-positive red cells were given to D-negative subjects at an interval of 6 months, six subjects formed serologically detectable anti-D only after the second injection. In four of these, red cell survival was clearly subnormal at 7 days, indicating that anti-D was present at the time of the second injection, even although it became detectable only later.

The effect on the survival of transfused red cells of a developing secondary response is illustrated in Figs 11.4–11.6 in Chapter 11.

Antibody never demonstrable despite shortened survival of transfused red cells

In subjects whose own red cells survive normally, shortened survival of transfused red cells in the absence of demonstrable alloantibodies is uncommon when therapeutic quantities of red cells are transfused, but relatively common when small volumes of red cells (less than 10 ml) are transfused. In subjects who have never been transfused, there may be an initial phase of normal survival lasting for 10 days or more, followed by a phase of accelerated destruction, suggesting that the transfusion has induced an immune response. This type of curve has been called a 'collapse' curve (Mollison 1961, p. 484); an example is shown in Fig. 10.20. Alternatively, random destruction may develop from the time of transfusion onwards, suggesting that the recipient is already immunized. Although survival curves can often be classified as showing either a collapse pattern or random destruction, in some cases lack of sufficient data leaves no alternative but to place them in a catch-all category of 'subnormal survival'.

It is convenient to consider results observed with large and small volumes of red cells separately, mainly because subnormal survival in the absence of demonstrable antibodies is much less common when large amounts of red cells are transfused.

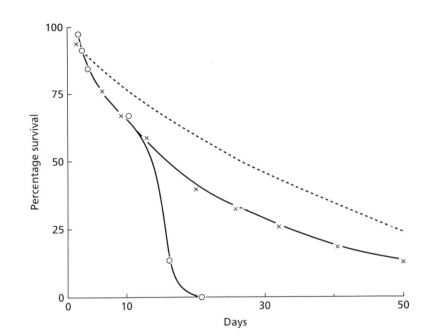

Fig 10.20 Survival of ^{51}Cr-labelled red cells from two newborn infants following injection into a previously untransfused adult. Small samples of blood were taken from two infants, the first aged 35 h and the second aged 50 h. The samples were mixed with acid–citrate–dextrose and then labelled with ^{51}Cr in the usual way. ○, Cr survival of red cells from the first infant; 2 ml of red cells were labelled. ×, Cr survival of red cells from the second infant: 8 ml of red cells were labelled. The interval between the two injections was 34 days. The dotted line shows the normal ^{51}Cr survival curve observed when red cells from normal adults are labelled with ^{51}Cr in the same way (ER Giblett, unpublished observations).

Subnormal survival of therapeutic amounts of transfused red cells in the absence of demonstrable antibodies

In 3 of 35 recipients of red cells stored in an acid–citrate–glucose solution, the rate of destruction was initially average but all the cells were eliminated within 40–60 days; further investigation suggested that some kind of incompatibility was involved (Loutit *et al.* 1943; Mollison 1951, p. 107). Similar cases were encountered in studying the survival of frozen red cells.

In one patient (a recently delivered woman), the survival of a therapeutic quantity of previously frozen red cells was zero at 6 weeks. Survival of red cells from the same donor, injected on two subsequent occasions 3 years later, was again grossly subnormal (Fig. 10.21). Red cell phenotyping of donor and recipient showed that incompatibility could not have been due to anti-D, -c, -C, -e, -K, -Fy^a, -Jk^a, -Jk^b, -S or -s; anti-E was a possibility, particularly because the red cells of another E-positive donor survived poorly and the red cells of one E-negative donor had only slightly subnormal survival, which might have been due to the recipient's menorrhagia. Nevertheless, repeated attempts to demonstrate anti-E in the recipient's serum were unsuccessful (Mollison 1959a).

More rapid destruction of transfused red cells without demonstrable antibodies was reported by Jandl and Greenberg (1957); in one case a first transfusion of the cells survived normally for 11 days, but by the seventeenth day had all been eliminated. The same recipient was transfused with blood from three other donors and in each instance destruction of red cells began immediately after transfusion and was complete within 5–10 days. On the other hand, the red cells of a fifth donor survived normally. In the second case the survival of transfused red cells was progressively shortened with each transfusion, although on each occasion survival was normal for a short period before the phase of accelerated destruction began. No antibodies could be demonstrated in either of these two cases.

Even more rapid destruction was observed by Stewart and Mollison (1959) in a patient who had developed haemoglobinuria following the transfusion of apparently compatible blood. As Fig. 10.22 shows, transfused red cells were eliminated within 24 h.

The patient was a woman aged 46 years suffering from reticulosarcoma who had been treated with irradiation. During the year in which she had been ill, she had received several transfusions. The second had been followed by jaundice, and the fourth and later transfusions by haemoglobinuria. Figure 10.22 shows the survival of red cells that were compatible *in vitro*

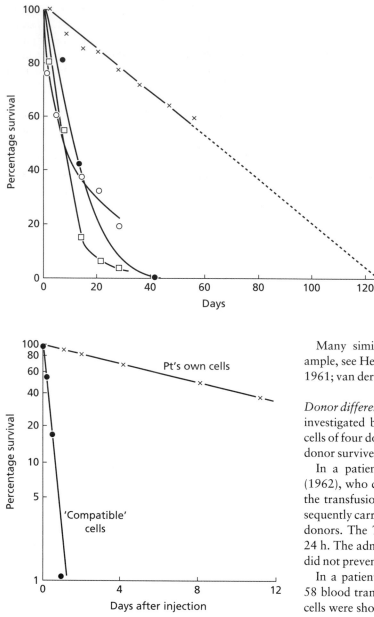

Fig 10.21 Accelerated red cell destruction in the absence of serologically demonstrable alloantibodies in a recipient. ●, Survival of previously frozen red cells from a normal donor, estimated by differential agglutination. ○, and □, Survival of red cells on two subsequent occasions, estimated with ^{51}Cr. ×, Survival of ^{51}Cr-labelled red cells in the donor's own circulation. All ^{51}Cr estimates corrected for Cr elution. For red cell phenotyping, see text (Mollison 1959a).

Fig 10.22 Rapid removal from the circulation of transfused cells, compatible by all the usual serological tests. For comparison, the survival of the patient's own red cells is shown (Stewart and Mollison 1959).

as judged by all tests available including the IAT against enzyme-treated red cells. The figure also shows that the patient's own red cells were removed from the circulation far more slowly, their average lifespan being about 11 days.

Many similar cases have been reported (for example, see Heisto *et al.* 1960; Kissmeyer-Nielsen *et al.* 1961; van der Hart *et al.* 1963).

Donor differences. As mentioned above, in one patient investigated by Jandl and Greenberg (1957) the red cells of four donors survived poorly, but those of a fifth donor survived normally.

In a patient described by Heisto and colleagues (1962), who developed haemoglobinuria 6 days after the transfusion of 2800 ml of blood, tests were subsequently carried out with red cells from eight different donors. The T_{50}Cr varied from 14 days to less than 24 h. The administration of large doses of prednisone did not prevent rapid red cell destruction.

In a patient with sickle cell disease, who had had 58 blood transfusions, many different samples of red cells were shown to be rapidly destroyed. Some specimens were completely removed within 24 h, whereas others survived normally for 1 week and were then rapidly eliminated. The only cells that survived well were obtained from two siblings (Chaplin and Cassell 1962). In a case of thalassaemia described by Vullo and Tunioli (1961), compatible red cells from the patient's father survived better than did those from an unrelated donor, although both were abnormally short.

Cases in which the specificity of an undetectable alloantibody may be inferred

A few cases have been described in which determination of the recipient's red cell phenotype has provided a valuable clue to the specificity of an undetectable alloantibody:

1 In investigating a delayed haemolytic transfusion reaction (DHTR), no evidence of the survival of transfused red cells was found on day 12; the only antigen possessed by all four donors but not by the recipient was c. Tests with ^{51}Cr-labelled red cells showed that c-positive cells underwent rapid destruction (48% survival at 3 h; less than 1% at 24 h) whereas c-negative cells had only slightly reduced survival (93% at 3 h, 80% at 48 h). The patient was transfused successfully with 8 c-negative units (Davey *et al.* 1980).

2 A patient who had previously received many transfusions received a further transfusion without incident. Two weeks later, another transfusion, this time of 2 units, later shown to be K positive, caused a haemolytic transfusion reaction characterized by haemoglobinuria and anuria. No alloantibodies could be found. One week later, another transfusion of 2 units, later shown to be K negative, caused another severe haemolytic transfusion reaction. Anti-K was now detected, but reacted only at room temperature and not at 37°C. Three days later, as the patient's Rh phenotype was found to be DccEe she was transfused with C-negative units. There was no untoward reaction and the PCV rose by the expected amount; C-negative cells continued to be demonstrable in further samples taken post transfusion. No antibodies other than anti-K could be detected at any time, despite the use of a wide range of sensitive methods (Halima *et al.* 1982).

3 A woman who had had previous pregnancies and, possibly, a previous transfusion developed a DHTR but did not produce detectable alloantibodies. Following a further transfusion of apparently compatible red cells, haemoglobinaemia and haemoglobinuria developed. The patient was found to have the probable Rh genotype *DcE/DcE*. On the chance that the patient might regard e-positive red cells as incompatible, survival studies were performed with both e-negative and e-positive cells. Whereas e-negative cells had a normal survival, e-positive red cells were cleared with a $T_{1/2}$ of 4.5–6 h on two separate occasions (Baldwin *et al.* 1983).

4 A man aged 55 years developed a DHTR after what appeared to be his first transfusion. The second transfusion, given 11 days after the first, produced immediate haemoglobinuria and so did a third transfusion given 2 days later. No red cell alloantibodies could be detected. The patient's probable Rh phenotype was DDcce. All 6 units that had been transfused to the patient were C positive. Tests with ^{99m}Tc-labelled red cells showed that cells from two different C-negative donors survived normally (uncorrected survival at 1 h = 93.9% and 98.6%) and these units were transfused without reaction. In contrast, cells from one C-positive donor had a survival of 71.1% at 1 h and 28.8% at 4 h (Harrison *et al.* 1986).

Subnormal survival of small amounts of transfused red cells without demonstrable antibodies

The fact that small amounts of ABO-compatible, Rh D-compatible red cells transfused to a previously untransfused recipient frequently survive subnormally was first recognized by Adner and Sjölin (1957). In estimating the survival of cord red cells transfused to adults they observed that in 5 out of 15 cases, a sudden increase in the rate of destruction ('collapse') occurred between 6 and 15 days after transfusion, and elimination of the red cells was complete within 1 month. A collapse curve had earlier been noted in studying a previously untransfused patient with thalassaemia–haemoglobin C disease. When a small volume of red cells was transfused, survival was normal for about 2 weeks but then the rate of destruction suddenly increased and all the cells were eliminated within 30–40 days. Red cells from two other donors survived normally in this patient (Mollison 1956).

The most thorough investigation of the collapse phenomenon was reported by Adner and co-workers (1963). Previously untransfused males were infused with 3–9 ml of red cells labelled with ^{51}Cr. In 31 cases, donor and recipient were matched by ABO and Rh D group (positive or negative). In 10 out of the 31 subjects a collapse curve was observed; nine of these subjects received a second injection of red cells from their first donor; in three cases rapid destruction occurred, but in the remaining six the survival of the red cells of the second injection was normal or only slightly subnormal. Of the three cases showing rapid destruction of the cells after the second injection, one had already formed anti-E and another formed anti-Fy[a].

Fourteen additional subjects, all of whom were K negative, were injected with K-positive blood. Four showed a collapse curve and all of these were given a second injection from their first donor: in two cases the red cells were more rapidly destroyed and one of the two formed anti-E; in the other two recipients the survival of a second injection was normal or only slightly subnormal. Eight out of the 14 who showed normal survival of the first lot of red cells were given a second injection; one showed rapid destruction and formed anti-K.

In summary, collapse curves were noted following 14 out of 45 first injections of red cells and occurred on average on the sixteenth day after injection (range 6–33 days). In 13 out of these 14 cases a second injection was given. Normal or only slightly subnormal survival was found in eight cases and in these no alloantibodies were found. In the remaining five, red cell destruction was observed following a second injection and in three of these, alloantibodies (two examples of anti-E and one of anti-Fy[a]) were detected.

Several other studies in humans have shown an incidence of collapse curves similar to that observed by Adner and co-workers (1963). For example, in one series the incidence was reported as 20% (Brown and Smith 1958). When further cases were added to the series the incidence of collapse curves became 15 out of 40 survival measurements in 32 subjects who had almost always received 10–20 ml of blood (5–10 ml of red cells). The diminished survival at first appeared to be related to passage of red cells through a pump oxygenator, but this factor was later deemed irrelevant (GS Eadie, personal communication). In a series studied by ER Giblett (1956, unpublished), red cells from 1–8 ml of blood obtained from the placenta of normal infants were labelled with ^{51}Cr and injected into normal adults. 'Collapse' was observed in three of nine cases and none of these cells was circulating at 20 days (see Fig. 10.20). In another series, 'collapse' occurred in 10 out of 41 crosstransfusions of small volumes of ^{51}Cr-labelled red cells, usually at about the fourteenth day after transfusion. The remaining cells were usually eliminated within the following week (Kaplan and Hsu 1961).

In summary, when transfusions of 1–10 ml of Rh D-compatible red cells are given to previously untransfused subjects, collapse curves are observed in approximately 30% of cases (Table 10.3).

When therapeutic amounts of blood are transfused to previously untransfused subjects, premature curtailment of survival is much less common. From a review of more than 100 cases in which the survival of transfused red cells had been followed for not less than 60 days after the transfusion of at least 400 ml of blood, unexpected shortening of survival was found in about 5% of cases (Mollison 1954). A similar incidence was apparent in a series described by Szymanski and Valeri (1971). Forty-four survival studies were carried out by automated differential agglutination in 39 subjects following a transfusion of 450 ml of blood. Two collapse curves were observed: accelerated destruction developed on about the tenth day after transfusion and all

Table 10.3 Incidence of collapse of the red cell survival curve following the transfusion of 1–10 ml of red cells to previously untransfused adult recipients.

Reference	Donors	Amount of red cells transfused (ml)	Incidence of collapse
Adner and Sjölin (1957)	Newborn infants	4–10	5/15
Unpublished observations made by ER Giblett	Newborn infants	1–8	3/9
Kaplan and Hsu (1961)	Newborn infants	2–7	10/41
Adner et al. (1963)*	Adults	3–9	14/45
			32/110 (29.1%)
GS Eadie (personal communication)	Adults	5–10	15/40[†]

* Following the red cell injections, alloantibodies were detected in three cases in the series of Adner et al. (1963) and in three cases in the series of Brown and Smith (1958), but in no cases in the other series.

[†] Not included in total above because 40 experiments were carried out in 32 recipients.

the cells had been eliminated by day 30. There is some evidence that collapse curves are less common in non-responders to Rh D than in responders, possibly indicating that non-responders to Rh D lack some recognition mechanism for allogeneic red cells (Mollison 1981).

What causes subnormal red cell survival without demonstrable antibodies?

It is tempting to suppose that collapse curves represent primary immunization. In support of this belief, the following observations can be cited: (1) in the series of Adner and co-workers (1963), a collapse curve following a first injection of red cells was sometimes followed by the rapid clearance of a second dose of red cells from the same donor with production of an alloantibody; (2) following a first injection of D-positive red cells to D-negative subjects, collapse curves are commonly observed in responders, whereas they are found rarely or not at all in non-responders (Mollison 1981). Evidence opposed to the hypothesis that collapse curves represent primary immunization is the following: (1) in the series of Adner and co-workers (1963), in about 50% of cases, a collapse curve following a first injection of red cells was followed by normal survival of a second dose of red cells from the same donor; (2) collapse curves are not found invariably during primary immunization to strong alloantigens, such as D and K – examples of the normal survival of a first dose of D-positive red cells at 28 days despite the formation of anti-D within the following 6 months were supplied by Samson and Mollison (1975), and an example of the normal survival of a first dose of K-positive red cells for at least 47 days in a subject who formed anti-K within 10 days of a second injection was described by Adner and co-workers (1963); and (3) in rabbits, when Hg (A+) red cells were transfused to Hg (A–) animals, the incidence of collapse curves was 41 out of 51 (Smith and Mollison 1974), but was also high (10 out of 16) when Hg (A–) red cells were transfused to Hg (A–) rabbits.

The possible role of cell-bound antibody in causing red cell destruction in the absence of detectable antibody in the serum

Griffiths and co-workers (1994) have suggested that in circumstances in which the ratio of specific antibody to non-specific plasma IgG is expected to be high, macrophages may become 'armed' with antibody in the spleen where antibody-secreting plasma cells and FcR-bearing macrophages are in close proximity. This idea is an extension of the previous suggestion that antibody-mediated destruction may be favoured in the spleen because plasma IgG has less of an opportunity to compete with IgG-coated red cells for binding to Fc receptors on macrophages (Engelfriet *et al.* 1981). The concept that there may be macrophages to which antibody has been bound would provide an explanation for the specific destruction of red cells in the absence of detectable antibody in the plasma.

Destruction of recipient's red cells by transfused antibodies

Passively acquired antibodies may destroy the recipient's own red cells or, when blood from more than one donor is transfused, the red cells of another donor. In either case, the mechanism of red cell destruction is similar to that brought about by actively produced antibodies, although the effects tend to be much less severe due to dilution of the transfused antibody by the recipient's plasma and, in the case of anti-A and anti-B, by the inhibiting effect of A and B substances in the plasma and in tissues other than red cells.

In this chapter, some experimental observations are described; haemolytic reactions arising accidentally are considered in the following chapter.

Destruction of recipient's red cells following the transfusion of plasma containing potent anti-A or anti-B

Ottenberg (1911) first suggested that persons of group O could be used as 'universal donors'. He argued that the anti-A and anti-B agglutinins in the donor's plasma, although theoretically capable of damaging the patient's red cells if the patient belonged to group AB, A or B, would in fact be so diluted in the recipient's plasma as to be harmless. The use of group O blood for transfusion to patients of all groups spread rapidly. Throughout the Second World War, enormous numbers of transfusions of group O blood were given to patients of all groups, without any preliminary matching tests. In the vast majority of cases there was no evidence of undesirable effects. Any risks that the procedure carried were considered small compared with the potential problems of attempting to group recipients and crossmatch blood under the extremely hazardous field conditions. Nevertheless, the transfusion of group O plasma to group A recipients sometimes causes severe red cell destruction. Acute haemolysis has been reported following ABO-incompatible single-donor platelet concentrates and may be more common than is appreciated (Larsson *et al.* 2000; see also Chapter 11).

Transfusion to human volunteers

The first systematic attempt to assess the effect of transfusions of incompatible plasma was made by Aubert and co-workers (1942), who transfused plasma containing potent anti-A alloagglutinins to volunteers of group A. By eliminating the complicating factor of the donor's red cells the investigators could be certain that any haemolysis was due to destruction of the patient's own cells. They observed varying degrees of haemoglobinaemia, 'intravascular agglutination' and hyperbilirubinaemia followed by a progressive reduction in red cell count. The lowest titre of anti-A agglutinin associated with signs of blood destruction was 512. In their hands, such anti-A titres were found in the plasma of 40% of group O donors and they concluded that only about 60% of group O individuals could be considered suitable as universal donors.

Similar findings were reported by Tisdall and co-workers (1946a). In their hands, about 23% of group O persons had anti-A or anti-B titres of 640 or higher. The transfusion of 250 ml of plasma with an alloagglutinin titre of 600–4000 frequently caused haemoglobinaemia. In one case, a volunteer who received plasma with a titre of only 600 developed a sufficient degree of haemoglobinaemia to produce haemoglobinuria. Many patients developed elevation of serum bilirubin, although none became jaundiced. Tisdall and co-workers also noted the phenomenon described by Aubert and co-workers (1942) as 'intravascular agglutination', the presence of agglutinates in saline suspensions of blood taken from patients immediately after the transfusions.

In a further series of experiments Tisdall and colleagues (1946b) took blood from a group B volunteer who had been immunized by the injection of group A substance, so that his anti-A titre was 2500. On one occasion, injection of as little as 25 ml of this plasma

into a group A volunteer produced haemoglobinuria. However, after the addition of group-specific substances to the plasma *in vitro*, as much as 250 ml could be injected without producing signs or symptoms. As the donor of the plasma was group B, the anti-A was probably mainly IgM. In a series of cases, 10 ml of the group-specific substances were added to 250-ml amounts of plasma containing potent agglutinins and transfused to volunteers. No signs of red cell destruction were observed in any of the recipients.

One of the difficulties in interpreting these observations is the uncertainty as to whether the high-titre agglutinins were IgM or IgG. IgM anti-A and anti-B are far more easily inhibited by soluble blood group substances than are IgG antibodies, so that it would be unwise to conclude that plasma from group O donors, containing potent anti-A and anti-B, can necessarily be rendered safe by the addition of blood group substances. In fact in at least one case a haemolytic transfusion reaction in a group A patient transfused with group O blood occurred despite the addition of AB substance to the plasma before transfusion (Ervin and Young 1950).

Observations made by Ervin and co-workers (1950) first called attention to the importance of 'immune' characteristics of anti-A and anti-B in causing red cell destruction *in vivo*. These authors investigated four severe haemolytic reactions in group A patients following the transfusion of group O blood and showed that in all four cases the donor's plasma contained anti-A, which was difficult to inhibit and had a higher indirect antiglobulin titre than saline–agglutinin titre. Signs of red cell damage persisted for relatively long periods after transfusion. Thus osmotic fragility was increased for 8–11 days and microspherocytes were seen on blood films for approximately 2 weeks after transfusion. The same authors reported the results of two transfusions of group O plasma to a group A volunteer. The first transfusion was of plasma with a moderate saline–agglutinin titre (640), which was readily inhibited by A substance *in vitro* and was presumably wholly or predominantly IgM. No signs of red cell destruction developed. By contrast, when the same volunteer received plasma that had a scarcely higher saline–agglutinin titre (1280) and probably contained a potent IgG antibody, as it was not readily inhibited by AB substance, the recipient developed severe intravascular haemolysis and his haematocrit fell from 43% to 24% in 5 days.

Summary of effects of incompatible plasma (anti-A and anti-B)

The following summary is based partly on the experimental work described above, partly on unpublished observations made with H Chaplin, H Crawford (Morton) and M Cutbush (Crookston) in 1952 and partly on various transfusion accidents described in the following chapter.

Haemoglobinaemia tends to be slight and haemoglobinuria is unusual.

Jaundice occurring within a few hours of transfusion has been noted occasionally; see, for example, the infants observed by Gasser (1945), referred to in the following chapter.

Progressive anaemia is the most commonly observed sign of red cell destruction; PCV may continue to fall for at least 1 week after transfusion; see Fig. 11.1.

Spontaneous agglutination of whole blood samples withdrawn from the recipient is an invariable feature. Agglutination occurs even when plasma containing relatively weak anti-A is transfused. (In a group A subject transfused over 20 min with 340 ml of blood from a donor whose serum had a saline–agglutinin titre of 64 and a haemolysin titre of 4, a sample of blood taken immediately after transfusion showed strong spontaneous agglutination; this was best demonstrated by spreading a drop of blood on an opal tile; 3 h later, the sign was still present but was weaker; the next day it was not present. In patients transfused with potent anti-A, spontaneous agglutination of blood samples *in vitro* may persist for more than 24 h.)

The direct antiglobulin test becomes positive in group A subjects transfused with plasma containing even weak immune anti-A. In the subject referred to in the paragraph above, the DAT was definitely positive immediately after transfusion, was weakly positive the next day and was negative thereafter. In patients transfused with potent immune anti-A the DAT may remain positive for as long as 1 week.

The osmotic fragility of the patient's red cells increases when incompatible plasma is transfused. After transfusion, maximal osmotic fragility occurs after 24 h and is almost maximal after 3 h (Ervin *et al.* 1950). It may remain elevated for at least 11 days and during this period peripheral blood films show microspherocytosis.

Destruction of recipient's red cells by transfused or injected anti-D

Only experimental observations are described in this section; for accidents in clinical practice see Chapter 11.

Transfusion of plasma containing anti-D

The transfusion, to D-positive subjects, of 200 ml of plasma containing anti-D with a titre of 256 (IAT) produced a positive DAT and spherocytosis within 24 h, and a fall in Hb concentration of 2.5 g/dl during the following week. In a second case, in which 250 ml of plasma with a titre of 128 was transfused, the recipient's bilirubin concentration rose to 2.5 mg/dl at the end of 5 h and the Hb concentration fell by 2.6 g/dl in 1 week. In several recipients who were transfused with plasma containing antibodies with titres between 8 and 16, no definite evidence of red cell destruction was detected (Jennings and Hindmarsh 1958).

In a series in which normal volunteers received 250 ml of plasma containing moderately potent anti-D (or anti-c or anti-K or anti-M), there were no definite signs of red cell destruction (Mohn *et al.* 1961). The blood volume of these recipients was considerably greater than that of the subjects studied by Jennings and Hindmarsh (1958). In one subject who was transfused with serum containing an exceptionally potent anti-D (indirect antiglobulin titre of 1000; serum albumin titre of 400 000), the PCV fell from 0.48 to 0.22 in 12 days, and spherocytosis and mild haemoglobinaemia persisted for 2 weeks (Bowman *et al.* 1961).

Injections of anti-D immunoglobulin

In one series of D-positive adults with AITP, who were injected with 750–4500 μg of intramuscular or intravenous anti-D over a period of 1–5 days, the red cells became coated with 3.2–7.7 μg of IgG/ml cells, but only minimal signs of red cell destruction developed (Salama *et al.* 1986). In another series, in which the AITP was related to AIDS, 13 μg of IgG anti-D/kg were given daily for 3 days, followed by 6–13 μg/kg weekly. In five out of six patients, Hb fell by 6–44 g/l (Cattaneo *et al.* 1989).

As described in Chapter 5, the intravenous injection of anti-D in doses between 10 and 15 μg/ml of red cells is sufficient to clear 200–600 ml of D-positive red cells from the circulation of D-negative subjects in 2–8 days. In a case in which approximately 3000 µg of anti-D were infused to a man with AITP over the course of 3 days, corresponding to a dose of less than 2 µg of anti-D/ml red cells, Hb concentration fell from 155 to 74 g/l and it was estimated that about 1600 ml of red cells had been destroyed. No cause could be determined for this surprising amount of red cell destruction (Barbolla *et al.* 1993), although in a patient with severe thrombocytopenia, internal haemorrhage is difficult to exclude.

IVIG preparations may contain potent anti-D (titre 64–256) and unexpected haemolytic reactions have been reported (Thorpe *et al.* 2003). Other red cell alloantibodies that cause sensitization but minimal haemolysis have been detected in these preparations as well (Moscow *et al.* 1987).

References

Adner PL, Sjölin S (1957) Unexpected blood group incompatibility revealed by Cr51-labelled red cells. Scand J Clin Lab Invest 9: 265

Adner PL, Foconi S, Sjölin S (1963) Immunization after intravenous injection of small amounts of ^{51}Cr-labelled red cells. Br J Haematol 9: 288

Akeroyd JH, O'Brien WA (1958) Survival of group AB red cells in a group A recipient. Vox Sang 3: 330

Anderson G, Gray LS, Mintz PD (1991) Red cell survival studies in a patient with anti-Tca. Am J Clin Pathol 95: 87–90

Andorka DW, Arosemena A, Harris JL (1974) Neutralization *in vivo* of Lewis antibodies. Report of two cases. Am J Clin Pathol 62: 47

Ashby W (1919) The determination of the length of life of transfused blood corpuscles in man. J Exp Med 29: 267

Athkambhira S, Chiewsilp P (1978) Neutralization of Lewis antibodies *in vivo*. Communications of the 17th Congress of the International Society of Hematology, Paris

Atkinson JP, Frank MM (1974a) Complement-independent clearance of IgG-sensitized erythrocytes: inhibition by cortisone. Blood 44: 629

Atkinson JP, Frank MM (1974b) Studies on the *in vivo* effects of antibody. Interaction of IgM antibody and complement in the immune clearance and destruction of erythrocytes in man. J Clin Invest 54: 339

Aubert EF, Boorman KE, Dodd BE (1942) The universal donor with high titre iso-agglutinins; the effect of anti-A iso-agglutinins on recipients of group A. BMJ i: 659.

Badakere SS, Vasantha K, Bhatia HM (1980) High frequency of Ina antigen among Iranians and Arabs. Hum Hered 30: 262–263

Baldwin ML, Barrasso C, Ness PM (1983) A clinically significant erythrocyte antibody detectable only by ^{51}Cr survival studies. Transfusion 23: 40–44

Baldwin ML, Ness PM, Barrasso C (1985) *In vivo* studies of the long-term 51Cr red cell survival of serologically incompatible red cell units. Transfusion 25: 34–38

Ballas SK, Sherwood WC (1977) Rapid *in vivo* destruction of Yt(a+) erythrocytes in a recipient with anti-Yta. Transfusion 17: 65–66

Ballas SK, Dignam C, Harris M (1985) A clinically significant anti-N in a patient whose red cells were negative for N and U antigens. Transfusion 25: 377–380

Barbolla L, Nieto S, Llamas P (1993) Severe immune haemolytic anaemia caused by intravenous immunoglobulin anti-D in the treatment of autoimmune thrombocytopenia. Vox Sang 64: 184–185

Basta M, Langlois PF, Marques M (1989a) High-dose intravenous immunoglobulin modifies complement-mediated *in vivo* clearance. Blood 74: 326–333

Basta M, Kirshbom P, Frank MM (1989b) Mechanism of therapeutic effect of high-dose intravenous immunoglobulin. J Clin Invest 84: 1974–1981

Basta M, Fries LF, Frank MM (1991) High doses of intravenous Ig inhibit *in vitro* uptake of C4 fragments onto sensitized erythrocytes. Blood 77: 376–380

Bettigole R, Harris JP, Tegoli J (1968) Rapid *in vivo* destruction of Yt(a+) red cells in a patient with anti-Yta. Vox Sang 14: 143

Blundell J (1824) Researches Physiological and Pathological. London: E Cox and Son

Borst-Eilers E (1972) Rhesusimmunisatie: onstaan en preventie. Thesis, University of Amsterdam.

Bowman HS, Brason FW, Mohn JF (1961) Experimental transfusion of donor plasma containing blood-group antibodies into compatible normal human recipients. II. Induction of iso-immune haemolytic anaemia by a transfusion of plasma containing exceptional anti-CD antibodies. Br J Haematol 7: 130

Brendemoen OJ, Aas K (1952) Hemolytic transfusion reaction probably caused by anti-Leª. Acta Med Scand 141: 458

Brown DJ (1988) A rapid method for harvesting autologous red cells from patients with hemoglobin S disease. Transfusion 28: 21–23

Brown DL, Lachmann PJ, Dacie JV (1970) The *in vivo* behaviour of complement-coated red cells: studies in C6-deficient, C3-depleted and normal rabbits. Clin Exp Immunol 7: 401

Brown E (1983) Studies in splenectomy. In: Immunoglobulin G Fc Receptor-mediated Clearance in Autoimmune Diseases. Ann Intern Med 98: 206–218

Brown I Jr, Smith WW (1958) Hematologic problems associated with the use of extra-corporeal circulation for cardiovascular subjects. Ann Intern Med 49: 1035

Buchholz DH, Bove JR (1975) Unusual response to ABO incompatible blood transfusion. Transfusion 15: 577

Burton MS, Mollison PL (1968) Effect of IgM and IgG iso-antibody on red cell clearance. Immunology 14: 861

Cattaneo M, Gringeri A, Capitanio AM *et al.* (1989) Anti-D immunoglobulins for treatment of HIV-related immune thrombocytopenic purpura. Blood 73: 357

Chaplin HJ (1959) Studies on the survival of incompatible cells in patients with hypo-gammaglobulinemia. Blood 14: 24

Chaplin HJ, Cassell M (1962) The occasional fallibility of *in vitro* compatibility tests. Transfusion 6: 375

Chaplin HJ, Coleman ME, Monroe MC (1983) *In vivo* instability of red-blood-cell-bound C3d and C4d. Blood 62: 965–971

Chaplin HJ, Hunter VL, Rosche ME (1985) Long-term *in vivo* survival of Rh(D)-negative donor red cells in a patient with anti-LW. Transfusion 25: 39–43

Christian RM, Stewart WB, Yuile CL (1951) Limitation of hemolysis in experimental transfusion reactions related to depletion of complement and isoantibody in the recipient. Blood 6: 142

Clancey M, Bond S, Van Eys J (1972) A new example of anti-Lan and two families with Lan-negative members. Transfusion 12: 106–108

Contreras M, Mollison PL (1981) Failure to augment primary Rh immunization using a small dose of 'passive' IgG anti-Rh. Br J Haematol 49: 371–381

Contreras M, Mollison PL (1983) Rh immunization facilitated by passively-administered anti-Rh? Br J Haematol 53: 153–159

Contreras M, De Silva M, Teesdale P (1987) The effect of naturally occurring Rh antibodies on the survival of serologically incompatible red cells. Br J Haematol 65: 475–478

Cooper AG, Brown DL (1971) Haemolytic anaemia in the rabbit following the injection of human anti-I cold agglutinin. Clin Exp Immunol 9: 99

Crawford DH, Azim T, Daniels GL *et al.* (1988) Monoclonal antibodies to the Rh antigen. In: Progress in Transfusion Medicine. Cash JD (ed.). Edinburgh: Churchill Livingstone, pp. 175–197

Crome P, Mollison PL (1964) Splenic destruction of Rh-sensitized and of heated red cells. Br J Haematol 10: 137

Cummings E, Pisciotto P, Roth G (1984) Normal survival of Rho(D) negative, LW(a+) red cells in a patient with allo-anti-LWa. Vox Sang 46: 286–290

Cutbush M, Mollison PL (1958) Relation between characteristics of blood-group antibodies *in vitro* and associated patterns of red cell destruction *in vivo*. Br J Haematol 4: 115

Cutbush M, Giblett ER, Mollison PL (1956) Demonstration of the phenotype Le(a+b+) in infants and in adults. Br J Haematol 2: 210

Dacie JV, Mollison PL (1943) Survival of normal erythrocytes after transfusion to patients with familial haemolytic anaemia (acholuric jaundice). Lancet i: 550

Davey RJ, Simpkins SS (1981) ^{51}Chromium survival of Yt(a+) red cells as a determinant of the *in vivo* significance of anti-Yta. Transfusion 21: 702–705

Davey RJ, Tourault MA, Holland PV (1978) The clinical significance of anti-H in an individual with the Oh (Bombay) phenotype. Transfusion 18: 738–742

Davey RJ, Gustafson M, Holland PV (1980) Accelerated immune red cell destruction in the absence of serologically detectable alloantibodies. Transfusion 20: 348–353

Davey RJ, Rosen SR, Holland PV (1982) *In vitro* thermal characteristics of anti-Leb antibodies as predictors of their *in vivo* significance. Abstracts of the 17th Congress of the International Society of Blood Transfusion, Budapest

Dobbs JV, Prutting DL, Adebahr ME *et al.* (1968) Clinical experience with three examples of anti-Yta1. Vox Sang 15: 216–221

Dzik WH, Blank J (1986) Accelerated destruction of radiolabelled red cells due to anti-Colton b. Transfusion 26: 246–248

Eckrich RJ, Mallory D, Sandler SG (1995) Correlation of monocyte monolayer assays and posttransfusion survival of Yt(a+) red cells in patients with anti-Yta. Immunohematology 11: 81–84

Eklund J, Nevanlinna HR (1971) Immuno-suppression therapy in Rh-incompatible transfusion. BMJ iii: 623

Engelfriet CP, von dem Borne AEGKr, Beckers T (1972) Autoimmune haemolytic anaemias. V. Studies on the resistance against complement haemolysis of red cells of patients with chronic cold agglutinin disease. Clin Exp Immunol 2: 255

Engelfriet CP, von dem Borne AEGKr, van der Meulen FW *et al.* (1981) Immune destruction of red cells. In: A Seminar on Immune-Mediated cell Destruction. Chicago, IL: Am Assoc Blood Banks

Ervin DM, Young LE (1950) Dangerous universal donors. 1. Observations on destruction of recipient's A cells after transfusion of group O blood containing high titer of A antibodies of immune type not easily neutralizable by soluble A substance. Blood 5: 61

Ervin DM, Christian RM, Young LE (1950) Dangerous universal donors. II. Further observations on the *in vivo* and *in vitro* behaviour of isoantibodies of immune type present in group O blood. Blood 5: 553

Evans RS, Turner E, Bingham M (1965) Studies with radio-iodinated cold agglutinins of ten patients. Am J Med 38: 378

Evans RS, Turner E, Bingham M (1967) Chronic hemolytic anaemia due to cold agglutinins: the mechanism of resistance of red cells to C' hemolysis by cold agglutinins. J Clin Invest 46: 1461

449

Evans RS, Turner E, Bingham M (1968) Chronic hemolytic anemia due to cold agglutinins. II. The role of C' in red cell destruction. J Clin Invest 47: 691

Fagge CH, Pye-Smith PH (1891) Textbook of the Principles and Practice of Medicine, vol. 2. London: J & A Churchill, p. 648

Fehr J, Hofman V, Kappeler U (1982) Transient reversal of thrombocytopenia in idiopathic thrombocytopenic purpura by high-dose intravenous gamma globulin. N Engl J Med 306: 1254–1258

Ferguson DJ, Gaal GD (1988) Some observations on the Inb antigen and evidence that anti-Inb causes accelerated destruction of radiolabeled red cells. Transfusion 28: 479–482

Fleer A, van Schaik MLJ, von dem Borne AEGKr (1978) Destruction of sensitized erythrocytes by human monocytes *in vitro*: effects of cytochalasin B, hydrocortisone and colchicine. Scand J Immunol 8: 515

Frank MM, Hamburger MI, Lawley TJ (1979) Defective Fc-receptor function in lupus erythematosus. N Engl J Med 300: 518–523

Fudenberg HH, Allen FJ (1957) Transfusion reactions in the absence of demonstrable incompatibility. N Engl J Med 256: 1180

Garratty G, Nance SJ (1990) Correlation between *in vivo* hemolysis and the amount of red cell-bound IgG measured by flow cytometry. Transfusion 30: 617–621

Garratty G, Arndt PA (1999) Applications of flow cytofluorometry to red blood cell immunology. Cytometry 38: 259–267

Gasser C (1945) Akute haemolytische Krisen nach Plasma-Transfusionen bei dystrophischtoxischen Saeuglingen. Helv Paediatr Acta 1: 38

Gesellius F (1874) Zur Thierblut-Transfusion beim Menschen. St Petersburg and Leipzig: Eduard Hoppe

Gobel U, Drescher KH, Pottgen W *et al.* (1974) A second example of anti-Yt^a with rapid *in vivo* destruction of Yt(a+) red cells. Vox Sang 27: 171–175

Gorick BD, Hughes-Jones NC (1991) Relative functional binding activity of IgG1 and IgG3 anti-D in IgG preparations. Vox Sang 62: 251–254

Greendyke RM, Chorpenning FW (1962) Normal survival of incompatible red cells in the presence of anti-Lu^a. Transfusion 2: 52

Griffin FM Jr, Mullinax PJ (1985) *In vivo* activation of macrophage C3 receptors for phagocytosis. J Exp Med 162: 352–357

Griffin GD, Lippert LE, Dow NS *et al.* (1994) A flow cytometric method for phenotyping recipient red cells following transfusion. Transfusion 34: 233–237

Griffiths HL, Kumpel BM, Elson CJ (1994) The functional activity of human monocytes passively sensitized with monoclonal anti-D suggests a novel role for FcγRI in the immune destruction of blood cells. Immunology 83: 370–377

Hadley A, Wilkes A, Poole J *et al.* (1999) A chemiluminescence test for predicting the outcome of transfusing incompatible blood. Transfusion Med 9: 337–342

Halima D, Postoway N, Brunt DEA (1982) Haemolytic transfusion reactions (HTR) due to a probable anti-C, not detectable by multiple techniques (Abstract). Transfusion 22: 405

Harrison CR, Hayes TC, Trow LL (1986) Intravascular hemolytic transfusion reaction without detectable anti-bodies: a case report and review of literature. Vox Sang 51: 96–101

van der Hart M, Engelfriet CP, Prins HK (1963) A haemolytic transfusion reaction without demonstrable antibodies *in vitro*. Vox Sang 8: 363

van der Hart M, Szaloky A, van der Berg-Loonen EM (1974) Présence d'antigènes HL-A sur les hématies d'un donneur normal. Nouv Rev Fr Hematol 14: 555

Hasse O (1874) Die Lammblut-Transfusion beim Menschen – Erste Reihe: 31 eigene Transfusionen umfassend. St Petersburg and Leipzig: Eduard Hoppe

Heistö H, Myhre K, Vogt E (1960) Haemolytic transfusion reaction due to incompatibility without demonstrable antibodies. Vox Sang 5: 538

Heistö H, Myhre K, Börresen W (1962) Another case of haemolytic transfusion reaction due to incompatibility without demonstrable antibodies. Vox Sang 7: 470

Hewitt WC Jr, Wheby M, Crosby WH (1961) Effect of prednisolone on incompatible blood transfusions. Transfusion 1: 184

Hopkins JG (1910) Phagocytosis of red blood-cells after transfusion. Arch Intern Med 6: 270

Hossaini AA (1972) Neutralization of Lewis antibodies *in vivo* and transfusion of Lewis incompatible blood. Am J Clin Pathol 57: 489

Howard JE, Winn LC, Gottlieb CE (1982) Clinical significance of the anti-complement component of antiglobulin sera. Transfusion 22: 269–272

Hsu TCS, Jagathambal K, Sabo BH (1975) Anti-Holley (Hy): characterization of another example. Transfusion 15: 604

Huchet J, Cregut R, Pinon F (1970) Immuno-globulines anti-D. Efficacitée, comparée des voies intra-musculaire et intra-veineuse. Rev Fr Transfusion 13: 231

Hughes-Jones NC, Mollison PL, Veall N (1957) Removal of incompatible red cells by the spleen. Br J Haematol 3: 125

Hughes-Jones NC, Mollison PL (1963) Clearance by the RES of 'non-viable' red cells. In: Role du Système Réticuloendothélial dans l'Immunit, antibacterienne et antitumorale. Paris: Edition du CNRS

Hughes-Jones NC, Mollison PL (1968) Failure of a relatively small dose of passively administered anti-Rh to suppress primary immunization by a relatively large dose of Rh-positive red cells. BMJ i: 150

450

ICSH (1980) Recommended methods for radioisotope red-cell survival studies. Br J Haematol 45: 659–666

Issitt PD, Valinsky JE, Marsh WL (1990) *In vivo* red cell destruction by anti-Lu6. Transfusion 30: 258–260

Jaffe CF, Atkinson JP, Frank MM (1976) The role of complement in the clearance of cold agglutinin-sensitized erythrocytes in man. J Clin Invest 58: 942

Jandl JH (1955) Sequestration by the spleen of red cells sensitized with incomplete antibody and with metallo-protein complexes (Abstract). J Clin Invest 34: 912

Jandl JH, Greenberg MS (1957) The selective destruction of transfused 'compatible' normal red cells in two patients with splenomegaly. J Lab Clin Med 49: 233

Jandl JH, Simmons RL (1957) The agglutination and sensitization of red cells by metallic cations: interactions between multivalent metals and the red-cell membrane. Br J Haematol 3: 19

Jandl JH, Kaplan ME (1960) The destruction of red cells by antibodies in man. III. Quantitative factors influencing the patterns of hemolysis *in vivo*. J Clin Invest 39: 1145

Jandl JH, Jones AR, Castle WB (1957) The destruction of red cells by antibodies in man. I. Observations on the sequestration and lysis of red cells altered by immune mechanisms. J Clin Invest 36: 1428

Jennings ER, Hindmarsh C (1958) The significance of the minor crossmatch. Am J Clin Pathol 30: 302

Jensen K, Freiesleben E, Sorensen SS (1965). The survival of red cells incompatible with Rh antibodies demonstrable only by enzyme technique. Communication of the 10th Congress of the European Society of Haematology, Strasbourg

Jouvenceaux A, Adenot N, Berthoux F (1969) Gamma-globuline anti-D lyophilisé intra-veineuse pour la prévention de l'immunisation anti-Rh. Rev Fr Transfusion 13 (Suppl.): 341.

Kaplan E, Hsu KS (1961) Determination of erythrocyte survival in newborn infants by means of Cr51-labelled erythrocytes. Pediatrics 27: 354

Kaplan ME, Jandl JH (1961) Inhibition of red cell sequestration by cortisone. J Exp Med 114: 921

Kelley CM, Karwal MW, Schlueter AJ et al. (1998) Outcome of transfusion of K:11 erythrocytes in a patient with anti-K11 antibody. Vox Sang 74: 205–208

Kissmeyer-Nielsen F, Jensen KB, Ersbak J (1961) Severe haemolytic transfusion reactions caused by apparently compatible red cells. Br J Haematol 7: 36

Kohan AI, Niborski RC, Rey JA et al. (1994) High-dose intravenous immunoglobulin in non-ABO transfusion incompatibility. Vox Sang 67: 195–198

Kumpel BM (1997) *In vitro* functional activity of IgG1 and IgG3 polyclonal and monoclonal anti-D. Vox Sang 72: 45–51

Kumpel BM, Judson PA (1995) Quantification of IgG anti-D bound to D-positive red cells infused into D-negative subjects after intramuscular injection of monoclonal anti-D. Transfusion Med 5: 105–112

Kumpel BM, Austin EB, Lee D et al. (2000) Comparison of flow cytometric assays with isotopic assays of (51)chromium-labeled cells for estimation of red cell clearance or survival *in vivo*. Transfusion 40: 228–239

Kumpel BM, De Haas M, Koene HR et al. (2003) Clearance of red cells by monoclonal IgG3 anti-D *in vivo* is affected by the VF polymorphism of Fcgamma RIIIa (CD16). Clin Exp Immunol 132: 81–86

Kurlander RJ, Rosse WF, Logue GL (1978) Quantitative influence of antibody and complement coating of red cells on monocyte-mediated cell lysis. J Clin Invest 61: 1309

Kurtz SR, Ouellet R, McMican A et al. (1983) Survival of MM red cells during hypothermia in two patients with anti-M. Transfusion 23: 37–39

Lachmann PJ, Pangburn MK, Oldroyd RG (1982) Breakdown of C3bi to C3c, C3d and a new fragment-C3g. J Exp Med 156: 205–216

Lampe TL, Moore SB, Pineda AA (1979) Survival studies of Lan-positive red blood cells in a patient with anti-Lan (Abstract). Transfusion 19: 640

Larsson LG, Welsh VJ, Ladd DJ (2000) Acute intravascular hemolysis secondary to out-of-group platelet transfusion. Transfusion 40: 902–906

Lau PYL, Jewlachow V, Leahy MF (1994) Successful transfusion of Yka-positive red cells in a patient with anti-Yka. Vox Sang 64: 254–255

Lawley TJ, Hall RP, Fauci AS (1981) Defective Fc-receptor function associated with the HLA-B8/DRw3 haplotype. Studies in patients with dermatitis herpetiformis and normal subjects. N Engl Med J 304: 185–192

Lee D, Remnant M, Stratton F (1984) 'Naturally occurring' anti-Rh in Rh(D) negative volunteers for immunization. Clin Lab Haematol 6: 33–38

Lewis SM, Dacie JV, Szur L (1960) Mechanism of haemolysis in the cold-haemagglutinin syndrome. Br J Haematol 6: 154

Lin-Chu M, Broadberry RE (1990) Blood transfusion in the para-Bombay phenotype. Br J Haematol 75: 568–572

van Loghem JJ (1965) Some comments on autoantibody induced red cell destruction. Ann NY Acad Sci 124: 465

Loutit JF, Mollison PL, Young IM (1943) Citric acid-sodium-citrate-glucose mixtures for blood storage. Quart J Exp Physiol 32: 183

MacKenzie FAF, Elliot DH, Eastcott HHG (1962) Relapse in hereditary spherocytosis with proven splenunculus. Lancet i: 1102

McSwain B, Robins C (1988) A clinically significant anti-Cra (Letter). Transfusion 28: 289–290

Maynard BA, Smith DS, Farrar RP (1988) Anti-Jka, -C and -E in a single patient, demonstrable only by the manual hexadimethrine bromide (polybrene) test, with incompatibilities confirmed by 51Cr-labelled red cell studies. Transfusion 28: 302–306

Mohn JF, Lambert RM, Bowman HS (1961) Experimental transfusion of donor plasma containing blood-group antibodies into incompatible normal human recipients. I. Absence of destruction of red-cell mass with anti-Rh, anti-Kell and anti-M. Br J Haematol 7: 112

Mollison PL (1943) The investigation of haemolytic transfusion reactions. BMJ i: 529–559

Mollison PL (1951) Blood Transfusion in Clinical Medicine. Oxford: Blackwell Scientific Publications

Mollison PL (1954) The life-span of red blood cells. Lectures on the Scientific Basis of Medicine 2: 269

Mollison PL (1956) Blood Transfusion in Clinical Medicine. Oxford: Blackwell Scientific Publications

Mollison PL (1959a) Blood group antibodies and red cell destruction. BMJ ii: 1035

Mollison PL (1959b) Factors determining the relative clinical importance of different blood group antibodies. Br Med Bull 15: 92

Mollison PL (1959c) Further studies on the removal of incompatible red cells from the circulation. Acta Haematol (Basel) 10: 495

Mollison PL (1961) Blood Transfusion in Clinical Medicine. Oxford: Blackwell Scientific Publications

Mollison PL (1962) Destruction of incompatible red cells in vivo in relation to antibody characteristics. In: Mechanism of Cell and Tissue Damage Produced by Immune Reactions. Basel: Schwabe, p. 267

Mollison PL (1970) The effect of isoantibodies on red-cell survival. Ann NY Acad Sci 169: 199

Mollison PL (1972) Blood Transfusion in Clinical Medicine. Oxford: Blackwell Scientific Publications

Mollison PL (1979) Blood Transfusion in Clinical Medicine. Oxford: Blackwell Scientific Publications

Mollison PL (1981) Determination of red cell survival using 51Cr. In: A Seminar on Immune-Mediated Cell Destruction. Chicago, IL: Am Assoc Blood Banks

Mollison PL (1983) Blood Transfusion in Clinical Medicine. Oxford: Blackwell Scientific Publications

Mollison PL (1985) Antibody-mediated destruction of foreign red cells. In: Antibodies; Protective, Destructive and Regulatory Role. F Milgrom, CJ Abeyounis, B Albini (eds). Basel: Karger, pp. 65–74

Mollison PL (1986) Survival curves of incompatible red cells. An analytical review. Transfusion 26: 43–50

Mollison PL (1989) Further observations on the patterns of clearance of incompatible red cells. Transfusion 29: 347–354

Mollison PL, Cutbush, M (1955) The use of isotope-labelled red cells to demonstrate incompatibility in vivo. Lancet i: 1290

Mollison PL, Hughes-Jones NC (1958) Sites of removal of incompatible red cells from the circulation. Vox Sang 3: 243

Mollison PL, Hughes-Jones NC (1967) Clearance of Rh positive cells by low concentration of Rh antibody. Immunology 12: 63

Mollison PL, Polley MJ, Crome P (1963) Temporary suppression of Lewis blood-group antibodies to permit incompatible transfusion. Lancet i: 909

Mollison PL, Crome P, Hughes-Jones NC (1965) Rate of removal from the circulation of red cells sensitized with different amounts of antibody. Br J Haematol 11: 461

Mollison PL, Frame M, Ross ME (1970) Differences between Rh(D) negative subjects in response to Rh(D) antigen. Br J Haematol 19: 257

Mollison PL, Johnson CA, Prior DM (1978) Dose-dependent destruction of A1 cells by anti-A1. Vox Sang 35: 149

Mollison PL, Engelfreit CP, Contreras S (1987) Blood Transfusion in Clinical Medicine. Oxford: Blackwell Scientific Publications

Moore HC, Issitt PD, Pavone BG (1975) Successful transfusion of Chido-positive blood to two patients with anti-Chido. Transfusion 15: 266

Morel PA, Garratty G, Perkins HA (1978) Clinically significant and insignificant antibodies in blood transfusion. Am J Med Technol 4L: 122

Moscow JA, Casper AJ, Kodis C et al. (1987) Positive direct antiglobulin test results after intravenous immune globulin administration. Transfusion 27: 248–249

Myllyla G, Furuhjelm U, Nordling S (1971) Persistent mixed field polyagglutinability. Electrokinetic and serological aspects. Vox Sang 20: 7

Nance SJ, Arndt P, Garratty G (1987) Predicting the clinical significance of red cell alloantibodies using a monocyte monolayer assay. Transfusion 27: 449–452

Nicholson-Weller A, Burge J, Fearon DT (1982) Isolation of a human erythrocyte membrane glycoprotein with decay accelerating activity for C3 convertases of the human complement system. J Immunol 129: 184–189

Niejadlik DC, Lozner EL (1974) Cooling mattress induced acute hemolytic anemia. Transfusion 14: 145–147

Nordhagen R, Aas M (1978) Association between HLA and red cell antigens. VII. Survival studies of incompatible red cells in a patient with HLA-associated haemagglutinins. Vox Sang 35: 319

Noyes WD, Bothwell TH, Finch CA (1960) The role of the reticulo-endothelial cell in iron metabolism. Br J Haematol 6: 43

Ottenberg R (1911) Studies in isoagglutination. I. Transfusion and the question of intravascular agglutination. J Exp Med 13: 425

Panzer S, Mueller-Eckhardt G, Salama A (1984) The clinical significance of HLA antigens on red cells. Survival studies in HLA-sensitized individuals. Transfusion 24: 486–489

Pelosi MA, Bauer JL, Langer A (1974) Transfusion of incompatible blood after neutralization of Lewis antibodies. Obstet Gynecol 4: 590

Perrault RA, Hogman CF (1972) Low concentration red cell antibodies. III. 'Cold' IgG anti-D in pregnancy: incidence and significance. Acta Univ Uppsaliensis 120

Peters B, Reid ME, Ellisor SS (1978) Red cell survival studies of Lu^b incompatible blood in a patient with anti-Lub (Abstract). Transfusion 18: 623

Polesky HF, Swanson JL (1966) Studies on the distribution of the blood group antigen Doa (Dombrock) and the characteristics of anti-Doa. Transfusion 11: 162

Ponfick P (1875) Experimentelle Beiträge zur Lehre von der Transfusion. Virchows Arch Pathol Anat 62: 273

Report from 9 Collaborating Laboratories (1991) Results of tests with different cellular bioassays in relation to severity of Rh D haemolytic disease. Vox Sang 60: 225–229

Rosenfield RE, Vitale B, Kochwa S (1967) Immune mechanisms for destruction of erythrocytes *in vivo*. II. Heparinization for protection of lysin-sensitized erythrocytes. Transfusion 7: 261

Sabo B, Moulds JJ, McCreary J (1978) Anti-JMH: another high titer-low avidity antibody against a high frequency antigen (Abstract). Transfusion 18: 387

Salama A, Kiefel V, Mueller-Eckhardt C (1986) Effect of IgG anti-Rho(D) in adult patients with chronic autoimmune thrombocytopenia. Am J Haematol 22: 241–250

Samson D, Mollison PL (1975) Effect on primary Rh immunization of delayed administration of anti-Rh. Immunology 28: 349

Sausais L, Krevans JR, Townes AS (1964) Characteristics of a third example of anti-Xga (Abstract). Transfusion 4: 312

Schanfield MS, Stevens JO, Bauman D (1981) The detection of clinically significant erythrocyte alloantibodies using a human mononuclear phagocyte assay. Transfusion 21: 571–576

Schmidt PJ, Nancarrow JF, Morrison EG (1959) A hemolytic reaction due to the transfusion of Ax blood. J Lab Clin Med 54: 38

Schneider J, Preisler O (1966) Untersuchungen zur serologischen Prophylaxe der Rh-Sensibilisierung. Blut 12: 1

Schreiber AD, Frank MM (1972) Role of antibody and complement in the immune clearance and destruction of erythrocytes. 1. *In vivo* effects of IgG and IgM complement-fixing sites. J Clin Invest 51: 575

Shirey RS, Oyen R, Heeb KN (1988) 51Cr radiolabelled survival studies in a patient with anti-Lu12. Transfusion 28: 375

Shirey RS, Boyd JS, King KE *et al.* (1998) Assessment of the clinical significance of anti-Dob. Transfusion 38: 1026–1029

Shore GM, Steane EA (1977) Survival of incompatible red cells in a patient with anti-Csa and three other patients with antibodies to high-frequency red cell antigens. Atlanta, GA: Commun Am Assoc Blood Banks

Sieg vW, Borner P, Pixberg HJ (1970) Die Elimination Rh-positiver fetaler Erythrozyten aus der Blutbahn Rh-negativer Erwachsener durch korpereigene Isoagglutinine. Blut 21: 69

Silvergleid A, Wells RF, Hafleigh EB (1978) Compatibility test using 51chromium-labelled red blood cells in cross-match positive patients. Transfusion 18: 8

Sistonen P, Nevanlinna HR, Virtaranta-Knowles K (1981) Nea, a new blood group antigen in Finland. Vox Sang 40: 352–357

Smith GN, Mollison PL (1974) Responses in rabbits to the red cell alloantigen HgA. Immunology 26: 865

Stewart JW, Mollison PL (1959) Rapid destruction of apparently compatible red cells. BMJ i: 1274

Strumia MM, Colwell LS, Dugan A (1958) The measure of erythropoiesis in anemias. I. The mixing time and the immediate post-transfusion disappearance of T-1824 dye and of Cr51-tagged erythrocytes in relation to blood volume determination. Blood 8: 128

Swisher SN, Young LE (1954) Studies of the mechanisms of erythrocyte destruction initiated by antibodies. Trans Assoc Am Phys 67: 124

Szymanski IO, Valeri CR (1971) Lifespan of preserved red cells. Vox Sang 21: 97

Thomson A, Contreras M, Gorick B (1990) Human monoclonal IgG3 and IgG1 anti-Rh D mediate clearance of D positive red cells. Lancet ii: 1147–1150

Thorpe SJ, Fox BJ, Dolman CD *et al.* (2003) Batches of intravenous immunoglobulin associated with adverse reactions in recipients contain atypically high anti-Rh D activity. Vox Sang 85: 80–84

Tilley CA, Crookston MC, Haddad SA (1977) Red blood cell survival studies in patients with anti-Cha, anti-Yka, anti-Ge and anti-Vel. Transfusion 17: 169

Tisdall LH, Garland DM, Szanto PB (1946a) The effects of the transfusion of group O blood of high iso-agglutinin titer into recipients of other blood groups. Am J Clin Pathol 16: 193

Tisdall LH, Garland DM, Wiener AS (1946b) A critical analysis of the value of the addition of A and B group-specific substances to group O blood for use as universal donor blood. J Lab Clin Med 31: 437

Todd C, White RG (1911) On the fate of red blood corpuscles when injected into the circulation of an animal of the same species: with a new method for the determination of the total volume of blood. Proc R Soc Lond B 84: 255

Tregellas WM, Moulds JJ, South SF (1978) Successful transfusion of a patient with anti-LW and LW positive blood (Abstract). Transfusion 18: 384.

453

Vogt E, Krystad E, Heisto H (1958) A second example of a strong anti-E reacting *in vitro* almost exclusively with enzyme-treated E-positive cells. Vox Sang 3: 118

Vullo C, Tunioli AM (1961) The selective destruction of 'compatible' red cells transfused in a patient suffering from thalassaemia major. Vox Sang 6: 583

Wallas CH, Tanley PC, Gorrell LP (1980) Recovery of autologous erythrocytes in transfused patients. Transfusion 20: 332–336

Wiener AS, Peters HR (1940) Hemolytic reactions following transfusions of blood of the homologous group, with three cases in which the same agglutinogen was responsible. Ann Intern Med 13: 2306

Wiener AS, Samwick AA, Morrison H (1953) Studies on immunization in man. II. The blood factor C. Exp Med Surg 11: 276

Wiener E, Jolliffe VM, Scott HCF (1988) Differences between the activities of human monoclonal IgG1 and IgG3 anti-D antibodies of the Rh blood group system in their abilities to mediate effector functions of monocytes. Immunology 65: 159–163

Williams BD, O'Sullivan MM, Ratanckaiyovong SS (1985) Reticuloendothelial Fc function in normal individuals and its relationship to the HLA antigen DR3. Clin Exp Immunol 60: 532–538

Winkelstein JA, Mollison PL (1965) The antigen content of 'inagglutinable' group B erythrocytes. Vox Sang 10: 614

Woodrow JC, Bowley CC, Gilliver BE *et al.* (1968) Prevention of Rh immunization due to large volumes of Rh-positive blood. BMJ i: 148

Woodrow JC, Finn R, Krevans JR (1969) Rapid clearance of Rh positive blood during experimental Rh immunization. Vox Sang 17: 349

Yates J, Howell P, Overfield J (1996) IgG Kidd antibodies are unlikely to fix complement. Transfusion Med 6 (Suppl. 2): 29

Zimmerman LM, Howell KM (1932) History of blood transfusion. Ann Med Hist (NS) 4: 415

11 Haemolytic transfusion reactions

A haemolytic transfusion reaction is one in which signs and symptoms of increased red cell destruction are produced by transfusion. A distinction is made between an immediate reaction (IHTR), in which destruction begins during transfusion, and a delayed reaction (DHTR), in which destruction begins only after there has been an immune response, provoked by the transfusion. Almost invariably, DHTRs are caused by secondary (anamnestic) immune responses. Although physicians assume as if by reflex that haemolysis in the setting of transfusion must be immune mediated, non-immune causes such as thermal, mechanical and osmotic stress, infection and intrinsic red cell defects should remain part of the differential diagnosis. Medication-associated autoimmune intravascular haemolysis may mimic an acute haemolytic reaction (Stroncek et al. 2000).

The previous chapter was concerned principally with patterns of removal of incompatible red cells from the circulation rather than with clinical signs and symptoms. The present chapter deals with the various syndromes produced by the transfusion of incompatible blood and also considers haemolytic reactions due to causes other than incompatibility.

Intravascular and extravascular destruction

By convention, red cell destruction is classified as either intravascular, characterized by rupture of red cells within the bloodstream and liberation of haemoglobin (Hb) into the plasma, or as extravascular, characterized by phagocytosis of red cells by macrophages of the mononuclear phagocyte system (MPS), with subsequent liberation of bilirubin into the plasma (Fairley 1940). Destruction of red cells throughout the circulation (intravascular haemolysis) is brought about by those antibodies that activate the entire classical complement cascade, leading to the production of pores in the red cell membrane followed by rupture of the cell (see Chapter 3). In contrast, antibodies that either fail to activate complement or activate it only to the C3 stage destroy red cells by mediating interaction with cells of the MPS. Traditional teachings attributed this reaction to phagocytosis alone, but when the interaction of antibody-coated red cells with monocytes was studied in vitro, red cell lysis outside of the monocyte was established. This finding explained previous observations that red cell destruction in vivo by a non-complement-activating antibody such as anti-Rh D might be accompanied by haemoglobinaemia. Thus, both Hb and bilirubin may be liberated into the plasma following 'extravascular destruction'. In this context 'extravascular' means 'outside the main blood vessels', for example within the hepatic and splenic sinusoids, and does not mean 'intracellular'. In describing red cell destruction caused by alloantibodies, 'C8–9 mediated' and 'macrophage mediated' are more accurate terms than are intravascular and extravascular, but this chapter will opt for the traditional terms instead of these awkward circumlocutions.

Intravascular destruction may be produced by antibodies such as anti-A and anti-B that are readily lytic in vitro, although not all of the red cells are lysed in the plasma; some are sensitized and removed from the circulation by erythrophagocytosis, mainly in the liver (see Chapter 10). Other causes of intravascular lysis include osmotic damage to red cells by preliminary contact with 5% dextrose during or prior to infusion

455

and the injection of water into the circulation. High levels of plasma Hb may be produced by the infusion of red cells that have been lysed *in vitro*, for example by accidental overheating, freezing or exposure to some microbial pathogens such as *Clostridium welchii*. Antibodies that are non-lytic *in vitro* bring about destruction that is predominantly extravascular, although, as mentioned above, the process may be accompanied by some degree of haemoglobinaemia. The destruction of non-viable stored red cells is a strictly intracellular process.

Intravascular destruction

Red cell destruction by anti-A, anti-B and other rapidly lytic antibodies

The importance of haemolysins as opposed to mere agglutinins was recognized very early in the practice of human transfusion. Indeed, Crile (1909) expressed the opinion that agglutinins could be disregarded. Similarly, crosstransfusion experiments in cats, some of which developed agglutinins and some lysins, demonstrated absolute correspondence between lysis *in vitro* and lysis *in vivo*. The authors concluded that 'similar tests for human transfusion can be relied on completely to prevent haemolytic accidents' (Ottenberg and Thalheimer 1915).

By far and away the most important lytic antibodies in human plasma are anti-A and anti-B. About three-quarters of all fatal acute haemolytic reactions are associated with ABO incompatibility. Haemolytic antibodies of other specificities, for example anti-PP_1P^k, anti-P_1 and anti-Vel, have been known to produce similar effects *in vivo*, but are rare. Lewis antibodies, which are relatively common, produce slow lysis *in vitro* and infrequently produce lysis *in vivo*. Kidd antibodies may also lyse untreated red cells, but usually extravascular destruction predominates; these antibodies are therefore considered in a later section. A number of other antibodies, including antibodies to HLA antigens (anti-Bg^a) have reportedly caused severe intravascular haemolysis and in some cases have not been detected by routine techniques (Benson *et al.* 2003). Haemolytic antibodies such as anti-A_1 and anti-P_1 may lyse enzyme-treated red cells *in vitro* but, even when active at 37°C, are usually non-lytic for untreated red cells. Haemolytic reactions caused by these antibodies are described in the section

on extravascular destruction, even although some instances of active intravascular haemolysis have been reported.

As described in the previous chapter, up to 90% of the cells may be lysed in the blood stream when a very small volume of incompatible red cells is injected, and 50% or more of the circulating transfused cells may be lysed when a relatively large volume of blood is transfused.

Examples of ABO-incompatible transfusions

Administration of ABO-incompatible red cells may trigger an abrupt, life-threatening syndrome characterized by anxiety (the ominous 'sense of impending doom'), flushing followed by cyanosis, fever, rigors, pain at the infusion site, lumbar spine and flanks, nausea, vomiting and shock. Coagulopathy with diffuse bleeding and renal failure complete the 'classic' description. Holmesian diagnostic acumen is not required when these signs and symptoms are present. However, reactions often present in a more subtle fashion, with little more than fever encountered during the course of transfusion.

In the following case, a plasmapheresis donor of group O was inadvertently given the red cells of a different donor, who was group A.

Mrs H was a regular plasmapheresis donor. On the day in question, after she had given blood and before her red cells were returned to her, she was asked to confirm that the signature on the unit was her own. She nodded in agreement, but afterwards admitted that although she had not seen the signature clearly, she felt that, in any case, she could trust the doctor. Within 2 min of the start of the red cell infusion she 'blacked out', felt very frightened and had pain all over, especially over the sternum and lower abdomen. The development of the symptoms was ascribed by the medical attendant to overly rapid infusion, the rate was slowed, and infusion completed in about 25 min. After a rest, Mrs H drove home.

One and a half hours later Mrs H felt very unwell and developed diarrhoea and vomiting. She passed a large amount of urine, but did not notice the colour. Three and a half hours after receiving the red cells she was visited by her own doctor, who administered an injection of furosemide. Six hours after receiving the red cells she passed a large volume (about 1 l) of red urine. The urine Hb concentration was 0.4 g/l and the plasma Hb concentration was 2.6 g/l. A blood specimen contained about 1.7% of group A red cells, the rest being group O. The concentration of fibrin degradation products in the serum was 80 μg/ml, suggesting a mild consumption coagulopathy. On the following morning plasma Hb was 0.55 g/l and the customary urine colour had returned. Three weeks after the episode, creatinine clearance was normal.

A change in the colour of urine may be the earliest or sole clue that a surgical patient under general anaesthesia has received an ABO-incompatible unit, and even this sign may be masked by haematuria in the patient undergoing genitourinary procedures. Early recognition is essential – to prevent transfusion of additional incompatible blood and to avoid possible administration of a second unit to other than the intended recipient.

As described later in this chapter, episodes of intravascular haemolysis following the transfusion of incompatible red cells are sometimes followed by renal failure and by the production of various other untoward signs. In patients whose serum contains non-lytic or only very weakly lytic anti-A or anti-B, following the transfusion of ABO-incompatible blood the level of plasma Hb may be less than 1 g/l and no Hb is passed in the urine. In fact, only when anti-A and anti-B are relatively potent is destruction predominantly intravascular.

After the transfusion of incompatible blood, erythrophagocytosis may be observed in samples of peripheral blood (Hopkins 1910; Ottenberg 1911). Striking leucopenia may result from the adherence of leucocytes to red cells and to one another. In one investigation, after the injection of 10 ml of ABO-incompatible red cells, the total leucocyte count sometimes fell from 9000 to 4000 per microlitre in 5 min. The principal effect was on the mature granulocytes and monocytes. In further experiments, the injection of as little as 0.05 ml of incompatible red cells (5×10^8 cells) caused a significant fall in leucocytes. A calculated 15 leucocytes per injected incompatible red cell was removed. Infusion of the stroma of compatible cells produced no effect, but the infusion of the stroma of incompatible cells produced leucopenia. Incidentally, the injection of A substance into O subjects produced leucopenia in six out of seven instances (Jandl and Tomlinson 1958).

Haemolysis with a unit from a chimera

A 61-year-old male patient typed as blood group O received two units of group O red cells after elective kidney surgery. Immediately following transfusion, he developed evidence of intravascular haemolysis (Pruss et al. 2003). Serological re-examination revealed a mixed-field pattern of agglutination of red cells in one of the two transfused units. The donor of this unit proved to be a 24-year-old man with a twin sister. Both siblings showed an identical mixture of roughly 95% group O and 5% group B red cells and chimerism was confirmed by genotyping.

Red cells present as 'contaminants'

When the donor is ABO incompatible, acute haemolysis may be provoked by red cells present in transfused platelet preparations, granulocyte concentrates or in bone marrow and progenitor cell suspensions, even when these suspensions have been treated with a sedimenting agent to remove the bulk of the red cells (Dinsmore et al. 1983). In the latter circumstance, significant reactions may develop when the recipient has a high-titre isoagglutinin and unmanipulated incompatible grafts are infused rapidly.

Transplacental haemorrhage

When the fetus is ABO incompatible, a large transplacental haemorrhage (TPH) may be associated with haemoglobinuria in the mother. In one such episode that followed an easy external cephalic version under general anaesthesia, the mother (group O) passed fetal Hb in the urine (0.2 g of Hb/dl). Four weeks later, a group A infant was born. The placenta showed a small area of separation. Of 14 further cases of external version, fetal cells were found in only one and in this case the mother's blood had not been examined before version (Pollock 1968).

In another case, abruptio placentae followed a car accident after which the mother (group A) gave birth to a stillborn group B infant. The mother exhibited haemoglobinaemia and haemoglobinuria (Glasser et al. 1970). In one more case, the group O mother of a B infant developed haemoglobinuria, acute tubular necrosis and disseminated intravascular coagulation (DIC) (Samet and Bowman 1961).

Frequency of ABO-incompatible transfusions

Data regarding the frequency of ABO-incompatible red cell transfusions are hard to come by. Almost all

457

surveys start with reported clinical episodes, such as haemoglobinuria following transfusion. For obvious reasons, such episodes are not always reported. Even then, the signs may be attributed to a cause other than the transfusion. Furthermore, transfusions of ABO-incompatible blood may not cause clinically obvious effects, particularly if the patient is anaesthetized. Therefore, the reported frequency with which ABO-incompatible blood is given must seriously underestimate the true frequency. Of course, the frequency with which the 'wrong' blood is given must be several-fold greater than that with which ABO-incompatible blood is given, as a random unit of blood will be ABO incompatible with a random patient about 36% of the time in Western nations (Linden et al. 1992).

Some estimates of the frequency of ABO-incompatible transfusion, based on the reporting of clinical episodes, are as follows: one in 10 000 units or one in 3000 patients (Wallace 1977); one in 18 000 transfusions, a figure based on almost half a million transfusions (Mayer 1982); one per 30 000 units transfused in a survey in which one-half of the participants relied on memory rather than written record (McClelland and Phillips 1994); and one in 33 000 transfusions (Linden et al. 1992). In an analysis of transfusion errors over a 10-year period in New York State (1990–99), Linden and co-workers (2000) documented erroneous blood administration as 1 in 19 000 red cell units, ABO-incompatible transfusions as 1 in 38 000, and acute haemolytic reactions or laboratory evidence of reactions as 1 in 76 000 red cell units transfused. This experience is similar to that of several national haemovigilance surveillance systems in Europe.

Another approach to discovering the incidence of giving the wrong blood is to start with records of blood issued by the laboratory and to discover from records to whom each unit was transfused. This may be described as the descending method of enquiry, contrasted with the ascending method already described. Of 2772 units, seven (0.25%) were transfused to unintended patients. Not a single one out of the seven had been reported, although at least three of the units were ABO incompatible (Baele et al. 1994). The estimate that one in 400 units is given to the wrong recipient may be atypically high; however, it does not include errors in labelling the sample taken from the patient or laboratory errors. Incredible as it sounds, the frequency of mislabelled and miscollected samples in an international survey of 62 hospitals (690 000 samples),

was 1 out of every 165 samples, and in a subset of hospitals, miscollected samples containing the wrong blood in the tube occurred in 1 out of every 1986 samples (Dzik et al. 2003). These appalling findings (including the failures of reporting) emphasize that estimates that start from clinical episodes must be far too low.

It has long been possible to devise systems of checking the identity of units and patients that lead to a very low error rate. At the Mayo Clinic, blood bank personnel have total control of blood units from the time when they are withdrawn from the donor to the time when they are given to the patient, the 'vein-to-vein' principle. Blood bank nurse transfusionists administer almost all blood that is transfused to patients in their rooms, and monitor all transfusions administered in operating theatres (Taswell et al. 1981, supplemented by personal communication from HF Taswell). In the period 1964–73, in the course of transfusing 268 000 units of blood, there was only one occasion on which ABO-incompatible blood was known to have been transfused (Pineda et al. 1978a). Systems approaches and evolving technology, from the lowly identification bracelet to bar codes and bedside computers, have reduced labour and improved safety and efficiency (Turner et al. 2003). The presence of national patient identification systems in Sweden and Finland has been associated with rates of miscollected samples that were too low to estimate (Dzik et al. 2003).

Mortality associated with ABO-incompatible transfusions

Statistics regarding frequency and mortality of early transfusions are incomplete and suspect. In the 25 years before frequent transfusion began in the Second World War, Kilduffe and DeBakey (1942) assembled a series of 43 284 transfusions with 80 haemolytic reactions (0.18%) and 32 deaths (0.07%) from haemolytic shock. An independent estimate from the same era quotes a mortality of 39 out of 19 275 for direct transfusions and 9 out of 8236 for transfusions of blood collected into citrate (Wiener and Moloney 1943). Some of these deaths may have resulted from volume overload rather than from acute haemolysis, so an accurate percentage cannot be calculated. Both approximations suffer at the very least from 'positive event' reporting bias. However, it is evident that from the time of these pre-modern era reports to the present, improved procedures, compatibility testing and positive identification methods have reduced dramatically the risk of acute haemolytic reactions and death. Unfortunately, progress in this area seems to have halted during the last several decades (see below).

Mortality estimates in the modern era

Three later estimates of the mortality of ABO-incompatible transfusion have been published: (1) in a hospital in the USA between 1960 and 1977, 0 out of 13; although three patients received 50 ml or less, five received 0.5 units or more, and five received 1 unit or more (sixth edition, p. 573); (2) in the State of New York in 1990–91, 3 out of 54 (Linden et al. 1992); and (3) in a series collected in London between 1940 and 1980, 0 out of 12; three patients received less than 50 ml, six received 200–600 ml, and three received 1–4 l (seventh edition, p. 649).

In December 1975, the USA FDA established mandatory reporting 'when a complication of blood collection and transfusion is confirmed to be fatal'. The information collected between 1976 and 1978 was reviewed by Schmidt (1980a,b) who considered that in only 39 out of the 69 cases could transfusion be regarded as the primary cause of death. In 24 out of the 39, death was due to an incompatible transfusion; 22 out of the 24 were immediate reactions due to transfusion of ABO-incompatible blood, and the remaining two were DHTRs associated with anti-c or anti-E. Almost the same series of cases was reviewed by Honig and Bove (1980), in an analysis that stressed the errors that had led to the transfusion of incompatible blood. They concluded that out of 44 acute haemolytic reactions, 38 were due to ABO incompatibility. Both reviews emphasized that the commonest cause of ABO-incompatible transfusion is failure to identify the recipient correctly and that the commonest place where incompatible blood is transfused is the operating theatre.

Deaths reported to the FDA in the 10-year period from 1976 to 1985 (inclusive) were reviewed by Sazama (1990). Of the cases attributed to red cell incompatibility, 158 were due to acute haemolysis (ABO incompatibility in 131) and 26 to delayed haemolysis (mainly anti-c and anti-Jk^a). Mortality calculated from the number of units of red cells transfused during this decade approximates 1 in 250 000 transfusions, although deaths are almost certainly under-reported. The previously referenced 10-year study of transfusion errors in New York State reported five deaths, 4% of all patients with acute haemolytic transfusion reactions, for an average of 0.5 events per year or 1 per 1.8 million transfusions (Linden et al. 2000). Although improved procedures and intensive care may have reduced the mortality since the reports of the 1940s, from the number of cases reported in the last 25 years, it is not possible to conclude that any significant reduction in these avoidable deaths has taken place.

Factors determining outcome

Two important factors in determining the outcome of an ABO-incompatible transfusion are the potency of the anti-A (or anti-B) in the patient's plasma and the volume of blood transfused. Rate of infusion may be a third. For example, in the case illustrated later in the text (see Fig. 11.6) in which virtually no ill-effects from the transfusion of A blood to an O subject occurred, the anti-A agglutinin titre before transfusion was 32 and the antibody was only very faintly lytic in vitro. Few adverse effects were noted in 12 carefully monitored patients who received entire units of incompatible red cells intentionally, albeit slowly, as part of a preparatory regimen for ABO-incompatible bone marrow transplantation (Nussbaumer et al. 1995) (see below).

Although striking reactions may develop during the first few minutes of transfusion with incompatible blood, the clinical severity generally depends on the amount of blood transfused. Most fatalities have been associated with transfusions of 200 ml or more, and mortality approaches 44% for infusions exceeding 1000 ml. However, volumes as small as 30 ml have been implicated (Honig and Bove 1980; Sazama 1990). Small volumes of ABO-incompatible blood may pose a higher risk for children and adolescents. This belief, although intuitive, finds little support in the published literature. One author (HGK) is aware of a mistransfusion of approximately 25 ml of group A red cells that proved fatal to a 6-year-old, group O, 28-kg child.

Role of disseminated intravascular coagulation

Transfusion of ABO-incompatible blood may prove lethal by precipitating a shock syndrome, initiating DIC or causing renal failure. In one series of 40

459

patients who received incompatible blood, four died as a direct result of the transfusion. This is the basis of the oft-quoted 10% mortality statistic. All four patients had been transfused during or immediately after major surgery. Severe and persistent hypotension was the main clinical manifestation. All four patients developed DIC; two died within 24 h from irreversible shock and two after about 4 days when evidence of acute uraemia appeared (Wallace 1977). The seriousness of DIC as a complication of ABO-incompatible transfusion is emphasized by an earlier series: of five patients transfused, who developed a haemorrhagic diathesis, all died (Binder *et al.* 1959). Nevertheless, in the majority of patients who receive ABO-incompatible blood, DIC is mild or undetectable and renal failure does not develop.

Destruction of recipient's own red cells by transfused anti-A or anti-B

On occasion, clinical signs of red cell destruction develop after the transfusion of group O blood or plasma to recipients of other ABO groups. As a rule, destruction is predominantly extravascular but, as these events are part of the spectrum of ABO haemolytic reactions, they will be discussed below.

Transfusion of group O blood to recipients of other ABO groups

Levine and Mabee (1923) coined the term 'dangerous universal donor' to describe group O donors whose plasma contained agglutinins of high titre. Nevertheless, in the early years of the Second World War, group O blood was used for all emergency transfusions in the UK, usually without any crossmatching or other serological testing. Adverse reactions were rare. In a series in the USA in which patients of groups A, B or AB were transfused with group O blood the frequency of frank haemolytic reactions was 1% (Ebert and Emerson 1946).

Experimental work on the transfusion of group O blood containing potent anti-A and anti-B to recipients of other groups has been described in the previous chapter. In the present section, a few examples will be given of accidental haemolytic transfusion reactions following the transfusion of ABO-incompatible plasma, either in the form of group O blood or as plasma alone.

The following case illustrates many of the features of a severe haemolytic transfusion reaction in a group A patient after the transfusion of blood from a 'dangerous' group O donor:

The patient was a woman aged 23, who had a postpartum haemorrhage, estimated at 800 ml of blood. The placenta was removed manually under anaesthesia. While the patient was recovering from the anaesthetic and during the transfusion of a second unit of group O blood, she developed seizures; her blood pressure was 80/40 mmHg. The transfusion was stopped after 800 ml had been given; the patient was treated conservatively and recovered rapidly. Investigation of a blood sample 12 h after transfusion showed that the patient was group A Rh D positive with approximately 0.9×10^9 group O red cells per litre. As Fig. 11.1 shows, over the following 9 days, the concentration of group O cells scarcely decreased, but PCV fell progressively due, evidently, to destruction of the patient's own red cells. The direct antiglobulin test (DAT) was strongly positive for about 48 h after transfusion and more weakly positive for the following week; the test was negative on the tenth day after transfusion. The plasma of the first unit of blood was shown to have an extremely high anti-A titre and to be strongly lytic for group

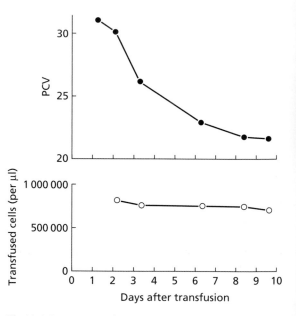

Fig 11.1 Destruction of recipient's own (group A) red cells following the transfusion of group O blood, the plasma of which contained potent anti-A. The transfused cells survived normally and the progressive fall in the recipient's packed cell volume (PCV) was therefore due entirely to the destruction of the patient's own cells.

A cells. The donor had received an injection of (horse) anti-tetanus serum contaminated with Hog A substance 38 days before giving blood (first edition, p. 286).

Plasma that has a comparatively low anti-A agglutinin titre (64–256) but contains potent IgG anti-A (IAT titre 1000–5000) may cause serious haemolytic reactions (Grove-Rasmussen *et al.* 1953; Stevens and Finch 1954).

Transfusion of red cells from group O blood to recipients of other ABO groups

The injection of as little as 25 ml of plasma containing potent anti-A may produce haemoglobinuria in a group A subject. It is therefore not surprising that haemoglobinuria may occur after the transfusion of a unit of O red cells to a group A, B or AB subject. In a case in which the recipient was group A, the unit, which had a packed cell volume (PCV) of 0.70, contained estimated 95 ml of plasma. After 'neutralization' by group A- and B-specific substances, the plasma had an anti-A indirect antiglobulin test (IAT) titre of 8192. Apart from developing haemoglobinuria, the patient suffered a rigor and vomited, but made an uneventful recovery (Inwood and Zuliani 1978). In another case, a group B newborn infant with *Escherichia coli* sepsis developed fever and haemoglobinuria after exchange transfusion with red cells from group O blood suspended in AB plasma. The IgG anti-B titre of the group O donor was 64 000 and was not neutralized by AB substance (Boothe *et al.* 1993).

Transfusions of group O plasma from single donors

In three group A (or AB) infants, weighing 3.5–4.5 kg, who received 50–90 ml of group O plasma, jaundice developed within a few hours. Examination of films of peripheral blood showed striking microspherocytosis. In one case an increase in osmotic fragility was demonstrated. An interesting point in two cases was that plasma from the same donor had been given on the previous day without producing reactions. This suggested that the capacity of the body to inhibit anti-A had been saturated by the first plasma transfusion so that a second transfusion within a short time had a more damaging effect (Gasser 1945).

Renal failure has been described in a 3-year-old haemophiliac given a transfusion of 300 ml of group O plasma before dental treatment. The patient vomited before and after the subsequent anaesthetic. By the following morning he was deeply jaundiced and had passed a small amount of almost black urine. His Hb concentration was about 60 g/l and the DAT was strongly positive. The patient recovered after treatment with peritoneal dialysis. The transfused plasma proved to have a haemolysin titre of 128 and an agglutinin titre of 256 (Keidan *et al.* 1966).

Transfusion of large amounts of low-titre or pooled plasma

In some patients with burns, haemoglobinuria developed 12–48 h after transfusion of an amount of pooled plasma equivalent to more than three times their plasma volume. More than 40% of the recipient's red cells were destroyed. The plasma used was prepared from the blood of 10 donors of different ABO groups (four group O, four group A and two group B or AB) and therefore had only low titres of anti-A and -B.

In a series of haemophiliacs who were transfused with large amounts of pooled plasma, haemolytic episodes characterized by an elevated serum bilirubin concentration and a positive DAT were common. Pooled plasma frequently had anti-A titres of 'immune' (non-inhibited) antibody as high as 64 (Delmas-Marsalet *et al.* 1969).

Anti-A or anti-B in factor VIII concentrates

A haemolytic reaction, characterized by a fall in the PCV to 0.20, microspherocytosis and haemoglobinaemia was caused by the administration of large amounts of a factor VIII concentrate to a group A patient (Rosati *et al.* 1970). In another group A patient, with a factor VIII inhibitor, who was given approximately 170 000 units of factor VIII, the DAT became positive, Hb fell to 50–60 g/l and the reticulocyte count rose to 54%; batches of the factor VIII preparation had anti-A IAT titres of 128–512 (Hach-Wunderle *et al.* 1989).

Anti-A and anti-B in immunoglobulin preparations for intravenous use

Episodes of severe intravascular haemolysis were observed in two group B recipients of bone marrow transplants following the infusion of an immuno-globulin preparation ('Gamimune'), later shown to contain anti-B with a titre of 32, as well as anti-A (Kim *et al.* 1988).

Anti-A or anti-B in platelet concentrates

A severe haemolytic reaction in a group A subject following the transfusion of 4 units of platelets from a group O donor suspended in 200 ml of the donor's plasma was shown to be due to anti-A in the donor's plasma with an IAT titre of 8192 and the ability to lyse A_1 red cells. The recipient developed haemoglobinuria and the PCV fell from 0.22 before transfusion to 0.16 8 h later; the DAT became positive (Siber *et al.* 1982). Severe haemolysis is a particular risk when platelet concentrates are administered to infants and children.

The increasing use of single-donor platelets collected by apheresis and containing 200–300 ml of plasma has resulted in reports of haemolysis during ABO-incompatible transfusions, even with low-titre agglutinins (Mair and Benson 1998; Larsson *et al.* 2000; Josephson *et al.* 2004). The frequency of such reactions is poorly documented. Platelet concentrates are not ordinarily screened for high-titre agglutinins:

A 44-year-old woman of blood group A received a unit of group O single-donor platelets for severe thrombocytopenia during induction chemotherapy for acute myeloid leukaemia. During this treatment, she had received several units of single-donor platelets of blood groups A and O as well as group A red cells. Five minutes after the beginning of the transfusion of group O platelets, the patient developed shortness of breath and felt 'flushed behind the ears'. The transfusion was stopped and the patient evaluated by a physician. After the administration of 50 mg of intravenous hydrocortisone, the transfusion was resumed. Forty minutes into the transfusion, the patient complained of back pain radiating into the legs and tingling of the fingers of both hands. The transfusion was again halted and the patient evaluated. After the infusion of 25 mg of diphenhydramine, the transfusion was resumed and completed without further incident. The 371-ml volume of the platelet unit was transfused over 55 min. Blood pressure, pulse and respirations all remained normal throughout the transfusion, and temperature did not increase.

The patient reported a transient feeling of nausea 1 h after the transfusion and at 2 h after transfusion passed 'bloody' urine. The patient's urine remained red for 24 h after the reaction. Despite transfusion of 2 units of compatible group A red cells, her Hb dropped by 23 g/l, from 77 g/l before the

transfusion to 54 g/l 6 h after the reaction. There was no impairment of renal function after the transfusion and no evidence of disseminated intravascular coagulation. The patient recovered without further difficulty (Larsson *et al.* 2000).

Haemolysis has also been reported with 'dry platelets', apheresis platelets that are resuspended in synthetic preservative media and contain no more than 25–30 ml of plasma (Valbonesi *et al.* 2000).

Destruction of transfused A_1 red cells by passively acquired anti-A

In an A_2 patient transfused with 5 units of A_1 blood, followed by 1 unit of group O blood containing immune anti-A, all the A_1 red cells were eliminated within about 2 days of transfusion and anti-A_1 could be demonstrated in the recipient's plasma (Ervin and Young 1950). In this case there was no evidence of adverse effects, but in another case in which a patient of subgroup A_2 was transfused with 3 units of group A_1 and 1 unit of group O blood, jaundice and anuria developed and the patient died (Grove-Rasmussen 1951).

Pathophysiology of acute haemolytic reactions

Haemoglobin release, complement activation and liberation of cytokines

Although clinical descriptions of acute haemolytic reactions were described in detail at the beginning of the twentieth century, and in fact as early as the seventeenth century (see below), the mechanisms remain incompletely understood. The reactions are triggered by the binding of antibody to the surface of the incompatible red cells, activation of complement and lysis of cells with release of Hb. Progression of the reaction then involves, to differing degrees, simultaneous activation of phagocytic cells, the coagulation cascade and the systemic inflammatory response involving both cellular and humoral components. The unpredictability of the response, the controlling factors of which remain maddeningly obscure, accounts for the differing signs and symptoms as well as the variable severity of these reactions.

Haemoglobin released into the bloodstream has cytotoxic and inflammatory effects (Wagener *et al.* 2001). Plasma haemoglobin has been associated with increased platelet adhesion and aggregation as well as vascular inflammation and obstruction *in vivo* (Simionatto *et al.* 1988). Nitric oxide binding by free haemoglobin may lead to smooth muscle dystonia with resultant hypertension, gastrointestinal contraction and vasoconstriction (Rother *et al.* 2005).

Activation of complement results in assembly of the membrane attack complex and liberation of the potent anaphylatoxins C3a and C5a, small polypeptides that increase vascular permeability, act directly on smooth muscle and interact with various cells. Complement fragments stimulate mast cells to degranulate and release vasoactive substances such as histamine and serotonin. Complement-coated cells bind to macrophages and other phagocytic cells, which, in turn, liberate interleukin 1 (IL-1) and other cytokines. Receptors for C3a and C5a are present on a wide variety of cells (leucocytes, macrophages, endothelial cells, smooth muscle cells), so that complement activation may be accompanied by production of free radicals and nitric oxide, release of leukotrienes and granule enzymes, and synthesis of interleukins (Butler *et al.* 1991; Davenport *et al.* 1994). C3a and C5a play a major role in producing the adverse effects of ABO-incompatible transfusions, but the release of cytokines may be equally important (Davenport 1995). Activation of the kallikrein system leads to further production of bradykinin with its powerful vascular effects (Capon and Goldfinger 1995).

In vitro, the incubation of A or B red cells with group O whole blood leads to the release of IL-8 and tissue necrosis factor (TNF) (Davenport *et al.* 1990, 1991). IL-8 has chemotactic and activating properties for neutrophils and is released by various cells, including monocytes. IL-8 production may be complement dependent (Davenport *et al.* 1990). TNF is one of the cytokines that plays a significant role in septic shock, a syndrome that shares many clinical characteristics with acute HTR. TNF activates the intrinsic coagulation cascade and may thus take part in initiating DIC (Davenport *et al.* 1991, 1992). TNF not only causes endothelial cells to increase tissue factor production but also decreases production of thrombomodulin, which, in turn, suppresses protein C activity. Thus, coagulation is promoted and anticoagulation inhibited (Capon and Goldfinger 1995).

The role of cytokines liberated from leucocytes in causing febrile transfusion reactions is discussed in Chapter 15.

Symptoms and signs associated with intravascular haemolysis

The symptoms and signs associated with the transfusion of ABO-incompatible red cells were vividly described by Oehlecker (1928). As a biological test for compatibility, he infused 5–20 ml of blood from a potential donor and observed the effects. The following is a rough translation of what he noted when the donor was ABO incompatible:

'After one or one and a half minutes the patient becomes restless, breathes deeply and complains of a feeling of oppression, perhaps also of sternal pain. The patient may also have abdominal discomfort and may vomit. The pulse becomes weaker and one often sees a characteristic change in colour; a pale patient may suddenly become strikingly red'.

Oehlecker pointed out that all symptoms usually subside rapidly, but that if more blood is infused the same symptoms recur within 1–2 min. The constricting pain in the chest may be due to a spasm of coronary vessels or to vascular occlusion by agglutinated cells.

Similar symptoms were noted in some of the early transfusions given to patients from animal donors. For example, the effects of transfusing calf blood to a human subject were reported as follows: after about 200 ml of blood had been transfused, the patient 'found himself very hot along his arm and under the armpits'. After a second larger transfusion on the following day (of about 450 ml of blood) 'he felt the like heat along his arm and under his armpits which he had felt before . . . and he complained of great pains in his kidneys and that he was not well in his stomach and that he was ready to choke unless they gave him his liberty' (Denis 1667).

Towards the end of the nineteenth century, lambs were in vogue as donors and a certain Dr Champneys (1880) reported that he had witnessed more than a dozen transfusions given directly from the carotid vessels of a lamb into the forearm veins of human subjects suffering from phthisis. After a short interval subjects developed difficult breathing along with a feeling of oppression, then flushing, followed by sweating. On the next day and for a few days subsequently, 'haematinuria' and, in nearly all cases, urticaria were noted.

Although constricting pain in the chest and pain in the lumbar region have been observed following the injection of 0.7 ml of A_1 red cells to a subject whose serum contained potent lytic anti-A (fifth edition, p. 549), the intravascular lysis of approximately 1 ml of ABO-incompatible red cells does not necessarily cause symptoms (tenth edition, p. 365). Similarly, when 10 ml of washed ABO-incompatible red cells were injected, only a few subjects developed transient symptoms: lumbar pain, dyspnoea, hyperperistalsis, flushing of the face and neck (Jandl and Tomlinson 1958). Several millilitres of incompatible cells are infused routinely with out-of-group allogeneic stem cell grafts, and are usually well tolerated (Braine et al. 1982; Dinsmore et al. 1983). These patients frequently undergo extensive plasmapheresis to reduce the antibody titre and receive heavy premedication, including corticosteroids, prior to the infusions. However, 12 patients received deliberately mismatched donor-type red cell transfusions (1 unit over 8 h on each of two consecutive days) to adsorb isoagglutinins from the recipient. The units were well tolerated, although one patient with pre-existing impaired renal function developed reversible renal failure after the stem cell transplant. Recipient antibody titre ranged from 32 to 1024 (Nussbaumer et al. 1995). Nevertheless, the experience with a relatively few cases may owe as much to good fortune as to low risk, and this procedure has not received wide acceptance (Davenport 1995).

In another series of experiments, an immediate reaction occurred only when intravascular red cell destruction occurred. In this series, ^{51}Cr-labelled group B red cells were injected into a group A patient with hypogammaglobulinaemia whose serum contained no detectable anti-B. The B red cells initially underwent only slow destruction corresponding to a T_{50}Cr of about 5 days. After 5 days, various amounts of anti-B were injected, and only when the amount of anti-B was sufficient to produce intravascular lysis were any symptoms noted; facial flushing began 2 min after injection, lasted 4 or 5 min, and was followed 7 min after injection by pain in the groin, thighs and lower back lasting 45 min. Subjects receiving small injections of red cells of incompatible ABO groups developed a small rise in body temperature but no chills (Jandl and Kaplan 1960).

Strongly lytic antibodies, other than anti-A and anti-B, which produce similar effects in vivo are rare. In the first subject in whom anti-PP$_1$P^k (-Tj^a) was identified, a test injection of 25 ml of incompatible blood was followed by an immediate severe reaction with haemoglobinaemia (Levine et al. 1951). In a subject with haemolytic anti-Vel, transfusion produced a rigor, lumbar pain and anuria (Levine et al. 1961).

As noted earlier, signs and symptoms of acute haemolysis may vary. The 'classic' presentation is a dramatic, life-threatening syndrome characterized by a feeling of dread, flushing, fever and chills, pain at the infusion site, lumbar spine and flanks, nausea, vomiting and shock. Patients may hyperventilate and develop cyanosis, or chest and abdominal pain may predominate, possibly as a result of occlusion and ischaemia in the microvasculature. Dyspnoea is common and the lung is an early, important, perhaps underappreciated target organ. Goldfinger and co-workers (1985) had the opportunity to observe a patient who received 20 ml of ABO-incompatible blood at the time of intensive haemodynamic monitoring. The earliest event, an increase in pulmonary vascular resistance, occurred within the circulation of the lung. Some patients will have minimal symptoms, and the first clues may be pallor, icterus and a fall in circulating Hb.

In patients who are anaesthetized or are heavily medicated during transfusion, the two signs that may call attention to the possibility that incompatible blood has been transfused are hypotension, despite apparently adequate replacement of blood, and abnormal bleeding.

Disseminated intravascular coagulation associated with intravascular haemolysis

In dogs, the infusion of autologous haemolysed red cells leads to intravascular coagulation (Rabiner and Friedman 1968). Thromboplastic substances in stroma appear to be responsible. In monkeys, the infusion of sonicated stroma, free of Hb, produces a fall in platelets, fibrinogen and factors II, V and VIII (Birndorf et al. 1971).

The fully developed syndrome of DIC is characterized by thrombocytopenia, a fall in the levels of factors V and VIII (particularly the latter), a low level of fibrinogen and deposition of fibrin thrombi in small vessels. Fibrin degradation products can be demonstrated in the serum.

In experiments in monkeys in which incompatible plasma was transfused, evidence of mild DIC was observed in two animals in which plasma Hb levels reached 6 g/l or more. No bleeding was observed in animals in which the plasma Hb level was below 1 g/l (Lopas et al. 1971). In other experiments in which incompatible allogeneic red cells were transfused, equivalent in amount to 250 ml of blood to a human adult, DIC was observed in three out of five cases in which intravascular haemolysis (average plasma Hb 6.5 g/l) associated with haemolytic antibodies. The main features were a fall in factors V, VIII and IX and a less consistent fall in fibrinogen concentration and in platelet count. Intravascular coagulation was not observed in two cases in which destruction was predominantly extravascular and associated with predominantly incomplete non-haemolytic antibodies; in these latter cases there was a slow rise of plasma Hb, reaching a peak of about 0.5 g/l in 4 h (Lopas and Birndorf 1971).

Following the transfusion of ABO-incompatible blood, a haemorrhagic state may develop after as little as 100 ml. If the patient is undergoing operation, uncontrollable bleeding from the wound develops; epistaxis and bleeding from the site of venepuncture have also been observed. A fibrinogen level as low as 15 mg/dl has been reported, with virtually incoagulable blood. Fibrin degradation products (FDPs) have been found in the serum, usually in concentrations in the range of 250 to 450 µg/ml, but as high as 1900 µg/ml in one case (Sack and Nefa 1970).

Various interactions have been demonstrated between the complement, kinin, coagulation and fibrinolytic systems (Kaplan *et al.* 2002). For example, low-molecular-weight fragments of factor XIIa (Hageman factor) may mediate C1 activity (Ghebrehiwet *et al.* 1981). The possible role of cytokines in precipitating DIC has been discussed above.

After predominantly extravascular destruction, DIC occurs only very occasionally. There are two reports in the literature of abnormal bleeding following incompatible transfusion due to antibodies that are not haemolytic *in vitro*: one due to anti-c (Wiener 1954) and one due to anti-Fy[a] (Rock *et al.* 1969).

Renal failure following intravascular haemolysis

Destruction of red cells within the bloodstream liberates Hb into the circulation and is sometimes followed by a decline in renal function The postulated direct nephrotoxicity of Hb itself, although widely taught, has not been unequivocally demonstrated, remains hotly debated (Viele *et al.* 1997) and probably does not exist outside of the vasoconstriction mediated by nitric oxide binding (see below). Of 41 cases of renal failure related to haemolytic reactions, 21 were related to ABO incompatibility (Bluemle 1965). Almost all instances of renal failure associated with ABO incompatibility

occur in group O patients, although only about 70% of ABO mismatched transfusions involve group O patients (Doberneck *et al.* 1964; Bluemle 1965).

The infusion of large volumes of stroma-free Hb has no effect on renal function in dogs and monkeys (Rabiner *et al.* 1970; Birndorf *et al.* 1971). On the other hand, when 250 ml of a preparation of Hb containing only 1.2% stromal lipid was administered at the rate of 4 ml/min to six well-hydrated healthy men, urinary output fell by 81%, mean creatinine clearance declined, and transient bradycardia and hypertension developed (Savitsky *et al.* 1978). In several studies, the infusion of Hb has been associated with vasoconstrictor effects such as increased blood pressure and reduced cardiac output (Hess *et al.* 1993; Thompson *et al.* 1994). Vasoconstriction may be produced by the interference of Hb with the action of nitric oxide. Hb is presumed to leak across the endothelial layer into the extravascular space. Hb is thought to interfere with nitric oxide function as nitric oxide diffuses from endothelial cells to smooth muscle, where it exerts its vasodilatory effects by regulating smooth muscle tone (Patel and Gladwin 2004). Hb breakdown products, for example metHb, may also play a role in generating damaging oxygen radicals (see also Ogden and MacDonald 1995).

Renal damage associated with intravascular destruction is relatively common when destruction is caused by potent lytic antibodies, and unusual when caused by non-lytic antibodies. Consumption coagulopathy with microvasculature clot deposition may compromise the function of several organs. In experiments in monkeys, in which haemolytic transfusion reactions were produced, fibrin thrombi were widespread and in at least one case were found in renal tufts (Lopas *et al.* 1971). Hypotension is doubtless another factor in precipitating renal failure. Potent complement activation leads to the release of large amounts of C3a and C5a, which, in turn, release vasoactive peptides from mast cells.

Renal failure following the infusion of stroma

There is evidence that the infusion of stroma from incompatible red cells is followed by renal failure. In one case, in an attempt to depress the titre of a panagglutinin in a patient's plasma, stroma from 4 units of red cells was infused. One hour later, the patient felt apprehensive and sustained a fall in blood pressure, a rapid decrease in urinary output, granulocytopenia and thrombocytopenia. Following an infusion of mannitol (25%), urinary flow was rapidly restored. In a second case, a patient whose serum contained anti-K was infused with stroma from 1 unit of K-positive red cells and 3 units of K-negative red cells. There followed a rigor and severe oliguria lasting 5 days. The authors stated that in 12 other cases in which stroma had been infused, no complications occurred (Schmidt and Holland 1967). These experiments reinforce the conclusion that transfusion of incompatible red cells produces its damaging effect on the kidney not by releasing Hb but by activating complement, liberating cytokines and triggering DIC.

Effect of incompatible transfusion in an anuric patient. A patient of group O with presumed tubular necrosis following severe injury 1 month earlier was given one-third of a unit of group AB blood over 4 min. The patient felt unwell and temporarily lost consciousness. At 1 h, plasma Hb had risen to 4.8 g/l, 1.82 g bound to haptoglobin (Hp) and the rest free. The plasma was cleared of Hb in about 10 h, during which time the patient excreted 8 ml of faintly orange urine. The episode may have delayed slightly the onset of diuresis, but ultimately renal function was only slightly impaired (Hoffsten and Chaplin 1969).

Management of suspected acute haemolytic transfusion reactions with intravascular haemolysis

Methods of diagnosing acute haemolytic transfusion reactions and the immediate steps to be taken when acute haemolysis is suspected are described later in this chapter; the serological investigations to be undertaken are discussed in Chapter 8.

Management of acute haemolytic reactions is both expectant and supportive. Early recognition and interdiction of further incompatible blood may be the single most important step. Although several treatment protocols have been proposed, there is no evidence that the supportive measures should differ from those administered for shock, renal failure and DIC from any cause. The degree of intensive medical support will depend on the severity of the reactions.

Hypotension is usually managed by aggressive fluid resuscitation, and when pressors are indicated, drugs that preserve renal blood flow, for example dopamine infused at 3–5 µg/kg per minute, are preferred. Timely

intervention may limit the degree of renal impairment. Both prophylaxis and immediate treatment of renal insufficiency traditionally include mannitol 20% (100 ml/m²) and diuretics to maintain a minimal urinary output of 0.5 ml/kg per hour, but little scientific evidence supports this recommendation. Further management depends on the clinical response. Alkalinization of the urine is routinely recommended, may be helpful and is unlikely to cause harm.

Appropriate management of the consumption coagulopathy in acute haemolytic transfusion reactions, as in other conditions, is fiercely debated. There is no evidence that prophylactic anticoagulation prevents or lessens the microvascular thrombosis or the bleeding. Heparin administration has been advocated by some once the diagnosis of DIC has been established, and if prescribed, a dose of 5000 units immediately, followed by a continuous infusion of 1500 units/hour for 6–24 h has been recommended (Goldfinger 1977). Heparin treatment carries the risk of exacerbating the bleeding. Few reports address the role of heparin during acute haemolytic transfusion reactions, although two apparent successes were reported by Rock and co-workers (1969). Use of blood components such as plasma, platelets and cryoprecipitate are equally controversial, but should in any case be limited to patients with life-threatening bleeding. As acute haemolytic transfusion reactions so often result from a transfusion error, special effort must be undertaken to ensure that any blood component selected has been determined to be compatible.

Non-immunological intravascular haemolysis

Haemolysis due to osmotic effects

Damage produced by exposure to 5% dextrose

Haemolytic transfusion reactions have been observed in patients receiving transfusions of whole blood passed through a bottle containing 5% dextrose and 0.225% saline [Ebaugh *et al.* 1958, cited by DeCesare and co-workers (1964)]. Similarly, red cells suspended in excess 5% dextrose or in 4.3% dextrose with 0.18% saline were almost completely lysed after 24 h at room temperature (Noble and Abbott 1959). On the other hand, when blood was mixed with 5% dextrose in normal saline, no lysis was found even after

15 h at 37°C (Ryden and Oberman 1975). The small number of agglutinates with negligible haemolysis that is sometimes observed in the intravenous tubing when a 5% dextrose solution follows transfusion of red cells is rapidly diluted in the patient's circulation and has not been associated with adverse events.

Injection of water into the circulation: best be a rabbit

Infusion of 100 ml of water into an adult produces only slight haemoglobinaemia (0.1–0.2 g/l), but the injection of 300–900 ml, infused over a period of 1–4 h, produces plasma Hb levels of 2–4 g/l. Water may gain entrance to the circulation if the bladder is irrigated with water rather than with saline during transurethral prostatectomy (TURP). Acute renal failure after TURP may be caused by hypotonicity and hypervolaemia with subsequent increased vascular leakage leading to hypotension and rapidly impaired renal function. Acute renal failure caused by haemolysis after TURP has been reported, but is rare (Gravenstein 1997). In patients who already have renal ischaemia, the entry of water into the circulation may precipitate renal failure (Landsteiner and Finch 1947).

Injection of water into the circulation can be lethal. Two patients who were accidentally given 1.5 and 2 l, respectively, of distilled water by rapid infusion developed rigors, haemoglobinuria and persistent hypotension, and both patients became oliguric and died (J Wallace, personal communication). Despite the evidence that infusion of large amounts of water is dangerous in humans, very large amounts have been given to rabbits without producing ill effects (Bayliss 1920).

Insufficiently deglycerolized red cells

Osmotic stress may cause lysis of red cells that have been cryopreserved with glycerol but inadequately washed free of the cryoprotectant after thaw. In most cases, haemolysis is minimal and patients may note a change in urine colour, but no other signs or symptoms.

A nine-year-old boy of blood group B with thalassaemia major was supported on a chronic outpatient transfusion programme with red cell transfusions at 3-week intervals. His Hb level prior to transfusion was 86 g/l and he received two units of frozen deglycerolized red cells (high-glycerol technique) that had been prepared according to a manual protocol. The patient had no atypical antibodies and the blood was compatible by a standard crossmatch technique. Transfusion was performed without incident and the patient was discharged. Three hours later, the parents called to report that the patient passed dark red urine, but had no fever or other signs or symptoms of illness. A post-transfusion specimen revealed an Hb of 111 g/l. The DAT was negative and no discrepancies were found after careful clerical check of transfusion records. The urine contained free Hb, but no red cells. Analysis of residual blood in one of the transfused red cell units revealed an osmolarity of > 2000 mOsm, suggesting incomplete removal of glycerol by washing, and haemolysis of a small amount of cells due to osmotic shock. The osmolarity of a specimen from the second unit was 310 mOsm. The patient suffered no clinical sequelae (HGK, personal observation).

Clinical symptoms of a haemolytic reaction occurred in one of two patients with sickle cell anaemia after in vivo haemolysis of transfused deglycerolized red cells (Bechdolt et al. 1986). Instrumentation that controls automated deglycerolization should reduce this risk in the future.

Transfusion of haemolysed blood

If enough free Hb is injected into the circulation the resultant haemoglobinaemia may be misinterpreted as a sign of intravascular haemolysis. Appreciable quantities of free Hb may be injected in any of the following circumstances.

Transfusion of overheated blood

Red cells are damaged and destroyed if warmed to a temperature of 50°C or more. Most heat-related accidents happen when a unit of blood is placed in a vessel containing hot water with the intention of warming the blood to body temperature. The transfusion of approximately 2.5 l of blood that had been accidentally overheated, and haemolysed, was associated with irreversible renal failure and death of the patient (J Wallace, personal communication). One of the authors (HGK) is aware of a similar tragic occurrence following transfusion of a unit of red cells that had been "warmed like a baked potato" in a commercial microwave oven. As discussed in Chapter 15, blood should not be warmed before transfusion except in special circumstances and using methods in which the temperature is carefully monitored.

Transfusion of blood haemolysed by accidental freezing

Blood may be accidentally frozen, either by storage in an unmonitored refrigerator or by inadvertent placement in a freezer. In one reported case, 3 units of autologous blood, donated 2–4 weeks previously, had been accidentally frozen at –20°C and were transfused during hip surgery. Six hours later, the patient's urine was noted to be dark red and oliguria developed. There were no signs of shock. The patient required repeated haemodialysis, but eventually recovered (Lanore *et al.* 1989).

Blood forced through a narrow orifice: easier to pass through the eye of a needle

Forcing blood through a narrow opening such as a narrow-gauge needle has been incriminated as the cause of haemolysis in several different circumstances:
1 Haemoglobinuria was observed in a 1-month-old infant, 1 h after a scalp vein transfusion of 55 ml of a partially packed suspension of red cells. The cells had been injected through a fine-gauge needle and considerable pressure was needed to infuse the blood. When stored blood was subsequently injected through a needle of similar gauge *in vitro*, substantial lysis occurred when the rate of injection exceeded about 0.3 ml/s (Macdonald and Berg 1959).
2 Haemoglobinuria was noted in a donor who was undergoing plateletpheresis on a continuous-flow cell separator as blood was pumped through partially obstructed tubing (Howard and Perkins 1976).
3 After the unexpected death of several infants following intrauterine transfusion, case analysis revealed that all deaths had occurred after the usual infusion catheter had been replaced with a model that had a much smaller side opening. When red cells were injected through the new type of catheter, substantial haemolysis occurred (Bowman and Pollack 1980).
4 Blood forced through a leucocyte reduction filter may haemolyse, and transfusion of such blood has been responsible for haemoglobinuria (Gambino *et al.* 1992; Ma *et al.* 1995).

Transfusion of infected blood – and of infected patients

Blood that has been contaminated with certain bacteria and stored may become grossly haemolysed. The transfusion of such blood does produce haemoglobinaemia and haemoglobinuria, but these signs pale into insignificance when compared with the very toxic effects of bacterial toxins (see Chapter 16). Haemolysis due to bacterial sepsis may mimic a haemolytic transfusion reaction (Felix and Davey 1987).

Transfusion of red cells with intrinsic defects – and of patients with red cell defects

Transfusion of cells with certain enzyme or membrane defects may result in acute haemolytic transfusion reactions, although in most instances haemolysis is asymptomatic, delayed or appreciated only in retrospect by a shortened interval between transfusions. Exchange transfusion with G6PD-deficient blood has resulted in acute haemolysis in infants (Kumar *et al.* 1994). Immediate post-transfusion haemolysis was documented in 6 out of 10 Israeli adults who received G6PD-deficient blood, although the degree of red cell destruction was minimal and no symptoms were noted (Shalev *et al.* 1993). The risk and degree of haemolysis depend on the particular enzyme variant and may be exacerbated by the concurrent administration of medications associated with oxidative stress (Beutler 1996; see also Chapter 1). Acute haemolysis related to enzyme deficiencies may mimic acute haemolytic transfusion reactions, particularly in the surgical setting (Sazama *et al.* 1980). Units from donors with hereditary spherocytosis and poikilocytosis may also result in haemolysis either during storage or post transfusion (Weinstein *et al.* 1997).

Autoimmune haemolytic anaemia

Haemoglobinuria following transfusion in autoimmune haemolytic anaemia (AIHA) seems most likely to be caused by increasing the red cell mass subject to autoimmune destruction in patients with a very severe haemolytic process (Chaplin 1979). Haemoglobinuria following transfusion in patients with complement-mediated AIHA may be due to the initial destruction of 'unprotected' red cells that, unlike the patient's own red cells, have little C3dg on them. Intravascular lysis due to the increased supply of complement in the transfused blood is probably an unusual cause of post-transfusion haemoglobinuria in patients with AIHA; however two possible cases, both in patients with cold haemagglutinin disease, were described by Evans and co-workers (1965).

Paroxysmal nocturnal haemoglobinuria: dispelling the washing myth

Patients with paroxysmal nocturnal haemoglobinuria (PNH) may develop haemoglobinuria after transfusion. The postulated mechanism involves activation of the complement cascade to which PNH red cells are abnormally sensitive (Rosse and Nishimura 2003). Customary practice for transfusing PNH patients has been to wash the red cells free of plasma in an effort to minimize complement and alloantibodies in the transfusion. However, in a 38-year experience at the Mayo Clinic, 23 patients with PNH were transfused with 556 blood components that included 94 units of whole blood, 208 units of red cells, 80 units of white cell-poor red cells, 38 units of washed red cells, 5 units of frozen red cells and 6 units of red cells salvaged during surgery. Only one documented episode of post-transfusion haemolysis related to PNH was confirmed. That episode was associated with the transfusion of a unit of group O whole blood with ABO-incompatible plasma to an AB-positive patient and probably involved antibody-mediated complement fixation on the red cell membrane (Brecher and Taswell 1989). This analysis suggests that the routine use of washed cells for PNH patients is unnecessary as long as ABO-identical blood components are transfused. But complement can be activated by antigen–antibody reactions not localized to the susceptible red cell membrane. Sporadic reports do suggest that leucocyte antibodies in transfused components may precipitate haemolysis in PNH recipients (Sirchia et al. 1970; Zupanska et al. 1999). If such antibodies are present, prudence dictates washing the cells free of plasma.

A recombinant humanized monoclonal antibody (eculizumab) that inhibits activation of terminal complement components has been shown to reduce haemolysis and transfusion requirement for six men and five women with chronic haemolysis of type II PNH cells (Hillmen et al. 2004). The long-term effects of such treatment are unknown.

Sickle-cell (SS) disease and sickle cell haemolytic transfusion reaction syndrome. Patients with SS disease may develop rapid destruction of transfused red cells consistent with either acute or delayed reactions. The classic description of this syndrome emphasized the presence of typical SS crisis pain and rapid destruction of large volumes of transfused cells despite compatible crossmatch results (Chaplin and Cassell 1962; Diamond et al. 1980). Symptoms suggestive of a sickle cell pain crisis develop or are intensified during the haemolytic reaction and may result in more severe anaemia after the transfusion than was present originally. Patients may have either marked reticulocytosis or severe reticulocytopenia. The syndrome(s) have been referred to collectively as the *sickle cell haemolytic transfusion reaction syndrome* (Petz et al. 1997). The pathophysiology of the so-called 'hyperhaemolysis' that appears to destroy autologous as well as transfused cells is not predictable (Petz et al. 1997), and the appropriate clinical management of this life-threatening complication is yet to be established (Telen 2001). Immune-mediated haemolysis is not always demonstrable when hyperhaemolysis occurs in the setting of recent transfusion (Aygun et al. 2002).

Bleeding into soft tissues

Massive but occult bleeding into soft tissues, typically retroperitoneal bleeding or haemorrhage into the thigh after femoral artery puncture, may mimic acute or DHTRs. Rapid fall in Hb concentration may be followed by elevation in serum bilirubin, lactate dehydrogenase and fibrin degradation products as clot is resorbed (HG Klein, personal observation).

Clearance of haemoglobin from the plasma (Fig. 11.2)

Haemoglobin liberated into the plasma dissociates into dimers that bind to haptoglobin (Hp) (see Bunn et al. 1969). Unbound Hb is partly processed by the liver and partly excreted (as dimers) in the urine. Free Hb is readily oxidized in the plasma to metHb; after dissociation from globin, haem binds preferentially to haemopexin. The globin split off from Hb is bound by Hp. Hb catabolism and other laboratory measurements during a representative acute haemolytic transfusion reaction are displayed in Fig. 11.2 (Duvall et al. 1974).

Haptoglobin (Hp) is a normal plasma protein, capable of binding about 1.0 g of Hb per litre of plasma. When amounts of Hb not exceeding this level are infused or liberated into the bloodstream, the Hb

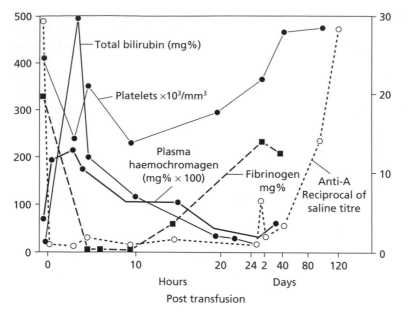

Fig 11.2 Time course of changes in anti-A titre, plasma Hb (mg/100 ml × 10), total bilirubin (mg/100 ml), platelets and fibrinogen following transfusion of 140 ml of incompatible (group A2) red blood cells to a group O patient. Modified from Duvall and co-workers (1974).

circulates as a complex with Hp. The molecular weight of Hp varies according to phenotype, and is about 100 kDa for Hp 1–1 and about 220 kDa for Hp 2–1 (Giblett 1969). Molecules of Hp tend to bind with dimers of Hb rather than with whole molecules (tetramers) of Hb to give a complex with a molecular weight (for Hp 1–1) of 135 kDa. When Hb tetramers are bound, the complex has a molecular weight (for Hp 1–1) of 169 kDa.

The complex Hb–Hp is taken up by hepatic parenchymal cells. When the amount of Hb liberated into the plasma corresponds to only a few grams per litre, the Hb complex is cleared exponentially with a half-time on the order of 20 min (Garby and Noyes 1959), but at higher Hb levels the clearance system is saturated and a constant amount of approximately 0.13 g of Hb per litre of plasma is cleared per hour (Laurell and Nyman 1957; Faulstick et al. 1962). After the injection of amounts of Hb calculated to suppress the Hp level to zero, the Hp level rose to 50% of the pre-injection level in 36 h and to 100% in 7–9 days (Noyes and Garby 1967).

Haemopexin (Hx) is a protein present in plasma in low concentration, to which methaem, derived from circulating free metHb, binds preferentially. Hx also binds haem from methaemalbumin and may provide the primary clearance route for haem complexed in this way (Muller-Eberhard et al. 1969).

Methaemalbumin is a pigment formed by haem (methaem) that is not bound to Hx, bound with albumin. Apart from acute haemolytic incidents, methaemalbumin is found in the plasma only when the amount of Hp has been reduced to a negligible level, less than 5 mg/dl (Nyman et al. 1959). The rapid infusion of 14 g of Hb into an adult will lead to the formation of sufficient methaemalbumin to give a positive Schumm's test, although about three times this amount of pigment must be present before it can be detected spectroscopically. Methaemalbumin can be detected about 5 h after injecting Hb and remains detectable for 24 h or more (Fairley 1940).

Haemoglobinuria

When the amount of Hb not bound by Hp reaches about 0.25 g/l, some is excreted in the urine. The clearance of Hb by the kidney is only 5% of that of water or 6 ml of plasma per minute per 1.73 m² of body surface compared with 100 ml plasma per minute for insulin (Lathem 1959). Some Hb is reabsorbed by the renal tubules (Lathem et al. 1960). At plasma Hb levels of approximately 1.8 g/l induced in normal males, the amount of Hb reabsorbed was approximately 1.4 mg/min, which was about one-third of the amount being filtered by the glomeruli (Lowenstein et al. 1961).

The fact that in most subjects haemoglobinuria occurs only when the plasma level exceeds about 1.5 g/l was known long before the role of Hp was appreciated (Ottenberg and Fox 1938; Gilligan et al. 1941). The latter investigators found that when the initial plasma Hb concentration was 0.4–0.6 g/l, the plasma was cleared in 5 h; when the initial level was 1.0–2.25 g/l the period was 8 h; and when the initial level was 2.8–3.0 g/l the plasma was not cleared for 12 h.

After the infusion or liberation of relatively large amounts of Hb into the circulation, up to one-third may be excreted in the urine. In six subjects receiving rapid injections of 12–18 g of Hb, the average amount excreted was about 18% of the amount injected (Amberson et al. 1949). In dogs transfused with incompatible blood in amounts equivalent to giving 200–1000 ml to an adult human, the amount of Hb excreted in the urine varied from 10% to 40% of the amount in the transfused red cells (Yuile et al. 1949).

Haemosiderinuria. When free Hb is filtered through the glomeruli, some or all of it is reabsorbed by the renal tubules and the iron released is stored as haemosiderin. If this process continues for a long period, iron-laden cells and free haemosiderin are found in the urine (see Bothwell and Finch 1962, p. 413). Haemosiderinuria is invariably found in adults whose plasma Hb concentration exceeds 0.25 g/l. Only microscopic amounts are found when the plasma Hb is below 0.20 g/l, but larger amounts are found when the level exceeds 0.50 g/l (Crosby and Dameshek 1951).

Bilirubinaemia following infusions of haemoglobin

The serum bilirubin concentration rises by about 0.5 mg/dl (1 mg/dl = 17 µmol/l) after an infusion of 14–21 g of Hb, and the maximum concentration is reached 3–6 h after injection (Fairley 1940). A similar rise was noted in a subject injected with 16 g in whom the maximum plasma Hb concentration was 3.8 g/l (Gilligan et al. 1941). One gram of Hb is converted to 40 mg of bilirubin (With 1949). Therefore the catabolism of 16 g of Hb should yield 640 mg of bilirubin. If this were liberated into the plasma of an adult who was incapable of excreting bilirubin, the plasma bilirubin concentration would rise by about 10 mg/dl (170 µmol/l), assuming that about one-half of the liberated bilirubin diffused rapidly into the extra-vascular fluid space (Weech et al. 1941). In practice the bilirubin is delivered to the circulation over a period of several hours and excretion almost keeps pace with production.

Extravascular destruction

Destruction by antibodies that are slowly lytic or only occasionally lytic *in vitro*

Lewis antibodies

Many examples of anti-Le[a] and a few examples of anti-Le[b] lyse untreated red cells *in vitro* although lysis occurs only slowly. When small amounts of Le(a+) red cells are injected into the circulation of a patient with potent anti-Le[a] the cells are normally cleared by the mononuclear phagocyte system (MPS) with the liberation of only traces of Hb in the plasma. Haemoglobinuria has been observed after the transfusion of relatively large amounts of Le(a+) red cells, perhaps because the amount of Hb released is greater, or possibly because, owing to slow clearance, the cells have time to undergo lysis in the circulation before clearance by the 'overloaded' MPS can occur.

In a patient, WB, whose serum contained anti-Le[a], capable of causing slow but appreciable lysis of Le(a+) red cells *in vitro*, 2 ml of Le(a+) red cells labelled with ^{51}Cr were infused and found to be cleared with a half-time of approximately 2 min. The maximum amount of ^{51}Cr found in the plasma during the following 40 min was 2% of the total injected as intact red cells. A few weeks previously, this same patient had developed haemoglobinuria following the transfusion of 250 ml of Le(a+) blood. It is possible that the haemoglobinuria developed because clearance of the large volume of Le(a+) red cells was substantially slower, so that there was time for intravascular haemolysis to occur. A second factor may have been the low Hp level in this patient, which would have led to haemoglobinuria at relatively low levels of haemoglobinaemia.

A similar phenomenon was observed during experiments with stored red cells in rabbits by Hughes-Jones and Mollison (1963). The red cells used for the experiments were rendered non-viable by storage at 37°C in trisodium citrate for 24 or 48 h. *In vitro* these red cells underwent rapid spontaneous haemolysis (5% per hour). When small numbers of red cells were infused, they were cleared rapidly by the MPS without liberation of Hb into the plasma. However when very large amounts of the red cells were transfused, so that the MPS was overloaded and complete clearance took more than 24 h, gross haemoglobinaemia and haemoglobinuria developed, presumably because the red cells were destroyed within the bloodstream before they could be phagocytosed by the MPS.

Other cold alloantibodies

As described in the previous chapter, cold alloantibodies cause *in vivo* red cell destruction only when they are active at 37°C *in vitro*. Because such antibodies should be detected in compatibility testing, it is not surprising that the literature contains only two examples of immediate haemolytic reactions due to anti-P_1 (Moureau 1945; Arndt *et al.* 1998) and only five due to anti-M (Broman 1944; Wiener 1950; Strahl *et al.* 1955) or anti-N (Yoell 1966; Delmas-Marsalet *et al.* 1967). In fact, in four out of the seven cases just referred to, no crossmatching at all was carried out before transfusion and in one of the remaining three (Strahl *et al.* 1955) only an agglutination test was carried out; subsequent testing showed that the antibody was readily detectable by IAT. The thermal range of cold alloantibodies occasionally increases after transfusion and in rare cases these antibodies have been the cause of DHTRs (see below).

Anti-Jk^a and anti-Jk^b

Anti-Jk^a and anti-Jk^b are occasionally weakly lytic *in vitro*. Although tests with small doses of incompatible red cells indicate that destruction is usually extravascular, incompatible transfusions due to these antibodies are sometimes characterized by haemoglobinuria and C8–9-mediated destruction is almost certainly involved. Haemolytic reactions due to anti-Jk^a are characterized by difficulty in detecting the antibody and by the occurrence of haemoglobinuria.

In one case, a woman who had been transfused twice previously (4–5 years earlier) received two transfusions at an interval of 9 days. The first of these two produced no obvious ill effects. However, 30 min after the start of the second unit, the patient developed nausea and shivering and passed red urine. A further blood transfusion 3 days later produced a similar clinical picture and this time haemoglobinaemia and methaemalbuminaemia were demonstrated. The

patient's serum contained a typical complement-binding anti-Jk^a (Kronenberg *et al.* 1958). In another case, a 60-year-old woman who had never been transfused before but had had five pregnancies was transfused with 300 ml of blood and developed a severe febrile reaction with haemoglobinuria. The blood had been screened as compatible but on repeat testing, a very weak anti-Jk^a was discovered (Degnan and Rosenfield 1965). In one case mentioned in Chapter 10, 50% of the radioactivity of an infusion of ^{51}Cr-labelled red cells was found in the plasma, clearly indicating intravascular lysis.

Destruction by antibodies that fail to activate complement or activate it only to the C3 stage

Antibodies that fail to activate complement include virtually all antibodies of the Rh, MNSs and Lu systems and some of the antibodies in the Kell, Fy, Di and various other systems. Conversely, some Kell, Fy, etc. antibodies activate complement, but only to the C3 stage. Although the binding of C3 determines destruction in the liver (and spleen) rather than in the spleen alone (see Chapter 10), it is not associated with 'intravascular lysis'. Release of Hb into the plasma in 'extravascular' lysis is caused by the destruction of red cells by lysozymes derived from macrophages. Factors that determine the extent of this lysis have yet to be determined. In the case of some antibodies such as Rh D in hyperimmunized subjects, there seems to be an association with *in vitro* antibody potency (Wiener and Peters 1940; Wiener 1941a; Vogel *et al.* 1943).

Some instances of haemoglobinuria following destruction by non-complement-binding antibodies are not well understood, as in the case of those associated with anti-C or -Ce of low titre.

Although the foregoing discussion has focused on the release of Hb into the circulation in extravascular destruction, most incompatible transfusions due to the antibodies considered in this section are not characterized by haemoglobinuria but by hyperbilirubinaemia.

Destruction of donor's red cells by passively acquired antibodies

Anti-Rh D. There is substantial experience with the effect of giving anti-D in an attempt to suppress primary RhD immunization of D-negative subjects who have been accidentally transfused with D-positive red cells. During the rapid destruction of D-positive red cells, some release of free Hb into the plasma occurs, but haemoglobinuria is observed only when the antibody is relatively potent, and even then not uniformly. Following the inadvertent transfusion of about 200 ml of D-positive red cells to a D-negative woman, anti-D was given intravenously, resulting in the destruction of almost all of the D-positive cells within 30 h. The plasma Hb concentration reached a maximum of 1.5 g/l at about 12 h after the onset of the red cell destruction (Eklund and Nevanlinna 1971).

Anti-K. Several cases have been reported in which reactions in K-negative subjects have been caused by the transfusion, either simultaneously or after an interval of only a few days, of K-positive red cells from one donor and of K-negative blood containing anti-K from a second donor: (1) a patient was transfused uneventfully with a K-positive unit but, following the transfusion of 1 unit of K-negative blood 12–24 h later, developed a severe febrile reaction; the patient was found to have a positive DAT. Serum from the K-negative donor was shown to contain anti-K with an IAT titre of 2048 (Zettner and Bove 1963); (2) a patient developed anuria after being transfused with 3 units of blood, two of which were K positive and a third K negative with potent anti-K (titre 2000) in the plasma (Franciosi *et al.* 1967); (3) a patient who was bleeding was transfused with 10 units of blood over a period of 24 h. During the transfusion of the tenth unit, chills and fever developed. A few hours later, haemoglobinaemia and signs of DIC were detected but the patient rapidly improved thereafter. One of the 10 units of blood was found to be K positive and another unit contained anti-K with a titre of more than 1000 (Abbott and Hussain 1970); and (4) a patient with acute leukaemia developed hypotension, malaise and a severe febrile reaction after the transfusion of a unit of granulocytes suspended in 400 ml of plasma with an anti-K titre of 128. Investigations showed that transfusions of granulocytes given during the previous 2 days contained about 30 ml of K-positive red cells (Morse 1978).

Destruction of recipient's red cells by passively acquired antibodies

Very few haemolytic transfusion reactions due to the accidental transfusion of plasma containing anti-D have been described. In one case, a patient who received 250 ml of fresh-frozen plasma following coronary artery bypass surgery developed a haemorrhagic syndrome 6 h later and was found to have a positive DAT. One of the units of fresh-frozen plasma contained anti-D with a titre of 1000. The patient developed renal failure and acute hepatic necrosis but eventually recovered (Goldfinger *et al.* 1979).

In 12 infants, injection of an IgM concentrate, containing about 10% IgM and 90% IgG, intended to protect against Gram-negative bacterial infections, produced mild jaundice and a positive DAT. The preparation was found to have an anti-D titre of 1000 (Ballowitz *et al.* 1981).

Several cases have been reported in which a dose of anti-D immunoglobulin that should have been given to a D-negative mother was in fact given to her D-positive infant. Details of one case are given in Chapter 12.

Febrile reactions associated with the extravascular destruction of antibody-coated red cells

The removal of relatively large numbers of non-viable (stored) red cells from the circulation is not associated with the production of fever or other symptoms. After transfusions of red cells that had been cryopreserved at –79°C in and then washed free of glycerol, no febrile reactions developed, even although in some cases as much as 50 ml of red cells were removed from the circulation within about 1 h (Chaplin *et al.* 1956). Similarly the injection of 50 ml of red cells rendered non-viable by storage at 37°C for 48 h did not produce chills, although 90% of the red cells were removed from the circulation within 20 min (Jandl and Tomlinson 1958).

In contrast, in subjects whose serum contained incomplete anti-D, the injection of 10 ml of washed D-positive red cells produced chills and fever after about 1 h in four out of four cases (Jandl and Kaplan 1960). A severe reaction, with shivering, has been observed in a volunteer injected with only 1 ml of anti-D-sensitized red cells; most of the cells were cleared within 1 h and the reaction, accompanied by generalized aching, developed about 2 h after the injection of the cells (fourth edition, p. 576). Similarly, a D-negative subject whose serum contained approximately 40 µg of anti-D /ml developed a feeling of malaise and coldness, shivering and back pain 2–3 h after the injection of 0.25 ml of red cells of the probable genotype *DcE/DcE*. The same subject had developed similar symptoms on a previous occasion following the injection of 0.5 ml of red cells of the probable genotype *Dce/dce*, when his anti-D concentration was only about 10 µg/ml. On the other hand, many other volunteers with anti-D levels of 40 µg/ml or more had no reactions following the injection of 0.5 ml of D-positive red cells (HH Gunson, personal communication). Similarly, no symptoms have been observed in some 30 subjects injected with 0.5–1.0 ml of red cells heavily coated with anti-D (PL Mollison, personal observations).

The fever that may develop in association with extravascular red cell destruction is presumed to result from liberation of cytokines into the circulation. In experiments in which human monocytes were incubated with anti-D-sensitized red cells, various cytokines became detectable in the culture supernatants. Cell-associated IL-1β, IL-8 and TNF were detectable at 2 h and clearly identifiable at 4 h. The level of TNF reached a peak at 6 h (Davenport *et al.* 1993). In view of the slight rise in temperature (0.3°C) and absence of chills after the injection of 10 ml of washed A or B red cells to subjects whose serum contains anti-A or anti-B Jandl and Tomlinson (1958) and Jandl and Kaplan (1960) some have suggested that the development of severe febrile reactions following red cell destruction by anti-D may be related to events that occur during splenic sequestration.

Oliguria associated with extravascular destruction

Oliguria is unusual after Rh-incompatible transfusions. In one series, oliguria developed in none out of four cases caused by anti-D and in only one out of six cases due to anti-c (Pineda *et al.* 1978a), and in another series in only 2 out of 10 cases due to anti-D (Vogel *et al.* 1943). The latter series was exceptional in that (1) most subjects were presumed to have had exceptionally potent anti-D following many transfusions of D-incompatible blood and (2) 7 out of 10 developed haemoglobinuria, an uncommon finding after transfusion of Rh D-incompatible blood. Anuria was not observed in any of the foregoing cases but occurred in 3 out of 10 cases due to anti-K and in 1 out of nine cases due to anti-Jk[a] in a Mayo Clinic series (Pineda *et al.* 1978a).

The cause of the renal damage when incompatibility is associated with antibodies other than anti-A and

anti-B is a matter of speculation. Some of the antibodies concerned activate complement but are either non-lytic or only weakly lytic *in vitro*, and bring about extravascular destruction *in vivo*. As these cases suggest an association between renal failure and haemoglobinuria, it is possible that circulating Hb triggers renal failure, possibly by binding nitric oxide. Alternatively, the release of endothelin following the generation of IL-1 may be a precipitating factor (Capon and Goldfinger 1995). The patients concerned are often already seriously ill and may have problems such as hypotension that contribute to the development of renal failure.

Destruction of red cells rendered non-viable by storage

The removal of non-viable red cells from the bloodstream is not associated with the liberation of any detectable amount of Hb into the plasma. This conclusion is based on observations with ^{51}Cr-labelled red cells (Jandl and Tomlinson 1958; see also Fig. 11.3) and on sensitive measurements of plasma Hb (Cassell

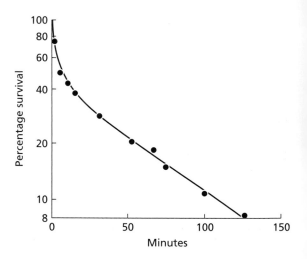

Fig 11.3 Rate of destruction of 'non-viable' stored red cells. A sample of blood was taken from a normal subject and stored at 4°C with trisodium citrate for 2 weeks. The red cells were then washed, labelled with ^{51}Cr, washed again and injected. As the figure shows, over 90% of the red cells were removed from the circulation in 2 h. The amount of radioactivity in the plasma never exceeded a level corresponding to 0.2% of the total dose injected.

and Chaplin 1961), and applies to red cells stored in the frozen as well as in the liquid state (Valeri 1965).

After transfusion of non-viable stored red cells, the serum bilirubin concentration normally reaches a peak about 5 h after transfusion (Mollison and Young 1942; Vaughan 1942). Jaundice is commonly observed in subjects with severe injuries who receive transfusions of large volumes of stored blood. In a series of 16 carefully studied cases, hyperbilirubinaemia reached a maximum about 5 days after the initial transfusion. All the subjects had bilirubin as well as elevated urobilinogen in the urine, indicating some interference with liver function. In these circumstances a transfusion of stored blood acts as a crude measure of liver function (Sevitt 1958).

Does loading of the mononuclear phagocyte system with non-viable red cells increase susceptibility to infection?

Experiments in mice suggest that loading with erythrocytes has some effect on the cells of the MPS, which makes them less effective in killing engulfed bacteria (Kaye and Hook 1963). It is not known whether this finding can be extrapolated to indicate that transfusion of large amounts of non-viable red cells is potentially harmful. However, a small number of observational studies of different patient populations have demonstrated a statistical association between prolonged storage of allogeneic blood and (1) rate of infection in trauma patients, (2) mortality in the intensive care unit and (3) postoperative pneumonia in open-heart surgery patients (Klein 2003).

Delayed haemolytic transfusion reactions

When incompatible red cells are transfused, the amount of antibody in the recipient's serum may be too low to effect rapid red cell destruction or even to be detected by sensitive compatibility tests. However, the transfusion may provoke an anamnestic immune response so that, a few days after transfusion, a rapid increase in antibody concentration develops and rapid destruction of the transfused red cells occurs.

Hédon (1902) was the first to describe a DHTR. After finding that rabbit serum that agglutinated and lysed red cells from pigs, horses and humans had scarcely any effect on dog red cells, he tried transfusing washed dog red cells to rabbits. After removing 120 ml of blood from a rabbit over a period of 1 h, he transfused it with 50 ml of a saline suspension of dog red cells. For the next 3 days the rabbit passed urine of a normal colour, but on the fourth day haemoglobinuria developed. By the fifth day the urine had turned black. On the sixth day the urine was deep yellow and by the eighth day after the transfusion had returned to a normal colour. Hédon noted that on about the fourth day after transfusion the serum of the rabbit became haemolytic and strongly agglutinating for dog red cells. When a second transfusion of dog red cells was given to rabbits immediate haemoglobinuria developed and, if a sufficient amount of red cells was transfused, rapid death ensued.

Virtually all DHTRs are due to secondary responses. Most commonly, the recipient has been immunized by one or more transfusions or pregnancies. Occasional DHTRs are observed following the transfusion of ABO-incompatible blood to a subject who has not been transfused previously, but subjects lacking A or B display typical secondary responses when exposed to these antigens and can be regarded as being always primarily immunized. In theory, a DHTR could be caused by a primary immune response but this event is expected to be rare. The most potent red cell alloantigen apart from A and B is Rh D. Following the transfusion of D-positive blood to a D-negative recipient, anti-D is seldom detectable before 4 weeks and even then is present only in low concentration. No case of a DHTR due to primary immunization to Rh D has been described but two suggestive cases involving immunization to K:6 and C, respectively, have been reported. In both, the interval between transfusion and the onset of red cell destruction was far longer than in the usual DHTR and, in one case at least, previous immunization was unlikely.

1 A white woman who had had four pregnancies by her K:6-negative husband, but who had had no earlier transfusions, developed a haemolytic syndrome 23 days after being transfused with 3 units of blood, one of which was K:6 positive. The unit was from a black donor; the frequency of the K:6 phenotype is 19% in black people but only 0.1% in white people. The patient's PCV, which, 5 days earlier had been 30%, fell to 25%, her reticulocyte count rose to 16% and her serum bilirubin to 2.1 mg/dl; spherocytosis was present. Her serum was found to contain anti-K6. Although the DAT was negative, anti-K6 was eluted from her red cells (Taddie et al. 1982).

2 A previously untransfused woman of probable Rh geno-type DcE/dce with a husband of probable genotype DCe/DCe was transfused with 12 units of blood after her first delivery. Five days later, her Hb concentration was 104 g/l. Four weeks later she developed haemoglobinuria; her Hb at that time was 80 g/l and her DAT was weakly positive with anti-complement only. After a further 5 days, the Hb was 89 g/l, the reticulocyte count was 17% but the haemoglobinuria had ceased. Eight weeks after delivery, anti-C was detectable in the plasma for the first time (Patten *et al.* 1982). Immuniza-tion to C during pregnancy may have played some role in this immune response (Mollison and Newland 1976).

Early descriptions of delayed haemolytic transfusion reactions in humans

The case described by Boorman and co-workers (1946) as a 'delayed blood-transfusion-incompatibility reaction' seems to be the first account of a DHTR in humans. The patient was a young woman with pul-monary tuberculosis and haemolytic anaemia; her blood group was A_2. She was given a transfusion of group O blood and, between 4 and 7 days afterward, 8 units of group A blood. At least 7 units were sub-sequently shown to be A_1. One week after the last transfusion she became severely jaundiced and anti-A_1, which had not previously been detected in her serum, was demonstrable (titre 32 at 37°C); some

20% of the group O transfused cells were still present in the circulation, but there were no circulating A_1 cells.

Other early descriptions of DHTR in humans include: (1) haemoglobinuria developing 8 days after transfusion shown to be due to anti-K [Collins, quoted by Young (1954)]; (2) accelerated destruction of Rh D-positive red cells starting on about the fourth day after transfusion (Mollison and Cutbush 1955; Fig. 11.4); and (3) jaundice and oliguria developing 10 days after the first of a series of transfusions, shown to be due to anti-k (Fudenberg and Allen 1957).

Clinical features of delayed haemolytic transfusion reactions

The most constant features are fever and a fall in Hb concentration (Pineda *et al.* 1978a). Other features that are often observed are jaundice and haemoglobinuria.

Jaundice

Jaundice does not appear before day 5 after trans-fusion. In nine reported cases in which adequate data were provided, jaundice was first noted at a mean of 6.9 days after transfusion (see fourth edition, p. 619). Jaundice may occur as late as 10 days after transfusion (Croucher *et al.* 1967).

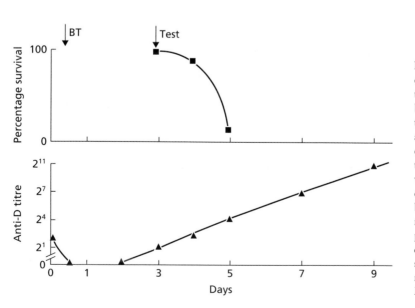

Fig 11.4 Delayed haemolytic reaction due to anti-D. The patient was transfused with 1 unit of D-positive blood on day 0 before it was realized that her serum contained a trace of anti-D. There were no signs of red cell destruction and 3 days later when a test dose of 1 ml of D-positive red cells was given, only 10% of the cells were destroyed within 24 h. However, between days 4 and 5 almost all the remaining labelled cells and presumably also the transfused red cells were destroyed; the anti-D titre started to increase on day 3 and reached 1000 on day 9 (data from Mollison and Cutbush 1955).

Haemoglobinuria

Haemoglobinuria is not uncommon in patients with DHTRs, and may occur in association with antibodies of many different specificities: anti-Jk^a (Rauner and Tanaka 1967); anti-Jk^b (Kurtides *et al.* 1966; Holland and Wallerstein 1968); anti-C (or Ce), in five cases described by Pickles and colleagues (1978); anti-c (Roy and Lotto 1962); anti-c plus anti-M (Croucher *et al.* 1967); anti-U (Meltz *et al.* 1971; Rothman *et al* 1976); anti-HI, -Jk^b, -S and -Fy^b (Giblett *et al.* 1965); anti-E, -K, -S and -Fy^a (Moncrieff and Thompson 1975); and anti-c, -E and -Jk^b (Joseph *et al.* 1964). In these 15 cases the mean interval between transfusion and haemoglobinuria was 7.9 days.

The association of anti-C (or -Ce) with haemoglobinuria is surprising. Apart from the five cases mentioned in the preceding paragraph, in all of which the antibody titre was relatively low, at least three cases have been encountered at the Puget Sound Blood Center, all characterized by intravascular haemolysis associated with anti-C reacting weakly *in vitro* (ER Giblett, personal communication, 1981).

DHTRs in patients with sickle cell disease frequently present with haemoglobinuria. An 11-year retrospective chart review of paediatric patients with a discharge diagnosis of sickle cell disease and transfusion reaction found seven patients who developed nine episodes of DHTR occurring 6–10 days after transfusion (Talano *et al.* 2003). Each presented with fever and haemoglobinuria. All but one patient experienced pain initially ascribed to vaso-occlusive crisis. The DAT was positive in only two out of the nine episodes. The presenting Hb was lower than pretransfusion levels in eight out of the nine events. Severe complications observed after the onset of DHTR included acute chest syndrome (3), pancreatitis (1), congestive heart failure (1), and acute renal failure (1). It is particularly important to consider this possibility in patients with apparent exacerbations of sickle cell syndromes within 10 days of transfusion, and to avoid additional transfusions when possible. When transfusion is necessary, red cells typed to avoid a variety of antigens known to provoke these reactions should be provided if the patient's extended phenotype is not available to assist with blood selection (Diamond *et al.* 1980).

Renal failure

DHTRs are only occasionally followed by renal failure. Moreover, when this complication does occur it is usually difficult to know what role, if any, has been played by the transfusion reaction, as the patients concerned often have concomitant failure of other systems. Although renal failure occurred in the case reported by Meltz and co-workers (1971) associated with anti-U, there was little evidence that the renal damage was due to intravascular lysis. In a case reported by Holland and Wallerstein (1968) due to anti-Jk^b, oliguria and uraemia developed about 2 weeks after the transfusion of 3 units of Jk(b+) blood; an additional unit of Jk(b+) blood was transfused at about the time of onset of oliguria. Renal failure has been reported in sickle cell patients with DHTR (Talano *et al.* 2003), but this is often in the setting of generalized sickling in patients with underlying renal disease.

Although renal failure was noted in 4 out of 23 DHTRs reported from the Mayo Clinic (Pineda *et al.* 1978a), all of the patients had serious underlying disease; in a later series from the same institution, not a single case of renal failure was reported in 37 patients (Moore *et al.* 1980).

Interval between transfusion and the time of maximal red cell destruction

As judged by the day after transfusion on which jaundice or haemoglobinuria occurs, increased red cell destruction does not begin before the fourth day after transfusion (see also Fig. 11.5).

When signs of red cell destruction develop within 24–48 h of transfusion, the patient has usually been transfused during the development of a secondary response to a transfusion given some days previously. A case described by Lundberg and McGinniss (1975) of an A$_2$B patient who developed anti-A$_1$ is a good example. The patient had been sensitized by an initial transfusion of A$_1$-positive blood and received a second transfusion of A$_1$-positive blood 6 weeks later. A third transfusion of A$_1$-positive blood, given 5 days after the second, was followed within 48 h by signs of red cell destruction, most likely because a secondary response to the second transfusion was developing. Anti-A$_1$ was not detected in the compatibility test at the time of the second transfusion, but was active at 37°C 4 days later.

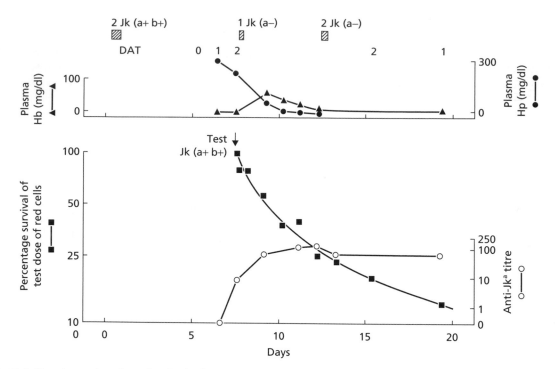

Fig 11.5 Slow destruction of transfused red cells in a delayed haemolytic transfusion reaction due to anti-Jkᵃ. The direct antiglobulin test (DAT) became weakly positive 6 days after an uneventful transfusion, but no alloantibodies could be detected in the plasma. On the same day that a dose of ^{51}Cr-labelled red cells was injected, anti-Jkᵃ was detected in the plasma. Although the titre of anti-Jkᵃ rose to 64 on day 9 and to 128 by day 12, the labelled red cells, and presumably the transfused red cells, were eliminated slowly, over a period of 3 weeks after the original transfusion. It may be relevant that the patient's spleen had been removed at the time of the original transfusion. The maximum rate of red cell destruction occurred between days 8 and 10 when mild haemoglobinaemia and a fall in plasma haptoglobin (Hp) were observed (from (Mollison and Newlands 1976).

In one exceptional case, signs of red cell destruction did not develop until about 3 weeks after a 6-unit transfusion given during a splenectomy. Anti-Fyᵇ was detected in the patient's serum. The late onset of red cell destruction might have been related to an altered immune response associated with the splenectomy (Boyland *et al.* 1982).

In DHTR, incompatible cells are not usually found in the recipient's circulation more than about 2 weeks after the transfusion, although in the case illustrated in Fig. 11.5 incompatible cells could still be detected 3 weeks after transfusion.

Occasionally, signs of an IHTR and of a delayed reaction are combined, such as when the recipient has a relatively low-titre antibody, so that there are only very mild signs of red cell destruction at the time of transfusion and further signs of destruction develop a few days later as the antibody reappears in the circulation. An example of such a reaction is shown in Fig. 11.6.

Haematological and serological features of delayed haemolytic transfusion reactions

Haematological findings

The regular occurrence of anaemia has already been described.

Spherocytosis is often noted in blood films taken from patients during DHTR and may be the first indication that red cell destruction is occurring. When large amounts of blood have been transfused, the majority of the red cells in the patient's blood may be involved in a subsequent DHTR, and a picture closely resembling AIHA may develop (Croucher *et al.* 1967).

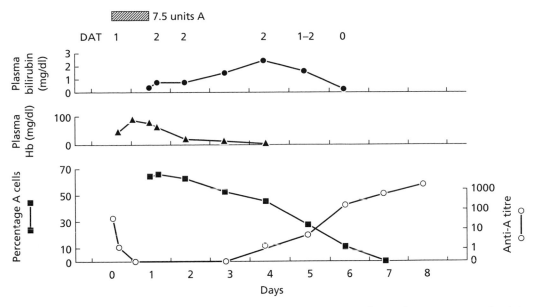

Fig 11.6 Mild immediate haemolytic reaction combined with a delayed haemolytic reaction following the transfusion of 7.5 units of group A blood to a group O subject whose plasma contained a relatively low-titre anti-A (32). The only sign of immediate red cell destruction was transient haemoglobinaemia. During the following 3 days, no anti-A could be detected in the plasma although appreciable destruction of group A red cells occurred from day 2 onwards and the serum bilirubin concentration reached a peak on day 4. Following the reappearance of anti-A, red cell destruction accelerated and was complete by day 7. Estimates of the survival of group A red cells were made by the differential agglutination/^{51}Cr method referred to on p. 347. As indicated, the direct antiglobulin test (DAT) turned negative by day 6. However, the results shown refer to tests with anti-IgG. With anti-C3d the test was still positive on day 11 (sixth edition 1979, p. 579, supplemented by unpublished data).

The patient had had two pregnancies and a blood transfusion between 16 and 18 years previously. On the present occasion she had been transfused with 9 units of blood in 6 days because of severe bleeding from fibroids. On day 6 she underwent a hysterectomy but, although the bleeding stopped, her Hb concentration continued to fall. From day 7 onwards, and up to about day 20, spherocytes were present on her peripheral blood films. Jaundice was noticed on day 9 and began to fade by day 13. Her urine contained 'blood' on day 10. On the same day her Hb concentration was found to have fallen to 62 g/l, the reticulocyte count was 13%, the serum bilirubin concentration 4.5 mg/dl, and the Hp concentration was nil. The DAT was strongly positive. A minor degree of red cell autoagglutination was observed and the serum reacted with all 30 samples tested. Based on the findings, the diagnosis of AIHA seemed possible. However, a sample composed largely of the recipient's own red cells was obtained by differential centrifugation and these cells were found to have a negative DAT and did not react with the patient's own serum. The patient's serum was found to contain the alloantibodies anti-Fy^a, anti-Ce and anti-e.

Serological findings

Positive direct antiglobulin test. Characteristically, the DAT becomes positive a few days after transfusion and remains positive until the incompatible transfused red cells have been eliminated (but see below). By making an eluate from the red cells it may be possible to identify the alloantibody responsible for the reaction at a time when antibody can be detected only with difficulty in the patient's plasma.

Antibody in plasma. It is typical of DHTRs that even when antibody has been present in the recipient's plasma immediately before transfusion, no free antibody is found for several days after transfusion. Typically, antibody becomes detectable between about 4 and 7 days after transfusion and reaches a peak value between 10 and 15 days after transfusion.

479

A D-negative patient was transfused with 6 units of D-positive blood during vascular surgery because insufficient D-negative blood was available and because no anti-D had been detected in his serum before transfusion. A routine blood film 5 days after transfusion showed striking microspherocytosis, which led to the discovery that the DAT was strongly positive and that potent anti-D was present in the serum. Retesting of the pretransfusion sample of serum showed a very low concentration of anti-D, estimated at 0.004 μg/ml; subsequent estimates were as follows: day 6, 90 μg/ml; day 9, 500 μg/ml; and day 12, 460 μg/ml.

In a case reported by Beard and co-workers (1971), the anti-D concentration was higher on day 14 (162 μg/ml) than on day 8 (95 μg/ml).

Some other serological findings in delayed haemolytic transfusion reactions

Persistent direct antiglobulin reactions following delayed haemolytic transfusion reaction. Some DHTRs are first diagnosed when the recipient requires a further blood transfusion and routine tests show that the previously negative DAT has turned positive. As the amount of the induced antibody increases in the recipient's plasma, the surviving incompatible red cells become coated with a sufficient amount of antibody to yield a positive DAT and the test will remain positive until the incompatible cells have been cleared from the circulation. In practice, the situation is even more complex, because the DAT may remain positive after all transfused cells have been cleared from the circulation.

In one series of DHTR, the DAT was found to be positive with anti-C3d 11 days or more after the last transfusion in at least 21 out of 26 cases. The DAT often remained positive for at least 3 months. In a minority of cases the red cells reacted with anti-IgG as well as with anti-C3d (Salama and Mueller-Eckhardt 1984). In another series mainly delayed serological transfusion reactions ('DSTR': see below), the DAT also remained positive for long periods after transfusion – for at least 25 days in 13 out of 15 cases. In this series, the red cells reacted with anti-IgG in 12 out of 15 cases, with anti-complement as well in five and with anti-complement alone in one (Ness *et al.* 1990). In both the foregoing series, in a minority of cases, alloantibody apparently having the same specificity as that in the serum could be eluted from circulating red cells many weeks after transfusion. These findings await explanation, although the pos-

sibility that they represent concurrently produced autoantibodies that either bind alloantibody or mimic alloantibody has substantial supportive evidence (Weber *et al.* 1979).

Development of warm autoantibodies in association with alloimmunization and delayed haemolytic transfusion reaction

Although alloimmunization to erythrocyte antigens is a recognized complication of heavily transfused patients, the frequency of concurrent autoantibody formation is an important but less well-appreciated occurrence. Dameshek and Levine (1943) first described this phenomenon more than 60 years ago in a case report of an alloimmunized patient who developed an autoantibody that resulted in a severe haemolytic episode. The clinical spectrum of these autoantibodies ranges from asymptomatic serological detection to severe life-threatening haemolysis. Chaplin and Zarkowsky (1981) described four patients with sickle cell anaemia who suffered severe autoimmune haemolysis after red blood cell transfusion. All four had previously been alloimmunized. These patients were treated with glucocorticosteroids with good clinical responses and the eventual reversion of their DAT results to negative. In a retrospective review, Castellino and colleagues (1999) described a series of 184 children with sickle cell anaemia, 14 (7.6%) of whom appeared to have transfusion-associated IgG warm-reactive red blood cell autoantibodies. Four of the 14 patients with autoantibodies developed clinically significant haemolysis.

Although most of the reported patients have been transfused for sickle cell disease, in a recent series, three of four patients had different disorders. In one case, the autoantibody found on routine screening had no clinical significance. In another case, the autoantibody made accurate blood typing and subsequent transfusion exceedingly difficult. Two patients experienced haemolysis as a consequence of the autoantibody (Zumberg *et al.* 2001). A typical patient is described below:

A 64-year-old woman with a history of stage IIB inflammatory carcinoma of the right breast underwent high-dose chemotherapy and autologous peripheral blood progenitor cell transplantation. Her blood type was A, Rh positive, and results of serum antibody screen were negative on eight separate occasions. During the 5-month treatment interval prior to the autologous stem cell transplantation, she had received 8 units of group A-compatible red blood cells without incident. The post-transplantation course was complicated by neutropenic fever, requiring intravenous antibiotics, and herpetic oesophagitis was treated successfully with famciclovir. She received an additional 6 units of red blood cells and 43 units of platelets, all gamma irradiated during the peritransplantation period. A DAT performed 6 days after transplantation was negative.

Ten weeks after discharge, the patient developed a low-grade fever nausea and mild diarrhoea. Her PCV had fallen from 0.34 to 0.28. Serological screening revealed anti-E and a weakly positive DAT with polyspecific antihuman globulin and anti-C3b-C3d reagents. The patient received 2 units of E-negative compatible red blood cells. Two weeks later, the PCV had fallen to 0.17, the lactate dehydrogenase level had risen to 542 units/l (normal range 113–226 units/l), and the bilirubin level had risen to 44 µmol/l (2.6 mg/dl) (normal range, 1.7–17 µmol/l (0.1–1.0 mg/dl). There was brisk haemolysis, with spherocytes on the blood film. During the next 2 weeks, serological studies confirmed the presence of an anti-E, a positive DAT with anti-IgG and anti-complement reagents, a panagglutinin in the eluate prepared from the coated red blood cells and serum reactivity consistent with a warm-reactive autoantibody. No other alloantibodies were identified. The patient required 15 additional compatible red blood cell transfusions for the management of her haemolysis. The possibility of drug-associated antibodies was investigated and eliminated. She was eventually treated with a short course of high-dose methylprednisolone sodium succinate, with resolution of autoimmune haemolysis over the next 2 weeks.

The mechanism of the allo/autoimmune response is unknown. It has been proposed that passively acquired erythrocyte alloantibodies bound to recipient antigen-positive red blood cells lead to a conformational change in surface antigen epitopes. These changes may increase the chance that the recipient red blood cells will be recognized as foreign by normal immune surveillance cells and lead to the subsequent formation of an autoantibody (Castellino *et al.* 1999).

The importance of recognizing this syndrome lies in the approach to treatment, which may favour corticosteroids and recombinant erythropoietin over additional transfusion.

Development of cold autoagglutinins. After repeated transfusion of rabbits, cold autoagglutinins may develop. It seems that, in humans also, potent cold autoagglutinins may sometimes develop in association with alloimmunization.

In a case described by Giblett and co-workers (1965), a 15-year-old boy with thalassaemia major who had received several previous transfusions was again transfused without immediate ill-effect, but 7 days later complained of back pain and passed red urine. During the following days, his liver enlarged rapidly, his PCV fell precipitously and methaemoglobinaemia was detectable; during a 3-day period his DAT was positive and a potent cold agglutinin of specificity 'pseudo-anti-IH' appeared in his serum. The authors concluded that the episode of red cell destruction was probably not due to this agglutinin but to other antibodies such as anti-S and anti-Fy[b] that later became detectable in the patient's plasma.

A similar case was encountered by GN Smith (personal communication). In a child aged 11 years with thalassaemia major, the transfusion of 2 units of blood produced an initially satisfactory response but 6 days after transfusion severe anaemia (Hb 3 g/dl) and jaundice developed. Anti-E, anti-Fy[b] and anti-Jk[b] were found in the serum together with a potent cold autoagglutinin of a specificity related to H. Although the autoagglutinin was active up to a temperature of about 30°C *in vitro* and was associated with a positive DAT (complement only) its contribution to the haemolytic process is uncertain.

Are the recipient's own red cells destroyed at an accelerated rate in some delayed haemolytic transfusion reaction?

The finding, referred to above, that following a DHTR the recipient's red cells may develop a positive DAT that persists for at least many weeks does not imply either that an autoantibody is involved or that the cells are undergoing accelerated destruction.

In a case described by Polesky and Bove (1964), there was good evidence of accelerated destruction of the patient's own red cells following a haemolytic transfusion reaction due to anti-Jk[a]. By a fortunate chance, the patient's own red cells had been labelled with ^{51}Cr for a red cell survival study and had been shown to be surviving normally for 1 week before the incompatible transfusion was given. After the haemolytic reaction due to anti-Jk[a], there was a rapid and substantial increase in the rate of destruction of the patient's own red cells. It has been suggested that the phenomenon of reactive lysis, the lysis of 'bystander' cells by C5b6 released from cells undergoing lysis by the membrane attack complex of complement, may explain the destruction of some of the recipient's red cells in haemolytic transfusion reactions (Greene *et al.* 1993).

Although little evidence supports this hypothesis, the phenomenon might account for red cell destruction in patients of groups A or B grafted with group O bone marrow, in whom transfused group O cells may be haemolysed (Gajewski *et al.* 1992).

Alloantibodies involved in delayed haemolytic transfusion reactions

In estimating the relative frequency with which different antibodies are involved, reviews of individual case reports are misleading because of the propensity to publish unusual cases. The best estimates can be obtained by analysing experience from particular centres over a relatively long period. Three such series are available for analysis: (1) Mayo Clinic, 1964–73, 23 cases (Pineda *et al.* 1978b); (2) Mayo Clinic, 1974–77, 37 cases (Moore *et al.* 1980); and (3) Toronto General Hospital 1974–78, 40 cases (Croucher 1979).

In each series there were cases in which more than one alloantibody was found in the patient's serum. In the following analysis, the published figures for the number of such cases have been revised slightly as follows: first, when both alloantibodies belonged to the same blood group system, for example anti-c and anti-E, the patient has been regarded as having only a single antibody; second, when one of the alloantibodies was known to be a common cause of a DHTR, such as anti-Jk^a, and the second alloantibody was a cold agglutinin such as anti-P_1, which hardly ever causes a DHTR, the case has again been regarded as having only one specificity, i.e. anti-Jk^a in this example. With these minor revisions the figures for the 100 cases were as follows: one alloantibody, 90 cases; two alloantibodies, 10 cases; of the cases in which only one antibody was found the specificities of the antibodies were as follows: Rh system, 31 (34.4%); Jk system, 27 (30%); Fy system, 13 (14.4%); Kell system, 12 (13.3%); MNSs system, 4 (4.4%); and others, 3 (3.3%). Among the 10 cases in which more than one specificity was found, the specificities were as follows: Rh, 8; Kell, 6; Jk 3; Fy, 2; and S, 1. In Chapter 3 (Table 3.6) these figures are compared with the relative frequencies with which the different red cell alloantibodies are found in random transfusion recipients and in patients who have had haemolytic transfusion reactions.

Further details of the figures given above are as follows: of the 90 cases in which only one antibody was involved, Rh system: anti-D or -D, -E, 3; -c, 5; -c, -E, 6; -E, 12; -C or -C^w, 3; -C, -E, 1; -e, 1; Jk system: 27 (-Jk^a, 24; -Jk^b, 23); Fy system: 13 (all -Fy^a); Kell system: 12 (all anti-K); MNSs system: 4 (-M, 2; -S, 1; -s, 1); anti-A_1, 1; anti-Le^a, -Le^b (see comment below), 1; and unidentified, 1.

As expected, anti-D is involved relatively infrequently, that is when, owing to a shortage of D-negative blood, D-positive blood is transfused to a D-negative subject whose plasma lacks detectable anti-D but who has been sensitized in the past by either previous transfusion or previous pregnancy.

Antibodies not mentioned in the above list but mentioned earlier in the chapter include anti-A, -B, -k, -Fy^b and -U. Others that have been implicated include anti-ce(f) (O'Reilly *et al.* 1985), anti-N (Ballas *et al.* 1985), anti-Lu^b (Greenwalt and Sasaki 1957), anti-Di^b (Thompson *et al.* 1967), anti-Do^b (Moheng *et al.* 1985) and anti-Co^b (Squires *et al.* 1985).

Cold alloantibodies have only very rarely been involved: anti-A_1 in five published cases (Boorman *et al.* 1946; Salmon *et al.* 1959; Perkins *et al.* 1964; Lundberg and McGinniss 1975; Pineda *et al.* 1978a); anti-P_1 in one (Dinapoli *et al.* 1977); and anti-M in one (Alperin *et al.* 1983).

Lewis antibodies have been believed to be responsible for a DHTR in two cases (Pineda *et al.* 1978b; Weir *et al.* 1987), but neither case is entirely convincing. The fact that transfused red cells rapidly assume the Lewis phenotype of the recipient makes it unlikely that Lewis antibodies can cause DHTR. For an example of a case in which, following the transfusion of Le(a+) red cells to an Le(a–b–) subject, a powerful secondary response failed to produce a DHTR, see Chapter 10.

DHTR associated with ABO-incompatible bone marrow transplantation

In the first case to be reported, a patient of group O was prepared for a transplant of bone marrow from a group AB donor by a plasma exchange of 11 l, which reduced the anti-A and anti-B titres of the plasma to low levels. Four units of group AB cells were then transfused without reaction, followed by the bone marrow. The total volume of AB cells transfused, including those in the transplanted marrow, was estimated at 1625 ml. On the sixth day after transplantation the patient became acutely dyspnoeic and was found to have a PCV of 0.18, a positive DAT and hyperbilirubinaemia with extensive agglutination of red cells on a blood smear. Anti-A and anti-B were eluted from circulating red cells. The patient was given group O red cells and corticosteroids and recovered rapidly (Warkentin *et al.* 1983).

Frequency of delayed haemolytic transfusion reactions

In three successive series from the Mayo Clinic over the period 1964–80, the frequency with which DHTRs were diagnosed, in relation to the numbers of units of blood transfused, increased as follows: 1964–73, 1 per 11 650; 1974–77, 1 per 4000; and 1978–80, 1 per 1500. The increase was attributed to a number of factors, including the introduction of more sensitive methods of antibody detection and a greater awareness of the syndrome, leading to an increasing tendency to include asymptomatic cases (Taswell *et al.* 1981). This latter point raises the question of the criteria for diagnosis.

The definition of a DHTR is accelerated destruction of transfused red cells after an interval, during which the recipient mounts an immune response to an antigen carried by the transfused cells. The problem is that, whereas it is relatively easy to demonstrate that a 'new' antibody has been produced following transfusion, it may be difficult to diagnose accelerated destruction of transfused red cells. The usual clinical criteria of increased destruction, fever and progressive anaemia, sometimes accompanied by jaundice or haemoglobinuria, have been discussed above, but the absence of all of these signs clearly does not exclude relatively minor increases in the rate of destruction. An example of a subclinical DHTR is given in Fig. 11.5.

Concept of delayed serological transfusion reaction

The term DSTR has been used to describe an anamnestic response following a transfusion but with no signs of haemolysis (Ness *et al.* 1990). The concept is not entirely satisfactory because there are bound to be differences in the assiduity with which signs of destruction are sought. For example, one observer might be satisfied to look for jaundice, whereas another would make daily estimations of serum bilirubin concentration. Furthermore, accelerated destruction of red cells

may be silent, detectable only by direct measurement of red cell survival (Fig. 11.5). Despite the absence of a clear-cut distinction from a DHTR, the concept of a DSTR is a useful one, as it recognizes the fact that anamnestic responses without overt signs or symptoms of haemolysis are common.

Frequency of delayed haemolytic transfusion reaction and delayed serological transfusion reaction

Between 1980 and 1992 more than half a million units of blood or red cells were transfused at the Mayo Clinic. Diagnoses of DHTR vs. DSTR were made while the patient was hospitalized or shortly after discharge. The frequency of DHTR was 1 in 5405 units and that of DSTR 1 in 2990 units (combined frequency 1 in 1899 units). Anti-Jk^a and anti-Fy^a were more likely to be associated with a DHTR than a DSTR, but the converse was true for antibodies belonging to the Rh and Kell systems (Vamvakas *et al.* 1995). In a much smaller series (about 50 000 units transfused to about 10 000 patients), the frequency of DSTR was similar (1 per 3000 units) but that of DHTR was less than one per 10 000 units (Pinkerton *et al.* 1992).

In a prospective study, 530 patients, 183 of whom had been pregnant or had been transfused previously, were tested 1 week after they had undergone cardiac surgery involving transfusion, most commonly of 2–6 units. Of the 530, 2% developed new antibodies but not one developed a positive DAT or signs of red cell destruction (Hewitt *et al.* 1988).

A high incidence of DHTR was reported in a small series of patients undergoing partial exchange transfusion in sickle cell disease. Of 18 patients, three developed a DHTR (Diamond *et al.* 1980). Similarly, in a series of 107 patients with sickle cell disease who received regular transfusions, 14 developed a DHTR (Vichinsky *et al.* 1990). This is much higher than the combined frequency of DSTR and DHTR (9%) in other series (Aygun *et al.* 2002).

Mortality associated with delayed haemolytic transfusion reactions

When patients die during the course of a DHTR, it is usually difficult to implicate the transfusion reaction as a cause of death. The series of Pineda and co-workers

(1978b) included three deaths, but the authors commented that there was serious underlying disease in all cases and that the 'hemolytic reaction merely complicated a tempestuous course that was undoubtedly lethal'. On the other hand, cases have been described in which the occurrence of a DHTR appears to have tipped the scale decisively against the patient's recovery. Perhaps the most clear-cut example was a case described by Bove (1968) in which a man aged 32 years was transfused with 10 units during an operation for the repair of a hiatus hernia. He progressed well until the seventh day after operation when chills and fever developed, the PCV fell from about 0.40 to 0.25 and haemoglobinuria was noted. Anti-Fy^b and anti-Jk^a were found in the serum and the DAT was strongly positive. The patient became anuric and progressively more anaemic, and died 8 days after the onset of the haemolytic syndrome. In a similar case, although in a man aged 72 years, sudden fever, cyanosis and acute respiratory distress developed on the sixth day after a partial gastrectomy and blood transfusion. There was haemoglobinuria and the DAT was positive. Anti-E and anti-c were found in the serum. The patient developed anuria and died (Hillman 1979).

Haemolytic syndrome after grafting due to an immune response by lymphocytes in a graft

Transplanted organs contain lymphocytes. Unless the organ is irradiated before transplantation the lymphocytes may survive and proliferate in the host, particularly when the host receives immunosuppressive treatment, and mount an immune response against host antigens. Haemolytic syndromes have frequently been observed 1–2 weeks after the transplantation of organs from group O donors to recipients of other blood groups. In the first reported case, 7 days after the transplantation of a lung from a group O donor to a group A recipient, potent anti-A was demonstrated in the recipient's serum. The authors speculated that the agglutinin might have been produced 'by lymphoreticular tissue transplanted with the lung' (Beck 1971). Many examples of haemolytic syndromes developing after grafting, associated with the development of antibodies outside the ABO system, have also been described. The fact that antibodies developing after grafting are alloantibodies (derived from the graft donor) and not autoantibodies has been demonstrated

by showing that they are of the same Gm type as the donor (Ahmed *et al.* 1987; Swanson *et al.* 1987).

Renal grafts

Numerous cases of severe haemolytic syndromes have been reported following transplantation of a kidney from a group O donor to a group A or B recipient. In reporting three cases, Mangal and co-workers (1984) stated that a retrospective analysis of their records showed that of four earlier cases in which an unirradiated kidney from a group O donor had been transplanted to a group A or B recipient receiving ciclosporin, three had developed 'pseudo-autoantibodies' (anti-A or anti-B). No such antibodies had been observed in 21 recipients of irradiated kidneys treated with either azathioprine or ciclosporin. Detailed studies on two further patients were reported by Bevan and co-workers (1985).

The production of Rh antibodies by lymphocytes in transplanted kidneys has also been described. In one case, cadaver kidneys from an O, D-negative donor with weak anti-D in the plasma were transplanted to two D-positive subjects. Both patients developed rejection episodes with anti-D in the serum and a positive DAT about 3 weeks later (Ramsey *et al.* 1986). Similarly, anti-c associated with immune red cell destruction developed in the recipient of a cadaver kidney from a donor whose serum contained anti-c (Herron *et al.* 1986). In another case of the development of anti-c, the donor was a D-positive subject who had been transfused with 4 units of D-positive blood 5–7 days before death and was presumed to have been thereby primarily immunized to c antigen (Hjelle *et al.* 1988).

In an e-positive patient who developed anti-e following a renal transplant from a living donor (the mother), a severe haemolytic anaemia lasted for 4 months (Swanson *et al.* 1985).

Bone marrow cannot, of course, be irradiated if the graft is to fulfil its desired function, and many haemolytic reactions have been observed in bone marrow-graft recipients due to donor lymphocyte-derived incompatible antibody. In a series of six cases, five were due to anti-A or anti-B and one to anti-D produced by donor lymphocytes. The maximum rate of red cell destruction was found 9–16 days after grafting. Although antibody against recipient red cell antigens was frequently produced after giving group O marrow to A or B recipients or D-negative marrow to D-positive recipients, only 10–15% of patients developed clinically significant red cell destruction (Hows et al. 1986). In a further retrospective series three of seven D-positive patients receiving D-negative marrow produced donor-derived anti-D (Gajewski et al. 1992). These subjects continued to produce anti-D for periods of up to 1 year after grafting. On the other hand, of 16 patients in whom donor-derived anti-A or anti-B was found, antibody production was only transient. The authors speculated that greater abundance of A and B antigens induced tolerance. Massive immune haemolysis due to donor-derived alloantibodies after myeloablative conditioning can prove fatal and may be even more common (25–30%) after dose-reduced conditioning. Patients not receiving methotrexate for graft-versus-host disease (GvHD) prophylaxis are at greatest risk of developing this complication (Bolan et al. 2001; Worel et al. 2002)

Heart–lung transplants

In 9 out of 84 cases, the donor was group O and the recipient group A, B or AB. Among these nine, six developed anti-A or anti-B or both after transplantation (Hunt et al. 1988).

Following a heart–lung transplant from an Rh D-negative donor to an Rh D-positive recipient, jaundice developed within a few days. Between days 7 and 13 the Hb fell from 107 g/l to 38 g/l, the DAT became strongly positive and anti-D was eluted from the red cells. Haemolysis persisted for 3 months and anti-D remained detectable for 10 months. Both donor and recipient lymphocytes could be demonstrated in the lungs at 57 days though not at 120 days. Serum taken from the donor contained anti-D (Knoop et al. 1993).

Liver grafts

Following the grafting of ABO-unmatched liver (donor plasma ABO incompatible with the recipient's red cells), anti-A or anti-B (of donor origin) were detected 8–16 days after grafting in 8 out of 29 (28%) evaluable recipients. IgG was detected on the patient's red cells in most cases and complement in all cases. Evidence of destruction of the recipient's red cells in five cases appeared 5–8 days after surgery, lasted 7–19 days and was characterized by hyperbilirubinaemia and a substantial fall in PCV (Ramsey et al. 1984).

In a larger series the findings were similar: anti-A and anti-B were detected in 22 out of 60 cases in which ABO-unmatched liver was transplanted, and a haemolytic syndrome developed in 13 out of 19 evaluable cases (Ramsey and Cornell 1989). In one reported case, in which a haemolytic syndrome developed in an A_2 subject following the transplant of a group O liver, red cell destruction was attributed to anti-A_1 (Brecher et al. 1989), but a more likely interpretation is that anti-A was responsible and that anti-A_1 was detected because it was not bound strongly by the A_2 red cells.

Investigation of haemolytic transfusion reactions

The need to search for signs of red cell destruction

As large numbers of red cells or Hb can be rapidly removed from the circulation without causing either haemoglobinuria or jaundice, the diagnosis of a haemolytic reaction cannot be excluded with certainty without laboratory tests. The following case is a striking example:

The patient was an elderly woman with carcinoma of the stomach who was transfused with a unit of citrated blood (equivalent to 420 ml of whole blood). By mistake she was given outdated blood that was awaiting return to the transfusion centre instead of the blood that had been selected for her. The unit of blood she received had been stored in a blood bank for 19 days and had then remained at room temperature for a further 4 weeks. The transfusion was completed in less than 3 h. After transfusion the patient developed a temperature of 38.3°C and a pulse rate of 135/min. A venous sample drawn an hour after transfusion revealed a plasma Hb of 1 g/l. A sample of urine passed 1 h after transfusion contained no free Hb. Differential agglutination tests showed no surviving donor cells. Two hours later, the degree of haemoglobinaemia had diminished but the serum bilirubin had risen considerably. The patient never became jaundiced. In summary, this elderly patient eliminated 400 ml of blood within 4 h without any overt signs of red cell destruction (Mollison 1943, case 10).

Some common difficulties in carrying out the investigation

Every haemolytic transfusion reaction must be extensively investigated. The difficulties of doing this are two-fold; first, many transfusion reactions that are in fact haemolytic do not produce obvious clinical signs of red cell destruction. Sometimes the only hint that a haemolytic reaction has occurred is a small increase in a patient's body temperature. It is good practice to record the temperature initially and at half-hourly intervals during the transfusion and for 2 h after its end, and to pay attention to any rise observed. Recurrent fevers related to the underlying illness, for example infections in pancytopenic oncology patients, should not eliminate ordinary vigilance.

The second difficulty in investigating DHTR is the absence of important sources of evidence. By the time that a haemolytic reaction is appreciated, the empty blood unit may have been discarded. A helpful practice is to retain the pack in a refrigerator for at least 24 h. It is equally important to retain a pretransfusion sample of blood from every patient. First, the patient's extended phenotype can be determined. This may prove important in the identification of a blood group antibody present in the serum: a patient who is found to be Fy(a+) cannot have formed anti-Fy^a. In a sample taken after transfusion, large numbers of transfused cells may complicate the analysis. Second, the presence of blood group antibodies can be determined with sensitive techniques. After the transfusion of incompatible blood, the antibody may be adsorbed onto the transfused cells. Finally, comparisons can be made between pre- and post-transfusion values of serum bilirubin, serum Hp, etc.

Methods of investigation

In investigating a haemolytic transfusion reaction the first concern is that the wrong blood may have been given. The first step should be a clerical check to ensure that the blood given was in fact the blood selected for the patient. If not, immediate action must be undertaken to prevent incorrect transfusion of a second patient.

Assuming that obviously incompatible blood has not been given, the investigation of a suspected haemolytic transfusion reaction falls conveniently into two parts: (1) obtaining evidence of increased red cell destruction; and (2) identifying the cause of the increased destruction.

Procedures in suspected haemolytic transfusion reactions

As soon as a haemolytic transfusion reaction is suspected the transfusion should be stopped (but the line kept open with saline) and a venous sample taken from the patient. Steps should be taken to secure the residues of all units of blood that have been transfused and any sample of serum or whole blood taken from the patient before transfusion.

Evidence of increased red cell destruction. The post-transfusion blood sample should be centrifuged and the supernatant plasma examined for Hb and for increased bilirubin. When there is sufficient pretransfusion plasma this may be used as a control. These steps can be taken immediately. The first sample of urine passed by the patient after transfusion should be obtained and examined for Hb and for urobilinogen. If the post-transfusion blood sample is taken some hours after transfusion, when the plasma may have been cleared of Hb, testing for methaemalbumin and estimating plasma Hp can be helpful. Serum lactate dehydrogenase (LDH) elevation provides the best semi-quantitative estimate of red cell haemolysis. Inappropriate rise in PCV may be a helpful finding if sufficient blood has been transfused.

Identifying the cause. The most important steps involve clerical checks and repeat compatibility testing. These and additional steps to discover a serological cause of a suspected haemolytic transfusion reaction are described in Chapter 8. When no serological cause can be found, suspicion should fall on the condition of the donor red cells at the time of transfusion.

Visual detection of haemoglobinaemia

In withdrawing blood samples, special precautions must be taken to prevent haemolysis. Blood must be drawn with a reasonably wide-bored needle and after the sample has been obtained, the needle should be removed from the syringe (if a self-contained unit is not used) before ejecting the sample slowly into a suitable container with anticoagulant. The top of the container can be covered with parafilm and the contents mixed gently. It is important not to allow any blood to dry on the walls of the container. Thus either the container should be filled almost to the top with blood or the container should be centrifuged immediately before any blood can dry on its walls. It is good practice to examine the part of the container above the level of the blood before centrifugation and to wipe away, with some cotton wool on a stick, any traces of blood. When these precautions are observed, the amount of free Hb in the plasma should not exceed 0.02 or 0.03 g/l.

A sample of plasma that contains about 0.2 g of Hb/l plasma will appear very faintly pink or light brown if examined in a thickness of about 1 cm. Even smaller amounts of Hb can be detected with a small spectroscope. Quantities of Hb of the order of 1 g/l make the plasma appear red. Quantitative determinations of plasma Hb are widely available.

Detection of methaemalbuminaemia

When the plasma contains Hb, detectable by the naked eye, it is usually pointless to look for methaemalbumin. However, if the sample has been obtained 12 h or more after transfusion and the plasma contains only traces of Hb, which might have been produced by careless sample handling, it is worth carrying out a spectroscopic examination. The α-band of methaemalbumin lies at 623–624 nm, whereas that of methaemoglobin lies at 630 nm. When methaemalbumin cannot be detected spectroscopically, Schumm's test, which is much more sensitive, should be used.

Estimation of serum haptoglobin

In theory, estimation of serum Hp concentration should be most useful a day or two after a suspected haemolytic reaction. Any appreciable amount of Hb that has been liberated into the plasma will have been cleared, but the plasma Hp level will be very low. Because occasional normal individuals have a very low level of plasma Hp, the finding of a low level following a suspected haemolytic episode is of limited value unless a pretransfusion sample is available for testing.

Detection of haemoglobinuria

When relatively low concentrations of oxyhaemoglobin are present in urine the sample appears red, but when high concentrations are present it may appear black when viewed by ordinary light: the red colour can be seen if the sample is examined against an intense source of light. The presence of Hb can be confirmed by using commercially available chemical tests.

Oxyhaemoglobin in urine may be converted to methaemoglobin; if desired, the two pigments can be distinguished by spectroscopy. The bands of oxyhaemoglobin lie at 578 nm (α) and 540 nm (β) in the yellow and green parts of the spectrum respectively; the α-band of methaemoglobin lies in the red at 630 nm. For the demonstration of this band, the urine must not be alkaline, as the band is not present in alkaline solution.

Detection of hyperbilirubinaemia

Following extravascular destruction, the serum bilirubin concentration increases, reaching a peak not less than 3–6 h after the episode of destruction. As mentioned above, when accelerated destruction of transfused red cells is suspected, the patient's plasma should be examined for Hb; if the plasma is not pink, tests for total and direct bilirubin should be undertaken. It may be helpful to compare the colour of the serum or plasma sample with that of one taken before transfusion. If the post-transfusion sample is definitely yellow, the bilirubin concentration should be recorded.

Tests for the survival of transfused red cells

Wiener (1941a,b, 1942a,b) was the first to insist on the importance of tests for red cell survival in demonstrating incompatibility, and he first used the term 'inapparent haemolysis' to describe those cases in which the red cells leave the circulation at a greatly increased rate despite the absence of clinical signs of blood destruction.

Differential agglutination. Quantitative estimates can be made if the donor lacks some red cell antigen which is present on the recipient's red cells, e.g. when group O blood has been transfused to a patient of group A, or M– blood has been transfused to a patient who is M+, and when a suitable potent agglutinating serum is available (i.e. anti-A or anti-M in the examples given).

As described in Appendix 7, differential haemolysis after ^{51}Cr labelling can be used to provide quantitative estimates of the proportion of red cells of different ABO groups in a sample, e.g. A and O. It is thus possible to estimate the survival of either group O cells in an A recipient or A red cells in a group O recipient; a case in which this method was applied to estimate the survival of a large volume of transfused A blood in an O recipient has been described above (see Fig. 11.6).

Flow cytometry. Flow cytometry can be used to estimate the survival of transfused red cells when there are antigenic differences between donor and recipient; for examples and brief discussion, see Chapters 9 and 10. Compared with differential agglutination and visual counting of cells, the method is more sensitive and more accurate.

Qualitative or semi-quantitative estimates of survival. These may be made in three ways: (1) by looking for agglutinates in a sample of blood taken from the recipient; (2) by performing a DAT; or (3) by applying the method of direct differential agglutination (see Appendix 7).

1 Agglutinates may be found in samples of the recipient's blood for a day or two after the transfusion of blood of the wrong ABO group.

Mrs D, an elderly blood group O woman with carcinoma of the lung, was inadvertently given 600 ml of group B blood. A sample of urine passed after transfusion was noted to be red but was not tested. The next day, the patient's blood contained a number of group B cells. These were apparent as small clumps visible microscopically in a saline suspension of the patient's blood; the clumps could be increased in size by the addition of anti-B serum. As anticipated, the titre of anti-B in the patient's serum on the day after transfusion was very low (Mollison 1943, case 4).

2 The DAT on samples taken from the recipient becomes positive when the recipient's serum contains an incomplete blood group antibody and incompatible red cells are present in the circulation. In D-negative patients whose serum contains potent anti-D, circulating D-positive red cells may sometimes be visualized as microspherocytes. Often some of these cells form small clumps, a not unexpected finding, as red cells heavily coated with anti-D tend to agglutinate in undiluted serum. If the circulation contains predominantly donor red cells, virtually all the cells may appear to be agglutinated by an antiglobulin serum and this may suggest that the recipient has developed AIHA (see above). When reticulocytes are present, the recipient's own cells can be separated from transfused cells by centrifugation (see Chapter 8) or flow cytometry (Griffin *et al.* 1994). Occasionally, a positive DAT following transfusion is due to the presence in the donor's plasma of an antibody that is incompatible with the recipient's red cells. For example, the transfusion of potent anti-A plasma to a group A recipient regularly produces a positive DAT (see Chapter 10).

3 Direct differential agglutination has a restricted scope and depends for its success on chance. Thus if the recipient happens to be group N and the transfused red cells happen to be group M, a test with anti-M can be used to discover whether or not any of the transfused cells are still present in the recipient's circulation (see Wiener 1941b).

Determination of the serological cause of a haemolytic transfusion reaction

See Chapter 8.

Tests when no serological cause can be demonstrated

Methods to detect immune-mediated haemolysis when no obvious serological evidence is found are discussed in Chapter 10. Non-immunological causes of haemolysis have been discussed above. To ensure that haemolysis has not occurred *ex vivo*, the supernatant plasma of the unit or units of transfused blood should be inspected for free Hb. If the concentration appears to be higher than expected for the period of storage, an attempt must be made to discover why the blood is haemolysed. The possibility that the blood is infected should be considered and cultures taken. In any case, enquiries about the conditions under which the blood was stored and subsequently handled must be made, to determine whether the red cells have been frozen, overheated or otherwise traumatized. Finally, conditions of transfusion should be investigated to assess the possibility that mechanical haemolysis might have occurred as a result of problems with the tubing, filter or needle.

References

Abbott D, Hussain S (1970) Intravascular coagulation due to inter-donor incompatibility. Can Med Assoc J 103: 752

Ahmed KY, Nunn G, Brazier SM (1987) Haemolytic anemia resulting from autoantibodies produced by the donor's lymphocytes after renal transplantation. Transplantation 34: 163–164

Amberson WR, Jennings JJ, Rhode CM (1949) Clinical experience with hemoglobin-saline solutions. J Appl Physiol 1: 469

Alperin JB, Riglin H, Branch DR (1983) Anti-M causing delayed hemolytic transfusion reaction. Transfusion 23: 322–324

Arndt PA, Garratty G, Marfoe RA et al. (1998) An acute hemolytic transfusion reaction caused by an anti-P^1 that reacted at 37 degrees C. Transfusion 38: 373–377

Aygun B, Padmanabhan S, Paley C et al. (2002) Clinical significance of RBC alloantibodies and autoantibodies in sickle cell patients who received transfusions. Transfusion 42: 37–43

Baele PL, De Bruyere M, Deneys V et al. (1994) Bedside transfusion errors. A prospective survey by the Belgium SAnGUI Group. Vox Sang 66: 117–121

Ballas SK, Dignam C, Harris M et al. (1985) A clinically significant anti-N in a patient whose red cells were negative for N and U antigens. Transfusion 25: 377–380

Ballowitz L, Beck C, Eibs G et al. (1981) Rh Antikoerper in kommerziellen Immunoglobulin-Konzentrat. Monatschr Kinderheilk 129: 537–540

Bayliss WM (1920) Is haemolysed blood toxic? Br J Exp Pathol 1: 1

Beard MEJ, Pemberton J, Blagdon J et al. (1971) Rh immunization following incompatible blood transfusion and a possible long-term complication of anti-D immunoglobulin therapy. Med Genet 8: 317

Bechdolt S, Schroeder LK, Samia C et al. (1986) In vivo hemolysis of deglycerolized red blood cells. Arch Pathol Lab Med 110: 344–345

Beck ML, Haines RF, Oberman HA (1971) Unexpected serologic findings following lung homotransplantation. Chicago, IL: Commun Am Assoc Blood Banks

Benson K, Agosti SJ, Latoni-Benedetti GF et al. (2003) Acute and delayed hemolytic transfusion reactions secondary to HLA alloimmunization. Transfusion 43: 753–757

Beutler E (1996) G6PD: population genetics and clinical manifestations. Blood Rev 10: 45–52

Bevan PC, Seaman M, Tolliday B et al. (1985) ABO haemolytic anaemia in transplanted patients. Vox Sang 49: 42–48

Binder LS, Ginsberg V, Harmel MH (1959) A six-year study of incompatible blood transfusions. Surg Gynecol Obstet 108: 19

Birndorf NL, Lopas H, Robboy SJ (1971) Disseminated intravascular coagulation and renal failure. Production in the monkey with autologous red blood cell stroma. Lab Invest 25: 314

Bluemle LW Jr (1965) Hemolytic transfusion reactions causing acute renal failure. Serologic and clinical considerations. Postgrad Med 38: 484–489

Bolan CD, Childs RW, Procter JL et al. (2001) Massive immune haemolysis after allogeneic peripheral blood stem cell transplantation with minor ABO incompatibility. Br J Haematol 112: 787–795

Boorman KE, Dodd BE, Loutit JF et al. (1946) Some results of transfusion of blood to recipients with 'cold' agglutinins. BMJ i: 751

Boothe G, Brecher M, Root M (1993) Acute hemolysis due to passive anti-B with spontaneous in vitro agglutination (Abstract). Transfusion 33(Suppl.): 550

Bothwell T, Finch CA (1962) Iron Metabolism. London: Churchill

Bove JR (1968) Delayed complications of transfusion. Connecticut Med 32: 36

Bowman JM, Pollack JM (1980) Haemolysis of donor red cells at fetal transfusion due to catheter trauma. Lancet ii: 1190

Boyland IP, Mufti GF, Hamblin TJ (1982) Delayed haemolytic transfusion reaction caused by anti-Fyb in a splenectomized patient (Letter). Transfusion 22: 402

Braine HG, Sensenbrenner LL, Wright SK et al. (1982) Bone marrow transplantation with major ABO blood group incompatibility using erythrocyte depletion of marrow prior to infusion. Blood 60: 420–425

Brecher ME, Taswell HF (1989) Paroxysmal nocturnal hemoglobinuria and the transfusion of washed red cells. A myth revisited. Transfusion 29: 681–685

Brecher ME, Moore SB, Reisner RK et al. (1989) Delayed hemolysis resulting from anti-A^1 after liver transplantation. Am J Clin Pathol 91: 232–235

Broman B (1944) The blood factor Rh in man. Acta Paediatr (Uppsala) 31(Suppl. 2): 128

Bunn FH, Esham WT, Bull RW (1969) The renal handling of hemoglobin. I. Glomerular filtration. J Exp Med 129: 909

Butler J, Parker D, Pillai R et al. (1991) Systemic release of neutrophil elastase and tumour necrosis factor alpha following ABO incompatible blood transfusion. Br J Haematol 79: 525–526

Capon SM, Goldfinger D (1995) Acute hemolytic transfusion reaction, a paradigm of the systemic inflammatory response: new insights into pathophysiology and treatment. Transfusion 35: 513–520

Cassell M, Chaplin H Jr (1961) Changes in the recipient's plasma hemoglobin concentration after transfusion with stored blood. Transfusion 1: 23

Castellino SM, Combs MR, Zimmerman SA et al. (1999) Erythrocyte autoantibodies in paediatric patients with sickle cell disease receiving transfusion therapy: frequency, characteristics and significance. Br J Haematol 104: 189–194

Champneys Dr (1880) In: Discussion of paper by AE Schaefer. Obstet Trans 21: 346

Chaplin H (1979) Special problems in transfusion management of patients with autoimmune hemolytic anemia. In: A Seminar on Laboratory Management of Hemolysis. Washington, DC: Am Assoc Blood Banks

Chaplin H Jr, Cassell M (1962) The occasional fallibility of in vitro compatibility tests. Transfusion 6: 375–384

Chaplin H Jr, Zarkowsky HS (1981) Combined sickle cell disease and autoimmune hemolytic anemia. Arch Intern Med 141: 1091–1093

Chaplin H, Crawford H, Cutbush M et al. (1956) The preservation of red cells at –79°C. Clin Sci 15: 27

Crile GW (1909) Hemorrhage and Transfusion: an Experimental and Clinical Research. New York: D Appleton

Crosby WH, Dameshek W (1951) The significance of hemoglobinuria and associated hemosiderinuria, with particular reference to various types of hemolytic anemia. J Lab Clin Med 38: 3

Croucher BEE (1979) Differential diagnosis of delayed transfusion reaction. In: A Seminar on Laboratory Management of Hemolysis. Las Vegas: Am Assoc Blood Banks

Croucher BEE, Crookston MC, Crookston JH (1967) Delayed transfusion reactions simulating auto-immune haemolytic anaemia. Vox Sang 12: 32

Dameshek W, Levine P (1943) Isoimmunization with Rh factor in acquired hemolytic anemia. N Engl J Med 228: 641–644

Davenport RD (1995) The role of cytokines in hemolytic transfusion reactions. Immunol Invest 24: 319–331

Davenport RD, Strieter RM, Standiford TJ et al. (1990) Interleukin-8 production in red blood cell incompatibility. Blood 76: 2439–2442

Davenport RD, Strieter RM, Kunkel SL (1991) Red cell ABO incompatibility and production of tumor necrosis factor-alpha. Br J Haematol 78: 540–544

Davenport RD, Burdick M, Kunkel SL (1992) Endothelial cell activation in hemolytic transfusion reactions. Transfusion 32(Suppl.): 535

Davenport RD, Burdick M, Moore SA et al. (1993) Cytokine production in IgG-mediated red cell incompatibility. Transfusion 33: 19–24

Davenport RD, Polak TJ, Kunkel SL (1994) White cell-associated procoagulant activity induced by ABO incompatibility. Transfusion 34: 943–949

DeCesare WR, Bove JR, Ebaugh EG Jr (1964) The mechanism of the effect of iso- and hyperosmolar dextrose-saline solutions on in vivo survival of human erythrocytes. Transfusion 4: 237

Degnan TJ, Rosenfield RE (1965) Hemolytic transfusion reaction associated with poorly detectable anti-Jkᵃ. Transfusion 5: 245

Delmas-Marsalet Y, Chateau G, Foissac-Gegoux P et al. (1967) Accident transfusionnel par iso-anticorps naturels de spécificite, anti-N. Transfusion (Paris) 4: 369

Delmas-Marsalet Y, Parquet-Gernez A, Bauters F (1969) Anemies hémolytiques dues à la plasmathérapie chez les hemophiles. Rev Fr Transfusion 12: 351

Denis J (1667–8) Letter to the Publishers. Philos Trans 32: 617

Diamond WJ, Brown FL Jr, Bitterman P et al. (1980) Delayed hemolytic transfusion reaction presenting as sickle-cell crisis. Ann Intern Med 93: 231–234

Dinapoli JB, Nichols ME, Marsh WL et al. (1977) Hemolytic transfusion reaction caused by IgG anti-P₁. Commun Amer Assoc Blood Banks, Atlanta, GA

Dinsmore RE, Reich LM, Kapoor N et al. (1983) ABH incompatible bone marrow transplantation: removal of erythrocytes by starch sedimentation. Br J Haematol 54: 441–449

Doberneck RC, Reiser MP, Yunis E (1964) Acute renal failure after hemolytic transfusion reaction. Surg Gynecol Obstet 119: 1069–1073

Duvall CP, Alter HJ, Rath CE (1974) Hemoglobin catabolism following a hemolytic transfusion reaction in a patient with sickle cell anemia. Transfusion 14: 382–387

Dzik WH, Murphy MF, Andreu G et al. (2003) An international study of the performance of sample collection from patients. Vox Sang 85: 40–47

Ebert RV, Emerson CP (1946) A clinical study of transfusion reactions. The hemolytic effect of group O blood and pooled plasma containing incompatible isoagglutinins. J Clin Invest 25: 627

Eklund J, Nevanlinna HR (1971) Immuno suppression therapy in Rh-incompatible transfusion. BMJ iii: 623

Ervin DM, Young LE (1950) Dangerous universal donors. I. Observations on destruction of recipient's A cells after transfusion of group O blood containing high titer of A antibodies of immune type not easily neutralizable by soluble A substance. Blood 5: 61

Evans RS, Turner E, Bingham M (1965) Studies with radio-iodinated cold agglutinins of ten patients. Am J Med 38: 378

Fairley NH (1940) The fate of extracorpuscular circulating haemoglobin. BMJ ii: 213

Faulstick DA, Lowenstein J, Yiengst MJ (1962) Clearance kinetics of haptoglobin-hemoglobin complex in the human. Blood 20: 65

Felix CA, Davey RJ (1987) Massive acute hemolysis secondary to Clostridium perfringens sepsis in a recently transfused oncology patient with multiple alloantibodies. Med Pediatr Oncol 15: 42–44

Franciosi R, Awer E, Santana M (1967) Interdonor incompatibility resulting in anuria. Transfusion 7: 297

Fudenberg HH, Allen F Jr (1957) Transfusion reactions in the absence of demonstrable incompatibility. N Engl J Med 256: 1180

Gajewski JL, Petz LD, Calhoun L et al. (1992) Hemolysis of transfused group O red blood cells in minor ABO-incompatible unrelated-donor bone marrow transplants in patients receiving cyclosporine without posttransplant methotrexate. Blood 79: 3076–3085

Gambino C, Craig D, Stiles M (1992) The effects of Pall RC-50 filtration under pressure on red cell hemolysis (Abstract). Transfusion 32(Suppl.): 27S

Garby L, Noyes WD (1959) Studies on hemoglobin metabolism. I. The kinetic properties of the plasma hemoglobin pool in normal man. J Clin Invest 38: 1479

Gasser C (1945) Akute haemolytische Krisen nach Plasma-Transfusionen bei dystrophischtoxischen Saeuglingen. Helv Paediatr Acta 1: 38

Ghebrehiwet B, Silverberg M, Kaplan AP (1981) Activation of the classical pathway of complement by Hageman factor fragment. J Exp Med 153: 665–676

Giblett ER (1969) Genetic Markers in Human Blood. Oxford: Blackwell Scientific Publications

Giblett FR, Hillman RS, Brooks LE (1965) Transfusion reaction during marrow suppression in a thalassemic patient with a blood group anomaly and an unusual cold agglutinin. Vox Sang 10: 448

Gilligan DR, Altschule MD, Katersky EM (1941) Studies of hemoglobinemia and hemoglobinuria produced in man by intravenous injection of hemoglobin solutions. J Clin Invest 20: 179

Glasser L, West JH, Hagood RM (1970) Incompatible feto-maternal transfusion with maternal intravascular lysis. Transfusion 10: 322

Goldfinger D (1977) Acute hemolytic transfusion reactions – a fresh look at pathogenesis and considerations regarding therapy. Transfusion 17: 85–98

Goldfinger D, Kleinman S, Connelly M (1979) Acute hemolytic transfusion reaction (HTR) with disseminated intravascular coagulation (DIC) and acute renal failure (ARF) due to transfusion of plasma containing Rh antibodies (Abstract). Transfusion 19: 639–640

Goldfinger D, O'Connell M, Ellrodt AG (1985) Pathogenesis and treatment of shock associated with hemolytic transfusion reactions (Abstract). Transfusion 25: 468

Gravenstein D (1997) Transurethral resection of the prostate (TURP) syndrome: a review of the pathophysiology and management. Anesth Analg 84: 438–446

Greene DL, Khan S (1993) Reactive lysis – a phenomenon of delayed hemolytic transfusion reactions. Immunohematology 9: 74–77

Greenwalt TJ, Sasaki T (1957) The Lutheran blood groups: a second example of anti-Lu[b] and three further examples of anti-Lu[a]. Blood 12: 998

Griffin GD, Lippert LE, Dow NS et al. (1994) A flow cytometric method for phenotyping recipient red cells following transfusion. Transfusion 34: 233–237

Grove-Rasmussen M, Soutter M, Marceau E (1951) The use of group O donors as 'universal' donors. Minneapolis, MN: Commun Am Assoc Blood Banks

Grove-Rasmussen M, Shaw RS, Marceau E (1953) Hemolytic transfusion reaction in group-A patient receiving group-O blood containing immune anti-A antibodies in high titer. Am J Clin Pathol 23: 828

Hach-Wunderle V, Texidor D, Zumpe P (1989) Anti-A in Factor VIII concentrate: a cause of severe hemolysis in a patient with acquired Factor VIII:C antibodies. Infusion Ther 16: 100–101

Hédon (1902) Archives de Médecine expérimentale et d'Anatomie pathologique 4: 297

Herron R, Clark M, Tate D (1986) Immune haemolysis in a renal transplant recipient due to antibodies with anti-c specificity. Vox Sang 51: 226–227

Hess JR, MacDonald VW, Brinkley WW (1993) Systemic and pulmonary hypertension after resuscitation with cell-free hemoglobin. J Appl Physiol 74: 1769–1778

Hewitt PE, MacIntyre EA, Devenish A (1988) A prospective study of the incidence of delayed haemolytic transfusion reactions following peri-operative blood transfusion. Br J Haematol 69: 541–544

Hillman NM (1979) Fatal delayed hemolytic transfusion reaction due to anti-c + E. Transfusion 19: 548–551

Hillmen P, Hall C, Marsh JC et al. (2004) Effect of eculizumab on hemolysis and transfusion requirements in patients with paroxysmal nocturnal hemoglobinuria. N Engl J Med 350: 552–559

Hjelle B, Donegan E, Cruz J (1988) Antibody to c antigen consequent to renal transplantation. Transfusion 28: 496–498

Hoffsten P, Chaplin HJ (1969) Hemolytic transfusion reaction occurring in a patient with acute renal failure. Blood 33: 234

Holland PV, Wallerstein RO (1968) Delayed hemolytic transfusion reaction with acute renal failure. JAMA 204: 1007

Honig CL, Bove JR (1980) Transfusion-associated fatalities: review of Bureau of Biologics Reports 1976–78. Transfusion 20: 653–661

Hopkins JG (1910) Phagocytosis of red blood-cells after transfusion. Arch Intern Med 6: 270

Howard JE, Perkins HA (1976) Lysis of donor RBC during plateletpheresis with a blood processor. JAMA 236: 289

Hows J, Beddow K, Gordon-Smith E (1986) Donor derived red blood cell antibodies and immune hemolysis after allogeneic bone marrow transplantation. Blood 67: 177–181

Hughes-Jones NC, Mollison PL (1963) Clearance by the RES of 'non-viable' red cells. In: Role du Système Réticuloendothelial dans l'Immunité, antibactérienne et antitumorale. Paris: Edition du CNRS

Hunt BJ, Yacoub M, Amin S (1988) Induction of red blood cell destruction by graft-derived antibodies after minor ABO mismatched heart and lung transplantation. Transplantation 46: 246–249

Inwood MJ, Zuliani B (1978) Anti-A hemolytic transfusion with packed O cells. Ann Intern Med 89: 515–516

Jandl JH, Kaplan ME (1960) The destruction of red cells by antibodies in man. III. Quantitative factors influencing the patterns of hemolysis in vivo. J Clin Invest 39: 1145

Jandl JH, Tomlinson AS (1958) The destruction of red cells by antibodies in man. II. Pyrogenic, leukocytic and dermal responses to immune hemolysis. J Clin Invest 37: 1202

Joseph JIJ, Awer E, Laulicht M (1964) Delayed hemolytic transfusion reaction due to appearance of multiple antibodies following transfusion of apparently compatible blood. Transfusion 4: 367

Josephson CD, Mullis NC, Van Demark C *et al.* (2004) Significant numbers of apheresis-derived group O platelet units have 'high-titer' anti-A/A,B: implications for transfusion policy. Transfusion 44: 805–808

Kaplan AP, Joseph K, Silverberg M (2002) Pathways for bradykinin formation and inflammatory disease. J Allerg Clin Immunol 109: 195–209

Kaye D, Hook EW (1963) The influence of hemolysis on susceptibility to salmonella infection: additional observations. J Immunol 91: 518

Keidan SE, Lohoar E, Mainwaring D (1966) Acute anuria in a haemophiliac due to transfusion of incompatible plasma. Lancet i: 179

Kilduffe RA, DeBakey M (1942) The Blood Bank and the Techniques and Therapeutics of Transfusion. St Louis, MO: CV Mosby

Kim HC, Park CL, Cowan JH III (1988) Massive intravascular hemolysis associated with intravenous immunoglobulin in bone marrow transplant recipients. Am J Pediatr Hematol/Oncol 10: 69–74

Klein HG (2003) Getting older is not necessarily getting better. Anesthesiology 98: 807–808

Knoop C, Andrien M, Antoine M (1993) Severe hemolysis due to a donor anti-D antibody after heart-lung transplantation. Am Rev Respir Dis 148: 504–506

Kronenberg H, Kooptzoff O, Walsh RJ (1958) Haemolytic transfusion reaction due to anti-Kidd. Aust Ann Med 7: 34

Kumar P, Sarkar S, Narang A (1994) Acute intravascular haemolysis following exchange transfusion with G-6-PD deficient blood. Eur J Pediatr 153: 98–99

Kurtides ES, Salkin MS, Widen AL (1966) Hemolytic reaction due to anti-Jk^b. JAMA 197: 816

Landsteiner EK, Finch CA (1947) Hemoglobinemia accompanying transurethral resection of the prostate. N Engl J Med 237: 310

Lanore JJ, Quarre MC, Audibert JD (1989) Acute renal failure following transfusion of accidentally frozen autologous red blood cells. Vox Sang 56: 293

Larsson LG, Welsh VJ, Ladd DJ (2000) Acute intravascular hemolysis secondary to out-of-group platelet transfusion. Transfusion 40: 902–906

Lathem W (1959) The renal excretion of hemoglobin. Regulatory mechanisms and the differential excretion of free and protein-bound hemoglobin. J Clin Invest 38: 652

Lathem W, Davis BB, Zweig PH (1960) The demonstration and localization of renal tubular reabsorption of hemoglobin by stop flow analysis. J Clin Invest 39: 840

Laurell C-B, Nyman M (1957) Studies on the serum haptoglobin level in hemoglobinemia and its influence on renal excretion of hemoglobin. Blood 12: 493

Levine P, Mabee JA (1923) Dangerous 'universal donor' detected by the direct matching of bloods. J Immunol 8: 425–431

Levine P, Bobbitt OB, Waller RK (1951) Isoimmunization by a new blood factor in tumor cells. Proc Soc Exp Biol (NY) 77: 403

Levine P, White JA, Stroup M (1961) Seven Ve^a (Vel) negative members in three generations of a family. Transfusion 1: 111–115

Linden JV, Paul B, Dressler KP (1992) A report of 104 transfusion errors in New York State. Transfusion 32: 601–606

Linden JV, Wagner K, Voytovich AE *et al.* (2000) Transfusion errors in New York State: an analysis of 10 years' experience. Transfusion 40: 1207–1213

Lopas H, Birndorf NI (1971) Haemolysis and intravascular coagulation due to incompatible red cell transfusion in isoimmunized monkeys. Br J Haematol 21: 399

Lopas H, Birndorf NI, Robboy SJ (1971) Experimental transfusion reactions and disseminated intravascular coagulation produced by incompatible plasma in monkeys. Transfusion 11: 196

Lowenstein J, Faulstick DA, Yiengst MJ (1961) The glomerular clearance and renal transport of hemoglobin in adult males. J Clin Invest 40: 1172

Lundberg WB, McGinniss MH (1975) Hemolytic transfusion reaction due to anti-A$_1$. Transfusion 15: 1

Ma SK, Wong KF, Siu L (1995) Hemoglobinemia and hemoglobinuria complicating concomitant use of a white cell filter and a pressure infusion device (Letter). Transfusion 35: 180

MacDonald WB, Berg RB (1959) Hemolysis of transfused cells during use of the injection (push) technique for blood transfusion. Pediatrics 23: 8

McClelland DB, Phillips P (1994) Errors in blood transfusion in Britain: survey of hospital haematology departments. BMJ 308: 1205–1206

Mair B, Benson K (1998) Evaluation of changes in hemoglobin levels associated with ABO-incompatible plasma in apheresis platelets. Transfusion 38: 51–55

Mangal AK, Growe GH, Sinclair M (1984) Acquired hemolytic anemia due to 'auto'anti-A or 'auto'anti-B induced by group O homograft in renal transplant recipients. Transfusion 24: 201–205

Mayer K (1982) A different view of transfusion safety – type and screen, transfusion of Coombs incompatible cells, fatal transfusion induced graft versus host disease. In: Safety in Transfusion Practices. HF Polesky, RH Walker (eds). Skokie, IL: College of American Pathologists

Meltz DJ, Bertles JF, David DS (1971) Delayed haemolytic transfusion reaction with renal failure. Lancet ii: 1348

Moheng MC, McCarthy P, Pierce SR (1985) Anti-Do[b] implicated as the cause of a delayed hemolytic transfusion reaction. Transfusion 25: 44–46

Mollison PL (1943) The investigation of haemolytic transfusion reactions. BMJ i: 529–559

Mollison PL (1951) Blood Transfusion in Clinical Medicine, 1st edn. Oxford: Blackwell Scientific Publications

Mollison PL (1967) Blood Transfusion in Clinical Medicine, 4th edn. Oxford: Blackwell Scientific Publications

Mollison PL (1972) Blood Transfusion in Clinical Medicine, 5th edn. Oxford: Blackwell Scientific Publications

Mollison PL (1979) Blood Transfusion in Clinical Medicine, 6th edn. Oxford: Blackwell Scientific Publications

Mollison PL (1983) Blood Transfusion in Clinical Medicine, 7th edn. Oxford: Blackwell Scientific Publications

Mollison PL, Newlands M (1976) Unusual delayed haemolytic transfusion reaction characterised by the slow destruction of red cells. Vox Sang 31: 54

Mollison PL, Young IM (1942) In vivo survival in the human subject of transfused erythrocytes after storage in various preservative solutions. Q J Exp Physiol 31: 359

Mollison PL, Cutbush M (1955) The use of isotope-labelled red cells to demonstrate incompatibility in vivo. Lancet i: 1290

Moncrieff RE, Thompson WP (1975) Delayed hemolytic transfusion reaction with four antibodies detected by pretransfusion tests. Am J Clin Pathol 64: 251

Moore SB, Taswell HF, Pineda AA (1980) Delayed hemolytic transfusion reactions. Evidence of the need for an improved pretransfusion compatibility test. Am J Clin Pathol 74: 94–97

Morse EE (1978) Interdonor incompatibility as a cause of reaction during granulocyte transfusion. Vox Sang 35: 215

Moureau F (1945) Les réactions post-transfusionnelles. Rev Belge Sci Med 16: 258

Muller-Eberhard U, Liem HH, Hanstein A (1969) Studies on the disposal of intravascular heme in the rabbit. J Lab Clin Med 73: 210

Ness PM, Shirey RS, Thoman SK (1990) The differentiation of delayed serologic and delayed hemolytic transfusion reactions: incidence, long-term serologic findings, and clinical significance. Transfusion 30: 688–693

Noble TC, Abbott J (1959) Haemolysis of stored blood mixed with isotonic dextrose-containing solutions in transfusion apparatus. BMJ ii: 865

Noyes WD, Garby L (1967) Rate of haptoglobin synthesis in normal man. Determination by the return to normal levels following hemoglobin infusion. Scand J Clin Lab Invest 20: 33

Nussbaumer W, Schwaighofer H, Gratwohl A et al. (1995) Transfusion of donor-type red cells as a single preparative treatment for bone marrow transplants with major ABO incompatibility. Transfusion 35: 592–595

Nyman M, Gydell K, Nosslin B (1959) Haptoglobin and Erythrokinetik. Clin Chim Acta 4: 82

Oehlecker F (1928) Haemolyse trotz Blutgruppenbestimmung. Anhang: experimentelle Studien ueber den Eintritt der Haemolyse. Arch Klin Chir 152: 477

Ogden JE, MacDonald SL (1995) Haemoglobin-based red cell substitutes: current status. Vox Sang 69: 302–308

O'Reilly RA, Lombard CM, Azzi RL (1985) Delayed hemolytic transfusion reaction associated with Rh antibody anti-f: first reported case. Vox Sang 49: 336–339

Ottenberg R (1911) Studies in isoagglutination. I. Transfusion and the question of intravascular agglutination. J Exp Med 13: 425

Ottenberg R, Fox CL (1938) Rate of removal of hemoglobin from the circulation and its renal threshold in human beings. Am J Physiol 123: 516

Ottenberg R, Thalheimer W (1915) Studies in experimental transfusion. J Med Res 33: 213

Patel RP, Gladwin MT (2004) Physiologic, pathologic and therapeutic implications for hemoglobin interactions with nitric oxide. Free Radical Biol Med 36: 399–401

Patten R, Reddi CR, Riglin H (1982) Delayed hemolytic transfusion reaction caused by a primary immune response. Transfusion 22: 248–250

Petz LD, Calhoun L, Shulman IA et al. (1997) The sickle cell hemolytic transfusion reaction syndrome. Transfusion 37: 382–392

Pickles MM, Jones MN, Egan J (1978) Delayed haemolytic transfusion reactions due to anti-C. Vox Sang 35: 32

Pineda AA, Brzica SM, Taswell HF (1978a) Hemolytic transfusion reaction. Recent experience in a large blood bank. Mayo Clin Proc 53: 378

Pineda AA, Taswell HF, Brzica SJ (1978b) Delayed hemolytic transfusion reaction. An immunologic hazard of blood transfusion. Transfusion 18: 1

Pinkerton PH, Coovadia AS, Goldstein J (1992) Frequency of delayed hemolytic transfusion reactions following antibody screening and immediate-spin crossmatching. Transfusion 32: 814–817

Polesky HF, Bove JR (1964) A fatal hemolytic transfusion reaction with acute autohemolysis. Transfusion 4: 285

Pollock A (1968) Transplacental haemorrhage after external cephalic version. Lancet i. 612

Pruss A, Heymann GA, Hell A et al. (2003) Acute intravascular hemolysis after transfusion of a chimeric RBC unit. Transfusion 43: 1449–1451

Rabiner SF, Friedman LH (1968) The role of intravascular haemolysis and the reticuloendothelial system in the production of a hypercoagulable state. Br J Haematol 14: 105

Rabiner SF, O'Brien K, Peskin GW (1970) Further studies with stroma-free hemoglobin solution. Ann Surg 171: 615

Ramsey G, Cornell FW (1989) Red cell antibody problems in 1000 liver transplants. Transfusion 29: 396–400

Ramsey G, Nusbacher J, Starzl TE (1984) Isohemagglutinins of graft origin after ABO-unmatched liver transplantation. N Engl J Med 311: 1167–1170

Ramsey G, Israel L, Gwenn D et al. (1986) Anti-Rho(D) in two Rh-positive patients receiving kidney grafts from an Rh-immunized donor. Transplantation 41: 67–69

Rauner RA, Tanaka KR (1967) Hemolytic transfusion reactions associated with the Kidd antibody (Jka). N Engl J Med 276: 1486

Rock RC, Bove JR, Nemerson Y (1969) Heparin treatment of intravascular coagulation accompanying hemolytic transfusion reactions. Transfusion 9: 57

Rosati LA, Barnes B, Oberman HA (1970) Hemolytic anemia due to anti-A in concentrated antihemophilic factor preparations. Transfusion 10: 139

Rosse WF, Nishimura J (2003) Clinical manifestations of paroxysmal nocturnal hemoglobinuria: present state and future problems. Int J Hematol 77: 113–120

Rother RP, Bell L, Hillmen P et al. (2005) The clinical sequellae of intravascular hemolysis and extravascular plasma hemoglobin. J Am Med Assoc 293: 1653–1662

Rothman IK, Alter HJ, Strewler GJ (1976) Delayed overt hemolytic transfusion reaction due to anti-U antibody. Transfusion 16: 357

Roy RB, Lotto WN (1962) Delayed hemolytic reaction caused by anti-c not detectable before transfusion. Transfusion 2: 342

Ryden SE, Oberman HA (1975) Compatibility of common intravenous solutions with CPD blood. Transfusion 15: 250

Sack ES, Nefa OM (1970) Fibrinogen and fibrin degradation products in hemolytic transfusion reactions. Transfusion 10: 317

Salama A, Mueller-Eckhardt C (1984) Delayed hemolytic transfusion reactions. Evidence for complement activation involving allogeneic and autologous red cells. Transfusion 24: 188–193

Salmon C, Schwartzenberg L, André R (1959) Anémie hémolytique post-transfusionelle chez un sujet A_3 à la suite d'un injection massive desang A_1. Sang 30: 223

Samet S, Bowman HS (1961) Fetomaternal ABO incompatibility: intravascular hemolysis, fetal hemoglobinemia and fibrinogenopenia in maternal circulation. Am J Obstet Gynecol 81: 49

Savitsky JP, Doczi J, Black J (1978) A clinical safety trial of stroma-free hemoglobin. Clin Pharmacol Ther 23: 73–80

Sazama K (1990) Reports of 355 transfusion-associated deaths: 1976 through 1985. Transfusion 30: 583–590

Sazama K, Klein HG, Davey RJ et al. (1980) Intraoperative hemolysis. The initial manifestation of glucose-6-phosphate dehydrogenase deficiency. Arch Intern Med 140: 845–846

Schmidt PJ (1980a) The mortality from incompatible transfusion. In: Immunobiology of the Erythrocyte. SG Sandler, J Nussbacher, MS Schanfield (eds). New York: Alan R Liss

Schmidt PJ (1980b) Transfusion mortality; with special reference to surgical and intensive care facilities. J Fla Med Assoc 67: 151–153

Schmidt PJ, Holland PV (1967) Pathogenesis of the acute renal failure associated with incompatible transfusion. Lancet ii: 1169

Sevitt S (1958) Hepatic jaundice after blood transfusion in injured and burned subjects. Br J Surg 46: 68

Shalev O, Manny N, Sharon R (1993) Posttransfusional hemolysis in recipients of glucose-6-phosphate dehydrogenase-deficient erythrocytes. Vox Sang 64: 94–98

Siber GR, Ambrosino DM, Gorgon BC (1982) Blood group A-like substance in a preparation of pneumococcal vaccine. Ann Intern Med 96: 580–586

Simionatta CS, Cabal R, Jones RL et al. (1988) Thrombophlebitis and disturbed hemostasis following administration of intravenous hematin in normal volunteers. Am J Med 85: 538–540

Sirchia G, Ferrone S, Mercuriali F (1970) Leukocyte antigen-antibody reaction and lysis of paroxysmal nocturnal hemoglobinuria erythrocytes. Blood 36: 334–336

Squires JE, Larison PJ, Charles WT (1985) A delayed hemolytic transfusion reaction due to anti-Co[b]. Transfusion 25: 137–139

Stevens AJ Jr, Finch CA (1954) A dangerous universal donor. Acute renal failure following transfusion of group O blood. Am J Clin Pathol 24: 612

Strahl M, Pettenkofer HJ, Hasse W (1955) A haemolytic transfusion reaction due to anti-M. Vox Sang (OS) 5: 34

Stroncek D, Procter JL, Johnson J (2000) Drug-induced hemolysis: cefotetan-dependent hemolytic anemia mimicking an acute intravascular immune transfusion reaction. Am J Hematol 64: 67–70

Swanson J, Sastamoinen R, Sebring E (1985) Rh and Kell antibodies of probable donor origin produced after solid organ transplantation (Abstract). Transfusion 25: 467

Swanson J, Sebring E, Sastamoinen R (1987) Gm allotyping to determine the origin of the anti-D causing hemolytic anemia in a kidney transplant recipient. Vox Sang 52: 228–230

Taddie SJ, Barrasso C, Ness PM (1982) A delayed transfusion reaction caused by anti-K6. Transfusion 22: 68–69

Talano JA, Hillery CA, Gottschall JL et al. (2003) Delayed hemolytic transfusion reaction/hyperhemolysis syndrome in children with sickle cell disease. Pediatrics 111: e661–e665

Taswell HF, Pineda AA, Moore SB (1981) Hemolytic transfusion reactions: frequency and clinical and laboratory aspects. In: A Seminar on Immune-mediated Cell Destruction. Chicago, IL: Am Assoc Blood Banks

Telen MJ (2001) Principles and problems of transfusion in sickle cell disease. Semin Hematol 38: 315–323

Thompson A, McGarry AE, Valeri CR (1994) Stroma-free hemoglobin increases blood pressure and GFR in the hypotensive rat: role of nitric oxide. J Appl Physiol 77: 2348–2354

Thompson PR, Childers DM, Hatcher DE (1967) Anti-Di[b] – first and second examples. Vox Sang 13: 314

Turner CL, Casbard AC, Murphy MF (2003) Barcode technology: its role in increasing the safety of blood transfusion. Transfusion 43: 1200–1209

Valbonesi M, De Luigi MC, Lercari G et al. (2000) Acute intravascular hemolysis in two patients transfused with dry-platelet units obtained from the same ABO incompatible donor. Int J Artif Organs 23: 642–646

Valeri CR (1965) Effect of resuspension medium on in vivo survival and supernatant hemoglobin of erythrocytes preserved with glycerol. Transfusion 5: 25

Vamvakas AA, Pineda AA, Reisner RR (1995) The differentiation of delayed hemolytic and delayed serologic transfusion reactions: incidence and predictors of hemolysis. Transfusion 35: 26–32

Vaughan JM (1942) Pigment metabolism following transfusion of fresh and stored blood. BMJ i: 548

Vichinsky EP, Earles A, Johnson RA (1990) Alloimmunization in sickle cell anaemia and transfusion of racially unmatched blood. N Engl J Med 322: 1617–1622

Viele MK, Weiskopf RB, Fisher D (1997) Recombinant human hemoglobin does not affect renal function in humans: analysis of safety and pharmacokinetics. Anesthesiology 86: 848–858

Vogel P, Rosenthal N, Levine P (1943) Hemolytic reactions as a result of iso-immunization following repeated transfusions of homologous blood. Am J Clin Pathol 13: 1

Wagener FA, Eggert A, Boerman OC et al. (2001) Heme is a potent inducer of inflammation in mice and is counteracted by heme oxygenase. Blood 98: 1802–1811

Wallace J (1977) Blood Transfusion for Clinicians. Edinburgh: Churchill Livingstone

Warkentin PI, Yomtovian R, Hurd D (1983) Severe delayed hemolytic transfusion reaction complicating an ABO-incompatible bone marrow transplantation. Vox Sang 45: 40–47

Weber J, Caceres VW, Pavone BG et al. (1979) Allo-anti-C in a patient who had previously made an autoantibody mimicking anti-C. Transfusion 19: 216–218

Weech AA, Vann D, Grillo RA (1941) The clearance of bilirubin from the plasma. A measure of the excretory power of the liver. J Clin Invest 20: 323

Weinstein R, Martinez R, Hassoun H et al. (1997) Does a patient with hereditary spherocytosis qualify for preoperative autologous blood donation? Transfusion 37: 1179–1183

Weir AB 3rd, Woods LL, Chesney C (1987) Delayed hemolytic transfusion reaction caused by anti-Le[bh] antibody. Vox Sang 53: 105–107

Wiener AS (1941a) Hemolytic reactions following transfusions of blood of the homologous group. II. Further observations on the role of property Rh, particularly in cases without demonstrable iso-antibodies. Arch Pathol 32: 227

Wiener AS (1941b) Subdivisions of group A and group AB. II Isoimmunization of A_2 individuals against A_1 blood; with special reference to the role of the subgroups in transfusion reactions. J Immunol 41: 181

Wiener AS (1942a) Hemolytic transfusion reactions. I. Diagnosis, with special reference to the method of differential agglutination. Am J Clin Pathol 12: 189

Wiener AS (1942b) Hemolytic transfusion reactions. III. Prevention, with special reference to the Rh and cross-match tests. Am J Clin Pathol 12: 302

Wiener AS (1950) Reaction transfusionnelle hémolytique due à une sensibiliation anti-M. Rev Hématol 5: 3

Wiener AS (1954) Newer blood factors and their clinical significance. NY State J Med 54: 3071

Wiener AS, Moloney WC (1943) Hemolytic transfusion reactions. IV. Differential diagnosis. 'Dangerous universal donor' or intragroup incompatibility. Am J Clin Pathol 13: 74

Wiener AS, Peters HR (1940) Hemolytic reactions following transfusions of blood of the homologous group, with three cases in which the same agglutinogen was responsible. Ann Intern Med 13: 2306

With TK (1949) On jaundice. Acta Med Scand (Suppl.): 234

Worel N, Greinix HT, Keil F et al (2002) Severe immune hemolysis after minor ABO-mismatched allogeneic peripheral blood progenitor cell transplantation occurs more frequently after nonmyeloablative than myeloablative conditioning. Transfusion 42: 1293–1301

Yoell JH (1966) Immune anti-N agglutinin in human serum. Report of apparent associated hemolytic reaction. Transfusion 6: 592

Young LE (1954) Blood groups and transfusion reactions. Am J Med 16: 885

Yuile CL, van Zandt TF, Ervin DM (1949) Hemolytic reactions produced in dogs by transfusion of incompatible dog blood and plasma. II. Renal aspects following whole blood transfusions. Blood 4: 1232

Zettner A, Bove JR (1963) Hemolytic transfusion reaction due to interdonor incompatibility. Transfusion 3: 48

Zumberg MS, Procter JL, Lottenberg R et al. (2001) Autoantibody formation in the alloimmunized red blood cell recipient: clinical and laboratory implications. Arch Intern Med 161: 285–290

Zupanska B, Uhrynowska M, Konopka L (1999) Transfusion-related acute lung injury due to granulocyte-agglutinating antibody in a patient with paroxysmal nocturnal hemoglobinuria. Transfusion 39: 944–947

495

12 Haemolytic disease of the fetus and the newborn

Definition

Haemolytic disease of the newborn (HDN) is a condition in which the lifespan of the infant's red cells is shortened by the action of specific antibodies derived from the mother by placental transfer. The disease begins in intrauterine life and is therefore correctly described as haemolytic disease of the fetus and newborn, but the simple term HDN has been used for a long time and can be taken to include haemolytic disease of the fetus (HDF).

An Rh D fetus carried by a D-negative mother whose serum contains anti-D may develop a positive direct antiglobulin test (DAT) by the eighth week of pregnancy, and severe anaemia and death *in utero* may occur as early as about the eighteenth week. However, in most cases, infants with a positive DAT are born alive. In such infants, the haemolytic process is maximal at the time of birth and thereafter diminishes as the concentration of maternal antibody in the infant's circulation declines. On the other hand, for reasons explained below, jaundice and anaemia become more severe after birth.

A positive DAT in a newborn infant does not establish the diagnosis of haemolytic disease. It is known that D-positive red cells may survive normally in a newborn infant with a positive DAT due to anti-D (first edition, p. 382) and that many infants with a positive DAT have no signs of increased red cell destruction. In practice it is often difficult to decide whether there is any increased red cell destruction because, in almost all newborn infants, serum bilirubin concentration rises during the first 2–3 days of life

(Davidson *et al*. 1941) and there is a progressive fall in Hb concentration, which continues for a period of about 2 months.

Transfer of antibodies from mother to fetus

In humans, the transfer of antibodies from mother to fetus takes place only via the placenta. The only immunoglobulin transferred is IgG, which is bound and transported by an Fc receptor. Substantial evidence supports the identification of this receptor as the neonatal Fc receptor (FcRn). The structure of FcRn is unlike other Fc receptors (see Chapter 3). It is a distant member of the MHC class 1 protein family and is dependent for function on dimerization with $\beta 2$ microglobulin. The $\alpha 2$ and $\beta 2$ microglobulin domains of FcRn interact with the $C\gamma 2$ and $C\gamma 3$ domains of the IgG molecule (Plate 12.1, shown in colour between pages 528 and 529). When male mice with a defective *FcRn* gene (FcRn–/–) were mated with an FcRn+/– female and the pregnant female given intravenous injection of anti-TNP IgG1 at 17 days of gestation, the resulting FcRn–/– pups had a minimum of 190-fold reduction in serum anti-TNP activity in comparison with her FcRn+/– pups at 3 days old (Roopenian *et al*. 2003). These results are not strictly transferable to man, as neonatal mice acquire most of their maternal IgG through transintestinal transport; however, studies of IgG transport in an *ex vivo* human placental model are entirely consistent with an essential role for FcRn. Firan and co-workers (2001) compared placental transport of a wild-type IgG1 and a humanized IgG1 with a His435Ala mutation (the mutant antibody did not react with human FcRn) and demonstrated defective transport of the mutant antibody. FcRn is not confined to placenta in man and is found in monocytes, macrophages and dendritic cells (Zhu et al. 2001). FcRn functions not only to transfer IgG from mother to fetus to provide passive protective immunity, but also to protect IgG from normal serum protein catabolism. As a consequence, the half-life of IgG is considerably longer than other immunoglobulins (22–23 days in humans; see Table 3.4). FcRn transports IgG in acidic vesicles (< pH 6.5) thereby preventing lysosomal degradation and releases IgG to the blood at pH 7.4. The pH-dependent interaction involves histidine residues on the Fc portion of IgG and residues on FcRn that are charged at acidic but not basic pH (Martin et al. 2001).

The transfer of IgG is an active process and takes place only from mother to fetus and not in the reverse direction. In the first 12 weeks of gestation, only small amounts of IgG are transferred, although when the mother's serum contains relatively potent anti-D the DAT on the fetal (D-positive) red cells may be positive as early as 6–10 weeks (Mollison 1951; Chown 1955). At about the twenty-fourth week of pregnancy, the mean IgG concentration in the fetus is 1.8 g/l and thereafter rises exponentially until term (Yeung and Hobbs 1968). At term, the IgG level in the infant tends to be higher than in its mother; only slight differences have been found in some series (e.g. Lee et al. 1986), but in one the differences in mean values were substantial, namely infants 15.12 g/l and mothers 12.60 g/l (Kohler and Farr 1966).

The rate of transfer of IgG from mother to fetus at term is relatively slow (DuPan et al. 1959). When labelled IgG was injected into pregnant women at various intervals before delivery, even after 12 days the concentration in the infant's serum was only about 40% of that in the mother's (Gitlin et al. 1964). The rate of transfer of anti-Rh D across the placenta may well be the rate-limiting step in the reaction between maternal anti-D and the fetal red cells (Hughes-Jones et al. 1971).

By giving large doses of IgG intravenously (IVIG) to a pregnant woman with hypogammaglobulinaemia throughout the third trimester, it has proved possible to increase the fetal serum IgG concentration substantially (Hammarström and Smith 1986). Evidence that large doses of IVIG given to mother or fetus diminish the severity of HDN is discussed later.

IgG subclasses

IgG1 levels begin to rise at an earlier stage of gestation than IgG3 levels (Morell et al. 1971; Schur et al. 1973). Although fetal to maternal ratios of all four IgG subclasses were found to be similar in cord serum by Morell and co-workers, others have found a relative deficiency of IgG2 (Wang et al. 1970; Hay et al. 1971). Whereas the relative concentration of IgG1 in fetal serum compared with maternal serum is 1.77, for IgG2 the figure is 0.99 (Einhorn et al. 1987). These findings are consistent with the observation that Fcγ receptors in placental tissue bind IgG1 with higher affinity than IgG2 (McNabb et al. 1976).

Persistence of anti-D in the infant after birth

In D-negative infants with passively acquired anti-D, the antibody titre declines with a $T_{1/2}$ of 2–3 weeks; owing to the growth of the infant, the titre declines a little more rapidly than expected from catabolism alone. As an example, when the titre at the time of birth is 128, the antibody will still be just detectable after 100 days. In D-positive infants not treated by exchange transfusion, the DAT may remain positive for at least 3 months.

IgG red cell alloantibodies causing haemolytic disease

The commonest IgG red cell antibodies in human serum are anti-A and anti-B, although, as described in Chapter 4, relatively high concentrations are found only in group O subjects. Although ABO haemolytic disease is common, relatively few infants are severely affected; the proportion is higher in some populations than in others.

Before the introduction of immunosuppressive therapy with anti-D Ig, the antibody involved in most cases of moderate or severe HDF was anti-D, and this antibody continues to be the commonest cause of death from haemolytic disease. Nevertheless, its importance relative to that of other alloantibodies has diminished substantially following the introduction of suppressive therapy with anti-D immunoglobulin. For example, the number of deaths registered in England and Wales from haemolytic disease due to anti-D fell from 106 in 1977 to 11 in 1990 (Clarke

497

and Whitfield 1979; Hussey and Clarke 1992). The number of deaths from haemolytic disease due to anti-c and -K was the same in 1977 and 1990, namely four. Similarly, if one compares the results of antenatal screening tests in periods before and after the introduction of suppressive therapy there has been a substantial change in the frequency with which anti-D is found in relation to anti-c. For example, in one series before the introduction of suppressive therapy the ratio was 74:1 (Giblett 1964) and in one series after the introduction of suppressive therapy it was 10:1 (Kornstad 1983).

Haemolytic disease due to anti-D tends to be more severe than haemolytic disease due to anti-c. As a cause of death from haemolytic disease, anti-K is next in importance after anti-c.

The presence of red cell alloantibodies in the serum of pregnant women is often the consequence of a previous transfusion rather than of pregnancy. For example, a history of transfusion is common in pregnant women whose serum contains anti-c, anti-K or anti-Fy^a.

The list of antibodies that have caused HDN includes most, but not all, of those that can occur as IgG, i.e. in the Rh system: anti-D -c, -C, -C^w, -C^X, -e, -E, -E^w, -ce, -Ce^s, -Rh29, -Rh32, -Go^a, -Be^a, -Evans, -Riv; in the Kell system: anti-K, -k, -Ku, -Kp^a, -Kp^b, -Js^a and -Js^b; in the Duffy system: anti-Fy^a and -Fy3; in the Kidd system: anti-Jk^a, -Jk^b and -Jk3; in the MNSs system: anti-M, '-N', -S, -s, -U, -Vw, -Far, -M^v, -Mit, -Mur, -Hil, -Hut and -En^a; in other systems: anti-PP$_1$P^k; anti-LW, -Di^a, -Di^b and -Wr^a; anti-Yt^a and -Yt^b; anti-Sc2; anti-Do^a; anti-Co^a and anti-Co3; anti-Ge; antibodies to the following low-frequency antigens: Bi, By, Fr^a, Good, Rd, Re^a Zd; and antibodies to the following high-frequency antigens: Jr^a and Lan. In the foregoing list, the only antibodies that have been associated with moderate or severe haemolytic disease are the following: all the Rh specificities mentioned, anti-K, -k, -Kp^a, -Kp^b, -Ku, -Js^a, -Js^b, -Jk^a, -Fy^a, -M, -U, -PP$_1$P^k, -Di^b, -Lan, -LW, -Far, -Good, -Wr^a, -Zd (for references, see Chapter 6 and Daniels 1995).

Failure of alloantibodies of some systems to cause HDN may be due to paucity of antigen sites on fetal red cells, for example Le, Lu, or to absorption by fetal antigen in the placenta, for example In (Longster and Robinson 1981), Cr (Reid *et al.* 1996) and Lu (Herron *et al.* 1996).

Haemolytic disease of the fetus and newborn due to anti-Rh D (Rh D haemolytic disease)

In a case described by Levine and Stetson (1939), a woman who had recently been delivered of a macerated stillborn fetus developed a severe reaction after receiving a transfusion from her husband. Her serum was found to contain an alloagglutinin reacting at 37°C and it was postulated that she had been immunized by 'products from her disintegrating fetus'. Although the fetal death was not attributed to the antibody, subsequently shown to be anti-Rh D, the role of anti-D in causing HDN was amply documented in a subsequent paper (Levine *et al.* 1941).

As Rh antigens are present only on red cells, Rh D immunization develops in D-negative subjects only after the i.v. or i.m. injection of D-positive red cells or following transplacental haemorrhage (TPH) from a D-positive fetus.

Immunization by pregnancy – transplacental haemorrhage

The fact that small numbers of fetal red cells very frequently cross the placenta was recognized only after the introduction of the 'acid-elution' method of differential staining, which permits the detection of very small numbers of fetal red cells in the mother's circulation.

Detection of fetal red cells by the acid-elution method

In this method, blood films are fixed in alcohol and then treated with an acid buffer (pH 3.3). Adult haemoglobin (Hb) but not fetal Hb is soluble at this pH so that (after counterstaining) fetal red cells stand out as dark cells in a field of ghosts (Kleihauer and Betke 1960). Details are given in Appendix 13.

In interpreting results obtained with the acid-elution method, the presence of an increased percentage of adult red cells containing fetal Hb (F cells) may cause difficulty. First, amongst the normal population, adults of both sexes may have some form of hereditary persistence of fetal Hb (HPFH), most commonly the so-called Swiss-type (heterocellular) HPFH; using the acid-elution method, F cells are found in small numbers in 1–2% of normal adults.

Second, in about 25% of pregnant women, the level of maternal Hb F rises above the upper limit of normal (0.9%), starting at about 8 weeks, and may reach 7%; the increase may persist until about the thirty-second week. When blood films from adults are examined by the acid-elution method, there are some cells that stain so darkly as to be indistinguishable from cells of fetal origin and there are many additional cells that give intermediate staining (Pembrey *et al.* 1973).

Using a very sensitive method employing fluorescein-labelled anti-Hb F, some F cells are found in all normal subjects, with an upper limit of 4.4% (Miyoshi *et al.* 1988; Sampietro *et al.* 1992), In a survey of normal adults in Japan, 11% of men and 20% of women had more than 4.4% of F cells, suggesting that the level of F cells in normal adults may be sex linked (Miyoshi *et al.* 1988). When the immunofluorescence method is used to examine the blood of pregnant women, an increase in F cells is always found in the second trimester; the increase starts at about 16 weeks and is usually maintained until 24–28 weeks (Popat *et al.* 1977).

Quantification of fetal red cells by the acid-elution method

Various methods have been used to estimate the amount of fetal red cells present in the maternal circulation. The best one is to express the number of fetal red cells present as a proportion of adult cells in the same sample, although in order to deduce the absolute amount of fetal red cells present, various points must be taken into account:

1 That fetal red cells are larger than adult cells so that the volume present will be greater than that indicated by the number present.
2 That not all fetal red cells stain darkly by the acid-elution method.
3 That an arbitrary figure for maternal red cell volume has to be assumed.

Making the following assumptions: (1) that fetal red cells have a volume about 22% larger than adult red cells; (2) that about 92% of fetal red cells stain darkly; and (3) that the average red cell volume of a recently delivered woman is 1800 ml, the volume of fetal red cells (ml) present in the maternal circulation is 2400 ÷ the ratio of darkly staining to normal staining red cells (Mollison 1972).

The method of estimating the size of TPH from the number of darkly staining cells per low-power field has been quite widely used but is very inaccurate. One important source of error is variability in the thickness of blood films; in one survey, the density of adult cells per square millimetre in different laboratories was found to vary from about 1000 to 16 000 (Mollison 1972).

If the number of adult red cells in a given area is determined, and the number of darkly stained cells expressed as a proportion of the total number of cells present, accuracy is improved. The accuracy of fetal cell counts in different laboratories was assessed by distributing samples of adult blood to which known amounts of fetal red cells had been added. Laboratories were asked to determine the ratio of fetal to adult red cells present. When the number of fetal red cells present was very small, for example corresponding to a ratio of 1:10 000 adult cells, there was an almost 10-fold difference between the lowest and highest estimates, but when the amount of red cells present corresponded to about 1:1000 or more, equivalent to a TPH of 2 ml or more, and the estimates were interpreted by the method described above, almost all values fell within 50–200% of the correct ones (Mollison 1972). A method of making quantitative estimates of the extent of TPH is described in Appendix 13. A simple modification of the method, which improves the accuracy of counting maternal cells, is described by Howarth and colleagues (2002). In this modification acid elution is performed on only one-half of the blood film and the maternal cells counted on the stained half of the film, rather than counted as red cell 'ghosts' after acid elution.

Detection of α-fetoprotein in maternal serum

α-Fetoprotein (α-FP), an analogue of albumin, has a concentration in fetal plasma of 3–4 mg/ml at about the thirteenth to fifteenth week of pregnancy, falling to about 50 µg/l at term. In pregnant women the plasma level is about 35 ng/ml in the first trimester, rising to a maximum of about 200 ng/ml at the end of pregnancy (Seppala and Ruoslahti 1972; Caballero *et al.* 1977). As the level of α-FP is so much higher in the fetus than in the mother, changes in maternal serum concentration have been used, although only in research, as an index of TPH.

499

Serological methods of detecting transplacental haemorrhage

Rosetting tests. In looking for small numbers of fetal D-positive red cells in the circulation of an Rh D-negative mother, the method is as follows: anti-D is added to a sample of red cells taken from the mother in order to coat any D-positive cells that may be present; the red cells are washed; D-positive 'detector' red cells (enzyme treated) are now added and form rosettes round any D-positive cells present in the original sample. In one study it was noted that when 15 ml or more of fetal cells was present in the mother's circulation they were detected by rosetting in 99–100% of cases. On the other hand, when the same maternal sample was incubated with anti-D and then tested by the indirect antiglobulin method (IAT) (a technique referred to in the past as a D^u test) the D-positive cells were missed in 15% of cases (Sebring 1984). By comparison with known mixtures of D-positive and D-negative red cells, an approximate estimate of the amount of fetal red cells present can be obtained.

Flow cytometry. In one method the maternal sample is first treated with anti-D and then with fluorescein-labelled anti-IgG. The smallest number of D-positive red cells in a D-negative population that can be detected with reasonable accuracy is about 1 in 1000; the coefficient of variation is approximately 13% (Nance *et al.* 1989a). Using the acid-elution method on the same samples, estimates were about twice as high, a result that could have been due only partly to the detection of HbF-containing maternal red cells and was otherwise unexplained (Nance *et al.* 1989a). Overestimates of TPH with the acid-elution method have been reported by others. In one series, no fetal cells were found by flow cytometry in 13 out of 43 cases that were positive by the acid-elution method, suggesting that the latter method was detecting fetal Hb in maternal red cells (Johnson *et al.* 1995). In another series, the acid-elution method was found to be more accurate when the TPH was less than 1 ml but to overestimate TPH when the amount was greater than this (Lloyd-Evans *et al.* 1996). Lloyd-Evans and co-workers used a monoclonal anti-D directly conjugated with fluorescein isothiocyanate (FITC-BRAD 3). Not all investigations have concluded that the acid-elution method overestimates the true proportion of fetal red cells present. From one comparison with flow cytometry on artificial mixtures it was concluded that 'acid elution is much more accurate and reliable than previously thought' (Bayliss *et al.* 1991). In a trial in which known mixtures of fetal and adult blood were distributed to many different centres, when the proportion of fetal red cells corresponded to a TPH of 1 ml or more the observed average values were virtually identical to the true values (Mollison 1972). Murine monoclonal anti-HbF conjugated to fluorescein iso-thiocyanate has been used to quantify fetal cells in adult blood in comparison with the Kleihauer–Betke method and a good correlation obtained (Davis *et al.* 1998). In this method, cells are fixed with glutaraldehyde and permeabilized by exposure to Triton X-100 prior to incubation with anti-HbF. Kennedy and co-workers (2003) provide evidence that using anti-HbF rather than anti-D underestimates the number of fetal cells detected when the TPH is equal to 1% of fetal cells per sample.

The lack of consensus in different studies seeking to compare the relative sensitivity of flow cytometry with the Kleihauer–Betke method is most likely a reflection of technical differences in the way the assays are performed in different laboratories. Direct measurement of the number of D-positive red cells in maternal circulation obviates concerns about false-positive measurement of adult cells containing HbF and, as flow cytometers become more widely available, it is likely that this will be the method of choice for measurement of transplacental haemorrhage. Nevertheless, careful standardization of the flow cytometry method is essential. One source of variation is the gating of total red cells for calculation of the size of the fetal bleed. In order to avoid errors in manual gating, the use of an antibody reactive with adult and fetal red cells has been proposed (Lloyd-Evans *et al.* 2000). In this method, phycoerythrin-conjugated murine monoclonal anti-glycophorin A (PE-BRIC-256) is used to label all red cells in the sample and fluorescein isothiocyanate-labelled human monoclonal anti-D (FITC-BRAD-3) is used to determine the proportion of D-positive (fetal) cells. Greiss and co-workers (2002) describe a semi-automated flow cytometry assay based on a standard-ized calibration curve created using artificial mixtures of D-positive red cells in D-negative red cells.

Transplacental haemorrhage measurement in the UK

At the end of 2004 there was a total of 250 registered

participating laboratories in the UK National External Quality Assessment Scheme for measurement of TPH; 23 were registered for screening only, 191 for quantification by acid elution only, 10 for quantification by flow cytometry only and 26 for quantification by both methods (C Milkins, personal communication).

Use of fluorescent microspheres

A minor population of D-positive red cells in a D-negative sample can be recognized by first adding anti-D, then fluorescent anti-IgG-coated microspheres. Using this method, one D-positive red cell per 10 000 D-negative cells could be detected, corresponding to a TPH of 0.2 ml. The frequency of TPH appeared to be much smaller than that found with the acid-elution method (van Dijk et al. 1994), but the sample was small and only TPHs of D-positive red cells in D-negative women were studied.

Frequency of transplacental haemorrhage

First two trimesters. The increase in HbF observed in about 25% of women between about the eighth and thirty-second weeks of pregnancy complicates the interpretation of counts of fetal cells made by the acid-elution method during this period. Nevertheless, some deductions can be made, particularly when findings in two different types of cases have been compared. For example, in women who had had ectopic gestations, blood samples taken 3 h or more after laparotomy contained substantially greater numbers of fetal red cells than samples taken from women with normal gestations at the same stage of pregnancy (Liedholm 1971). Incidentally, in the women with ectopic gestations, blood had been found in the abdominal cavity in almost every case.

In another comparison HbF cells were found in 35% of women who had spontaneous abortions in the first or second trimester but in only 13% of women with normal pregnancies at the same stage. The amount of red cells in the circulation was never more than about 0.05 ml. In women undergoing therapeutic abortions, comparisons of blood samples before and after the operation showed an increase in the number of HbF cells in 17%. The extent of the haemorrhage was greater than 0.05 ml of red cells in 5% and greater than 0.5 ml in 2% (Jorgensen 1975).

Third trimester. The proportion of women in whom fetal red cells can be detected is greater towards the end of pregnancy than in the earlier stages. In one series, cells were found almost twice as frequently in the third trimester as in the second (Cohen et al. 1964); in another, fetal cells were found only rarely in the first and second trimesters, but commonly in the third (Krevans et al. 1964). Quantitative estimates have varied widely. Some figures for the frequency with which fetal cells can be identified in the maternal circulation are as follows: at 28–30 weeks, 0.40% and at 30–39 weeks, 1.84% (Bowman and Pollock 1987); at 28 weeks, 5.8% and at 34 weeks 7.0% (Huchet et al. 1988) and in the last trimester, 3.5% (Woodrow and Finn 1966). As one might expect, the discrepancies arise from the number of women estimated to have very small TPHs, which are difficult to determine with certainty. For TPHs of 2.5 ml or more of red cells, the discrepancies were relatively minor, namely at 30–39 weeks, 0.94% (Bowman and Pollock 1987) and at 34 weeks, 0.5% (Huchet et al. 1988).

Amniocentesis. The use of methods, particularly ultrasonography, for localizing the placenta has greatly reduced but has not abolished the risk of causing TPH during amniocentesis. In one retrospective survey covering the period 1981–84, of almost 1000 women on whom amniocentesis had been performed at 16–18 weeks' gestation for diagnosing genetic disorders, 2.6% had a TPH > 0.1 ml of fetal red cells due, presumably, to placental trauma. In 1.6% of the women, the TPH was estimated to be 1 ml or more. In approximately 1200 women having an amniocentesis between 32 and 38 weeks' gestation to assess Rh D haemolytic disease, 2.3% had a TPH of > 0.1 ml and 1.8% of > 1 ml (Bowman and Pollock 1985).

The risk of Rh D immunization following amniocentesis is greater than these figures imply. In one series of D-negative women with D-positive infants, anti-D developed in 3 out of 58 who were not given anti-D, even although no fetal cells had been detected following amniocentesis; of 59 women who were given anti-D Ig after the amniocentesis, not one became immunized (MRC 1978). Rapid rises in maternal anti-D concentration following amniocentesis were observed in several cases in another series (Grant et al. 1983).

Chorionic villus sampling. This can be carried out as early as 8–11 weeks' gestation for the diagnosis of chromosomal abnormalities and genetically determined diseases or for determining fetal blood groups.

Using a solid-phase microfluorescence technique, fetal red cell antigens could be detected in all of 11 cases in which they carried an antigen (A, B, c or E) not present on the maternal cells (Gemke *et al.* 1986).

In 161 patients undergoing chorionic villus sampling (CVS) at 7–14 weeks, no fetal red cells could be detected by the acid-elution method. On the other hand, the maternal α-FP level rose significantly in 49%; the chance of an increase was correlated with the number of attempts at biopsy. It was concluded that as few attempts as possible should be made and that in any case, when the mother was D negative, a dose of anti-D Ig should be given (Warren *et al.* 1985).

During normal delivery. TPH is relatively common. In one series in which fetal red cells were detected in the blood of 59 out of 200 women immediately after delivery, it was concluded that in 40 of the cases the TPH had occurred during delivery (Woodrow *et al.* 1965).

If the placental blood is allowed to drain freely, immediately after the cord has been tied and the infant separated, the incidence and magnitude of TPH are substantially reduced (Terry 1970; Ladipo 1972).

Following normal delivery. In three series, in each of which the blood of between 2000 and 5000 recently delivered women was examined, estimates of the extent of TPH were similar (Fig. 12.1).

In Fig. 12.1, the magnitude of TPH on a logarithmic scale is plotted against cumulative frequency, also on a logarithmic scale. The fact that the data can be reasonably well fitted by a straight line is convenient, as it is easy to read off the expected frequency of interpolated values. As the figure shows, about 1% of women have 3.0 ml or more of fetal red cells in their circulation at the time of delivery and 0.3% have 10 ml or more. The latter estimate agrees closely with other estimates, for example more than about 10 ml of fetal red cells in 0.2% of recently delivered women (Bartsch 1972) and 15 ml or more in 0.3%, based on about 8000 cases from seven different centres (Zipursky 1971).

The data plotted in Fig. 12.1 suggest that the fact that fetal red cells can be detected in the circulation of only about 50% of recently delivered women, using the acid-elution method, is due simply to the relative insensitivity of the method.

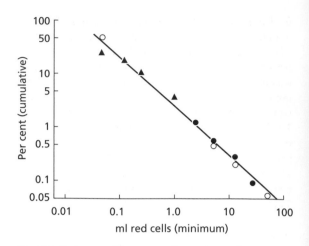

Fig 12.1 Estimates of the extent of transplacental haemorrhage at the time of delivery in three different series: 1 (▲), Woodrow and Donohoe (1968); 2 (○), E Borst-Eilers (personal communication); 3 (●), Poulain and Huchet (1971).

Only women with ABO-compatible infants were included in the first series; in the other two series, the cases were unselected. Each point indicates the percentage of women found to have x ml or more of fetal red cells in their circulation immediately after delivery.

Effect of ABO incompatibility. When the fetus is ABO incompatible with the mother, fetal red cells are less frequently detected in her circulation and then only in small numbers.

In two large series, when the fetus was ABO incompatible, fetal red cells were found in 19% and 24.7% of cases, respectively, compared with 50% and 56%, respectively, when the fetus was ABO compatible (Cohen and Zuelzer 1967; Woodrow and Donohoe 1968). Moreover, when the fetus was ABO incompatible, the amount of fetal red cells was usually very small, for example 0.1 ml or more in only 1.9% of cases when the fetus was ABO incompatible, compared with 18.5% when it was compatible (Woodrow and Donohoe 1968). In another series, 0.05 ml or more of red cells were found in 0.5% of cases when the fetus was ABO incompatible but in 23.1% of cases in which it was ABO compatible (Schneider 1969).

Caesarean section and manual removal of placenta. These are associated with a considerable increase in the number of fetal red cells found in the maternal circulation: in one series the incidence of those with fetal cells was 23.5% compared with only 5.2% in mothers who had had a normal labour (Finn *et al.* 1963), and in another series the number of women with more than 0.5 ml of fetal blood in the circulation was about 11% after a caesarean section or manual removal of the placenta compared with less than 1% in women with uncomplicated deliveries (Zipursky *et al.* 1963a,b). Similarly, of women with a TPH corresponding to 5 ml or more of fetal red cells, 12% had had the placenta removed manually compared with 1% of those who had not; fetal distress during labour was also significantly more frequent when there was a TPH of 5 ml or more (Li *et al.* 1988).

'Late' entry of fetal red cells into the maternal circulation, via the peritoneal cavity. There seem to be two possible routes by which fetal red cells may reach the mother's peritoneal cavity and thence make their way into her circulation. First, if they are spilled into the uterine cavity, they may pass into the peritoneal cavity by the fallopian tubes. Occasionally this can be observed after vaginal termination of pregnancy, when this is followed immediately by tubal ligation or diathermy. Second, fetal red cells may be spilt into the peritoneal cavity at hysterotomy or caesarean section. In one series of 46 women who underwent caesarean section, fetal cells were not detected in any maternal samples at 4 h but were found in six cases at 6 days (Hindemann 1966).

Massive transplacental haemorrhage. A massive TPH may be arbitrarily defined as one of more than 25 ml of red cells (50 ml of blood). TPHs of this magnitude occur in approximately one per 1000 pregnancies (Renaer *et al.* 1976) (see also Fig. 12.1). If the blood volume of an infant at term is taken as 270 ml plus 120 ml in the placental circulation, i.e. 390 ml, a haemorrhage of 50 ml is equivalent to 13% of the circulating blood volume.

The cause of most massive TPHs is unknown, but can occasionally be identified, as when there is maternal trauma, for example a fall or a car accident, or when there is a placental chorioangioma (Sims *et al.* 1976) or a uterine choriocarcinoma (Blackburn 1976). From a review of the literature and from 64 personally observed cases, it was concluded that more than 50% of women with a TPH of 15 ml or more of fetal red cells have no history of any of the risk factors commonly believed to be important, for example intrapartum

manipulation or placenta praevia. The few risk factors that were associated with large TPHs included premature separation of the placenta, manual removal of the placenta and fetal death (Sebring and Polesky 1990). Dziegiel and co-workers (2005) describe a case of massive TPH from an ABO-compatible fetus, which demonstrated the lifespan of some fetal red cells in the adult circulation to be the same as that of adult red cells (but see Chapter 9, p. 358).

When the fetus is ABO incompatible, a large TPH may be masked. In two cases in which infants were born with Hb concentrations of 3.5 and 6.9 g/dl, respectively, the percentage of fetal red cells demonstrable in the mother's circulation was 0.6% and 1.9% respectively. As these infants must have lost amounts of red cells of the order of 100 ml, at least 6% of the cells in the mother's circulation would have been expected to have been of fetal origin if they had survived normally, i.e. had been ABO compatible (Cohen and Zuelzer 1967).

Effect on fetus. Of women who had had a stillbirth, 4.5% were found to have the equivalent of 25 ml or more of fetal red cells in their circulation (Huchet *et al.* 1975). This incidence is far higher than in a random series, leading to the conclusion that some stillbirths are caused by a massive TPH.

When a massive TPH occurs during delivery, the infant may be in a condition of oligaemic shock at birth but with a more or less normal Hb concentration, as there has been too little time for haemodilution. On the other hand, when there has been chronic severe bleeding the infant may be born with severe anaemia with signs of intense blood regeneration (Huchet *et al.* 1975; Renaer *et al.* 1976; Sims *et al.* 1976); very occasionally, hydrops has been observed (e.g. Weisert and Marstrander 1960; Renaer *et al.* 1978). In one case, diagnosed from reduced fetal movements, haemorrhage was estimated as 350 ml of blood; the fetal PCV was 0.056. Following two intrauterine transfusions, the hydrops resolved and the infant was born alive. After further transfusions, the infant's progress was normal (Konugres *et al.* 1994).

Chronic fetal–maternal bleeding may be responsible for iron deficiency anaemia in the fetus (Pearson and Diamond 1959; Miles *et al.* 1971).

Effect on the mother. When the fetus is ABO incompatible, a large TPH may be associated with haemoglobinuria in the mother. One such episode fol-lowed an easy external cephalic version under general anaesthesia. The mother (group O) passed fetal Hb in the urine (0.2 g Hb/dl). Four weeks later, a group A infant was born; the placenta showed a small area of separation (Pollock 1968). In 14 further cases of exter-nal version, fetal cells were found in only one, and in this case the mother's blood had not been examined before version.

The passage of red cells from mother to fetus

The passage of red cells from mother to fetus is far less common than traffic in the reverse direction. Using a rosetting test, maternal red cells were detected in 70% of infants, but the total volume of maternal red cells in the infant exceeded 0.01 ml in only 2 out of 92 cases (Helderweirt 1963). With a new cytological method, the Kleihauer immunogold-silver-staining technique, 73 newborn infants were tested; the mothers had been selected as having an Rh antigen (D, c or E) absent from the infant's red cells so that their cells could be recognized serologically; maternal red cells equivalent to 1 μl or more of blood were detected in only three infants; the amount was about 1 μl in two cases and about 100 μl in the third (Brossard et al. 1996). A very rare case in which a massive materno-fetal haemor-rhage was associated with non-immunological hydrops fetalis is described on p. 508.

Frequency of opportunities for Rh D immunization in pregnancy

In about one of every 10 pregnancies in white people, the mother is D negative and the fetus is D positive. The calculation is as follows: 17% of women are D negative; 83% of their partners are D positive of whom 35 are DD and 48 Dd. All children born to the homozygous (DD) fathers will be D positive but only one-half of those born to the heterozygous (Dd) fathers will be D positive. Thus, of every 100 pregnan-cies, the number in which the fetus is D positive and the mother is D negative will be:

$$17\left(\frac{35}{100} + \frac{0.5 \times 48}{100}\right) = 10 \qquad (12.1)$$

When primary Rh D immunization is induced in a first pregnancy, the amount of anti-D produced is almost always too small to produce haemolytic disease in the fetus. In considering the opportunities for pro-ducing Rh D haemolytic disease, one must therefore calculate how frequently a D-negative woman gives birth to two D-positive infants. As family size is often restricted to two children, one may consider how often a D-negative woman has two D-positive infants in suc-cession. When her partner is DD, all her infants will be D positive, but when he is Dd, the chance that he will pass on D twice in succession is only one in four.

Thus, of every 100 second pregnancies, the number in which a D-negative woman is carrying her second D-positive infant is given by:

$$17\left(\frac{35}{100} + \frac{0.25 \times 48}{100}\right) = 8 \qquad (12.2)$$

In calculating the frequency of opportunities for immunization to Rh D, account must be taken of the fact that primary immunization to Rh D is rare when the fetal red cells are ABO incompatible with the mother's serum, as occurs, in white people, in about 20% of pregnancies. Thus, the figure '8' must be multi-plied by 0.8 (80%) to give an estimate of the number, i.e. about 6, of second pregnancies in every 100 in which a D-negative mother would be expected to have an infant with Rh D haemolytic disease if: (1) every first pregnancy with an ABO-compatible, D-positive infant induced primary immunization to Rh D; and (2) every subsequent pregnancy with a D-positive infant resulted in haemolytic disease. The frequency of Rh D haemolytic disease in the era before immunoprophy-laxis was about one-sixth of this, i.e. 1 per 100 of second pregnancies. The main reasons why, in five out of six cases, in the absence of immunoprophylaxis, the second infant is not affected with haemolytic dis-ease are, first, that the amount of TPH is often too small to induce primary immunization and, second, that even when the amount is large enough to induce primary immunization in some subjects, in others (non-responders) it is not.

In the preceding paragraph, for convenience, a positive DAT has been regarded as diagnostic of haemolytic disease. As discussed above, some infants with a positive DAT due to maternally derived alloan-tibody have no signs of increased red cell destruction. However, in practice there is no way of distinguishing in a newborn infant between no increased red cell destruction and a slight increase in red cell destruction and so, in calculating the frequency of the disease, all infants with a positive DAT have to be included.

Primary Rh D immunization caused by pregnancy in the absence of immunosuppressive therapy

Abortion

There is evidence that significant TPH occurs only after curettage and does not occur after either threatened or incomplete spontaneous abortions (Katz 1969; Matthews and Matthews 1969; Jørgensen 1975). In fact, evidence that spontaneous abortion occurring in the first trimester can cause primary Rh D immunization scarcely exists. In one series of women who had not been given anti-D Ig after an abortion occurring in the first 12 weeks of pregnancy and who developed anti-D during the following pregnancy, there were eight in whom the abortion had been spontaneous. In these eight cases, anti-D developed only during the last weeks of the succeeding pregnancy, and immmunization might well have been initiated by TPH occurring during the second pregnancy rather than by the previous abortion (LAD Tovey, personal communication).

Following induced abortion in D-negative primiparae, anti-D was found within the first 3 months of the following pregnancy in 1.5% and by term in 3.1% of the women (Simonovits et al. 1980). A similar frequency was found in another series, in which termination in the second month of pregnancy seemed to carry about the same risk of inducing immunization as termination carried out later (Hočevar and Glonar 1974). As 40% of fetuses carried by D-negative women are expected to be D positive, the frequency with which immunization to Rh D occurs following the induced abortion of a D-positive fetus must be higher than 3%. Even after making allowance for the fact that some women must become primarily immunized during the following pregnancy, the overall risk of immunization following the termination of pregnancy in a D-negative woman seems to be at least 4%.

Anti-D present by the end of a first full-term pregnancy

In D-negative women with no history of previous transfusion who are tested at the end of their first pregnancy with a D-positive infant, anti-D is found in approximately 1%, for example 0.8%, deduced from

the data of Hartmann and Brendemoen (1953); 0.71%, (Eklund 1973); and 0.9%, i.e. 18 in 2000 (Tovey et al. 1983). An apparently much higher incidence, namely 62 in 3533, or 1.8%, was reported in a Canadian series (Bowman et al. 1978). However, the series included some women who had been pregnant previously and some in whom anti-D was not present at delivery although present 3 days later. If only primiparae are considered and only those in whom anti-D was found by the time of delivery, the figures become 34 in 2767, or 1.2% (excluding one woman in whom anti-D was detected at 11 weeks). The remaining discrepancy between this figure and those (0.7–0.9%) reported by others can be explained by the fact that, in almost one-third of the Canadian cases, the anti-D was detectable only in the autoanalyzer or by enzyme methods. If only cases in which the antibody was detectable by IAT are included, the figures become the same as those reported by others.

When anti-D develops during a first pregnancy, it is most commonly first detectable in the last few weeks: in one series, antibody was detected between 36 weeks and term in 50% (Eklund 1971); in another, antibody was detected in about 40% at 34 weeks, although not at 28 weeks, and in the remaining 60% was found for the first time at delivery, having been undetectable at 34 weeks (Tovey et al. 1983). In the Canadian series, among the 34 primiparae (see above), anti-D was first detected by 28 weeks in two, by 34 weeks in three more, between 35 and 40 weeks in 15 more, and immediately after delivery in the remaining 14; antibody was found in a further 10 for the first time 3 days after delivery (Bowman et al. 1978).

Cases in which anti-D was detected 8 days after delivery, having been undetectable at the time of delivery, were originally reported by Bishop and Krieger (1969) and were also noted by Jørgensen (1975).

The evidence that, in a substantial number of D-negative women, primary immunization to Rh D occurs during pregnancy indicates that anti-D Ig must be given antenatally as well as postnatally if Rh D haemolytic disease is to be prevented in as many cases as possible.

Anti-D first detected 3–6 months after a first pregnancy, or during or after a subsequent pregnancy. Estimates of the incidence of anti-D in D-negative women 6 months after the birth of a first D-positive, ABO-compatible infant range from 4.3% in 1012 mothers (Eklund and Nevanlinna 1973) through 7.7% in 337 mothers (Borst-Eilers 1972) and 8.2% in about 400 mothers (Woodrow 1970) to 9.0% in 106 mothers (Jørgensen 1975). When antibody is present at 6 months it can almost always be detected at 3 months (Eklund and Nevanlinna 1973).

After the birth of a first D-positive infant to a D-negative mother, a relationship can be demonstrated between the number of fetal red cells demonstrable in the mother's circulation at the time of delivery and the chance that anti-D will appear. When no fetal cells are detectable, anti-D is found in only about 3% of cases, whereas when the amount is 0.1 ml or more anti-D is found in about 31% of cases (Woodrow 1970). In the series of Woodrow (1970) in which 8.2% of D-negative mothers had anti-D in their plasma 6 months after their first pregnancy with a D-positive fetus, by the end of a second pregnancy with a D-positive fetus the frequency of anti-D was 17% (or one in six). The appearance of anti-D in a further 9% of women during the second pregnancy must have been due, in the great majority of cases, to a secondary response during the second pregnancy, so that the conclusion is that, for every woman who develops serologically detectable anti-D following a first pregnancy, there is another who has been primarily immunized but who requires a further stimulus to produce sufficient anti-D to be detectable serologically.

Anti-D developing during or following a second or later pregnancy may of course be due to primary Rh D immunization initiated during that pregnancy. Anti-D detected only during the last few weeks of pregnancy or after the pregnancy is likely to be due to primary immunization occurring during that pregnancy, whereas anti-D detected early in a pregnancy is likely to represent secondary Rh D immunization.

After delivery it is not uncommon for the titre of anti-D to increase, reaching a peak 1–3 weeks post-partum (Boorman *et al.* 1945).

Fetal factors that may affect Rh D immunization

There is evidence that R_2r infants are more effective in sensitizing their mothers to Rh D than are infants of other phenotypes (Murray 1957).

There is also evidence which suggests that the D-positive infant that initiates Rh D immunization is more frequently male than female. The sex ratio, M/F, in one series was 1.44:1, control 1.05 (Renkonen and

Seppälä 1962), in another was 1.74 (Renkonen and Timonen 1967), and in another 1.5 (Woodrow 1970). In one more series, 18 out of 21 D-positive infants who initiated Rh D immunization in their mothers were male (Scott 1976).

Influence of ABO incompatibility on Rh D immunization in pregnancy

The fact that immunization to Rh D during pregnancy is less common when the father is ABO incompatible with the mother was noted by Levine (1943). In a series of matings between D-positive fathers and D-negative mothers who had given birth to infants affected with HDN, 25% were ABO incompatible (father's red cells vs. mother's serum) compared with 35% of ABO-incompatible matings expected in the general population (for later reviews, see Nevanlinna 1965 and Levine 1958.) It has been estimated that (in white people) group A incompatibility between infant and mother gives 90% protection, and B incompatibility gives 55% protection against Rh D immunization (Murray *et al.* 1965).

Do Rh D-negative infants get immunized by maternal Rh D-positive red cells?

Although it has been claimed that some D-negative infants born to D-positive mothers develop anti-D within the first 6 months of life, the data have never seemed convincing (for references and discussion, see eighth edition, p. 653). Incidentally, tests on the maternal grandmothers of infants with HDN have failed to show any significant excess of D positives amongst them (Booth *et al.* 1953; Owen *et al.* 1954; Ward *et al.* 1957).

Clinical manifestations of Rh D haemolytic disease

Haemolytic disease due to anti-D shows a wide spectrum of severity. In some D-positive infants whose red cells are coated with anti-D, as demonstrated by a positive DAT, there are no signs of red cell destruction. In infants in whom signs of red cell destruction are present, they may be so mild as to be recognized only by the development of mild jaundice on the first day or two of life and a slightly more rapid than normal fall in Hb concentration during the first 10 days or so (Fig. 12.2). (In all newborn infants, the Hb concentration falls because red cell production decreases rapidly

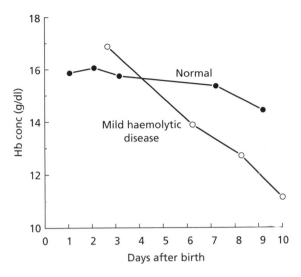

Fig 12.2 Rate of fall of haemoglobin (Hb) concentration in an infant mildly affected with haemolytic disease of the newborn, contrasted with the changes in a normal infant (from first edition, p. 385).

after birth, in association with a fall in erythropoietin levels, and remains depressed until the Hb concentration falls to about 10 g/dl.)

In more severely affected infants, jaundice may develop very rapidly (icterus gravis neonatorum). Unless the infant is treated promptly by exchange transfusion it may develop kernicterus, a syndrome characterized by lethargy, spasticity and opisthotonos, followed by irregular respiration. Of infants who develop kernicterus, about 70% die between about the second and fifth days of life and are found at autopsy to have yellow staining of the basal ganglia of the brain. Those who survive have permanent cerebral damage, characterized by choreoathetosis and spasticity; some infants show high-frequency deafness as the only sign. There is a close relationship between the peak serum bilirubin concentration and the development of kernicterus. In mature infants, kernicterus seldom, if ever, develops in association with serum bilirubin concentrations of less than 18 mg/dl (306 μmol/l) (Mollison and Cutbush 1951, 1954), although in premature infants there is some evidence that kernicterus develops at lower bilirubin levels (Ackerman et al. 1970).

In infants with a still more severe haemolytic process, profound anaemia develops and the infants may die *in utero* at any time from about the seventh week of gestation onwards.

In a series in which blood samples were obtained by fetoscopy at 18–24 weeks from 29 fetuses with severe haemolytic disease there were 14 with Hb values of less than 4 g/dl and 10 of these had the syndrome of hydrops fetalis (Nicolaides et al. 1985a). In this syndrome there is ascites and generalized oedema together with gross enlargement of the liver and spleen and, in many cases, of the heart. The oedema has been ascribed to the low serum albumin concentration that is almost always found (Phibbs et al. 1974). The finding of a relatively high concentration of albumin in the ascitic fluid suggests that damage to vascular endothelium, secondary to chronic hypoxia, may be an important feature in lowering the serum albumin concentration (Nicolaides et al. 1985b).

Severe hydrops fetalis is complicated by intravascular coagulation with widespread pulmonary haemorrhage and, in many cases, subarachnoid haemorrhage (Ellis et al. 1979). The outlook for infants with established or threatened hydrops due to haemolytic disease has been dramatically improved by the introduction of intravascular transfusion *in utero* (see below).

Non-immunological hydrops occurs in about 1 in 3500 births (MacAfee et al. 1970; Hutchinson et al. 1982). The list of causes is very long; among the commonest are cardiac abnormalities, chromosomal abnormalities and the twin-to-twin transfusion syndrome (Holzgreve et al. 1985). A single case has been described of hydrops due to a massive transfer, estimated at 470 ml of blood, from the maternal into the fetal circulation (Bowman et al. 1984).

The mortality rate of non-immunological hydrops is over 80% (Holzgreve et al. 1985). The subsequent infant is almost always normal (MacAfee et al. 1970).

Before the introduction of immunoprophylaxis with anti-D Ig, more than 80% of cases of fetal hydrops were due to haemolytic disease (MacAfee et al. 1970). Now, the percentage is less than 20.

Pattern of haemolytic disease in successive siblings

When anti-D develops during the first pregnancy it is only very seldom detected as early as the twenty-eighth week and is most commonly first detected during the last few weeks of pregnancy (see above). Moreover, when anti-D does develop during a first pregnancy, the concentration of the antibody is usually low. Accordingly, a D-positive infant born following a first pregnancy in a previous unimmunized woman very seldom shows clinical signs of haemolytic disease, and may simply have a positive DAT. When severe haemolytic disease is observed in a first-born infant it must always be suspected that the mother was immunized before the pregnancy.

In the first affected infant (i.e. in most cases born to a mother following a second or later pregnancy) haemolytic disease tends to be less severe than in subsequent affected siblings. For example, in first affected infants the stillbirth rate is 6% (Walker *et al.* 1957) but in second affected and later infants is about 29% (sixth edition, p. 677). After the second affected infant there is no tendency for the disease to become progressively more severe (HR Nevanlinna, personal communication, 1964; for further details, see previous editions of this book). Accordingly, in women who have had an affected infant the history is very helpful in giving a prognosis for any future infants. For example, the risk of stillbirth in a woman who has previously had a mildly affected infant is of the order of 2%, whereas in a woman who has had one previous stillbirth the risk of a subsequent stillbirth is as high as 70% (Walker *et al.* 1957). However, exceptions are known to occur. In one mother to whom a mildly affected infant was born after one fatally affected infant and two moderately affected ones, Fc receptor blocking antibodies were demonstrated in the mother's serum (see below).

Significance of a previous transfusion to the mother

Although the prognosis for infants of women who have previously been transfused with D-positive blood is not essentially different from that of other affected infants (Nevanlinna 1953), this generalization does not seem to apply if only first affected infants are considered (Levine *et al.* 1953; Mollison and Cutbush 1954). The greater severity of the disease in first affected infants born to previously transfused mothers is presumably due simply to the fact that a transfusion is a better primary stimulus than a small TPH.

Routine tests to detect Rh D immunization

All so far unimmunized women should have their Rh D group determined on at least two occasions during pregnancy: at their first antenatal visit and at about 32 weeks.

Tests for anti-D

The sera of all D-negative women should be tested for anti-D at the time of their first antenatal visit, i.e. at about the twelfth week of gestation. In women believed to be pregnant for the first time, anti-D will be found only occasionally, namely in those who have been immunized either by a previous transfusion of D-positive blood or by a previous unrecognized or undisclosed abortion. In women known to have been pregnant before, the presence of anti-D at 12 weeks will usually be due to the fact that they have not been given anti-D Ig following an earlier pregnancy or, if it has been given, the dose has been too small or given too late. In women without anti-D at their first antenatal visit, it is sufficient to make the next test at 28–32 weeks. As discussed later, there is a strong case for beginning immunoprophylaxis with anti-D Ig at 28 weeks. In women who have not formed anti-D when tested at 28–32 weeks, no further tests need be made until the time of delivery when, as soon as the infant is born, cord blood should be taken for determination of the D group and the DAT.

Changes in anti-D concentration when the infant is D negative. Significant rises in anti-D concentration in women carrying a D-negative fetus were found in 4 out of 239 cases in one series (Hopkins 1970) and in 13 out of 300 in another (Fraser and Tovey 1976).

Antenatal tests for alloantibodies in D-positive women

When D-positive women form antibodies such as anti-c or anti-E, or alloantibodies outside the Rh system such as anti-K, there may be serious delay in diagnosing haemolytic disease in their infant after birth unless antenatal tests have revealed the presence of the antibody. The serum of all pregnant women should be screened for alloantibodies at the time of their first antenatal visit. If a clinically significant antibody is found, monthly tests until about 32 weeks are indicated, with two-weekly tests until term and a DAT on the infant's cord blood at the time of delivery. If no alloantibodies are found at the first antenatal visit, it is sufficient to make a second test at 32 weeks.

Determination of D group of fetus in utero

The D group of the fetus can be determined prenatally, by polymerase chain reaction (PCR) amplification of that region of fetal DNA encoding *RHD*. Initially, fetal DNA for this purpose was obtained from amniotic fibroblasts. Only 1–2 ml of amniotic fluid is needed and can be obtained late in the first trimester or early in the second. The test can also be done on a chorionic villus sample but this carries greater risks for the fetus and is also a cause of TPH (Bennett *et al.* 1993). The preferred method utilizes fetal DNA present in maternal plasma, as this poses no risk to the pregnancy or of TPH and thereby the possibility of sensitizing the mother to fetal antigens. This method can be undertaken from the beginning of the second trimester (Lo *et al.* 1998).

Methods for the determination of the D group of a fetus require very careful design. *RHD* and *RHCE* are highly homologous genes and the D-negative phenotype can arise from a large number of different genetic mechanisms (see Chapter 5). Early methods of D typing from DNA were based on the assumption that *RHD* was absent from the DNA of D-negative individuals and primers for PCR were designed around regions of significant difference between *RHD* and *RHCE*, most notably in exon 7, the 3′ untranslated region of exon 10 and a 600-bp size difference in intron 4 (Arce *et al.* 1993; Bennett *et al.* 1993; Wolter *et al.* 1993). It soon became clear that although complete absence of *RHD* is by far the commonest cause of the D-negative phenotype in white people this is not true of other races (Chapter 5). A particular problem is detection of the so-called pseudo *RHD* frequently found in black people with D-negative red cells. About 67% of D-negative black people have the pseudo *RHD*. It can be detected by amplification of exon 4 which contains a 37-bp insert in the pseudo *RHD* and so can be diagnosed from the size of the PCR fragment obtained (Singleton *et al.* 2000). These authors describe a multiplex PCR based on exon 4 and exon 7 that can be used for routine diagnostic purposes (Fig. 12.3). Others have devised multiplex assays in which all *RHD*-specific coding exons are amplified in a single tube (Maaskant-van Wijk *et al.* 1998) and in which all *RHD* exons are amplified specifically and sequenced (Legler *et al.* 2001). The last two methods require optimal standardized conditions and are not so easily introduced into routine diagnostic laboratories (Van der Schoot *et al.* 2003).

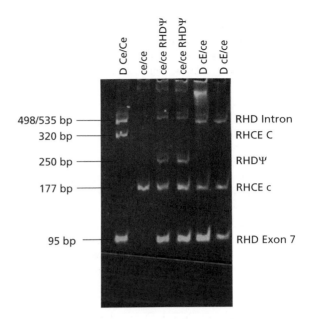

Fig 12.3 Fetal D typing by PCR (Singleton *et al.* 2000).

The D group of a fetus can also be determined using real-time PCR. This method requires two sequence specific oligonucleotide primers to amplify the region of interest and a third oligonucleotide (probe) that anneals to a region within the amplicon. The probe has fluorescent dyes attached at its 5′-end (reporter dye) and its 3′-end (quencher dye). When the probe is intact, the proximity of the two dyes causes the emission spectrum of the reporter dye to be quenched. As the PCR progresses, the 5′ exonuclease activity of the Taq DNA polymerase causes cleavage of the reporter dye from the probe and the reporter dye fluorescence is detected by a laser. As the release of reporter dye fluorescence is directly proportional to the target amplification the method is quantitative (Fig. 12.4). The method is extremely sensitive and, provided the PCR is designed to take account of common forms of D-negative phenotype where *RHD* is not completely absent such as the pseudo *RHD* discussed above, can be used to provide a very effective diagnostic service (Finning *et al.* 2002; Daniels *et al.* 2004). One problem with this method concerns the availability of controls to ensure fetal DNA is present in cases where the D type is D negative. This is easily solved when the fetus is male by amplifying the Y chromosome-specific gene *SRY*, but suitable markers when the fetus is female are

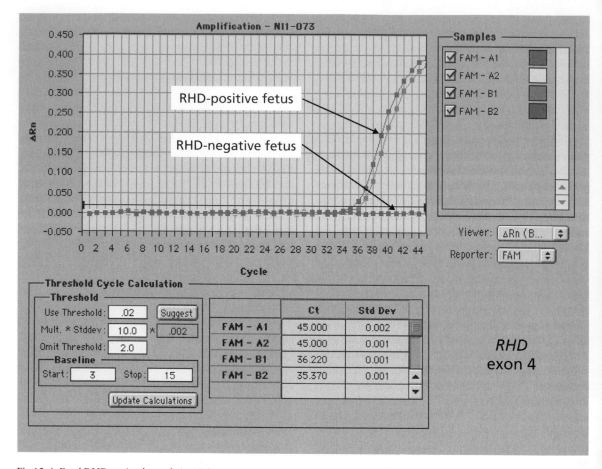

Fig 12.4 Fetal RHD typing by real-time PCR using maternal plasma as a source of fetal DNA.

not available. One approach is to test maternal DNA (derived from buffy coat cells) for a number of insertion/deletion polymorphisms and then look for the presence of polymorphisms in fetal DNA that are absent from the mother's DNA (Finning *et al.* 2004). Quantification of total plasma DNA can be obtained by amplification of *CCR5* and reference to a calibration curve. If total DNA is greater than 125 ng/ml, white cell lysis may have occurred and the assay may be compromised by excessive maternal DNA. Quantification of total plasma DNA is also valuable for avoiding the problem of a D-negative mother with pseudo *RHD*, as quantification of the maternal gene will give values approaching the total DNA value, far higher than that found for fetal DNA sequences (Finning *et al.* 2004).

Determination of RHD zygosity

Knowledge of the genotype of the father can be helpful when anti-D is found in maternal serum or when a previous pregnancy has resulted in HDN. Serological methods are of limited value in this respect but several molecular methods have been described (reviewed in Van der Schoot *et al.* 2003). Real-time PCR can be used to compare the amount of *RHD* product with that of a reference gene provided more than one *RHD*-specific region is amplified (to take account of pseudo *RHD* and other aberrant *RHD* alleles). Another approach targets the so-called Rhesus box sequences upstream and downstream of *RHD* and *RHCE* respectively (see Fig. 5.2). When *RHD* is deleted by an unequal crossover event, the crossover point occurs within the Rhesus boxes creating a hybrid Rhesus box comprising parts of the upstream and downstream boxes (Wagner and Flegel 2000). Assays that target the hybrid Rhesus box can therefore be used to determine zygosity (Chiu *et al.* 2001; Van der Schoot *et al.* 2003).

Antenatal assessment of severity

The severity of haemolytic disease can be assessed most reliably by fetal blood sampling but the procedure carries a small risk to the fetus and may provoke a TPH, followed by an increase in maternal antibody concentration. Accordingly, various non-invasive methods of assessment are used in the first instance and fetal blood sampling is used only in selected cases.

Estimation of maternal antibody concentration

Estimations of antibody concentration, using an autoanalyzer, are useful in two ways. First, a low value almost always indicates that the infant will be mildly affected, or unaffected. In one series, in 78 cases in which the maternal anti-D concentration remained below 4 iu/ml (0.8 µg/ml), no infant had a cord Hb concentration of less than 100 g/l and only three infants needed an exchange transfusion (Bowell *et al.* 1982). Unfortunately, though, antibody levels of 6 iu/ml or more, predicting moderately severe disease, are quite commonly found when the infant is unaffected (Hadley *et al.* 1993).

Second, an increase in anti-D concentration is a warning that the severity of the haemolytic process may be increasing. In 11 cases in which fetal blood sampling had shown that the fetus was not anaemic, and in which maternal anti-D concentration rose to more than 15 iu/ml within the following 2–3 weeks, a further fetal sample showed that the fetus had become moderately or severely anaemic (Nicolaides and Rodeck 1992). In interpreting apparent changes in antibody concentration, it is essential to compare the latest sample with earlier samples by testing the samples together.

Relation between IgG subclass of anti-D and severity

When only IgG3 anti-D was present, severity was less than when IgG1 alone or IgG1 + IgG3 were present (Zupanska *et al.* 1989; Pollock and Bowman 1990;

Alie-Daren *et al.* 1992). In one investigation, when both IgG1 and IgG3 were present, IgG1 was usually preponderant and most severe disease correlated with IgG1, particularly G1m(3) (Alie-Daran *et al.* 1992). In other investigations, when only IgG1 was detected disease was more severe (Parinaud *et al.* 1985), less severe (Zupanska *et al.* 1989) or no different (Pollock and Bowman 1990) than when both IgG1 and IgG3 were present. These apparent discrepancies are probably due to the fact that when both IgG1 and IgG3 are present, the fraction of IgG1 may vary from 11% to 99% (Garner *et al.* 1995). Correlation of the amount of IgG1 and the severity of HDN is substantially better than that of IgG3 and severity (Garner *et al.* 1995; Lambin *et al.* 2002).

Cellular bioassays in the assessment of severity

Bioassays are substantially more cumbersome to perform than estimates of antibody concentration but are expected on theoretical grounds to give better predictions of severity. Monocyte monolayer assays (MMAs), applied to maternal serum, have been found to distinguish between mildly and severely affected infants (Nance *et al.* 1989a; Zupanska *et al.* 1989). MMAs were more reliable than amniotic fluid measurements in predicting the need for treatment (Nance *et al.* 1989b).

In a series in which the results of an antibody-dependent, cell-mediated, monocyte-dependent cytotoxicity [ADCC(M)] assay were compared with IAT titres, either at 32 weeks or at term, severe disease was correctly predicted in 75% by ADCC(M) but only in 15% by IAT titre (Engelfriet and Ouwehand 1990). In a small series in which an ADCC assay with lymphocytes (ADCC(L) assay) was used, of 10 women, all of whom had anti-D concentrations of 20 iu/ml or more, three had low assay values and these were the only ones whose infants did not require exchange transfusion (Urbaniak *et al.* 1984).

In a study in which samples were tested 'blind' by several different laboratories, the frequency of results with various assays that correctly predicted the severity of HDN was as follows: ADCC(M), 60%; ADCC(L), 57%; chemiluminescence (CL), 50%; adherence and phagocytosis with peripheral blood monocytes, 41% and with U937 cells or cultured macrophages, 32%. In many cases, maternal samples were taken only some time after delivery, which may

511

explain why the frequencies of correct results were not higher (Report from Nine Collaborating Laboratories 1991).

In perhaps the most decisive investigation so far, sera from 44 D-negative women with D-positive infants were tested extensively; the series included approximately equal numbers of unaffected, moderately affected, severely affected and very severely affected infants. The tests used were the monocyte monolayer assay (MMA), antibody-dependent cellular cytotoxicity (ADCC) assay (with monocytes), estimation of anti-D concentration in the autoanalyzer and measurement of the number of IgG1 and IgG3 molecules bound to target cells. ADCC correctly predicted severity in 39 out of 44 cases, autoanalyzer quantification in 35 cases and MMA in 32 cases. ADCC activity and HDN severity were correlated with the number of IgG1 molecules bound to target cells but MMA activity was most closely correlated with the number of IgG3 molecules bound, thus explaining the superior predictive value of ADCC compared with MMA (Garner et al. 1995).

Unfortunately, cellular bioassays are cumbersome and are unsuitable for routine use.

False-positive results in cellular bioassays

In three circumstances, the fetus may be unaffected or only mildly affected despite a strongly positive result in a cellular bioassay:

1 Fetus Rh D negative. For examples, see Urbaniak et al. (1984) and Nance et al. (1989b).

2 Presence of Fc receptor blocking antibodies. In about 4% of second or later pregnancies, the mother forms an antibody that blocks the Fc receptor on fetal monocytes, thus interfering with the binding of IgG-coated red cells to the monocytes and reducing or even preventing the haemolytic process (Engelfriet and Ouwehand 1990). Fc receptor blocking antibodies were present in seven of 13 cases in which, despite the presence of potent anti-D in the mother's serum (ADCC(M) test giving > 80% lysis), the infant was very mildly affected or unaffected, and were not found in any of 14 infants suffering from severe HDN. In six out of seven cases, Fc receptor blocking antibodies had anti-HLA-DR specificity (Dooren et al. 1992). Further evidence of the role of FcR blocking antibodies was provided by successive infants born to the same mothers: in one family, protection was afforded to an infant whose monocytes reacted with the mother's antibody but not to a subsequent infant whose monocytes did not react. In a second family, at a time when a mother had no FcR blocking antibody, her infant was severely affected but subsequently, after such an antibody had developed, the infant was only mildly affected (Dooren et al. 1993).

3 Diminished transport of maternal IgG to fetus. In a case in which the ADCC(M) assay on the maternal serum became strongly positive by the thirty-fifth week of pregnancy, the infant was born at 39 weeks with a positive DAT but without definite signs of HDN. Whereas the mother's serum IgG concentration was normal (8.7 g/l), that of the infant was greatly reduced (2.9 g/l); it was postulated that diminished transport of IgG anti-D to the fetus had protected it from HDN (Dooren and Engelfriet 1993). After binding to Fc receptors on the syncitiotrophoblast, IgG is transported from mother to fetus through the formation of complexes of placental alkaline phosphatases (PLAPs) with IgG, which are transported to the fetus by coated placental vesicles that then dissociate in the fetal circulation. A determinant on the Fab portion of some IgG antibodies causes binding to PLAP in the maternal circulation and thus blocks placental transport, not only of anti-D, but also of total IgG. The presence of PLAP–IgG complexes in the maternal serum was found to be associated with a reduction of fetal serum IgG to about one-half of the normal level (Grozdea et al. 1995).

Amniocentesis in estimating the severity of haemolytic disease

Estimation of the amount of bile pigment in amniotic fluid is performed by measuring the difference in optical density at 450 nm (OD_{450}) between the observed density and an extrapolated baseline (Fig. 12.5). The optical density of amniotic fluid falls during the last 13 weeks of pregnancy so that the stage of pregnancy has to be taken into account when interpreting the findings. Figure 12.6 shows a chart produced by Liley (1961) to indicate the approximate severity of disease for a particular OD_{450} at any stage of pregnancy from 27 weeks onwards.

If the lines in Liley's chart are extrapolated to earlier stages of pregnancy, misleading results are obtained. For example, in one series, if results had been interpreted in this way, 10 out of 31 severely anaemic

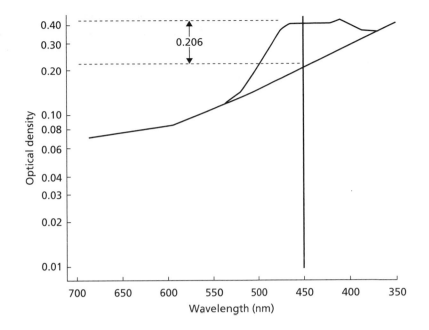

Fig 12.5 Plot of optical density readings of amniotic fluid from an Rh D immunized woman at the thirty-fifth week of pregnancy. The optical density at 450 nm (OD_{450}) is expressed as the height (in this case 0.206) above the conjectural baseline (slightly modified from Bowman and Pollock 1965).

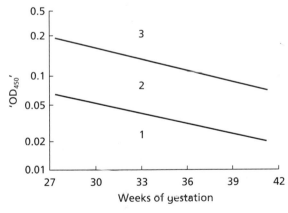

Fig 12.6 Liley's three zones, indicating the approximate severity of haemolytic disease, from readings of the OD_{450} of amniotic fluid (see Fig. 12.3) during the last trimester of pregnancy. Zone 1 indicates a mildly affected or unaffected infant, whereas zone 3 indicates a high probability of hydrops and fetal death; the significance of zone 2 is intermediate. In the original paper the chart begins, as here, at 27 weeks 1 day, i.e. at the start of the twenty-eighth week of gestation (Liley 1961). Subsequently, the lines were extrapolated to 20 weeks but then provided a far less reliable guide (see text).

fetuses (Hb < 6 g/dl) would not have received an intrauterine transfusion, whereas many mildly affected fetuses would have been treated unnecessarily (Nicolaides *et al.* 1986).

Examination of the fetus by ultrasonography and fetal Doppler blood flow velocity

Ultrasonography can be used to diagnose hydrops fetalis as indicated by ascites, pleural or pericardial effusions and skin oedema (Bowman 1983). In fetuses of 18–24 weeks, ascites diagnosed in this way is always associated with Hb levels of less than 4 g/dl (Nicolaides *et al.* 1985a). Repeated examination of the fetus by ultrasonography can detect early signs of cardiac decompensation, i.e. a small pericardial effusion or dilatation of cardiac chambers.

Combined with monitoring of the fetal heart rate, sonographic examination makes conservative management of the fetus possible and helps to avoid unnecessary intervention (Frigoletto *et al.* 1986). In a study of 50 Rh-immunized pregnancies at 18–20 weeks' gestation, when ultrasound was compared with fetal blood sampling, ultrasound was found unreliable in predicting fetal anaemia in the absence of hydrops (Nicolaides *et al.* 1988a).

513

Many studies report the value of Doppler velocimetry measurement of fetal middle cerebral artery peak systolic velocity in detecting moderate to severe fetal anaemia in red blood cell alloimmunized pregnancies. Mari and co-workers (2000) report an increase in peak systolic velocity to have a predictive value of 100% in moderate to severe anaemia in the presence or absence of hydrops. Others report similar findings (Dukler et al. 2003; Pereira et al. 2003). However, a systematic review of non-invasive techniques (fetal ultrasonography and Doppler blood flow velocity) to predict fetal anaemia, published in 2001, concluded 'the literature reporting non-invasive techniques to predict fetal anaemia is methodologically poor and a standard approach to the evaluation of these techniques is lacking. A recommendation for practice cannot be generated without further rigorous research' (Divakaran et al. 2001). Abdel-Fattah and Soothill (2002, cited in Petz and Garratty (2004), p. 524) conclude that careful attention to obstetric history and serial antibody quantitation is equally as important as Doppler velocimetry.

Fetal blood sampling

The preferred method of obtaining blood from the fetus in utero is by inserting a needle percutaneously and guiding it by ultrasonographic monitoring into the umbilical or hepatic vein. This procedure is described as cordocentesis or percutaneous umbilical vein sampling (PUBS). In 394 women in whom 606 fetal samplings were carried out by this method before the twenty-fourth week, the pregnancy loss rate was 0.8% (Daffos et al. 1985).

It is essential to confirm that the sample obtained is of pure fetal blood. A rapid method is to determine the mean cell volume (MCV) in an automated blood counter; fetal values are 118–135 µ3. Examination of a blood film stained by the Kleihauer–Betke method (see Appendix 13) is a more accurate method of excluding the presence of maternal red cells but takes substantially longer. Another reliable method is to visualize the streaming of microbubbles in the umbilical vein during the infusion of saline (King and Sacher 1989).

It is now routine practice to determine the fetal PCV or Hb concentration before intrauterine transfusion. Figure 12.7 shows the Hb concentration from 17 weeks to term of 106 non-hydropic and 48 hydropic infants with Rh D haemolytic disease. The figure also shows the range of values in 200 normal fetuses and 10 cord samples obtained at the time of delivery. As the figure shows, the Hb concentration of normal fetuses was found to increase from 11 g/dl at 17 weeks' gestation to about 13.5 g/dl at 32 weeks and to 15.0 g/dl at term, although this latter value is somewhat lower

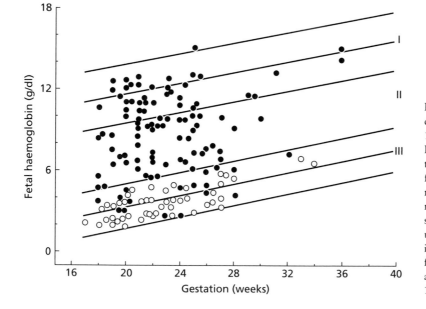

Fig 12.7 Haemoglobin concentrations of 48 hydropic (○) and 106 non-hydropic (●) fetuses with HDN due to anti-D, at the time of taking the first sample from each fetus. Zone I indicates the zone of normal values (the lines mark the mean and limits of ± 2SD), based on samples from 200 normal fetuses undergoing prenatal tests. Zone III indicates the mean ± 2SD for hydropic fetuses, and zone II is that of moderate anaemia (from Nicolaides et al. 1988a).

than the generally accepted value of about 16.5 g/dl for the cord blood of normal mature infants.

A paper giving more details of the 110 fetuses in this series sampled between 15 and 21 weeks gave the following values before 22 weeks: for Hb, between 12.3 and 13.0 Hb g/dl, and for PCV, 0.373–0.393; there was no obvious trend towards higher values during this period although values for six fetuses at 15 weeks were slightly lower (Millar *et al.* 1985). In another series, of 163 fetuses of 18–30 weeks' gestation, Hb increased from 11.47 g/dl at 18–20 weeks to 13.35 g/dl at 26–30 weeks; corresponding figures for PCV were 0.359–0.415 (Forestier *et al.* 1986).

The severity of haemolytic disease *in utero* can be assessed from the deviation of the observed Hb from the normal mean for the period of gestation. Normal fetal Hb can be predicted from: [85 + (1.4 × gestational weeks)] g/l, based on cordocentesis results in 726 pregnancies in which the fetus proved to be normal (Nicolaides and Rodeck 1992); a deficit of 2 g/dl is diagnosed as mild, of 2–7 g/dl as moderate, and of > 7 g/dl as severe (Nicolaides *et al.* 1988b).

Routine antenatal determination of fetal D type

The availability of molecular methods for the determination of fetal D type using cell-free fetal DNA in maternal blood (see above) makes it feasible to consider the use of automated DNA typing of antenatal patients so that only those carrying a D-positive fetus are given prophylactic anti-D (Van der Schoot *et al.* 2004).

Assessment of severity in the newborn infant

Although many infants born with a positive DAT require no treatment, others need exchange transfusion or phototherapy if they are to be prevented from developing kernicterus. It is therefore essential to assess severity at the earliest possible moment. As explained below, there is a special advantage in testing cord blood rather than blood obtained from the infant after birth.

The best single criterion of severity of haemolytic disease is the cord Hb concentration, although in practice other criteria are always taken into account. The reason for preferring to test cord blood to blood obtained from the infant after birth is simply that

during the few minutes after delivery a variable amount of blood is transferred from the placenta to the infant (Budin 1875; DeMarsh *et al.* 1942; Yao *et al.* 1969). Accordingly, interpreting Hb values in infants shortly after birth presents just the same difficulties as interpreting the significance of Hb values in any other subject who has recently been transfused with an unknown amount of red cells. The postnatal rise in Hb concentration has the effect of widening the normal range of values. Whereas the normal range (mean ± 2 SD) of Hb values in cord blood is approximately 13.6–19.6 g/dl, the range in samples taken on the first day of life is approximately 14.5–22.5 g/dl (Mollison and Cutbush 1949a). These figures refer to venous samples. In newborn infants, skin-prick samples tend to give distinctly higher values (for references, see third edition, pp. 579–80). The practical importance of Hb changes in the immediate postnatal period is illustrated in Fig. 12.8. In the case shown, an infant with moderately severe haemolytic disease had a cord Hb concentration of 12.8 g/dl, a value definitely below the lower limit of normal, whereas a sample taken a few hours after birth was within the normal range.

Before the introduction of immunoprophylaxis, almost 50% of affected infants had cord Hb concentrations of 14.5 g/dl or more, 30% had cord Hb values between 10.5 and 14.4 g/dl, and about 20% had Hb values of between 3.4 and 10.4 g/dl (second edition, p. 464). The probability of survival diminishes as the cord Hb concentration falls (Mollison and Cutbush 1951; Armitage and Mollison 1953); there is also a correlation between cord bilirubin concentration and severity, although the relation is less close than that between cord Hb concentration and severity (Mollison and Cutbush 1949a).

Indications for exchange transfusion and phototherapy are described below.

Estimation of the amount of antibody on red cells of affected infants

In one series, the amount of anti-D on the cord red cells varied from 0.4 to 18.0 μg/ml of cells. The amount of antibody on the red cells was not highly correlated with either the infant's cord Hb concentration or the cord serum bilirubin concentration (correlation coefficient about 0.6). All 13 infants with more than 8 μg of anti-D per millilitre of red cells required treatment, but even at a level of 2 μg of anti-D per millilitre,

515

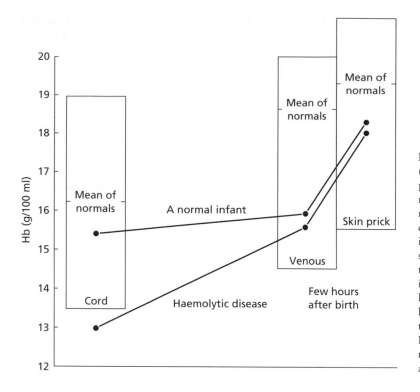

Fig 12.8 Changes in haemoglobin (Hb) concentration produced by the placental transfer of blood tend to mask mild degrees of anaemia in newborn infants. Often the Hb concentration of skin-prick samples is much higher than that of venous samples and this is a second factor that may mask anaemia. In the case illustrated here, an infant with haemolytic disease of the newborn has a cord Hb concentration below the normal range, but after birth its Hb concentration is as high as that of many normal infants (from Mollison and Cutbush 1949a).

6 out of 14 infants required treatment (Hughes-Jones *et al.* 1967). In cases in which, due to a misunderstanding, a dose of 150–300 μg of anti-D has been given to a D-positive infant, instead of to its D-negative mother, only a very mild haemolytic syndrome has as a rule been produced. In one such case the infant's red cells were shown to be coated with approximately 1.5 μg of anti-D per millilitre (Marsh *et al.* 1970; Fig. 12.9).

Antenatal treatment of haemolytic disease

Plasma exchange in the mother

Although at first sight intensive plasma exchange in women immunized to Rh D seems entirely rational and might be expected to lead to a substantial lowering of the concentration of anti-D, to the benefit of the D-positive fetus *in utero*, results of this treatment have in fact been very variable. In one series of Rh-immunized women in whom a mean volume of 3.5 1 of plasma was exchanged on average twice a week, the anti-D level was rapidly lowered and maintained at a lower level than previously in 15 out of 35 cases. In the

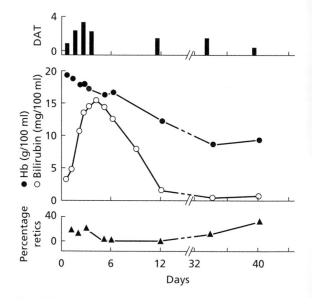

Fig 12.9 Changes in haemoglobin (Hb) concentration (●—●); serum bilirubin concentration (○—○); reticulocyte count (▲—▲); and direct antiglobulin test (DAT; positive reactions graded from 0 to 4) in a D-positive infant injected, 5 h after birth, with 200 μg of anti-D (from Marsh *et al.* 1970).

remaining 20, the anti-D level remained high despite intensive plasma exchange or was lower only until the thirtieth week of pregnancy, after which an uncontrollable rise occurred (Robinson 1984). Animal experiments indicate that one reason for lack of success is the fact that temporary lowering of antibody levels tends to provoke a rebound, suggesting that plasma antibody levels play an important part in regulating antibody production (Bystryn et al. 1970). The ability to maintain normal concentrations of serum IgG is critically dependent on FcRn, which maintains a balance between recycling of IgG and catabolism of IgG (Roopenian et al. 2003). It seems likely that removal of IgG by plasma exchange is compensated by an increase in IgG recycling through FcRn and a consequent reduction in the rate of catabolism.

In centres with a large experience of intravascular transfusion of the fetus in utero, plasma exchange has a very limited application because deaths in utero from haemolytic disease are believed not to occur before about 17 weeks, and i.v. transfusion becomes possible as early as the eighteenth week of gestation (Nicolaides and Rodeck 1985). It has been suggested that plasma exchange should be reserved for the woman with a previous history of hydrops developing before 24–26 weeks' gestation, with a homozygous (DD) partner. Intensive plasma exchange should then be begun at 10–12 weeks, with fetal blood sampling at 19–22 weeks (Bowman 1990).

Absorption of alloantibodies on to red cells

As mentioned in Chapter 1, one method of removing alloantibodies is to withdraw plasma, absorb the plasma with appropriate red cells and return it to the donor. In a case in which this method was used in an Rh-immunized woman there was a dramatic increase in anti-D concentration, which may well have been due to the presence of red cells or stroma in the plasma (Robinson 1981). To prevent this hazard, plasma can be passed through a microfilter (Yoshida et al. 1981).

Intravenous immunoglobulin given to the mother

A single course totalling 2 g/kg over 5 days or repeated weekly injections of 1 g/kg have been tried in conjunction with plasma exchange or with intravascular trans-

fusion of the fetus in two very small series. There was apparent benefit in one but not in the other (Rubo and wahn 1990; Chitkara et al. 1990). In two much larger series, there was suggestive evidence that the severity of haemolytic disease in the fetus was reduced (Margulies et al. 1991; C De la Camera and R Arrieta, personal communication). However, because there was great variability in previous obstetric histories, in the stage of pregnancy at which treatment was started and in the number of courses of Ig given, definite conclusions cannot yet be reached.

IVIG might act by saturating FcRn and thereby inhibiting placental transfer of anti-D to the fetus: in perfusion experiments with a lobule of human placenta, a plasma level of 20 g/l IgG in the maternal circulation, produced by injecting commercial IVIG, inhibited the transfer of the alloantibody anti-Pl^{A1} (HPA-1a) (Morgan et al. 1991). Inhibition of placental anti-D IgG transfer was also observed at similar levels of maternal IgG (Urbaniak et al. 1999).

IVIG given to the fetus

In a small randomized trial, severely affected fetuses were treated with intravascular transfusions with, or without, IVIG in a mean dose of 85.7 mg/kg/body weight determined by ultrasound. IVIG conferred no apparent benefit, but the largest dose that could be given was too small and the average number of treatments was only two or three (Dooren et al. 1994).

Transfusion of the fetus in utero

Intraperitoneal transfusion was the first method to be used (Liley 1963): red cells are injected into the peritoneal cavity of the fetus, whence they are taken up into the bloodstream via the subdiaphragmatic lacunae and right lymphatic duct. Uptake is dependent on diaphragmatic movements (Menticoglou et al. 1987) and intraperitoneal transfusions are therefore useless in those hydropic fetuses who have no such movements. Although intraperitoneal transfusion has been largely superseded by intravascular transfusion, it still has a place. It is easy to perform and may also be used in combination with intravascular transfusion to increase the total volume of blood given to the fetus, thus prolonging the interval between transfusions (Nicolini and Rodeck 1988; Rodeck and Letsky 1989).

Intravascular transfusion is performed through a needle inserted into the umbilical vein by ultrasonographic guidance. Results obtained with this method have been spectacular. In one early series of 29 fetuses severely affected with Rh D haemolytic disease (10 with hydrops) treated at 18–24 weeks, 25 survived (Rodeck *et al.* 1984). In another series, 16 out of 22 hydropic fetuses survived and three of the six deaths were at 19–22 weeks in the fetuses of i.v. drug abusers (Bowman 1990). In a third series, the survival rate of fetuses developing hydrops before 26 weeks was 61%, and of those developing hydrops later was 100% (Grannum and Copel 1988).

In 10 published series of fetuses with severe haemolytic disease treated by intravascular transfusion *in utero*, of those with hydrops 66 out of 96 (69%) survived, compared with 114 out of 134 (85%) of those without hydrops. Hydrops was reversed in 60% of cases and in these, the survival rate was 92%, compared with 43% in those cases in which hydrops was not reversed (Tannirandorn and Rodeck 1990). Even in very experienced hands, a single intravascular transfusion has a mortality rate of 2% (Rodeck and Letsky 1989). In a retrospective study of pregnancy outcome following intrauterine transfusion for fetal anaemia due to red cell alloimmunization in the Netherlands during the period 1988–99, 210 fetuses from 208 pregnancies received 593 transfusions. Survival rate in fetuses without hydrops was 92% compared with 78% in those with hydrops. In maternal D immunizations, 89% of fetuses survived. The overall fetal loss rate was 4.8% (Van Kamp *et al.* 2004).

It is customary to use blood that is less than 72 h old. The red cells should be group O, D negative, K negative and should be compatible with the mother's serum; the PCV of the red cell preparation should be 0.70–0.85. To avoid the risk of graft-versus-host disease, the red cells should be irradiated. The white cells should be removed by filtration to avoid possible immunomodulatory effects of transfusion and the transmission of cell-associated viruses such as cytomegalovirus (CMV) and human T-lymphotropic virus (HTLV). In addition to being submitted to all the mandatory tests, the blood should be screened for HBs and anti-CMV. The usual transfusion volume is 50 ml per kg estimated non-hydropic weight, reduced to 30–40 ml/kg estimated non-hydropic weight for hydropic fetuses (Bowman 1994). Red cells suspended in non-protein solutions such as SAG-M or Adsol should not be used for transfusion to the fetus *in utero*.

Alloimmunization of the mother may follow intrauterine sampling or transfusion of the fetus. Fetal or donor red cells may enter the maternal circulation, either by being shed into the mother's peritoneal cavity or by entering maternal blood vessels in the placenta, and may stimulate the formation of 'new' alloantibodies or increase the concentration of existing ones.

In two series of Rh D-immunized women managed differently, when fetal blood sampling was used, other alloantibodies were found during pregnancy in 3 out of 63 cases and in a further 2 out of 38 examined after delivery; in contrast, when only amniotic fluid examinations were used, other antibodies were found during pregnancy in 1 out of 52 cases and in 1 out of 22 examined after delivery (Pratt *et al.* 1989). The development of alloantibodies within 2–4 weeks of giving intraperitoneal transfusions to fetuses has been recorded in three cases: anti-Fy[b] in a woman who had already formed anti-Ce (Contreras *et al.* 1983), and anti-Jk[a] and a combination of anti-Fy[b], -Jk[b] and -S in two other women (Barrie and Quinn 1985).

Following a series of 68 fetal intravascular transfusions, TPH, as judged by an increase of at least 50% in the level of maternal α-FP, occurred in 27 cases (40%). The frequency was much higher (66%) in women with an anterior placenta than in those in whom the placenta was posterior or fundal (frequency of TPH, 17%). The mean estimated volume of TPH was 2.4 ml (blood). When the volume of TPH following the first intravascular transfusion exceeded 1 ml, the mother's anti-D titre rose by more than 150% within the following 3 weeks (Nicolini *et al.* 1988).

Donor red cells are less frequently the source of immunization than fetal red cells. Among 91 women, following 280 intrauterine transfusions (IUTs), additional antibodies appeared in 24 (26%). The immunizing source could be identified in 14; in 11 of these, the antibodies were directed against fetal antigens and in three, against donor antigens (Viëtor *et al.* 1994).

Induction of GvHD. In occasional infants transfused *in utero*, a subsequent postnatal exchange transfusion induces GvHD. The cells causing the GvHD have the HLA group of the donor used in the exchange transfusion and it is presumed that the IUT has an immunomodulatory effect (Williamson and Warwick 1996).

Premature delivery

At a time when premature delivery was being practised only occasionally, it was found that approximately 50% of all stillbirths due to haemolytic disease occurred after 35 weeks' gestation (Allen 1957; Walker *et al.* 1957). Because of the high mortality rate in premature infants at that time, there was reluctance to carry out premature delivery before about the thirty-fifth week of pregnancy but, with the steadily increasing success in the care of premature infants, delivery is now carried out as early as 30–32 weeks with high survival rates.

Postnatal treatment of haemolytic disease

Exchange transfusion

Exchange transfusion with D-negative blood greatly increases the survival rate and almost removes the risk of kernicterus (Allen *et al.* 1950; Mollison and Walker 1952). In the method introduced by Diamond (1947), blood is withdrawn and injected, intermittently, through a plastic catheter passed up the umbilical vein. The primary object of exchange transfusion is to remove D-positive red cells which, in a severe case of HDN, may have a survival time as short as 2 or 3 days (Mollison 1943). (In contrast, D-negative red cells almost always survive normally (Mollison 1951, p. 398).) The secondary object of exchange transfusion is to remove bilirubin already present in the plasma.

It is possible to predict accurately the volume of D-positive red cells remaining in the infant's circulation if the infant's initial PCV and body weight are known: a nomogram was published by Veall and Mollison (1950). However, the amount of bilirubin removed is more difficult to calculate, as during exchange transfusion bilirubin enters the plasma from the extravascular space. For this reason most clinicians like to exchange relatively large volumes of blood, for example 200 ml/kg, and to spend some time, for example 60–90 min, over the exchange transfusion.

Plasma-reduced blood with a PCV of at least 0.60 should be used for exchange transfusion; the blood should be group O, D negative and K negative, and should be compatible with the mother's serum; it should be less than 7 days old. The blood should be screened for HbS and for anti-CMV, as well as being submitted to all the usual tests.

Erythropoiesis may be suppressed for many months after exchange transfusion and infants may be misdiagnosed as having red cell aplasia.

Indications for exchange transfusion. When the fetus has been transfused prenatally for severe disease, exchange transfusion is not usually required after birth and phototherapy (see below) is, in 80% of cases, adequate to control hyperbilirubinaemia. Exchange transfusion is carried out only if the serum bilirubin concentration threatens to reach or exceed 340 µmol/l.

Infants who have been transfused *in utero* and who do not require exchange transfusion after birth invariably require one or more simple 'booster' transfusions during the first 6–8 weeks of life. Hb concentration should be estimated at 10- to 14-day intervals until it stops falling. If the concentration falls towards 70 g/l, a transfusion of 20 ml of packed red cells/kg body weight should be given (JM Bowman, personal communication). In newborn infants who have not been transfused prenatally, a cord Hb concentration of 110 g/l is an indication for exchange transfusion. Before the introduction of improved methods of phototherapy, a cord serum bilirubin concentration of 60–70 µmol/l (in an infant with a cord Hb of 110 g/l or less) was also an indication for exchange transfusion but, now, phototherapy is tried first (JM Bowman, personal communication, 1996).

Phototherapy to reduce serum bilirubin concentration

On exposure to light, particularly in the region of 420–480 nm, bilirubin is converted to the non-toxic pigment, biliverdin. Exposing jaundiced newborn infants to a suitable fluorescent light lowers serum bilirubin concentration (Cremer *et al.* 1958; Costa *et al.* 1960), an effect that was confirmed in a controlled trial (Tabb *et al.* 1972).

Phototherapy, when applied early enough and with sufficient intensity, can avoid the need for exchange transfusion in many infants. One recent improvement in the efficacy of phototherapy has been the introduction of a fibreoptic blanket that delivers phototherapy to the anterior and posterior surfaces of the infant simultaneously. With this device the hourly decline in serum bilirubin concentration in low-birthweight infants with hyperbilirubinaemia was almost doubled (Holtrop *et al.* 1991).

519

Intravenous IgG to reduce the need for exchange transfusion

In a trial, infants with Rh HDN were randomly assigned as soon after birth as possible to receive phototherapy alone or phototherapy plus high-dose IgG (500 mg/kg over a 2-h period). Serum bilirubin was monitored 6-hourly. Exchange transfusion was required in 11 out of 16 infants receiving only phototherapy but in only 2 out of 16 who also received IgG (Rubo and Wahn 1991). A systematic review of randomized and quasi-randomized controlled trials comparing the effectiveness of high-dose intravenous immunoglobulin and phototherapy with phototherapy alone in neonates with Rh and/or ABO incompatibility concluded that significantly fewer infants required exchange transfusion in the intravenous immunoglobulin group (Gottstein and Cooke 2003).

Suppression of Rh D immunization that would otherwise follow pregnancy

As pointed out in Chapter 5, Rh D immunization can be prevented by giving 20 µg or more of anti-D immunoglobulin for every 1 ml of D-positive red cells introduced into the circulation. So far as Rh D immunization by pregnancy is concerned there are two causes of failure to prevent immunization when anti-D immunoglobulin is given: either the dose of anti-D is insufficient or it is given too late, that is to say after primary Rh D immunization has been induced.

When anti-D immunoglobulin was first used to prevent Rh D immunization associated with pregnancy, it was injected immediately following delivery. It was assumed that if given during pregnancy it would harm the fetus and that, in any case, TPH occurred mainly during delivery so that treatment immediately after delivery would be effective. It eventually became clear that in a minority of cases primary Rh D immunization occurs during pregnancy so that when anti-D is injected only postnatally there is a regular, although small, failure rate.

The results of giving anti-D only postnatally will be considered first.

Administration of anti-D only postnatally

Failure rates at 6 months. When 100–300 µg of anti-D Ig is injected immediately after delivery, the number of

D-negative women who develop anti-D within the following 6 months is 0.1–0.5%. For example, 34 out of 33 260 (0.1%) in Finland, where women were treated with 250 µg of anti-D (Eklund, 1978); 55 out of 16 142 (0.34%) women treated in Scotland with either 100 or 200 µg of anti-D (I Cook, personal communication), and 16 out of 3113 (0.51%) in an Australian series. The somewhat higher failure rate in the Australian series does not seem to have been due to the inclusion of women already immunized before being treated, as anti-D was detected in 0.71% at delivery and these women were excluded (Davey 1976a).

Failure rates at the end of a second D-positive pregnancy. From what has been said already, the minimum failure rate expected is about 1.5%, i.e. an incidence of 0.7% in each of the two pregnancies due to primary immunization occurring during the pregnancy and an additional 0.2% or so for failures due to a TPH at the time of the first delivery too large to be covered by a dose of 300 µg of anti-D or less. In fact, failure rates of the order expected have been observed in many series; for example, 1.86% [see Davey (1976a), supplemented by personal communication]; approximately 1.5% (Eklund 1978); and approximately 1.5% in women treated with 50, 100 or 200 µg of anti-D in a controlled trial (see Table 12.1).

When anti-D is detected for the first time during a second pregnancy in a woman who has been given anti-D Ig after her first pregnancy, there are two possible explanations: (1) sensitization to D occurred by

Table 12.1 Controlled trials of anti-D dosage in suppressing Rh D immunization (MRC 1974).

| Dose* (µg) | % of women with anti-D[†] | |
	6 months after first pregnancy	At the end of second pregnancy
200	0.2	1.5
100	0.2	1.1
50	0.4	1.5
20	1.4	2.9

All women D negative with two D-positive infants, the first being ABO compatible.
* Anti-D injected i.m. within 36 h of delivery of first infant.
[†] Detected by indirect antiglobulin test.

the time of the first delivery but anti-D was produced in detectable amounts only after the further stimulus of a second pregnancy; (2) primary immunization to D occurred only during the second pregnancy. It seems that the second explanation is usually the right one; the evidence is that in these cases the antibody develops only towards the end of the second pregnancy, for example in the last 4 weeks in 50% of the cases in one series (Eklund 1978).

Effect of different amounts of anti-D given immediately after delivery. In a 'blind' trial conducted by a working party of the Medical Research Council (MRC) and begun in 1967 in the UK, different doses of anti-D were given to four groups of women (about 450 women in each group). Over the dose range 200 to 20 μg there was a significant, although small, trend towards an increase in the failure rate 6 months after a first pregnancy (see Table 12.1). Approximately 200 women in each of the four groups were followed through a second pregnancy with a D-positive infant; the differences in the failure rates in the different groups were not statistically significant, although failures were suggestively more frequent with the 20-μg dose than with the larger doses.

Doses of anti-D for postpartum injection

Evidence that 20 μg of anti-D/ml red cells is effective in suppressing primary immunization has been reviewed earlier. To allow a margin of safety, 25 μg/ml has been recommended (WHO 1971). A dose of 300 μg of anti-D has long been the standard postpartum dose in the USA and many other countries, although 100 μg has been used in the UK. A dose of 300 μg covers TPHs of about 15 ml or less, that is to say the amounts found in approximately 99.8% of women at the time of delivery, whereas 100 μg covers TPHs of 4 ml or less, as found in about 99% of women. The dose of 300 μg was chosen to cover the vast majority of TPHs and to make screening tests for the occasional very large TPH inessential; nevertheless, a screening test capable of testing TPHs of 15 ml or more of red cells is mandatory in the USA (AABB 1991). With the 100-μg dose, the screening test is obviously even more important and must detect TPHs of 4 ml or more. Furthermore, when screening tests are positive, an estimate must be made of the size of the TPH so that an appropriate extra dose of anti-D can be given.

Flow cytometry can be used both to detect TPHs of 2 ml or more (see above) and to provide an accurate estimate of their size, but this technique is not widely available. In detecting TPHs of 15 ml or more, the rosetting test is probably the most convenient and can be used to provide semi-quantitative estimates. The acid-elution technique can also be used to provide quantitative estimates (Appendix 13).

In women in whom an unusually large TPH has been detected and who have been given extra anti-D Ig, tests are sometimes done to confirm that an adequate dose has been given. One practice is to look for the presence of anti-D in the maternal plasma but this is unsound in principle, as even when the antigen concentration is low, not all the antibody will be bound, however little is given. Furthermore, the method has been shown to be of no practical value (Ness and Salamon 1986). The method that seems most likely to be worthwhile is to test for clearance of fetal red cells from the maternal circulation, for example by using a rosetting test. Although a relationship between clearance and immunosuppression has yet to be firmly established, the two seem at least to be associated; see Chapter 3 for further discussion.

Doses of anti-D following premature termination of pregnancy

In women undergoing termination of pregnancy, usually at about 3 months, a common practice is to give 50 μg of anti-D. In a series of 3080 women treated with this dose following therapeutic abortion, only 13 (0.42%) were found to be immunized during a second pregnancy (I Simonovits, personal communication), suggesting a very low failure rate of suppression.

The dose which should be given between about 12 and 20 weeks is uncertain; some give the same amount as for a termination at 12 weeks and others give the same dose as would be given at 28 weeks. There is general agreement that from 20 weeks onwards the dose used should be that normally used at 28 weeks (e.g. in the USA, 300 μg).

Antenatal administration of anti-D

As described above, a single pregnancy with a D-positive, ABO-compatible infant initiates primary Rh D immunization in about one in six (17%) of D-negative women. When anti-D immunoglobulin is given postnatally, the incidence of primary Rh D immunization falls to about 1.5%, as judged by the development of anti-D by the time of delivery of a second D-positive infant. Thus, in some 90% of cases Rh D immunization that would otherwise follow pregnancy can be prevented by giving anti-D postnatally. As described below, it seems likely that most of the remaining 10% of cases can be prevented by antenatal treatment.

Safety of antenatal treatment. Although it was at first believed that injecting anti-D into a D-negative woman pregnant with a D-positive fetus was potentially dangerous, further consideration and practical experience show that the fear is groundless.

In D-positive infants born to mothers who are actively immunized to Rh D, the total amount of anti-D in the infant is only about 10% of that in the mother (Hughes-Jones *et al.* 1971). Accordingly, when 300 μg of anti-D is injected into the mother, even if equilibration across the placenta occurred immediately, not more than about 30 μg would be expected to be in the infant. In fact, as discussed earlier, IgG is transferred relatively slowly across the placenta. Accordingly, by the time that equilibrium is reached a considerable amount of the anti-D which has been injected into the mother will have been catabolized and the total amount reaching the infant will be less than 30 μg.

In trials in which 300 μg of anti-D were given to D-negative women at the twenty-eighth week and again at the thirty-fourth week of pregnancy, although as many as 28% of ABO-compatible D-positive infants had a weakly positive DAT the cord serum bilirubin concentration never exceeded 3.4 mg/dl (58 μmol/l) and no infant developed hyperbilirubinaemia severe enough to require phototherapy (Bowman *et al.* 1978). In a few cases in which D-negative women were given four doses of 300 μg of anti-D between about the twelfth and thirty-fourth weeks of pregnancy in an attempt to turn off the immune response following the discovery of low concentrations of maternal anti-D reacting only with enzyme-treated cells, not all the D-positive infants born subsequently had a positive DAT (JM Bowman, personal communication).

Results observed with antenatal treatment

A review of 11 published trials (seven non-randomized trials with historical or geographical controls, one

randomized control trial, one quasi-randomized controlled trial, one community intervention trial and one retrospective before-and-after study) concluded that routine antenatal anti-D prophylaxis is effective in reducing the number of D-negative women who are sensitized during pregnancy (Chilcott *et al.* 2003). These authors suggest that introduction of routine antenatal anti-D prophylaxis in England and Wales would reduce the sensitization rate from 0.95% to 0.35%. Furthermore, such an intervention is cost-effective, at least in the UK (Chilcott *et al.* 2004). In one series in which almost 10 000 D-negative women carrying D-positive fetuses were given an injection of anti-D at 28 weeks (either 300 μg i.m. or 240–300 μg i.v.), less than 0.1% developed anti-D by full term, whereas previous experience indicated that without antenatal anti-D the incidence would have been 1.8% (Bowman 1984). As explained on p. 505, the figure of 1.8% is substantially greater than that reported by others, but the discrepancy can be explained.

In another series in which, unlike the one just referred to, only primiparae were included, of 1238 D-negative women carrying D-positive fetuses who were injected at both 28 and 34 weeks with 100 μg of anti-D, only 0.16% developed anti-D by the time of delivery. In an earlier series from the same centre in which women were given anti-D only after delivery, 0.9% formed anti-D by the end of pregnancy (Tovey *et al.* 1983). The foregoing figures give a slightly too favourable impression of the success of antenatal immunoprophylaxis with anti-D because in both series a few additional women developed anti-D either 6 months after delivery or during a second pregnancy. In the first series, in which most of the women were tested at 6 months, there were two in whom anti-D was detected for the first time, an incidence of very approximately 0.02%; of an unknown number who had a second D-positive pregnancy there were another two who developed anti-D before the twenty-eighth week (Bowman 1984). In the second of the two series quoted above anti-D developed during a second pregnancy with a D-positive infant in 2 out of 325 women, but in neither case did the antibody appear to cause clinically significant haemolytic disease.

Amount of anti-D for antenatal injection. From the data of Bowman and co-workers (1978) it appears that treatment should be given as early as 28 weeks. In the USA and some other countries, the only antenatal dose of anti-D is 300 µg, injected at 28 weeks. In nine women who had received this dose, plasma levels of anti-D 9–10 weeks later were between 0.7 and 2.6 ng/ml, corresponding to a total residue of 6–21 µg of anti-D. At term, some women had no detectable anti-D (Bowman and Pollock 1987). Better survival of injected IgG anti-D, indicating that an average of 19 µg should remain 12 weeks after a dose of 250 µg, was found in another investigation, although there was substantial variation between different women (Eklund et al. 1982). It must be concluded that a single dose of 300 µg given at 28 weeks may be too small to protect all women (Bowman and Pollock 1987). The administration of 300 µg of anti-D at 28 weeks is convenient in countries where 300 µg of or thereabouts is the standard dose to be given postpartum, as the same preparation can then be given on the two occasions. On the other hand, in countries where the standard postpartum dose is 100 µg it is convenient to give two doses of 100 µg during pregnancy, at 28 weeks and 34 weeks respectively. This dosage will in fact result in a rather higher concentration of anti-D in the mother's plasma immediately before delivery than when a single dose of 300 µg is given at 28 weeks (seventh edition, p. 395), will result in a certain saving of anti-D and, again, will avoid the confusion of having two different sized doses to be administered antenatally and postnatally.

When anti-D is given antenatally, the serum concentration at term may still be high enough to be detectable by the IAT. In women who have been given anti-D Ig antenatally, the finding of a positive IAT at the time of delivery must not be regarded as a contraindication to giving the usual postpartum dose.

Intravenous administration of anti-D. As discussed in Chapter 5, it is possible that when anti-D is given intravenously at the same time as an injection of D-positive red cells, the dose of antibody required for the suppression of primary Rh D immunization may be smaller than when the anti-D is injected intramuscularly. There is therefore a potential advantage in giving anti-D intravenously rather than intramuscularly immediately following delivery when it is likely that any D-positive red cells in the circulation have arrived there only recently. In practice, because of the increased risk of transmitting viral infections when Ig is given intravenously (see Chapter 16) and because the methods used for viral inactivation in some

preparations are suspect, the i.m. route should be used whenever possible. When giving anti-D antenatally there does not seem to be any potential advantage in i.v. administration, as the object is to protect against Rh D immunization over a period of many weeks and, within 3 days of giving anti-D, plasma levels are the same whether the injection has been given intravenously or intramuscularly.

Occasional reactions have been reported following the i.v. injection of anti-D immunoglobulin prepared by fractionation on DEAE Sephadex (Hoppe et al. 1973); at one centre, only seven reactions, two of which were severe enough to require treatment, were noted following injections to 80 000 women (H Hoppe, personal communication). In another series, transient marked flushing and mild chest discomfort were noted in 2 out of 2792 women. The reactions were thought to be due to aggregated material in vials that had too high a moisture content (Bowman et al. 1980). In a third series, not a single untoward reaction was reported amongst 120 000 recipients (JR O'Riordan, personal communication). In a fourth series involving 261 women no adverse reactions were reported (MacKenzie et al. 2004).

Monoclonal/recombinant anti-D for prophylaxis

Although human monoclonal anti-D derived from Epstein–Barr virus (EBV)-transformed B lymphocytes has been available since 1984 (Crawford 1983), it has not yet emerged as a licensed product capable of replacing the tried and tested polyclonal product described above. Two monoclonal antibodies, one IgG1 (BRAD5) and one IgG3 (BRAD3), have been used as a blend in trials and shown to be capable of protecting D-negative male volunteers from D immunization (Kumpel et al. 1995; Smith et al. 2000). BRAD5 can be quantified in human serum using a monoclonal anti-BRAD5 idiotype by ELISA (Austin et al. 2001). Monoclonal anti-D produced by EBV transformation of B lymphocytes can be manipulated using recombinant DNA technology to optimize affinity and Fc effector functions (Proulx et al. 2002) and expressed in alternative expression systems for manufacture (Edelman et al. 1997; Miescher et al. 2000). A recombinant IgG1 anti-D produced in CHO cells was shown to prevent D immunization in male volunteers (Miescher et al. 2004).

Immunosuppression of D sensitization by induction of tolerance

Successful induction of tolerance to peptides corresponding to regions of the D polypeptide in transgenic mice presages the development of a new approach to prevention of haemolytic disease resulting from D immunization (Hall *et al.* 2005; see also Chapter 3).

Paternal leucocyte therapy

Lam and co-workers (2003) investigated the feasibility of isolating paternal mononuclear cells free of red cell contamination with a view to using these cells as a treatment for severe D alloimmunization.

Changes in the incidence and mortality of haemolytic disease

As described in Chapter 3, before the introduction of immunoprophylaxis of Rh D haemolytic disease, the frequency of the disease, both in England and in North America was about 1 per 170 births. Assuming an average family size of more than two children, this figure is close to expectation: the frequency of the disease in first pregnancies is very low (less than one per 1000 births), in second pregnancies is about one per 100 births, and in subsequent pregnancies is somewhat greater.

Immunoprophylaxis became available in 1968–70. In one North American hospital (dealing with a predominantly white population), in which postnatal anti-D was introduced in 1968, and antenatal anti-D added in 1985, the frequency with which (immune) anti-D was found in pregnant women declined from 1 in 238 in 1974 (Walker 1984) to 1 in 963 in 1988 (Walker and Hartrick 1991) and to 1 in 1663 in 1990–92; in the last period, HDN was diagnosed in only 1 in 2419 births (Walker *et al.* 1993).

In one English region (East Anglia), the figures for 1993–95 were as follows: anti-D was found in one per 584 pregnant women but in almost 80% of cases the anti-D was not detected at the time of the first antenatal visit and was subsequently present at a concentration of less than 1 iu/ml (0.2 μg/ml). Less than one infant per 2000 had clinical signs of HDN (A Rankin, personal communication). It should be noted that anti-D is given antenatally in only approximately 12% of hospitals in England and Wales (Chilcott *et al.* 2003).

The decline in the death rate from Rh haemolytic disease has been substantially greater than the decline in the incidence of the disease. In England and Wales, registered deaths fell from 1 in 2180 births in 1953 (Walker 1958) to 1 in 5400 in 1977 and to 1 in 62 500 in 1990 (Clarke and Mollison 1989; Hussey and Clarke 1992). It must be emphasized that these figures are not for total deaths, as up to September 1992 deaths occurring before the twenty-eighth week of pregnancy were not registered in England and Wales. (Since October 1992, deaths from 24 weeks onward have been registered.) Chilcott and co-workers (2003) put the figure at one death in every 20 800 births.

The most important steps in preventing Rh D immunization by pregnancy

First, in order to minimize the risk that, due to a technical or clerical error, a D-negative woman will be reported as D positive and thus not be given anti-D immunoglobulin after delivery, the D group of all so far unimmunized women should be determined (using two different anti-Ds) on at least two separate occasions: (1) at the time of the first antenatal visit (booking); and (2) at 28–34 weeks. In addition, the following steps are recommended for all so far unimmunized D-negative women:

1 As anti-D immunoglobulin is sometimes withheld because a report on the infant's D group has not yet been received, anti-D immunoglobulin (100 μg or more) should be given to all D-negative women within 72 h of delivery, unless the infant has been shown to be D negative.

2 After delivery, if the infant is D positive, a screening test for fetal red cells should be made on a sample of the mother's blood; if this is positive a quantitative estimate of the number of cells present should be made (see Appendix 13) and extra anti-D Ig given if indicated.

All D-negative women should be given a dose of anti-D immunoglobulin after induced abortion. The case for giving anti-D after spontaneous abortions in the first trimester is not strong (see p. 505) and practice varies.

After obstetric interference, for example amniocentesis or other potentially sensitizing event, anti-D immunoglobulin should be given, whether or not fetal red cells can be demonstrated in the mother's blood.

In women who are 20 or more weeks' pregnant, a test for fetal red cells should be made and extra anti-D immunoglobulin given when indicated. If the pregnancy continues, further anti-D should be given, for example 300 µg at 28 weeks or 100 µg at 28 weeks and again at 34 weeks.

Women with partial D

A woman with partial D may develop anti-D as a result of a pregnancy with a fetus whose red cells carry the D epitopes which she lacks. In two reported cases (Davey 1976b; Lacey *et al.* 1983), the mother's red cells belonged to category VI and, in both, the mother had apparently been immunized by pregnancy alone. In the second of the two cases, the infant was severely affected and died, although mild HDN is the rule. In the years 1976–85, 28 pregnant D-positive women with anti-D in their serum were tested at various centres of the National Blood Service in the UK; most of the women either belonged to category VI or had red cells which reacted too weakly with anti-D to be categorized; 26 out of the 28 infants were normal or only mildly affected; in most of these cases the titre of anti-D in the mother's serum was low although in a few cases it was in the range 20–256; of the remaining two infants, one required an exchange transfusion and one died *in utero* at 37–38 weeks (maternal anti-D titre in this case was 128).

When a woman is grouped as weak D (D^u) for the first time after delivery it is essential to do a screening test for fetal red cells, as she may in fact be D negative with a substantial number of D-positive fetal red cells in her circulation and not only need anti-D immunoglobulin but require more than the standard dose.

Administration of anti-D Ig to women with partial D

Most partial D red cells absorb little anti-D. Accordingly, after the injection of anti-D Ig to a woman with partial D recently delivered of a D-positive fetus, there should be enough circulating antibody to suppress Rh D immunization (Lubenko *et al.* 1989). Incidentally, in subjects with 'high-grade D^u' red cells injected with D-positive red cells, followed by IgG anti-D, clearance was about twice as slow as in D-negative subjects (Schneider 1976).

D-negative woman with a partial-D infant

A D-negative woman, whose infant was typed as D positive, was given 100 µg of anti-D immunoglobulin after it had been estimated that her circulation contained approximately 4 ml of fetal red cells. Despite a second dose of 100 µg of anti-D 72 h later, the fetal red cells were not cleared from the maternal circulation and it was then shown that the infant's red cells not only reacted weakly with anti-D but failed altogether to react with some anti-D sera, indicating that they were partial D. *In vitro*, the red cells reacted relatively weakly with the anti-D Ig that had been injected (Revill *et al.* 1979, supplemented by personal communication from P Tippett).

Haemolytic disease due to antibodies other than anti-D, anti-A and anti-B

A list of the various red cell alloantibodies that can cause haemolytic disease is given near the beginning of this chapter; after anti-D, anti-c and anti-K are easily the most important.

Rh antibodies other than anti-D

Haemolytic disease due to anti-c

Of all deaths from HDN not due to anti-D registered in England and Wales for the years 1977–90, 32 out of 49 were associated with anti-c, with or without anti-E (Clarke and Mollison 1989, supplemented by personal communication from CA Clarke). Anti-c, with or without anti-E, is found in about 0.7 per 1000 pregnant women, for example 177 out of 280 000 (Bowell *et al.* 1986); 65 in about 90 000 (Tovey 1986). The frequency of haemolytic disease due to anti-c is substantially lower than this for two reasons: first, as 40–50% of pregnant women with anti-c have been immunized by transfusion (Astrup and Kornstad 1977; Bowell *et al.* 1986), the fetus is relatively often c negative; and second, as the antibody is often present in low titre, a substantial number of c-positive infants have a negative DAT. For example, of 42 c-positive infants born to mothers with anti-c, 10 had a negative DAT; in 3 out of the 10 the antibody was detectable only with enzyme-treated red cells. In 24 out of 42 infants, including the 10 with a negative DAT, the titre of anti-c was 8 or less (Astrup and Kornstad 1977). In

525

another series, the titre of anti-c was 8 or less in 129 out of 177 (Bowell *et al.* 1986). In two series, only about 20% of c-positive infants born to mothers with anti-c required exchange transfusion (Astrup and Kornstad 1977; Hardy and Napier 1981). In the several series referred to above no stillbirths and only one neonatal death were recorded. In contrast, in another series, of 62 c-positive infants born to c-immunized women over a 40-year period, 20 required transfusion and eight were either stillborn (with hydrops) or died in the neonatal period (Wenk *et al.* 1985). In a study from the USA, covering the period 1967 to 2001, fetuses from 46 out of 55 pregnancies with anti-c had a positive direct antiglobulin test and eight of the affected neonates had HDN requiring fetal transfusion. An antibody titre of 1:32 or greater or the presence of hydrops identified all affected fetuses. There were no perinatal deaths in this study (Hackney *et al.* 2004). In England and Wales in 1977–87, among approximately 7 000 000 births, there were 26 infants recorded as dying from HDN due to anti-c (Clarke and Mollison 1989), that is approximately one per 250 000 births; even at the end of this period, that is in 1987, the death rate from HDN due to anti-D was still very much higher, i.e. one per 25 600 births. Several reliable methods for c typing of fetal DNA are available, based on the polymorphism at nucleotide 307 of *RHCE* (reviewed in Van der Schoot *et al.* 2003; see Chapter 5). Quantitative real-time PCR can be used for c typing of cell-free fetal DNA from maternal blood in pregnancies at risk from HDN due to anti-c [Finning K, Martin P, Daniels G, cited in Daniels *et al.* (2004)].

Other Rh antibodies

Anti-C was found in 38 out of 280 000 pregnancies (0.14 per 1000); it was about five times commoner in DccEE than in DccEe women; of infants tested at birth, two out of three had a negative DAT and there were no deaths from HDN (Bowell *et al.* 1988).

Anti-Cʷ is almost always associated with unaffected or mildly affected infants, although it has caused kernicterus (Lawler and van Loghem 1947); the incidence of HDN due to anti-Cʷ is probably less than 1 in 50 000 pregnancies (Bowman and Pollock 1993).

Anti-E alone is the Rh antibody found most commonly after anti-D. In one series, it was present in 97 of about 90 000 pregnancies (Tovey 1986). The antibody is often naturally occurring and is then sometimes detectable only with enzyme-treated red cells. Anti-E very seldom causes haemolytic disease. In a review of 283 pregnancies affected by anti-E alone during the period from 1959 to 2004 there was one perinatal death attributable to anti-E HDN (Joy *et al.* 2005).

Anti-e is a very rare cause of HDN; the disease is usually mild (Moncharmont *et al.* 1990).

Anti-Rh29 in Rh-null pregnant women has been associated with both mild (Bruce *et al.* 1985) and severe HDN (Lubenko *et al.* 1992).

Anti-Rh17 in D–/D– women has been associated with both moderate (Lenkiewicz and Zupanska 2000; Brumit *et al.* 2002) and severe HDN (Denomme *et al.* 2004). In the case described by Denomme and co-workers, maternal ABO-mismatched blood was successfully used for intrauterine transfusion.

Kell antibodies

Anti-K is found in about one per 1000 pregnant women, for example 127 out of 127 000 (Caine and Mueller–Heubach 1986); 27 out of 40 000 (Tovey 1986, estimates for 1982 only); 407 out of 350 000 (Mayne *et al.* 1990). The frequency of HDN due to anti-K is much lower, as in most cases the mother has been immunized by a transfusion of K-positive blood and not by pregnancy and the fetus is K negative. A history of previous transfusion was elicited from 88% of K-immunized pregnant women in one series (Mayne *et al.* 1990) and from 80% in another (Pepperell *et al.* 1977). In one more series, of 396 infants born to women with anti-K, only 20 were K positive, with a positive DAT. In the period concerned there were somewhat more than 800 000 deliveries, giving an overall incidence of HDN due to anti-K of about one in 40 000 births (Bowman 1994, supplemented by personal communication). From this figure the incidence of HDN due to anti-K can be deduced as approximately 1 in 20 000 pregnancies.

As the finding of anti-K during pregnancy is due in most cases to immunization by a previous transfusion rather than immunization by TPH from the fetus, and in most cases the fetus is K negative, the fetal genotype (i.e. *Kk* or *kk*) should be determined. The results of PCR-based tests on DNA obtained from amniotic fluid or chorionic villi were in complete agreement with those of subsequent tests on red cells after birth (Lee *et al.* 1996). Several PCR assays for K typing of fetuses have been described (reviewed by Van der Schoot *et al.*

2003; see also Chapter 8). Quantitative real-time PCR can be used for K typing of cell-free fetal DNA from maternal blood in pregnancies at risk of HDN from anti-K [Finning K, Martin P, Daniels G, cited in Daniels *et al.* (2004)].

The frequency of very severe haemolytic disease (stillbirth or hydrops) in K-positive infants born to mothers with anti-K was 5 out of 13, 2 out of 10 and 3 out of 20 in three series (Caine and Mueller-Heubach 1986; Mayne *et al.* 1990; Bowman 1994), giving an approximate mortality rate of one per 100 000 births for HDN due to anti-K. This estimate agrees very poorly with registered deaths. Over the period 1977–90, there were approximately 9 000 000 births in England and Wales and 15 deaths from HDN in which the mother's serum contained anti-K, either alone (11 cases) or with antibodies other than anti-D, giving a mortality of one in 600 000. The discrepancy between this figure and the one deduced above can only partly be explained by the fact that deaths before the twenty-eighth week of pregnancy were not recorded.

HDN due to anti-K has been found to be more severe when immunization is due to a previous pregnancy rather than a previous transfusion, even when the mother has had no previously affected infant (Pepperell *et al.* 1977; Caine and Mueller-Heubach 1986).

There is evidence that fetal anaemia caused by anti-K is due partly to suppression of erythropoiesis. More than one observer has noted that the levels of reticulocytes and of amniotic fluid bilirubin are lower than expected in relation to the degree of anaemia (see eighth edition, p. 685). In 11 cases of HDN due to anti-K with moderate or severe anaemia, levels of reticulocytes, erythroblasts and amniotic bilirubin levels were significantly lower than in 11 matched cases due to anti-D (Vaughan *et al.* 1994). Kell antigens are present on early erythroblasts [J Valinsky, cited by Marsh and Redman (1990); Southcott *et al.* (1999)]. Both monoclonal and polyclonal anti-K inhibit K-positive red cell progenitors but, with anti-D, there is no consistent inhibition of D-positive progenitors (Vaughan *et al.* 1998). Inhibition of erythropoiesis by anti-K may result from immune destruction of the erythroid precursors (Daniels *et al.* 1999). As D is expressed much later than K during erythropoiesis the lack of inhibition of erythropoiesis in cases of HDN caused by anti-D (and other Rh antibodies) can be explained.

Inhibition of myeloid and platelet progenitors by anti-K *in vitro* has also been reported and correlated with thrombocytopenia in three cases of HDN attributable to anti-K (Wagner *et al.* 2000a,b). The mechanism for these effects is unclear.

Another feature of haemolytic disease due to anti-K, which has been noted occasionally, is a poor correlation between the severity of the disease and the titre of antibody in the mother's serum. In one case, hydrops fetalis occurred despite an anti-K titre of only two at the thirty-seventh week of pregnancy (L McDonnell, personal communication). In another, hydrops at 23 weeks, associated with an Hb concentration of 22 g/l, was associated with a maternal anti-K titre of 8 (Bowman *et al.* 1989; see also Fleetwood *et al.* 1996). A quantitative method for the measurement of anti-K in the serum of alloimmunized women is described by Ahaded and co-workers (2002). The method is based on elution of anti-K from K-positive red cells at acid pH and quantification of the antibody (and subclass) by enzyme-linked immunosorbent assay (ELISA).

Anti-k is a very rare cause of HDN. As in HDN due to anti-K, the disease may be severe despite a low maternal antibody titre. For example, in a case in which the mother's anti-k titre was 16, the infant's Hb concentration at 31 weeks was only 60 g/l and three intravascular transfusions were given to the infant *in utero* (Bowman *et al.* 1989). In another case, despite a maternal anti-k titre of only 8–16, the infant, after being born spontaneously at 33 weeks, had an Hb concentration of 76 g/l (Anderson *et al.* 1990).

Other antibodies of the Kell system. Anti-Kp[a], -Js[a] and -Ku have been implicated in HDN of varying severity (for references, see Daniels 2002); anti-Js[b] has caused hydrops fetalis (Gordon *et al.* 1995). In two cases of severe HDN due to anti-Kp[b], the mother had presumably been primarily immunized by transfusion in childhood (Dacus and Spinnato 1984; Gorlin and Kelly 1994).

Other antibodies

Anti-Fy[a]. Anti-Fy[a] usually causes mild haemolytic disease, although among 11 cases reviewed by Greenwalt and colleagues (1959) there were two deaths. In a more recent study of 68 pregnancies when anti-Fy[a] was detected, three severely anaemic fetuses were identified, two of which required intrauterine transfusions (Goodrick *et al.* 1997). These authors suggest that pregnancies in which anti-Fy^a is detected at titres > 1:64 should be closely monitored. Mild haemolytic disease due to anti-Fy3 has been reported (Albrey *et al.* 1971).

Anti Jk^a. Anti Jk^a very rarely causes severe HDN; kernicterus has once been reported (Matson *et al.* 1959) and the authors know of a single case of hydrops fetalis: a grossly oedematous infant born by caesarean section at 36 weeks, with a positive DAT and a cord Hb of 39 g/l. The mother, who had had two previous infants, had an anti-Jk^a titre that varied from 16 to 128 (SL Barron, E Hey and M Reid, personal communication).

Haemolytic disease due to anti-M. When anti-M develops during pregnancy, it may fail to affect the fetus (see Bowley and Dunsford 1949; De Young-Owens *et al.* 1997). In rare cases, haemolytic disease develops and is occasionally responsible for hydrops fetalis (Stone and Marsh 1959; Matsumoto *et al.* 1981). In both of these cases, the anti-M in the mother's serum was very potent. In cases in which the infant is mildly or moderately affected with haemolytic disease due to anti-M there are two features that resemble ABO haemolytic disease rather than Rh haemolytic disease: first, the DAT is only weakly positive but unwashed red cells agglutinate spontaneously in a colloid medium, and second, the osmotic fragility of the red cells may be greatly increased (Stone and Marsh 1959; Freiesleben and Jensen 1961).

In a pregnant woman with relatively potent anti-M and a history of stillbirths, plasma to a total volume of 51 l was withdrawn, absorbed with M-positive red cells and reinfused. Although there was only a small fall in antibody titre, the woman was delivered of a normal infant (Yoshida *et al.* 1981).

Haemolytic disease due to anti-S and anti-s. This is very occasionally severe or even fatal (Levine *et al.* 1952; Issitt 1981, p. 43).

Haemolytic disease due to anti-U. This may be severe or even fatal (Bürki *et al.* 1964). In a review of 15 cases, severe HDN occurred only when the maternal anti-U had a titre of 1:512 or more. However, titres as high as 1:4000 were not necessarily associated with significant haemolysis (Smith *et al.* 1998).

Haemolytic disease due to anti-PP$_1$P^k. HDN of varying severity has been reported. In one case the IgG component of the antibody in the mother's serum had a titre of 16 (Hayashida and Watanabe 1968). In another, in which the infant had an Hb concentration of 8.7 g/dl, the DAT was only weakly positive (Levene *et al.* 1977).

Antibodies to low-frequency antigens. These have occasionally caused HDN but very few severe cases have been reported. In a case due to anti-ELO, exchange transfusion was needed (Better *et al.* 1993).

Haemolytic disease of the newborn due to anti-A and anti-B (ABO haemolytic disease)

Anti-A and anti-B occurring in group B and A subjects are predominantly IgM, but in O subjects are at least partly IgG. In 15% of all pregnancies in white people, the mother is O and her infant is A or B, but clinically obvious haemolytic disease is comparatively rare. There seem to be two main reasons for this finding: first, the A and B antigens are not fully developed at birth, and second, A and B substances are not confined to the red cells so that only a small fraction of IgG anti-A and anti-B which crosses the placenta combines with the infant's red cells. The protective effect of A and B determinants in fluids and tissues other than red cells was discussed by Tovey (1945) and Wiener and co-workers (1949).

Using sensitive methods, small amounts of IgG anti-A or anti-B are commonly found on the red cells of group A and B infants born to group O mothers (Hsu *et al.* 1974). Although severe HDN due to anti-A and anti-B is relatively rare, minor degrees of red cell destruction are common, as shown by the incidence of neonatal jaundice and by the slight lowering of the Hb concentration in ABO-incompatible infants compared with ABO-compatible infants.

Incidence

ABO haemolytic disease must be defined before its incidence can be estimated. For example, taking the criterion of the development of jaundice within 24 h of birth, the incidence was estimated to be one in 180 (Halbrecht 1951); taking the faintest trace of

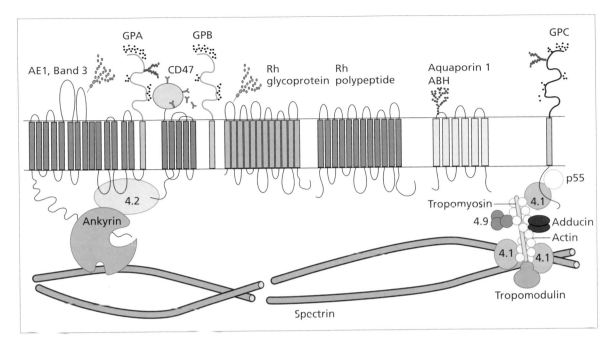

Plate 3.1 The red cell membrane, showing some of the major transmembrane proteins and attachment sites to the underlying red cell skeleton. Carbohydrate molecules with their side-chains are also shown (N-glycans(Y) or O-glycans). There are two major attachment sites between the membrane and the skeleton. One is mediated through the amino-terminal cytoplasmic domain of band 3 and also involves protein 2.1 (ankyrin), protein 4.2 (pallidin) and CD47. The other involves the cytoplasmic domain of glycophorin C, band 4.1, actin and p55. The heterodimer adducin binds to actin and spectrin, and promotes the binding of spectrin to actin. Dematin (protein 4.9) and tropomodulin are also involved in the spectrin–actin junction. Modified from Issitt PD and Anstee DJ (1998) Applied Blood Group Serology, 4th edn, Montgomery Scientific Publications, and Durham NC, Lux SE, Palek J (1995) Disorders of the red cell membrane, in: Handin R, Lux SE, Stossel T (eds) Principles and Practice of Hematology, Philadelphia, PA: JB Lippincott Co.

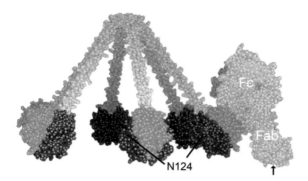

Plate 3.4 The interaction of C1q with IgG1. The black arrow indicates the antigenic site. N124 indicates the position of the carbohydrate attached to the C1qA subunit. From Gaboriaud *et al.* (2003).

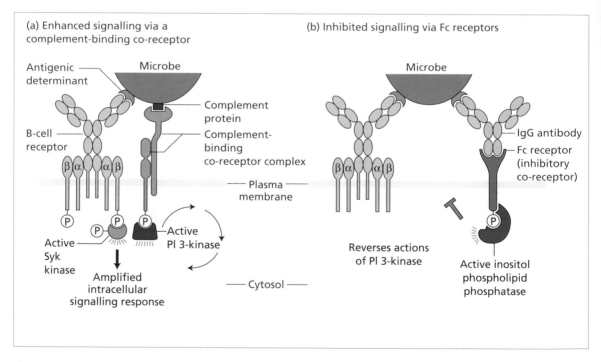

Plate 3.5 Influence of B-cell co-receptors on B-cell signalling. From Alberts *et al.* (2002, p. 1417). (a) The binding of microbe–complement complexes to a B cell crosslinks the antigen receptors to complement-binding co-receptor complexes amplifying the intracellular signalling response. (b) IgG antibodies bound to antigen bind to FcγreceptorIIB and cause inhibition of B-cell signalling.

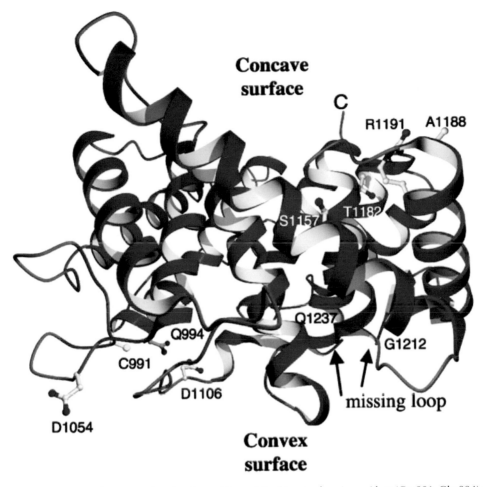

Plate 3.6 Side view of the C4Ad structure showing the positions of the thioester forming residues (Cys991, Gln 994) and the polymorphic amino acids Ser 1157, Thr 1182, Ala 1188 and Arg 1191. From van den Elsen (2002).

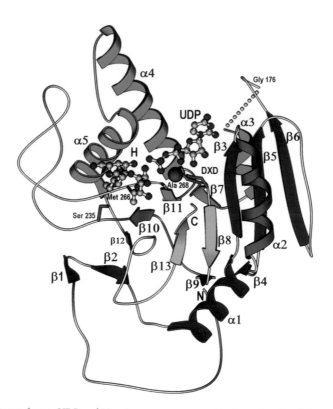

Plate 4.1 Structure of the B transferase. UDP and H antigen are represented in the active site of the enzyme by ball and stick models. Mn^{2+} is represented by the large circle in the active site. Also indicated are the four critical amino acids that distinguish the B and A transferases (Gly176Arg; Ser235Gly; Met266Leu; Ala268Gly). From Patanaude *et al.* 2002.

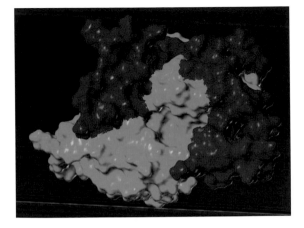

Plate 5.1 Orthogonal surface view of Rh D cat VI type III. Regions derived from Rh CE are coloured green, regions derived from Rh D are coloured magenta. The view is from the outside of the cell, showing the putative extracellular surface. Model produced by 'Modeller' web server, based on the structure of Amt B (Khademi *et al.* 2004). Only helices 3–12 (standard Rh numbering) are shown. Courtesy of N. Burton.

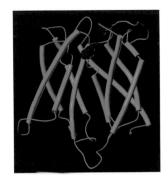

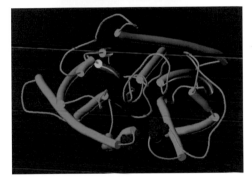

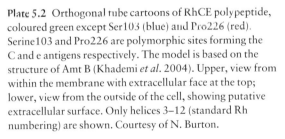

Plate 5.2 Orthogonal tube cartoons of RhCE polypeptide, coloured green except Ser103 (blue) and Pro226 (red). Serine103 and Pro226 are polymorphic sites forming the C and e antigens respectively. The model is based on the structure of Amt B (Khademi *et al.* 2004). Upper, view from within the membrane with extracellular face at the top; lower, view from the outside of the cell, showing putative extracellular surface. Only helices 3–12 (standard Rh numbering) are shown. Courtesy of N. Burton.

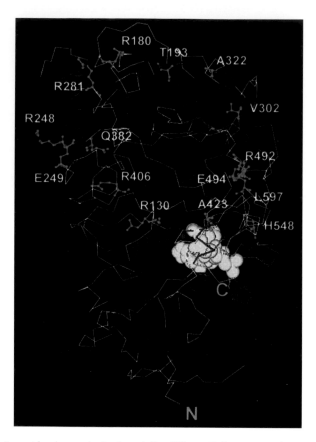

Plate 6.1 Locations of the amino acids whose substitutions define different Kell antigens. The amino acids whose mutations result in different Kell phenotypes are labelled (green) and are shown on a backbone structure of a model of the Kell ectodomain. Met193Thr defines Kk, Pro597Leu defines Js^a/Js^b and Trp281Arg or Gln defines Kp^a/Kp^b/Kp^c. The active and substrate binding sites are marked by the locations of zinc (pink ball) and of the inhibitor, phosphoramidon (yellow). N marks the amino terminus of the ectodomain. From Lee *et al.* (2003b) with permission.

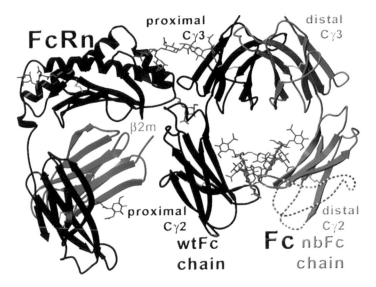

Plate 12.1 Structure of FcRn interaction with IgG. Ribbon diagrams of the structure of the extracellular domain of rat FcRn [blue and green (β2 microgobulin domain)] interacting with a heterodimeric Fc (hdFc) comprising wild-type Fc (red) and nbFc (yellow) (nbFc is engineered to lack an FcRn binding site). N-linked carbohydrates are shown in ball-and-stick representation. FcRn uses its α2- and β2-microglobulin domains and carbohydrate to interact with the Fc Cγ2–Cγ3 interface. From Martin *et al.* (2001).

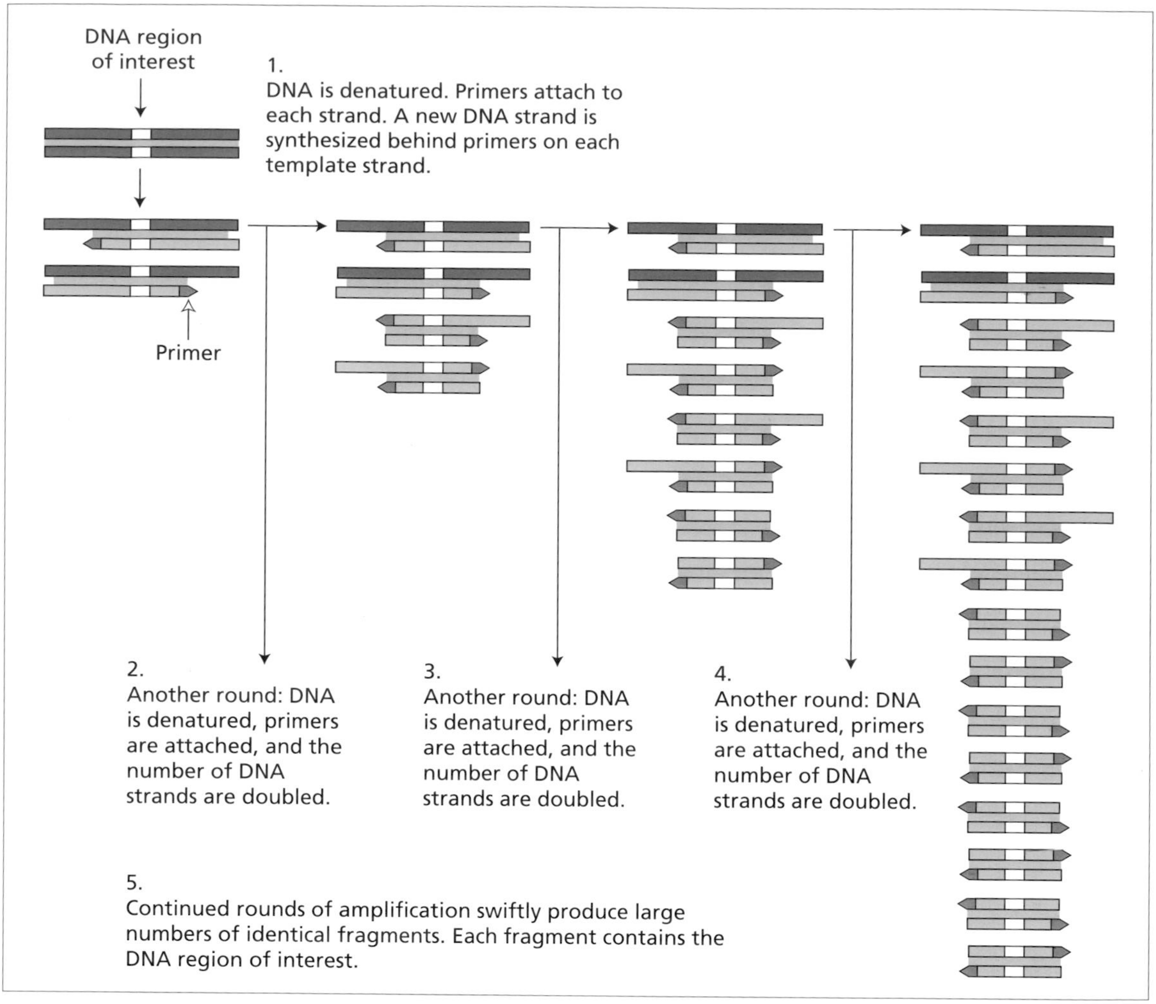
DNA region
of interest
1.
DNA is denatured. Primers attach to each strand. A new DNA strand is synthesized behind primers on each template strand.
Primer
2.
Another round: DNA is denatured, primers are attached, and the number of DNA strands are doubled.
3.
Another round: DNA is denatured, primers are attached, and the number of DNA strands are doubled.
4.
Another round: DNA is denatured, primers are attached, and the number of DNA strands are doubled.
5.
Continued rounds of amplification swiftly produce large numbers of identical fragments. Each fragment contains the DNA region of interest.

Plate 16.1 The polymerase chain reaction (PCR). A fragment of double-stranded DNA has the specific gene sequence for amplification flanked by two vertical lines. The two DNA strands separate (heat denaturation) and are then allowed to reassociate (anneal) with their primers (dark bars) that mark the ends of the target sequence. The primers then synthesize two new chains complementary to the original strands starting from the 5'-end in the presence of *Taq* polymerase and the four deoxyribonucleotide triphosphates. Each cycle doubles the DNA and is repeated 25–35 times with a final enrichment of the target sequence of 10^5–10^6.

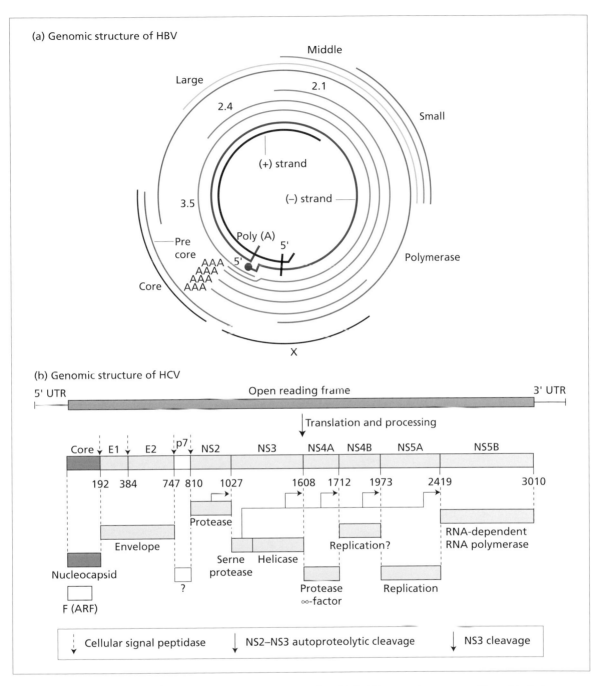

(a) Genomic structure of HBV

Middle

Large

2.1

2.4

Small

(+) strand

3.5

(−) strand

Pre core

Poly (A)

5'

5'

AAA
AAA
AAA
AAA

Core

Polymerase

X

(b) Genomic structure of HCV

5' UTR   Open reading frame   3' UTR

Translation and processing

Core   E1   E2   p7   NS2   NS3   NS4A   NS4B   NS5A   NS5B

192   384   747 810   1027   1608   1712   1973   2419   3010

Protease

RNA-dependent
RNA polymerase

Envelope

Serne   Helicase
protease

Replication?

Nucleocapsid

?

Protease
∞-factor

Replication

F (ARF)

| Cellular signal peptidase | NS2–NS3 autoproteolytic cleavage | NS3 cleavage |

Plate 16.2a The genomic structure of hepatitis B virus (HBV). The inner circles represent the full-length minus (−) strand with the terminal protein attached to its 5'-end and the incomplete plus (+) strand of the HBV genome. The thin black lines represent the 3.5, 2.4, 2.1 and 0.7-kb mRNA transcripts. The outermost lines indicate the translated HBV proteins, the surface proteins, polymerase protein, and core and pre-core proteins.

Plate 16.2b The genomic structure of hepatitis C virus (HCV). A long open reading frame (ORF) encodes a polyprotein of 3010 amino acids. The numbers below the polyprotein indicate the amino acid positions of the cleavage sites for cellular and viral proteases. An F (frameshift) protein is translated from a short alternative reading frame (ARF). E, envelope protein; NS, non-structural protein; UTR, untranslated region. From Rehermann and Nascimbeni 2005 with permission.

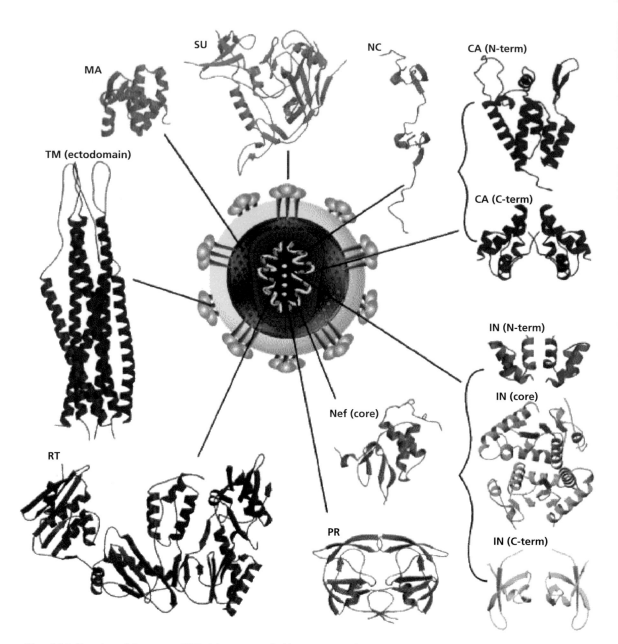

Plate 16.3 Drawing of the mature HIV virion surrounded by ribbon representations of the structurally characterized viral proteins and protein fragments. The protein structures have been drawn to the same scale. The virus enveloped is a lipid bilayer (yellow) that is derived from the membrane of the host cell. Exposed surface glycoproteins (SU, gp120; cyan) are anchored to the virus via interactions with the transmembrane protein (TM, gp41; violet). The lipid bilayer also contains several cellular membrane proteins derived from the host cell, including major histocompatibility antigens, actin and ubiquitin. A matrix shell comprising approximately 2000 copies of the matrix protein (MA, p17; green) lines the inner surface of the viral membrane, and a conical capsid core particle comprising around 2000 copies of the capsid protein (CA, p24; red) is located in the centre of the virus. The capsid particle encapsidates two copies of the unspliced viral genome, which is stabilized as a ribonucleoprotein complex with around 2000 copies of the nucleocapsid protein (NC, p7; blue), and also contains three essential virally encoded enzymes: protease (PR; pink), reverse transcriptase (RT; purple) and integrase (IN; olive). Virus particles also package the accessory proteins, Nef (orange), Vif and Vpr (not shown). Three additional accessory proteins that function in the host cell, Rev, Tat and Vpu, do not appear to be packaged. Adapted from Turner and Summers 1999.

Table 12.2 Effect of ABO incompatibility between infant's red cells and mother's serum on cord blood findings (from Rosenfield and Ohno 1955).

	No. of cord blood samples*	Mean values		
		Haemoglobin concentration (g/dl)	Reticulocytes (%)	Bilirubin concentration (mg/dl)[†]
A Infant's red cells compatible with mother's serum	2256	16.05	4.34	2.11
B Infant's red cells incompatible with mother's serum: infant's direct antiglobulin test negative	558	15.82	4.53	2.22
C As B, but direct antiglobulin test positive	89	14.85	5.94	2.96

* Haemoglobin estimates were made on all samples, and reticulocyte counts and bilirubin estimates on almost all samples.
[†] 1 mg/dl = 17 µmol/l.

jaundice in the first 24 h as the criterion, the incidence was as high as one in 70 in another series (Valentine, 1958).

In two series in which the Hb concentration and bilirubin concentration of cord blood were measured in ABO-compatible and ABO-incompatible infants born to group O mothers, it was found that values for Hb concentration were slightly lower, and those for bilirubin concentration slightly higher, in ABO-incompatible infants. In the first of these series the DAT was positive in 14% of the ABO-incompatible infants and in these the Hb concentration was distinctly lower and the bilirubin concentration distinctly higher than in the infants with a negative antiglobulin test (Table 12.2). In the second series, a positive DAT was found in as many as 32.8% of the ABO-incompatible infants and anti-A or anti-B could be eluted from the infant's red cells in a further 38%, but clinically significant disease, judged by a peak bilirubin concentration of more than 12 mg/dl (204 µmol/l) together with anaemia and reticulocytosis, was diagnosed in only 27 out of the 680 infants, i.e. in 1 in 125 of all newborn infants or 1 in 25 ABO-incompatible infants (Desjardins *et al.* 1979).

Cases of HDN due to anti-A or anti-B that are severe enough to need exchange transfusion are relatively rare, for example none amongst 1500 newborn infants (Rosenfield 1955); 3 out of 14 000 consecutive births (second edition, p. 505); 3 out of 8000 births (Ames and Lloyd 1964); and 6 out of 5704 infants born to group O mothers (Voak and Bowley 1969).

The foregoing figures are from Europe or North America; a higher incidence has been found in some other populations.

Higher incidence in certain populations

Black people. There is apparent disagreement about the relative frequency of ABO haemolytic disease in black people and in white people. The disease was found to be commoner in black people by Kirkman (1977), but in another series, although a positive DAT was commoner in black than in white infants, there was no difference in bilirubin levels or in the need for phototherapy (Peevy and Wiseman 1978).

In assessing the relative frequency of ABO haemolytic disease in black people and white people, a complication is introduced by the fact that in ABO-compatible infants hyperbilirubinaemia is commoner in white than in black people. Accordingly, if, for example, all ABO-incompatible infants whose serum bilirubin concentration exceeds 170 µmol/l are considered to have ABO haemolytic disease, the disease will appear to be much commoner in white people than it really is. One way of assessing the effect of ABO incompatibility is to compare various indices, i.e. the DAT, the age at the onset of jaundice and the maximum recorded serum bilirubin concentration, in ABO-incompatible and ABO-compatible infants. When this was done, in a very careful study in which black and white infants were being treated in the same nursery, ABO haemolytic disease was found to be clearly commoner in black than in white people, the relative frequency being between 2 and 6:1, depending on the particular criteria chosen for diagnosis (Kirkman 1977).

In a survey in Nigeria, the serum of about one-third of group O subjects was found to have strong lytic activity for A or B cells, anti-B lytic activity being commoner than anti-A lytic activity; moderate or severe jaundice, defined as a serum bilirubin concentration exceeding 10 mg/dl (170 µmol/l with a positive DAT was found to develop in about one-third of infants whose red cells were lysed *in vitro* by their mother's serum (Worlledge *et al.* 1974). These figures indicate that the frequency of ABO HDN in Nigeria is about 5% of births.

A factor that might be expected to produce relatively severe HDN in black people is the relatively strong expression of A and B that they have (see Chapter 4). Although the relative potency of anti-A and anti-B has in the past been suspected of being racially determined, recent work indicates that environmental factors may be more important (see Chapter 4).

Arabs. From a survey of almost 3000 newborn Arab infants it was concluded that ABO haemolytic disease was about as common in Arabs as in black people and that the disease tended to be more severe in Arabs than in Europeans: exchange transfusion for ABO haemolytic disease was carried out in one in every 500 newborn Arab infants (Al-Jawad *et al.* 1985).

Selected populations in Central and South America. In a comparison between populations in Puerto Rico and North Carolina, the incidence of ABO HDN was found to be substantially higher in Puerto Rico (Huntley *et al.* 1976); a similar increase has been found in Venezuela, i.e. about 30% of ABO-incompatible infants have signs of haemolytic disease compared with 20% or less in European and North American populations (Cariani *et al.* 1995). About one in 300 of all newborn infants in Venezuela need exchange transfusion (Romano *et al.* 1994). The higher incidence and greater severity of ABO HDN in Venezuela may be due to raised anti-A titres associated with infestation with Ascaris (Romano *et al.* 1988).

Relative frequency in group A and B infants

If group A and B infants were equally liable to the disease, the ratio A/B in white affected infants should be

approximately 2.7:1. In the series of Fischer (1961) the ratio was 3.7:1, suggesting that, in white people, group B infants are slightly less liable than group A infants to develop haemolytic disease. On the other hand, in another study a positive DAT was found to be relatively commoner in group B than in group A infants, in both white and black people (Peevy and Wiseman 1978).

Familial incidence

In about 50% of families in which ABO haemolytic disease is diagnosed, the first ABO-incompatible infant in the family is affected (first edition, p. 391).

In families in which ABO haemolytic disease is mild, an affected infant may be followed by a clinically unaffected infant. On the other hand, when severe disease occurs it is likely to be followed by similarly severe disease in subsequent infants of the same blood group.

Mrs Bak: First infant born February 1960; rapidly developed jaundice and found to have erythroblastaemia; diagnosed as having haemolytic disease due to anti-A; exchange transfusion given but infant died. Second infant born April 1961; cord Hb 11.6 g/dl, DAT weakly positive; blood film showed numerous normoblasts and microspherocytes; osmotic fragility: 50% lysis in 0.590% NaCl (grossly increased). The infant was given one exchange transfusion and made excellent progress. Third infant born November 1962; cord blood findings almost identical to those of the second infant, for example cord Hb 11.8 g/dl; DAT weakly positive, infant was treated by exchange transfusion and recovered uneventfully. As the findings indicate, the degree of severity of the haemolytic process appeared to be almost identical in the second and third infants. The titre of IgG anti-A in the mother's serum, estimated by the method of Polley and co-workers (1965), was virtually the same at the time of birth of these two infants, namely 4096 and 8192 respectively.

Serological findings in mothers

ABO group

Mothers of infants with ABO haemolytic disease almost invariably belong to group O (Rosenfield 1955), evidently because IgG anti-A and anti-B occur far more commonly in group O than in group B and A mothers (Rawson and Abelson 1960; Kochwa *et al.* 1961). In one series of 45 cases the mother was group O in 43 instances and subgroup A_2 in the remaining two; A_2 mothers produced much stronger 'incomplete' anti-B than A_1 mothers (Munk-Andersen 1958).

IgG anti-A and anti-B

The simplest and most satisfactory test is to treat the mother's serum with a reducing agent (e.g. DTT) to inactivate IgM antibodies and then determine the anti-A or anti-B titre by IAT using an anti-IgG serum (Voak and Bowley 1969). Using this method, a titre of 512 or more was found to be very suggestive of haemolytic disease. An earlier study, using a modification of the partial neutralization test of Witebsky, had shown that in ABO haemolytic disease the indirect antiglobulin titre was almost always in the range 64–16 000, and was 1000 or more in 13 out of 18 cases in which an infant needed an exchange transfusion (Polley et al. 1965).

IgG subclasses of anti-A and anti-B. Anti-A and anti-B from pregnant women are at least partly IgG2 (see Chapter 4). Macrophages carrying the high-affinity FcIIa receptor mediate lysis of red cells sensitized with IgG2 anti-A, although not that of cells sensitized with IgG2 anti-Rh D (Kumpel et al. 1996). Presumably, therefore, IgG2 anti-A and -B play a part in red cell destruction in those infants with ABO HDN whose macrophages carry the high-affinity FcRIIa receptor.

Antibody-dependent cell-mediated cytotoxicity assays with monocytes

In a large number of cases in which an ADCC(M) assay gave negative results, i.e. < 10% lysis, the infant never showed signs of red cell destruction; in three cases in which the ADCC assay was strongly positive, i.e. > 45% lysis, the infant was severely affected and needed more than one exchange transfusion. In cases in which there was 10–45% lysis in the assay, the degree of affection could not be predicted. The discrepancy between the results of the assay and the severity of red cell destruction in the infant appeared to be due to using standard adult red cells in the assay. When the infant's red cells were used, the degree of lysis was strongly affected by the number of A or B sites on the red cells (Brouwers et al. 1988a).

Serological findings in infants

The direct antiglobulin test using anti-IgG

In infants with relatively severe ABO haemolytic disease the amount of antibody on the cells was found to be less than 220 molecules per cell (0.6 µg IgG/ml red cells) in 10 of 15 cases (Romano et al. 1973). As, when the spin-tube antiglobulin test is used, the minimum number of antibody molecules that can be detected is about 100–150 (see Chapter 8), it is not surprising that in mildly affected infants the DAT may be negative. When a very sensitive method is used some anti-A or anti-B can be demonstrated on the red cells of virtually all ABO-incompatible infants. When the DAT was carried out in an autoanalyzer, using a low-ionic-strength medium with enhancing agents, the red cells of 13 A_1 and eight B infants, all apparently healthy, gave positive results. The authors calculated that there were between eight and 85 molecules of IgG per red cell (Hsu et al. 1974). Incidentally, the DAT was positive in only one of seven A_2 infants.

It is evident that there is an apparent substantial discrepancy between the findings in haemolytic disease due to anti-D, on the one hand, and to anti-A and anti-B, on the other. In Rh D haemolytic disease, infants may have a strongly positive DAT without showing any clinical signs of disease, whereas in ABO haemolytic disease they may be clinically affected but have a negative or only very weakly positive test. It has been suggested that in ABO haemolytic disease the findings in DATs do not indicate correctly the amount of antibody bound to the red cells *in vivo*. Romans and co-workers (1980) showed, for single examples of IgG anti-A and anti-B, that these antibodies must be bound by both combining sites (monogamous bivalency) to be detectable in the antiglobulin test.

The presence of A antigen sites on unbranched chains of glycolipids or glycoproteins on the surface of the red cells of newborn infants would make it difficult for molecules to bind bivalently because the sites on unbranched chains are not close enough together. Incidentally it would also make it difficult for molecules binding univalently to co-operate in activating C1 (see also Chapter 3).

Although the foregoing explanation is intellectually satisfying, it may not be correct. For one thing, the claim that the binding of anti-A to adult group A red cells is predominantly bivalent has been challenged by

Romano and co-workers (1983), who found that the binding constants of anti-A and its Fab derivative were similar with both adult and newborn group A red cells. Other observations that appear to be incompatible with the hypothesis of Romans and co-workers (1980) have been discussed previously (seventh edition, p. 695). To take one example, if cord group A_1 red cells are coated with ^{125}I-labelled human IgG anti-A, some 90% of the antibody appears to be firmly bound by the red cells (NC Hughes-Jones, personal communication, 1981). It seems that further experimental work is needed to define precisely the extent and nature of the binding of IgG anti-A and anti-B to the red cells of newborn infants.

The direct antiglobulin test using anti-C3d

Even in severe ABO haemolytic disease the infant's red cells do not react with anti-C3d (Mollison 1983, p. 694). This finding is due partly to the weak expression of A and B antigens on the red cells of newborn infants but also to the relatively low level of complement in the serum of newborn infants (Brouwers et al. 1988b).

Elution of antibody from infant's red cells

In ABO haemolytic disease, when the DAT is only weakly positive or even negative, eluates from the infant's red cells may give strong indirect antiglobulin reactions with adult A_1 red cells (Voak and Bowley 1969). The explanation for the finding seems to be that the elution procedure results in a considerable concentration of antibody (Voak and Williams 1971; Romano et al. 1973).

There is a relation between crossreactivity of eluates, for example reaction of an eluate from group A cells with B cells as well as with A cells, and severity, simply because there is a relation between crossreactivity and potency (see Chapter 4).

Spontaneous agglutination of red cells

Red cells from infants with ABO haemolytic disease tend to clump spontaneously when suspended in plasma (Wiener et al. 1949). Similarly, in observations on a series of moderately severely affected infants it was noticed that 'blood freshly drawn from the infant formed large clumps which were easily seen when the

blood was allowed to flow down the side of a tube or was examined on an opal glass tile'; the authors pointed out that if blood is taken from a patient of group A_1 who has received a transfusion of plasma containing potent anti-A, it behaves in the same way (Crawford et al. 1953).

The tendency of red cells taken from infants with ABO haemolytic disease to clump spontaneously was re-investigated by Romano and Mollison (1975). Red cells coated with small amounts IgG anti-A and then washed were found to be almost as readily agglutinated by ABO-compatible plasma as by anti-IgG. Plasma was very much more effective than serum in potentiating agglutination. In a series of infants suspected of having ABO haemolytic disease, a test for autoagglutination, performed by mixing red cells with their own plasma on a slide, was positive in 23 out of 25 cases, whereas the DAT was positive in only 20 of the cases (Romano et al. 1982).

The observation described by Lewi and Clarke (1960) presumably also demonstrates some change in the surface charge of the red cells of affected infants. Washed red cells from infants suspected of having HDN due to ABO incompatibility were suspended in polyvinyl pyrrolidone (PVP) and were found to sediment far more rapidly than similarly treated red cells from normal infants.

Reactivity of infant's red cells with anti-A and anti-B in vitro

As described in Chapter 4, the red cells of newborn infants react relatively weakly with anti-A and anti-B in vitro. HDN due to anti-A is observed only in infants who are genetically A_1 (Zuelzer and Kaplan 1954). At the time of birth the red cells of such infants may fail to react with anti-A_1, although samples taken when the infant is a few months old do react (Crawford et al. 1953). No case of HDN due to anti-A in an infant unequivocally belonging to subgroup A_2, as shown by tests at least many months after birth, has yet been described.

One puzzling observation is that, whereas the red cells of healthy infants who are genetically A_1 are agglutinated at the time of birth by an extract of Dolichos biflorus, red cells from genetically A_1 infants with haemolytic disease due to anti-A may fail to be agglutinated by an extract of Dolichos (Gerlini et al. 1968). The cause of this finding has never been demonstrated but blocking of antigen sites by bound IgG anti-A seems to be a possibility.

Premature infants seem to be protected from ABO haemolytic disease, presumably because there are fewer A and B sites on the red cells than on the cells of full-term newborn infants (Schellong 1964).

Secretor status of infant

It seems that the secretor status of the infant plays little or no part in protecting it against ABO haemolytic disease. In fact, the ratio of secretors to non-secretors is slightly higher than expected; see Voak (1969) who also quotes several earlier papers in support. The excess of secretors may be related to the fact that secretor infants are more prone to induce immune responses in their mothers (see Chapter 4).

Haematological findings

Haemoglobin concentration

In moderately severe ABO haemolytic disease, the Hb concentration of cord blood may be below normal limits (Mollison and Cutbush 1949b; see also the cases described above). After birth, due to the wider range of normal Hb values that then prevail, it is unusual to find infants who are definitely anaemic. Compared with Rh D haemolytic disease, ABO haemolytic disease is a shortlived affair and it is unusual for anaemia to be found after the first 2 weeks or so of life.

Reticulocytosis and erythroblastaemia

A slight increase in reticulocytes is a common feature in HDN due to ABO incompatibility (Rosenfield 1955). In the series of fairly severe cases collected by Crawford and co-workers (1953), the reticulocyte count exceeded 15% in 6 out of 11 cases. In five of these cases there were 30 or more nucleated red cells per 100 leucocytes.

Spherocytosis and changes in osmotic fragility

Microspherocytes are frequently prominent in blood films from infants with ABO haemolytic disease (Grumbach and Gasser 1948). Similarly, red cell osmotic fragility is almost always above normal limits, at least in moderately severe cases, whereas in Rh D haemolytic disease, even in severe cases, only minor increases in osmotic fragility are found and spherocytosis is unusual (Crawford et al. 1953). In ABO haemolytic disease, the changes in osmotic fragility may persist for as long as 2 or 3 weeks after birth.

Changes in bilirubin concentration

Although the rise in serum bilirubin concentration is usually only moderate and can be controlled by phototherapy, occasional cases of kernicterus have been reported (Grumbach and Gasser 1948) so that, as mentioned above, early exchange transfusion is occasionally indicated.

Management of ABO haemolytic disease

Routine antenatal tests not indicated

ABO incompatibility seldom causes severe haemolytic disease and routine antenatal tests to assess the potency of anti-A and anti-B are not indicated. In women who have a history suggesting that a previous infant has been affected with ABO haemolytic disease, cord blood should be taken and tested as soon as possible after birth.

The authors of the tenth edition of this book report finding only two convincing cases of hydrops fetalis due to ABO incompatibility. In both, abnormal swelling of the mother's abdomen at 32–34 weeks prompted an examination of the fetus by ultrasonography and revealed fetal hydrops. In the first case, the infant was born by caesarean section at 32 weeks and found to be group A with a strongly positive DAT; haemoglobinuria was noted. The cord PCV was reported to be 0.43, but 1 h after birth was 0.30. Packed group O red cells were transfused but the infant died at 20 h. Two previous infants had had severe neonatal jaundice. The mother's IgG anti-A titre was 4000 (Gilja and Shah 1988). In the second case, the infant was born by caesarean section at 34 weeks and found to be group B with a positive DAT. The cord blood PCV was 0.20, identical to that of an umbilical sample taken while the infant was still in utero. At the time of the report the infant remained gravely ill. The mother's anti-B titre was reported as 65 536 (Sherer et al. 1991).

Exchange transfusion in ABO haemolytic disease

As severe anaemia is very uncommon, the main indication for exchange transfusion is the threat of serious hyperbilirubinaemia, leading to kernicterus. Moderate hyperbilirubinaemia can be controlled by phototherapy.

When exchange transfusion is judged to be necessary, group O blood should be used. Provided that the donor's plasma has been screened so as to exclude donors with potent anti-A or anti-B, the antibodies in the transfused plasma are unlikely to exacerbate the haemolytic process. A better solution is to use group O red cells suspended in group AB plasma, preferably from an ABH secretor.

Phototherapy

The mode of action of phototherapy in lowering serum bilirubin concentration is described briefly on p. 519. In those full-term infants with ABO haemolytic disease whose serum bilirubin concentrations threaten to rise to dangerous levels, phototherapy is often sufficient to control the situation. Some recommendations about monitoring bilirubin levels and indications for phototherapy were given as follows: if the cord serum bilirubin concentration is known to have been > 4 mg/dl, estimate bilirubin every 4 h; otherwise, estimate bilirubin 6-hourly. Phototherapy should be begun if the bilirubin level reaches 10 mg/dl within 12 h, or 12 mg/dl (68 μmol/l) within 18 h, or 14 mg/dl within 24 h or 15 mg/dl thereafter (Osborn et al. 1984). Of 44 infants diagnosed by these authors as having ABO haemolytic disease, only four required phototherapy.

Use of intravenous immunoglobulin

In a study from Saudi Arabia, the value of phototherapy plus intravenous immunoglobulin G (IVIG) was compared with phototherapy alone (control group) in reducing the requirement for exchange transfusion of babies with hyperbilirubinaemia due to ABO haemolytic disease. Each group comprised 56 babies. Exchange transfusion was carried out on four babies in the study group compared with 16 babies in the control group. No adverse effects of IVIG were reported in the study group (Miqdad et al. 2004).

Alternatives to exchange transfusion

A case in which an ABO-incompatible term infant with hyperbilirubinaemia was successfully treated with oral D-penicillamine (300 mg/kg per day divided in three doses for 3 days), phototherapy, intravenous fluids and recombinant human erythropoietin (200 units/kg subcutaneously on every second day for 2 weeks) is described by Lakatos and co-workers (1999). This alternative treatment regime was undertaken because the infant's parents were Jehovah's Witnesses and would not agree to exchange transfusion.

Thirteen infants with ABO HDN, with a pretreatment serum bilirubin level of 14.6 mg/dl, were treated with A or B trisaccharides, usually in a dose of 45 mg. Within 5–6 days bilirubin levels were normal in 10 out of 13. A comparable group not treated with trisaccharides showed no fall in bilirubin levels after 5 days (Romano et al. 1994).

Haemolytic reactions after transfusing A or B red cells

When red cells from adult group A or group B donors are transfused, the red cells will almost always have more A and B sites than the infant's own red cells and are likely to undergo more rapid destruction.

In one case in which an infant with HDN was given an exchange transfusion with A_1 blood, the infant developed haemoglobinuria and died (Carpentier and Meersseman 1956). In two other group A infants with haemolytic disease due to anti-A, the use of group A blood, for exchange transfusion in the first case, and for a simple transfusion in the second, led to a substantial increase in jaundice and the development of kernicterus. The authors noted that the DAT became positive only after the transfusion of group A blood and then gave a mixed-field appearance, evidently because only the transfused group A red cells from adult donors were agglutinated (Sender et al. 1971).

Danger of transfusing A or B red cells from adult donors to A or B premature infants born to group O mothers

As described above, A and B antigens are particularly weak in premature infants; maternal IgG anti-A or anti-B may therefore be present without causing a haemolytic syndrome. However, a haemolytic transfusion reaction may be produced if group A or B red cells from adult donors are transfused. In three cases described by Falterman and Richardson (1980), haemolytic reactions were observed in infants with birthweights of between 1280 and 1560 g (30–32 weeks' gestation). In all three infants the DAT was negative in the first 2 days of life but, after transfusion of red cells of the infant's ABO group, hyperbilirubinaemia developed in all three cases and haemoglobinuria occurred in two. The authors described the infants as suffering from unrecognized ABO haemolytic disease, but to the present authors that seems to be a misconception.

Haemolytic disease due to anti-H

Following the birth of an unaffected group B infant, two successive group O infants were born to an Oh mother, whose serum contained lytic IgG anti-H. Both infants had cord bilirubin levels of 45 µmol/l and needed exchange transfusion; lytic anti-H was demonstrated in cord serum (Moores et al. 1994). Exchange transfusion is not always necessary when group O infants are born to an Oh mother. In a case described by Battacharya and co-workers (2002) an Oh lady with potent anti-H gave birth to two group O children in consecutive pregnancies and neither child was affected by HDN. These authors suggest the low expression of H antigen on cord blood and/or absorption of anti-H by H antigen on the placenta may account for the lack of disease in this case.

References

AABB (1991) Standards for Blood Banks and Transfusion Services, 14th edn. Arlington, VA: Am Assoc Blood Banks

Ackerman BD, Dyer GY, Leydorf MM (1970) Hyperbilirubinemia and kernicterus in small premature infants. Pediatrics 45: 968

Ahaded A, Brossard Y, Debbia M et al. (2002) Quantitative determination of anti-K (KEL1) IgG and IgG subclasses in the serum of severely alloimmunized pregnant women by ELISA. Transfusion 40: 1239–1245

Albrey JA, Vincent EER, Hutchinson J et al. (1971) A new antibody, anti-Fy3, in the Duffy blood group system. Vox Sang 20: 29–35

Alie-Daran SJ, Dugoujon J-M, Fournie A (1992) Gm typing, IgG subclasses of anti-Rh (D) and severity of hemolytic disease of the newborn. Vox Sang 62: 127–128

Al-Jawad ST, Keenan P, Kholeif S (1985) Incidence of ABO haemolytic disease in a mixed Arab population. Saudi Med J 7: 41–45

Allen FH Jr (1957) Induction of labor in the management of erythroblastosis fetalis. Q Rev Pediat 12: 1

Allen FH Jr, Diamond LK, Vaughan VC III (1950) Erythroblastosis fetalis, VI. Prevention of kernicterus. Am J Dis Child 80: 779

Ames AC, Lloyd RS (1964) A scheme for the ante-natal prediction of ABO haemolytic disease of the newborn. Vox Sang 9: 712

Anderson NA, Tandy A, Westgate J et al. (1990) Haemolytic disease of the newborn caused by anti-k (Abstract). Transfus Med 1(Suppl. 1): 58

Arce MA, Thompsen ES, Wagner S et al. (1993) Molecular cloning of RhD cDNA derived from a gene present in RhD-positive, but not RhD-negative individuals. Blood 82: 651–655

Armitage P, Mollison PL (1953) Further analysis of controlled trials of treatment of haemolytic disease of the newborn. J Obstet Gynaecol Br Emp 60: 605

Astrup J, Kornstad L (1977) Presence of anti-c in the serum of 42 women giving birth to c positive babies: serological and clinical findings. Acta Obstet Gynecol Scand 56: 185

Austin EB, Smith LC, Walker RY (2001) An anti-idiotopic antibody-based enzyme-linked immunosorbent assay for the quantification of the monoclonal anti-D BRAD-5. Vox Sang 80: 179–183

Barrie JV, Quinn MA (1985) Selection of donor red cells for fetal intravenous transfusion in severe haemolytic disease of the newborn (Letter). Lancet i: 1327–1328

Bartsch FK (1972) Fetale Erythrozyten im mütterlichen Blut und Immunprophylaxe der Rh-Immunisierung. Klinische und experimentelle Studie. Acta Obstet Gynecol Scand 20: (Suppl.): 1–128

Battacharya S, Makar Y, Laycock RA et al. (2002) Outcome of consecutive pregnancies in a patient with Bombay (Oh) blood group. Transfus Med 12: 379–382

Bayliss KM, Kueck BD, Johnson ST et al. (1991) Detecting fetomaternal hemorrhage: a comparison of five methods. Transfusion 31: 303–307

Bennett PR, Le Van Kim C, Colin Y et al. (1993) Prenatal determination of fetal RhD type by DNA amplification. N Engl J Med 329: 607–610

Better PJ, Ford DS, Frascarelli A et al. (1993) Confirmation of anti-ELO as a cause of haemolytic disease of the newborn. Vox Sang 65: 70

Bishop GJ, Krieger VI (1969) The timing of rhesus immunization and the prevention of antibody response using anti-Rh immune globulin. Aust NZ J Obstet Gynaecol 9: 228

Blackburn GK (1976) Massive fetomaternal haemorrhage due to choriocarcinoma of the uterus. J Pediatr 89: 680

Boorman KE, Dodd BE, Mollison PL (1945) Iso-immunisation to the blood-group factors A, B and Rh. J Pathol Bact 57: 157

Booth PB, Dunsford I, Grant J et al. (1953) Haemolytic disease in first-born infants. BMJ ii: 41

Borst-Eilers E (1972) Rhesusimmunisatie: onstaan en preventie. MD Thesis, University of Amsterdam, Amsterdam

Bowell PJ, Wainscot JS, Peto TEA et al. (1982) Maternal anti-D concentrations and outcome in rhesus haemolytic disease of the newborn. BMJ 285: 327–329

Bowell PJ, Brown SE, Dike AE et al. (1986) The significance of anti-c alloimmunization in pregnancy. Br J Obstet Gynaecol 93: 144–1048

Bowell PJ, Inskip MJ, Jones MN (1988) The significance of anti-C sensitization in pregnancy. Clin Lab Haematol 10: 251–255

Bowley CC, Dunsford I (1949) The agglutinin anti-M associated with pregnancy. BMJ ii: 681

Bowman JM (1983) Blood group immunization in obstetric practice. Curr Probl Obstet Gynecol 7: 4–61

Bowman JM (1984) Controversies in Rh prophylaxis. In: Hemolytic Disease of the Newborn. G. Garratty (ed.), pp. 67–85. Arlington, VA: Am Assoc Blood Banks

Bowman JM (1990) Treatment options for the fetus with alloimmune hemolytic disease. Transfus Med Rev 4: 191–207

Bowman JM (1994) Intrauterine and neonatal transfusion. In: Scientific Basis of Transfusion Medicine. KC Anderson, PM Ness (eds). Philadelphia, PA: WB Saunders

Bowman JM, Pollock JM (1965) Amniotic fluid spectrophotometry and early delivery in the management of erythroblastosis fetalis. Pediatrics 35: 815

Bowman JM, Pollock JM (1985) Transplacental fetal hemorrhage after amniocentesis. Obstet Gynecol 66: 749–754

Bowman JM, Pollock JM (1987) Failures of intravenous Rh immune globulin prophylaxis; an analysis of the reasons for such failures. Transfus Med Rev 1: 101–112

Bowman JM, Pollock J (1993) Maternal C^w alloimmunization. Vox Sang 64: 226–230

Bowman JM, Chown B, Lewis M et al. (1978) Rh-immunization during pregnancy, antenatal prophylaxis. Can Med Assoc J 118: 623

Bowman JM, Friesen AD, Pollack JM et al. (1980) WinRho: Rh immune globulin prepared by ion exchange for intravenous use. Can Med Assoc J 123: 1121–1125

Bowman JM, Lewis M, De Sa DJ et al. (1984) Hydrops fetalis caused by massive maternofetal transplacental haemorrhage. J Pediatr 104: 769–772

Bowman JM, Harman FA, Manning CR et al. (1989) Erythroblastosis fetalis produced by anti-k. Vox Sang 56: 187–189

Brossard Y, Pons JC, Jrad I et al. (1996) Maternal-fetal hemorrhage: a reappraisal. Vox Sang 71: 103–107

Brouwers HAA, Overbeeke MAM, van Ertbruggen I et al. (1988a) What is the best predictor of the severity of ABO haemolytic disease of the newborn? Lancet ii: 641–644

Brouwers HAA, Overbeeke MAM, Huiskes E et al. (1988b) Complement is not activated in ABO-haemolytic disease of the newborn. Br J Haematol 68: 363–366

Bruce M, Watt AH, Gabra GS et al. (1985) Rh null with anti-Rh29 complicating pregnancy: the first example in the United Kingdom. Commun Br Blood Transfus Soc, Oxford

Brumit MC, Carnahan GE, Stubbs JR et al. (2002) Moderate hemolytic disease of the newborn (HDN) due to anti-Rh17 produced by a black female with an e variant phenotype. Immunohematology 18: 40–42

Budin P (1875) A quel moment doit-on pratiquer la ligature du cordon ombilical? Progr Méd (Paris) 3: 750 (see also (1876) 4: 2 and 36)

Bürki U, Degnan TJ, Rosenfield RE (1964) Stillbirth due to anti-U. Vox Sang 9: 209

Bystryn J-C, Graf MW, Uhr JW (1970) Regulation of antibody formation by serum antibody. II. Removal of specific antibody by means of exchange transfusion. J Exp Med 132: 1279

Caballero C, Vekemans M, Lopez del Campo JG et al. (1977) Serum alpha-fetoprotein in adults, in women during pregnancy, in children at birth, and during the first week of life: a sex difference. Am J Obstet Gynecol 127: 384

Caine ME, Mueller-Heubach E (1986) Kell sensitization in pregnancy. Am J Obstet Gynecol 154: 85–90

Cariani L, Romano EL, Martinez N et al. (1995) ABO-haemolytic disease of the newborn (ABO-HDN): factors influencing its severity and incidence in Venezuela. J Trop Pediatr 41: 14–21

Carpentier M, Meersseman F (1956) Considération sur le traitement, à propos d'un cas d'isoimmunisation gravidique vis-à-vis du facteur A. Bull Soc Roy Belge Gynécol Obstet 26: 374

Chilcott J, Lloyd Jones M, Wight J et al. (2003) A review of the clinical effectiveness and cost-effectiveness of routine anti-D prophylaxis for pregnant women who are rhesus-negative. Health Technol Assess 7(4)

Chilcott J, Tappenden P, Lloyd Jones M et al. (2004) The economics of routine antenatal anti-D prophylaxis for pregnant women who are rhesus negative. Br J Gynaecol 111: 903–7

Chitkara U, Bussel J, Alvarez M et al. (1990) High dose intravenous gamma globulin: does it have a role in the treatment of severe erythroblastosis fetalis. Obstet Gynecol 76: 703–708

Chiu RW, Murphy MF, Fidler C et al. (2001) Determination of RhD zygosity: Comparison of a double amplification refractory mutation system approach and a multiplex real-time quantitative PCR approach. Clin Chem 47: 667–672

Chown B (1955) On a search for rhesus antibodies in very young foetuses. Arch Dis Child 30: 237

Clarke CA, Mollison PL (1989) Deaths from Rh haemolytic disease of the fetus and newborn, 1977–87. J R Coll Phys 23: 181–184

Clarke SC, Whitfield AGW (1979) Deaths from rhesus haemolytic disease in England and Wales in 1977: accuracy of records and assessment of anti-D prophylaxis. BMJ i: 1665–1669

Cohen F, Zuelzer WW (1967) Mechanisms of isoimmunization. II. Transplacental passage and postnatal survival of fetal erythrocytes in heterospecific pregnancies. Blood 30: 796

Cohen F, Zuelzer WW, Gustafson DC et al. (1964) Mechanisms of iso-immunisation. I. The transplacental passage of fetal erythrocytes in homospecific pregnancies. Blood 23: 621

Contreras M, Gordon H, Tidmarsh E (1983) A proven case of maternal alloimmunization due to Duffy antigens in donor blood used for intrauterine transfusion (Letter). Br J Haematol 53: 355–356

Costa FH, Cardim WH, Mellone O (1960) Fototerapia. Novo recurso terapeutico na hiperbilirubinemia do recemnascido. J Pediatr 25: 347–391

Crawford DH, Barlow MJ, Harrison JF et al. (1983) Production of human monoclonal antibody to rhesus D antigen. Lancet 1(8321): 386–388

Crawford H, Cutbush M, Mollison PL (1953) Hemolytic disease of the newborn due to anti-A. Blood 8: 620

Cremer RJ, Perryman P, Richards DH (1958) Influence of light on the hyperbilirubinaemia of infants. Lancet i: 1094

Dacus JV, Spinnato JA (1984) Severe erythroblastosis secondary to anti-Kp^b sensitization. Am J Obstet Gynecol 150: 888–889

Daffos F, Capella-Pavlovsky M, Forrestier F (1985) Fetal blood sampling during pregnancy with use of a needle guided by ultrasound: a study of 606 consecutive cases. Am J Obstet Gynecol 153: 655–660

Daniels G (1995) Human Blood Groups. Oxford: Blackwell Science

Daniels GL (2002) Human Blood Groups, 2nd edn. Oxford: Blackwell Science

Daniels GL, Hadley AG, Green CA (1999) Fetal anaemia due to anti-Kell may result from immune destruction of early erythroid progenitors. Transfus Med 9(Suppl.): 16

Daniels GL, Finning K, Martin P et al. (2004) Fetal blood group genotyping from DNA from maternal plasma: an important advance in the management and prevention of haemolytic disease of the fetus and newborn. Vox Sang 87: 225–232

Davey MG (1976a) Antenatal administration of anti-Rh: Australia 1969–1975. In: Proceedings of Symposium on Rh Antibody Mediated Immunosuppression. Raritan, NJ: Ortho Research Institute

Davey MG (1976b) Epidemiology of failures of Rh immune globulin and ABO protection. In: Proceedings of Symposium on Rh Antibody Mediated Immunosuppression. Raritan, NJ: Ortho Research Institute

Davidson LT, Merritt KT, Weech AA (1941) Hyperbilirubinemia in the newborn. Am J Dis Child 61: 958

Davis BH, Olsen S, Bigelow NC et al. (1998) Detection of fetal red cells in fetomaternal hemorrhage using a fetal hemoglobin monoclonal antibody by flow cytometry. Transfusion 38: 749–756

DeMarsh QB, Windle WF, Alt HL (1942) Blood volume of newborn infants in relation to early and late clamping of the umbilical cord. Am J Dis Child 63: 1123

Denomme GA, Ryan G, Seaward PG et al. (2004) Maternal ABO-mismatched blood for intrauterine transfusion of severe hemolytic disease of the newborn due to anti-Rh17. Transfusion 44: 1357–1360

Desjardins L, Blajchman MA, Chintu C et al. (1979) The spectrum of ABO hemolytic disease of the new born infant. J Pediatr 95: 447–449

De Young-Owens A, Kennedy M, Rose RL et al. (1997) Anti-M isoimmunization: management and outcome at the Ohio State University from 1969–1995. Obstet Gynecol 90: 962–996

Diamond LK (1947) Erythroblastosis foetalis or haemolytic disease of the newborn. Proc R Soc Med 40: 546

van Dijk BA, de Man AJM, Kunst VAJM (1994) Quantitation of fetomaternal hemorrhage by a fluorescent microsphere method (Abstract). Vox Sang 67 (Suppl. 2): 34

Divakaran TG, Waugh J, Clark TJ et al. (2001) Noninvasive techniques to detect fetal anemia due to red cell alloimmunization: a systematic review. Obstet Gynecol 98: 509–517

Dooren MC, Engelfriet CP (1993) Protection against Rh D-haemolytic disease of the newborn by a diminished transport of maternal IgG to the fetus. Vox Sang 65: 59–61

Dooren MC, Kuijpers RWAM, Joekes EC et al. (1992) Protection against immune haemolytic disease of newborn infants by maternal monocyte-reactive IgG alloantibodies (anti-HLA-DR). Lancet i: 1067–1070

Dooren MC, van Kamp IL, Kanhai HHH et al. (1993) Evidence for the protective effect of maternal Fc-R blocking IgG alloantibodies HLA-DR in Rh-D haemolytic disease of the newborn. Vox Sang 65: 55–58

Dooren MC, Kamp IL, Scherpenisse JW et al. (1994) No beneficial effect of low-dose fetal intravenous gammaglobulin administration in combination with intravascular transfusions in severe RhD haemolytic disease. Vox Sang 66: 253–257

Dukler D, Oepkes D, Seaward G et al. (2003) Noninvasive tests to predict fetal anemia: a study comparing Doppler and ultrasound parameters. Am J Obstet Gynecol 188: 1310–1314

DuPan RM, Wenger P, Koechli S et al. (1959) Étude du passage de la γ-globuline marquée à travers le placenta humain. Clin Chim Acta 4: 110

Dziegiel MH, Koldkjaer O, Berkowicz A (2005) Massive antenatal fetomaternal hemorrhage: evidence for long-term survival of fetal red blood cells. Transfusion 45: 539–544

Edelman L, Margaritte C, Chaabihi H *et al.* (1997) Obtaining a functional recombinant anti-rhesus (D) antibody using the baculovirus-insect cell expression system. Immunology 91: 13–19

Einhorn MS, Granoff DM, Nahm MH *et al.* (1987) Concentration of antibodies in paired maternal and infant sera: relationship to IgG subclass. J Pediatr 111: 783–788

Eklund J (1978) Prevention of Rh immunization in Finland. A national study, 1969–1977. Acta Paediatr Scand 274 (Suppl.): 1–57

Eklund J, Nevanlinna HR (1971) Immuno-suppression therapy in Rh-incompatible transfusion. BMJ iii: 623

Eklund J, Nevanlinna HR (1973) Rh prevention: a report and analysis of a national programme. J Med Genet 10: 1

Eklund J, Hermann M, Kjellman H *et al.* (1982) Turnover rate of anti-D IgG injected during pregnancy. BMJ 284: 854–855

Ellis MI, Hey EN, Walker W (1979) Neonatal death in babies with Rhesus isoimmunization. Q J Med (NS) 48: 211–225

Engelfriet CF, Ouwehand WH (1990) ADCC and other cellular bioassays for predicting the clinical significance of red cell alloantibodies. In: Blood Transfusion: the Impact of New Technologies. M Contreras (ed.). Baillière's Clinical Haematology 3: 321–337

Falterman CG, Richardson J (1980) Transfusion reaction due to unrecognized ABO hemolytic disease of the newborn infant. J Pediatr 97: 812–814

Finn R, Harper DT, Stallings SA *et al.* (1963) Transplacental hemorrhage. Transfusion 3: 114

Finning KM, Martin PG, Soothill PW *et al.* (2002) Prediction of fetal D status from maternal plasma: introduction of a new noninvasive fetal *RHD* genotyping service. Transfusion 42: 1079–1085

Finning K, Martin P, Daniels G (2004) A clinical service in the UK to predict fetal Rh (Rhesus) D blood group using free fetal DNA in maternal plasma. Ann NY Acad Sci 1022: 119–23

Firan M, Bawdon R, Radu C *et al.* (2001) The MHC class I-related receptor, FcRn, plays an essential role in the maternofetal transfer of gammaglobulin in humans. Int Immunol 13: 993–1002

Fischer K (1961) Morbus Haemolyticus Neonatorum im ABO-System. Stuttgart: Georg Thieme Verlag

Fleetwood P, De Silva PM, Knight RC (1996) Clinical significance of red cell antibody concentration in pregnancy (Abstract). Br J Haematol 93 (Suppl 1.): 13

Forestier F, Daffos F, Galacteaos F *et al.* (1986) Hematological values of 163 normal fetuses between 18 and 30 weeks gestation. Pediatr Res 20: 342–346

Fraser ID, Tovey GH (1976) Observations on Rh isoimmunisation: past, present and future. Clin Haematol 5: 149

Freiesleben E, Jensen KG (1961) Haemolytic disease of the newborn caused by anti-M. The value of the direct conglutination test. Vox Sang 6: 328

Frigoletto FD, Greene MF, Benaceraff BR *et al.* (1986) Ultrasonographic fetal surveillance in the management of the isoimmunized pregnancy. N Engl J Med 315: 430–432

Garner SF, Gorick BD, Lai WYY *et al.* (1995) Prediction of the severity of haemolytic disease of the newborn. Vox Sang 68: 169–176

Gemke RJ, Kanhai HH, Overbecke MA *et al.* (1986) ABO and Rhesus phenotyping of fetal erythrocytes in the first trimester of pregnancy. Br J Haematol 64: 689–697

Gerlini G, Ottaviano S, Sbraccia C *et al.* (1968) Reattività dell'antigene A_1 e suoi rapporti con la malattia emolitica del neonato da incompatibilità ABO. Haematologica 53(Suppl.): 1019

Giblett ER (1964) Blood group antibodies causing hemolytic disease of the newborn. Clin Obset Gynecol 7: 1044

Gilja BK, Shah VP (1988) Hydrops fetalis due to ABO incompatibility. Clin Pediatr (Phila) 27: 210–212

Gitlin D, Kumate J, Urrusti J *et al.* (1964) The selectivity of the human placenta in the transfer of plasma proteins from mother to fetus. J Clin Invest 43: 1938

Goodrick MJ, Hadley AG, Poole G (1997) Haemolytic disease of the fetus and newborn due to anti-Fy(a) and the potential clinical value of Duffy genotyping in pregnancies at risk. Transfus Med 7: 301–304

Gordon MC, Kennedy MS, O'Shaughnessy RW *et al.* (1995) Severe hemolytic disease of the newborn due to anti-Js[b]. Vox Sang 69: 140–141

Gorlin JB, Kelly L (1994) Alloimmunization via previous transfusion places female Kp[b]-negative recipients at risk for having children with clinically significant hemolytic disease of the newborn. Vox Sang 66: 46–48

Gottstein R, Cooke RW (2003) Systematic review of intravenous immunoglobulin in haemolytic disease of the newborn. Arch Dis Child Fetal Neonatal Ed 88: F6–F10

Grannum PAT, Copel JA (1988) Prevention of Rh isoimmunization and treatment of the compromised fetus. Semin Perinatol 12: 324–335

Grant CJ, Hamblin TJ, Smith DS *et al.* (1983) Plasmapheresis in Rh hemolytic disease: the danger of amniocentesis. Int J Artif Organs 6: 83–86

Greenwalt TJ, Sasaki T, Gajewski M (1959) Further examples of haemolytic disease of the newborn due to anti-Duffy (anti-Fy[a]). Vox Sang 4: 138

Greiss MA, Armstrong-Fisher SS, Perera WS *et al.* (2002) Semiautomated data analysis of flow cytometric estimation of fetomaternal hemorhagge in D-women. Transfusion 42: 1067–1078

Grozdea J, Alie-Daram S, Vergnes H *et al.* (1995) About diminished transport of maternal IgG (RhD alloimmunization) to the fetus. Vox Sang 68: 134–135

Grumbach A, Gasser C (1948) ABO-inkompatibilitäten und Morbus haemolyticus neonatorum. Helv Paediatr Acta 3: 447

Hackney DN, Knudtson EJ, Rossi KQ et al. (2004) Management of pregnancies complicated by anti-c isoimmunisation. Obstet Gynecol 103: 24–30

Hadley AG, Garner SF, Taverner JM (1993) AutoAnalyzer quantification, monocyte-mediated cytotoxicity and chemiluminescence assays for predicting the severity of haemolytic disease of the newborn. Transfus Med 3: 195–200

Halbrecht I (1951) Icterus precox: further studies on its frequency, etiology, prognosis and the blood chemistry of the cord blood. J Pediatr 39: 185

Hall AM, Cairns LS, Altmann DM et al. (2005) Immune responses and tolerance to the RhD blood group protein in HL-A transgenic mice. Blood 105: 2175–2179

Hammerström L, Smith CIE (1986) Placental transfer of intravenous immunoglobulin (Letter). Lancet i: 681

Hardy J, Napier JAF (1981) Red cell antibodies detected in antenatal tests on Rhesus positive women in south and mid Wales 1948–1978. Br J Obstet Gynaecol 88: 91–100

Hartmann O, Brendemoen OJ (1953) Incidence of Rh antibody formation in first pregnancies. Acta Paediatr (Uppsala) 42: 20

Hay FC, Hull MGR, Torrigiani G (1971) The transfer of human IgG subclasses from mother to foetus. Clin Exp Immunol 9: 355–358

Hayashida Y, Watanabe A (1968) A case of a blood group p Taiwanese woman delivered of an infant with hemolytic disease of the newborn. Jap J Legal Med 22: 10

Helderweirt G (1963) Le passage de globules foetaux et maternels à travers le placenta. Ann Soc Belge Méd Trop 43: 575

Herron B, Reynolds W, Northcott M et al. (1996) Data from two patients providing evidence that the placenta may act as a barrier to the maternal fetal transfer of anti-Lutheran antibodies (Abstract). Transfus Med 6(Suppl. 2): 24

Hindemann P (1966) Experimentelle und klinische Untersuchungen über eine transabdominale Späteinschwemmung fetaler Erythrozyten in den mütterlichen Kreislauf. Gerburtsh Frauenheilk 26: 1359

Hočevar M, Glonar L (1974) Rhesus factor immunization. In: The Ljubljana Abortion Study 1971–1973. L Ardolsek (ed.). Maryland: National Institute of Health Center for Population Research

Holtrop PC, Ruedisueli K, Regan R et al. (1991) Double vs. single phototherapy in low-birth-weight infants. Pediatr Res 29: 218A

Holzgreve W, Holzgreve B, Curry CJ et al. (1985) Nonimmune hydrops fetalis: diagnosis and management. Semin Perinatol 9: 52–67

Hopkins DF (1970) Maternal anti-Rh(D) and the D-negative fetus. Am J Obstet Gynecol 108: 268

Hoppe HH, Mester T, Hennig et al. (1973) Prevention of Rh immunisation. Modified production of IgG anti-Rh for intravenous application by ion exchange chromatography (IEC). Vox Sang 25: 308

Howarth DJ, Robinson FM, Williams M et al. (2002) A modified Kleihauer technique for the quantitation of fetomaternal haemorrhage. Transfus Med 12: 373–378

Hsu TCS, Rosenfield RE, Rubinstein P (1974) Instrumented PVP-augmented antiglobulin tests. III. IgG-coated cells in ABO incompatible babies: depressed hemoglobin levels in type A babies of type O mothers. Vox Sang 26: 326

Huchet J, Crégut R, Pinon F et al. (1975) Les hémorragies foeto-maternelles et leur importance dans la pathologie perinatale. Rev Fr Transfus Immunohématol 18: 361

Huchet J, Defossez Y, Brossard Y (1988) Detection of transplacental haemorrhage during the last trimester of pregnancy (Letter). Transfusion 28: 506

Hughes-Jones NC, Hughes MIJ, Walker W (1967) The amount of anti-D on red cells in haemolytic disease of the newborn. Vox Sang 12: 279

Hughes-Jones NC, Ellis M, Ivona J et al. (1971) Anti-D concentration in mother and child in haemolytic disease of the newborn. Vox Sang 21: 135

Huntley CC, Lyerley AD, Littlejohn MP et al. (1976) ABO hemolytic disease in Puerto Rico and North Carolina. Pediatrics 57: 875

Hussey R, Clarke CA (1992) Deaths from haemolytic disease of the newborn in 1990 (Letter). BMJ 304: 444

Hutchinson AA, Drew JH, Yu VYH et al. (1982) Nonimmunologic hydrops fetalis: a review of 61 cases. Obstet Gynecol 59: 347–352

Issitt PD (1981) The MN Blood Group System. Cincinnati, OH: Montgomery Scientific Publications

Johnson PRE, Tait RC, Austin EB et al. (1995) Flow cytometry in diagnosis and management of large fetomaternal haemorrhage. J Clin Pathol 48: 1005–1008

Jørgensen J (1975) Foeto-maternal blødning. MD Thesis, University of Copenhagen, Copenhagen

Joy SD, Rossi KQ, Krigh D et al. (2005) Management of pregnancies complicated by anti-E alloimmunisation. Obstet Gynecol 105: 24–28

Katz J (1969) Transplacental passage of fetal red cells in abortion; increased incidence after curettage and effect of oxytoxic drugs. BMJ 4: 84

Kennedy GA, Shaw R, Just S et al. (2003) Quantification of feto-maternal haemorrhage (FMH) by flow cytometry: anti-fetal haemoglobin labelling potentially underestimates massive FMH in comparison to labelling with anti-D. Transfus Med 13: 25–33

King JC, Sacher RA (1989) Percutaneous umbilical blood sampling. In: Contemporary Issues in Pediatric Transfusion Medicine. RA Sacher, RG Strauss (eds), pp. 33–53. Arlington, VA: Am Assoc Blood Banks

Kirkman NN (1977) Further evidence for a racial difference in frequency of ABO hemolytic disease. J Pediatr 90: 717

Kleihauer E, Betke K (1960) Praktische Anwendung des

Nachweises von Hb F-haltigen Zellen in fixierten Blutaus-strichen. Internist 1: 292

Kochwa S, Rosenfield RE, Tallal L et al. (1961) Isoagglutinins associated with erythroblastosis. J Clin Invest 40: 874

Kohler PF, Farr RS (1966) Elevation of cord over maternal IgG immunoglobulin: evidence for an active placental IgG transport. Nature (Lond) 210: 1070

Konugres AA, Fontain DK, Thiet M-P et al. (1994) Intrauterine transfusion to prevent fetal demise in a case of fetal-maternal hemorrhage. Vox Sang 67(Suppl. 2): 145

Kornstad L (1983) New cases of irregular blood group antibodies other than anti-D in pregnancy: frequency and clinical significance. Acta Obstet Gynecol Scand 62: 431–436

Krevans JR, Woodrow JC, Nosenzo C et al. (1964) Patterns of Rh-immunization. Commun 10th Congr Int Soc Haematol, Stockholm

Kumpel BM, Goodrick J, Pamphilon DH et al. (1995) Human Rh D monoclonal antibodies (BRAD-3 and BRAD-5) cause accelerated clearance of Rh D+ red blood cells and suppression of Rh D immunization in Rh D– volunteers. Blood 86: 1701–1709

Kumpel BM, van de Winkel JGJ, Westerdaal NAC et al. (1996) Antigen topography is critical for interaction of IgG2 anti-red-cell antibodies with Fcγ receptors. Br J Haematol 94: 175–183

Lacey PA, Caskey CR, Werner OJ et al. (1983) Fatal hemolytic disease of a newborn due to anti-D in an Rh-positive Du variant mother. Transfusion 23: 91–94

Ladipo OA (1972) Management of third stage of labour, with particular reference to reduction of fetomaternal transfusion. BMJ i: 721

Lakatos L, Csathy L, Nemes E (1999) 'Bloodless' treatment of a Jehovah's Witness infant with ABO hemolytic disease. J Perinatol 19: 530–2

Lam GK, Subramanyam L, Orton S et al. (2003) Minimizing red blood cell contamination while isolating mononuclear cells from whole blood: the next step for the treatment of severe hemolytic disease of the fetus/newborn. Am J Obstet Gynecol 189: 1012–6

Lambin P, Debbia M, Puillandre P et al. (2002) IgG1 and IgG3 anti-D in maternal serum and on the RBCs of infants suffering from HDN: relationship with severity of the disease. Transfusion 42: 1537–1546

Lawler SD, Vanloghem JJ (1947) The rhesus antigen Cw causing haemolytic disease of the newborn. Lancet ii: 545

Lee SI, Heiner DC, Wara D (1986) Development of serum IgG subclass levels in children. Monogr Allergy 19: 108–121

Lee S, Bennett PR, Overton T et al. (1996) Prenatal diagnosis of Kell blood group (genotypes: KEL1 and KEL2). Am J Obstet Gynecol 175: 455–459

Legler TJ, Maas JH, Kohler M et al. (2001) RHD sequencing: A new tool for decision making on transfusion therapy and provision of Rh prophylaxis. Transfus Med 11: 383–388

Lenkiewicz B, Zupanska B (2000) Moderate hemolytic disease of the newborn due to anti-Hr0 in a mother with the D–/D-phenotype. Immunohematology 16: 109–111

Levene C, Sela R, Rudolphson Y et al. (1977) Hemolytic disease of the newborn due to anti-PP1Pk(anti-Tja). Transfusion 17: 569

Levine P (1943) Serological factors as possible causes in spontaneous abortions. J Hered 34: 71

Levine P (1958) The influence of the ABO system on hemolytic disease. Hum Biol 30: 14

Levine P, Stetson R (1939) An unusual case of intragroup agglutination. JAMA 113: 126

Levine P, Burnham L, Katzin EM et al. (1941) The role of iso-immunization in the pathogenesis of erythroblastosis fetalis. Am J Obstet Gynecol 42: 925

Levine P, Ferraro LR, Koch E (1952) Hemolytic disease of the newborn due to anti-S. Blood 7: 1030

Levine P, Vogel P, Rosenfield RE (1953) Hemolytic disease of the newborn. Adv Pediatr 6: 97

Lewi S, Clarke TK (1960) A hitherto undescribed phenomenon in ABO haemolytic disease of the newborn. Lancet, ii: 456

Li TC, Bromham DR, Balmer BM (1988) Fetomaternal macrotransfusion in the Yorkshire region. 1. Prevalence and obstetric factors. Br J Obstet Gynaecol 95: 1144–1151

Liedholm P (1971) Feto maternal haemorrhage in ectopic pregnancy. Acta Obstet Gynecol Scand 50: 367

Liley AW (1961) Liquor amnii analysis in management of pregnancy complicated by rhesus sensitization. Am J Obstet Gynecol 82: 1359

Liley AW (1963) Intrauterine transfusion of foetus in haemolytic disease. BMJ ii: 1107

Lloyd-Evans P, Kumpel BM, Bromelow I et al. (1996) Use of a directly conjugated monoclonal anti-D (BRAD-3) for quantification of foetomaternal haemorrhage by flow cytometry. Transfusion 36: 432–437

Lloyd-Evans P, Guest AG, Austin EB et al. (2000) Use of a phycoerythrin-conjugated anti-glycophorin A monoclonal antibody as a double label to improve the accuracy of FMH quantification by flow cytometry. Transfus Med 9: 155–160

Lo YM, Hjelm NM, Fidler C et al. (1998) Prenatal diagnosis of fetal RhD status by molecular analysis of maternal plasma. N Engl J Med 339: 1734–1738

Longster GH, Robinson EAE (1981) Four further examples of anti-Inb detected during pregnancy. Clin Lab Haematol 3: 351–356

Lubenko A, Contreras M (1989) A review: low-frequency red cell antigens. Immunohematology 5: 7–14

Lubenko A, Contreras M, Habash J (1989) Should anti-Rh

immunoglobulin be given to D variant women? Br J Haematol 72: 429–433

Lubenko A, Contreras M, Portugal CL (1992) Severe haemolytic disease in an infant born to an Rh$_{null}$ proposita. Vox Sang 63: 43–47

Maaskant-van Wijk PA, Faas BH, de Ruijter JA et al. (1998) Genotyping of RHD by multiplex polymerase chain reaction analysis of six RHD-specific exons. Transfusion 38: 1015–1021

MacAfee CAJ, Fortune DW, Beischer NA (1970) Non-immunological hydrops fetalis. J Obstet Gynaecol Br Cwlth 77: 226

MacKenzie IZ, Bichler J, Mason GC et al. (2004) Efficacy and safety of a new, chromatographically purified rhesus (D) immunoglobulin. Eur J Obstet Gynecol Reprod Biol 117: 154–161

McNabb T, Koh T-Y, Dorrington KJ et al. (1976) Structure and function of immunoglobulin domains. V. Binding of immunoglobulin G and fragments to placental membrane preparations. J Immunol 117: 882

Margulies M, Voto LS (1991) High dose intravenous gamma globulin: does it have a role in the treatment of severe erythroblastosis fetalis. Obstet Gynecol 77: 804–806

Mari G, Deter RL, Carpenter RL et al. (2000) Noninvasive diagnosis by Doppler ultrasonography of fetal anemia due to maternal red cell alloimmunisation. N Engl J Med 342: 9–14

Marsh GW, Stirling Y, Mollison PL (1970) Accidental injection of anti-D immunoglobulin to an infant. Vox Sang 19: 468

Marsh WL, Redman CM (1990) The Kell blood group system: a review. Transfusion 30: 158–167

Martin WL, West AP Jr, Gan L et al. (2001) Crystal structure at 2.8A of an FcRn/heterodimeric Fc complex: mechanism of pH-dependent binding. Mol Cell 7: 867–877

Matson GA, Swanson J, Tobin JD (1959) Severe haemolytic disease of the newborn due to anti-Jk^a. Vox Sang 4: 144

Matsumoto H, Tamaki Y, Sato S et al. (1981) A case of hemolytic disease of the newborn caused by anti-M: serological study of maternal blood. Acta Obstet Gynaecol Japan 33: 525–528

Matthews CD, Matthews AEB (1969) Transplacental haemorrhage: spontaneous and induced abortion. Lancet i: 694

Mayne KM, Bowell PJ, Pratt GA (1990) The significance of anti-Kell sensitization in pregnancy. Clin Lab Haematol 12: 379–385

Menticoglou SM, Harman CR, Manning FA et al. (1987) Intraperitoneal fetal transfusion: paralysis inhibits red cell absorption. Fetal Therapy 2: 154

Miescher S, Zahn-Zabal M, De Jesus M et al. (2000) CHO expression of a novel human recombinant IgG1 anti-RhD antibody isolated by phage display. Br J Haematol 111: 157–166

Miescher S, Spycher MO, Amstutz H et al. (2004) A single recombinant anti-RhD IgG prevents RhD immunization: association of RhD-positive red blood cell clearance rate with polymorphisms in the FcγRIIA and FcγIIIA genes. Blood 103: 4028–4035

Miles RM, Maurer HM, Valdes OS (1971) Iron-deficiency anaemia at birth. Two examples secondary to chronic fetal-maternal hemorrhage. Clin Pediatr 10: 223

Millar DS, Davis LR, Rodeck CH et al. (1985) Normal blood cell values in the early mid-trimester fetus. Prenatal Diagn 5: 367–373

Miqdad AM, Abdelbasit OB, Shaheed MM et al. (2004) Intravenous immunoglobulin G (IVIG) therapy for significant hyperbilirubinemia in ABO hemolytic disease of the newborn. J Matern Fetal Neonatal Med 16: 163–166

Miyoshi K, Kaneto Y, Lawai H et al. (1988) X-linked dominant control of F-cells in normal adult life: characterization of the Swiss type as hereditary persistence of fetal hemoglobin regulated dominantly by gene(s) on X chromosome. Blood 72: 1854–1860

Mollison PL (1943) The survival of transfused red cells in haemolytic disease of the newborn. Arch Dis Child 18: 161

Mollison PL (1951) Blood Transfusion in Clinical Medicine. Oxford: Blackwell Scientific Publications

Mollison PL (1972) Quantitation of transplacental haemorrhage. BMJ iii: 31 and 115

Mollison PL (1983) Blood Transfusion in Clinical Medicine, 7th edn. Oxford: Blackwell Scientific Publications

Mollison PL, Cutbush M (1949a) Haemolytic disease of the newborn: criteria of severity. BMJ i: 123

Mollison PL, Cutbush M (1949b) Haemolytic disease of the newborn due to anti-A antibodies. Lancet ii: 173

Mollison PL, Cutbush M (1951) A method of measuring the severity of a series of cases of hemolytic disease of the newborn. Blood 6: 777

Mollison PL, Cutbush M (1954) Haemolytic disease of the newborn. In: Recent Advances in Paediatrics. D Gairdner (ed.). London: J & A Churchill

Mollison PL, Walker W (1952) Controlled trials of the treatment of haemolytic disease of the newborn. Lancet i: 429

Mollison PL, Engelfriet CP, Contreras M (1987) Blood Transfusion in Clinical Medicine, 8th edn. Oxford: Blackwell Scientific Publications

Moncharmont P, Juron-Dupraz F, Rigal M et al. (1990) Haemolytic disease of two newborns in a rhesus anti-e alloimmunised woman. Review of literature. Haematologia 23: 97–100

Moores PP, Smart E, Gabriel B (1994) Hemolytic disease of the newborn in infants of an O$_h$ mother (Letter). Transfusion 34: 1015–1016

Morell A, Skvaril F, van Loghem E *et al.* (1971) Human IgG subclasses in maternal and fetal serum. Vox Sang 21: 481

Morgan CL, Cannell GR, Addison RS *et al.* (1991) The effect of intravenous immunoglobulin on placental transfer of a platelet-specific antibody: anti-Pl^{A1}. Transfus Med 1: 209–216

MRC (1978) An assessment of the hazards of amniocentesis (Report of a Working Party). Br J Obstet Gynaecol 85 (Suppl. 2): 1

Munk-Andersen G (1958) Excess of group O-mothers in ABO-haemolytic disease. Acta Pathol Microbiol Scand 42: 43

Murray S (1957) The effect of Rh genotypes on severity in haemolytic disease of the newborn. Br J Haematol 3: 143

Murray S, Knox EG, Walker W (1965) Rhesus haemolytic disease of the newborn and the ABO groups. Vox Sang 10: 6

Nance SJ, Nelson JM, Arndt *et al.* (1989a) Quantitation of fetal-maternal hemorrhage by flow cytometry. A simple and accurate method. Am J Clin Pathol 91: 288–292

Nance SJ, Nelson JM, Horenstein J *et al.* (1989b) Monocyte monolayer assay: an efficient noninvasive technique for predicting the severity of haemolytic disease of the newborn. Am J Clin Pathol 92: 89–92

Ness PM, Salamon JL (1986) The failure of postinjection Rh immune globulin titers to detect large fetalmaternal hemorrhages. Am J Clin Pathol 85: 604–606

Nevanlinna HR (1953) Factors affecting maternal Rh immunization. Ann Med Exp Fenn 31(Suppl. 2): 1–80

Nevanlinna HR (1965) ABO protection in Rh immunization. Commun 10th Congr Eur Soc Haematol, Strasbourg

Nicolaides KH, Rodeck C (1992) Maternal serum anti-D antibody concentration and assessment of rhesus isoimmunization. BMJ 304: 1155–1156

Nicolaides KH, Rodeck CH, Millar DS *et al.* (1985a) Fetal haematology in rhesus isoimmunization. BMJ 290: 661–663

Nicolaides KH, Warenski JC, Rodeck CH (1985b) The relationship of fetal plasma protein concentration and hemoglobin level to the development of hydrops in rhesus isoimmunization. Am J Obstet Gynaecol 152: 341–344

Nicolaides KH, Rodeck CH, Mibashan RS *et al.* (1986) Have Liley charts outlived their usefulness? Am J Obstet Gynecol 155: 90–94

Nicolaides KH, Fontanarosa M, Gabbe SG *et al.* (1988a) Failure of ultrasonographic parameters to predict the severity of fetal anaemia in rhesus isoimmunisation. Am J Obstet Gynecol 158: 920–6

Nicolaides KH, Soothill PW, Clewell WH *et al.* (1988b) Fetal haemoglobin measurement in the assessment of red cell immunisation. Lancet i: 1073–1075

Nicolini U, Rodeck CH (1988) A proposed scheme for planning intrauterine transfusion in patient with severe Rh-immunisation. J Obstet Gynecol 9: 162–163

Osborn LM, Lenarsky C, Oakes RC *et al.* (1984) Phototherapy in full-term infants with hemolytic disease secondary to ABO incompatibility. Pediatrics 74: 371–374

Owen RD, Woon HR, Foord AG *et al.* (1954) Evidence for actively acquired tolerance to Rh antigens. Proc Natl Acad Sci USA 40: 420

Parinaud J, Blanc M, Grandjean H *et al.* (1985) IgG subclasses and Gm allotypes of anti-D antibodies during pregnancy: correlation with the gravity of the fetal disease. Am J Obstet Gynecol 151: 1111–1115

Pearson HA, Diamond LK (1959) Fetomaternal transfusion. Am J Dis Child 97: 267

Peevy KJ, Wiseman HJ (1978) ABO hemolytic disease of the newborn: evaluation of management and identification of racial and antigenic factors. Pediatrics 61: 475

Pembrey ME, Weatherall DJ, Clegg JB (1973) Maternal synthesis of haemoglobin F in pregnancy. Lancet i: 1350

Pepperell RJ, Barrie JU, Fliegner JR (1977) Significance of red-cell irregular antibodies in the obstetric patient. Med J Aust ii: 453

Pereira L, Jenkins TM, Berghella V (2003) Conventional management of maternal red cell alloimmunization compared with management by Doppler assessment of middle cerebral artery peak systolic velocity. Am J Obstet Gynecol 189: 1002–1006

Petz LD, Garratty G (2004) Immune Hemolytic Anemias, 2nd edn. New York: Churchill Livingstone

Phibbs RH, Johnson P, Tooley WH (1974) Cardiorespiratory status of erythroblastic newborn infants. II. Blood volume, hematocrit, and serum albumin concentration in relation to hydrops fetalis. Pediatrics 53: 13

Polley MJ, Mollison PL, Rose J *et al.* (1965) A simple serological test for antibodies causing ABO-haemolytic disease of the newborn. Lancet i: 291

Pollock A (1968) Transplacental haemorrhage after external cephalic version. Lancet i: 612

Pollock JM, Bowman JM (1990) Anti-Rh(D) subclasses and severity of Rh hemolytic disease of the newborn. Vox Sang 59: 176–179

Popat N, Wood WG, Weatherall DJ (1977) Pattern of maternal F-cell production during pregnancy. Lancet ii: 377

Poulain M, Huchet J (1971) Appréciation de l'hémorragie foeto-maternelle après l'accouchement en vue de la prévention de l'immunisation anti-D (Bilan de 5.488 tests de Kleihauer). Rev Fr Transfus 14: 219

Pratt GA, Bowell PJ, MacKenzie IZ *et al.* (1989) Production of additional atypical antibodies in Rh(D)-sensitised pregnancies managed by intrauterine investigation method. Clin Lab Haematol 11: 241–248

Proulx C, Boyer L, St-Amour I *et al.* (2002) Higher affinity human D MoAB prepared by light-chain shuffling and selected phage display. Transfusion 42: 59–65

Ranasinghe E, Goodyear E, Burgess G (2003) Anti-Ce complicating two consecutive pregnancies with increasing severity of haemolytic disease of the newborn. Transfus Med 13: 53–55.

Rawson AJ, Abelson NM (1960) Studies of blood group antibodies. IV. Physico-chemical differences between iso-anti-A,B and iso-anti-A or iso-anti-B. J Immunol 85: 640

Reid ME, Chandrasekaran V, Sausais L et al. (1996) Disappearance of antibodies to Cromer blood group system antigens during mid pregnancy. Vox Sang 71: 48–50

Renaer M, van de Putte I, Vermylen C (1976) Massive feto-maternal hemorrhage as a cause of perinatal mortality and morbidity. Eur J Obstet Gynecol Reprod Biol 6: 125

Renaer M, van der Putte I, Vermylen C (1976) Massive feto-maternal hemorrhage as a cause of perinatal mortality and morbidity. Eur J Obstet Gynecol Reprod Biol 6: 125

Renkonen KO, Seppälä M (1962) The sex of the sensitizing Rh-positive child. Ann Med Exp Fenn 40: 108

Renkonen KO, Timonen S (1967) Factors influencing the immunization of Rh-negative mothers. J Med Genet 4: 166

Report from 9 Collaborating Laboratories (1991) Results of tests with different cellular bioassays in relation to severity of Rh D haemolytic disease. Vox Sang 60: 225–229

Revill JA, Emblin KF, Hutchinson RM (1979) Failure of anti-D immunoglobulin to remove fetal red cells from maternal circulation. Vox Sang 36: 93–96

Robinson AE (1981) Unsuccessful use of absorbed autologous plasma in Rh-incompatible pregnancy (Letter). N Engl J Med 305: 1346

Robinson AE (1984) Principles and practice of plasma exchange in the management of Rh hemolytic disease of the newborn. Plasma Therapy 5: 7–14

Rodeck CH, Letsky E (1989) How the management of erythroblastosis fetalis has changed (Commentary). Br J Obstet Gynaecol 96: 759–763

Rodeck CH, Nicolaides KH, Warshof SL et al. (1984) The management of severe rhesus isoimmunization by feto-scopic intravascular transfusions. Am J Obstet Gynecol 150: 769–774

Romano EL, Mollison PL (1975) Red cell destruction in vivo by low concentrations of IgG anti-A. Br J Haematol 29: 121

Romano EL, Hughes-Jones NC, Mollison PL (1973) Direct antiglobulin reaction in ABO-haemolytic disease of the newborn. BMJ i: 524

Romano EL, Linares J, Suarez G (1982) Plasma fibrinogen concentration in ABO-hemolytic disease of the newborn. Int Arch Allergy Appl Immunol 67: 74–77

Romano EL, Zabner-Oziel P, Soyano A et al. (1983) Studies on the binding of IgG and F(ab) anti-A to adult and newborn group A red cells. Vox Sang 45: 378–383

Romano EL, Rossi DML, Hagel I et al. (1988) Infestacion por Ascaris: una posible explicacion para los altos niveles de IgG anti-A observados en la poblacion Venezolana. Acta Cient Venezol 39: 75–78

Romano EL, Soyano A, Montano RF et al. (1994) Treatment of ABO hemolytic disease with synthetic blood group trisaccharides. Vox Sang 66: 194–199

Romans DG, Tilley CA, Dorrington KJ (1980) Monogamous bivalency of IgG antibodies. I. Deficiency of branched ABHI-active oligosaccharide chains on red cells of infants causes the weak antiglobulin reactions in hemolytic disease of the newborn due to ABO incompatibility. J Immunol 124: 2807–2811

Roopenian DC, Christianson GJ, Sproule TJ et al. (2003) The MHC Class I-like IgG receptor controls perinatal IgG transport, IgG homeostasis and fate of IgG-Fc-coupled drugs. J Immunol 170: 3528–3533

Rosenfield RE (1955) A-B hemolytic disease of the newborn. Analysis of 1480 cord blood specimens, with special reference to the direct anti-globulin test and to the group O mother. Blood 10: 17

Rosenfield RE, Ohno G (1955) A-B hemolytic disease of the newborn. Rev Hématol 10: 231

Rubo J, Wahn V (1990) A trial with high-dose gamma globulin therapy in 3 children with hyperbilirubinemia in rhesus incompatibility. Monatsschr Kinderheilkd 138: 216

Rubo J, Wahn V (1991) High-dose intravenous gammaglobulin in rhesus-haemolytic disease (Letter). Lancet 337: 914

Sampietro M, Thein SL, Contreras M et al. (1992) Variation of HbF and F-cell number with the G-gamma Xmn l (C-T) polymorphism in normal individuals (Letter). Blood 79: 832–833

Schellong G (1964) Über den Einfluss mütterlicher Antikörper des ABO-systems auf Reticulocyten-zahl und Serumbilirubin bei Frühgeborenen. Commun 10th Congr Int Soc Blood Transfus, Stockholm

Schneider J (1969) Prophylaxe der Rh-Sensibilisierung durch Anti-D-Applikation, in Ergebnisse der Bluttransfusions-forschung. Bibl Haematol (Basel) 32: 113

Schneider J (1976) German Trials. In: Proceedings of Symposium on Rh Antibody Mediated Immunosuppression. Raritan, NJ: Ortho Research Institute

Schur PH, Alpert E, Alper C (1973) Gamma G subgroups in human fetal, cord, and maternal sera. Clin Immunol Immunopathol 2: 62

Scott JR (1976) Immunologic risks to fetuses from maternal to fetal transfer of erythrocytes. In: Proceedings of Symposium on Rh antibody Mediated Immunosuppression. Raritan, NJ: Ortho Research Institute

Sebring ES (1984) Fetomaternal hemorrhage – incidence and methods of detection and quantitation. In: Hemolytic Disease of the Newborn. G Garratty (ed.), pp. 87–117. Arlington, VA: Am Assoc Blood Banks

Sebring ES, Polesky HF (1990) Fetomaternal hemorrhage:

incidence, risk factors, time of occurrence, and clinical effects. Transfusion 30: 344–357

Sender A, Maigret P, Poulain M *et al.* (1971) La règle de compatibilité transfusionnelle A.B.C. à la période néonatale. Bull Feb Soc Gynecol Obstet 23: 560

Seppola M, Ruoslahti E (1972) Alpha fetoprotein in amniotic fluid: an index of gestational age. Am J Obstet Gynecol 114: 595–598

Sherer DM, Abramowicz JS, Ryan RM *et al.* (1991) Severe fetal hydrops resulting from ABO incompatibility. Obstet Gynecol 78: 897–899

Simonovits I, Timár I, Bajtai G (1980) Rate of Rh immunization after induced abortion. Vox Sang 38: 161–164

Sims DG, Barron SL, Wadehra V *et al.* (1976) Massive chronic feto-maternal bleeding associated with placental chorioangiomas. Acta Paediatr Scand 65: 271

Singleton BK, Green CA, Avent ND *et al.* (2000) The presence of an RHD pseudogene containing a 37 base pair duplication and a nonsense mutation in Africans with the RhD-negative blood group phenotype. Blood 95: 12–18

Smith G, Knott P, Rissik J *et al.* (1998) Anti-U and haemolytic disease of the fetus and newborn. Br J Obstet Gynaecol 105: 1318–1321

Smith NA, Ala FA, Lee D *et al.* (2000) A multi-centre trial of monoclonal anti-D in the prevention of Rh-immunisation of RhD negative male volunteers by RhD+ red cells Transfus Med 10 (Suppl. 1): 8

Southcott MJ, Tanner MJ, Anstee DJ. (1999) The expression of human blood group antigens during erythropoiesis in a cell culture system. Blood 93: 4425–4435

Stone B, Marsh WL (1959) Haemolytic disease of the newborn caused by anti-M. Br J Haematol 5: 344

Tabb PA, Inglis J, Savage DCL *et al.* (1972) Controlled trial of phototherapy of limited duration in the treatment of physiological hyperbilirubinaemia in low-birth-weight infants. Lancet 2: 1211

Tannirandorn Y, Rodeck CH (1990) New approaches in the treatment of haemolytic disease of the fetus. In: Blood Transfusion: the Impact of New Technologies. M Contreras (ed.). Baillière's Clinical Haematology 3: 289–320

Terry MF (1970) A management of the third stage to reduce feto-maternal transfusion. J Obstet Gynaecol Br Cwlth 77: 129

Tovey GH (1945) A study of the protective factors in heterospecific group pregnancy and their role in the prevention of haemolytic disease of the newborn. J Pathol Bact 57: 295

Tovey LAD (1986) Haemolytic disease of the newborn: the changing scene. Br J Obstet Gynaecol 93: 960–966

Tovey LAD, Townley A Stevenson BJ *et al.* (1983) The Yorkshire antenatal anti-D immunoglobulin trial in primigravidae. Lancet 2: 244–246

Urbaniak SJ, Greiss MA, Crawford RJ *et al.* (1984) Prediction of the outcome of rhesus haemolytic disease of the newborn: additional information using an ADCC assay. Vox Sang 46: 323–329

Urbaniak SJ, Duncan JI, Armstrong-Fisher SS *et al.* (1999) Variable inhibition of placental IgG transfer in vitro with commercial IvgG preparations. Br J Haematol 107: 815–817

Valentine GH (1958) ABO incompatibility and haemolytic disease of the newborn. Arch Dis Child 33: 185

Van der Schoot CE, Tax GHM, Rijnders RJP *et al.* (2003) Prenatal typing of Rh and Kell blood group system antigens: the edge of a watershed. Transfus Med Rev 17: 31–44

Van der Schoot CE, Soussan AA, Dee R *et al.* (2004) Screening for fetal RHD-genotype by plasma PCR in all D-negative pregnant women is feasible. Vox Sang 87(Suppl. 3): 9

Van Kamp IL, Klumper FJ, Meerman RH *et al.* (2004) Treatment of fetal anemia due to red cell alloimmunization with intrauterine transfusions in the Netherlands, 1988–1999. Acta Obstet Gynecol Scand 83: 731–737

Vaughan JI, Warwick R, Letsky E *et al.* (1994) Erythropoietic suppression in fetal anemia because of Kell alloimmunization. Am J Obstet Gynecol 171: 247–252

Vaughan JI, Manning M, Warwick RM *et al.* (1998) Inhibition of erythroid progenitor cells by anti-Kell antibodies in fetal alloimmune anemia. N Engl J Med 338: 798–803

Veall N, Mollison PL (1950) The rate of red cell exchange in replacement transfusion. Lancet ii: 792

Viëtor HE, Kanhai HHH, Brand A (1994) Induction of additional red cell antibodies after intrauterine transfusions. Transfusion 34: 970–974

Voak D (1969) The pathogenesis of ABO haemolytic disease of the newborn. Vox Sang 17: 481

Voak D, Bowley CC (1969) A detailed serological study on the prediction and diagnosis of ABO haemolytic disease of the newborn (ABO HD). Vox Sang 17: 321

Voak D, Williams MA (1971) An explanation of the failure of the direct antiglobulin test to detect erythrocyte sensitization in ABO haemolytic disease of the newborn and observations on pinocytosis of IgG anti-A antibodies in infant (cord) red cells. Br J Haematol 20: 9

Wagner FF, Flegel WA (2000) RHD gene deletion occurred in the Rhesus box. Blood 95: 3662–3668

Wagner T, Berer A, Lanzer G *et al.* (2000a) Kell is not restricted to erythropoietic lineage but is also expressed on myeloid progenitor cells. Br J Haematol 110: 409–411

Wagner T, Bernaschek G, Geissler K (2000b) Inhibition of megakaryopoiesis by Kell-related antibodies. N Engl J Med 343: 72

Walker RH (1984) Relevance in the selection of serologic tests for the obstetric patient. In: Hemolytic Disease of the

Newborn. G Garratty (ed.), pp. 173–200. Arlington, VA: Am Assoc Blood Banks

Walker RH, Hartrick MB (1991) Non-ABO clinically significant erythrocyte alloantibodies in Caucasian obstetric patients (Abstract). Transfusion 31(Suppl.): 52S

Walker RH, Batten DG, Morrison MM (1993) The current rarity of Rh D hemolytic disease of the newborn in a community hospital. Am J Clin Pathol 100: 340–341

Walker W (1958) The changing pattern of haemolytic disease of the newborn (1948–1957). Vox Sang 3: 225, 236

Walker W, Murray S, Russell JK (1957) Stillbirth due to haemolytic disease of the newborn. J Obstet Gynaecol Br Emp 44: 573

Wang AC, Faulk WP, Stuckey MA et al. (1970) Chemical differences of adult, fetal and hypogammaglobulinemic IgG immunoglobulins. Immunochemistry 7: 703

Ward HK, Walsh RJ, Kooptzoff O (1957) Rh antigens and immunological tolerance. Nature (Lond) 179: 1352

Warren RC, Butler J, Morsman JM et al. (1985) Does chorionic villus sampling cause fetomaternal haemorrhage? Lancet i: 691

Weisert O, Marstrander J (1960) Severe anemia in a newborn caused by protracted feto-maternal 'transfusion'. Acta Paediatr 49: 426

Wenk RE, Goldstein P, Felix JK (1985) Kell alloimmunization, hemolytic disease of the newborn, and perinatal management. Obstet Gynecol 66: 473–476

WHO (1971) Prevention of Rh sensitization. Technical Report Series 468

Wiener AS, Wexler LB, Hurst JG (1949) The use of exchange transfusion for the treatment of severe erythroblastosis due to A-B sensitization with observations on the pathogenesis of the disease. Blood 4: 1014

Williamson LM, Warwick RM (1995) Transfusion-associated graft-versus-host disease and its prevention. Blood Rev 9: 251–261

Walport MJ, Lachmann PJ (1993) Complement. In: Clinical Aspects of Immunology, 5th edn. PJ Lachmann, K Peters, FS Rosen et al. (eds). Oxford: Blackwell Scientific Publications, pp. 347–375

Wolter LC, Hyland CA, Saul A (1993) Rhesus D genotyping using polymerase chain reaction. Blood 82: 1682–1683

Woodrow JC (1970) Rh immunization and its prevention. Ser Haematol 3: no. 3

Woodrow JC, Donohoe WTA (1968) Rh-immunization by pregnancy: results of a survey and their relevance to prophylactic therapy. BMJ iv: 139

Woodrow JC, Finn R (1966) Transplacental haemorrhage. Br J Haematol 12: 297

Woodrow JC, Clarke CA, Donohoe WTA et al. (1965) Prevention of Rh-haemolytic disease: a third report. BMJ i: 279

Worlledge S, Ogiemudia SE, Thomas CO et al. (1974) Blood group antigens and antibodies in Nigeria. Ann Trop Med Parasitol 68: 249

Yao AC, Moinian M, Lind J (1969) Distribution of blood between infant and placenta after birth. Lancet ii: 871

Yeung CY, Hobbs JR (1968) Serum-γG-globulin levels in normal, premature, post-mature, and 'small-for-dates' newborn babies. Lancet ii: 1167

Yoshida Y, Yoshida H, Tatsumi K et al. (1981) Successful antibody elimination in severe M-incompatible pregnancy. N Engl J Med 305: 460–461

Zhu X, Meng G, Dickinson BL et al. (2001) MHC class I-related neonatal Fc receptor for IgG is functionally expressed in monocytes, intestinal macrophages and dendritic cells. J Immunol 166: 3266–3276

Zipursky A (1971) The universal prevention of Rh immunization. Clin Obstet Gynecol 14: 869

Zipursky A, Pollock J, Neelands P et al. (1963a) The transplacental passage of foetal red blood-cells and the pathogenesis of Rh immunization during pregnancy. Lancet ii: 489

Zipursky A, Pollock J, Chown B et al. (1963b) Transplacental foetal hemorrhage after placental injury during delivery or amniocentesis. Lancet ii: 493

Zuelzer WW, Kaplan E (1954) ABO heterospecific pregnancy and hemolytic disease. IV. Pathologic variants. Am J Dis Child 88: 319

13 Immunology of leucocytes, platelets and plasma components

Antigens expressed on leucocytes and platelets include HLA class I and II molecules as well as those that are specific for particular cells and those that are shared with red cells. In this chapter, these antigens, their structure, function and corresponding antibodies are described, together with methods for detecting them. The chapter includes an account of the clinical relevance of these systems and effects owing to related incompatibilities.

The human leucocyte antigen (HLA) system

The human leucocyte antigens (HLAs), coded by genes of the major histocompatibility complex (MHC) are cell surface glycoproteins that are critical in determining the compatibility of tissue grafts, in selecting donor–recipient pairs for transfusion and transplantation and in designing epitope-specific cellular immunotherapy. HLA antibodies are commonly formed after blood transfusion and pregnancy. The name is misleading. HLA molecules are expressed on a wide range of cells in addition to leucocytes, and although these molecules prove 'alloantigenic' to gravid women and to transfusion and graft recipients, they function not as antigens but as peptide chaperones crucial to the process of adaptive immunity (Paul 2003; Wang *et al.* 2005). HLA molecules play a key role in host defences by presenting foreign antigens to the immune.

The first HLA antigen to be clearly defined was HLA-A2, first named MAC (Dausset 1958). Early work on the definition of HLA antigens was complicated by the poor reproducibility of the leucoagglutination assay and by the fact that the early seroreagents

contained mixtures of several antibodies. This problem was partly overcome by applying extensive statistical analysis to the results (van Rood and van Leeuwen 1963) in order to define single specificities. Progress became more rapid with (1) the replacement of leucoagglutination by lymphocytotoxicity tests and (2) the realization that HLA antibodies are frequently formed in pregnancy, particularly as these antibodies, in contrast with those formed after blood transfusion are directed against a limited number of HLA antigens (Payne and Rolfs 1958; van Rood 1958) and (3) the organization of international histocompatibility workshops in which different laboratories were able to compare results by sharing reagents and typing common panels of cells. These workshops, which continue on a regular basis, have been instrumental in the orderly development of the HLA system and its nomenclature (Bodmer 1997). The HLA antigens first detected were found to be encoded by three closely linked genes: HLA-*A*, -*B* and C, subsequently named class I genes.

The observation that lymphocytes from two unrelated individuals can stimulate each other to blast formation when cultured together (mixed lymphocyte culture (MLC) assay), and that the antigens responsible for this stimulation are inherited together with HLA antigens, led to the discovery of HLA-D antigens (Bach and Hirschhorn 1964; Bain *et al.* 1964), which were later detected serologically on B cells and named DR antigens (van Rood *et al.* 1975, 1976; van Rood and van Leeuwen 1976). HLA-DR molecules together with HLA-DQ and HLA-DP constitute the classical class II molecules.

The ability to study HLA genes and their alleles at the molecular level has enormously advanced the knowledge of the HLA genes. Not only is the region now known 'nucleotide by nucleotide' at the genome level, but also hundreds of alleles of the different loci have been sequenced in the population. Most HLA typing is now done at the DNA level.

Human leucocyte antigen: the human major histocompatibility complex

The name MHC refers to the ability of the genes of this genomic region to determine graft rejection between individuals of the same species. In the 1960s, the HLA genes, first discovered through leucocyte agglutination, were established as the genes responsible for graft rejection in man. The physiologic function of these molecules was determined during the following decade: presentation of antigens to T cells (Zinkernagel and Doherty 1974). The mechanism of this 'HLA restriction' was first explained by Townsend and co-workers (1986), who showed that synthetic peptides could be presented to the T cell. The final explanation of how this peptide could be presented to the T cell awaited the discovery of the structure of the HLA molecules in 1987 and the crystallization of a T-cell receptor bound to an MHC molecule.

The extremely polymorphic, closely linked genes of the HLA system are located in a region that spans about 4000 kilobases (kb) on the short arm of chromosome 6 (Breuning et al. 1977). Moving from centromere to telomere, the class II genes are separated from the class I genes by a number of functionally unrelated genes (and pseudogenes) that encode the complement factors C2, C4a and C4b heat shock proteins, cytokines and enzymes (class III genes) (Fig. 13.1).

After three decades of maps of ever increasing elaboration, the complete sequence of the human MHC was published in 1999 by the MHC Sequencing Consortium (1999).

Class I region

HLA-A, -B and -C code for the heavy chain of the MHC class I molecules expressed on most cells. HLA-F, -G and -E code for the heavy chain of non-classical class I molecules, with highly specialized functions. The MIC genes or human MHC class I chain-related genes encode stress-inducible proteins implicated in the regulation of NK cell activity. HFE is a class I-like

gene located approximately 4 Mb telomeric of HLA-F and responsible for most hereditary haemochromatosis.

Class III region

TNFB and -A code for tumour necrosis factors, HSP genes for heat shock proteins, C2, Bf and C genes for proteins of the complement system, and P450-C21B for a steroid 21-hydroxylase.

Class II region

The HLA-DRBA1, -DQA1 and -DPA1 genes code for alpha chains of the DR, DQ and DP class II molecules. HLA-DRB1, -DQB1 and -DPB1 code for the beta chain of the DR, DQ and DP class II molecules. In addition to HLA-DRB1, which codes for the primary HLA specificities such as DR1, DR2, DR4, etc., other DRB genes code for the beta chain of the specificities DR52 (DRB3), DR53 (DRB4) and DR51 (DRB5) not present in all haplotypes. The DO and DM molecules regulate the loading of exogenous peptides into class II molecules. LMP2 and LMP7, which encode the subunits of the proteasome, and TAP1 and TAP2, which encode a peptide transporter, are involved in the processing and presentation of antigens by class I molecules.

HLA class I and II molecules: structure and function

HLA molecules engage two distinct arms of the T-cell-mediated immune response. MHC class I molecules present antigen to cytotoxic T cells (CTLs), whereas MHC class II present to helper T cells. Antigens are not presented by HLA molecules as intact proteins. The antigen must first be degraded to peptide fragments and presented in the context of the HLA molecule to the T-cell receptor.

HLA class I molecules

HLA-A, -B and -C genes produce a transmembrane glycosylated polypeptide of molecular weight 4300 (the α or heavy chain) linked non-covalently to $\beta2$-microglobulin, a non-polymorphic and non-glycosylated polypeptide of molecular weight 1200 (the β or light chain), which is encoded by a gene on chromosome 15 (Snary et al. 1977a; Barnstable et al.

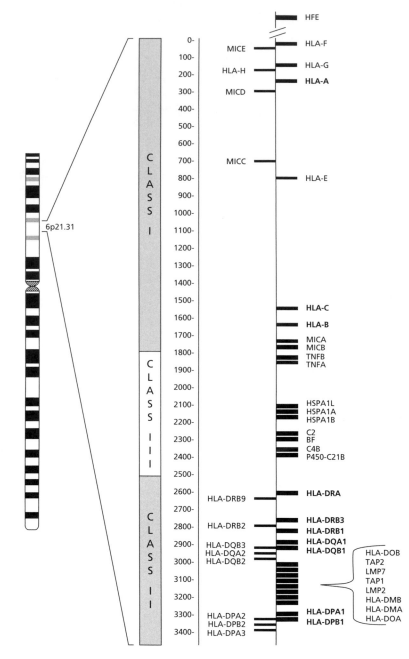

Fig 13.1 The segment of the small arm of chromosome 6 that contains the HLA complex is shown in detail. The first bar shows the division of the complex into class I, II and III regions. The ruler indicates the number of kilobases. The genomic map shows the approximate positions of the gene loci mentioned in the text. Bars to the right show expressed genes and to the left, pseudogenes (not expressed). In bold

are shown the genes coding for the heavy chain of the classical class I molecules and the alpha and beta chains of the class II molecules. *Class I region*: HLA-A, B and C code for the heavy chain of the MHC class I molecules expressed on most cells. HLA-F, G and E code for the heavy chain of non-classical class I molecules, with highly specialized functions. The MIC genes or human MHC class I

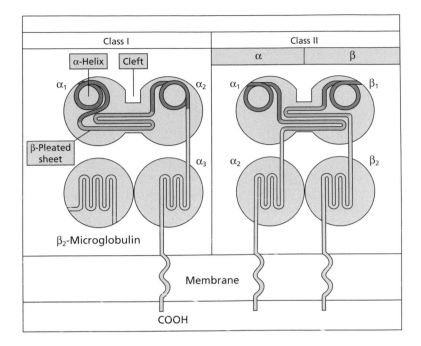

Fig 13.2 Structure of class I and class II HLA molecules showing domains and transmembrane segments. From Roitt and Delves (2001).

1978). The extracellular part of the heavy chain consists of three domains: $\alpha 1$, $\alpha 2$ and $\alpha 3$ (Fig. 13.2).

The three-dimensional structure of class I molecules has been revealed by X-ray crystallographic analysis, first of HLA-A2 (Fig. 13.3) and subsequently of HLA-A68 and HLA-B27 (Bjorkman *et al.* 1987; Garretti *et al.* 1989; Madden *et al.* 1991). The $\alpha 3$ and $\beta 2m$ domains have tertiary structures similar to domains in the constant region of the immunoglobulins. The top of the molecule is formed by pairing the $\alpha 1$ and $\alpha 3$ domains, which together form the antigen peptide-binding groove. The majority of the polymorphic determinants in class I molecules occur on the floor of this cleft (Bjorkman *et al.* 1987) (see Fig. 13.3). The class I molecules specifically bind peptides of defined length, usually 6–10 residues (Falk *et al.* 1991). All

peptides bind similarly with their N- and C-termini sequestered in the binding groove by a network of hydrogen bonds to residues conserved in all class I glycoproteins (Madden and Wiley 1992). In addition, there are allele-specific binding pockets with a strong preference for a few side-chains at some positions of the peptide. This explains the correlation between class I polymorphism and the affinity of peptide binding (Falk *et al.* 1991). Generally, these peptides derive from self-proteins, but in virus-infected cells the peptides from the pathogen may be processed in the cytosol and migrate with the HLA molecules to the cell surface (Pamer and Cresswell 1998). Tumour antigens can be detected in the same way. Class I molecules are expressed on most cells and they inform the scanning CTL about the status of potential target cells for

---

Fig 13.1 *(cont.)*

chain-related genes encode stress-inducible proteins implicated in the regulation of NK cell activity. HFE is a class I-like gene located approximately 4 Mb telomeric of HLA-F and responsible for hereditary haemochromatosis. *Class III region*: TNFB and A code for tumour necrosis factors, HSP genes for heat shock proteins, C2, Bf and C genes for proteins of the complement system, and P450-C21B for a steroid 21-hydroxylase. *Class II region*: The HLA-DRBA1, -DQA1 and -DPA1 genes code for alpha chains of the DR, DQ and DP class II molecules.

HLA-DRB1, -DQB1 and -DPB1 code for the beta chain of the DR, DQ and DP class II molecules. In addition to HLA-DRB1, which codes for the primary HLA specificities such as DR1, DR2, DR4, etc., other DRB genes code for the beta chain of the specificities DR52 (DRB3), DR53 (DRB4) and DR51 (DRB5) not present in all haplotypes. The DO and DM molecules regulate the loading of exogenous peptides into class II molecules. LMP2 and LMP7, which encode the subunits of the proteasome, and TAP1 and TAP2, which encode a peptide transporter, are involved in the processing and presentation of antigens by class I molecules.

(a)

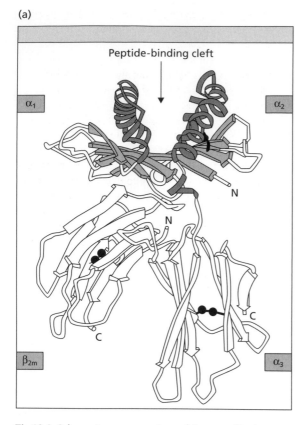

Peptide-binding cleft

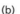

(b)

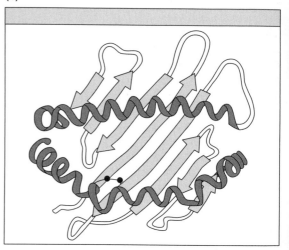

Fig 13.3 Schematic representations of the crystallized structure of the HLA-A2 molecule. (a) The four domains, with the α_1 and α_2 domains forming a putative peptide-binding region. (b) Top surface of the molecule. The putative antigen-binding groove is shown, made up of a β-pleated sheet flanked by two α-helices (Bjorkman *et al.* 1987).

destruction. Peptide epitopes presented by them can only be recognized by CTL if these (1) have a specific receptor for the antigen and (2) the same HLA class antigens as the target cell. This phenomenon, known as HLA restriction, was first described in the mouse (Zinkernagel and Doherty 1974). The HLA-A, -B and -C antigens are expressed on all nucleated cells except spermatozoa and placental trophoblast. The antigens are also found on platelets and some class I antigens have been detected on red cells. The number of class I molecules on various cells differs and, particularly on platelets, some of the antigens are weakly expressed.

HLA class II molecules

All typical class II molecules consist of two transmembrane glycoprotein chains of molecular weight 33 kDa (the heavy or α-chain) and 28 kDa (the light or β-chain) respectively (Snary *et al.* 1977b). The extracellular component of both chains consists of two distinct domains: $\alpha1$, $\alpha2$ and $\beta1$, $\beta2$. The domains distal to the cell surface carry most of the polymorphic determinants. The constant domain near the cell surface is very similar to the constant domain of the immunoglobulin heavy chains (Shackelford *et al.* 1982; see also Fig. 13.2).

The crystal structure of class II molecules (DR1) is similar to that of class I molecules; polymorphic determinants of class II molecules are also clustered in the antigen peptide-binding groove (Brown *et al.* 1993). In contrast with class I molecules, class II molecules bind longer peptides with no apparent restriction on peptide length (Rudensky *et al.* 1991). The peptides bind to the groove as a straight extended chain with a single pronounced twist. Hydrogen bonds along the main chain of all peptides interact with residues from the α-helical regions and the β-sheet in the peptide-binding groove and thus provide a binding component that is independent of the sequence of the peptide. Twelve hydrogen bonds on the peptide bind to determinants encoded by residues conserved in most class II alleles and this suggests that peptides bind to class II molecules by a universal mode. However, particular side-chains of the peptide are accommodated in polymorphic pockets in the binding groove that determine specific binding of peptides and thus the affinity of the peptide class II molecule bond (Stern *et al.* 1994). The expression of class II antigen is restricted to B cells and to antigen-presenting cells such as macrophages, dendritic cells and Langerhans cells. Class II antigens are also present on activated T lymphocytes and some tumour cells (Winchester and Kunkel 1979).

The cells that express class II molecules, specialized antigen-presenting cells (APCs), such as dendritic cells, mononuclear phagocytes and B cells, bind exogenously derived peptides of 9–22 residues. In the case of macrophages and B cells, the HLA molecule–antigen complex is assembled within intracellular organelles. With all APCs the antigen peptides are held in a groove in HLA class II molecules, and this plasma membrane-bound compound antigen is recognized by helper T lymphocytes via their T-cell receptors during immunosurveillance. The polymorphic HLA determinants in the peptide-binding groove of the class II molecule strongly influence peptide binding.

Dendritic cells, which express HLA class II antigens particularly well, are the APCs that present antigen to helper T cells to induce a primary immune response. Memory T cells can be stimulated by macrophages, B cells and even by free antigens (Berg *et al.* 1994). Class II antigen complexes instruct the helper T-cell system to initiate the humoral immune response and assist in the cellular immune process; for this reason, class II genes are often referred to as 'immune response genes'.

HLA genes and antigens

The linkage between the HLA genes is so strong that crossing over between them is rare; therefore the alleles of the HLA genes present on one chromosome usually segregate together within a family. The two alleles of each individual gene are expressed co-dominantly (e.g. HLA-A1, -A11). The set of HLA alleles present on a single chromosome is known as a haplotype. Siblings

who inherit the same haplotypes from their parents are thus HLA identical, unless crossing over between HLA genes has occurred.

As crossing over within the HLA region is rare, with random assortment equilibrium should be reached in a population over a long period of time; particular combinations of alleles at, for example, the *A* and *B* loci or at the loci of the *D* region should not be more common than predicted from the product of their relative frequencies in the population. However, in any given population, certain combinations of alleles or haplotypes are more frequent than expected, a phenomenon known as 'linkage disequilibrium'. For example, the frequency of HLA-A1-B8 in European white people is 8.8%, whereas the expected frequency of this haplotype, based on the individual frequencies of A1 and B8, is 1.6%. Selective pressures that affect survival or reproductive capacity usually drive linkage disequilibrium. Patterns of linkage disequilibrium vary in different populations.

Nomenclature

A history of the development of HLA system nomenclature has been compiled by Boolmer (1997). Nomenclature for the HLA genes and antigens is regularly updated by the WHO Nomenclature Committee for factors of the HLA system (Marsh 2003). For the non-aficionado, nomenclature remains a challenge, because two systems remain in general use. The older serological nomenclature relies on identification of antigens on the leucocyte surface (HLA antigens) (Tiercy *et al.* 2002). The following terms are used for the 'classical' HLA antigens: for class I, the capital letters -A, -B -C are appended to identify the locus; for class II, the prefix *D* followed by a letter (-DR, -DQ, -DP) for the subregion and by the letters A or B to indicate whether the gene codes for the α- or β-chain, for example DRA, DQB, etc. The letters are followed by a number that identifies epitopes determined by alloantibodies or less often alloreactive cytotoxic T cells.

Sequence-based nomenclature separates the HLA locus with an asterisk (*) followed by four digits used to designate the alleles of a particular gene; the first two digits describe the serologically defined antigen with which the allele is (or alleles are) most closely associated, and the last two or three digits complete the number of the allele as defined by molecular

551

techniques (DNA typing, oligonucleotide typing, nucleotide and amino acid sequencing, cloning), for example HLA-*A*0101* for the allele that encodes the A1 antigen and *A*0201*, *A*0202*, etc. for the alleles associated with the antigen A2; the serologically defined antigens encoded by alleles of each gene are also numbered: A1, A2 etc.; w ('workshop') was used to indicate that the specificity was provisional, but in the future all serological specificities will be named on the basis of correlation with an identified sequence. The letter 'w' can therefore be dropped with three sets of exceptions: (1) Bw4 and Bw6 to distinguish them as epitopes from those encoded by other alleles of the *HLA-B* gene; (2) the C antigens for which the w is retained throughout to avoid confusion with the nomenclature of the complement system; and (3) the Dw specificities defined by the MLC assay; and the DP specificities defined by a secondary response of T lymphocytes that had been primed by a first step in the MLC (primed lymphocyte typing) (Bodmer *et al.* 1992).

One of the non-classical HLA class I genes, the HLA-G gene, encodes a non-polymorphic α-chain with a shortened cytoplasmic segment. The HLA-G molecule is expressed only on the trophoblast, which suggests that it may have a role in embryonic development or fetal–maternal immune interactions, or both (Geraghty *et al.* 1987; Kovats *et al.* 1991). Class I antigens are detected in a lymphocytotoxicity test, using either alloantibodies or human or murine monoclonal antibodies.

Some 250 alleles of the class I *A* gene, about twice this number of *B* alleles and 119 *C* alleles are recognized by the WHO Nomenclature Committee. The numbers have been increasing rapidly. For a list of these and of class I antigens, see Marsh (2003).

Class II genes and antigens

The polymorphism of the class II genes is much greater than detected on their products by serological typing and by the MLC assay. Studies at the DNA level have shown that, in addition to the classical *DR*, *DQ* and *DP* series of genes, there are several other non-classical class II genes in the D region: *DOA*, *DOB*, *DNA* and the *DMA* and *DMB* genes. In addition, in the class II chromosomal region, there are four genes, *TAP1* and *TAP2*, and *LMP2* and *LMP7*, which encode molecules involved in antigen processing (see below).

In the DR subregion there is a single α-chain gene (*DRA*) with two alleles that, however, do not encode a polymorphism on the α-chain. There are nine *DRB* genes, five of which are pseudogenes (*DRB2*, *DRB6*, *DRB7*, *DRB8* and *DRB9*). Seven of the *DRB* genes (except *DRB1* and *DRB9*) are restricted to certain DR haplotypes. The genomic organization of the DR region is shown in Figure 13.4. The *DRB1*, *DRB3*, *DRB4* and *DRB5* genes encode four separate β-chains. *DRB1* encodes the major DR antigens, whereas the *DRB3* gene codes for *DR52*, and the *DRB5* gene for DR51.

In the DQ subregion there are two α genes: *DQA1*, which encodes an α-chain and *DQA2*, which is not known to be expressed. There are three *B* genes: *DQB1*, which encodes a β-chain and *DQB2* and *DQB3*, not known to be expressed. *DQA1* and *DQB1* are polymorphic but only the products of the *DQB1* alleles have been serologically recognized (DQ antigens).

In the DP subregion there are two α and two β genes: *DPA1*, *DPA2*, *DPB1* and *DPB2*. *DPA1* and *DPB1* encode an α- and a β-chain respectively, whereas *DPA2* and *DPB2* are pseudogenes.

Additional HLA class II genes

The genes *DOB* and *DNA* located between the DP and DQ subregions encode a β- and α-chain, respectively, whose function is as yet unknown. The genes *DMA* and *DMB* encode an α- and a β-chain, which associate to form a class II molecule that contains a peptide-binding groove involved in antigen presentation (Kelly *et al.* 1991). The *DM* genes are polymorphic, but the polymorphism is limited and the resulting antigenic determinants occur only on the area of the extracellular portion of the protein that is proximal to the cell membrane. They therefore do not occur in the peptide-binding groove and thus do not affect antigen presentation, in which the DM molecule probably has a specialized function (Sanderson *et al.* 1994).

Non-HLA genes involved in antigen processing

The *TAP1* and *TAP2* genes, located between *DBO* and *DNA*, do not encode typical class II proteins but instead encode an important peptide transporter molecule involved in the endogenous processing of antigen (Spies *et al.* 1991). The TAP genes are polymorphic (Colonna *et al.* 1992; Powis *et al.* 1992a,b,

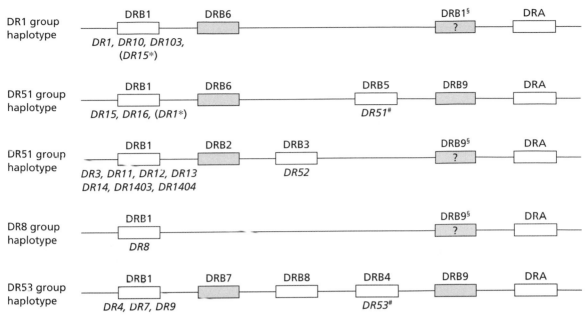

Fig 13.4 Genomic organization of the HLA-DR region and encoded products (specificities) (Bodmer *et al.* 1992). Pseudogenes are indicated by shaded boxes, expressed genes by open boxes. The serological specificity encoded by a gene is shown underneath in italics. *, rarely observed haplotypes; #, DR51 and DR53 may not be expressed on certain haplotypes; §, the presence of DRB9 in these haplotypes needs confirmation.

1993). This polymorphism may affect antigen processing and thus the immune response, but at present this is speculation. The *LMP2* and *LMP7* genes, located near the *TAP* genes, encode proteasomes that affect the degradation of antigen molecules to peptides (Cerundolo *et al.* 1995).

The class II antigens are detected by alloantibodies and, in some cases, also by monoclonal antibodies, using a complement-dependent cytotoxicity test on isolated B lymphocytes or a two-colour immunofluorescence test on unseparated cells (van Rood *et al.* 1976).

As mentioned above, a polymorphism (Dw) encoded by the *D* region has been defined by using homozygous typing cells in the mixed lymphocyte culture (MLC). The exact relationship between Dw determinants and the polymorphic determinants encoded by the *DR*, *DP* genes is not known. However, a strong correlation has been observed between matching and mismatching for *DR* polymorphic DNA sequences and reactivity in the MLC. The lymphocytes of all DR mismatched pairs were reactive and 37% of the matched pairs were nonreactive in the MLC. The MLC reactivity of 63% of the matched pairs may be due to unrecognized *DR*

alleles (Baxter-Lowe *et al.* 1992), but incompatibility for HLA-DP specificities has also been found to induce significant proliferation in the primary MLC in HLA-A, -B, -DR and -DQ identical subjects (Olerup *et al.* 1990). *HLA-DQA1* or *-DQB1* allele differences are not important in the primary MLC among otherwise HLA identical, unrelated subjects (Termijtelen *et al.* 1991).

For a list of the very numerous class II alleles, antigens and determinants agreed by the WHO Nomenclature Committee, see Marsh (2003).

Other genes in the HLA region

As the products of these genes are not leucocyte antigens and are not involved in antigen presentation by HLA molecules, they will not be discussed further.

Crossreactions in the HLA system

Sera from subjects alloimmunized against HLA antigens are frequently crossreactive, as shown by the following example: a given serum may react with two different serologically defined antigens, for example

HLA-B51 and HLA-B52, but antibodies recognizing these two specificities individually cannot be separated from the serum. The antibodies in such a serum are in fact directed against a different antigen, HLA-B5 in this example, which occurs together with B51 and B52. Thus the antibodies (anti-B5) crossreact with B51- and B52-positive cells.

This kind of crossreactivity is explained by the multiple mutations within the HLA genes. A single allele of a gene may code for different, separate polymorphisms on the single HLA molecule it produces. The frequencies of the epitopes encoded by these different polymorphisms within a single allele differ greatly. Some have a very high frequency, for example HLA-B4 and HLA-B6, and are called supratypic or 'public' antigens. At the other end of the scale are antigens with a very low frequency (1–2%) that are called 'private' antigens. Thus, epitopes with different frequencies in the population, and against which separate alloantibodies can be made, occur on a single HLA molecule and are the basis of the crossreactivity: antibodies against public antigens (also called crossreactive antigens) react with cells carrying different private antigens. Particular public antigens occur together with particular private antigens that are said to form crossreactive groups (CREGs) of (private) antigens. The higher the frequency of the public antigen in the population, the more important are antibodies against the antigen for crossreactivity. Thus, anti-HLA-B4 and -B6 are responsible for much of the crossreactivity among the HLA-B antigens.

The occurrence of crossreactive antigens is also responsible for what are called 'splits' of HLA antigens. Frequently, a crossreactive antigen, for example the antigen B5 in the above example, was defined before the two private antigens B51 and B52, together with which it occurs. Later, when antibodies recognizing B51 and B52 were found, the B5 antigen was 'split' into B51 and B52 (see Table 13.2).

Soluble HLA class I antigens in plasma

Using monoclonal antibodies coated on to immunobeads and one-dimensional isoelectric focusing, followed by immunoblotting using specific class I antisera, all antigens defined to date have been detected in plasma (Doxiadis and Grosse-Wilde 1989).

Soluble HLA class I antigens (sHLA) may have important immunological effects. sHLA have been shown to inhibit alloreactive cytotoxic T cells (Zavazava *et al.* 1991) and to block specifically the induction of HLA alloantibody formation (Grumet *et al.* 1994). Allogeneic sHLA alone or complexed with antibody induces prolongation of allograft survival (Sumimoto and Kamada 1990; Wang *et al.* 1993a). When a graft is rejected, sHLA is shed from it and thus graft rejection episodes can be identified by serial measurements of donor-specific sHLA (Claas *et al.* 1993; Puppo *et al.* 1994).

HLA antibodies

Mechanisms of alloimmunization

The high density of HLA molecules on the cell surface renders allogeneic leucocytes highly immunogenic following transfusion or pregnancy. Sensitization depends upon both donor and recipient factors. Two recipient T-cell recognition mechanisms have been shown to be critical for the initiation of alloimmunity (Semple and Freedman 2002). The direct pathway occurs when recipient helper T cells interact with MHC molecules on donor APCs. The indirect pathway is more analogous to the normal immune response. Indirect recognition involves processing of allogeneic donor molecules by recipient APCs and presentation to recipient helper T cells. With indirect allorecognition, interactions between donor antigen and recipient APCs are essential for T-cell activation and subsequent antibody formation. For both pathways, the MHC molecules are expressed on the surface of the APC and are available for presentation to circulating T cells. If a T cell has a receptor with sufficient affinity for the peptide–MHC combination (first signal) and various co-stimulatory (second signal) events occur, the T cell will be activated and differentiate into an effector cell. Cytokines such as interleukin 2 (IL-2), IL-4 and alpha-interferon (IFN-α) secreted from the activated helper cells stimulate donor MHC class I-primed B cells to differentiate into the plasma cells that secrete IgG antibodies and helper T cells (Weiss and Samuelsen 2003).

Development of HLA antibodies after transfusion

Unless measures are taken to reduce the number of transfused leucocytes (see below), a high incidence of HLA antibodies will be encountered in patients who receive multiple transfusions from different donors. However, even in subjects exposed to the blood of a single donor, the incidence of HLA antibodies is high. In a series in which patients awaiting renal grafting were given three transfusions at 2-weekly intervals from a potential donor, who in each case had a haplotype identical with one of the recipient's haplotypes, HLA antibodies developed in some 30% of recipients (Salvatierra *et al.* 1980).

After the massive blood transfusion that used to be associated with open heart surgery, lymphocytotoxic antibodies and/or leucoagglutinins could be found in almost all subjects, provided that repeated tests are made, as some of the antibodies can be detected only transiently. In a series in which patients were tested at 1 week and usually also at 2, 4 and 12 weeks after open heart surgery, 52 out of 54 developed leucocyte antibodies; 12 weeks after transfusion antibodies were present in only 62.5% of the subjects (Gleichmann and Breininger 1975). The majority of HLA antibodies formed after blood transfusion are directed against class I antigens. HLA antibodies are the most important cause of antibody-mediated refractoriness to platelet transfusions (see later), of febrile transfusion reactions prior to leucoreduction and of transfusion-associated acute lung injury (see Chapter 15).

Some patients never become immunized despite repeated transfusions of blood or of platelets. Such subjects are considered to be non-responders to HLA.

Development of HLA antibodies in pregnancy

In primiparous women, lymphocytotoxic class I antibodies may be found as early as the twenty-fourth week of pregnancy and are present by the last trimester in 10% of women (Overweg and Engelfriet 1969). Estimates of the incidence of lymphocytotoxic antibodies after a first pregnancy vary widely: 4.3% (Ahrons 1971), 9.1% (Nymand 1974), 13% (Overweg and Engelfriet 1969) and 25% (Goodman and Masaitis 1967). The discrepancies may well be due to the varying extent of the panels of lymphocytes with which the sera were tested and the sensitivity of the techniques applied. The majority of HLA antibodies developed in pregnancy are directed against class I antigens.

Women tend to make antibodies against only certain of the HLA antigens to which they are exposed during pregnancy. In multiparous women who had had at least four pregnancies, and were therefore likely to have been exposed to antigens encoded by both of their partner's haplotypes, the frequency of women with antibodies against only a single paternal antigen was the same as that in primiparous women (Tongio *et al.* 1985). Both maternal and paternal (fetal) HLA antigens play a role in the class I differential immunogenicity (Dankers *et al.* 2003).

Although HLA antibodies are usually IgG, they produce no obvious damage to the fetus, presumably because they are absorbed by fetal cells in the placenta.

Monoclonal HLA antibodies

Most murine monoclonal HLA antibodies are directed against non-polymorphic determinants of the HLA molecules (Brodsky *et al.* 1979; Trucco *et al.* 1980; 1979); some antibodies detect a polymorphism that is different from those detected by alloantisera (Quaranta 1980). However, many murine monoclonals which recognize HLA antigens as defined by alloantisera have been described, particularly anti-DR and anti-DQ (Marsh and Bodmer 1989).

In addition, many human monoclonal HLA antibodies against both class I and class II antigens have now been described.

Some features of HLA antibodies

HLA antibodies formed after blood transfusion or pregnancy are characteristically IgG. They are complement activating and have cytotoxic properties and, like most granulocyte-reactive IgG antibodies, are leucoagglutinins (see below). HLA antibodies may be naturally occurring. Using very sensitive techniques, weak HLA antibodies, particularly anti-B8, have been demonstrated in the serum of about 1% of normal donors who had had no known pregnancies or transfusions (Tongio *et al.* 1985). These antibodies are usually IgM and, in the cytotoxicity test, react only with B cells, on which class I antigens are more strongly expressed than on T cells.

HLA and haematopoietic progenitor cell grafts

Graft-versus-host-disease and graft-versus-tumour or -leukaemia

Haematopoietic cell (marrow, umbilical cord blood or mobilized peripheral blood) transplantation is performed to replace inadequate or defective blood cell production, for example in aplastic anaemia, sickle cell disease and thalassaemia (Walters *et al.* 2000; La Nasa *et al.* 2002; Ades *et al.* 2003; Atkins and Walters 2003), for adoptive immunotherapy of malignancy (Landsteiner and Levine 1929; Landsteiner 1931; Barrett 2003; Chakrabarti and Childs 2003) and for reconstitution of 'normal' immune function as in treatment of severe combined immunodeficiency (SCID) and Wiskott–Aldrich syndrome (Filipovich *et al.* 2001). The role of HLA 'compatibility' falls into four different areas: (1) sufficient compatibility to permit engraftment and prevent late rejection (with appropriate preparative and immunosuppressive regimens); (2) enough compatibility to minimize graft-versus-host-disease (GvHD); (3) ample immune reconstitution to permit immuno-surveillance; and (4) sufficient immune potency to effect adoptive immune therapy of neoplasia. HLA identity is neither necessary nor sufficient to ensure these effects, but serological and molecular similarities are the best available surrogate assays to guide related and unrelated transplants. Both GvHD and graft-versus-tumour (GvL) occur in the presence of a full HLA match, suggesting that the classical HLA molecules themselves are not targets of allosensitization, but rather present polymorphic molecules expressed by recipient cells that are recognized by the grafted immune cells.

Graft-versus-host disease: the dark cloud of haematopoietic cell grafts

Donor lymphocytes engraft, replicate and react against the normal tissues of the recipient, resulting in a syndrome known as GvHD. Myeloablative conditioning administered before transplant effectively minimizes graft rejection. The art of post-transplant immunosuppression consists of achieving a balance between graft immunocompetence and GvHD without allowing rejection of the graft. The risk of GvHD increases with genetic disparity between donor and recipient. HLA identical twins have the least chance of developing GvHD, followed by HLA identical siblings, minor degrees of mismatching among siblings, and unrelated donors of differing degrees of similarity at the MHC locus (Longster and Major 1975; Hansen *et al.* 1999). However, while the genetic homogeneity between donor and recipient generally decreases the risk of GvHD, it lessens the therapeutic benefit and increases the chance of tumour relapse as well (Weiden *et al.* 1981).

Graft-versus-tumor effect: a silver lining of graft-versus-host disease?

One possibly beneficial effect of GvHD, or perhaps an immunological activity difficult to separate from GvHD, is rejection of recipient tumour cells by the donor immune system (graft-versus-leukaemia (GvL) effect) (Mavroudis and Barrett 1996; Mavroudis *et al.* 1998). The GvL effect has long been recognized to play a powerful therapeutic role in the treatment of chronic myelocytic leukaemia and more recently recognized as treatment of refractory malignant disorders including some solid tumours (graft-versus-tumour, GVT) (Childs and Barrett 2002). GVT may be the most potent form of tumour immunotherapy currently in clinical use, but its mechanism(s) of action is still poorly understood. Allogeneic T cells clearly play a fundamental role in the initiation and maintenance of the effect on neoplastic cells (Kolb *et al.* 1990). The risk of relapse increases markedly for patients with chronic myelogenous leukaemia who received a T-cell-depleted graft compared with a subset of patients who had received a T-cell-replete one, although the former patients avoided significant GvHD (Leak *et al.* 1990; Champlin *et al.* 2000). These results suggest that GvHD is a biological entity different from the GvL effect. In addition, upon leukaemia relapse, administration of donor lymphocyte infusion can induce clinical and molecular remission. Donor T cells may target not only tumour-specific antigens but also allelic variants of these antigens, minor histocompatibility antigens and, in the case of HLA-mismatched transplants, HLA antigens disparate from the donor but expressed by the tumour cells (Leddy and Bakemeier 1967; Lederman *et al.* 1983; Marijt *et al.* 2003). Although several theories about the mechanisms of the GvL effect have been proposed, the reasons that allogeneic T cells seem superior to native tumour immunity for some leukaemias and solid tumours remain to be clarified.

Effect of previous transfusion on success of bone marrow grafting

Previous transfusions, particularly from close relatives, prejudice the success of subsequent bone marrow grafting (Storb *et al.* 1980). The chance of rejection of the graft increases with the number of transfusions. If future recipients of a bone marrow graft need to be transfused, they should receive leucocyte-depleted blood or blood components from random donors and not from relatives. The discrepancy between the effect of transfusion of blood containing white cells on grafted bone marrow and the apparent mitigating effect on renal grafts has not been explained. The development of GvHD after the transfusion of allogeneic leucocytes is described in Chapter 15.

HLA and organ grafting

Renal grafts

Significance of HLA antibodies. When HLA alloantibodies directed against antigens expressed on the donor kidney are present in the serum of a renal graft recipient, acute or hyperacute rejection of the graft will occur. It is therefore necessary to perform a crossmatch between the patient's serum and the B and T lymphocytes of the donor. Not all antibodies detected in the crossmatch are harmful. Cold-reacting IgM autoantibodies directed against B and T cells may be present in the serum of dialysis patients and do not appear to be harmful (Ting 1983).

Significance of matching for HLA. The extent to which matching for HLA improves renal graft survival remains controversial. In many studies, matching has had no obvious benefit due, perhaps, to the small numbers of cases studied, interference of the many factors influencing graft survival and incomplete tissue typing. Furthermore, the survival of mismatched kidneys has improved greatly following the discovery of the beneficial effect of previous blood transfusion and of the value of ciclosporin A as an immunosuppressive drug. Nevertheless, in some large studies, a significant beneficial effect of HLA matching on long-term graft survival has been observed.

In a study in which 240 laboratories participated, the results of 30 000 first cadaver kidney transplants were analysed. Cases in which the donor and recipient were typed for all known 'splits' of HLA-A and -B antigens and those in which typing was restricted to the broad antigens were analysed separately. At 3 years, an 18% difference in survival rates between grafts with zero and four mismatches typed for A and B antigen splits was found, but only a 2% difference when typing was restricted to broad antigens. When A, B and DR antigens were considered together, the differences in rates of survival were 31% and 6%, respectively, in the

two groups. It was concluded that typing for antigen splits is important (Opelz 1992). Molecular typing of DR alleles revealed an error rate in serological typing of about 25% (Mytelineos *et al.* 1990). The impact of DR matching is particularly significant if patients and donors are typed at the DNA level (Opelz *et al.* 1993).

In a recent study, complete matching for serologically determined HLA-A, B and DR antigens was found to have a significant and clinically important impact on short- and long-term graft survival (Opelz *et al.* 1999). On the other hand, partial matching provided little benefit (Held *et al.* 1994). The advantage of complete matching was diminished by the negative influence of longer periods of organ preservation and by the fact that in practice only 50% of perfectly matched kidneys were actually transplanted into the identified recipient. An analysis of more than 150 000 renal transplants between 1987 and 1997 in the Collaborative Transplant Study indicates that a first cadaver graft with a 6-locus mismatch has a 17% lower 10-year survival than a graft with no mismatch at these sites (Opelz *et al.* 1999). In the latter study, the matching effect is even more striking in patients with highly reactive preformed lymphocytotoxic antibodies. Among first cadaver transplant recipients with antibody reactivity against > 50% of the test panel, the difference in graft survival at 5 years between patients with zero or six mismatches reached 30%. Once again, correction of serological HLA typing errors by more accurate DNA typing resulted in a significantly improved HLA matching effect, and matching for the class II locus HLA-DP, a locus that can be typed reliably only by DNA methods, showed a significant effect for cadaver kidney re-transplants. Non-HLA transplant immunity may be more important for long-term graft survival (Opelz *et al.* 2005).

For brief discussions of the importance of ABO as a major histocompatibility system and of the possible effects of Lewis groups on renal transplantation, see Chapter 4.

Liver grafts and heart–lung grafts

The survival of liver grafts is reportedly improved with HLA matching and is worse when the T-cell crossmatch is positive (Nikaein *et al.* 1994). However, this finding could not be confirmed in the Collaborative Transplant analysis (Opelz *et al.* 1999). Matching for HLA-DR diminished the frequency of rejection episodes after heart transplantation from 34% to 16%, and at

3 months there was an additional beneficial effect of HLA-B matching (Sheldon *et al.* 1994). An independent study of heart transplants showed a highly significant impact of HLA compatibility on graft outcome (*P* < 0.0001) (Opelz *et al.* 1999). In practice, matching for HLA is much more difficult in the transplantation of liver and heart than of kidney, mainly because there is no large pool of HLA-typed recipients to choose from.

Immunomodulatory effect(s) of transfusion

As knowledge about the mechanisms of immune responsiveness and tolerance evolves, and as tools to measure alterations in immunity become available, additional immunological consequences of blood transfusion are being detected. Numerous variations in circulating blood cells have been reported in patients transfused with allogeneic blood (see below). Some of these changes persist for months or even longer after transfusion. The lingering question has been whether these observations represent no more than laboratory curiosities, or whether they reflect some clinically relevant alteration in the recipient's immune status, the so-called 'immunomodulatory effects' of blood transfusion. Based on the sum of clinical evidence (see below) immunomodulation seems likely to be added to the list of unintended consequences of allogeneic blood transfusion. The magnitude and importance of these effects, the causative agents, the biological mechanisms and the patients or patient groups that are at particular risk have yet to be defined (Klein 1999).

Dzik (2003) has suggested that there may be two categories of immunosuppressive transfusion effect: one that is HLA dependent and directed against adaptive immunity and a second that is mild, non-specific and directed against innate immunity. The non-specific effect might result from the infusion of blood cells that undergo apoptosis during refrigerated storage. The infusion of apoptotic cells has been shown to be immunosuppressive in animal models. Immunosuppression resulting from the infusion of apoptotic cells may be linked to transforming growth factor beta (TGF-β) (Dzik 2003).

Changes in recipient's lymphocytes after blood transfusion

Following the transfusion of large amounts of fresh or stored blood, changes develop in the recipient's lymphocytes after an interval of about 1 week. Atypical lymphocytes increase by a factor of five or more and lymphocytes may incorporate ^{3}H-thymidine *in vitro* at an increased rate. Values return to the pretransfusion level by about 3 weeks. Changes are not seen after transfusion of frozen and washed (leucocyte-depleted) red cells (Schechter *et al.* 1972). Confirmatory observations were published by Hutchinson and co-workers (1976). The changes are interpreted as a response to donor HLA antigens (presumably of the Dw series) and may be regarded as those of an MLC *in vivo*. A number of other alterations of immune cells including a decrease in NK function and delayed hypersensitivity have been published (Tartter *et al.* 1986, 1989; Jensen *et al.* 1992). Blood transfusion alters immune cell antigen expression in premature neonates and may initially be immunostimulatory and later immunosuppressive (Wang-Rodriguez *et al.* 2000). Donor lymphocytes may circulate for prolonged periods in some patient groups, such as trauma victims, whereas in others such as patients infected with HIV, microchimerism appears to be transient (Kruskall *et al.* 2001; Lee *et al.* 1995, 1999, 2001). The immunomodulatory role of persistent microchimerism post transfusion and its relationship to the HLA system are areas of active investigation. For the relationship of microchimerism and transfusion-associated GVHD, see Chapter 15.

Effect of previous transfusion on success of renal graft

Patients who have antibodies against HLA antigens of the donor undergo acute rejection of renal allografts. On the other hand, blood transfusion has been shown to have a striking effect in improving the survival of subsequent renal grafts in subjects who have not developed cytotoxic antibodies, or who have done so and have received renal grafts from HLA-compatible donors (Opelz *et al.* 1973; van Hooff *et al.* 1976). Leucocytes in the donor blood have been found to be essential for the beneficial effect (Persijn 1984).

After the introduction of more potent immunosuppression with ciclosporin, transfusions before cadaver grafting were found to confer little additional benefit (Kaban *et al.* 1983; Lundgren *et al.* 1986; Opelz 1987), although a single-centre randomized study attributed pretransplant transfusion benefit to reduced mortality related to immunosuppression (Vanrenterghem *et al.* 1994). However, transfusions improved the 1-year graft survival rate by 8% ($P < 0.01$) in recipients of a one-DR mismatched graft and by 10% ($P < 0.01$) in recipients of a two-DR mismatched graft (Iwaki *et al.* 1990). Two to four transfusions from random donors were sufficient to obtain this effect. This study concluded that despite the use of ciclosporin, the practice of giving deliberate transfusions before grafting should not be abandoned. In a randomized, controlled multicentre trial, cadaver graft survival rate was significantly higher in the 205 recipients who underwent three pretransplant transfusions than in the 218 patients who did not receive transfusions (Opelz *et al.* 1997).

When a kidney from a live donor is used, it is possible to give both transfusion and graft from the same donor. Donor-specific blood transfusions (DSTs) lead to increased graft survival rates (Salvatierra *et al.* 1981, 1986; Kaplan 1984). A disadvantage of DST is that the patient may develop lymphocytotoxic antibodies against donor HLA antigens. In animal models it was found that heat treatment of the donor blood (Martinelli *et al.* 1987), or pre-treatment of the recipient with donor leucocytes coated with anti-lymphocyte antibody, diminished the chance of such immunization (Susal *et al.* 1990). Treatment of the patient with azathioprine also had this effect (Anderson *et al.* 1982).

Several mechanisms have been suggested to explain the beneficial effect of previous blood transfusions on renal graft survival: (1) the induction of increased suppressor cell activity (Marquet and Heystek 1981; Quigley *et al.* 1989); (2) decreased natural killer cell activity (Gascon *et al.* 1984); (3) specific unresponsiveness due to idiotype antibodies, which inactivate T-cell clones (Woodruff and van Rood 1983; Kawamura *et al.* 1989); (4) impairment of the function of the mononuclear phagocyte system (MPS) by iron loading (Akbar *et al.* 1986; de Sousa 1989); (5) deletion of clones of cells, which are first activated by blood transfusion and then killed or inactivated by high-dose immunosuppressive therapy during the anamnestic response after transplantation (Terasaki 1984); and (6) the production of non-cytotoxic, Fc receptor-blocking antibodies (MacLeod *et al.* 1985; Petranyi *et al.* 1988).

Sharing of MHC antigens between donor and recipient has been found to determine the extent of the blood transfusion effect. The survival of kidney grafts in recipients who were given transfusions, and who shared one HLA-DR antigen with the donors, was significantly better (81% at 5 years) than in recipients who were given transfusions from donors mismatched for both DR antigens (57% at 5 years), or in recipients who were not transfused (45%). Immunization occurred less frequently in the recipients who shared one DR antigen with the donor (Lagaaij *et al.* 1989). In another study, sharing of one HLA haplotype (or at least one HLA B and DR antigens) between donor and recipients had a mitigating effect because it led to a specific suppression of the formation of cytotoxic T lymphocytes (CTLs), i.e. to CTL non-responsiveness; recipients of blood from fully identical donors remained CTL responders (van Twuyver *et al.* 1991). Furthermore, transfusion of blood from HLA-identical donors induces the generation of suppressor cell-independent, high-affinity CTL against donor antigens (van Twuyver *et al.* 1994). These mitigating and immunizing effects are donor specific, but the beneficial effect of blood transfusion on kidney survival is also due to a non-specific effect. Transfusion of blood from donors who share one HLA haplotype induces a general decrease in the usage of T-cell Vβ families (Munson *et al.* 1995). These effects are probably due to the survival of donor lymphocytes in the recipient. Studies in mice have shown that sharing of H2 antigens between donor and recipient of a blood transfusion facilitates the persistence of donor lymphoid cells in the recipient, which is associated with tolerance for donor alloantigens. Donor lymphocytes can be detected 10–20 years after transplantation in patients in whom the graft survives for long periods of time. Such chimerism may be important in modulating the immune response (Starzl *et al.* 1992).

Effect of transfusion on tumour growth and recurrence of cancer

A retrospective analysis of the recurrence rate of carcinoma of the colon after surgical resection first suggested that the 5-year disease-free survival rate was reduced by blood transfusion given at the time of surgery (Burrows and Tartter 1982). However, despite numerous subsequent reports, including more than 100 observational studies and three controlled trials, and several meta-analyses, the relationship between blood transfusion, cancer growth and cancer-free survival remains murky and contradictory (Klein 2001). The numerous variables including different tumours, locations, extent of disease, histological grade and modes of treatment make this a particularly difficult area to evaluate.

Prospective randomized clinical studies have been conducted with patients undergoing surgery for colorectal carcinoma. In one large multicentre randomized trial, patients who were operated on because of colorectal cancer and who needed blood transfusion were randomized to an autologous or allogeneic transfusion regimen. At study conclusion, patients received allogeneic blood only (133), autologous and allogeneic blood (66), autologous blood only (112) or no blood at all (164). There were no significant differences between the groups receiving allogeneic blood or autologous blood only: at 4 years, survival rates were 67% and 62%, respectively, and in survivors, no recurrence of cancer in 63% and 66% respectively. On the other hand, many patients did not receive the 'treatment' specified by their prospective treatment assignment, and cancer recurred significantly more frequently in the transfused than in the non-transfused patients. This difference may have been associated with the circumstances that necessitated transfusion (Klein 1999). The red cells transfused in the allogeneic arm were buffy coat depleted as was the routine in the Netherlands at the time. In a second controlled study of colorectal cancer in the Netherlands, leucoreduced red cells were compared with buffy coat-reduced red cells. No significant differences were found between the two trial transfusions in survival, disease-free survival or cancer recurrence rate after an average follow-up of 36 months. Patients who had a curative resection and who received blood of any sort had a lower 3-year survival than non-transfused patients (69% vs. 81%, $P = 0.001$). These observations confirm an association between blood transfusion and poor patient survival, but suggest that the relation is not due to promotion of cancer (Houbiers et al. 1994). The third prospective study of colorectal cancer from a single centre in Germany found that blood transfusion was an independent factor associated with tumour recurrence, and that survival of transfused patients tended to be shorter although the difference was not statistically significant (Heiss et al. 1994). There may well be some subset of patients, perhaps defined by immune status or tumour subtype, that is particularly susceptible to the effects of allogeneic transfusion. Demonstration of such a difference will probably require a large, carefully controlled, prospective study.

Effect of transfusion on postoperative infections

As is the case with cancer, a large number of observational studies find an association between allogeneic blood transfusion and postoperative bacterial infection, while a few do not (Vamvakas and Blachman 2001). For example, Carson and co-workers (1999) conducted a retrospective cohort study of 9598 consecutive patients with hip fracture who underwent surgical repair between 1983 and 1993 at 20 hospitals across the USA. Bacterial infection, defined as bacteraemia, pneumonia, deep wound infection or septic arthritis/osteomyelitis was the primary endpoint and numerous variables were included in the statistical model; a highly significant association was found between serious postoperative infection and transfusion. Chang and co-workers (2000) analysed a database of 1349 patients undergoing elective colorectal surgery for any disease of the colon or rectum at 11 university hospitals across Canada. To adjust for confounding effects associated with remote infections such as pneumonia and urinary tract infections, the study limited the analysis to postoperative wound infection. Allogeneic blood transfusion was a highly significant independent predictor of postoperative wound infection. Vamvakas and Carven (1998) reported a retrospective cohort study of 416 coronary artery bypass graft patients admitted to one hospital. The endpoints were limited to postoperative wound infection or pneumonia, and adjustment was made for the effects of chronic systemic illness and specific risk factors for wound infection or pneumonia. The risk of postoperative wound infection or pneumonia increased by 6% per unit of allogeneic red blood cells (RBCs) and/or platelets transfused, or by 43% for a patient receiving the mean transfusion dose of 7.2 units of either component. Nevertheless, these analyses are inevitably flawed, despite meticulous multivariate testing, by the numerous variables that predispose to postoperative infection (comorbidities, catheters, respirator time, impaired consciousness, etc.), not to mention factors related to the blood components such as storage time and method of preparation (Vamvakas and Carven 1998).

Seven randomized controlled trials compare the incidence of postoperative infection between recipients of buffy coat-reduced (Heiss et al. 1993; Busch et al. 1994; Houbiers et al. 1994; Jensen et al. 1996; van de Watering et al. 1998) or standard allogeneic red cells (Tartter et al. 1998) or whole blood (Jensen et al. 1992) and recipients of autologous or WBC-reduced, buffy coat-reduced allogeneic red cells or whole blood. Two studies (Jensen *et al.* 1992, 1996) reported a significant effect, two studies (Heiss *et al.* 1993; van de Watering *et al.* 1998) reported a marginal effect, and three studies (Busch *et al.* 1994; Houbiers *et al.* 1994; Tartter *et al.* 1998) did not detect an effect. The strengths and weakness of these studies have been analysed exhaustively (Vamvakas and Blachman 2001). However, insufficient data are available to perform the kind of meta-analysis that might help draw conclusions from these studies.

Postoperative mortality

In addition to the possible association between allogeneic transfusion and postoperative infection, van de Watering and co-workers (1998) detected an unexpected association between WBC-containing allogeneic blood transfusion and postoperative mortality from causes other than postoperative infection. In total, 24 out of 306 patients (7.8%) transfused with buffy coat-reduced red cells died, compared with 11 out of 305 patients (3.6%) receiving buffy coat-reduced red cells that were leucoreduced before storage, and 10 out of 303 patients (3.3%) receiving buffy coat-reduced red cells that were leucoreduced after storage ($P = .015$). The overall difference in 60-day mortality was due to a highly significant difference among the three randomization arms. The number of RBC units transfused was the most significant predictor of postoperative mortality. The association between leucocyte-containing allogeneic blood and increased mortality may be limited to cardiac surgery and should not be extended to other clinical settings. At the very least, the finding requires confirmation by a study designed with mortality as the primary endpoint.

Possible role of HLA in habitual abortion

Parental sharing of HLA antigens has been thought to be a cause of habitual abortion. In such cases, noncytotoxic antibodies that are normally produced in the mother and that protect the fetus are absent (Adinolfi 1986; Scott *et al.* 1987).

Immunization of women with leucocytes has been employed with the object of correcting the immunological unresponsiveness (Taylor and Falk 1981; Beer *et al.* 1985). One problem in assessing the benefit of such immunization is that the definition of habitual

abortion varies. Furthermore the chance of a successful pregnancy after three abortions is about 60% (Regan 1991). One prospective randomized trial (Mowbray *et al.* 1987) has shown an apparent benefit; in another trial, no clear advantage of leucocyte injection was observed, and the authors expressed their concern about severe growth retardation seen in some fetuses (Beer *et al.* 1985). The Recurrent Miscarriage Study enrolled women who had had three or more spontaneous abortions of unknown cause in a double-blind, multicentre, randomized clinical trial (Ober *et al.* 1999). In total, 91 women were assigned to immunization with paternal mononuclear cells (treatment) and 92 to immunization with sterile saline (control). The primary endpoints were the inability to achieve pregnancy within 12 months of randomization, or a pregnancy that terminated before 28 weeks of gestation (failure); and pregnancy of 28 or more weeks of gestation (success). Immunization with paternal mononuclear cells did not improve pregnancy outcome in women with unexplained recurrent miscarriage. However, it is possible that a subset of responders might be identified by using some as yet unrecognized laboratory determination or susceptibility factor. Until this is possible, immune therapy in women with habitual abortion should be restricted to clinical trials (Moloney *et al.* 1989).

Tests for HLA alleles, antigens and antibodies

HLA alleles

HLA alleles can be determined directly at the DNA level. The resolution of DNA-based typing is limited only by the available allele-specific probes. The relevant techniques are based on several different principles (see Chapter 3). While the heterogeneity of the MHC has made high-resolution typing problematic for matching donor and recipient for transplantation (Petersdorf *et al.* 2001), the stringency of the HLA role in antigen presentation has made high resolution increasingly desirable for immunotherapy trials.

Anthony Nolan HLA informatics group publishes up-to-date online HLA Class I and II Sequence Alignments (http://www.anthonynolan.com/HIG/data.html).

Sequence-specific oligonucleotides. DNA is amplified in the polymerase chain reaction (PCR) and a set of sequence-specific oligonucleotides (SSOs) is used in a dot-blot or reverse dot-blot hybridization technique to detect allelic sequences (Saiki *et al.* 1986, 1989; Ng *et al.* 1993). Several modifications of this technique have been described (Bidwell 1994). In one, a strand of heat-denatured, amplified DNA is ligated with SSOs by an added ligase. Ligation only occurs when the sequences of the DNA and SSO are identical. The ligated product is detected by enzyme-linked immunosorbent assay (ELISA) (Fischer *et al.* 1995). The techniques permit the identification of alleles, even of those differing from each other by a single nucleotide.

Sequence-specific primers. PCR is performed with a set of sequence-specific primers (SSPs) that will only amplify DNA with sequences complementary to the primers (Olerup *et al.* 1993; Olerup 1994; Bunce *et al.* 1995). A simple and quick SSP test in microplates has been described (Chia *et al.* 1994).

The limitations of both SSO and SSP are requirements for a large number of PCRs to include the known alleles, and the inability to identify polymorphisms unless the variation happens to lie within the region spanned by the assay. These limitations are addressed by nucleotide sequencing of PCR-amplified DNA, the method of choice for 'high-resolution' typing that is required in the selection of an unrelated stem cell donor (Spurkland *et al.* 1993). High-throughput robotic sequence-based typing allows daily sequencing of hundreds of genomic fragments, and high-density array technology promises to permit extensive typing of polymorphisms, both known and unknown, on microchips (Adams *et al.* 2001; Wang *et al.* 2003).

HLA antigens and antibodies

Class I antigens are determined using the lymphocytotoxicity test. Crossreactivity and the lack of specific antisera led to difficulties in HLA typing; several antisera must be used in typing for a particular antigen. In serological typing for DR and DQ antigens, the two-colour fluorescence test or the lymphocytotoxicity test on B cells is applied (see below). These same techniques are used for the detection of class I and class II antibodies respectively. Lymphocytotoxicity is declining in interest in the USA as most laboratories switch to easier, higher resolution molecular methods. However, immunological methods remain valuable to characterize functional aspects of HLA as molecular methods cannot

define whether an HLA allele is expressed or how a sequence correlates with empirically determined antigen importance.

Lymphocytotoxicity test

Complement-dependent cytotoxicity remains the standard test for determining HLA class I antigens. Lymphocytes are incubated with antibody and rabbit complement, and a dye (Trypan blue or eosin) is then added. If the lymphocytes carry an antigen corresponding to the antibody, complement is fixed, the cell membrane is damaged and dye enters and stains the cell (blue or red). The percentage of stained cells is counted. Live cells are unstained, smaller and refractile. It is essential to use a pure lymphocyte suspension, as platelets carry A, B and C antigens and granulocytes are always killed in the cytotoxic assay and stain non-specifically. Details of the NIH-recommended lymphocytotoxicity test, using microdroplets, were published by Terasaki and co-workers (1973).

For the determination of DR and DQ antigens by lymphocytotoxicity, B lymphocytes can be isolated: (1) by removing the T lymphocytes from a lymphocyte suspension by rosetting with Z-aminoethylisothiouronium bromide-treated sheep red cells and centrifugation on Ficoll-hypaque (density 1.077) (Pellegrino *et al.* 1976); (2) by the use of nylon fibre columns (Wernet *et al.* 1977); or (3) by the use of magnetic beads coated with monoclonal antibodies specific for class II epitopes (Vartdal *et al.* 1986).

In the two-colour fluorescence tests the IgG on the B cells is capped with FITC-labelled anti-IgG followed by a cytotoxicity test. The B cells can be distinguished from the T cells by the green IgG cap on their surface. For a description of the technique, see van Rood and van Leeuwen (1976).

The mixed lymphocyte culture

This test was described by Bain and co-workers (1964). The principle is to irradiate or add a substance such as mitomycin C to one sample, usually the donor's, and to mix these lymphocytes with those from another subject such as a potential recipient. Irradiation, or treatment with mitomycin C, prevents lymphocytes from transforming to blast cells but does not destroy their ability to stimulate other lymphocytes. Blast transformation of the untreated lymphocytes indicates that they have recognized a foreign antigen on the treated lymphocytes (Bach and Voynow 1966), and this transformation can be assessed by measuring the incorporation of tritiated thymidine (one-way MLC).

In the MLC, the cells that stimulate are B cells and monocytes carrying Dw determinants and class II antigens. Those that respond are T cells (Potter and Moore 1977).

If irradiated or mitomycin C-treated stimulator cells, homozygous for a Dw determinant (homozygous typing cells, or HT), are used they can only stimulate untreated lymphocytes that do not carry the Dw determinant for which they are homozygous. Thus, panels of HTC are used to identify Dw determinants (Bradley *et al.* 1972).

The two-way MLC, in which the lymphocytes in both samples are able to respond by blast formation, has been used as a final test for HLA identity of donors and recipients of bone marrow who are serologically identical.

HLA antibody detection

Typed repository cell lines are used in a complement-dependent cytotoxicity assay to identify alloantibodies in sera of sensitized subjects. The percentage of cell lines killed by the sera is used as a rough measure of the degree of sensitization or 'panel reactive antibody' (PRA) reactivity. Some antibodies activate complement, yet kill cells inefficiently, a phenomenon known as 'cytotoxicity negative absorption positive' (CYNAP) (Lublin and Grumet 1982). The CYNAP phenomenon may result in underestimation of sensitization. However, augmentation of the assay to increase sensitivity may implicate innocuous antibodies and thus overestimate clinically relevant sensitization. Another method of identifying alloantibodies uses (Le Pendu *et al.* 1986; Le Pont *et al.* 1995) flow cytometry of a variety of microbeads loaded with known HLA alleles (Guertler *et al.* 1984; Moses *et al.* 2000). An interlaboratory comparison of techniques suggests that considerable inconsistencies in serum screening and crossmatching exist among laboratories participating in the American Society for Histocompatibility and Immunogenetics/College of American Pathologists surveys (Duquesnoy and Marrari 2003). The lack of uniformity in test results may limit the usefulness of these methods in a clinical setting.

Other antigens found on leucocytes

Some red cell antigens are also found on leucocytes; see Chapters 4 and 6.

Antigens located on granulocytes (human neutrophil antigens)

Nomenclature: confusion, controversial and evolving

Neutrophil antigens were first characterized using sera collected from neutropenic patients who formed clinically important allo- and autoantibodies. Although the presence of the first granulocyte-specific antigen, NA1, was inferred from the presence of an antibody in a case of neonatal neutropenia in 1960, the antigen was not identified until 1966 (Lalezari *et al.* 1960; Lalezari and Bernard 1966a). As new antigens were discovered, nomenclature threatened to assume some of the quirky randomness that characterized red cell blood group antigens. A new nomenclature was proposed in 1998 by an International Society of Blood Transfusion (ISBT) Working Party to permit separate notations for the phenotype associated with the glycoprotein location and for the alleles, according to the guidelines for human gene nomenclature (Bux 1999). Although the proposed nomenclature has been criticized for including antigens found on cells other than granulocytes, the ISBT proposal represents a sound first attempt at standardization.

In the ISBT nomenclature, antigen systems are referred to as human neutrophil antigens (HNA). The antigen systems, the polymorphic forms of the immunogenic proteins, are indicated by integers and specific antigens within each system are designated alphabetically by date of publication. Alleles of the coding genes are named according to the Guidelines for Human Gene Nomenclature. Neutrophil antigens NA1 and NA2 became HNA-1a and HNA-1b in the new nomenclature and the third antigen reported, NB1 became HNA-2a (Table 13.1).

The HNA-1 system

The neutrophil-specific antigens HNA-1a and -1b (NAl and NA2) are products of alleles that form a biallelic system confined to granulocytes (Lalezari *et al.* 1960; Lalezari and Radel 1974) and NK cells.

Table 13.1 ISBT Human Neutrophil Antigen (HNA) nomenclature.

Antigen system	Antigens	Location	Former name	Alleles
HNA-1	HNA-1a	FcγRIIIb	NA1	FCGR3B*1
	HNA-1b	FcγRIIIb	NA2	FCGR3B*2
	HNA-1c	FcγRIIIb	SH	FCGR3B*3
HNA-2	HNA-2a	CD177 (NB1 gp)	NB1	CD177*1
HNA-3	HNA-3a	70–95 kDa gp	5b	Not defined
HNA-4	HNA-4a	CD11b (CR3)	Mart[a]	CD11B*1
HNA-5	HNA-5a	CD11a (LFA-1)	Ond[a]	CD11A*1

CR3, C3bi receptor; gp, glycoprotein; HNA, human neutrophil antigen; ISBT, International Society of Blood Transfusion; LFA-1, leukocyte function antigen-1.

From Wang E, Marincola FM, Stroncek D. Human leukocyte antigen (HLA) and human neutrophil antigen (HNA) systems. In: Hematology: Basic Principles and Practice (2005), Philadelphia, PA: Elsevier Churchill Livingstone.

Exceptions to the inheritance of the NA antigens first suggested the possibility of a silent allele at the NA locus (Lalezari *et al.* 1975; Clay 1985). The HNA-1 antigens are located on the FcγRIIIb of neutrophils (Huizinga *et al.* 1990). FcγRIIIb on neutrophil membranes is a phosphatidylinositol-linked glycoprotein with a molecular weight of 50–80 kDa (Huizinga *et al.* 1989, 1990).

FcγRIIIb and the HNA-1 antigens are encoded by the FCGR3B gene located on chromosome 1q23–24 within a cluster of two families of the FcγR genes, FcγR2 and FcγR3. The FcγR3 family is made up of FCGR3A and FCGR3B. FCGR3B is highly homologous to FCGR3A, which encodes FcRIIIa. The most important difference between the two genes is a C-to-T change at 733 in FCGR3B, which creates a stop codon in FcγRIIIb. As a result, FCGR3A has 21 more amino acids than FCGR3B, and FCGR3A is a transmembrane rather than a GPI-anchored glycoprotein (Ory *et al.* 1989; Ravetch and Perussia 1989; Huizinga *et al.* 1990; Trounstine *et al.* 1990). FcγRIIIa is expressed only by NK cells and FcRIIIb only by neutrophils (Trounstine *et al.* 1990).

HNA-1a, -1b and –1c polymorphisms. The HNA-1 antigen system consists of the three alleles HNA-1a, -1b and -1c (Bux *et al.* 1997). The antigens are also known as NA1, NA2 and SH (Table 13.1). The gene frequencies of the three alleles vary widely among different racial groups (Hessner *et al.* 1999; Matsuo *et al.* 2001). Among white people, the frequency of the gene encoding HBA-1a, FCGR3B*1, is between 0.30 and 0.37, and the frequency of the gene encoding HNA-1b, FCGR3B*2, is from 0.63 to 0.70. In Japanese and Chinese populations, the FCGR3B*1 gene frequency is from 0.60 to 0.66, and the FCGR3B*2 gene frequency is from 0.30 to 0.33. The gene frequency of the gene encoding HNA-1c, FCGR3B*3, also varies among racial groups. FCGR3B*3 is expressed by neutrophils from 4% to 5% of white people and 25 to 38% of African Americans (Kissel *et al.* 2000).

The FCGR3B*1 gene differs from the FCGR3B*2 gene by only five nucleotides in the coding region at positions 141, 147, 227, 277 and 349 (Ory *et al.* 1989; Ravetch and Perussia 1989; Huizinga *et al.* 1990; Trounstine *et al.* 1990). Four of the nucleotide changes result in changes in amino acid sequence between the HNA-1a and the HNA-1b forms of the glycoprotein. The fifth polymorphism at site 147 is silent. The glycosylation pattern differs between the two antigens because of the two nucleotide changes at bases 227 and 277. The HNA-1a form of FcγRIIIb has six N-linked glycosylation sites and the HNA-1a form has four glycosylation sites.

The gene encoding the HNA-1c form of FγcRIIIb, FCGR3B*3, is identical to FCGR3B*2 except for a C-to-A substitution at amino acid 78 of FcRIIIb (Bux *et al.* 1997). In many cases, FCGR3B*3 exists on the same chromosome with a second or duplicate FCGR3B gene (Koene *et al.* 1998).

Several other sequence variations in FCGR3B have been described. These chimeric alleles have single-base substitutions involving one of the five SNPs that distinguish FCGRB3B*1 and FCGR3B *2. FCGR3B alleles that more closely resembled FCGR3B*2 were found more often in African Americans than in white people or Japanese people (Matsuo et al. 2001).

Function of HNA-1 antigens. The low-affinity FcγRIIIb receptors link humoral and cellular immune function. The FcγRIIIb on effector cells bind cytotoxic IgG molecules and immune complexes containing IgG. Polymorphisms in FcγRIIIb affect neutrophil function. Neutrophils that are homozygous for HNA-1a have a greater affinity for IgG3 than do those that are homozygous for HNA-1b (Nagarajan et al. 1995). Neutrophils from subjects homozygous for HNA-1b phagocytize erythrocytes sensitized with IgG1 and IgG3 anti-Rh monoclonal antibodies and bacteria opsonized with IgG1 less efficiently than do granulocytes homozygous for HNA-1a (Bredius et al. 1994).

FcγRIIIb deficiency. Blood cells from patients with paroxysmal nocturnal haemoglobinuria (PNH) lack the GPI-linked glycoproteins and their granulocytes express reduced amounts of FcγRIIIb and the HNA-1 antigens (Huizinga et al. 1990). Genetic deficiency of granulocyte FcγRIIIb and the HNA-1 antigens has been reported. With inherited deficiency of FcγRIIIb, the FCGR3B gene is deleted along with an adjacent gene, *FCGR2C* (De Haas et al. 1995). Despite the primary role of FcγRIIIb in neutrophil function, deletion of the entire *FcγRIIIB* gene results in no obvious clinical abnormality. Although most subjects who lack FcγRIIIb appear healthy, too few have been studied to ensure that no subtle alteration in immune function is present. In a study of 21 *Fc*γRIIIb subjects with FcγRIIIb deficiency, two were found to have autoimmune thyroiditis and four had sustained multiple episodes of bacterial infections (De Haas et al. 1995).

FCGR3B polymorphisms and disease associations

Several studies suggest that FCGR3B polymorphisms affect the incidence and outcome of some autoimmune and inflammatory diseases. Children with chronic immune thrombocytopenic purpura were more likely to be FCGR3B*1 homozygous than were control subjects (Foster et al. 2001), but Spanish patients with systemic lupus erythematosus were more likely to be FCGR3B*2 homozygous (Gonzalez-Escribano et al.

2002). Myasthenia gravis is more severe in FCGR3B*1 homozygous patients (Raknes et al. 1998), but multiple sclerosis is more benign in FCGR3B*1 homozygous patients (Myhr et al. 1999). Patients with chronic granulomatous disease who are FCGR3B*1 homozygous are less likely to develop major gastrointestinal or urinary tract infectious complications compared with those who are heterozygous or FCGR3B*2 homozygous (Foster et al. 1998). As FCGR3B is clustered with FCGR3BA and FCGR2B on chromosome 1q22, some of these findings may reflect in part linkage disequilibrium among Fc receptors.

The HNA-2 system

The HNA-2 system has one well-described allele, HNA-2a (NB1) expressed only on neutrophils, metamyelocytes and myelocytes (Stroncek et al. 1998a). The 58- to 64-kDa glycoprotein that carries HNA-2a (NB1 gp) is located on neutrophil plasma membranes and in secondary granules, and is linked to the plasma membrane by a glycosylphosphatidylinositol (GPI) anchor. HNA-2a is expressed on 45–65% of circulating neutrophils; expression is greater on neutrophils from women than from men (Stroncek et al. 1996; Matsuo et al. 2001). Pregnant women express HNA-2a more strongly than do healthy female blood donors (Caruccio et al. 2003). Expression of HNA-2a decreases with age in women, but remains constant in men. Administration of G-CSF to healthy subjects can increase the proportion of neutrophils expressing HNA-2a to near 90% (Stroncek et al. 1998b). Monoclonal antibodies specific to HNA-2a have been clustered as CD177. The role of CD177 in neutrophil function is unknown. Women who lack NB1 gp are healthy. Although the expression of HNA-2a is reduced on neutrophils from patients with PNH and chronic myelocytic leukaemia (CML), no clinical significance has been attributed to this observation.

HNA-2 polymorphisms. HNA-2a is expressed on neutrophils by approximately 97% of white people, 95% of African Americans and 89–99% of Japanese people (Matsuo et al. 2000; Taniguchi et al. 2002). HNA-2a has been reported to have an allele, NB2, but the product of this gene cannot be identified reliably with alloantisera, and no monoclonal antibody specificity for NB2 has been identified (Stroncek et al. 1993a). The HNS-2a-negative neutrophil phenotype is due to a CD177 transcription defect Kissel. HNA-2a genes from two women with HNA-2a-negative neutrophils, who produced HNA-2a-specific alloantibodies have been studied and CD177 cDNA sequences were present in both women. Sequencing of cDNA prepared from neutrophil mRNA demonstrated accessory sequences in the lengths coding CD177.

The HNA-3 system

The HNA-3 antigen system has one antigen HNA-3a that was previously known as 5b. HNA-3a is expressed by neutrophils, lymphocytes, platelets, endothelial cells, kidney, spleen and placental cells (van Rood and Ernisse 1968) and weakly expressed on red cells (Rosenfield *et al.* 1967). The gene encoding HNA-3a is located on chromosome 4 (van Kessel *et al.* 1983), but has not yet been cloned. The nature and function of the 70–95 kDa gp is unknown. Potent anti-HNA-3a agglutinins in transfused plasma can cause transfusion-related acute lung injury (TRALI) (see Chapter 15).

HNA-4 and HNA-5 systems

The HNA-4 and HNA-5 antigens are located on the β_2 integrins. Each system contains only a single antigen, HNA-4a and HNA-5a. The HNA-4a antigen, previously known as Mart[a], has a phenotype frequency of 99.1% in white people (Kline *et al.* 1982). HNA-4a is expressed on granulocytes, monocytes and lymphocytes, but not on platelets or red blood cells. HNA-4a has been located on the αM chain (CD11b) of the receptor CR3. Neonatal alloimmune neutropenia has been caused by antibody to HNA-4a, but this is the exception rather than the rule (Fung *et al.* 2003). A second polymorphism of the β_2 integrins, HNA-5a, previously Ond[a] with a frequency of 95%, is located on the α-chain of the leucocyte function-associated antigen (LFA-1, CD11a) molecule (Simsek *et al.* 1996).

Other granulocyte-specific antigens

Other granulocyte-specific antigens are ND1, NE1 and LAN (Lalezari and Radel 1974; Verheugt *et al.* 1978; Claas *et al.* 1979; Rodwell *et al.* 1991). Like the NA antigens, LAN is located on the FcγRIIIb (Metcalfe and Waters 1992). Another high-frequency antigen,

also located on the FcγRIIIb, was described by Bux and colleagues (1994). The antigen NC1 (Lalezari and Radel 1974) is identical with HNA-1b (Bux *et al.* 1995a). Most granulocyte-specific antigens have been defined by alloantibodies, but ND1 and NE1 were defined by autoantibodies. These granulocyte-specific antigens appear to be true differentiation antigens, as they appear at the myelocyte or metamyelocyte stage or even later (Lalezari 1977; Evans and Mage 1978).

Antigens on granulocytes and monocytes

The following antigens have been shown to be present on granulocytes and monocytes: HGA-1 (Thompson *et al.* 1980) and the HMA-1 and HMA-2 antigens, products of a biallelic gene (Jager *et al.* 1986). The AYD antigen is shared by granulocytes, monocytes and endothelial cells (Thompson and Severson 1980). The 9a antigen, which was first thought to be granulocyte specific, is also expressed on monocytes (Jager *et al.* 1986).

Antibodies to neutrophil antigens

Antibodies to neutrophil antigens may be responsible for five different clinical syndromes: (1) neonatal allo- and isoimmune neutropenia; (2) autoimmune neutropenia; (3) transfusion-related alloimmune neutropenia; (4) pulmonary infiltrates following transfusion (TRALI); and (5) febrile reactions following transfusion. The last two conditions are discussed in detail in Chapter 15. Transfusion-related alloimmune neutropenia is probably a variant of TRALI and appears to be rare (Wallis *et al.* 2002).

Neonatal alloimmune neutropenia

This syndrome, analogous to haemolytic disease of the newborn (HDN), is usually recognized when infection in a newborn infant is found to be accompanied by severe neutropenia. Neutrophil antigens in the fetus that are inherited from the father but foreign to the mother provoke formation of maternal IgG antibodies that cross the placenta and react with the neonate's neutrophils (Lalezari and Bernard 1966b). Absolute neutrophil counts typically range from 0.100 to 0.200 $\times$ 10^9/l. Bone marrow examination reveals myeloid hyperplasia. The syndrome is self-limited, but may persist from days to weeks as passive antibody is cleared (Bux *et al.* 1992). Treatment with IVIG or recombinant cytokines such as granulocyte colony-stimulating factor (G-CSF) has met with variable success (Maheshwari *et al.* 2002).

In reviewing the syndrome, Lalezari and Radel (1974) described results in 19 infants from 10 families. The specificity of the antibody in three families was anti-HNA-1a; in two, anti-HNA-1b; in four, anti-HNA-2a; and in one, not determined. In four of the families the first-born infant was affected. Antibodies of other specificities have been implicated, but much less frequently (Stroncek 2002).

A prospective survey of some 200 pregnant women, either primiparae at term or multiparae, in which the woman's serum was tested against her partner's granulocytes and lymphocytes, indicated that the incidence of neutrophil antibodies was about 3% (Verheugt *et al.* 1979). The incidence of diagnosed cases of neonatal alloimmune neutropenia is much lower.

Neonatal isoimmune neutropenia

Subjects who lack a membrane glycoprotein due to deletion of the gene encoding the glycoprotein may form strong antibodies (named isoantibodies) against non-polymorphic determinants on the glycoprotein. Severe neonatal neutropenia caused by maternal isoantibodies may occur in infants from mothers with a deletion of the FcγRIIIb gene (Huizinga *et al.* 1990; Stroncek *et al.* 1991; Cartron *et al.* 1992; Fromont *et al.* 1992).

Autoantibodies to granulocytes

The first convincing case that implicated autoantibodies as the cause of neutropenia involved a female infant who had severe infections and was found at the age of 7 months to have a neutrophil count of $1.0 \times 10^9/l$. The peripheral blood contained fewer than 3% mature neutrophils and the bone marrow revealed virtually no mature granulocytes, although it did contain normal granulocyte precursors. The patient's serum contained the neutrophil-specific autoantibody anti-HNA-1b with a titre of 16–256. The antibody was mainly IgG and the patient was HNA-1b positive. After steroid therapy, the granulocyte count rose to $310 \times 10^9/l$ and the leucoagglutinin titre fell to 2, but the patient relapsed when steroids were discontinued (Lalezari

et al. 1975). The syndrome is now well established (McCullough 1988; Bux *et al.* 1998).

Autoimmune neutropenia (AIN) in children is traditionally divided into two forms. In so-called 'primary' AIN, neutropenia is the sole abnormality and, although neutrophil counts may fall below 0.500/l, bacterial infections, when they occur, are generally benign. Primary AIN is commonly diagnosed between the ages of 5 and 15 months, but has been observed as early as day 33 of life (Bux *et al.* 1998). Spontaneous remission occurs in 95% of the patients within 7–24 months. A high percentage of autoantibodies (35–86%) bind preferentially to granulocytes from HNA-1a and HNA-1b homozygous donors, but other specificities have been found (Bux *et al.* 1998; Bruin *et al.* 1999). The bone marrow is typically normocellular or hypercellular, with a variably diminished number of segmented granulocytes. For severe infections or prior to surgery, G-CSF, corticosteroids and IVIG (19 mg/kg per day) can effect neutrophil increases of 50–100% and each has been used successfully in many cases (Pollack *et al.* 1982; Bussel and Lalezari 1983; Bux *et al.* 1998).

Secondary AIN occurs in association with other autoimmune diseases. In contrast with primary AIN, infections are usually more severe and the autoantibody is more commonly directed against FcγRIIIb (Shastri and Logue 1993; Bruin *et al.* 1999).

Drug-induced immune granulocytopenia

Mechanisms responsible for drug-induced immune neutropenia are similar to those involving red cells (see Chapter 7). The classic case of pyramidon-induced granulocytopenia described by Moeschlin and Wagner (1952) is an example of the mechanism in which the drug does not bind firmly to the cells, but in which drug, antibody and a determinant on the cell membrane form a trimolecular complex. Although quinine is usually implicated in drug-induced thrombocytopenia, it may be involved rarely in cases of drug-induced neutropenia in which the quinine antibodies react with the same glycoprotein as anti-HNA-2a, and/or an 85-kDa glycoprotein (Stroncek *et al.* 1994). Drug-induced neutrophil antibodies may be directed against a metabolite of the drug (Salama *et al.* 1989). Recombinant G-CSF has reportedly shortened the period of granulocytopenia in some of these cases.

Reactions to granulocyte transfusions

Granulocyte transfusion recipients sometimes produce antibodies specific to HNA-1a, HNA-1b and HNA-2a (see also Chapters 14 and 15). Further transfusion of granulocytes to patients with these antibodies may lead to severe febrile and pulmonary transfusion reactions (Stroncek 1996). Haematopoietic progenitor cell transplant recipients who produce HNA-2a antibodies as a result of granulocyte transfusions have experienced marrow graft failure (Stroncek *et al.* 1993b).

Tests for granulocyte antibodies and antigens

The following techniques are used in detecting granulocyte-specific antibodies: (1) granulocyte agglutination; (2) immunofluorescence; (3) chemiluminescence; and (4) monoclonal antibody-specific immobilization of granulocyte antigen assays.

The granulocyte agglutination technique

Pure granulocyte suspensions are prepared by dextran sedimentation followed by centrifugation of the supernatant on Ficoll-hypaque (density 1.077). The contaminating red cells in the granulocyte pellet at the bottom of the tube are lysed with ammonium chloride or distilled water. Alternatively, granulocytes can be isolated by double-density gradient centrifugation. Agglutination techniques are carried out in microplates.

Granulocytes, in contrast to red cells and platelets, are agglutinated by two different mechanisms:

1 Like red cells and platelets granulocytes are agglutinated by crosslinking of cells by IgM antibodies.

2 An entirely different mechanism is responsible for agglutination of granulocytes by IgG antibodies. In this case, agglutination results from a response to sensitization by an antibody that requires active cell participation. Sensitization does not lead to immediate agglutination but to the formation of pseudopods. The granulocytes migrate towards each other until membrane contact is established (Lalezari and Radel 1974). This process is time and temperature (37°C) dependent. Agglutination may be due to changes in membrane-bound molecules that cause granulocytes to adhere to each other, or to IgG antibodies on one granulocyte that adhere to Fc receptors on other granulocytes. In any case, both IgM and IgG antibodies can

be detected by the granulocyte agglutination test. Both granulocyte-specific and HLA-A, -B and -C antibodies are detected, but HLA antibodies are better detected by the lymphocytotoxicity test.

Granulocyte immunofluorescence technique

Purified suspensions of granulocytes are prepared as described above. The granulocytes are fixed with paraformaldehyde, incubated with the serum to be tested, then washed and finally incubated with fluorescein isothiocyanate-labelled anti-Ig serum. The Fab or F(ab')$_2$ fragments of the IgG fraction of anti-human Ig are used because whole IgG anti-Ig tends to bind to the Fc receptor on granulocytes. With the above modifications, the fluorescein-labelled anti-globulin test is more sensitive than granulocyte agglutination for the detection of IgG antibodies (Verheugt *et al.* 1977).

Using flow cytometry for the granulocyte immunofluorescence technique (GIFT) instead of microscopy, there is no need for isolating granulocytes, as granulocytes can be identified according to light scatter patterns. Furthermore, granulocytes, platelets and lymphocytes can be tested simultaneously (Robinson *et al.* 1987). Flow cytometry has been found to be slightly more sensitive for the detection of granulocyte antibodies than the GIFT (Sintnicolaas *et al.* 1991).

Both granulocyte-specific and HLA-A, -B and -C antibodies are detected in the GIFT. The lymphocytotoxicity test (LCT) and the immunofluorescence test are more sensitive for the detection of HLA class I antibodies. If a serum is negative in these tests but positive in the GIFT, the serum is very likely to contain granulocyte-specific antibodies. If the tests on lymphocytes are positive and if it is necessary to ascertain whether granulocyte-specific antibodies are present, the serum should be absorbed with pooled platelets to remove any HLA class I antibodies or the serum must be tested with a granulocyte panel typed for granulocyte-specific antigens. Unfortunately, positive reactions with lymphocytes particularly in the immunofluorescence test may be due to lymphocyte-specific antibodies, in which case it may be difficult to ascertain the presence of granulocyte-specific antibodies, unless a known specificity is detected.

With the GIFT, not only antibodies but also pre-formed immune complexes cause positive reactions, due to adherence to Fc and complement receptors (Camussi *et al.* 1979; Engelfriet *et al.* 1984). There are three possible ways of distinguishing between antibodies and fixed immune complexes:

1 Preparation of an eluate from positively reacting granulocytes. Eluted antibodies will again react with granulocytes while immune complexes are usually dissociated by the elution procedure (Helmerhorst *et al.* 1982).

2 Testing the serum under investigation in an ADCC assay on granulocytes.

3 Blocking Fc receptors on target granulocytes with monoclonal antibodies (Engelfriet *et al.* 1984). In practice, it is difficult to distinguish between autoantibodies and bound immune complexes, because there are seldom enough cells to prepare an eluate and because the results of the ADCC assay on patients' granulocytes are difficult to interpret.

Chemiluminescence test

To prepare suspensions of mononuclear cells and granulocytes, fresh EDTA blood is centrifuged on Ficoll-hypaque (density 1.077). The mononuclear cell fraction is washed three times. The red cell/granulocyte fraction is resuspended in PBS and mixed 1:4 with dextran solution. After sedimentation (30 min) the granulocytes in the supernatant are packed and then washed twice in PBS. The granulocytes are resuspended in PBS and transferred to a glass tube pre-located in a waterbath at 52°C and after 2 min are allowed to cool in another tube at room temperature. The purpose of the heat treatment is to render the granulocytes incapable of responding to immunoglobulin aggregates in the sera to be tested which would lead to non-specific generation of chemiluminescence.

For the assay, granulocytes are incubated with serum and then washed in phosphate-buffered solution (PBS) and resuspended in Hanks' BSS. The granulocytes are then incubated with freshly prepared mononuclear cells from the peripheral blood and with luminol. Chemiluminescence is generated as a result of phagocytosis of sensitized granulocytes, which leads to the formation of oxygen radicals and oxidation of luminol. Chemiluminescence is measured in a luminometer (Hadley and Holburn 1984). The sensitivity of the chemiluminescence (CL) test is similar to that of the GIFT (Lucas 1994).

Phenotyping and genotyping of neutrophil antigens

Phenotyping. By tradition, neutrophil antigen typing has been performed using human alloantibodies in the granulocyte agglutination or GIFT assay. However, alloantisera are difficult to obtain. Monoclonal antibodies specific to HNA-1a, HNA-1b and HNA-2a have been described and are available commercially. These reagents have been used to phenotype neutrophils by flow cytometry. This method is faster and easier than manual methods with alloantibodies, as whole blood rather than isolated neutrophils can be used.

Genotyping. As alloantibodies are difficult to obtain and monoclonal antibodies are not available for all neutrophil antigens, genotyping assays have gained importance. Genotyping assays are performed with DNA isolated from whole blood, thus eliminating the need to isolate granulocytes. Furthermore, leucocyte DNA can be stored for months before testing is performed. The characterization of the genes encoding HNA-1 antigens has led to the development of assays for these antigens (Bux *et al.* 1995b; Hessner *et al.* 1996). Genotyping of HNA-1 antigens is particularly valuable given the rarity of alloantibodies to HNA-1c and the absence of monoclonal antibodies. Genotyping for FCGR3B alleles is complicated by the high degree of homology between FCGR3B and FCGR3A. Among the five nucleotides that differ between FCGR3A*1 and FCGR3A*2, FCGR3A is the same as FCGR3A*1 at three nucleotides and the same as FCGR3A*2 at two nucleotides. As a result, most laboratories use PCR and sequence-specific primers to distinguish FCGR3A alleles. A unique set of primers is used to amplify each of the three alleles.

Unfortunately, HNA-2a genotyping reagents are not available. The HNA-2a-negative phenotype is caused by CD177 mRNA splicing defects (Kissel *et al.* 2002). However, no mutations have been detected in the CD177 genomic DNA from subjects with HNA-2a-negative neutrophils. It may be possible to distinguish positive and negative phenotypes by analysing CD177 mRNA for accessory sequences, but this is a highly sophisticated methodology.

Antigens found only on lymphocytes

In addition to HLA antigens (see above) to some red

cell antigens (see Chapter 5), 5a and HNA-3a antigens, and antigens also present on granulocytes and monocytes, lymphocytes carry antigens that do not occur on other cells.

Two biallelic systems, one on Tγ cells with the antigens TCA1 and TCA2, and one on Tμ cells with the antigens TCB1 and TCB2 have been defined (van Leeuwen *et al.* 1982a). Non-HLA antigens only expressed on activated T cells have been described (Gerbase *et al.* 1981; Wollman *et al.* 1984). The clinical significance of alloantibodies against lymphocyte-specific antigens is uncertain, but a case of alloimmune lymphocytopenia of the newborn, due to maternal alloantibodies and resulting in severe combined immune deficiency has been reported (Bastian *et al.* 1984).

Cold autoantibodies to lymphocytes

Anti-I and anti-i. See Chapter 4.

Lymphocyte autoantibodies reactive at 37°C in vitro

Single cases of (1) hypogammaglobulinaemia with cytotoxic autoantibodies against B cells reactive at 37°C and (2) acquired hypogammaglobulinaemia with autoantibodies specific for T-helper cells, leading to increased activity of T-suppressor cells, have been described (Tursz *et al.* 1977).

Antibodies against various subsets of lymphocytes have been described in patients with AIDS and may contribute to the decline in the CD4+ T-cell count.

Antigens found only on monocytes

In addition to HLA class I and class II antigens, and the antigens shared by monocytes and granulocytes mentioned above, monocytes carry alloantigens that do not occur on other blood cells. Some of these antigens (EM antigens) are also present on endothelial cells (Moraes and Stastny 1977; Claas *et al.* 1980; Cerilli *et al.* 1981; Stastny and Nunez 1981); others are monocyte specific (Cerilli *et al.* 1981; Baldwin *et al.* 1983; Paul 1984). Antibodies against EM antigens are detrimental to transplanted kidneys and may be involved in GvHD. EM antibodies and antibodies reacting with monocytes, tubular endothelium and kidney cells in the cortex can be eluted from rejected kidneys

(Joyce *et al.* 1988). The significance of monocyte-specific alloantibodies needs further evaluation.

Antigens of platelets

Antigens shared with other cells

HLA antigens

Platelets possess mRNA encoding HLA class I molecules and are capable of synthesizing them. Only a small proportion of the A, B and C antigens on platelets are absorbed from the plasma (Santoso *et al.* 1993a). The number of some of the class I antigens on platelets varies greatly in different subjects. Class II antigens are not detectable on platelets but HLA-DR antigens can be induced at the platelet surface by stimulation with cytokines, for example gamma-interferon, both *in vitro* and *in vivo* (Boshkov *et al.* 1992).

Red cell antigens also found on platelets

ABH, Lewis, I, i and P antigens on platelets are described in Chapter 4. Using a sensitive two-stage radioimmunoassay the major antigens of the Rh, Duffy, Kell, Kidd and Lutheran systems have been shown to be absent from platelets (Dunstan *et al.* 1984).

Antigens found only on platelets (platelet-specific antigens)

Several systems have been defined whose antigens are found on glycoproteins of platelets. Some of these antigens are found on other cells such as endothelial cells as well. The human platelet antigen (HPA) nomenclature system was adopted in 1990 (von dem Borne and Decary 1990). The HPA nomenclature categorizes all alloantigens expressed on the platelet membrane, except those encoded by genes of the major histocompatibility complex. A platelet-specific alloantigen is called a HPA when its molecular basis has been defined. The different HPAs are grouped in systems based on having alloantibodies defining a given alloantigen and its 'antithetical' alloantigen. A large number of antigens have been described and the molecular basis of many has been resolved. To date, 24 platelet-specific alloantigens have been defined by immune sera, of which 12 are grouped into six biallelic systems (HPA-1, -2, -3, -4, -5, -15) (Table 13.2 and Metcalfe *et al.*

Table 13.2 Human platelet antigens (HPAs).

System	Antigen	Original names	Glycoprotein	CD
HPA-1	HPA-1a	Zw^a, Pl^{A1}	GPIIIa	CD61
	HPA-1b	Zw^b, Pl^{A2}		
HPA-2	HPA-2a	Ko^b	GPIb$^\alpha$	CD42b
	HPA-2b	Ko^a, Sib^a		
HPA-3	HPA-3a	Bak^a, Lek^a	GPIIb	CD41
	HPA-3b	Bak^b		
HPA-4	HPA-4a	Yuk^b, Pen^a	GPIIIa	CD61
	HPA-4b	Yuk^a, Pen^b		
HPA-5	HPA-5a	Br^b, Zav^b	GPIa	CD49b
	HPA-5b	Br^a, Zav^a, Hc^a		
	HPA-6bw	Ca^a, Tu^a	GPIIIa	CD61
	HPA-7bw	Mo^a	GPIIIa	CD61
	HPA-8bw	Sr^a	GPIIIa	CD61
	HPA-9bw	Max^a	GPIIb	CD41
	HPA-10bw	La^a	GPIIIa	CD61
	HPA-11bw	Gro^a	GPIIIa	CD61
	HPA-12bw	Iy^a	GPIb$^\beta$	CD42c
	HPA-13bw	Sit^a	GPIa	CD49b
	HPA-14bw	Oe^a	GPIIIa	CD61
HPA-15	HPA-15a	Gov^b	CD109	CD109
	HPA-15b	Gov^a		
	HPA-16bw	Duv^a	GPIIIa	CD61

From Metcalfe *et al.* (2003).

2003). For the remaining 12 antibodies, alloantibodies against the antithetical antigen have yet to be discovered. The molecular basis of 22 out of the 24 serologically defined antigens has been resolved. In all but one, the difference involves a single amino acid substitution generally caused by a single nucleotide polymorphism (SNP) in the gene encoding the relevant membrane glycoprotein. The systems are numbered in the order of the date of publication and the antigens are designated alphabetically in the order of their frequency in the population. This nomenclature has been criticized, the main objection being that HPA-1a, HPA-4a, HPA-6a, HPA-7a and HPA-8a are five different names for identical GPIIIa molecules carrying these high-frequency antigens. Only the GPIIIa molecules that carry the low-frequency antigens of these systems differ from each other due to amino acid substitutions at different positions of the molecule (Newman 1994).

HPA-1 system (Zw, Pl^A)

The first system to be described was recognized by van Loghem and co-workers (1959) when a serum was found that agglutinated some samples of platelets but not others; the antigen was named Zw^a when an antithetical antigen (Zw^b) was recognized (van der Weerdt *et al.* 1962, 1963). Anti-Pl^{A1} (Shulman *et al.* 1961) was subsequently shown to have the same specificity as anti-Zw^a. The system is now named HPA-1 and the antigens, HPA-1a and HPA-1b. Ninety-eight per cent of white people are HPA-1(a+) and 27% HPA-1 (b+).

The HPA-1 gene has two alleles, HPA-1a and HPA-1b. Anti-HPA-1a is associated with most cases of post-transfusion purpura and neonatal alloimmune thrombocytopenia (NATP).

HPA-1a and -1b antigen sites are situated on the membrane glycoprotein IIIa (Kunicki and Aster 1979; van der Schoot and von dem Borne 1986). The HPA-1 polymorphism results from the substitution of a single basepair in the coding DNA at position 33, coding for leucine in HPA-1a and for proline in HPA-1b (Newman *et al.* 1989). Patients with Glanzmann's thrombocytopenia type I have no detectable membrane glycoprotein IIIa (or IIb) on their platelets and are therefore unable to express the HPA-1 antigens (Kunicki *et al.* 1981; van Leeuwen *et al.* 1981).

The HPA-1 polymorphism is not found in Japanese people (Shibata *et al.* 1986b).

HPA-2 system (Ko)

A second biallelic system, Ko (HPA-2), was described by van der Weerdt and co-workers (1962). In total, 16% of subjects were found to be HPA-2(b+) (Ko(a+)) and 99% were HPA-2(a+) (Ko(b+)). Like anti-HPA-1a, anti-HPA-2a and -2b were detected by platelet agglutination. The HPA-2 antigens are situated on GPIb/IX (Kuijpers *et al.* 1989). The polymorphism involves substitution of a single nucleotide in the DNA at position 434, which codes for the β-chain of GPIb, to give methionine in HPA-2b and threonine in HPA-2a at position 145 (Kuijpers *et al.* 1992a). A platelet antigen Sib^a, described by Saji and co-workers (1989), was shown to be identical to Ko^a (Kuijpers *et al.* 1989).

HPA-3 system (Bak, Lek)

The platelet antigen, Bak^a (HPA-3a) is present in about 90% of the Dutch population (von dem Borne *et al.* 1980). The first example of anti-HPA-3a was responsible for NATP. An antigen, Lek^a, at first found to be closely associated serologically with Bak^a (Boizard 1984) was subsequently shown to be identical (von dem Borne and van der Plas-van Dalen CM 1985). HPA-3a is present on glycoprotein IIb (Kieffer *et al.* 1984; van der Schoot and von dem Borne 1986). The antigen HPA-3b, antithetical to HPA-3a, was described independently by Kickler and co-workers (1988a) and Kiefel and co-workers (1989a). In both cases, anti-HPA-3b was responsible for post-transfusion purpura. The HPA-3 polymorphism is also due to the substitution of a single basepair in the coding DNA, to give isoleucine at amino acid residue 843 in HPA-3a and serine in HPA-3b (Lyman and Aster 1990).

HPA-4 system (Pen, Yuk)

Another biallelic system, Yuk (HPA-4) was described by Shibata and co-workers (1986a,b). Both the low-frequency antigen Yuk^a (HPA-4b) and the high-frequency antigen Yuk^b (HPA-4a) were detected with antibodies that caused NATP.

The antigen, Pen^a, that had been described by Friedman and Aster (1985), proved to be identical to Yuk^b (RH Aster and Y Shibata, unpublished observation). HPA-4a is present on GPIIIa (Furihata *et al.* 1987; Santoso *et al.* 1987). The HPA-4 polymorphism has not been found in white people (Friedman and Aster 1985; Kiefel *et al.* 1988). The Yuk polymorphism involves substitution of a single nucleotide in the DNA which encodes the GPIIIa protein, coding for arginine at position 526 in HPA-4a and for glutamine in HPA-4b (Wang *et al.* 1991).

HPA-5 system (Br, He, Zav, Tu^a, Ca^a Mo^a, Sr^a, Max^a, La^a, Gro^a, Iy^a, Sit^a, Oe^a)

The antigens Br^a (HPA-5b) and Br^b (HPA-5a) were described by Kiefel and co-workers (1988, 1989a). The HPA-5 antigens are present on glycoprotein Ia (Kiefel *et al.* 1989a; Santoso *et al.* 1989). Anti-HPA-5a and -5b have been responsible for NATP.

Most HPA-5 antibodies are non-reactive in the immunofluorescence test because of the low number of antigenic sites (Kiefel *et al.* 1989b). HPA-5 antibodies can best be detected by the MAIPA, a glycoprotein-specific assay (see below). The polymorphism involves substitution of a single nucleotide in the cDNA at position 1648, to give glutamine in HPA-5a and lysine in HPA-5b at position 505 (Santoso *et al.* 1993b). The biallelic Zav system described by Smith and co-workers (1989) is identical with the HPA-5 system and the antigen Hca is the same as HPA-5b (Woods *et al.* 1989). Tu/Ca (HPA-6bw), a low-frequency antigen located on GPIIIa and involved in NATP was at first named Tu^a (HPA-6b) (Kekomaki *et al.* 1993). It is identical to Ca^a described by McFarland and co-workers (1993). The polymorphism involves a single nucleotide substitution at position 1564 to give 489 glutamine in HPA-6a and 489 arginine in HPA-6b (Wang *et al.* 1993b). The antigen Mo (HPA-7bw), involved in NATP, is located on GPIIIa and due to a C–G substitution at position 1267 in the cDNA, resulting in a substitution of proline by alanine at position 407 (Kuijpers *et al.* 1993). Sr^a (HPA-8b) has so far been detected in only one family, in which it was involved in NATP. The antigen is located on GPIIIa and is due to the substitution at position 636 of cysteine (in HPA-8b) for arginine (normally present in GPAIIIa) (Kroll *et al.* 1990; Santoso *et al.* 1994). Max^a (HPA-9bw), a low-frequency alloantigen responsible for NATP, is located on GPIIb and the polymorphism is due to a single nucleotide substitution G→A at position 2603 (Noris et al. 1995). HPA-11bw (Gro[a]) is located on GPIIIa and involved in NATP. It has so far been found in only a single family. A guanine for adenine mutation was found, predicting an arginine→histidine substitution at position 633 of the mature glycoprotein (Simsek et al. 1997). The antigen ly (HPA-12 bw) is a low-frequency antigen located on the glycoprotein Ib/IX complex. Anti-Iy[a] was the cause of severe NATP (Kiefel et al. 1995). Sit[a] (HPA-13bw), a low-frequency antigen in the German population, was identified in a severe case of neonatal alloimmune thrombocytopenia. Sit(a) epitopes reside on platelet GPIa. A threonine→methionine substitution at the 799 position is responsible for formation of the Sit(a) alloantigen, and diminished platelet aggregation responses of Sit(a)(+) individuals indicate that the Thr(799)Met mutation affects the function of the GPIa–IIa complex (Santoso et al. 1999). Oe[a] (HPA-14bw), a low-frequency alloantigen responsible for a case of neonatal NATP, has been assigned to platelet GPIIIa. Molecular studies suggest that Oe[a] arose as a result of a mutational event from an already mutated GPIIIa allele (Santoso et al. 2002).

HPA-15 system (Gov, Duv)

A biallelic system with the alleles Gov[a] (HPA-15b) and Gov[b] (HPA-15a) was reported by Kelton and co-workers (1990). Anti-Gov[a] was found in a patient with post-transfusion purpura. The Gov antigens are expressed on the CDw 109 protein (Smith et al. 1995). Anti-Duv(a+), directed against an antigen HPA-16bw (Duv[a]) on glycoprotein GPIIIa has been implicated in a case of neonatal thrombocytopenia. Sequencing of the exons 2–15 of GPIIIa revealed a single base substitution 517C→T (complementary DNA) present in a heterozygous state in DNA from the father leading to amino acid substitution of threonine for isoleucine at position within the Arg-Gly-Asp binding domain of GPIIIa (Jallu et al. 2002).

Obsolete systems and systems not yet included in the HPA nomenclature

DUZO. Moulinier (1957), using the antiglobulin consumption technique, demonstrated a platelet antibody in the serum of a woman whose four children had died from neonatal purpura. The corresponding antigen was termed 'DUZO'. However, no second example of anti-DUZO has been found and this antigen has therefore become obsolete.

PlE system. The two alleles of this system (Pl[E1] and Pl[E2]) were defined by Shulman and co-workers (1964). This system has not been included in the HPA nomenclature because anti-Pl[E1] was probably an isoantibody from a patient with Bernard–Soulier syndrome and anti-Pl[E2] is no longer available (Shulman 1987).

PlT antigen. An antigen, Pl[T], with a very high frequency was described by Beardsley and co-workers (1987). It is present on glycoprotein V.

Nak[a]. The antigen Nak[a] is absent in 3–11% of Japanese people and is present on GPIV (Ikeda et al. 1989). However, the Nak antigen appears to be a non-polymorphic determinant of GPIV, Nak(a–) subjects being deficient for GPIV. Anti-Nak therefore is not an alloantibody, but an isoantibody (Yamamoto et al. 1990).

Va[a]. The low-frequency antigen Va[a], involved in NATP, is located on GPIIIa (Kekomaki et al. 1992).

Presence of platelet-'specific' antigens on other cells

The antigens of the HPA-1 system are present on endothelial cells (Leeksma et al. 1987; Giltay et al. 1988a). HPA-1a has also been detected on vascular smooth muscle cells and fibroblasts (Giltay et al. 1988b).

As mentioned above, the HPA-5 antigens are present on the Ia–IIa glycoprotein complex, which is also expressed on activated T cells (Santoso et al. 1989; Woods et al. 1989). This GP complex is also known as VLA2 (very late activation antigens 2) (Pischel et al. 1988). The HPA-5 antigens are probably also present on endothelial cells, which express VLA-2.

Alloimmunization to platelet antigens

Role of HLA class I antibodies in refractoriness to platelet transfusions

When no measures are taken to reduce the number

of leucocytes in red cell or platelet concentrates, 80–100% of patients, depending upon the disease, may develop HLA antibodies; only 40–70% patients treated with immunosuppressive regimens become immunized (Howard and Perkins 1978; Dutcher *et al.* 1980, 1981). In the great majority of immunized patients, the alloantibodies are directed against HLA class I antigens (Schiffer *et al.* 1976). Primary immunization occurs as early as 10 days after transfusion, although 3–4 weeks is more usual; reappearance of lymphocytotoxic antibodies appeared as early as 4 days in previously sensitized subjects. In total, 62% of women with acute myelocytic leukaemia and previous pregnancies became alloimmunized following transfusion during cytoreductive therapy (Trial to Reduce Alloimmunization to Platelets Study Group 1997). HLA alloimmunization does not necessarily correlate with the number or schedule of transfusions, at least when multiple transfusions are administered. When the number of leucocytes in the transfused cell concentrate is reduced, the percentage of immunized patients decreases, and at levels of $1–5 \times 10^6$ or fewer, primary immunization against HLA class I antigens is prevented (see below).

The presence of HLA class I antibodies in a patient's serum does not equate with refractoriness to platelet transfusions. The frequency of most HLA antigens is low and antibodies against them may not react with the platelets of any randomly chosen donors or may react with only a few of them. Furthermore, some class I antigens may be expressed so weakly on the donor platelets that they survive normally, or nearly normally, in a patient with antibodies against them. Furthermore, patients with alloantibodies against HLA class I antibodies may form anti-idiotype antibodies that react with and inactivate the class I antibodies. For this reason refractoriness to platelet transfusions may be overcome in spite of continued transfusions of incompatible platelets (Atlas *et al.* 1993). In a significant percentage of alloimmunized patients, evidence of alloimmunization declines or disappears with time (Lee and Schiffer 1987; Murphy *et al.* 1987). Nevertheless, 10–20% of patients in large prospective and retrospective series of thrombocytopenic patients treated for malignancy become alloimmune refractory following transfusion therapy (Trial to Reduce Alloimmunization to Platelets Study Group 1997; Seftel *et al.* 2004).

Role of platelet-specific antibodies

Even when HLA-matched platelets, either from close relatives or from random donors, are transfused, 19% of recipients became refractory (Schiffer 1987). In most cases refractoriness was probably related to HLA incompatibilities that went undetected rather than to antibodies to platelet-specific antigens, because the latter occur almost exclusively in patients who are strongly immunized to HLA class I antigens. Using the MAIPA, platelet-specific antibodies were found in 25% (9 out of 36) of patients with high levels of HLA immunization (Schnaidt *et al.* 1996). This figure corresponds well with the observation that transfusions of HLA-compatible platelets are unsuccessful in about 20% of HLA-immunized patients (Saji *et al.* 1989).

Prevention of alloimmunization to HLA class I antigens

There is strong evidence that the leucocytes in the platelet concentrate rather than the platelets evoke the formation of antibodies against histocompatibility antigens (Welsh *et al.* 1977; Claas *et al.* 1981; van Marwijk *et al.* 1991). Formation of such antibodies occurs if the platelets are contaminated with leucocytes, but platelets alone are capable of inducing a secondary immune response (Gouttefangeas *et al.* 2000). Although foreign antigen is presented to helper T cells by the subject's own HLA class II-positive antigen-presenting cells (APCs), the induction of a primary immune response to foreign class I antigens must be presented by class II-positive APCs of the donor (Lechler and Batchelor 1982; Sherwood *et al.* 1986). Dendritic cells are probably the class II-positive donor cells responsible for antigen presentation (Deeg *et al.* 1988). Thus alloimmunization against class I antigens should be prevented when class II-positive cells have been either removed from red cell or platelet concentrates or inactivated.

Removal of leucocytes

An early study showed that patients transfused with platelet concentrates from which most of the leucocytes have been removed, for example by passage through cotton wool filters, were substantially less likely to become refractory to transfusion of platelets

(Eernisse and Brand 1981). This observation has been frequently confirmed (Murphy *et al.* 1986; van Marwijk *et al.* 1991). A multi-institutional, randomized, blinded trial was conducted to determine whether transfusion of platelets from which leucocytes had been removed by a filter before storage would prevent the formation of platelet alloantibodies and refractoriness to platelet transfusions. Patients who were receiving induction chemotherapy for acute myeloid leukaemia were randomly assigned to receive one of four types of platelet transfusions: unmodified, pooled platelet concentrates from random donors (control); filtered, pooled platelet concentrates from random donors (F-PC); ultraviolet B-irradiated, pooled platelet concentrates from random donors (UVB PC); or filtered platelets obtained by apheresis from single random donors (F-AP). All patients received transfusions of filtered, leucocyte-reduced red cells. Of 530 patients with no alloantibodies at the trial initiation, 13% of those in the control group produced lymphocytotoxic antibodies and their thrombocytopenia became refractory to platelet transfusions, compared with 3% in the F-PC group, 5% in the UVB-PC group and 4% in the F-AP group ($P = 0.03$ for each treated group compared with the control subjects). Lymphocytotoxic antibodies were found in 45% of the controls, compared with 17–21% in the treated groups ($P < 0.001$ for each treated group compared with the control subjects). Reduction of leucocytes by filtration and ultraviolet B irradiation of platelets was equally effective in preventing alloantibody-mediated refractoriness to platelets during chemotherapy for acute myeloid leukaemia. Platelets obtained by apheresis from single random donors provided no additional benefit compared with pooled platelet concentrates from random donors (Trial to Reduce Alloimmunization to Platelets Study Group 1997). Universal pre-storage leucoreduction (ULR) of red cell and platelet products has been performed in Canada since August 1999. In a retrospective analysis of 13 902 platelet transfusions in 617 patients undergoing chemotherapy for acute leukaemia or stem cell transplantation before ($n = 315$) and after ($n = 302$) the introduction of ULR, alloimmunization was significantly reduced (19–7%) in the post-ULR group. Alloimmune platelet refractoriness was similarly reduced (14–4%). Fewer patients in the post-ULR group received HLA-matched platelets (14% vs. 5%). Thus leucocyte reduction (see below) reduces

alloimmunization, refractoriness and requirements for HLA-matched platelets when applied as routine transfusion practice to patients receiving chemotherapy or stem cell transplant (Seftel *et al.* 2004). While the total number of platelet transfusions was also reduced after ULR, this was probably related to other factors such as a reduction in the platelet transfusion trigger.

As might be expected, following the transfusion of leucocyte-poor platelet concentrates, the development of platelet refractoriness is much more common in patients who have been transfused previously or have been pregnant, which confirms the suspicion that secondary immune responses to HLA class I antigens cannot be prevented (Brand *et al.* 1988; Novotny *et al.* 1995; Sintnicolaas *et al.* 1995). However, in the two large studies, alloimmunization and alloimmune refractoriness in patients who were previously pregnant or transfused were also reduced after ULR (Trial to Reduce Alloimmunization to Platelets Study Group 1997; Seftel *et al.* 2004).

Counting small numbers of leucocytes

The small numbers of residual leucocytes in filtered concentrates (1–3 cells/μl) can be determined accurately either by flow cytometry, after staining the nucleated cells with propidium iodide (Wenz *et al.* 1991), or by using a large-volume counting chamber, for example the Nageotte chamber (Masse *et al.* 1991). In trials in 20 laboratories, the detection limits for the flow cytometry and NC techniques were 0.1 and 1 leucocyte/μl respectively. Both methods are suitable for assessing the adequacy of leucodepletion filters. Sampling error and instrument precision remain hurdles for all proposed methods. Issues involving counting technique and guidelines for process control of leucoreduced blood components have been published (Dumont *et al.* 1996; Dzik 2000).

Filters for whole blood and red cell concentrates

There is ample evidence that primary HLA immunization does not occur, or occurs only rarely, when fewer than 5×10^6 leucocytes are transfused (Sirchia *et al.* 1982; Saarinen *et al.* 1990; Novotny *et al.* 1995). To avoid primary immunization, the total number of leucocytes transfused in a red cell or platelet concentrate must therefore be less than this number. For red cells and whole blood collections, the only practical method of achieving this level is by filtration, using cotton wool, cellulose acetate, porous polycarbonate or polyester. Current high-performance leucocyte reduction filters can decrease contaminant leucocytes by 4–5 logs (van der Meer *et al.* 1999).

Filtration is a complicated process that is influenced by factors such as temperature (Beaujean *et al.* 1992), the speed of the blood flow through the filter (Sivakumaran *et al.* 1993) and the prefiltration white cell count (Sirchia *et al.* 1982). Lymphocytes and monocytes are captured passively in the small pores of the filter network, but granulocytes are removed by both adherence, particularly by interaction with platelets adhering to the filter, and trapping (Steneker and Biewenga 1991; Steneker *et al.* 1992). These variables explain why results of filtration, even with the same filter, may vary considerably (Pietersz *et al.* 1998).

The quality of filters has improved progressively and results obtained in three studies confirm that numerous commercially available filters are capable of achieving levels of residual leucocytes that qualify blood components as leucoreduced (Rebulla *et al.* 1993; Bontadini *et al.* 1994; van der Meer *et al.* 1999). Red cell concentrates filtered through any of these filters contain $< 5 \times 10^6$ residual leucocytes and even $< 1 \times 10^6$. Unexpectedly, no clear correlation emerged between the original and the residual number of leucocytes. The results with current filters are far better than those with earlier filters (Table 13.3). Despite the reliability of filters and careful attention to laboratory technique, no combination of filter and technique eliminates alloimmunization (Kao *et al.* 1995a).

Filters for platelet concentrates

Platelet transfusion components may be leucoreduced during apheresis collection with blood cell processors licensed for this purpose (Gambro Spectra; Baxter Amicus) or by filtration. Platelets tend to adhere to polyester and cellulose acetate and these substances must be specially treated if platelet recovery after filtration is to be satisfactory. In a multicentre study of filtration at the bedside, 11–39% of platelets were lost from apheresis concentrates and 11–29% from pooled platelet concentrates. The number of residual leucocytes exceeded 5×10^6 in 7% of apheresis concentrates and in 5% of pooled concentrates. The number correlated with the prefiltration leucocyte count (Kao *et al.* 1995b).

Platelet function does not appear to be adversely affected by filtration (Holme *et al.* 1989; Bertolini *et al.* 1990; Dumont *et al.* 2001).

Should red cell concentrates and platelet concentrates be leucodepleted as a routine?

The removal of leucocytes not only reduces primary immunization against HLA class I antigens but prevents most febrile transfusion reactions as well. Leucocyte reduction effectively reduces the load of cytomegalovirus in platelet concentrates and leucoreduction is used in many institutions to reduce the risk of cytomegalovirus transmission to susceptible patients (see Chapter 15). Although some physicians prefer to use units that test seronegative for cytomegalovirus (CMV) for cytomegalovirus-seronegative haematopoietic

Table 13.3 Results obtained with polyester flat-bed filters.

Filter	No. of residual leucocytes ($\times 10^6$) in red cell concentrates		Authors
	Standard	Buffy coat-poor	
Sepacell R-500	2–4		Reverberi and Menini (1990)
	8		Korner *et al.* (1992)
	1.5 (0.65–35)	0.3 (0.02–6)	Mass *et al.* (1992)
		9.1 (4.6–13.6)	Pietersz *et al.* (1992)
Leukostop	1–4		Reverberi and Menini (1990)
	12		Koerner *et al.* (1991)
		11.3 (1.5–12.1)	Pietersz *et al.* (1992)
Pall RC 50	4		Koerner *et al.* (1991)
	2.7 (0.02–47)	0.3 (0.02–6)	Masse *et al.* (1992)
		8.8 (3.9–13.7)	Pietersz *et al.* (1992)

progenitor transplant recipients, neither testing nor leucoreduction eliminates transmission and both result in equivalently 'safe' components (Bowden *et al.* 1995; Nichols *et al.* 2003). Leucocyte reduction may also reduce red cell alloimmunization and the postulated immunosuppressive effect of transfusion (Blumberg and Heal 1996; Vamvakas and Blajchman 2001; Blumberg *et al.* 2003). On the other hand, filters are expensive, they do not prevent secondary immunization in patients who have been primarily immunized by previous pregnancy or transfusion and result in a 10–15% loss of the processed component. Furthermore, the presence of HLA antibodies does not always render patients refractory to transfusions from randomly chosen donors, nor does CMV transmission injure the vast majority of blood recipients. Several European countries and Canada have adopted universal leucoreduction of blood components, whereas the USA and Japan have opted to target this therapy to patients with specific indications.

A prospective case–control study was implemented in which all patients admitted over a 1-year period for open heart surgery at a single hospital were given leucoreduced blood components. Clinical outcomes were measured prospectively and compared to a historical cohort of patients from the previous year when leucoreduced blood components were not used routinely. A highly significant reduction in the mean postoperative length of stay was seen in the study group ($n = 645$ vs. control group $n = 501$; 10.1 vs. 9.5 days; $P = 0.005$). No significant changes were seen in the rate of mediastinitis, operative mortality or length of stay in the intensive care unit. The postoperative length of stay among study patients who did not receive transfusion was the same as that of control patients who received no transfusion. The reason for the shortened hospital stay is unexplained (Fung *et al.* 2004).

Using a retrospective, before-and-after design shortly after universal leucocyte reduction was mandated in Canada, Hébert and co-workers (2003) studied patients who had undergone cardiovascular or hip surgery or who were in an intensive care unit after surgical intervention. In a parallel study, Fergusson and co-workers (2003) studied neonates with birthweights of less than 1250 g in a neonatal intensive care unit. The former study demonstrated that the introduction of universal leucoreduction was associated with modest reductions in fever, antibiotic usage and mortality, although these outcomes did not result from

any decrease in serious infections. The latter study found a modest improvement in morbidity associated with the introduction of universal leucoreduction in neonates, but no significant reductions in bacteraemia or in neonatal intensive care unit mortality.

In contrast, a prospective, controlled clinical trial of conversion to universal leucocyte reduction was conducted in a large tertiary care hospital in the USA. Patients with established medical indications for leucocyte-reduced blood, some 11%, were excluded from randomization. All other patients who required transfusion were assigned at random to receive either unmodified blood components or stored leucocyte-reduced red cells and platelets. All eligible patients (2780) were enrolled. The three specified primary outcome measures did not differ between the two groups: (1) in-hospital mortality (8.5% control; 9.0% WBC reduced); (2) hospital length of stay after transfusion (median number of days, 6.4 for control and 6.3 for leucocyte reduced); and (3) total hospital costs (median, $19 500 for control and $19 200 for leucocyte reduced). Nor did the several secondary outcomes (intensive care length of stay, postoperative length of stay, antibiotic usage and readmission rate) differ between the two groups (Dzik *et al.* 2002). The reasons for the disparity in results between this study and the studies by Hébert and co-workers and Fergusson and co-workers are unclear, but may involve differences in the patient groups or study designs.

In summary, leucocyte reduction produces superior quality blood components, albeit at a significant cost and some loss of component during processing. Some patients benefit from leucoreduced transfusions and many of these, such as the anaemic patient who will eventually require transplantation for leukaemia, will not be identified before several transfusions are administered. Inadvertent immunization or exposure to CMV might be avoided with universal leucoreduction. For the majority of patients, benefits are difficult to measure, yet disadvantages are few, and no physician is likely to insist upon leucoreplete blood. Arguments against universal application emphasize the high cost and meagre improvement in health outcome measures (Corwin and AuBuchon 2003).

Preparation of leucoreduced components: best to avoid the bedside

When leucodepletion filters are used, the case for

preparing red cell or platelet concentrates in the laboratory ('pre-storage') rather than at the bedside ('post storage') is overwhelming. Routine filtration at the bedside is unreliable. In a multicentre study the use of red cell concentrates filtered in this way, and therefore not controlled for the number of residual leucocytes, resulted in only a small, statistically insignificant reduction in the incidence of HLA class I antibodies (Williamson *et al.* 1994). In a comparison of 30 procedures carried out by each method, 13% of red cell concentrates filtered at the bedside had more than 5×10^6 leucocytes compared with none of the concentrates prepared in the laboratory (Sprogoe-Jakobsen *et al.* 1995). Pre-storage leucoreduction, performed under controlled conditions in the blood collection centre, should reduce the filtration failures, documented at about 5% in clinical trials (Novotny *et al.* 1995b; Kao *et al.* 1995; Popovsky 1996). Hypotensive reactions associated with post-storage leucocyte reduction are described in Chapter 15.

One author's (HGK) personal experience with bedside filtration includes the discovery of unused filters in the nursing station (post transfusion) and the revelation that some outpatient personnel use syringes to force blood through the filters to reduce transfusion time – an innovative but impermissible practice that results in unsatisfactory, leucocyte-replete transfusions.

Inactivation of HLA class II-positive cells

HLA class II-positive cells, notably donor dendritic cells, which are essential for the induction of a primary alloimmunization against HLA class I antigens, can be inactivated by exposure to ultraviolet B (UV-B) irradiation (Lindahl-Kiessling and Safwenberg 1971). Dogs that received three transfusions of blood from a bone marrow donor before transplantation invariably rejected the marrow graft, but marrow grafts were not rejected by dogs that had received UV-B irradiated donor blood (Deeg *et al.* 1986). Furthermore, of 12 dogs that received eight weekly transfusions of UV-B irradiated platelet concentrates from random donors, only one became refractory, whereas 18 out of 21 dogs that received non-irradiated platelets became refractory (Slichter *et al.* 1987). Addition of non-irradiated dendritic cells to UV-B irradiated blood restored the ability to immunize canine recipients. UV-B irradiated dendritic cells had no such effect (Deeg 1989). In clinical trials, UV-B has been found to be as effective as

leucocyte reduction in reducing HLA sensitization (Trial to Reduce Alloimmunization to Platelets Study Group 1997). No instrument has been licensed for UV-B irradiation of blood.

Use of single donor platelets collected by apheresis

Platelets from single donors have not been clearly established as superior to platelets from random donors in delaying alloimmunization. In dogs that are given weekly transfusions of platelet pools derived from six animals, refractoriness occurred earlier than in dogs that received platelets from each of the six animals separately (Slichter *et al.* 1986). In two clinical studies, alloimmunization occurred less frequently with single donor platelets (Sintnicolaas *et al.* 1981; Gmur *et al.* 1983). On the other hand, single donor platelets did not delay alloimmunization in acute leukaemia patients in a separate study (Vicariot *et al.* 1984). When leucocyte-reduced components are used, single donor platelets do not appear superior to pooled platelet concentrates for the prevention of alloimmunization (Trial to Reduce Alloimmunization to Platelets Study Group 1997).

Management of alloimmunized patients

Poor response to platelet transfusion (refractoriness) is not always caused by immune incompatibility. A less than anticipated *in vivo* platelet recovery and survival may be caused by a variety of recipient-related factors such as infection, splenomegaly, intravascular coagulation, massive transfusion, medications (particularly heparin), as well as by a platelet component of poor quality (see also Chapter 14). These causes should be excluded while the question of platelet compatibility is being investigated.

As mentioned above, alloimmunization is not equivalent to refractoriness. Furthermore, even when a patient is alloimmunized and refractory, alloantibodies frequently become undetectable over the course of time; tests for antibodies should therefore be repeated periodically. If the antibodies disappear, the patient may again respond to platelets from random donors (see above). Because patients may have a poor increment to a single transfusion but respond well to subsequent transfusions, a diagnosis of refractoriness to platelet transfusion should be withheld until two or more ABO-compatible transfusions, stored less than 72 h, result in poor increments. Patients who are refractory to platelet transfusions as defined above and express antibodies associated with platelet destruction are considered to be 'immune refractory' (Schiffer *et al*. 2001).

Use of ABO-compatible platelets

In dealing with immune refractoriness, the first step is to use fresh (< 72 h old), single donor, ABO-compatible platelets (Lee and Schiffer 1989). Platelets, like red cells and other tissues, express ABH antigens on surface glycoproteins and glycosphingolipids (Mollicone *et al*. 1988). An early study showed that recovery averaged 67% with ABO-compatible platelets but only 19% with ABO-incompatible platelets, and that the subsequent survival of the incompatible platelets was shortened (Aster 1965). In a series of thrombocytopenic patients who had become refractory to platelet transfusion, a relatively small difference was found between the survival of all ABO-compatible and -incompatible platelets, but the authors pointed out that such factors as the recipients' anti-A or -B titres and the amount of A and B on the platelets probably affect the results (Duquesnoy *et al*. 1979). By way of illustration, ABO-incompatible platelets were rapidly destroyed in group O recipients with potent IgG anti-A or -B (Brand *et al*. 1986). However, platelets of A_2 donors were not destroyed in O recipients (Skogen *et al*. 1988). When the A and B antigen expression on platelets of 100 group A_1 and group B blood donors was measured, 7% and 4%, respectively, expressed A and B antigen levels consistently beyond two standard deviations of the mean ('high expressers'). Serum A_1- and B-glycosyltransferase levels of A and B high expressers were significantly higher than those of group A_1 and B individuals with normal expression. Immunochemical studies demonstrated high levels of A antigen on various glycoproteins from high-expresser platelets, especially GPIIb and PECAM (CD31) (Curtis *et al*. 2000). Among A_1 platelet donors, ABH expression varies significantly, although for any given donor expression is stable (Cooling *et al*. 2004). Unlike A_2 red cells, A_2 platelets express a Bombay-like phenotype with low or undetectable A and H antigens, which makes these donors, along with the 5% A_1 low expressers, an additional resource for alloimmunized recipients (Cooling *et al*. 2004). When a group O

Japanese patient responded poorly to 2 out of 12 ABO-incompatible, HLA-matched platelet transfusions, 20-fold levels of group B substance were measured on the platelets of the incompatible donors. Seven per cent of 313 Japanese donors have been characterized as high expressers of A or B antigen (Ogasawara *et al*. 1993).

In patients given ABO-identical platelets from the start, the platelet count increment was significantly higher than with ABO-incompatible platelets, and fewer patients became refractory (Heal *et al*. 1993a). These favourable results were not seen with platelets that were merely ABO compatible, probably due to the effect of passively acquired anti-A and -B from the donor plasma (Heal *et al*. 1993b).

Use of HLA-matched platelets

Because most alloantibodies responsible for refractoriness in immunized patients have HLA specificity, the use of HLA-compatible platelets improves the results of transfusion in most refractory patients. Because of the weak expression of HLA-C antigens on platelets, matching is performed for HLA-A and HLA-B antigens only; matching for HLA-C antigens does not further improve the increment (Duquesnoy *et al*. 1977). If the specificity of the recipient's HLA-A or HLA-B antibodies (or both) can be determined, the incompatible antigens can be avoided. Unfortunately, it is often impossible to define the specificity, which leaves the use of HLA-matched platelets as the only alternative.

Improved results when using HLA-matched platelets have been demonstrated repeatedly. The first such study demonstrated that HLA-alloimmunized refractory patients responded well to platelets from matched, related donors (Yankee *et al*. 1969). In one large prospective study of refractory patients, 16 out of 22 transfusions of HLA-matched platelets were successful, compared with 10 out of 21 with HLA-mismatched transfusion. The number of mismatches (1–4) made no difference (Moroff *et al*. 1992). Nevertheless, adequate increments are achieved in only 50–60% of alloimmunized refractory patients when HLA-matched platelets are used (Engelfriet *et al*. 1997).

The enormous polymorphism of the HLA-A and -B antigens implies that a very large number of HLA-typed plateletpheresis donors must be available. Some 2500 typed donors are needed to ensure that HLA-matched platelets are available for most refractory patients (Bolgiano *et al.* 1989). Even so, for unusual HLA types, identifying a perfectly matched unrelated donor is often impossible. Other strategies have been adopted to find the best possible match. To expand the search, matching criteria of donor–recipient pairs are based on shared public epitopes assigned to crossreacting groups (CREGS, see above) or shared amino acid polymorphisms defined through sequence information (Duquesnoy *et al.* 1990; Duquesnoy and Marrari 1997). Highly sensitized recipients represent a particularly challenging problem. Mismatching for one or two crossreactive HLA class I antigens was found to have no adverse effect in one study (Duquesnoy *et al.* 1977). However, in another, results with platelets mismatched for one crossreactive antigen were no better than with platelets mismatched for an HLA-A or -B antigen, due presumably to antibodies against the crossreactive antigen (Moroff *et al.* 1992). An alternative approach to the exclusion of alloreactive determinants is the inclusion of 'acceptable' antigen mismatches expressed in panels of cells that give negative reactions with the recipient sera, a technique developed for organ transplantation to extend the repertoire of possible donors (Claas *et al.* 1999).

Recently, Duquesnoy (2002) described a molecular-based algorithm to identify histocompatible pairs called HLAMatchmaker. This method focuses on the structural basis of HLA class I polymorphism, so that compatible HLA mismatches can be identified without extensive serum screening. This algorithm is based on the principle that short amino acid sequences (triplets) characterizing polymorphic sites of the HLA molecules are critical components of allosensitizing epitopes. As each HLA molecule expresses a characteristic string of these determinants each molecule can be characterized according to the linear sequence of amino acid triplets present on its surface. Based on the assumption that patients cannot be immunized by triplets in their own HLA repertoire, donors with HLA alleles different from the recipient's, but containing shared triplets are identified. These HLA alleles should be compatible, as they do not contain any epitope absent in the recipient.

Most HLA molecules span conserved domains so that only 142 different polymorphic triplets designate serologically defined HLA-A, -B and -C antigens. Triplet polymorphism can occur in 30 locations on HLA-A, 27 in HLA-B and 19 in HLA-C chains. Using the HLAMatchmaker, it is possible to broaden significantly the number of 'molecularly matched' HLA alleles and increase the chances of identifying a compatible platelet donor particularly in those cases when the recipient has a rare HLA phenotype. Preliminary results in a retrospective series of allo-immunized platelet recipients confirm the algorithm's usefulness (Nambiar *et al.* 2003).

Selection of compatible donors by crossmatching

Several techniques have proved suitable for crossmatching. In 14 patients who did not respond to transfusions of random platelets, satisfactory increments were observed in 95% of transfusions of platelets compatible by ELISA (see below) and in 91% of transfusions compatible by platelet immunofluorescence test (PIFT) (see below). In 11 patients with broadly reacting HLA antibodies, the increments after platelets that were compatible in a crossmatch by a radiolabelled antiglobulin test were about eight times greater at 1 h and some 30 times greater at 24 h than with crossmatch incompatible platelets (Kickler *et al.* 1988b). Another satisfactory technique is the mixed red cell adherence assay (see below). Using this technique, none of 11 transfusions of crossmatch-positive platelets produced a satisfactory increment, contrasted with 20 out of 21 transfusions of crossmatch-negative platelets (Rachel *et al.* 1988). Satisfactory results with this technique have been reported by others (O'Connel and Schiffer 1990; O'Connell *et al.* 1992). The results of using this method of crossmatching correlated sufficiently with the post-transfusion increment in one study that when crossmatch-negative platelets were available, the use of HLA-matched platelets produced no further benefit (Friedberg *et al.* 1994).

Two rapid methods of crossmatching have been described: in the first platelets are incubated with the patient's serum, then washed and incubated on microtitre plates with anti-IgG-coated latex particles. After centrifugation of the plates, a pellet indicates a negative reaction and smooth coating of the wells, a positive reaction (Ramos *et al.* 1992). In the second assay, donor platelets are solubilized with detergent and the glycoproteins in the lysate are absorbed onto polystyrene latex beads that are agglutinated by a serum that contains antibodies to the donor platelets. The coated beads can be stored at −70°C for long periods. Results obtained with this test correlate well with post-transfusion increment (Ogden *et al.* 1993).

In summary, compatible platelets that produce a satisfactory increment may be found for immunized patients even when antibodies react broadly. If cross-matching is to be applied, the most practical solution is to establish a large panel of plateletpheresis donors whose platelet samples can be stored and cross-matched with the serum of immunized patients in need of platelet transfusions. The choice of HLA-matched or HLA-compatible donors and donors selected by crossmatching, or donors selected by both methods, for the management of alloimmunized patients depends on the resources available to the laboratory.

Use of acid-treated platelets

Platelets were treated with citric acid according to Sugawara and co-workers (1987) to remove HLA class I antigens. *In vivo* recovery of acid-treated platelets in two healthy subjects was excellent and the survival time was 6.25 days compared with 7.95 days for untreated platelets. In alloimmunized patients the post-transfusion increment was comparable to that of HLA-compatible platelets (Shanwell *et al.* 1991).

Treatment with IVIG, RhIg and splenectomy: alloimmune differs from autoimmune

The administration of high-dose IVIG or RhIg and splenectomy may increase the platelet count in ITP (see Chapter 14). For the occasional immunologically refractory patient, high-dose IVIG appears to improve platelet increments, especially after transfusion of HLA-compatible platelets (Zeigler *et al.* 1991; Chen *et al.* 1995). However, most refractory patients will derive little or no benefit from this manoeuvre (Schiffer *et al.* 1984; Kickler *et al.* 1990). Rh immune globulin in a dose of 20 µg/kg neither improved platelet response nor prevented alloimmunization in acute leukaemia undergoing induction chemotherapy (Heddle *et al.* 1995). Splenectomy is equally ineffective (Slichter *et al.* 2005). In a study of splenectomy on the response to random donor platelet transfusion in 15 multi-transfused thrombocytopenic patients, eight patients responded poorly, with low corrected platelet count increments at 1 and 24 h post transfusion. These patients were clinically refractory and had lymphocy-totoxic antibody in their sera. All eight responded well

to HLA-matched transfusions. In contrast, of seven splenectomized patients who responded well to random donor platelets, five had no evidence of alloimmunization and two had 'weak' antibody reactivity.

Neonatal thrombocytopenia

From 17 weeks' gestation, fetal platelet count normally exceeds $150 \times 10^9/l$. However, almost one-quarter of pre-term infants may have a lower count (Castle *et al.* 1986). The platelet count usually reaches a nadir by day 4 and resolves by day 10. The frequency of thrombocytopenia in full-term infants is less than 1%, and few of these neonates suffer adverse events unless a maternal alloantibody is directed against fetal platelet-specific antigens (Burrows and Kelton 1993). The numerous causes of neonatal thrombocytopenia include allo- and autoimmune disease, infections and a variety of congenital chromosomal and non-chromosomal disorders. The most serious consequence of thrombocytopenia in the fetus and neonate is intracranial haemorrhage, which can occur *in utero* as early as 18 weeks' gestation. The secret to perinatal prevention of intracranial haemorrhage is early diagnosis and treatment, occasionally *in utero* (see below). Cordocentesis under ultrasonic guidance and platelet transfusions have revolutionized the management of thrombocytopenia for neonates suspected to be at risk. Maintenance of a 'normal' platelet count following delivery does not reduce neonatal morbidity and mortality (Andrew *et al.* 1993). However, aggressive management of the bleeding neonate, prophylaxis of the neonate whose count falls to $20 \times 10^9/l$ or below and transfusion prior to invasive procedures are generally accepted tenets of treatment for neonatal thrombocytopenia.

Neonatal alloimmune thrombocytopenia

This syndrome, first described by Moulinier (1957), was attributed to destruction of platelets of the fetus or the newborn by maternal IgG alloantibodies specific for platelet antigens by van Loghem and co-workers (1959). Neonatal alloimmune thrombocytopenia is the platelet equivalent of hae-molytic disease of the newborn. In large prospective studies, neonatal alloimmune thrombocytopenia (NATP) has been identified at a frequency of 1 in 350 to 1 in 1800 births (Durand-Zaleski *et al.* 1996; Uhrynowska *et al.* 2000).

NATP is the commonest cause of severe thrombocytopenia in the first few days of life, resulting in 400–600 cases in the UK each year (Burrows and Kelton 1993). Unlike HDN, it often occurs in first-born infants. The typical picture is of a generalized petechial rash developing minutes to hours after birth. Haematomas are common and bleeding from the gastrointestinal, upper respiratory or urinary tracts may occur. Intracranial haemorrhage develops in 15–40% of cases and may result in death (10%) or persistent neurological damage (25%), which may become apparent only after a period of time (McIntosh et al. 1973; Naidu 1983; Mueller-Eckhardt et al. 1989a). The severity of the thrombocytopenia often increases in the first 48 h of life, possibly as a result of rapid postnatal maturation of the monocyte macrophage system (Shulman et al. 1964). Nevertheless, severe thrombocytopenia may occur early during gestation and intracranial haemorrhage may develop in utero (see below). The thrombocytopenia usually lasts for a few weeks after birth, but may persist much longer.

In principle, demonstration of platelet-specific (IgG) alloantibodies in the maternal serum is essential in diagnosis. However, the antibodies may not be detectable at the time of delivery and, in any case, because of the insensitivity of available tests, negative results do not exclude their presence. When no antibodies can be detected, tests for relevant platelet-specific antigens in the father, the mother and the infant may help to make the diagnosis. Genotyping of the infant is now possible by molecular techniques even if no platelets are available. In some cases, antibodies that are undetected in the maternal serum at delivery may become detectable after 3–6 months. It is important to ascertain that the mother is not thrombocytopenic, as maternal platelet autoantibodies may also cause neonatal thrombocytopenia.

In white patients, the majority of severe cases are caused by anti-HPA-1a (Shulman et al. 1964; von dem Borne et al. 1981; Durand-Zaleski et al. 1996; Uhrynowska et al. 2000). In one series, this antibody was detected in the serum of 147 (73.9%) of 199 HPA-1(a–) mothers who gave birth to an infant suspected of having NATP. In contrast, platelet-specific alloantibodies were detected in only 19 (5.5%) out of 348 HPA-1(a+) mothers whose children were thrombocytopenic at the time of birth. In 15 out of the 19, anti-HPA-5b was detected. This antibody is therefore the second most frequently responsible for NATP (Mueller-Eckhardt 1991). Thirty-nine cases of NATP due to anti-HPA-5b have been described (Kaplan et al. 1991).

Most other platelet-specific antibodies have occasionally been involved. In a prospective study the incidence of platelet-specific antibodies was studied in 933 mothers and their infants who were typed for the HPA-1, -2, -3 and -5 antigens. Anti-5b was found by far the most frequently (17 cases) but none of the infants had NATP. Evidently anti-HPA-5b only rarely causes NATP presumably due to the low number of antigenic sites on the platelet membrane (Panzer et al. 1995).

HLA class I antibodies are often detected in the serum of mothers of infants with NATP but it seems unlikely that HLA antibodies cause NATP. Most class I antibodies are adsorbed onto fetal cells in the placenta and, if they reach the fetal circulation at all, they react not only with platelets but with all nucleated cells.

A strong association has been observed between the HLA class II antigen DR3 and alloimmunization against HPA-1a (Reznikoff-Etievant et al. 1981; Taaning et al. 1983; Mueller-Eckhardt et al. 1985). Association with DR52 appeared to be even stronger (de Waal et al. 1986), and was found to be with DR52a, which is in linkage disequilibrium with DR3 (Valentin et al. 1990; Decary et al. 1991). A very strong association was also found with the DQB1*0201 allele. The relative risk for immunization is 39.7 for DQB1*0201 and 24.9 for DR52a (L'Abbé et al. 1992). Interestingly, no association with HLA was observed in women who had made anti-HPA-lb. The explanation is probably that the affinity of the DR52a-positive class II molecule for the HPA-1 polypeptide is far greater when leucine is present as in HPA-1a than if proline is present in the same position as in HPA-1b, thus facilitating presentation of the antigen to T-helper cells in DRw52a subjects (Kuijpers et al. 1992b). Similarly the affinity of the product of the DBQ1*0201 allele is much greater than that of the product of other DBQ1 alleles. DR52a- and DBQ1*0201-negative women are at very low risk of becoming immunized against HPA-1a. In fact, none of 36 immunized women was found to be negative for both markers (L'Abbé et al. 1992). A strong association has also been observed between alloimmunization against HPA-5b and DR6 (Mueller-Eckhardt et al. 1989b).

Treatment of neonatal alloimmune thrombocytopenia

Prenatal treatment

In NATP, thrombocytopenia does not, as a rule, become severe before the twentieth week of gestation (Daffos *et al.* 1988). Intracranial haemorrhage does occur before the twentieth week (De Vries *et al.* 1988), and bleeding often occurs in the last trimester. As thrombocytopenia almost invariably occurs in susceptible fetuses during subsequent pregnancies, prenatal diagnosis and treatment are critical for women who have delivered one affected fetus or neonate (Bussel *et al.* 1997). Molecular typing and intrauterine fetal blood sampling make this possible. However, *in utero* transfusion of compatible platelets must accompany fetal blood sampling to reduce the risk of bleeding. Even with this precaution, the procedure carries the risk of fetal death or morbidity.

When a woman who has previously delivered an infant with NATP becomes pregnant again, the father's phenotype should be ascertained. If the father is heterozygous for the antigen involved, the genotype of the fetus should be determined using DNA from nucleated cells obtained by amniocentesis The circumstances in which fetal blood sampling should be performed are not well established (Reesink and Engelfriet 1993). In some centres, fetal sampling is performed at about the twentieth week in all cases in which there has been a previous affected fetus, or even whenever platelet-specific antibodies are detected in the maternal serum (Flug *et al.* 1994; Kaplan *et al.* 1995). In other centres, fetal sampling is done only if a previous infant has suffered from intrauterine haemorrhage and even then only after 4–6 weeks of treatment (Decary and Goldman 1993).

Three forms of prenatal therapy and combinations have been tried:

1 High-dose IVIG administered to the mother (1 g/kg per week) has proved effective (Bussel *et al.* 1988; Lynch *et al.* 1992a), but not invariably so (Silver *et al.* 2000). The initial fetal platelet count, at least with NATP caused by anti-HPA-1a, may predict a favourable response (Gaddipati *et al.* 2001). Inhibition, by IgG, of the transfer of anti-HPA-1a across the placenta has been studied experimentally.

2 Success after treatment of the mother with low-dose corticosteroids has been reported in a few cases, but has not been confirmed (Daffos *et al.* 1988). Corticosteroid administration does not appear to increase the effectiveness of antenatal IVIG (Bussel *et al.* 1996).

3 Transfusions of irradiated compatible allogeneic platelets or washed, irradiated maternal platelets can be given to the fetus.

The application of these therapeutic measures differs from centre to centre. In one regimen, if fetal thrombocytopenia is diagnosed at 20 weeks, the mother is treated either with corticosteroids (0.5 mg of prednisone/kg per day) or with IVIG (1g/kg per week). A further fetal blood sample is obtained at 28 weeks. If the treatment appears to have been successful, it is continued until a final sample is taken just before delivery. If the platelet count is $> 50 \times 10^9/l$, vaginal delivery is allowed. If it is $< 5 \times 10^9/l$, a transfusion of washed, irradiated maternal platelets is given. If the initial treatment of the mother with either corticosteroids or IVIG is unsuccessful, both treatments are given from 28 weeks onwards. With this regimen, no intracranial haemorrhage was seen in two centres (Kaplan *et al.* 1992; Lynch *et al.* 1992b).

In another centre, the mother is given IVIG from the twentieth week onwards if a previous child had NATP. A first fetal sample is taken after 4–6 weeks to determine whether the treatment has been successful. If it was not, corticosteroids are added to IVIG. If an intracranial haemorrhage is detected, weekly transfusions of compatible platelets are administered to the fetus (Décary and Goldman 1993). In a third centre, weekly transfusions of compatible platelets are given to the fetus if the platelet count is $< 2 \times 10^9/l$ at 20 weeks; otherwise IVIG or corticosteroids are given to the mother (Mueller-Eckhardt *et al.* 1993).

In addition to being ABO compatible, platelet donors must be negative in all the usual screening tests and must also be anti-CMV negative unless leucocyte-depleted platelet concentrates are used. Platelet concentrates must be irradiated. This is particularly important when maternal platelets are used because the mother shares one HLA haplotype with the fetus (see Chapter 15). If an infant who received intrauterine platelet concentrates needs platelet transfusions after birth, the concentrates must also be irradiated because of evidence that intrauterine platelet transfusions predispose to neonatal transfusion-related GvHD (N Mode and R Warwick, unpublished observation). The survival of transfused donor platelets may be adversely affected by maternal HLA antibodies (Murphy *et al.* 1993).

Postnatal treatment

Thrombocytopenia in an otherwise healthy infant should be considered NATP until proved otherwise. The immediate treatment of a neonate with severe thrombocytopenia ($< 20 \times 10^9$ platelets/litre), and a probable diagnosis of neonatal alloimmune thrombocytopenia is urgent correction of the platelet count. Transfusion of a neonatal dose of ABO, Rh D-compatible and HPA-1a (and HPA-5b)-negative cells will be compatible in approximately 95% of cases with an alloimmune cause. In the UK, HPA-1a (and HPA-5b)-negative platelets can be obtained from the National Blood Service; treatment should be started as soon as practically feasible. If no compatible donors are available, washed, irradiated maternal platelets can be used. An alternative therapy is high-dose IVIG (1 g/kg body weight/day for two consecutive days), but the delay in achieving a safe platelet count is significantly longer than with platelet transfusion. Of 12 infants with NATP due to anti-HPA-1a, who were treated with IVIG (doses between 1 and 9 g), 10 responded, often with an immediate and sustained increase in the platelet count (Mueller-Eckhardt and Kiefel 1989). Transfusion of HPA-incompatible platelets should only be considered when compatible platelets are unavailable. Corticosteroids for the neonate have no value.

Neonatal thrombocytopenia due to maternal autoantibodies

Unwarranted confusion arises regarding two pathophysiologically similar, but fundamentally different diseases, neonatal autoimmune thrombocytopenia caused by passive transfer of maternal autoantibodies (neonatal thrombocytopenia due to maternal autoantibodies, NAITP) and NATP. The former is caused by maternal autoantibody that crosses the placenta, whereas the latter is due to maternal alloantibody directed against a platelet-specific antigen on the fetal platelets. The two disorders differ in clinical course, diagnostic approach and therapy.

Immune thrombocytopenia (ITP) affects both mother and fetus, but neonatal disease is typically benign. The diagnosis of NAITP can be suspected from a low maternal platelet count; this contrasts with the normal maternal value found in NATP. Only 10% of neonates delivered of women with ITP develop significant thrombocytopenia and only 10% of those (at most), or 1% overall, suffer an intracranial haemorrhage (ICH) (Samuels *et al.* 1990; Burrows and Kelton 1993). Although maternal antibody studies can predict NATP, the only clear predictor of NAITP is a previous neonate with neonatal thrombocytopenia. Antenatal diagnosis is further complicated by the lack of an assay that unequivocally distinguishes the mild thrombocytopenia of pregnancy ('gestational thrombocytopenia') from ITP (Lescale *et al.* 1996). Maternal platelet number and indices do not correlate reliably with the fetal platelet count (Cines *et al.* 1982; Kaplan *et al.* 1990). The risk of thrombocytopenia in the offspring is greater in mothers with known chronic ITP than in cases of asymptomatic thrombocytopenia detected during pregnancy (Kaplan *et al.* 1990). Fetal blood sampling and fetal scalp sampling to determine the fetal platelet count before delivery have been used in cases in which the mother has ITP or thrombocytopenia of unknown origin with a count $< 100 \times 10^9$/l (Kaplan *et al.* 1990). However, because these procedures are not without risk, and morbidity from maternal autoantibody is minimal, invasive obstetrical procedures are indicated for few if any mothers with ITP (Copplestone 1990; Burrows and Kelton 1993). Unlike NATP, antenatal IVIG and platelet transfusions are rarely necessary or effective, and far less experience supports their use. The postnatal treatment of choice of thrombocytopenia due to maternal autoantibodies is high-dose IVIG (Blanchette *et al.* 1989).

Tests for platelet alloantibodies

Techniques for the detection of platelet antibodies used at present are based on the detection of platelet-bound Ig.

The classical antiglobulin test cannot be applied to platelets because of their tendency to aggregate spontaneously, particularly when they are washed. However, all of the more successful techniques for the detection of platelet antibodies are based on the antiglobulin principle in various ways, for example the immunofluorescence test, ELISA and the mixed red cell adherence assay (solid phase). A general problem in these techniques is the presence on platelets of Fc receptors for IgG that bind inert IgG. Methods have been developed to detect antibody binding to particular platelet membrane glycoproteins: radioimmunoprecipitation, immunoblotting and antigen capture assays using solubilized glycoproteins in platelet lysates that are captured by monoclonal antibodies.

Of the numerous techniques that have been described, the following are advised for the detection of platelet alloantibodies.

Platelet immunofluorescence test (PIFT)

The improved method described by von dem Borne and co-workers (1978) depends on pre-treatment of platelets with paraformaldehyde (PFA). The advantages of this treatment are a diminished uptake of aggregated IgG and immune complexes together with swelling of the platelets with expulsion of platelet-associated Ig, which overcomes the problem of non-specific fluorescence (Helmerhorst et al. 1983). PFA-treated platelets are incubated with serum, washed, incubated with antiglobulin serum labelled with fluorescein isothiocyanate, then washed again and examined under a fluorescence microscope. Advantages of this test are: (1) because the fluorescence of single platelets is assessed, non-specific reactions due to cell fragments (see below) are avoided (Shulman et al. 1982); and (2) a polyspecific anti-Ig reagent for the recognition of IgG, IgM and IgA antibodies can be used.

A disadvantage of the test is its relative insensitivity; at least 1000 molecules of IgG must be bound to a platelet to produce a positive reaction (Tijhuis et al. 1991).

The immunofluorescence test described by von dem Borne and co-workers (1978) has been chosen as the standard technique by the ISBT/ICSH working party on platelet serology. An efficient modification of this technique in microplates has been described by Andersen and co-workers (1981).

An alternative to the 'microscopic' immunofluorescence test is the flow cytometric immunofluorescence test (FCIT) of Rosenfeld and Bodensteiner (1986), which has been used to detect alloantibodies reactive with platelets and for platelet crossmatching (Freedman et al. 1991; Worfolk and McPherson 1991; Skogen et al. 1995). The FCIT has been found to be slightly more sensitive than the 'microscopic' test (Sintnicolaas et al. 1991).

The enzyme-linked immunosorbent assay

The use of enzyme (peroxidase-labelled) antiglobulin for detecting platelet antibodies was first described by Tate and co-workers (1977). After incubation of sensitized platelets with enzyme-linked antiglobulin serum, substrate is added and the coloured reaction product is quantified spectrophotometrically. The platelets can be coated onto slides or the wells of microplates, and various other enzyme conjugates can be used. A drawback of solid-phase ELISAs is that with some sera IgG is bound strongly, and non-specifically, to plastic. A quick and simple ELISA has been developed (Bessos et al. 2001).

Mixed red cell adherence assay (solid-phase technique)

In this assay, platelets are fixed to the wells of a microplate coated with immune monoclonal anti-platelet antibody, incubated with the serum under investigation and washed. Anti-IgG-coated red cells are then added. If the platelets have been sensitized by antibody, the red cells will cover the platelet monolayers; otherwise the indicator cells will collect in a tight button in the centre of the well. A modification of this technique, in which low-ionic-strength medium is used in sensitizing the platelets, has been described (Rachel et al. 1985). In another modification, IgG anti-D-sensitized red cells together with anti-IgG are used to detect platelet-bound antibodies. This test was found to be as sensitive as the PIFT (Lown and Ivey 1991). A kit for this modified assay is commercially available.

Monoclonal antibody-specific immobilization of platelet antigens assay

In this assay (MAIPA), target platelets are incubated with a serum under investigation, then washed once and incubated with monoclonal antibodies against a particular platelet glycoprotein (Kiefel et al. 1987). The platelets are then solubilized and the lysate is incubated in the wells of microtitre plates coated with polyclonal antimouse Ig. Human antibodies in the complex of antigen (i.e. glycoprotein), human antibody and murine monoclonal antibody are then detected with alkaline phosphatase-labelled anti-human Ig and substrate. This assay has the following advantages: the technique is more sensitive than the immunofluorescence test; the glycoprotein against which the platelet anti-bodies are directed is automatically defined; and contaminating antibodies which may be present in the serum, for example anti-HLA class I, do not interfere. Disadvantages of the assay are that, in the detection of unknown antibodies, a panel of monoclonal antibodies must be used and monoclonals to all glycoproteins may not yet be available. Furthermore, if a human antibody is directed against the same epitope as the monoclonal antibody (or an adjacent epitope), false-negative results may be obtained. A rapid and sensitive modification of this technique in which glycoprotein-coated immunomagnetic beads are used instead of platelet-coated microtitre plates has been described (Loeliger *et al.* 1993).

Distinction between platelet-specific and HLA antibodies

In the diagnosis of NATP and post-transfusion purpura (Chapter 15), detection and definition of platelet-specific alloantibodies are essential. Definition of specificity is often hampered by the presence of strong HLA class I antibodies present in many of the sera under investigation. The problem can be overcome by treating platelets with chloroquine to remove HLA-A and HLA-B antigens (Blumberg *et al.* 1984). Chloroquine-treated platelets do not react with HLA antisera in the platelet immunofluorescence test, although they react with anti-HPA-1a and anti-HPA-3a. After 20 min of incubation with chloroquine, 80% of HLA antigens are removed whereas GPIIb/IIIa and GPIb/IX are unaffected. However, after 1 h of incubation, approximately 50% of these glycoproteins are removed (Langenscheidt *et al.* 1989). An alternative method of removing HLA class I antigens from platelets is treatment with a citric acid–phosphate buffer (Kurata *et al.* 1989). A method in which the two above principles are combined, and in which acidified chloroquine diphosphate is used, has been found to be effective; fewer platelets are damaged and lost than in the above methods (Srivastava *et al.* 1993). As mentioned above, if the MAIPA is used to detect platelet-specific allo-antibodies, HLA antibodies do not interfere.

Use of frozen platelets in serology

Platelets, frozen in microplates with 6% dimethyl sulphoxide and stored at −80°C for 12 months, give satisfactory results in the PIFT. Concordant reactions were obtained with both HLA antisera and platelet-specific antibodies with frozen and fresh platelets from the same donors (Porretti *et al.* 1994).

Genotyping for platelet-specific polymorphisms

Reliable typing sera for most platelet-specific antigens are available in only a few specialized laboratories. Furthermore, under certain circumstances, for example when fetal platelets must be typed, insufficient platelets may be available for serological typing. Geno-typing for platelet-specific polymorphisms is therefore an important alternative because cDNA from any source can be used, for example from amniocytes. Several DNA techniques have been applied. For the HPA1, -2, -3, -4 and -7 systems, the RFLP technique can be used because one of the two alleles of the responsible genes contains a specific restriction site (Newman *et al.* 1989; Williamson *et al.* 1992; Kuijpers *et al.* 1993). Allele-specific oligonucleotides or allele-specific primers can be used for all systems of which the molecular basis is known and have been successfully applied to type for, for example the HPA1–4 systems (Bray *et al.* 1994) and the HPA1–6 systems (Skogen *et al.* 1994) respectively. In general, the results of phenotyping and DNA typing are identical, but a few discrepancies have been found in families with Glanzmann's disease (Morel-Kopp *et al.* 1994). An extended, streamlined PCR-SSP protocol for simultaneous genotyping of HPA-1 to HPA-13w suitable for large-scale genetic population studies has been reported (Lyou *et al.* 2002). The method allows fast and reliable diagnosis of alloimmune thrombocytopenia.

Detection of alloantibodies in neonatal alloimmune thrombocytopenia

When thrombocytopenia is detected in a newborn infant, the maternal serum can be tested first with paternal platelets, or, if paternal platelets are not available, with platelets from typed donors. If the result is positive a distinction must be made between HLA class I and platelet-specific antibodies, using chloroquine- or acid-treated platelets. If platelet-specific antibodies are detected, their specificity must be determined using a panel of phenotyped platelets. If the mother is thrombocytopenic the presence of platelet autoantibodies must be excluded (see below).

A negative immunofluorescence test with the maternal serum does not exclude the presence of platelet-specific antibodies because of the relative insensitivity of the test. A more sensitive test, for example the MAIPA (see above), must then be applied. Most anti-HPA-5[a] and -5[b] antibodies are not detected by the PIFT but are readily detected by the MAIPA (Kiefel et al. 1987). The specificity of maternal platelet-specific antibodies can be confirmed by phenotyping the maternal and paternal platelets.

If there has been a previous affected child and if the father is heterozygous for the antigen involved, the genotype of the fetus should be determined using amniocytes (see above). If fetal platelets have been obtained by fetal blood sampling, their phenotype can be determined.

Detection of alloantibodies in post-transfusion purpura

In the diagnosis of post-transfusion purpura (PTP) (Chapter 15), the detection of platelet-specific alloantibodies in the patient's serum is essential. As the great majority of cases of PTP are caused by anti-HPA-1a, it is expedient to first type the patient for this antigen and if the patient is negative, to test the serum which nearly always also contains HLA antibodies, for anti-HPA-1a in the MAIPA. If the patient is HPA-1(a+), the serum must be tested with a panel of phenotyped and chloroquine- or acid-treated platelets in the fluorescence test. If all reactions are negative, it is advisable to test the serum in the MAIPA using a panel of monoclonal antibodies again platelet glycoproteins.

If thrombocytopenia has developed during or immediately after a transfusion, the serum of the donor must be investigated (see Chapter 15).

(Auto)immune thrombocytopenia

The presence of an antiplatelet factor in the plasma of patients with 'idiopathic' thrombocytopenic purpura was first demonstrated by Harrington and co-workers (1951): plasma from a patient transfused to a normal subject produced an immediate and profound fall in the recipient's platelet count. The effect proved to be dose dependent, reactive with both autologous and allogeneic platelets and resident in the IgG fraction of plasma (Shulman et al. 1965). Autoantibodies can be demonstrated on the platelets of most patients with ITP, and hence the term 'immune' thrombocytopenia (ITP) is now preferred. In ITP, the platelet lifespan is shortened due to random destruction of antibody-sensitized platelets by cells of the MPS. In some patients platelet production is also decreased because the autoantibodies bind to megakaryocytes that carry the same antigens as platelets (Vinci et al. 1984; Nagasawa et al. 1995).

Using the platelet immunofluorescence test, autoantibodies were detected on the platelets of 69 out of 75 (92%) patients with ITP. In 92% of these 69 cases, antibodies were also detected in an eluate from the patient's platelets. The platelet-bound autoantibodies were IgG in 92%, IgM in 42% and IgA in 9% of cases. IgG1 was detected in 82%, IgG2 in 11%, IgG3 in 50% and IgG4 in 20% of the patients with IgG autoantibodies. Complement was never detected on the platelets of these patients (von dem Borne et al. 1986a). Patients with complement-binding autoantibodies have been described but such autoantibodies seem to be very rare (Tsubakio et al. 1986; Lehman et al. 1987).

Specificity of platelet autoantibodies

The majority of autoantibodies are directed to epitopes on either glycoprotein GPIIb-IIIa (van Leeuwen et al. 1982b; Beardsley et al. 1984; Woods et al. 1984; McMillan et al. 1987) or GPIb-IX (Woods et al. 1984; Szatkowski et al. 1986). Autoantibodies may also react with non-polymorphic epitopes on GPIb/IIa and IV (Kiefel et al. 1989c) or on GPV (Beardsley 1989).

The newer antigen-specific autoantibody assays are capable of detecting both platelet-associated and plasma autoantibodies and are useful in the diagnosis of immune thrombocytopenia, particularly of severe, chronic ITP (McMillan 2003). A positive assay provides strong evidence for the presence of immune thrombocytopenia; however, a negative assay does eliminate the diagnosis of ITP. The large number of patients who have negative assays is somewhat disconcerting. Some patients may not have chronic ITP (e.g. patients with mild ITP pre-splenectomy, who have platelet counts > 50 000/μl). Platelet antigens or Ig subtypes other than those screened may be involved. Patients may have received therapy that suppresses autoantibody prior to the assay (Fujisawa et al. 1993), or there may be technical or sensitivity problems with the available assays. Recent studies have localized some ITP autoepitopes to specific regions of GPIIb-IIIa and GPIb-IX. Most autoepitopes on GPIIb-IIIa are conformational, in view of their dependence on divalent cations, and are localized to the N-terminal portion of GPIIb, whereas the GPIb-IX autoepitopes that have been identified are localized to GPIb amino acids 333–341.

Pseudothrombocytopenia and autoantibodies against cryptantigens

In pseudothrombocytopenia the platelet count is spuriously low in EDTA-anticoagulated blood, because of EDTA-induced platelet agglutination. This phenomenon is caused by platelet autoantibodies that bind to platelets after removal of Ca^{2+} (Pegels *et al.* 1982; von dem Borne *et al.* 1986b). The antibodies are directed against non-polymorphic cryptantigens on the GPIIb–IIIa complex that are exposed by conformational changes induced by the absence of Ca^{2+}.

Autoantibodies against cryptantigens exposed by fixation with PFA also occur (Magee 1985; von dem Borne *et al.* 1986b). Neither of these two kinds of autoantibodies causes thrombocytopenia *in vivo*, but they cause misleading positive reactions in techniques in which EDTA- and/or PFA-fixed platelets are used.

Tests for platelet autoantibodies

A simple technique for detecting these antibodies is the direct immunofluorescence test on the patient's platelets; if the result is positive and sufficient platelets are available, an eluate can be made (see below) to confirm the presence of autoantibodies. As mentioned above, however, the immunofluorescence test is relatively insensitive. Therefore, if the direct immunofluorescence test is negative, a more sensitive test should be applied, for example a radioimmunoassay (RIA) to measure platelet-bound Ig (PBIg). Many different versions of this assay have been described. The amount of PBIg found with these techniques is often remarkably high and probably reflects non-specific binding of plasma proteins. An important source of non-specific binding is the presence of platelet fragments in the platelet suspension (Shulman *et al.* 1982). A more specific assay in which monoclonal anti-IgG is used has been described (Lo Buglio *et al.* 1983). The improvement was considered to be due to the restricted specificity and the single binding affinity of the monoclonal reagent, as well as to removal of platelet

fragments by centrifugation of the platelet suspension over a discontinuous Percoll gradient.

A slightly modified assay, the monoclonal antibody radioimmunoassay (MARIA), in which a sucrose gradient is used to separate platelets from fragments has been adapted for the use of monoclonal anti-IgM and anti-IgG subclass reagents (Tijhuis *et al.* 1991). A positive reaction in the MARIA was found in 21% of 55 patients with ITP in whom the direct fluorescence test was negative (Tijhuis *et al.* 1991).

Two capture assays are useful in the clinical setting: the immunobead assay and the MAIPA assay (Kiefel *et al.* 1987; Millard *et al.* 1987). Both assays are technically simple and can measure both platelet-associated and plasma antibodies. A prospective study of 282 patients with adult chronic ITP and 289 patients with thrombocytopenia associated with other illnesses found a sensitivity of between 31% and 87%, depending on the subgroup of ITP, and a specificity in the range of 90% (McMillan *et al.* 2003).

Elution of antibodies from platelets

Ether-elution method. This is a modification of the method described for red cells by Rubin (1963). Platelets from EDTA blood are washed and suspended in phosphate-buffered saline with 2% bovine serum albumin (PBS-BSA) to a final concentration of 0.5×10^9 cells/μl; one volume of this suspension is mixed with two volumes of ether and shaken vigorously for 2 min. The mixture is incubated for 30 min at 37°C in a waterbath and shaken frequently. After centrifugation of the mixture, three layers can be distinguished: the stroma, ether and the eluate, which is removed with a pipette (von dem Borne *et al.* 1980).

Acid-elution technique. A volume of platelets from EDTA blood is washed three times in PBS-BSA and the supernatant discarded. A volume of citric acid, pH 2.8, equal to that of the cell pellet, is added. The mixture is incubated for 7 min at room temperature and then centrifuged at 1000 g for 5 min. A volume of NaOH is added to adjust the final pH to 7.2.

Drug-induced immune thrombocytopenia

Mechanisms responsible for drug-induced immune thrombocytopenia are similar to those involving red cells (see Chapter 7) and granulocytes. In the classical example of sedormid-induced thrombocytopenia, the drug does not bind firmly to the cell, the antibodies being demonstrable only when tested against a mixture of the drug and platelets (Ackroyd 1954). In quinine- or quinidine-induced thrombocytopenia, the mechanism is similar. The interaction between the quinine- (or quinidine-) dependent antibody, and in fact many drug-induced antibodies and platelets, involves glycoprotein IX or the β-subunit of glycoprotein 1b or both (Berndt et al. 1985). Two residues, Gln115 and Arg110, play an important role in the structure of the antigenic site on GPIX recognized by anti-GPIX antibodies (Asvadi et al. 2003). In gold-induced thrombocytopenia, true autoantibodies, reacting independently of the drug, are formed (von dem Borne et al. 1986c): the mechanism is thus similar to that in aldomet-induced autoimmune haemolytic anaemia and levamisole-induced granulocytopenia.

Heparin-induced thrombocytopenia (HIT) represents a particularly important example of drug-related immune thrombocytopenia because of its frequency, singular mechanism and devastating effects. Between 1% and 5% of patients receiving unfractionated heparin develop thrombocytopenia or a 50% decline in platelet count from the pre-treatment value (Babcock et al. 1976). Frequency appears to be lower when low-molecular-weight heparin is used or when low doses, such as those used to keep central venous lines patent, are used. HIT typically develops in patients 5–10 days after starting heparin therapy, but can occur sooner with recent heparin exposure and delayed onset up to 3 weeks after exposure to heparin has been reported (Warkentin and Kelton 2001a,b). The platelet count typically drops below $150 \times 10^9/l$ (average $60 \times 10^9/l$), but bleeding seldom occurs, even with very low counts. On the contrary, patients may experience progressive venous and arterial thromboses that result in loss of limb in up to 10% and up to a 30% mortality.

Platelet factor 4 (PF4), a small positively charged peptide released from the platelet alpha granules during activation, is expressed on the platelet surface and binds the highly negatively charged heparin molecules. IgG_1 antibodies directed against the surface complex activate platelets by binding to the Fc receptors and releasing procoagulant-active, platelet-derived microparticles (Amiral et al. 1992; Hughes et al. 2000). Two functional assays, a platelet aggregation test and a serotonin release assay, are sensitive and specific, but problematic for the average clinical laboratory: an enzyme immunoassay that recognizes the IgG antibody is slightly less sensitive and specific (Greinacher et al. 1994).

Management of drug-induced immune thrombocytopenia

The primary treatment for all instances of drug-induced thrombocytopenia is prompt discontinuation of the implicated medication. Most drug-related cases require nothing more. The recognition that HIT involves intense thrombin generation dictates the use of antithrombin agents such as argatroban and hirudin in HIT therapy (Kelton 2002). Oral anticoagulation with warfarin, which induces rapid decline in the naturally occurring anticoagulant protein C, is not indicated as immediate treatment and may contribute to extension of thrombosis. Platelet transfusions are rarely useful, even for severe drug-induced immune thrombocytopenia and may exacerbate thrombosis in HIT.

Serum protein antigens and antibodies

There are a few antibodies to serum proteins that are relevant to blood transfusion. Antibodies to factor VIII may seriously impair the response to transfused factor VIII but are of IgG4 subclass (Anderson and Terry 1968) and do not bind complement, and perhaps for this reason, do not provoke transfusion reactions. Antibodies to determinants on immunoglobulin molecules may interfere with the interpretation of serological tests. Although antibodies to serum lipoproteins are also recognized, they have no known clinical significance.

IgG

Antibodies with several different specificities are found, reacting with determinants on native IgG molecules (anti-Gm), with determinants exposed following the combination of antigen with antibody ('anti-antibodies') and with determinants exposed by pepsin digestion.

IgG allotypes

These are defined by polymorphic antigenic determinants carried on γ-chains, i.e. the heavy chains of IgG. The existence of Gm groups was first demonstrated by showing that Rh D-positive red cells coated with selected examples of 'incomplete' anti-D were agglutinated by the serum of some patients with rheumatoid arthritis and that the reactions could be inhibited by selected normal sera (Grubb 1956). Four different determinants are recognized on the heavy chains of IgG1 and 13 on IgG3; only one determinant has been recognized so far on IgG2 and none on IgG4.

In Gm typing, red cells coated with selected Rh antibodies can be used to identify IgG1 and IgG3 markers, for example G1m(f) and G3m; however, in identifying other markers, such as G2m(n), which are not found, or at least not commonly, on red cell alloantibodies, selected myeloma proteins bound to red cells must be used.

Nomenclature (WHO 1976). The subclass designation, for example (Ig) G1, is followed by m for marker and then (in brackets) a number or a letter, as unfortunately, both numeric and 'alphameric' terminologies are still allowed. Here, the alphameric notation is used, for example G1m(a) rather than G1m(1). Some symbols in the alphameric notation consist of letters and numbers, for example G3m(b1). The phenotype is written in the numerical order of subclasses, for example for a person with G1m(a), G1m(f), G2m(n), G3m(b1) and G3m(g), the phenotype is Gm(af; n; b1g).

Some Gm allotypes are associated with replacement of one amino acid residue by another in the same position of an otherwise identical polypeptide chain, for example G1m(z) and G1m(f). The alternative to some Gm allotypes is an antigenic determinant that is not limited to molecules of the subclass concerned but also occurs on other subclasses. Such determinants are described as isoallotypes, as they are allotypic in one subclass and isotypic in one or more of the other subclasses.

Anti-Gm may be found in the following circumstances:

1 In patients with rheumatoid arthritis; these sera, known as 'Raggs' (Rheumatoid agglutinators), are autoantibodies, usually have multiple specificities and exhibit prozones so that few are useful as typing reagents.

2 In normal subjects, some of whom have been transfused or have been pregnant, these sera, known as 'SNaggs' (Serum Normal agglutinators), are usually less potent than Raggs but are usually monospecific and do not exhibit prozones. Moreover, their titre

usually remains the same for years. These are the reagents normally used in Gm typing.

3 In normal subjects, usually children, in whom the stimulus for anti-Gm formation can often be shown to have been maternal IgG transferred across the placenta.

4 Polyclonal and monoclonal anti-Gm reagents of animal origin are now available.

Serum from patients with rheumatoid arthritis usually contains a whole family of autoantibodies reacting with many epitopes on the IgG molecule, some of which are revealed only when the IgG is altered in some way, either by being denatured or by reacting with an antigenic site.

Formation of anti-Gm following transfusion

Antibodies, often of recognizable specificities, have been found in patients who have received multiple blood transfusions, particularly children (Allen and Kunkel 1963, 1966; Stiehm and Fudenberg 1965).

In adults, prolonged stimulation is usually required for the production of anti-Gm. A single injection of immunoglobulin produces a scarcely significant increase in the incidence of antibodies against immunoglobulins in parous women (Sturgeon and Jennings 1968). Similarly, no anti-Gm was detected after a single transfusion followed by an injection of immunoglobulin (Auerswald *et al.* 1967).

Anti-Gm has also been produced by deliberate immunization of volunteer recipients with plasma of incompatible types. Following an initial intravenous transfusion of 125 ml of Gm-incompatible plasma, weekly subcutaneous injections of 0.1 ml of the same plasma were given. By about 2 months after the first transfusion three out of three recipients had formed anti-Gm (Fudenberg *et al.* 1964).

In one large study in which sera from patients who had been transfused repeatedly were tested against various monoclonal IgGs, evidence was obtained that anti-Gm was frequently not allotype specific but rather resembled rheumatoid factor (Salmon *et al.* 1973).

Formation of anti-Gm after pregnancy

Fudenberg and Fudenberg (1964) reported the finding of anti-G1m(a) in the serum of a pregnant woman whose infant was subsequently shown to be G1m(a); they pointed out that cord serum contains a small amount (1% or less) of endogenous IgG so that there is no theoretical reason why the mother should not be stimulated when the infant's IgG carries determinants that are foreign to the mother.

Response of newborn infants to maternal IgG allotypes

Speiser (1964) postulated that, during the first few months of life, infants regularly became immunized to maternal Gm allotypes; he demonstrated the presence of anti-G1m(a) in G1m(a−) infants born to G1m(a+) mothers. Similarly, Steinberg and Wilson (1963) showed that the specificity of anti-Gm antibodies in children corresponded to that of the mother's Gm antigens.

IgA

In approximately 50% of IgA-deficient patients, anti-IgA antibodies of various specificities are found, i.e. class specific (anti-α), subclass specific (anti-α_1 or anti-α_2) or allotype specific (anti-A2m(1) or anti-A2m(2)). In patients who are not IgA deficient, antibodies of limited specificity may be found, including antibodies reacting with the recognized allotype markers just mentioned.

Class-specific anti-IgA

The prevalence of subjects who are apparently lacking in serum IgA varies according to the sensitivity of the test used. For example, in tests on healthy Finnish blood donors, using a gel-diffusion method that could not detect less than 10 µg of IgA/ml, 1 out of 396 subjects appeared to lack IgA, but with a radio-immunoassay capable of detecting 0.015 µg/ml, only 1 out of 800 lacked IgA (Koistinen 1975). Similarly, Vyas and co-workers (1975) found that the incidence of IgA deficiency was 1 in 650 using gel diffusion, which in their hands did not detect less than 100 µg of IgA/ml, but was only 1 in 886 using haemagglutination inhibition, with a sensitivity of 0.5 µg of IgA/ml. The findings of Holt and co-workers (1977) were broadly similar: 1 in 522 subjects had less than 40 µg of IgA/ml and 1 in 875 had less than 0.5 µg of IgA/ml.

Class-specific anti-IgA is found only in IgA-deficient subjects and is then found quite often, even in patients without a history of pregnancy or blood transfusion or injections of blood products. In the series of Vyas and

co-workers (1975), 20 out of 83 IgA-deficient subjects had anti-IgA, and 13 of these had an anti-IgA titre of more than 256. Only two subjects had a history of transfusion of blood components. Of seven subjects with anti-IgA interviewed by Koistinen and Sarna (Koistinen 1975), only one had received a transfusion. Of 15 IgA-deficient subjects reported by van Loghem (1974), eight had anti-IgA but several of these had not been pregnant or received IgA-containing preparations. Anti-IgA was found in one 5-year-old child lacking IgA; the child had not been transfused but evidently might have been immunized by maternal IgA during intrauterine life (Vyas et al. 1970).

In the series of Holt and co-workers (1977) 10 out of 34 IgA-deficient subjects had antibodies for IgA. Six antibodies were class specific, three were subclass specific (Strauss et al. 1983) and one had allotypic specificity for A2m(2).

The role of class-specific anti-IgA in causing transfusion reactions, and the use of IgA-deficient donors for the transfusion of subjects whose serum contains anti-IgA, is discussed in Chapter 15.

Subclass-specific anti-IgA

Anti-α_1 and anti-α_2 antibodies may be present in addition to class-specific anti-α in the serum of IgA-deficient subjects (van Loghem 1974). Selective deficiency for IgA2 was described in a patient who developed a severe reaction following transfusion and who was found to have IgG anti-α_2 in her serum (van Loghem et al. 1983). Selective absence of IgA1 was detected in six and selective absence of IgA2 in 15 out of 93 020 normal donors investigated by Ozawa and co-workers (1985). No anti-α_1 or anti-α_2 was detected in the serum of any of these subjects, none of whom had been transfused or had been pregnant.

Anti-IgA of limited specificity

The term anti-IgA of limited specificity is used for antibodies that react with some, but not all, IgA myeloma proteins. Some examples of anti-IgA of limited specificity may have been anti-α_1 or anti-α_2 and some have been identified as anti-A2m(2) or anti-A2m(1), reacting with one or other of the two allotypes of IgA2. No allotypes of IgA1 have yet been recognized.

Anti-IgA of limited specificity is found mainly in patients who have been transfused or have received an injection of immunoglobulin, or in women who have had one or more pregnancies. Of a series of examples of anti-IgA of limited specificity, 19 reacted with one particular myeloma protein, indicating the importance of this particular specificity in alloimmunization and in transfusion reactions (Vyas *et al.* 1969). The possible role of anti-IgA of limited specificity in causing transfusion reactions is discussed in Chapter 15.

Determinants on light chains

Antibodies analogous to anti-Gm but directed to determinants on k-chains are termed anti-Km (previously Inv). Three markers, Km(1), Km(2) and Km(3), are recognized. No allotype markers are recognized on λ-chains.

Tests for immunoglobulin allotypes

Agglutination inhibition method

A volume of 25 µl of test serum, diluted appropriately, is mixed in a well of a microtitre plate with an equal volume of anti-Gm, -Am or -Km serum in optimal dilution. An equal volume of a 0.2% suspension of red cells sensitized with incomplete anti-D carrying the corresponding allotype is added. After careful mixing the plate is incubated overnight at 4°C or for 1 h at room temperature and centrifuged. The plates are tilted at an angle of about 60° and reactions are read. If the allotype is present in the serum, agglutination of the sensitized red cells by the anti-allotype serum is inhibited.

Method of passive haemagglutination

The term 'passive agglutination' is used for a reaction in which antigen is attached to a carrier particle (e.g. red cells), which plays a passive role in that it does not itself react with the antibody. Red cells treated with various agents will adsorb protein antigens 'non-specifically'. The following method can be used to couple proteins to red cells.

Chromic chloride. To one volume of 0.1% $CrCl_3$ in 0.9% NaCl add one volume of protein antigen and then immediately add one volume of three-times

washed red cells. After 4 min of continuous shaking at 20°C, wash the red cells three times in 20–40% BSA. Coated cells suspended in red cell preservation fluid can be kept for 4–6 weeks without loss of activity. The coated cells are mixed on slides or in the wells of microplates with the antisera to be tested (Gold and Fudenberg 1967). The coating proteins, as well as the saline solution, should be phosphate free (Schanfield 1986).

References

The MHC sequencing consortium (1999) Complete sequence and gene map of a human major histocompatibility complex. Nature 401: 921–923

Ackroyd JF (1954) The role of sedormid in the immunological reaction that results in platelet lysis in sedormid purpura. Clin Sci 13: 409

Adams SD, Barracchini KC, Simonis TB *et al.* (2001) High throughput HLA sequence-based typing (SBT) utilizing the ABI Prism 3700 DNA Analyzer. Tumori 87: S40–S43

Ades L, Mary JY, Robin M *et al.* (2003) Long-term outcome after bone marrow transplantation for severe aplastic anemia. Blood 103: 2490–2497

Adinolfi M (1986) Recurrent habitual abortion. HLA sharing and deliberate immunization with partner's cells; a controversial topic. Hum Reprod 1: 45–48

Ahrons S (1971) HL-A antibodies: Influence on the human foetus. Tissue Antigens 1: 129

Akbar AN, Fitzgerald-Bocarsly PA, de Sousa M *et al.* (1986) Decreased natural killer activity in thalassemia major: a possible consequence of iron overload. J Immunol 136: 1635–1640

Allen JC, Kunkel HG (1963) Antibodies to genetic types of gamma globulin after multiple transfusions. Science 139: 418

Allen JC, Kunkel HG (1966) Antibodies against globulin after repeated blood transfusions in man. J Clin Invest 45: 29

Amiral J, Bridey F, Dreyfus M *et al.* (1992) Platelet factor 4 complexed to heparin is the target for antibodies generated in heparin-induced thrombocytopenia. Thromb Haemost 68: 95–96

Andersen E, Bashir H, Archer GT (1981) Modification of the platelet suspension immunofluorescence test. Vox Sang 40: 44–47

Anderson BR, Terry WD (1968) Gamma G4-globulin antibody causing inhibition of clotting Factor VIII. Nature (Lond) 217: 174

Anderson CB, Sicard GA, Etheredge EE (1982) Pretreatment of renal allograft recipients with azathioprine and donor specific blood products. Surgery 92: 315–321

Andrew M, Vegh P, Caco C et al. (1993) A randomized, controlled trial of platelet transfusions in thrombocytopenic premature infants. J Pediatr 123: 285–291

Aster RH (1965) Effect of anticoagulant and ABO incompatibility on recovery of transfused human platelets. Blood 26: 732

Asvadi P, Ahmadi Z, Chong BH (2003) Drug-induced thrombocytopenia: localization of the binding site of GPIX-specific quinine-dependent antibodies. Blood 102: 1670–1677

Atkins RC, Walters MC (2003) Haematopoietic cell transplantation in the treatment of sickle cell disease. Expert Opin Biol Ther 3: 1215–1224

Atlas E, Freedman J, Blanchette V (1993) Down regulation of the anti-HLA alloimmune response by variable region reactive (anti-idiotype) antibodies in leukemic patients transfused with platelet concentrates. Blood 81: 538–542

Auerswald VW, Bodis-Wollner I, Kiesewetter E (1967) Zur Frage der Antikörperbildung Erwachsener gegen Gm nach wiederholter parenteraler Zufuhr von homologem Gammaglobulin. Wien Med Wochenschr 117: 1006

Babcock RB, Dumper CW, Scharfman WB (1976) Heparin-induced immune thrombocytopenia. N Engl J Med 295: 237–241

Bach FH, Voynow NK (1966) One-way stimulation in mixed leukocyte cultures. Science 153: 545

Bach P, Hirschhorn K (1964) Lymphocyte interaction: a potential histocompatibility test in vitro. Science 143: 813–815

Bain BV, Magdalene R, Lowenstein L (1964) The development of large immature mononuclear cells in mixed leukocyte cultures. Blood 23: 108

Baldwin WM, Claas FHJ, Paul LC (1983) All monocyte antigens are not expressed on renal endothelium. Tissue Antigens 21: 254–259

Barnstable CJ, Jones EA, Crumpton MJ (1978) Isolation, structure and genetics of HLA-A, -B, -C and -DRw (Ia) antigens. Br Med Bull 34: 241

Barrett J (2003) Allogeneic stem cell transplantation for chronic myeloid leukemia. Semin Hematol 40: 59–71

Bastian JF, Williams RA, Ornelas W (1984) Maternal isoimmunisation resulting in combined immunodeficiency and fatal graft-versus-host disease in an infant. Lancet i: 1435–1437

Baxter-Lowe LA, Eckels DD, Ash R (1992) The predictive value of HLA-DR oligotyping for MLC responses. Transplantation 53: 1352–1357

Beardsley DS (1989) Platelet autoantigens. In: Platelet Immunobiology. TJ Kunicki and JN George (eds). Philadelphia, PA: JP Lippincott

Beardsley DS, Spiegel JE, Jacobs MM (1984) Platelet membrane glycoprotein IIIa contains target antigens that bind anti-platelet antibodies in immune thrombocytopenias. J Clin Invest 74: 1701–1707

Beardsley DS, Ho JS, Moulton T (1987) A new platelet specific antigen on glycoprotein V. Blood 70 (Suppl.) 347a

Beaujean F, Sieger JM, Le Forestier C (1992) Leukocyte depletion of red cell concentrates by filtration: influence of blood product temperature. Vox Sang 62: 242–244

Beer AE, Semprini AE, Ziaoyu Z (1985) Pregnancy outcome in human couples with recurrent spontaneous abortions; HLA antigen profiles; HLA antigen sharing; female serum MLR blocking factors; and paternal leukocyte immunization. Exp Clin Immunogenet 2: 137–153

Berg SF, Mjaaland S, Fossum S (1994) Comparing macrophages and dendritic leucocytes as antigen-presenting cells for humoral responses in vivo by antigen targeting. Eur J Immunol 24: 1262–1268

Berndt MC, Chong BH, Bull HA et al. (1985) Molecular characterization of quinine/quinidine drug-dependent antibody platelet interaction using monoclonal antibodies. Blood 66: 1292–1301

Bertolini F, Rebulla P, Porretti L (1990) Comparison of platelet activation and membrane glycoprotein Ib and IIb-IIIa expression after filtration through three different leukocyte removal filters. Vox Sang 59: 201–204

Bessos H, Drummond O, Prowse C et al. (2001) The release of prion protein from platelets during storage of apheresis platelets. Transfusion 41: 61–66

Bidwell J (1994) Advances in DNA-based HLA-typing methods. Immunol Today 15: 303–307

Bjorkman PJ, Saper MA, Samraoui B et al. (1987) Structure of the human class I histocompatibility antigen, HLA-A2. Nature (Lond) 329: 506–511

Blanchette V, Andrew MMI, Perlman M (1989) Neonatal autoimmune thrombocytopenia: role of high-dose intravenous immunoglobulin G therapy. Blut 59: 139–144

Blumberg N, Heal JM (1996) Immunomodulation by blood transfusion: an evolving scientific and clinical challenge. Am J Med 101: 299–308

Blumberg N, Heal JM, Gettings KF (2003) WBC reduction of RBC transfusions is associated with a decreased incidence of RBC alloimmunization. Transfusion 43: 945–952

Blumberg N, Masel D, Mayer TH (1984) Removal of HLA-A, B antigens from platelets. Blood 63: 448–450

Bodmer JC, Marsh SGE, Albert ED (1992) Nomenclature for factors of the HLA system. Tissue Antigens 39: 161–173

Bodmer WF (1997) HLA: what's in a name? A commentary on HLA nomenclature development over the years. Tissue Antigens 49: 293–296

Boizard B, Wautier JL (1984) Lek^a, a new platelet antigen absent in Glanzmann's thrombasthenia. Vox Sang 46: 47–54

Bolgiano DC, Larson EB, Slichter SJ (1989) A model to determine required pool size for HLA-typed community donor apheresis programs. Transfusion 29: 306–310

Bontadini A, Fruet F, Tazzari PL (1994) Comparative analysis of six different white cell-reduction filters for packed red cells. Transfusion 34: 531–535

von dem Borne AE, Décary F (1990) Nomenclature of platelet-specific antigens. Transfusion 30: 477

von dem Borne AEGK, van der Plas-van Dalen CM (1985) Further observations on posttransfusion purpura (Letter). Br J Haematol 61: 374–375

von dem Borne AEGK, Verheught FWA, Oosterhof F (1978) A simple immunofluorescence test for the detection of platelet antibodies. Br J Haematol 39: 195

von dem Borne AEGK, von Riesz E, Verheught FWA (1980) Baka, a new platelet-specific antigen involved in neonatal alloimmune thrombocytopenia. Vox Sang 39: 113–120

von dem Borne AEGK, van Leeuwen EF, von Riesz LE (1981) Neonatal alloimmune thrombocytopenia: detection and characterization of the responsible antibodies by the platelet immunofluorescence test. Blood 57: 649–656

von dem Borne AEGK, Vos JJE, van de Lelie J (1986a) Clinical significance of a positive immunofluorescence test in thrombocytopenia. Br J Haematol 64: 767–776

von dem Borne AEGK, van der Lelie J, Vox JJE (1986b) Antibodies against cryptantigens of platelets. Characterization and significance for the serologist. In: Platelet Serology, Research Progress and Clinical Implications. FD Cary, GA Rock (eds). Basel: SA Karger

von dem Borne AEGK, Pegels JG, van der Stadt RJ (1986c) Thrombocytopenia associated with gold therapy: a drug-induced autoimmune disease? Br J Haematol 63: 509–516

Boshkov KL, Kelton JG, Halloran PE (1992) HLA-DR expression by platelets in acute idiopathic thrombocytopenic purpura. Br J Haematol 81: 552–557

Bowden RA, Slichter SJ, Sayers M et al. (1995) A comparison of filtered leukocyte-reduced and cytomegalovirus (CMV) seronegative blood products for the prevention of transfusion-associated CMV infection after marrow transplant. Blood 86: 3598–3603

Bradley BA, Edwards JM, Durm DC (1972) Quantitation of mixed lymphocyte reaction by gene dosage phenomenon. Nature (Lond) 240: 54

Brand A, Sintnicolaas K, Claas FHJ (1986) ABH antibodies causing platelet transfusion refractoriness. Transfusion 26: 463–366

Brand A, Claas FHJ, Voogt PL (1988) Alloimmunization after leukocyte depleted multiple random donor platelet transfusions. Vox Sang 54: 160–166

Bray PF, Jin Y, Kickler T (1994) Rapid genotyping of the five major platelet alloantigens by reverse dot-blot hybridization. Blood 84: 4361–4367

Bredius RG, Fijen CA, De Haas M et al. (1994) Role of neutrophil Fc gamma RIIa (CD32) and Fc gamma RIIIb (CD16) polymorphic forms in phagocytosis of human IgG1- and IgG3-opsonized bacteria and erythrocytes. Immunology 83: 624–630

Breuning MH, van den Berg-Loonen EM, Bernini LF (1977) Localization of HLA on the short arm of chromosome 6. Hum Genet 37: 131–139

Brodsky FM, Parham P, Barnstable CJ et al. (1979) Monoclonal antibodies for analysis of the HLA system. Immunol Rev 47: 3–61

Brown JH, Jardetzky TS, Gorg LJ (1993) 3-dimensional structure of the human class-II histocompatibility antigen DRI. Nature (Lond) 364: 33–39

Bruin MC, von dem Borne AEGK, Tamminga RY et al. (1999) Neutrophil antibody specificity in different types of childhood autoimmune neutropenia. Blood 94: 1797–1802

Bunce M, O'Neill CM, Barnardo MC et al. (1995) Phototyping: comprehensive DNA typing for HLA-A, B, C, DRB1, DRB3, DRB4, DRB5 & DQB1 by PCR with 144 primer mixes utilizing sequence-specific primers (PCR-SSP). Tissue Antigens 46: 355–367

Burrows L, Tartter P (1982) Effects of blood transfusion on colonic malignancy recurrence rate (Letter). Lancet ii: 662

Burrows RF, Kelton JG (1993) Fetal thrombocytopenia and its relation to maternal thrombocytopenia. N Engl J Med 329: 1463–1466

Busch OR, Hop WC, Marquet RL et al. (1994) Autologous blood and infections after colorectal surgery. Lancet 343: 668–669

Bussel J, Lalezari PH (1983) Reversal of neutropenia with intravenous gammaglobulin in autoimmune neutropenia of infancy. Blood 62: 398–400

Bussel J, Berkowitz R, McFarland J (1988) In-utero platelet transfusion for alloimmune thrombocytopenia. Lancet ii: 1307–1308

Bussel JB, Berkowitz RL, Lynch L et al. (1996) Antenatal management of alloimmune thrombocytopenia with intravenous gamma-globulin: a randomized trial of the addition of low-dose steroid to intravenous gamma-globulin. Am J Obstet Gynecol 174: 1414–1423

Bussel JB, Zabusky MR, Berkowitz RL et al. (1997) Fetal alloimmune thrombocytopenia. N Engl J Med 337: 22–26

Bux J (1999) Nomenclature of granulocyte alloantigens. ISBT Working Party on Platelet and Granulocyte Serology, Granulocyte Antigen Working Party. International Society of Blood Transfusion. Transfusion 39: 662–663

Bux J, Jung KD, Kauth T et al. (1992) Serological and clinical aspects of granulocyte antibodies leading to alloimmune neonatal neutropenia. Transfusion Med 2: 143–149

Bux J, Hartmann C, Mueller-Eckhardt C (1994) Alloimmune neonatal neutropenia resulting from immunization to a high-frequency antigen on the granulocyte Fcγ receptor III. Transfusion 34: 608–611

Bux J, Behrens G, Leist M (1995a) Evidence that the granulocyte-specific antigen NC1 is identical with NA2. Vox Sang 68: 46–49

Bux J, Stein EL, Santoso S et al. (1995b) NA gene frequencies in the German population, determined by polymerase chain reaction with sequence-specific primers. Transfusion 35: 54–57

Bux J, Stein EL, Bierling P et al. (1997) Characterization of a new alloantigen (SH) on the human neutrophil Fc gamma receptor IIIb. Blood 89: 1027–1034

Bux J, Behrens G, Jaeger G et al. (1998) Diagnosis and clinical course of autoimmune neutropenia in infancy: analysis of 240 cases. Blood 91: 181–186

Camussi G, Tetta C, Caligaris-Cappio FC (1979) Detection of immune complexes on the surface of polymorphonuclear neutrophils. Int Arch Allerg Appl Immunol 58: 135–139

Carson JL, Altman DG, Duff A et al. (1999) Risk of bacterial infection associated with allogeneic blood transfusion among patients undergoing hip fracture repair. Tranfusion 39: 694–700

Cartron J, Celton JL, Cane P (1992) Iso-immune neonatal neutropenia due to an anti-Fc receptor III (CD16) antibody. Eur J Pediatr 151: 438–441

Caruccio L, Bettinotti M, Matsuo K et al. (2003) Expression of human neutrophil antigen-2a (NB1) is increased in pregnancy. Transfusion 43: 357–363

Castle V, Andrew M, Kelton J et al. (1986) Frequency and mechanism of neonatal thrombocytopenia. J Pediatr 108: 749–755

Cerilli GJ, Brasile L, Gazoulis T (1981) Clinical significance of anti-monocyte antibody in kidney transplant recipients. Transplantation 32: 495–497

Cerundolo V, Kelly A, Elliott T (1995) Genes encoded in the major histocompatibility complex affecting the generation of peptides for TAP transport. Eur J Immunol 25: 554–562

Chakrabarti S, Childs R (2003) Allogeneic immune replacement as cancer immunotherapy. Expert Opin Biol Ther 3: 1051–1060

Champlin RE, Passweg JR, Zhang MJ et al. (2000) T-cell depletion of bone marrow transplants for leukemia from donors other than HLA-identical siblings: advantage of T-cell antibodies with narrow specificities. Blood 95: 3996–4003

Chang H, Hall GA, Geerts WH et al. (2000) Allogeneic red blood cell transfusion is an independent risk factor for the development of postoperative bacterial infection. Vox Sang 78: 13–18

Chen SH, Liang DC, Lin M (1995) Treatment of platelet alloimmunization with intravenous immunoglobulin in a child with aplastic anemia. Am J Hematol 49: 165–166

Chia D, Terasaki P, Chan H (1994) A new simplified method of gene typing. Tissue Antigens 44: 300–305

Childs R, Barrett J (2002) Nonmyeloablative stem cell transplantation for solid tumors: expanding the application of allogeneic immunotherapy. Semin Hematol 39: 63–71

Cines DC, Dusak B, Tomaski A (1982) Immune thrombocytopenia and pregnancy. N Engl J Med 306: 826–831

Claas FH, Langerak J, Sabbe LJ et al. (1979) NE1: a new neutrophil specific antigen. Tissue Antigens 13: 129–134

Claas FHJ, Paul LC, van Es LA (1980) Antibodies against donor antigens on endothelial cells and monocytes in eluates of rejected kidney allografts. Tissue Antigens 15: 19–24

Claas FHJ, Smeenk RJT, Schmidt R (1981) Alloimmunization against the MHC antigens after platelet transfusions is due to contaminating leukocytes in the platelet suspension. Exp Hematol 9: 84–89

Claas FHJ, Jakowska-Gan E, De Vito LD (1993) Monitoring of heart transplant rejection using a donor-specific soluble HLA class I ELISA (Abstract). Hum Immunol 37: 121

Claas FH, De Meester J, Witvliet MD et al. (1999) Acceptable HLA mismatches for highly immunized patients. Rev Immunogenet 1: 351–358

Clay ME, Kline WE (1985) Detection of granulocyte antigens and antibodies. In: Current Concepts in Transfusion Therapy. Arlington, VA: Am Assoc Blood Banks

Colonna M, Bresnahan M, Bahran S (1992) Allelic variants of the human putative peptide transporter involved in antigen processing. Proc Natl Acad Sci USA 89: 3932–3936

Cooling LL, Kelly K, Barton J et al. (2005) Determinants of ABH expression on human blood platelets. Blood 105: 3356–3364

Copplestone JA (1990) Fetal platelet counts in thrombocytopenic pregnancy (Letter). Lancet ii: 1375

Corwin HL, AuBuchon JP (2003) Is leukoreduction of blood components for everyone? JAMA 289: 1993–1995

Curtis BR, Edwards JT, Hessner MJ et al. (2000) Blood group A and B antigens are strongly expressed on platelets of some individuals. Blood 96: 1574–1581

Daffos F, Forestier F, Kaplan C (1988) Prenatal diagnosis and management of bleeding disorders with fetal blood sampling. Am J Obstet Gynecol 158: 939–946

Dankers MKA, Roelen DL, Korfage L et al. (2003) Differential immunogenicity of paternal class I antigens in pregnant women. Hum Immunol 64: 600–606

Dausset J (1958) Iso-leuco-anticorps. Acta Haemutol 20: 156

De Haas M, Kleijer M, van Zwieten R et al. (1995) Neutrophil Fc gamma RIIIb deficiency, nature, and clinical consequences: a study of 21 individuals from 14 families. Blood 86: 2403–2413

Décary F, Goldman M (1993) Prenatal management of fetal alloimmune thrombocytopenia. Vox Sang 65: 181–182

Décary F, L'Abbé D, Tremblay L (1991) The immune response to the HPA-1a antigen: association with HLA-DRw52a. Transfusion Med 1: 55–63

Deeg HJ (1989) Transfusion with a tan. Prevention of allosensitization by ultraviolet irradiation. Transfusion 29: 450–455

Deeg HJ, Aprile J, Graham TC (1986) Ultraviolet irradiation of blood prevents transfusion-induced sensitization and marrow graft rejection in dogs. Blood 76: 537–539

Deeg HJ, Aprile J, Starb R (1988) Functional dendritic cells are required for transfusion-induced sensitization in canine marrow graft recipients. Blood 71: 1138–1140

De Vries LS, Connell J, Bydder GM (1988) Recurrent intracranial haemorrhage in utero in an infant with alloimmune thrombocytopenia. Br J Obstet Gynaecol 95: 299–302

Doxiadis I, Grosse-Wilde H (1989) Typing for HLA class I gene products using plasma as a source. Vox Sang 56: 196–200

Dumont LJ, Dzik WH, Rebulla P et al. (1996) Practical guidelines for process validation and process control of white cell-reduced blood components: report of the Biomedical Excellence for Safer Transfusion (BEST) Working Party of the International Society of Blood Transfusion (ISBT). Transfusion 36: 11–20

Dumont LJ, Luka J, VandenBroeke T et al. (2001) The effect of leukocyte-reduction method on the amount of human cytomegalovirus in blood products: a comparison of apheresis and filtration methods. Blood 97: 3640–3647

Dunstan RA, Simpson MB, Rosse WF (1984) Erythrocyte antigens on human platelets. Absence of the Rhesus, Duffy, Kell, Kidd, and Lutheran antigens. Transfusion 24: 243–246

Duquesnoy RJ (2002) HLAMatchmaker: a molecularly based algorithm for histocompatibility determination. I. Description of the algorithm. Hum Immunol 63: 339–352

Duquesnoy RJ, Marrari M (1997) Determination of HLA-A,B residue mismatch acceptability for kidneys transplanted into highly sensitized patients: a report of a collaborative study conducted during the 12th International Histocompatibility Workshop. Transplantation 63: 1743–1751

Duquesnoy RJ, Marrari M (2003) Multilaboratory evaluation of serum analysis for HLA antibody and crossmatch reactivity by lymphocytotoxicity methods. Arch Pathol Lab Med 127: 149–156

Duquesnoy RJ, Filip DJ, Rodney GE (1977) Successful transfusion of platelets 'mismatched' for HLA antigens to alloimmunized thrombocytopenic patients. Am J Hematol 2: 219–226

Duquesnoy RJ, Anderson AJ, Tomasulo PA (1979) ABO compatibility and platelet transfusions of alloimmunized thrombocytopenic patients. Blood 54: 595–599

Duquesnoy RJ, White LT, Fierst JW et al. (1990) Multiscreen serum analysis of highly sensitized renal dialysis patients for antibodies toward public and private class I HLA determinants. Implications for computer-predicted acceptable

and unacceptable donor mismatches in kidney transplantation. Transplantation 50: 427–437

Durand-Zaleski I, Schlegel N, Blum-Boisgard C et al. (1996) Screening primiparous women and newborns for fetal/neonatal alloimmune thrombocytopenia: a prospective comparison of effectiveness and costs. Immune Thrombocytopenia Working Group. Am J Perinatol 13: 423–431

Dutcher JP, Schiffer CA, Aisner J et al. (1980) Alloimmunization following platelet transfusion: the absence of a dose response relationship. Blood 57: 395–398

Dutcher JP, Schiffer CA, Aisner J (1981) Long-term follow-up of patients with leukemia receiving platelet transfusion: identification of a large group of patients who do not become alloimmunized. Blood 58: 1007–1011

Dzik WH (2000) Leukocyte counting during process control of leukoreduced blood components. Vox Sang 78 (Suppl. 2): 223–226

Dzik WH (2003) Apoptosis, TGF beta and transfusion-related immunosuppression: Biologic versus clinical effects. Transfusion Apheresis Sci 29: 127–129

Dzik WH, Anderson JK, O'Neill EM et al. (2002) A prospective, randomized clinical trial of universal WBC reduction. Transfusion 42: 1114–1122

Eernisse JG, Brand A (1981) Prevention of platelet refractoriness due to HLA antibodies by administration of leukocyte-poor blood components. Exp Hematol 9: 77–83

Engelfriet CP, Tetteroo PAT, van der Veen JPW et al. (1984) Granulocyte-specific antigens and methods for their detection. In: Advances in Immunology: Blood Cell Antigens and Bone Marrow Transplantation. Progress in Clinical and Biological Research. J McCullough, SG Sandler (eds). New York: Alan R Liss, pp. 121–154

Engelfriet CP, Reesink HW, Aster RH et al. (1997) Management of alloimmunized, refractory patients in need of platelet transfusions. Vox Sang 73: 191–198

Evans WH, Mage M (1978) Development of surface antigen during maturation of bone marrow neutrophil granulocytes. Exp Hematol 6: 37–42

Falk K, Rötzchke O, Stevanovic S (1991) Allele-specific motifs revealed by sequencing of self-peptides eluted from MHC molecules. Nature (Lond) 351: 290–296

Fergusson D, Hébert PC, Lee SK et al. (2003) Clinical outcomes following institution of universal leukoreduction of blood transfusions for premature infants. JAMA 289: 1950–1956

Filipovich AH, Stone JV, Tomany SC et al. (2001) Impact of donor type on outcome of bone marrow transplantation for Wiskott–Aldrich syndrome: collaborative study of the International Bone Marrow Transplant Registry and the National Marrow Donor Program. Blood 97: 1598–1603

Fischer GF, Faée I, Petrasek M (1995) A combination of two distinct in vitro amplification procedures for DNA typing of HLA-DRB and PQBI alleles. Vox Sang 69: 328–335

Flug F, Karkapkin M, Karpatkin S (1994) Should all pregnant women be tested for their platelet PlA (Zw, HPA-1) phenotype. Br J Haematol 86: 1–5

Foster CB, Lehrnbecher T, Mol F et al. (1998) Host defense molecule polymorphisms influence the risk for immune-mediated complications in chronic granulomatous disease. J Clin Invest 102: 2146–2155

Foster CB, Zhu S, Erichsen HC et al. (2001) Polymorphisms in inflammatory cytokines and Fcgamma receptors in childhood chronic immune thrombocytopenic purpura: a pilot study. Br J Haematol 113: 596–599

Freedman J, Blanchette V, Hornstein A (1991) Utility of antiplatelet antibody detection methods (Abstract). Blood 78 (Suppl.): 351a

Friedberg RC, Donnelly SF, Mintz PD (1994) Independent roles for platelet crossmatching and HLA in the selection of platelets for alloimmunized patients. Transfusion 34: 215–220

Friedman JM, Aster RH (1985) Neonatal alloimmune thrombocytopenic purpura and congenital porencephaly in two siblings associated with a 'new' maternal anti-platelet antibody. Blood 65: 1412–1415

Fromont P, Bettaieb A, Skouri H (1992) Frequency of the polymorphonuclear neutrophil Fc gamma receptor III deficiency in the French population and its involvement in the development of neonatal alloimmune neutropenia. Blood 79: 2131–2134

Fudenberg HH, Fudenberg BR (1964) Antibody to hereditary human gamma-globulin (Gm) factor resulting from maternal-fetal incompatibility. Science 145: 170

Fudenberg HH, Franklin EC, Meltzer M et al. (1964) Antigenicity of hereditary human gamma-globulin (Gm) factors – biological and chemical aspects. Cold Spring Harbor Symp Quart Biol 29: 463

Fujisawa K, Tani P, Piro L et al. (1993) The effect of therapy on platelet-associated autoantibody in chronic immune thrombocytopenic purpura. Blood 81: 2872–2877

Fung MK, Rao N, Rice J et al. (2004) Leukoreduction in the setting of open heart surgery: a prospective cohort-controlled study. Transfusion 44: 30–35

Fung YL, Pitcher LA, Willett JE et al. (2003) Alloimmune neonatal neutropenia linked to anti-HNA-4a. Transfusion Med 13: 49–52

Furihata K, Nugent DJ, Bissonette A (1987) On the association of the platelet-specific alloantigen, Pena, with glycoprotein IIIa. Evidence for the heterogeneity of glycoprotein IIIa. J Clin Invest 80: 1624–1630

Guertler LG, Wernicke D, Eberle J (1984) Increase in prevalence of anti-HTLV-III in haemophiliacs. Lancet ii: 1275–1276

Gaddipati S, Berkowitz RL, Lembet AA et al. (2001) Initial fetal platelet counts predict the response to intravenous gammaglobulin therapy in fetuses that are affected by PLA1 incompatibility. Am J Obstet Gynecol 185: 976–980

Garretti TPJ, Saper MA, Bjorkman PJ (1989) Specificity pockets for the side chains of peptide antigens in HLA-Aw68. Nature (Lond) 342: 692–696

Gascon P, Zoumbos NC, Young NS (1984) Immunologic abnormalities in patients receiving multiple blood transfusions. Ann Intern Med 100: 173–177

Geraghty DE, Koller DH, Orr HT (1987) A human histocompatibility complex class I gene that encodes a protein with a shortened cytoplasmic sequence. Proc Natl Acad Sci USA 84: 9145–9149

Gerbase DL, Wollman EE, Lepage V (1981) Alloantigens expressed on activated human T cells different from HLA-A, B, C and DR antigens. Immunogenetics 13: 529–537

Giltay JC, Leeksma OC, dem Borne AEGK (1988a) Alloantigenic composition of the endothelial vitronectin receptor. Blood 72: 230–233

Giltay JC, Brinkman HJM, dem Borne AEGK (1988b) Expression of alloantigen Zwa (or PLA1) on human vascular smooth muscle cells and foreskin fibroblasts. A study on normal individuals and a patient with Glanzmann's thrombasthenia. Blood 74: 965–970

Gleichmann H, Breininger J (1975) Over 95% sensitization against allogeneic leukocytes following single massive blood transfusion. Vox Sang 28: 66

Gmur J, van Elten A, Osterwalder B (1983) Delayed alloimmunization using random single donor platelet transfusion: a prospective study in thrombocytopenic patients with acute leukemia. Blood 62: 473–479

Gold ER, Fudenberg HH (1967) Chromic chloride: a coupling reagent for passive hemagglutination reactions. J Immunol 99: 859

Gonzalez-Escribano MF, Aguilar F, Sanchez-Roman J et al. (2002) FcgammaRIIA, FcgammaRIIIA and FcgammaRIIIB polymorphisms in Spanish patients with systemic lupus erythematosus. Eur J Immunogenet 29: 301–306

Goodman HS, Masaitis L (1967) Analysis of the isoimmune response to leucocytes. I. Maternal cytotoxic leucocyte isoantibodies formed during the first pregnancy. Vox Sang 16: 97

Gouttefangeas C, Diehl M, Keilholz W et al. (2000) Thrombocyte HLA molecules retain nonrenewable endogenous peptides of megakaryocyte lineage and do not stimulate direct allocytotoxicity in vitro. Blood 95: 3168–3175

Greinacher A, Amiral J, Dummel V et al. (1994) Laboratory diagnosis of heparin-associated thrombocytopenia and comparison of platelet aggregation test, heparin-induced platelet activation test, and platelet factor 4/heparin enzyme-linked immunosorbent assay. Transfusion 34: 381–385

597

Grubb R (1956) Agglutination of erythrocytes coated with 'incomplete' anti-Rh by certain rheumatoid arthritic sera and some other sera despite dilution. The existence of human serum groups. Acta Path Microbiol Scand 39: 105

Grumet FC, Krishnaswaney S, See-Tho K (1994) Soluble form of an HLA-B7 class I antigen specifically suppresses humoral alloimmunisation. Hum Immunol 40: 228–234

Hadley A, Holburn AM (1984) The detection of anti-granulocyte antibodies by chemiluminescence. Clin Lab Haematol 6: 351–361

Hansen JA, Yamamoto K, Petersdorf E et al. (1999) The role of HLA matching in hematopoietic cell transplantation. Rev Immunogenet 1: 359–373

Harrington WJ, Minnich V, Hollingsworth JM (1951) Demonstration of a thrombocytopenic factor in the blood of patients with thrombocytopenic purpura. J Lab Clin Med 38: 1

Heal JM, Rowe JM, McMican A (1993a) The role of ABO matching in platelet transfusion. Eur J Haematol 50: 100–117

Heal JM, Rowe JM, Blumberg N (1993b) ABO and platelet transfusion revisited. Am Haematol 66: 309–314

Hebert PC, Fergusson D, Blajchman MA et al. (2003) Clinical outcomes following institution of the Canadian universal leukoreduction program for red blood cell transfusions. JAMA 289: 1941–1949

Heddle NM, Klama L, Kelton JG (1995) The use of anti-D to improve post-transfusion platelet response: a randomized trial. Br J Haematol 89: 163–168

Heiss MM, Mempel W, Jauch KW et al. (1993) Beneficial effect of autologous blood transfusion on infectious complications after colorectal cancer surgery. Lancet 342: 1328–1333

Heiss MM, Mempel W, Delanoff C et al. (1994) Blood transfusion-modulated tumor recurrence: first results of a randomized study of autologous versus allogeneic blood transfusion in colorectal cancer surgery. J Clin Oncol 12: 1859–1867

Held JP, Kahan BD, Lawrence G (1994) The impact of HLA mismatching on the survival of first cadaveric kidney transplants. N Engl J Med 331: 765–770

Helmerhorst FM, Smeenk RJT, Hack CE (1983) Interference of IgG, IgG aggregates and immune complexes in tests for platelet autoantibodies. Br J Haematol 55: 533

Helmerhorst FM, van Oss CJ, Bruynes ECE (1982) Elution of granulocyte and platelet antibodies. Vox Sang 43: 196–204

Hessner MJ, Curtis BR, Endean DJ et al. (1996) Determination of neutrophil antigen gene frequencies in five ethnic groups by polymerase chain reaction with sequence-specific primers. Transfusion 36: 895–899

Hessner MJ, Shivaram SM, Dinauer DM et al. (1999) Neutrophil antigen (FcgammaRIIIB) SH gene frequencies in six racial groups. Blood 93: 1115–1116

Holme S, Ross D, Heaton WA (1989) In vitro and in vivo evaluation of platelet concentrates after cotton wool filtration. Vox Sang 57: 112–115

Holt PDJ, Tandy NP, Anstee DJ (1977) The screening of blood donors for IgA deficiency: a study of the donor population of South-West England. J Clin Pathol 30: 1007

van Hooff JP, Kalff MW, van Poelgeest AE (1976) Blood transfusions and kidney transplantation. Transplantation 22: 306

Houbiers JG, Brand A, van de Watering LM et al. (1994) Randomised controlled trial comparing transfusion of leucocyte-depleted or buffy-coat-depleted blood in surgery for colorectal cancer. Lancet 344: 573–578

Howard JE, Perkins HA (1978) The natural history of allo-immunization to platelets. Transfusion 18: 496–503

Hughes M, Hayward CP, Warkentin TE et al. (2000) Morphological analysis of microparticle generation in heparin-induced thrombocytopenia. Blood 96: 188–194

Huizinga TWJ, Kerst JM, Nuyens JH (1989) Binding characteristics of dimeric IgG subclass complexes to human neutrophils. J Immunol 142: 2359–2364

Huizinga TWJ, Kleijer M, Tettroo PAT (1990) Biallelic neutrophil NA-antigen system is associated with a polymorphism on the phospho-inositol-linked Fc-gamma receptor III (CD16). Blood 75: 213–217

Hutchinson RM, Sejeny SA, Fraser ID (1976) Lymphocyte response to blood transfusion in man: a comparison of different preparations of blood. Br J Haematol 33: 105

Ikeda H, Mitani T, Ohnuma M et al. (1989) A new platelet specific antigen, Nak^a involved in the refractoriness of HLA-matched platelet transfusion. Vox Sang 57: 213

Iwaki Y, Cecka JM, Terasaki PI (1990) The transfusion effect in cadaver kidney transplants, yes or no. Transplantation 49: 56–59

Jager MJ, Claas FHJ, Witvliet M (1986) Correspondence of the monocyte antigen HMA-1 to the non-HLA antigen 9a. Immunogenetics 23: 71–78

Jallu V, Meunier M, Brement M et al. (2002) A new platelet polymorphism Duv(a+), localized within the RGD binding domain of glycoprotein IIIa, is associated with neonatal thrombocytopenia. Blood 99: 4449–4456

Jensen LS, Andersen AJ, Christiansen PM et al. (1992) Postoperative infection and natural killer cell function following blood transfusion in patients undergoing elective colorectal surgery. Br J Surg 79: 513–516

Jensen LS, Kissmeyer-Nielsen P, Wolff B et al. (1996) Randomised comparison of leucocyte-depleted versus buffy-coat-poor blood transfusion and complications after colorectal surgery. Lancet 348: 841–845

Joyce S, Wayne FW, Mohanakumar T (1988) Characterization of kidney cell-specific, non-major histocompatibility complex alloantigen using antibodies eluted from rejected human renal allografts. Transplantation 46: 362–369

Kaban BD, van Buren CT, Flechner SM (1983) Cyclosporine immunosuppression mitigates immunologic risk factors in renal allotransplantation. Transplant Proc 15: 2469–2479

Kao KJ, Mickel M, Braine HG et al. (1995) White cell reduction in platelet concentrates and packed red cells by filtration: a multicenter clinical trial. The TRAP Study Group. Transfusion 35: 13–19

Kaplan C (1984) Donor-specific blood transfusion and renal graft survival: a 3 year experience in pediatrics. In: Histocompatibility Testing. ED Albert, MP Baur, WR Mayr (eds). Berlin: Springer-Verlag

Kaplan C, Daffos F, Forestier F (1990) Fetal platelet counts in thrombocytopenic pregnancy. Lancet ii: 979–982

Kaplan C, Morel-Kopp MC, Clemenceau S (1992) Fetal and neonatal alloimmune thrombocytopenia: current trends in diagnosis and therapy. Transfusion Med 2: 265–271

Kaplan C, Daffos F, Forestier F (1995) Management of fetal and neonatal alloimmune thrombocytopenia. Vox Sang 67, S3: 85–88

Kaplan C, Morel-Kopp MC, Kroll H et al. (1991) HPA-5b (Bra) neonatal alloimmune thrombocytopenia; clinical and immunological analysis of 39 cases. Br J Haematol 78: 425–430

Kawamura T, Sakagami K, Haisa M (1989) Induction of antiidiotypic antibodies by donor-specific blood transfusions. Transplantation 48: 459–463

Kekomaki R, Raivio P, Kers P (1992) A new low-frequency platelet alloantigen, Vaa, on glycoprotein IIb/IIIa associated with neonatal alloimmune thrombocytopenia. Transfusion Med 2: 27–33

Kekomaki R, Suomalainen M, Ollikainen J (1993) A new low frequency platelet alloantigen Tu(a) on glycoprotein IIIa associated with neonatal alloimmune thrombocytopenia. Br J Haematol 83: 306–310

Kelly AP, Monaco JJ, Cho S (1991) A new human class II related locus, DM. Nature (Lond) 353: 571–573

Kelton JG (2002) Heparin-induced thrombocytopenia: an overview. Blood Rev 16: 77–80

Kelton JG, Smith JW, Horsewood P (1990) Gova/b alloantigen system on human platelets. Blood 75: 2172–2176

van Kessel AHMG, Stoker K, Claas FHJ (1983) Assignment of the leucocyte group five surface antigens to human chromosome 4. Tissue Antigens 21: 213–218

Kickler T, Braine HG, Piantadosi S et al. (1990) A randomized, placebo-controlled trial of intravenous gammaglobulin in alloimmunized thrombocytopenic patients. Blood 75: 313–316

Kickler TS, Herman JH, Furihata K (1988a) Identification of Bak(b), a new platelet-specific antigen associated with posttransfusion purpura. Blood 71: 894–898

Kickler TS, Ness PM, Braine HG (1988b) Platelet crossmatching. A direct approach to the selection of platelet transfusions for the alloimmunized thrombocytopenic patient. Am J Clin Pathol 90: 69–72

Kiefel V, Santoso S, Weisheit M et al. (1987) Monoclonal antibody-specific immobilization of platelet antigens (MAIPA): a new tool for the identification of platelet-reactive antibodies. Blood 70: 1722–1726

Kiefel V, Santoso S, Katzmann B (1988) A new platelet-specific alloantigen Br(a). Report on four cases with neonatal alloimmune thrombocytopenia. Vox Sang 54: 101–106

Kiefel V, Santoso S, Glockner B (1989a) Post-transfusion purpura associated with an antibody against an allele of the Bak^a antigen. Vox Sang 56: 93–97

Kiefel V, Santoso S, Katzmann B (1989b) The Br(a)/Br(b) alloantigen systems on platelets. Blood 73: 2219–2223

Kiefel V, Santoso S, Mueller-Eckhardt C (1989c) Autoimmune thrombocytopenic purpura: diversity of glycoprotein specificity of autoantibodies determined with monoclonal antibodies. Blood 74 (Suppl.) 1: 147a

Kiefel V, Vicariot M, Giovangrandy Y (1995) Alloimmunization against Iy, a low frequency antigen on platelet glycoprotien Ib/IX as cause for severe neonatal alloimmune thrombocytopenic purpura. Vox Sang 69: 250–255

Kieffer N, Boizard B, Didry D (1984) Immunochemical characterization of the platelet-specific alloantigen Lek^a, a comparative study with the Pla^1 alloantigen. Blood 64: 1212–1219

Kissel K, Hofmann C, Gittinger FS et al. (2000) HNA-1a, HNA-1b, and HNA-1c (NA1, NA2, SH) frequencies in African and American Blacks and in Chinese. Tissue Antigens 56: 143–148

Kissel K, Scheffler S, Kerowgan M et al. (2002) Molecular basis of NB1 (HNA-2a, CD177) deficiency. Blood 99: 4231–4233

Klein HG (1999) Immunomodulatory aspects of transfusion: a once and future risk? Anesthesiology 91: 861–865

Klein HG (2001) The immunomodulatory effects of blood transfusion. Tumori 87: S17–S19

Kline WE, Press C, Clay ME (1982) Studies of sera defining a new granulocyte antigen (Abstract). Transfusion 22: 428

Koene HR, Kleijer M, Roos D et al. (1998) Fc gamma RIIIB gene duplication: evidence for presence and expression of three distinct Fc gamma RIIIB genes in NA(1+,2+)SH(+) individuals. Blood 91: 673–679

Koistinen J (1975) Selective IgA deficiency in blood donors. Vox Sang 29: 192

Kolb HJ, Mittermuller J, Clemm C et al. (1990) Donor leukocyte transfusions for treatment of recurrent chronic myelogenous leukemia in marrow transplant patients. Blood 76: 2462–2465

Kovats S, Main E, Librach C (1991) A class I antigen expressed in human trophoblasts. Science 248: 220–223

Kroll H, Kiefel V, Santoso S (1990) Srᵃ, a private platelet antigen on glycoprotein IIIa associated with neonatal alloimmune thrombocytopenia. Blood 76: 2296–2302

Kruskall MS, Lee TH, Assmann SF et al. (2001) Survival of transfused donor white blood cells in HIV-infected recipients. Blood 98: 272–279

Kuijpers RWAM, Modderman PW, Bleeker PMM (1989) Localization of the platelet specific Ko-system antigen Koa/Kob in GP/1b/1x. Blood 74 Suppl. I: 226a

Kuijpers RWAM, Faber NM, Cuypers HM (1992a) The N-terminal globular domain of human platelet glycoprotein Ibx has a methionine145/threonine145 amino-acid polymorphism, which is associated with the HPA-2 (Ko) alloantigens. J Clin Invest 89: 381–384

Kuijpers RWAM, dem Borne AEGK, Kiefel V (1992b) Leucine33-proline33 substitution in human platelet glycoprotein IIIa determines the HLA DRw52a (Dw24) association of the immune response against HPA-1a (Zwa/Pla¹) and HPA-1b(Zwb/Pla²). Hum Immunol 34: 253–256

Kuijpers RWAM, Simsek S, Faber NM (1993) Single point mutation in human glycoprotein IIIa is associated with a new platelet-specific alloantigen (Mo) involved in neonatal alloimmune thrombocytopenia. Blood 81: 70–76

Kunicki TJ, Aster RH (1979) Isolation and immunologic characterization of the human platelet alloantigen, Pla¹. Mol Immunol 16: 353–360

Kunicki TJ, Pidard D, Cazenave J-P (1981) Inheritance of the human platelet alloantigen, Pla¹, in Glanzmann's thrombasthenia. J Clin Invest 67: 712–724

Kurata Y, Oshida M, Take H et al. (1989) New approach to eliminate HLA class I antigens from platelet surface without cell damage: acid treatment at pH 3.0. Vox Sang 57: 199–204

L'Abbé D, Trumblay L, Filion M (1992) Alloimmunization to platelet antigen HPA-1a (Pla¹) is strongly associated with both HLA-DRB3*0101 and HLA-DQB*0201. Hum Immunol 34: 107–114

Lagaaij EL, Hennemann IP, Ruigrok M et al. (1989) Effect of one-HLA-DR-antigen-matched and completely HLA-DR-mismatched blood transfusions on survival of heart and kidney allografts. N Engl J Med 321: 701–705

Lalezari P (1977) Neutrophil antigens: immunology and clinical implications. In: The Granulocyte: Function and Clinical Utilization. Progress in Clinical and Biological Research. TJ Greenwalt, GA Jamieson (eds). New York: Alan R Liss, p. 209

Lalezari P, Bernard GE (1966a) An isologous antigen-antibody reaction with human neutrophiles, related to neonatal neutropenia. J Clin Invest 45: 1741–1750

Lalezari P, Bernard GE (1966b) A new neutrophile-specific antigen. Its role in the pathogenesis of neonatal neutropenia. Fed Proc 25: 371

Lalezari P, Radel E (1974) Neutrophil-specific antigens: immunology and clinical significance. Semin Hematol 11: 281

Lalezari P, Nussbaum M, Gelman S (1960) Neonatal neutropenia due to maternal isoimmunization. Blood 15: 236

Lalezari P, Jiang AF, Yegen L (1975) Chronic autoimmune neutropenia due to anti-NA2 antibody. N Engl J Med 293: 744

La Nasa G, Giardini C, Argiolu F et al. (2002) Unrelated donor bone marrow transplantation for thalassemia: the effect of extended haplotypes. Blood 99: 4350–4356

Landsteiner K (1931) Individual differences in human blood. Science 73: 405

Landsteiner K, Levine P (1929) On isoagglutinin reactions of human blood other than those defining the blood groups. J Immunol 17: 1

Langenscheidt F, Kiefel V, Santoso S (1989) Quantitation of platelet antigens after chloroquine treatment. Eur J Haematol 42: 186–192

Leak M, Poole J, Kaye T (1990) The rare MkMk phenotype in a Turkish antenatal patient and evidence for clinical significance of anti-Enᵃ (Abstract). Transfusion Med (Suppl. 1): 26:

Lechler RJ, Batchelor JR (1982) Restoration of immunogenicity to passenger cell depleted kidney allografts by the addition of donor strain dentritic cells. J Exp Med 155: 31–41

Leddy JP, Bakemeier RF (1967) A relationship of direct Coombs test pattern to autoantibody specificity in acquired hemolytic anemia. Proc Soc Exp Biol (NY) 125: 808

Lederman MM, Ratnoff OD, Scillian JJ (1983) Impaired cell-mediated immunity in patients with classic haemophilia. N Engl J Med 308: 79–83

Lee EJ, Schiffer CA (1987) Serial measurement of lymphocytotoxic antibody and response to nonmatched platelet transfusions in alloimmunized patients. Blood 70: 1727–1729

Lee EJ, Schiffer CA (1989) ABO compatibility can influence the results of platelet transfusion. Results of a randomized trial. Transfusion 29: 384–389

Lee TH, Donegan E, Slichter S et al. (1995) Transient increase in circulating donor leukocytes after allogeneic transfusions in immunocompetent recipients compatible with donor cell proliferation. Blood 85: 1207–1214

Lee TH, Paglieroni T, Ohto H et al. (1999) Survival of donor leukocyte subpopulations in immunocompetent transfusion recipients: frequent long-term microchimerism in severe trauma patients. Blood 93: 3127–3139

Lee TH, Reed W, Mangawang-Montalvo L et al. (2001) Donor WBCs can persist and transiently mediate immunologic function in a murine transfusion model: effects of irradiation, storage, and histocompatibility. Transfusion 41: 637–642

Leeksma OC, Giltay JC, Zandbergen-Spaargaren J (1987) The platelet alloantigen Zw^a or Pla^1 is expressed on cultured endothelial cells. Br J Haematol 66: 369–373

van Leeuwen A, Festenstein H, van Rood JJ (1982) Di-allelic alloantigenic systems on subsets of T-cells. Hum Immunol 4: 109–121

van Leeuwen EF, von dem Borne AEGK, von Riesz LE (1981) Absence of platelet-specific alloantigens in Glanzmann's thrombasthenia. Blood 57: 49–54

van Leeuwen EF, van der Ven JT, Engelfriet CP (1982) Specificity of autoantibodies in autoimmune thrombocytopenia. Blood 59: 23–26

Lehman HA, Lehman LO, Rustagi PK (1987) Complement-mediated autoimmune thrombocytopenia. Monoclonal IgM antiplatelet antibody associated with lymphoreticular malignant disease. N Engl J Med 316: 194–198

Lescale KB, Eddleman KA, Cines DB et al. (1996) Anti-platelet antibody testing in thrombocytopenic pregnant women. Am J Obstet Gynecol 174: 1014–1018

Lindahl-Kiessling K, Safwenberg J (1971) Inability of UV-irradiated lymphocytes to stimulate allogeneic cells in mixed lymphocyte culture. Int Arch Allerg Appl Immunol 41: 670–678

Lo Buglio AF, Court WS, Vincour L (1983) Immune thrombocytopenic purpura. Use of 121I-labeled anti-human IgG monoclonal antibody to quantify platelet-bound IgG. N Engl J Med 309: 459–463

Loeliger C, Ruhlmann E, Kuhnl P (1993) A rapid and sensitive immunoassay for antibodies against alloantigens on human platelet glycoproteins (BIPA). J Immunol Methods 158: 197–200

van Loghem E (1974) Familial occurrence of isolated IgA deficiency associated with antibodies to IgA. Evidence against a structural gene defect. Eur J Immunol 4: 56

van Loghem E, Zegers BJM, Blast EJEG (1983) Selective deficiency of IgA2. J Clin Invest 72: 1918–1923

van Loghem JJ, Dorfmeijer H, Hart M van der (1959) Serological and genetical studies on a platelet antigen (Zw). Vox Sang 161–169

Longster GH, Major KE (1975) Anti-Kell (K1) in ascitic fluid. Vox Sang 28: 253

Lown JAG, Ivey JG (1991) Evaluation of a solid-phase red cell adherence technique for platelet antibody screening. Transfusion Med 1: 163–167

Lublin DM, Grumet FC (1982) Mechanisms of the CYNAP phenomenon: evidence in the Bw49/Bw50 model for epitopes with different spatial orientation of antibody. Hum Immunol 4: 137–145

Lucas CF (1994) Prospective evaluation of the chemiluminescence test for the detection of granulocyte antibodies: comparison with the granulocyte immunofluorescence test. Vox Sang 66: 141–147

Lundgren G, Groth CG, Albrechtsen D (1986) HLA-matching and pretransplant blood transfusions in cadaveric renal transplantation – a changing picture with cyclosporin. Lancet ii: 66–69

Lyman S, Aster RH, Visentin GP et al. 1990) Polymorphism of human platelet membrane glycoprotein IIb associated with the Baka/Bakb alloantigen system. Blood 75: 2343–2348

Lynch L, Bussel JB, McFarland JG et al. (1992a) Antenatal treatment of alloimmune thrombocytopenia. Obstet Gynecol 80: 67–71

Lynch L, Bussel JB, McFarland JG (1992b) Antenatal treatment of alloimmune thrombocytopenia. Obstet Gynecol 80: 67–71

Lyou JY, Chen YJ, Hu HY et al. (2002) PCR with sequence-specific primer-based simultaneous genotyping of human platelet antigen-1 to -13w. Transfusion 42: 1089–1095

McCullough J (1988) Granulocyte Serology: A Clinical and Laboratory Guide. Chicago, IL: American Society of Clinical Pathologists Press

McFarland JG, Blanchett V, Collins J (1993) Neonatal alloimmune thrombocytopenia due to a new platelet-specific alloantibody. Blood 81: 3318–3322

McIntosh S, O'Brien R, Schwartz A (1973) Neonatal isoimmune purpura. Response to platelet infusions. J Pediatr 82: 1020

MacLeod A, Catto G, Mather A (1985) Beneficial antibodies in renal transplantation developing after blood transfusion: evidence for HLA linkage. Transplant Proc 27: 1057–1058

McMillan R (2003) Antiplatelet antibodies in chronic adult immune thrombocytopenic purpura: assays and epitopes. J Pediatr Hematol Oncol 25 Suppl. 1: S57–S61

McMillan R, Tani P, Milland F (1987) Platelet-associated and plasma anti-glycoprotein autoantibodies in chronic ITP. Blood 70: 1040–1145

McMillan R, Wang L, Tani P (2003) Prospective evaluation of the immunobead assay for the diagnosis of adult chronic immune thrombocytopenic purpura (ITP). J Thromb Haemost 1: 485–491

Madden DR, Wiley DC (1992) Peptide binding to the major histocompatibility complex molecules. Curr Opin Struct Biol 2: 300–304

Madden DR, Gorga JC, Strominger JL (1991) The structure of HLA-B27 reveals nonamer self-peptides bound in an extended conformation. Nature (Lond) 352: 321–325

Magee JM (1985) A study of the effects of treating platelets with paraformaldehyde for use in the platelet suspension immunofluorescence test. Br J Haematol 61: 513–516

Maheshwari A, Christensen RD, Calhoun DA (2002) Resistance to recombinant human granulocyte colony-stimulating factor in neonatal alloimmune neutropenia associated with anti-human neutrophil antigen-2a (NB1) antibodies. Pediatrics 109: e64

Marijt WA, Heemskerk MH, Kloosterboer FM *et al.* (2003) Hematopoiesis-restricted minor histocompatibility antigens HA-1- or HA-2-specific T cells can induce complete remissions of relapsed leukemia. Proc Natl Acad Sci USA 100: 2742–2747

Marquet RL, Heystek GA (1981) Induction of suppressor cells by donor-specific blood transfusion and heart transplantation in rats. Transplantation 31: 272–274

Marsh SG (2003) Nomenclature for factors of the HLA system, update, September 2002. Hum Immunol 64: 572–573

Marsh SGE, Bodmer JG (1989) HLA-DR and -DQ epitopes and monoclonal antibody specificity. Immunol Today 10: 305–312

Martinelli GP, Horowitz C, Chiang K (1987) Pretransplant conditioning with donor-specific transfusions using heated blood and cyclosporine. Transplantation 43: 140–145

van Marwijk KM, van Prooijen HC, Moes M *et al.* (1991) Use of leukocyte-depleted platelet concentrates for the prevention of refractoriness and primary HLA alloimmunization: a prospective, randomized trial. Blood 77: 201–205

Masse M, Andreu G, Angue M (1991) A multicenter study on the efficacy of white cell reduction by filtration of red cells. Transfusion 31: 792–797

Matsuo K, Lin A, Procter JL *et al.* (2000) Variations in the expression of granulocyte antigen NB1. Transfusion 40: 654–662

Matsuo K, Procter JL, Chanock S *et al.* (2001) The expression of NA antigens in people with unusual Fcgamma receptor III genotypes. Transfusion 41: 775–782

Mavroudis D, Barrett J (1996) The graft-versus-leukemia effect. Curr Opin Hematol 3: 423–429

Mavroudis DA, Dermime S, Molldrem J *et al.* (1998) Specific depletion of alloreactive T cells in HLA-identical siblings: a method for separating graft-versus-host and graft-versus-leukaemia reactions. Br J Haematol 101: 565–570

van der Meer PF, Pietersz RN, Nelis JT *et al.* (1999) Six filters for the removal of white cells from red cell concentrates, evaluated at 4 degrees C and/or at room temperature. Transfusion 39: 265–270

Metcalfe P, Waters AH (1992) Location of the granulocyte-specific antigen LAN on the Fc-receptor 111. Transfusion Med 2: 283–287

Metcalfe P, Watkins NA, Ouwehand WH *et al.* (2003) Nomenclature of human platelet antigens. Vox Sang 85: 240–245

Millard FE, Tani P, McMillan R (1987) A specific assay for anti-HLA antibodies: application to platelet donor selection. Blood 70: 1495–1499

Moeschlin S, Wagner K (1952) Agranulocytosis due to the occurrence of leucocyte agglutinins (pyramidon and cold agglutinins). Acta Haematol 8: 29

Mollicone R, Caillard T, Le Pendu J *et al.* (1988) Expression of ABH and X (Lex) antigens on platelets and lymphocytes. Blood 71: 1113–1119

Moloney MD, Bulmer JN, Scott JS (1989) Maternal immune responses and recurrent miscarriage (Letter). Lancet i: 46

Moraes JR, Stastny P (1977) Human endothelial cell antigens: molecular independence from HLA and expression in blood monocytes. Transplant Proc 9: 605

Morel-Kopp MC, Clemenceau S, Aurousseau MH (1994) Human platelet alloantigen typing. PCR analysis is not a substitute for serological methods. Transfusion Med 4: 9–14

Moroff G, Garratty G, Heal IM (1992) Selection of platelets for refractory patients by HLA matching and prospective crossmatching. Transfusion 32: 633–640

Moses LA, Stroncek DF, Cipolone KM *et al.* (2000) Detection of HLA antibodies by using flow cytometry and latex beads coated with HLA antigens. Transfusion 40: 861–866

Moulinier J (1957). Iso-immunisation maternelle antiplaquettaire et purpura néo-natal. Le système de groupe plaquettaire 'Duzo'. Proc 6th Congr Europe Soc Haem Copenhagen, p. 817

Mowbray JF, Underwood JC, Michel M (1987) Immunization with paternal lymphocytes in women with recurrent spontaneous abortion. Lancet ii: 679–680

Mueller-Eckhardt C (1991) Platelet allo- and autoantigens and their clinical implications. In: Transfusion Medicine in the 1990s. ST Nance (ed.). Arlington, VA: American Association of Blood Banks

Mueller-Eckhardt C, Kiefel VG (1989) High dose IgG treatment for neonatal autoimmune thrombocytopenia. Blut 59: 145–146

Mueller-Eckhardt C, Mueller-Eckhardt G, Willen-Ohff H (1985) Immunogenicity of, and immune response to, the human platelet antigen Zw^a is strongly associated with HLA-B8 and -DR3. Tissue Antigens 26: 71–76

Mueller-Eckhardt C, Kiefel V, Grubert A *et al.* (1989a) 348 cases of suspected neonatal alloimmune thrombocytopenia. Lancet 1: 363–366

Mueller-Eckhardt C, Kiefel V, Kroll H (1989b) HLA-Drw6, a new immune response marker for immunization against the platelet alloantigen Br^a. Vox Sang 57: 90–91

Mueller-Eckhardt C, Giers G, Bold R (1993) Prenatal management of fetal alloimmune thrombocytopenia. Vox Sang 65: 186–187

Munson JL, van Twuyver E, Mooijaart RJD (1995) Missing T cell receptor V beta families following blood transfusion. Hum Immunol 42: 43–54

Murphy ME, Metcalf P, Thomas H (1986) Use of leucocyte-poor blood components and HLA-matched platelet donors to prevent HLA-alloimmunization. Br J Haematol 62: 529–534

Murphy MF, Metcalfe P, Ord J et al. (1987) Disappearance of HLA and platelet-specific antibodies in acute leukaemia patients alloimmunized by multiple transfusions. Br J Haematol 67: 255–260

Murphy MF, Metcalfe P, Waters AH (1993) Antenatal management of severe fetomaternal alloimmune thrombocytopenia: HLA incompatibility may affect responses to fetal platelet transfusions. Blood 81: 2174–2179

Myhr KM, Raknes G, Nyland H et al. (1999) Immunoglobulin G Fc-receptor (FcgammaR) IIA and IIIB polymorphisms related to disability in MS. Neurology 52: 1771–1776

Mytelineos J, Scherer S, Opelz G (1990) Comparison of RFLP-DRP and serological DR typing in 1500 individuals. Transplantation 50: 870–873

Nagarajan S, Chesla S, Cobern L et al. (1995) Ligand binding and phagocytosis by CD16 (Fc gamma receptor III) isoforms. Phagocytic signaling by associated zeta and gamma subunits in Chinese hamster ovary cells. J Biol Chem 270: 25762–25770

Nagasawa T, Hasegawa Y, Korneno T (1995) Simultaneous measurement of megakaryocyte-associated IgG (MAIgG) and platelet-associated IgG (PAIgG) in chronic idiopathic thrombocytopenic purpura. Eur J Haematol 54: 314–320

Naidu S (1983) Central nervous system lesions in neonatal isoimmune thrombocytopenia. Arch Neurol 40: 552–554

Nambiar A, Adams S, Reid J et al. (2003) Hlamatchmaker-driven analysis of response to HLA matched platelet transfusions. Hum Immunol 64: S77

Newman PJ (1994) Nomenclature of human platelet alloantigens: a problem with the HPA system? Blood 83: 1447–1451

Newman PJ, Derbes RS, Aster RH (1989) The human platelet alloantigens PlA1 and PlA2 are associated with a leucine33/proline33 amino acid polymorphism in membrane glycoprotein IIIa and are distinguishable by DNA typing. J Clin Invest 83: 1778–1781

Ng J, Hurley LA, Baxter-Lowe LA (1993) Large-scale oligonucleotide typing for HLA-DRBl/3/4 and HLA-DQB1 is highly accurate, specific and reliable. Tissue Antigens 42: 473–479

Nichols WG, Price TH, Gooley T et al. (2003) Transfusion-transmitted cytomegalovirus infection after receipt of leukoreduced blood products. Blood 101: 4195–4200

Nikaein A, Backman L, Jennings L (1994) HLA compatibility and liver transplant outcome. Transplantation 58: 786–792

Noris P, Simsek S, Bruyne-Admiraal LG (1995) Mana, a new low frequency platelet-specific antigen localized on glycoprotein IIb, is associated with neonatal alloimmune thrombocytopenia. Blood 86: 1019–1026

Novotny VMJ, van Doorn R, Witvliet MD (1995) Occurrence of allogeneic HLA and non-HLA antibodies after transfusion of prestorage filtered platelets and red blood cells: a prospective study. Blood 85: 1736–1741

Nymand G (1974) Complement-fixing and lymphocytotoxic antibodies in serum of pregnant women at delivery. Vox Sang 27: 322

Ober C, Karrison T, Odem RR et al. (1999) Mononuclear-cell immunisation in prevention of recurrent miscarriages: a randomised trial. Lancet 354: 365–369

O'Connel BA, Schiffer CA (1990) Donor selection for alloimmunized patients by platelet crossmatching of random donor platelet concentrates. Transfusion 30: 314–317

O'Connell BA, Lee ES, Rothko K (1992) Selection of apheresis platelet donors by crossmatching random donor platelet concentrates. Blood 79: 527–531

Ogasawara K, Ueki J, Takenaka M et al. (1993) Study on the expression of ABH antigens on platelets. Blood 82: 993–999

Ogden PM, Astour A, Koller C (1993) Platelet crossmatches of single-donor platelet concentrates using a latex agglutination assay. Transfusion 33: 644–650

Olerup O (1994) HLA-B27 typing a group-specific PCR amplification. Tissue Antigens 43: 253–256

Olerup O, Möller E, Persson U (1990) HLA-DP incompatibilities induce significant proliferation in primary mixed lymphocyte cultures in HLA-A, -B, -DR and -DQ compatible individuals: implications for allogeneic bone marrow transplantation. Tissue Antigens 36: 194–202

Olerup O, Aldenes A, Fogdell A (1993) HLA-DQB1 and -DQA1 typing by PCR amplification with sequence-specific primers (PCR-SSP) in 2 hours. Tissue Antigens 41: 119–134

Opelz G (1987) Improved kidney graft survival in non-transfused recipients. Transplant Proc 19: 149–153

Opelz G (1992) Collaborative Transplant Study. Newsletter 1992, University of Heidelberg, Heidelberg

Opelz G (2005) Collaborative Transplant Study. Non-HLA transplant immunity revealed by lymphocytotoxic antibodies. Lancet 365: 1570–1576

Opelz G, Sengar DPS, Mickey MR (1973) Effect of blood transfusions on subsequent kidney transplants. Transplant Proc 5: 253

Opelz G, Mytilineos J, Scherer S (1993) Analysis of HLA-DR matching in DNA-typed cadaver kidney transplants. Transplantation 55: 782–785

Opelz G, Vanrenterghem Y, Kirste G et al. (1997) Prospective evaluation of pretransplant blood transfusions in cadaver kidney recipients. Transplantation 63: 964–967

Opelz G, Wujciak T, Dohler B et al. (1999) HLA compatibility and organ transplant survival. Collaborative Transplant Study. Rev Immunogenet 1: 334–342

Ory PA, Clark MR, Kwoh EE et al. (1989) Sequences of complementary DNAs that encode the NA1 and NA2 forms of Fc receptor III on human neutrophils. J Clin Invest 84: 1688–1691

603

Overweg J, Engelfriet CP (1969) Cytoxic leucocyte isoanti-bodies formed during the first pregnancy. Vox Sang 16: 97

Ozawa N, Shimiza M, Imai M (1985) Selective absence of immunoglobulin A1 or A2 among blood donors and hospital patients. Transfusion 26: 73–76

Pamer E, Cresswell P (1998) Mechanisms of MHC class I-restricted antigen processing. Annu Rev Immunol 16: 323–358

Panzer S, Auerbach L, Chechova E (1995) Maternal alloim-munization against fetal platelets: a prospective study. Br J Haematol 90: 655–660

Paul LC, Baldwin WM, Klaas HJ et al. (1984) Monocyte alloantigens in man: genetics and expression on the renal endothelium. In: Mononuclear Phagocyte Biology. A Volkmann (ed.). New York: M Dekker

Paul WC (ed.) (2003) Fundamental Immunology. Philadel-phia, PA: Lippincott, Williams & Wilkins

Payne R, Rolfs MR (1958) Fetomaternal leucocyte incompat-ibility. J Clin Invest 37: 1756

Pegels JG, dem Borne AEGK, Bruynes ECE (1982) Pseudothrombocytopenia: an immunological study on platelet antibodies dependent on ethylene diamine tetra-acetate. Blood 59: 157

Pellegrino MA, Ferrone S, Theofilopoulos AN (1976) Isolation of human T and B lymphocytes by rosette forma-tion with 2-aminoethyliso thiouronium bromide (AET)-treated sheep red blood cells and with monkey red blood cells. J Immunol Methods 11: 273

Persijn GG, Henriks GFJ, van Rood JJ (1984) HLA matching, blood transfusion and renal transplantation. In: Clinical Immunology and Allergy. JJ van Rood, RRP de Vries (eds). London: WB Saunders

Petersdorf EW, Hansen JA, Martin PJ et al. (2001) Major-histocompatibility-complex class I alleles and antigens in hematopoietic-cell transplantation. N Engl J Med 345: 1794–1800

Petranyi CC, Padanyi A, Horuzsko A (1988) Mixed lympho-cyte culture evidence that pretransplant transfusion with platelets induces FcR and blocking antibody production similar to that induced by leucocyte transfusion. Trans-plantation 45: 823–824

Pietersz RN, van der Meer PF, Seghatchian MJ (1998) Update on leucocyte depletion of blood components by filtration. Transfusion Sci 19: 321–328

Pischel KD, Bluestein HG, Woods WL (1988) Platelet glyco-protein Ia, Ic and IIa are physicochemically indistinguish-able from the very late activation adhesion-related proteins of lymphocytes and other cell types. J Clin Invest 81: 505–513

Pollack S, Cunningham-Rundles C, Smithwick EM (1982) High dose intravenous gamma globulin in autoimmune neutropenia. N Engl J Med 307: 253

Popovsky MA (1996) Quality of blood components filtered before storage and at the bedside: implications for trans-fusion practice. Transfusion 36: 470–474

Porretti L, Marangoni F, Rebulla P (1994) Frozen platelets for platelet antibody detection and crossmatch. Vox Sang 67: 52–57

Potter ML, Moore M (1977) Human mixed lymphocyte culture using separated lymphocyte preparations. Immunol 32: 359

Powis SH, Mockridge I, Kelly PA (1992a) Effect of polymor-phism of an MHC-linked transporter gene on the peptides assembled in a class I molecule. Proc Natl Acad Sci USA 89: 71

Powis SH, Mockridge I, Kelly PA (1992b) Polymorphism in a second ABC transporter gene located within the class II region of the human major histocompatibility complex. Proc Natl Acad Sci USA 89: 71463–71467

Powis SH, Tonks S, Mockridge I (1993) Alleles and haplo-types of the MHC-encoded ABC transporters TAP1 and TAP2. Immunogenetics 37: 373–380

Puppo F, Pellicci R, Brenci S (1994) HLA class-I soluble antigen serum levels in liver transplantation: a predictor marker of acute rejection. Hum Immunol 40: 166–171

Quaranta V (1980) Manufacture of monoclonal antibodies to human melanoma associated and histocompatibility antigens. In: Immunology, Clinical Laboratory Techniques for the 1980s. RM Nakamura, WR Dito, ES Tucjer (eds). New York: Alan R Liss

Quigley RL, Wood KJ, Morris PJ (1989) Transfusion induces blood donor-specific suppressor cells. J Immunol 142: 463–470

Rachel JM, Sinor LT, Tawfik DW (1985) Solid-phase red cell adherence test for platelet cross-matching. Med Lab Sci 42: 194–195

Rachel JM, Summers TC, Sinor LT (1988) Use of a solid phase red blood cell adherence method for pretransfusion platelet compatibility testing. Am J Clin Pathol 90: 63–68

Raknes G, Skeie GO, Gilhus NE et al. (1998) Fc gamma RIIA and Fc gamma RIIIB polymorphisms in myasthenia gravis. J Neuroimmunol 81: 173–176

Ramos RR, Curtis BR, Chaplin H (1992) A latex particle assay for platelet-associated IgG. Transfusion 32: 235–238

Ravetch JV, Perussia B (1989) Alternative membrane forms of Fc gamma RIII(CD16) on human natural killer cells and neutrophils. Cell type-specific expression of two genes that differ in single nucleotide substitutions. J Exp Med 170: 481–497

Rebulla P, Porretti L, Bertolini F (1993) White cell-reduced red cells prepared by filtration: a critical evaluation of cur-rent filters and methods for counting residual white cells. Transfusion 33: 128–133

Reesink HW, Engelfriet CP (1993) Prenatal management of fetal alloimmune thrombocytopenia (Int. Forum). Vox Sang 65: 180–189

Regan L (1991) Recurrent miscarriage. BMJ 302: 543–544

Reznikoff-Etievant MF, Dangu C, Lobet R (1981) HLA-B8 antigen and anti-PlA1 alloimmunization. Tissue Antigens 18: 66–68

Robinson JP, Duque RE, Boxer LA (1987) Measurement of antineutrophil antibodies by flow cytometry: simultaneous detection of antibodies against monocytes and lymphocytes. Diagn Clin Immunol 5: 163–170

Rodwell RL, Tudehope PI, O'Regan P (1991) Alloimmune neutropenia in Australian aboriginals: an unrecognized disorder? Transfusion Med 1: 63–67

Roitt IM, Delves PJ (2001) Roitt's Essential Immunology. Oxford: Blackwell Scientific Publications

van Rood JJ (1958) Leucocyte antibodies in sera from pregnant women. Nature (Lond) 181: 1735

van Rood JJ, Ernisse JG (1968) The detection of transplantation antigens in leukocytes. Semin Hematol 5: 2

van Rood JJ, van Leeuwen A (1963) Leukocyte grouping. A method and its application. J Clin Invest 42: 1382

van Rood JJ, van Leeuwen AT (1976) B-cell antibodies, Ia-like determinants, and their relation to MLC-determinants in man. Transplant Rev 30: 122

van Rood JJ, van Leeuwen A, Keuning JJ (1975) The serological recognition of the human MLC determinants using a modified cytotoxicity technique. Tissue Antigens 5: 73

van Rood JJ, van Leeuwen A, Ploem JS (1976) Simultaneous detection of two cell populations by two-colour fluorescence and application to the recognition of B-cell determinants. Nature (Lond) 262: 795

Rosenfeld CS, Bodensteiner DC (1986) Detection of platelet alloantibodies by flow cytometry. Am J Clin Pathol 85: 207

Rosenfield RE, Schmidt PJ, Calvo RC et al. (1967) Hemagglutination by human anti-leukocyte serums. Vox Sang 13: 461

Rubin H (1963) Antibody elution from red blood cells. J Clin Pathol 16: 70

Rudensky AY, Preston-Hurlburt P, Hong SC (1991) Sequence analysis of peptides bound to MHC class II molecules. Nature (Lond) 353: 622–627

Saarinen UM, Kekomaki R, Siimes MA (1990) Effective prophylaxis against platelet refractoriness in multitransfused patients by use of leucocyte-free blood components. Blood 75: 512–517

Saiki RK, Bugawan TL, Horn GT (1986) Analysis of enzymatically amplified beta-globin and HLA-DQ alpha DNA with allele-specific oligonucleotide probes. Nature (Lond) 324: 163–166

Saiki RK, Walsh PS, Levenson CH (1989) Genetic analysis of amplified DNA with immobilized sequence-specific oligonucleotide probes. Proc Natl Acad Sci USA 86: 6230–6234

Saji H, Maruya E, Fujii H (1989) New platelet antigen, Sib[a] involved in platelet transfusion refractoriness in a Japanese man. Vox Sang 56: 283

Salama A, Schutz B, Kiefel V (1989) Immune-mediated agranulocytosis related to drugs and heterogeneity of antibodies. Br J Haematol 72: 127–132

Salmon C, Ropars C, Gerbal A (1973) Quelques aspects des anti-immunoglobulines chez les polytransfuses. Rev Fr Transfusion 16: 373

Salvatierra O, Vincent F, Amend W (1980) Deliberate donor-specific blood transfusions prior to living related renal transplantation. Ann Surg 192: 543–552

Salvatierra Oj, Iwaki Y, Vincenti F (1981) Incidence, characteristics and outcome of recipients sensitized after donor-specific blood transfusions. Transplantation 32: 528–531

Salvatierra O, Melzer J, Potter D (1986) A seven-year experience with donor-specific blood transfusions. Results and considerations for maximum efficacy. Transplantation 40: 654–659

Samuels P, Bussel JB, Braitman LE et al. (1990) Estimation of the risk of thrombocytopenia in the offspring of pregnant women with presumed immune thrombocytopenic purpura. N Engl J Med 323: 229–235

Sanderson F, Powis SH, Kell AP (1994) Limited polymorphism in HLA-DM does not involve the peptide binding grove. Immunogenetics 39: 56–58

Santoso S, Shibata Y, Kiefel VC (1987) Identification of the Yukb alloantigen on platelet glycoprotein IIIa. Vox Sang 53: 48–51

Santoso S, Kiefel V, Mueller-Eckhardt C (1989) Human platelet alloantigens Bra/Brb are expressed on the very late activation antigen 2 (VLA-2) of T lymphocytes. Hum Immunol 25: 237–246

Santoso S, Kalb R, Kiefel V (1993a) The presence of messenger RNA for HLA class I in human platelets and its capacity for protein biosynthesis. Br J Haematol 84: 451–456

Santoso S, Kalb R, Walka M (1993b) The human platelet alloantigen, Bra and Brb, are associated with a single amino acid polymorphism on glycoprotein Ia (integrin subunit 2). J Clin Invest 92: 2427–2432

Santoso S, Kalb R, Kroll H (1994) A point mutation leads to an unpaired cysteine residue and a molecular weight polymorphism of a functional platelet α3 integrin subunit. J Biol Chem 269: 8439–8444

Santoso S, Amrhein J, Hofmann HA et al. (1999) A point mutation Thr(799)Met on the alpha(2) integrin leads to the formation of new human platelet alloantigen Sit(a) and affects collagen-induced aggregation. Blood 94: 4103–4111

Santoso S, Kiefel V, Richter IG et al. (2002) A functional platelet fibrinogen receptor with a deletion in the cysteine-rich repeat region of the beta(3) integrin: the Oe(a) alloantigen in neonatal alloimmune thrombocytopenia. Blood 99: 1205–1214

605

Schanfield MS, van Loghem E (1986) Human immunoglobulin allotypes. In: Handbook of Experimental Immunology. Genetics and Molecular Immunology. Oxford: Blackwell Scientific Publications, pp. 94

Schechter GP, Soehlen F, McFarland W (1972) Lymphocyte response to blood transfusion in man. N Engl J Med 28: 1169

Schiffer CA (1987) Management of patients refractory to platelet transfusion. An evaluation of methods of donor selection. Prog Hematol 15: 91

Schiffer CA, Lichtenfeld JL, Wiernik PH (1976) Antibody response in patients with acute nonlymphocytic leukemia. Cancer 37: 2177

Schiffer CA, Hogge DE, Aisner J et al. (1984) High-dose intravenous gammaglobulin in alloimmunized platelet transfusion recipients. Blood 64: 937–940

Schiffer CA, Anderson KC, Bennett CL et al. (2001) Platelet transfusion for patients with cancer: clinical practice guidelines of the American Society of Clinical Oncology. J Clin Oncol 19: 1519–1538

Schnaidt M, Northoff H, Wernet D (1996) Frequency and specificity of platelet-specific alloantibodies in HLA-immunized haematologic-oncologic patients. Transfusion Med 6: 111–114

van der Schoot CE, WMM von dem Borne AEGKr (1986) Characterization of platelet-specific alloantigens by immunoblotting: localization of Zw and Bak antigens. Br J Haematol 64: 715–723

Scott JR, Rote NS, Branch DW (1987) Immunologic aspects of recurrent abortion and fetal death. Obstet Gynecol 70: 645–656

Seftel MD, Growe GH, Petraszko T et al. (2004) Universal prestorage leukoreduction in Canada decreases platelet alloimmunization and refractoriness. Blood 103: 333–339

Semple JW, Freedman J (2002) Recipient antigen-processing pathways of allogeneic platelet antigens: essential mediators of immunity. Transfusion 42: 958–961

Shackelford DA, Kaufman JF, Korman AJ et al. (1982) HLA-DR antigens: structure, separation of subpopulations, gene cloning and function. Immunol Rev 66: 133–187

Shanwell H, Sallander S, Olsson I (1991) An alloimmunised, thrombocytopenic patient successfully transfused with acidtreated random donor platelets. Br J Haematol 79: 462–465

Shastri KA, Logue GL (1993) Autoimmune neutropenia. Blood 81: 1984–1995

Sheldon S, Hasleton PS, Yonan NA (1994) Rejection in heart transplantation strongly correlates with HLA-DR antigen mismatch. Transplantation 58: 719–722

Sherwood RA, Brent L, Rayfield LS (1986) Presentation of alloantigens by host cells. Eur J Immunol 16: 574–596

Shibata Y, Miyaji T, Ischikawa Y (1986a) A new platelet antigen system, Yuk^a/Yuk^b. Vox Sang 51: 334–337

Shibata Y, Miyaji T, Ischikawa Y (1986b) Yuka, a new platelet antigen involved in two cases of neonatal alloimmune thrombocytopenia. Vox Sang 50: 177–181

Shulman NR JJ (1987) Platelet immunobiology. In: Haemostasis and Thrombosis. RW Colman, J Hirsch, VG Marder et al. (eds). Philadelphia, PA: Lippincott, pp. 452–529

Shulman NR, Aster RH, Leitner A (1961) Immunoreactions involving platelets. V. Post-transfusion purpura due to a complement-fixing antibody against a genetically controlled platelet antigen. A proposed mechanism for thrombocytopenia and its relevance in 'autoimmunity'. J Clin Invest 40: 1597

Shulman NR, Marder VJ, Hiller MC (1964) Platelet and leukocyte isoantigens and their antibodies: serologic, physiologic and clinical studies. Progr Hematol 4: 222

Shulman NR, Marder VJ, Weinrach RS (1965) Similarities between known antiplatelet antibodies and the factor responsible for thrombocytopenia in idiopathic purpura. Physiologic, serologic and isotopic studies. Ann NY Acad Sci 124: 499–542

Shulman NR, Leissinger CA, Hotchkiss A (1982) The nonspecific nature of platelet-associated IgG. Trans Assoc Am Phys 14: 213–220

Silver RM, Porter TF, Branch DW et al. (2000) Neonatal alloimmune thrombocytopenia: antenatal management. Am J Obstet Gynecol 182: 1233–1238

Simsek S, van der Schoot CE, Daams M (1996) Molecular characterisation of antigenic polymorphisms (Ond^a and Mart) of the β2 family recognised by human leucocyte alloantibodies. Blood 88: 1350–1359

Simsek S, Folman C, van der Schoot CE et al. (1997) The Arg633His substitution responsible for the private platelet antigen Gro(a) unravelled by SSCP analysis and direct sequencing. Br J Haematol 97: 330–335

Sintnicolaas K, Sizoo W, Haye WG (1981) Delayed immunization by random single donor platelet transfusions. Lancet i: 750

Sintnicolaas K, Vries W, van der Linden R (1991) Simultaneous flow cytometric detection of antibodies against platelets, granulocytes and lymphocytes. J Immunol Methods 142: 215–222

Sintnicolaas K, van Marwijk KM, van Prooijen HC (1995) Leukocyte depletion of random single-donor platelet transfusions does not prevent secondary human leukocyte antigen-alloimmunization and refractoriness: a randomized prospective study. Blood 85: 824–828

Sirchia G, Parravicini A, Rebulla P (1982) Effectiveness of red blood cells filtered through cotton wool to prevent antileukocyte antibody production in multitransfused patients. Vox Sang 42: 190–197

Sivakumaran M, Norfolk DR, Major KE (1993) A new method to study the efficiency of third generation blood filters. Br J Haematol 84: 175–177

Skogen B, Rossebo HB, Husebekk A (1988) Minimal expression of blood group A antigen on thrombocytes from A2 individuals. Transfusion 28: 456–459

Skogen B, Bellissimo DB, Hessner MJ (1994) Rapid determination of platelet alloantigen genotypes by polymerase chain reaction using allele specific primers. Transfusion 34: 955–960

Skogen B, Christiansen D, Husebekk A (1995) Flow-cytometric analysis in platelet crossmatching using a platelet suspension immunofluorescence test. Transfusion 35: 832–836

Slichter SJ, O'Dormell MR, Weiden FL (1986) Canine platelet alloimmunization: the role of donor selection. Br J Haematol 63: 713–727

Slichter SJ, Deeg HJ, Kennedy MS (1987) Prevention of platelet alloimmunization in dogs with systemic cyclosporine and by UV-irradiation of cyclosporine-loading of donor platelets. Blood 69: 414–418

Slichter SJ, Davis K, Enright H et al. (2005) Factors affecting post-transfusion platelet increments, platelet refractoriness, and platelet transfusion intervals in thrombocytopenic patients. Blood 105: 4106–4114

Smith JW, Kelton JG, Horsewood P (1989) Platelet specific alloantigens on the platelet glycoprotein Ia/IIa complex. Br J Haematol 72: 534–538

Smith JW, Hayward CPM, Horsewood P (1995) Characterization and localization of the Gova/b alloantigens to the glycosylophosphatidyl-inositol-anchored protein CDw109 on human platelets. Blood 86: 2807–2814

Snary D, Barnstable C, Bodmer WF (1977a) Human Ia antigens – purification and molecular structure. Cold Spring Harb Symp Quant Biol 41: 379

Snary D, Barnstable CJ, Bodmer WF (1977b) Molecular structure of human histocompatibility antigens: the HLA-C series. Eur J Immunol 8: 580

de Sousa M (1989) Immune cell functions in iron overload. Clin Exp Immunol 75: 1–6

Speiser P (1964) Anti-Koerperbildung von Kindern gegen die Gm-Gruppe ihrer Mutter (Weitere Beobachtungen). Commun 10th Congr Int Soc Blood Transfus, Stockholm

Spies T, Bresnahan M, Bahram S (1991) A gene in the human major histocompatibility complex class II region controlling the class I antigen presenting pathway. Nature (Lond) 348: 744–747

Sprogoe-Jakobsen U, Saetre AM, Georgsen J (1995) Preparation of white cell-reduced red cells by filtration: comparison of a bedside filter and two blood bank filter systems. Transfusion 35: 421–426

Spurkland A, Knutsen I, Markussen G (1993) HLA matching of unrelated bone marrow transplant pairs: direct sequencing of in vitro amplified HLA-DRB1 and DQB1 genes using magnetic beads as solid support. Tissue Antigens 41: 155–164

Srivastava A, Pearson H, Bryant J (1993) Acidified chloroquine treatment for the removal of class I HLA antigens. Vox Sang 65: 146–150

Starzl T, Demetris A, Murase N (1992) Cell migration, chimerism and graft acceptance. Lancet 339: 1579–1582

Stastny P, Nunez G (1981) The role of endothelial and monocyte antigens in kidney transplantation. Transplant Clin Immunol 13: 133–139

Steinberg AG, Wilson J (1963) Hereditary globulin factors and immune tolerance in man. Science 140: 303

Steneker I, Biewenga J (1991) Histological and immuno-histochemical studies on the preparation of leukocyte-poor red cell concentrates by filtration. The filtration process using three different filters. Transfusion 31: 40–46

Steneker I, van Luijn MJA, van Wachem PB (1992) Electronmicroscope examination of white cell depletion of four leukocyte depletion filters. Transfusion 32: 450–457

Stern J, Brown JH, Jardetzky TS (1994) Crystal structure of the human class II MHC protein HLA-DR1 complexed with an influenza virus peptide. Nature (Lond) 368: 215–221

Stiehm ER, Fudenberg HH (1965) Antibodies to gamma globulin in infants and children exposed to isologous gamma-globulin. Pediatrics 35: 229

Storb R, Thomas ED, Buckner CD et al. (1980) Marrow transplantation in thirty 'untransfused' patients with severe aplastic anemia. Ann Intern Med 92: 30–36

Strauss RA, Gloster E, Shanfield MS (1983) Anaphylactic transfusion reaction associated with a possible anti-A2m(1). Clin Lab Haematol 5: 371–377

Stroncek D (2002) Neutrophil alloantigens. Transfusion Med Rev 16: 67–75

Stroncek DF, Skubitz KM, Plachta LB (1991) Alloimmune neonatal neutropenia due to an antibody to the neutrophil Fc-gamma receptor III with maternal deficiency of CD16 antigen. Blood 77: 1572–1580

Stroncek DF, Shankar RA, Plachta LB et al. (1993a) Polyclonal antibodies against the NB1-bearing 58- to 64-kDa glycoprotein of human neutrophils do not identify an NB2-bearing molecule. Transfusion 33: 399–404

Stroncek DF, Shapiro RS, Filipovich AH et al. (1993b) Prolonged neutropenia resulting from antibodies to neutrophil-specific antigen NB1 following marrow transplantation. Transfusion 33: 158–163

Stroncek DF, Herr GP, Magnire RB (1994) Characterization of the neutrophil molecules identified by quininedependent antibodies from two patients. Transfusion 34: 980–985

Stroncek DF, Shankar RA, Noren PA et al. (1996a) Analysis of the expression of NB1 antigen using two monoclonal antibodies. Transfusion 36: 168–174

Stroncek DF, Leonard K, Eiber G et al. (1996b). Alloimmunization after granulocyte transfusions. Transfusion 36, 1009–1015

Stroncek DF, Shankar R, Litz C et al. (1998a) The expression of the NB1 antigen on myeloid precursors and neutrophils from children and umbilical cords. Transfusion Med 8: 119–123

Stroncek DF, Jaszcz W, Herr GP et al. (1998b) Expression of neutrophil antigens after 10 days of granulocyte-colony-stimulating factor. Transfusion 38: 663–668

Sturgeon P, Jennings ER (1968) Anti-gamma-globulins in women treated with anti-RhoD-globulin. Transfusion 8: 343

Sugawara S, Abo T, Kumagai K (1987) A simple method to eliminate the antigenicity of surface class I MHC molecules from the membrane of viable cells by acid treatment at pH3. J Immunol Methods 100: 83–90

Sumimoto R, Kamada N (1990) Specific suppression of allograft rejection of soluble class I antigen and complexes with monoclonal antibody. Transplantation 50: 678

Susal C, Terness P, Opelz G (1990) An experimental model for preventing alloimmunization against platelet transfusions by pretreatment with antibody-coated cells. Vox Sang 59: 209–215

Szatkowski NS, Kunicki TJ, Aster RH (1986) Identification of glycoprotein Ib as a target of autoantibody in idiopathic (autoimmune) thrombocytopenic purpura. Blood 67: 310–315

Taaning E, Antonsen H, Peterson S et al. (1983) HLA antigens and maternal antibodies in allo-immune neonatal thrombocytopenia. Tissue Antigens 21: 351–360

Taniguchi K, Kobayashi M, Harada H et al. (2002) Human neutrophil antigen-2a expression on neutrophils from healthy adults in western Japan. Transfusion 42: 651–657

Tartter PI, Heimann TM, Aufses AH Jr (1986) Blood transfusion, skin test reactivity, and lymphocytes in inflammatory bowel disease. Am J Surg 151: 358–361

Tartter PI, Steinberg B, Barron DM et al. (1989) Transfusion history, T cell subsets and natural killer cytotoxicity in patients with colorectal cancer. Vox Sang 56: 80–84

Tartter PI, Mohandas K, Azar P et al. (1998) Randomized trial comparing packed red cell blood transfusion with and without leukocyte depletion for gastrointestinal surgery. Am J Surg 176: 462–466

Tate Y, Sorensen RL, Gerrard JM (1977) An immunoenzyme histochemical technique for the detection of platelet antibodies from the serum of patients with idiopathic (autoimmune) thrombocytopenic purpura. Br J Haematol 37: 265

Taylor C, Falk WP (1981) Prevention of recurrent abortion with leucocyte transfusions. Lancet ii: 68–70

Terasaki P (1984) The beneficial transfusion effect on kidney graft survival attributed to clonal deletion. Transplantation 37: 119–125

Terasaki PI, McClelland JC, Park MS (1973) Microdroplet lymphocyte cytotoxicity test. In: Manual of Tissue Typing Techniques. DHEW publ. (NIH) 74545. Washington, DC: Government Printing Office

Termijtelen A, Erlich HA, Brins LA (1991) Oligonucleotide typing is a perfect tool to identify antigens stimulatory in the mixed lymphocyte culture. Hum Immunol 31: 241–245

Thompson JS, Severson CD (1980) Granulocyte Antigens in Blood Cells and Body Fluids. Washington, DC: Am Assoc Blood Banks, pp. 151–187

Thompson JS, Overlin V, Severson CD (1980) Demonstration of granulocyte, monocyte, and endothelial cell antigens by double fluorochromatic microcytotoxicity testing. Transplant Proc 12 (Suppl. 1): 26–31

Tiercy JM, Marsh SG, Schreuder GM et al. (2002) Guidelines for nomenclature usage in HLA reports: ambiguities and conversion to serotypes. Eur J Immunogenet 29: 273–274

Tijhuis GJ, Klaassen RJL, Modderman PW (1991) Quantification of platelet-bound immunoglobulins of different class and subclass using radiolabelled monoclonal antibodies: assay conditions and clinical application. Br J Haematol 77: 93–101

Ting A (1983) The lymphocytotoxic crossmatch test in clinical renal transplantation. Transplantation 35: 403–407

Tongio MM, Falkenrodt A, Mitsuishi Y (1985) Natural HLA antibodies. Tissue Antigens 26: 271–285

Townsend AR, Rothbard J, Gotch FM et al. (1986) The epitopes of influenza nucleoprotein recognized by cytotoxic T lymphocytes can be defined with short synthetic peptides. Cell 44: 959–968

Trial to Reduce Alloimmunization to Platelets Study Group (1997) Leukocyte reduction and ultraviolet B irradiation of platelets to prevent alloimmunization and refractoriness to platelet transfusions. N Engl J Med 337: 1861–1869

Trounstine ML, Peltz GA, Yssel H et al. (1990) Reactivity of cloned, expressed human Fc gamma RIII isoforms with monoclonal antibodies which distinguish cell-type-specific and allelic forms of Fc gamma RIII. Int Immunol 2: 303–310

Trucco M, de Petris S, Garrotta G (1980) Quantitative analysis of cell surface HLA structures by means of monoclonal antibodies. Hum Immunol 3: 233–243

Tsubakio T, Tani P, Curd JR (1986) Complement activation in vitro by anti platelet antibodies in chronic immune thromboyctopenic purpural. Br J Haematol 63: 293–300

van Twuyver E, Mooijaart RJD, Ten BI (1991) Pretransplantation blood transfusion revisited. N Engl J Med 325: 1210–1213

van Twuyver E, Mooijaart RID, ten Berge R (1994) High affinity cytotoxic T lymphocytes after non-HLA-sharing blood transfusion: the other side of the coin. Transplantation 57: 1246–1251

Tursz T, Preud'Homme J-L, Labanne S *et al.* (1977) Autoantibodies to B lymphocytes in a patient with hypo-immunoglobulinemia. Characterization and pathogenic role. J Clin Invest 60: 405–410

Uhrynowska M, Niznikowska-Marks M, Zupanska B (2000) Neonatal and maternal thrombocytopenia: incidence and immune background. Eur J Haematol 64: 42–46

Valentin N, Vergracht A, Bignon JD (1990) HLA-DRw52a is involved in alloimmunization against Pl-A1 antigen. Hum Immunol 27: 73–80

Vamvakas EC, Carven JH (1998) Transfusion of white-cell containing allogeneic blood components and postoperative wound infection: effect of confounding factors. Transfusion Med 8: 29–36

Vamvakas EC, Blachman MA (2001) Deleterious clinical effects of transfusion-associated immunomodulation: fact or fiction? Blood 97: 1180–1195

Vanrenterghem Y, Waer M, Roels L *et al.* (1994) A prospective, randomized trial of pretransplant blood transfusions in cadaver kidney transplant candidates. Leuven Collaborative Group for Transplantation. Transplant Int 7 (Suppl. 1): S243–S246

Vartdal F, Gaudernack G, Funderud S (1986) HLA class I and II typing using cells positively selected from blood by immunomagnetic isolation – a fast and reliable technique. Tissue Antigens 28: 301–312

Verheugt FWA, dem Borne AEGK, Décary F (1977) The detection of granulocyte alloantibodies with an indirect immunofluorescence test. Br J Haematol 36: 533

Verheugt FWA, von dem Borne AEGK, van NoordBokhorst IC (1978) ND1, a new neutrophil granulocyte antigen. Vox Sang 35: 13

Verheugt FWA, Noord-Bokhorst JC, von dem Borne AEGK (1979) A family with allo-immune neonatal neutropenia: group-specific pathogenicity of maternal antibodies. Vox Sang 36: 1–8

Vicariot M, Abgroll IF, Dutel JL *et al.* (1984) Alloimmunization anti-leuco-plaquettaire en reanimation hematologique. Les transfusions de plaquettes de donneurs uniques presentent-elles un avantage sur les pla quettes de donneurs multiples. Rev Fr Transfusion Immunol 27: 35–43

Vinci G, Tabilio A, Deschamps IF (1984) Immunologic study of *in vivo* maturation of human megakaryocytes. Br J Haematol 56: 589–605

Vyas GN, Holmdahl L, Perkins HA (1969) Serological specificity of human anti-IgA and its significance in transfusion. Blood 34: 573

Vyas GN, Levin AS, Fudenberg HH (1970) Intrauterine isoimmunization caused by maternal IgA crossing the placenta. Nature (Lond) 225: 275

Vyas GN, Perkins HA, Yang YM (1975) Healthy blood donors with selective absence of immunoglobulin A:

prevention of anaphylactic transfusion reactions caused by antibodies to IgA. J Lab Clin Med 85: 838

Wallis JP, Haynes S, Stark G *et al.* (2002) Transfusion-related alloimmune neutropenia: an undescribed complication of blood transfusion. Lancet 360: 1073–1074

Walters MC, Storb R, Patience M *et al.* (2000) Impact of bone marrow transplantation for symptomatic sickle cell disease: an interim report. Multicenter investigation of bone marrow transplantation for sickle cell disease. Blood 95: 1918–1924

Wang E, Adams S, Zhao Y *et al.* (2003) A strategy for detection of known and unknown SNP using a minimum number of oligonucleotides applicable in the clinical settings. J Transplant Med 1: 4

Wang E, Marincola FM, Stroncek D (2005) Human leukocyte antigen and human neutrophil antigen systems. In: Hematology. Basic Principles and Practice. R Hoffman, EJ Benz, SJ Shattil *et al.* (eds). Philadelphia, PA: Elsevier Churchill Livingstone

Wang J, Geissler E, Knechtle SJ (1993a) *In vivo* transfer of gene encoding soluble MHC class I prolongs heart transplant survival (Abstract). Hum Immunol 37: 121

Wang J, McFarland JG, Keko KR (1993b) Amino acid 489 is encoded by a mutational 'Hot Spot' on the α3 integrin chain: the Ca/Tu human platelet alloantigen system. Blood 82: 3386–3391

Wang L, Juji T, Shibata Y (1991) Sequence variation of human platelet membrane glycoprotein IIIa associated with the Yuk^a/Yuk^b alloantigen system. Proc Jap Acad 67: 102–106

Wang-Rodriguez J, Fry E, Fiebig E *et al.* (2000) Immune response to blood transfusion in very-low-birthweight infants. Transfusion 40: 25–34

Warkentin TE, Kelton JG (2001a) Delayed-onset heparin-induced thrombocytopenia and thrombosis. Ann Intern Med 135: 502–506

Warkentin TE, Kelton JG (2001b) Temporal aspects of heparin-induced thrombocytopenia. N Engl J Med 344: 1286–1292

van de Watering LM, Hermans J, Houbiers JG *et al.* (1998) Beneficial effects of leukocyte depletion of transfused blood on postoperative complications in patients undergoing cardiac surgery: a randomized clinical trial. Circulation 97: 562–568

van der Weerdt CM, Wiel-Dorfmeyer H, Engelfriet CP (1962) A new platelet antigen. Proc 8th Congr Europ Soc Haemat, Vienna, 1961, p. 379

van der Weerdt CM, Veenhoven V, Nijenhuis LE (1963) The Zw blood group system in platelets. Vox Sang 8: 513

Weiden PL, Sullivan KM, Flournoy N *et al.* (1981) Antileukemic effect of chronic graft-versus-host disease: contribution to improved survival after allogeneic marrow transplantation. N Engl J Med 304: 1529–1533

Weiss A, Samuelson LE (2003) T-lymphocyte activation. In: Fundamental Immunology. WE Paul (ed.). Philadelphia, PA: Lippincott Williams & Wilkins, p. 231

Welsh KJ, Burgoss H, Batchelor R (1977) Immune response to allogeneic rat platelets: Ag-B antigens in matrix lacking I[a]. Eur J Immunol 7: 267–272

Wenz B, Burns ER, Lee V (1991) A rare event analysis model for quantifying white cells in white cell-depleted blood. Transfusion 31: 156–159

Wernet C, Klouda PT, Carrea MC (1977) Isolation of B and T lymphocytes by nylon filter columns. Tissue Antigens 9: 227

WHO (1976) Review of the notation for the allotypic and related markers of human immunoglobulins. Amended report of WHO meeting, 1974. J Immunol 117: 1056

Williamson L, Wimperis JZ, Williamson P (1994) Bedside filtration of blood products in the prevention of HLA immunization – a prospective randomized study. Blood 83: 3028–3035

Williamson LM, Bruce D, Lubenko A (1992) Molecular biology for platelet alloantigen typing. Transfusion Med 2: 255–264

Winchester RJ, Kunkel HG (1979) The human Ia system. Adv Immunol 28: 221–293

Wollman EE, Guilherme L, Lepage V (1984) Non HLA antigenic determinants expressed on activated T and B human lymphocytes. Tissue Antigens 23: 1–11

Woodruff MFA, van Rood JJ (1983) Possible implication of the effect of blood transfusion on allograft survival. Lancet i: 1202

Woods VL, Kurata Y, Montgomery RR (1984) Auto-antibodies against platelet glycoprotein I[b] in patients with chronic ITP. Blood 64: 156–160

Woods VL, Pischel ED, Avery ED (1989) Antigenic polymorphism of human very late activation protein-2 (platelet glycoprotein Ia-IIa): platelet alloantigen Hc[a]. J Clin Invest 83: 978–985

Worfolk LA, McPherson BR (1991) The detection of platelet alloantibodies by flow cytometry. Transfusion 31: 340–344

Yamamoto N, Ikeda H, Tandon NN (1990) A platelet membrane glycoprotein (GP) deficiency in healthy blood donors: Nak[a]-platelets lack detectable GPIV (CD36). Blood 76: 1698–1703

Yankee RA, Grumet FC, Rogentine GN (1969) Platelet transfusion. The selection of compatible platelet donors for refractory patients by lymphocyte HL-A typing. N Engl J Med 281: 1208–1212

Zavazava N, Hausmann R, Mueller-Rucholtz W (1991) Inhibition of anti-HLAB7 alloreactive CTL by affinity-purified soluble HLA. Transplantation 51: 838

Zeigler ZR, Shadduck RK, Rosenfeld CS et al. (1991) Intravenous gamma globulin decreases platelet-associated IgG and improves transfusion responses in platelet refractory states. Am J Hematol 38: 15–23

Zinkernagel RM, Doherty PC (1974) Restriction of in vitro T cell mediated cytotoxicity in lymphocyte choriomeningitis within a syngeneic or semi-allogeneic system. Nature (Lond) 248: 701

14 The transfusion of platelets, leucocytes, haematopoietic cells and plasma components

Transfusion of platelets

The transfusion of platelets to patients with impaired haematopoiesis, with bone marrow aplasia induced by chemotherapy and with a variety of miscellaneous disorders of platelet number and function has provided life-saving supportive therapy. The preparation and preservation of platelet concentrates and indications for platelet transfusions are discussed below.

Preparation of platelet concentrates from single units of whole blood

The first platelet concentrates derived from whole blood were prepared as platelet-rich plasma, a component containing relatively few platelets (3.0×10^{11}/l) in an impractically large volume of plasma (> 200 ml) (Freireich *et al.* 1963). Efforts to reduce volume by high-speed centrifugation resulted in a pellet of irreversibly clumped cells, and the alternative use of the low-volume anticoagulant, ethylenediamenetetraacetate (EDTA) caused the transfused platelets to undergo rapid hepatic sequestration (Aster and Jandl 1964). Technical modifications that included acidification of the suspension medium and room temperature preparation eventually led to the current method of preparing platelet concentrates (Mourad 1968).

Meticulous attention to numerous small steps in the preparation and storage of platelet concentrates from whole blood is necessary to ensure the maximum number of viable and functional platelets. Early empirical studies defined in detail the anticoagulant, storage container plastic, initial 'soft spin' (1000 *g* for 9 min), subsequent 'hard spin' (3000 *g* for 20 min), resuspension technique, storage volume and storage conditions to achieve platelets with 46% *in vivo* recovery and 7.9-day survival following 72 h of storage (81% of fresh platelet viability) (Slichter and Harker 1976a,b,c). In addition, the temperature at which the blood is maintained before and during processing, the interval between collection and preparation of the platelet concentrate, the white cell and red cell contamination, and the temperature and mode of agitation during storage are all important considerations (Slichter 1985).

Two methods for preparing platelet concentrates are described in Appendix 1; one method involves an initial gentle centrifugation to obtain platelet-rich plasma (PRP) and concentration of platelets by further centrifugation and the second method involves a more vigorous initial centrifugation to obtain buffy coats from whole blood and the subsequent recovery of the platelets by gentle centrifugation. Single or previously pooled, resuspended buffy coats (4–7 units) can be stored for up to 5 days to provide an adult platelet dose of 3×10^{11} platelets in approximately 300 ml of plasma (Pietersz *et al.* 1985; Wildt-Eggen *et al.* 1996). Two types of instruments, the Optipress or Biopack, using two outlets in the primary collection pack ('bottom and top'), and the Compomat or Ex30, using traditional multiple packs, have been developed to automate buffy coat platelet collection and plasma separation. Platelet concentrates prepared under these conditions have 0.09 ± 0.04 leucocytes $\times 10^8$/unit. The full adult dose of approximately 3×10^{11} platelets in 300 ml of plasma prepared with Optipress contains the same number of leucocytes. Platelet concentrates from PRP should contain at least 5.5×10^{10} platelets in 50 ml of plasma or an appropriate platelet suspension medium. Storage of pooled PRP-derived platelet concentrates is not licensed at present, although *in vitro* studies suggest that component quality is maintained for 5 days (Snyder *et al.* 1989a; Moroff *et al.* 1993).

The principles of platelet storage (see below) are probably identical regardless of the method of preparation. The pH should not be allowed to fall below 6.4 or rise above 7.4 throughout the shelf-life of any platelet concentrate. Leucocyte-reduced buffy coat platelet pools can be prepared either by filtration or by centrifugation (Wildt-Eggen *et al.* 2001). Leucodepletion filters especially designed for platelet concentrates remove more than 90% of leucocytes from pooled platelets or platelet concentrates collected with cell separators (Chapter 17) with a loss of less than 15% of platelets.

The survival of platelets *in vivo*

^{51}Cr and ^{111}In as labels

The introduction of ^{51}Cr as a label for platelets (Aas and Gardner 1958) provided an objective means of defining the kinetics of platelet transfusion. Because uptake of ^{51}Cr by platelets is poor, ^{51}Cr has now been replaced by ^{111}In ($T_{1/2}$ 2.8 days) or ^{113}In ($T_{1/2}$ 100 min), complexed with a suitable chelating agent as the label of choice for platelet studies. Although oxine (8-hydroxyquinoline) was used originally (Thakur *et al.* 1976), tropolone proved a more convenient chelator because indium tropolonate, unlike indium oxinate, labels cells effectively in the presence of plasma. Results using the two methods do not differ significantly (Kotze *et al.* 1991). Optimal labelling with ^{111}In is achieved using a tropolone concentration of 2×10^{-4} mol/l and a plasma concentration of 50% (Danpure *et al.* 1990). Under these conditions, autologous platelets can be used in patients with platelet counts as low as 4×10^9/l. Conditions may need to be altered when labelling platelets stored in plasma-free synthetic media (see below). Compared with ^{51}Cr, ^{111}In is less radiotoxic and far more suitable for quantitative scintillation camera imaging.

Storage of platelets does not appear to affect the uptake of ^{51}Cr or ^{111}In. Therefore radiolabelled platelet recovery and survival studies can be used to define optimal conditions for storage. The lifespan of two populations of platelets in the same subject can be compared by using ^{51}Cr for one population and ^{111}In

for the other (Keegan *et al.* 1992). However, the $T_{1/2}$ and mean lifespan of stored platelets are significantly longer with ^{51}Cr than with ^{111}In labelling, indicating that estimates of viability of stored platelets may be influenced by the choice of label (Wadenvik and Kutti 1991) or even by the use of different methods using the same the label (Rock and Tittley 1990). Other factors that obscure comparisons between labelling studies are differences in sampling and curve fitting, which substantially affect estimates of mean platelet lifespan (Wadenvik and Kutti 1991). Comparisons of results from different laboratories are valid only when identical methods have been used. Detailed methods for conducting survival studies with radiolabelled platelets have been published (Snyder *et al.* 1986).

Use of biotin

Platelets labelled with biotin can be detected in a blood sample by adding streptavidin–phycoerythrin prior to flow cytometry. By labelling platelets in two populations at different strengths, the lifespan of the two populations can be compared (Franco *et al.* 1994).

Normal survival of platelets in vivo: venting the spleen and other issues

Although *in vivo* characterization of platelet recovery and survival was derived initially from measurements made with ^{51}Cr, most studies in the last 20 years have been made with ^{111}In and γ-scintillation camera computer systems that are capable of dynamic imaging.

Initial survival ('recovery'). If fresh platelets from a normal subject are labelled with ^{111}In, the initial rapid fall in the plasma concentration of platelets, which is also seen with ^{51}Cr-labelled platelets (Kotilainen 1969), is complete in 20 min; at 10 min the value is about 5% above the 20-min value (Peters *et al.* 1980). The term *recovery* is used for the number remaining in the circulation after this phase of rapid disappearance, and is expressed as a percentage of the number expected if all the transfused platelets were in the circulation.

Platelet recovery has been determined as follows: with ^{111}In, 71% (Heaton *et al.* 1979) and 72% (Heyns *et al.* 1980); with ^{51}Cr, 66% (Aster and Jandl 1964); 67% (Aster 1965) and 64.6% (Harker and Finch 1969). In splenectomized subjects, about 90% of injected platelets are recovered (Harker and Finch 1969; Kotilainen 1969). Conversely, with splenomegaly, low values have been found (7–27% in congestive splenomegaly; Harker and Finch 1969). When the spleen is extremely enlarged, seven times as many platelets may be sequestered as circulate in the blood (Penny *et al.* 1966).

Although a fraction of total circulating platelets normally pools in the spleen (see below), recovery of labelled platelets from splenectomized subjects rarely exceeds 90%. The rapid disappearance of a proportion of labelled platelets from the bloodstream soon after injection may reflect damage that occurs during the labelling process.

The *disappearance curve* may be obtained by plotting the number of circulating labelled platelets against time after injection. In normal subjects the number decreases rapidly in the first 10–20 min but falls much more slowly thereafter. The survival time is defined as the time after injection at which survival falls to zero. Estimates of survival time using ^{111}In-labelled platelets are 9 days (Heyns *et al.* 1980) and 8–10 days (Bautista *et al.* 1984), findings identical to those established with ^{51}Cr-labelled platelets (Kotilainen 1969; Abrahamsen 1970). Platelet survival values obtained with ^{111}In fit linear kinetics (Heyns *et al.* 1980; Bautista *et al.* 1984). Several mathematical models of data analysis have been investigated; however, the multiple-hit method and the weighted mean technique yield similar results (Lotter *et al.* 1986).

In normal subjects, two mechanisms of platelet removal have been identified: (1) a fixed number of platelets is consumed for daily vascular maintenance and (2) platelet ageing determines the remaining lifespan (Hanson and Slichter 1985). Platelet survival correlates directly with platelet count in the thrombocytopenic patients. Platelet lifespan is modestly reduced in patients with counts in the range of 50 000–100 000/µl, but markedly reduced when the count falls below 50 000/µl. The recovery of autologous platelets is normal when the platelet count exceeds 50 000/µl, but reduced in patients with lower counts because the number of platelets required for vascular maintenance becomes an increasing percentage of the total count. All patient and normal data correlate well with a model that predicts a fixed requirement for 7100 platelets per microlitre of blood per day, or about 18% of the normal rate of platelet turnover (41 200 platelets per microlitre per day on average) (Hanson and Slichter 1985). If the population of newly formed platelets is labelled with ^{51}Cr and followed after an episode of rapid platelet destruction, a plateau type of disappearance curve is observed with 50% survival at 7 days, followed by almost complete disappearance of the labelled population by 9 days, thus demonstrating the relationship between platelet ageing and survival (Harker 1977). In addition to the physiological requirement for platelets, thrombocytopenic patients who are febrile, infected and undergoing cytoreductive therapy require additional platelets to maintain haemostasis (Harker and Slichter 1972a).

Platelets can be separated by centrifugation into 'heavy' cells, with a mean survival time of about 314 h, and 'light' cells, with a mean survival time of 75 h. The total population lifespan is about 190 h (Corash 1978). Cohort experiments confirm that the heavy platelets are the younger ones. In the same study, platelets from platelet-rich plasma had a survival time of 155 h, presumably because a percentage of young platelets were spun down with the red cells and leucocytes and excluded from the platelet-rich plasma. Examples of platelet survival curves obtained with ^{111}In are presented in Fig. 14.1.

[51]Cr labelling studies indicate that about one-third of the total circulating platelets are concentrated in the spleen, exchanging freely with platelets circulating in the periphery (Aster 1966; Harker and Finch 1969). Using ^{111}In-labelled platelets, a scintillation camera and computer-assisted imaging, Heyns and co-workers (1980) estimated the splenic pool to be 29.6% of the total circulating platelets. Measurements of intrasplenic platelet transit time arrive at a similar figure (Peters *et al.* 1984). Some pooling of platelets may occur in the liver (Heyns *et al.* 1980). The liver and spleen account for the clearance of 72.3% of the total radioactivity, a figure that corresponds closely to values obtained using [51]Cr (Aster 1966). Most of the activity not in the liver or spleen remains in the thorax and lower abdomen indicating that these regions contain sites that sequester platelets.

Radiolabelling to assess viability of transfused platelets

Isotopic studies are used to predict the circulation of stored platelets that are transfused to amegakaryocytic, thrombocytopenic patients. Recovery and viability are

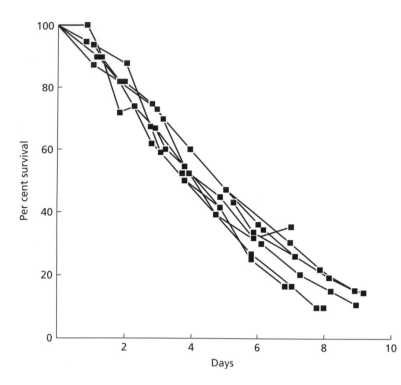

Fig 14.1 Survival curves of autologous platelets labelled with ^{111}In in seven normal subjects. The values at equilibrium after injection were defined as 100% and correspond to a mean value of 72% (SD 16%) of that expected if all the labelled platelets had been in the circulation. The slopes are best fitted by a linear function and mean survival is 9.0 days (SD 0.71 days). Elution of label from the platelets is negligible. Modified from Heyns *et al.* (1980).

reasonable surrogates for the post-transfusion increment that is used by clinicians, although none of these measurements ensures haemostatic efficacy *in vivo*. Unlike the case of the red cell, no generally accepted standard for survival after 24 h has been set for the radiolabelled platelet (Murphy 2002). As a result, studies that propose extending storage tend to use isotopic studies of platelets stored for currently licensed maximum periods, rather than fresh platelet values, as a control (Hogge *et al.* 1986; Simon *et al.* 1987). A recent proposal to use two-thirds survival and 50% recovery of fresh platelets (< 24 h post collection) as the 'gold standard' has been validated for current 5-day platelet storage (AuBuchon *et al.* 2004; Murphy 2004).

Relation between platelet count and bleeding time

In patients with thrombocytopenia due to underproduction, the bleeding time is prolonged when the platelet count falls below about $100 \times 10^9/l$. Below this level, the relation between the bleeding time, as determined by the template method of Mielke (Mielke *et al.* 1969), and the platelet count is roughly linear to a count of about $20 \times 10^9/l$ as described by the following equation (Harker and Slichter 1972b):

$$\text{Bleeding time (minutes)} = 30.5 - \frac{\text{platelet count}}{3850} \quad (14.1)$$

so that for a platelet count of 10 000/μl

$$\text{bleeding time} = 30.5 - \frac{10\,000}{3850} = 28 \text{ minutes}$$

In patients with immune thrombocytopenic purpura (ITP), the bleeding time is shorter than that predicted from the platelet count, whereas in conditions in which platelet function is disturbed, as in uraemia or in von Willebrand disease, bleeding time is prolonged even when the platelet count is normal (Harker and Slichter 1972b).

This relationship can be used to measure *in vivo* function of stored platelets both at the time of transfusion and several hours later (Fig. 14.2).

Storage of platelets in the liquid state

Preparation of platelet concentrates

Platelet-rich plasma (PRP) method. In this method, the PRP is centrifuged at high speed and, after storage

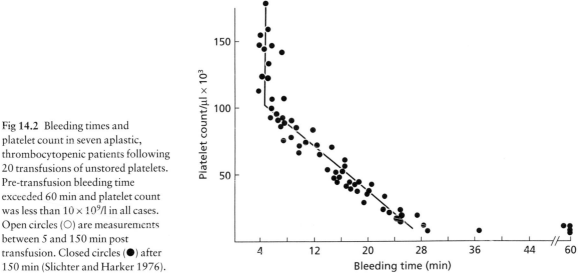

Fig 14.2 Bleeding times and platelet count in seven aplastic, thrombocytopenic patients following 20 transfusions of unstored platelets. Pre-transfusion bleeding time exceeded 60 min and platelet count was less than $10 \times 10^9/l$ in all cases. Open circles (O) are measurements between 5 and 150 min post transfusion. Closed circles (●) after 150 min (Slichter and Harker 1976).

at room temperature for 1–1.5 h, the platelets in the pellet are resuspended in about 60 ml of autologous plasma or synthetic medium (see Appendix 1).

The buffy coat (BC) method. With this method, whole blood is centrifuged at high speed, after which first the plasma and then the buffy coat is removed. To the buffy coat, 60 ml of plasma or synthetic medium is added and, by centrifugation at low speed, the platelets are separated from the remaining red cells and the leucocytes. Then, 25 ml or so of red cells from the collected unit are lost during the buffy coat preparation. Pooling of platelets from four donations provides a therapeutic platelet dose (see Appendix 1).

The BC method has several advantages over the PRP method. More plasma becomes available for fractionation; BC-PC contain fewer leucocytes than PRP-PC (Pietersz *et al.* 1987). Furthermore, buffy coat platelets are less activated than PRP platelets (Fijnheer *et al.* 1990; Bertolini *et al.* 1992). Activation of platelets may decrease viability *in vivo* (see below). Initially, a disadvantage of the BC method was a lower platelet yield (Hirosue *et al.* 1988), but automated systems for preparing BC have improved the yield (Högman *et al.* 1989; Pietersz *et al.* 1989). The yield improves further when the blood from which the BC is prepared is kept at 20°C for 12–24 h before centrifugation (Fijnheer *et al.* 1990).

Plateletpheresis. This is used to obtain an adult therapeutic dose (or more) of platelets from a single donor. For further details, see Chapter 17.

Platelet metabolism

In plasma, platelets derive 85% of their energy from oxidative metabolism using as substrates exogenous glucose, free fatty acids, acetate and amino acids (Kilkson *et al.* 1984; Bertolini *et al.* 1992; Shimizu and Murphy 1993). Only 15% of energy is derived from anaerobic glycolysis (Kilkson *et al.* 1984). The carbon dioxide produced in the oxidative pathway may be converted to bicarbonate, the major buffer in plasma. During anaerobic glycolysis, lactate is produced, which, unless neutralized by bicarbonate, causes a rapid fall in pH. Lack of oxygen switches the metabolism to anaerobic glycolysis, whereas addition of acetate to the preservation medium may direct metabolism to oxidative metabolism, thus decreasing lactate formation (Guppy *et al.* 1990; Bertolini *et al.* 1992).

Storage temperature

Originally platelets were stored at 4°C, but at that temperature platelets lose their discoid shape and survive poorly after transfusion. Platelets retain viability well

615

when stored at 20–24°C (Murphy and Gardner 1969, 1971, 1976). Recovery and survival time are similar after storage for 72 h at 22°C in CPD, ACD, CPD-A1 or CPD-A2 plasma (Slichter and Harker 1976c; Scott and Slichter 1980; Holme *et al.* 1987). After storage at 4°C for 24 and 72 h, platelet viability drops to 18% and 9%, respectively, compared with that of fresh controls (Slichter and Harker 1976c; Murphy and Gardner 1969). Loss of viability is a function of both degree of chilling and length of exposure. Exposure of platelets, even for short periods of time (17 h), to 12°C or 16°C, or even to 18°C for 96 h, significantly reduces *in vivo* viability (Gottschall *et al.* 1986; Moroff and George 1994). Although chilled storage is associated with a morphological disc to sphere transformation in the platelet (White and Krivit 1967), shape change does not appear to cause the loss of viability (see below).

After storage of platelets at 22°C for 24 h, glycogen stores become depleted, toxic metabolites accumulate and the cells develop impaired aggregation and adhesion responses. These functions are well preserved at 4°C (Shively *et al.* 1970; Murphy and Gardner 1971; Rock and Figueredo 1976). The storage abnormalities reverse *in vivo* after transfusion, although the exact interval required for recovery is not known (Murphy and Gardner 1971; Becker *et al.* 1973). These observations have led some to suggest that an inventory of 'activated' refrigerated platelets be maintained to treat bleeding thrombocytopenic patients, while a separate stock of room temperature platelets with superior survival characteristics is kept for prophylactic transfusion (Valeri 1976), an imaginative if impractical proposal.

Storage lesion: is platelet activation partly to blame?

Glycolysis during storage at 22°C results in an increased lactate production and a fall in pH (Murphy *et al.* 1970). When pH reaches 6.8, platelet morphology begins to change and shape change becomes striking when pH reaches 6.0 and viability is lost. The rate of change in pH is affected by the platelet concentration and by the availability of oxygen. Therefore the gas permeability of the plastic container for carbon dioxide diffusion and the preservative solution are critical factors. When too few platelets are stored in gas-permeable plastics, excess carbon dioxide may be

lost and pH may rise too high. A pH rise above 7.3 is also accompanied by platelet shape change, and at a pH above 7.5 (at 22°C), platelet viability deteriorates (Murphy 1985).

Even at normal pH, platelet function and integrity decline during storage. Activation is considered the main culprit for the storage lesion of 22°C-stored platelets, although the evidence is largely circumstantial. A negative correlation has been found between platelet viability and the expression of activation-dependent antigens such as P-selectin (Keegan *et al.* 1992), CD62 and lysome-associated membrane proteins 1 and 2 (Divers *et al.* 1995). A correlation has also been found between the amount of glycoprotein (GPIb and GPIIb/IIIa) on the platelet surface and platelet survival. The amount of these GPs decreases during storage, apparently as a consequence of platelet activation (Fijnheer 1991). Finally, addition to the anticoagulant of inhibitors of platelet activation and an inhibitor of thrombin improves the condition of platelets after 5 days of storage (Bode and Miller 1988, 1989). However, the amount of membrane GPIb and IIb/IIIa does not correlate well with platelet injury (Murphy *et al.* 1994). Furthermore platelets activated by thrombin *ex vivo* circulate well in animal models (see below). In any case, the decreased aggregation and adhesion capacity of stored platelets cannot easily be attributed to activation.

Effect of different plastics

The permeability of the plastic to oxygen is of great significance for oxidative metabolism and thus for the quality of stored platelets. The following 'second generation' plastics have been found to be satisfactory: (1) a blend of polyolefin plastic constituents without a plasticizer (PL-732, Baxter Healthcare) (Murphy *et al.* 1982); (2) polyvinyl chloride (PVC) plasticized with tri-(2-ethylhexyl) trimellate (CLX Cutter) (Murphy *et al.* 1982); (3) PVC plasticized with the conventional di-(2-ethylhexyl) phthalate (DEHP) but with a reduced thickness and a larger surface area (Teruflexa, Terumo) (Holme *et al.* 1989); (4) PVC with the phthalate ester analogue tri-(2-ethylhexyl)-1,2,4 benzene tricarboxylate as plasticizer (F720-BIOtrans) (Koerner 1984); (5) PVC plasticized with butyryl-n-trihexyl citrate (BTHC) (PL-2209, Baxter Healthcare). BTHC has the advantage of being suitable for both platelets and red cells and, unlike DEHP, does not leach into blood components during storage (Gullikson *et al.* 1991; Högman *et al.* 1991a). DEHP has been cited as a potential toxin (see Chapter 15); and (6) polyvinyl chloride plasticized with di-n-decyl phthalate (DNDP) (Murphy *et al.* 1995).

The effects of agitation

When platelet concentrates are not agitated during storage, pH falls rapidly (Murphy and Gardner 1976). Agitation facilitates gas exchange, which is usually cited as its mode of action, although diffusion of metabolites and maintenance of platelets in a mobile liquid medium may be an added benefit (Sweeney *et al.* 1995). The method of agitation makes a difference; a flat-bed agitator was found to be more effective than a rotary agitator (Murphy *et al.* 1982). Vertical and horizontal agitation appear equally effective (Gunson *et al.* 1983). Flat-bed shakers with 1.5-inch lateral movement are preferable to shakers with a 1.0-inch lateral movement because, with more rapid acceleration and deceleration, platelet buttons formed after centrifugation are resuspended more efficiently (Snyder *et al.* 1985). Before agitation is begun, the platelets should remain undisturbed for 1 h. When platelets are stored in polyolefin bags, discontinuation of agitation, even for 24 h, has hardly any effect on pH (Moroff and George 1990; Hunter *et al.* 2001). Platelets that are shipped, even with land and air transport lasting 12 h, result in adequate viability, post-transfusion increments and apparent *in vivo* function, equivalent to cells that are kept in storage with agitation (Simon and Sierra 1982, 1989; SA Haddad and HG Klein, personal observations).

A 34-year-old woman with transfusion-dependent aplastic anaemia was supported for 6 years with single-donor platelet transfusions. Over time, she became more broadly alloimmunized until platelet transfusion support relied upon 12 closely matched unrelated donors. She was subsequently transferred to a distant hospital for stem cell transplantation. Seventeen HLA-matched apheresis collections from the same 12 matched donors were shipped by ground and air transport that required interruption of agitation for 6–11 h. Post-transfusion corrected count increments (CCI, see below) for the transported platelets were clinically acceptable and not different from increments recorded at her initial treatment facility with platelets that were collected from the same donors and stored at 22°C with constant agitation (Fig. 14.3).

Effect of contamination with leucocytes

When platelet concentrates are stored in thick plastic containers, the oxygen supply is limited. Under these circumstances, leucocytes in the concentrate compete with platelets for available oxygen; anaerobic glycolysis and lactate production in the platelets are stimulated, leading to an accelerated fall in pH (Gottschall *et al.* 1984). When the more oxygen-permeable containers are used, a marked decrease in pH is rarely seen, regardless of the leucocyte content of the concentrate (Moroff and Holme 1991). However, proteolytic enzymes produced by monocytes and released from neutrophils during storage, may remove glycoproteins from the platelet membrane (Sloand and Klein 1990). The loss of glycoproteins may affect platelet viability (see below).

Concern has been expressed that removal of leucocytes before storage might increase the danger of bacterial growth. However, when the buffy coat is maintained for 1 h at 22°C before the platelet concentrate is prepared, most of the bacteria are ingested and removed with the leucocytes, thus considerably reducing the danger of bacterial contamination (Högman *et al.* 1991b).

Plasma versus synthetic media for storage of platelets

Advantages of storage in synthetic media include the removal of plasma proteins such as thrombin, plasmin and C3a that are involved in platelet activation and, depending on the composition of the medium, less accumulation of lactate and a smaller fall in pH. The viability of platelets after storage in a plasma-free electrolyte medium containing glucose, with bicarbonate to buffer lactic acid, was substantially better than after storage in plasma (survival after 7 days' storage 144.1 ± 15.9 h and 100 ± 32 h respectively) (Holme *et al.* 1987). Unfortunately, the bicarbonate has to be sterilized and stored at an alkaline pH in a separate container (Holme *et al.* 1987). Replacement of bicarbonate by phosphate buffer is not effective because phosphate stimulates glycolysis and the formation of lactic acid (Murphy *et al.* 1991). Excellent results have been obtained with glucose-free crystalloid media such as plasmalyte-A. The essential constituent of these media is acetate, which is oxidized to bicarbonate by platelets (Bertolini *et al.* 1992; Shimizu and Murphy

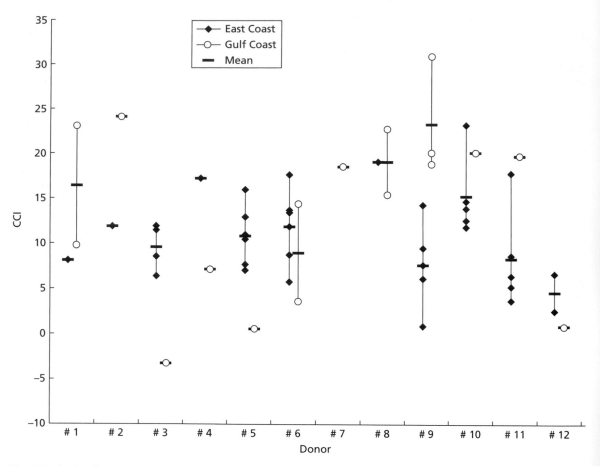

Fig 14.3 Platelets from 12 HLA-matched donors given to the same patient. Corrected count increment (CCI) at site of collection and storage at a hospital on the east coast of the USA (closed diamonds). CCI after surface and air transport to a hospital on the Gulf Coast, USA (open circles); transport time (without agitation) was 6–11 h.

1993; Murphy *et al.* 1995). Metabolism of platelets stored in solutions containing acetate is significantly different from that of platelets stored in plasma. If the oxygen supply is adequate, less glucose is metabolized and less lactic acid is produced and an adequate pH is maintained for 15 days unless the number of stored platelets is exceptionally large (Bertolini *et al.* 1992). Acetate has been confirmed as a useful fuel for platelet metabolism (Whisson *et al.* 1993). Pyruvate suppresses lactic acid production to the same extent as does acetate (Murphy *et al.* 1995). Storage of platelets for 7 days or longer is now possible (Dumont *et al.* 2002; Sweeney *et al.* 2004), although measures must be taken to reduce the risk of bacterial growth (see Chapter 16).

Relation between in vitro *platelet assays and in vivo recovery and survival*

The response of platelets to hypotonic shock, also called the 'osmotic reversal reaction', was first described by Fantl (1968). The results of this test correlate well with viability (Murphy *et al.* 1991). The test is based on the observation that light transmission through platelet-containing plasma increases abruptly after addition of hypotonic solutions, because the influx of water into the platelets leads to swelling and a dilution of cytoplasmic contents. Healthy platelets regain their initial volume and initial concentration of cytoplasmic colloids. Water and electrolytes are pumped out of the platelets and light transmission returns to normal values.

Morphological changes in platelets stored at 20°C correlate with post-transfusion viability; concentrates with the highest proportion of discoid platelets have the best survival (Kunicki *et al.* 1975). Similarly, the shape of platelets, or their change in shape and lactate production, correlate with viability (Moroff *et al.* 1990). The shape change is also associated with a decrease in the amount of ATP and ADP in platelets (de Korte *et al.* 1990).

The percentage of discoid platelets has been assessed by light-scattering measurements (Fratantoni *et al.* 1984) and a method has been devised for assessing platelet viability by visual inspection. If a bag containing platelet concentrate is held near a light source and given a twist, an appearance of swirling, caused by light scattering indicates that the platelets have retained their discoid shape. The swirling does not occur when platelets have been stored at 4°C and when the pH has fallen to 6.2. A scoring system to assess the magnitude of the swirling phenomenon has been devised (Fijnheer *et al.* 1989; George *et al.* 1989). In a study conducted with 11 laboratories, the reproducibility of swirling as a measure of platelet quality proved promising (Murphy *et al.* 1994).

Refrigerated storage of platelets

Storage lesion: what's activation got to do with it?

Refrigerated storage compromises platelet recovery and survival following transfusion. Although platelets stored in the cold have better *in vitro* function than platelets stored at room temperature (Becker *et al.* 1973; Snyder *et al.* 1989b), the markedly shortened survival of chilled platelets offsets any functional advantage. Recent studies suggest that the storage lesion is not one of activation (Hoffmeister *et al.* 2001).

Biochemical analyses indicate that platelet cytoskeletal alterations and increased responsiveness to agonists are detectable as the temperature falls below 37°C (Hoffmeister *et al.* 2001). Cooling below 15°C induces extensive platelet shape changes mediated by intracellular cytoskeletal rearrangements. These alterations can be partially reversed by rewarming. Rewarmed concentrates contain more spherical than discoid platelet forms. Conventional teaching aside, platelets activated *ex vivo* by thrombin, despite extensive shape

changes, continue to circulate and function in mice and in non-human primates (Michelson *et al.* 1996; Berger *et al.* 1998). Chilled and rewarmed platelets, preserved as discs with pharmacological agents, are cleared with the same speed as are untreated chilled platelets; misshapen chilled and rewarmed platelets circulate just like 22°C platelets in a mouse model (Hoffmeister *et al.* 2003a). The cold storage lesion appears to be something other than or in addition to shape change.

The quantities of IgG or IgM bound to chilled or room temperature human platelets are identical, implying that binding of platelet-associated antibodies to Fc receptors does not mediate the clearance of cooled platelets. Chilling of platelets does not induce detectable phosphatidyl serine on the platelet surface *in vitro*, so that phosphatidyl serine exposure and the involvement of scavenger receptors in the clearance of chilled platelets seem unlikely. Complement type 3 (CR3) receptors on hepatic macrophages are responsible for the recognition and clearance of chilled platelets. Chilled platelets develop clustered von Willebrand (vWF) surface receptors (GP1b), enhancing recognition of mouse and human platelets by hepatic macrophage CR3 receptors. The extracellular domain of the GPIbα molecule, isolated by proteolysis from intact platelets, binds avidly to CR3 *in vitro*, and when immobilized on a surface, supports the rolling and firm adhesion of THP-1 cells (Simon *et al.* 2000). Cleavage of the extracellular domain of murine GPIbα results in normal survival of chilled platelets transfused into mice. GPIbα depletion of human chilled platelets greatly reduces ingestion of the treated platelets by macrophage-like cells *in vitro*. The normal clearance of chilled platelets lacking the N-terminal portion of GPIbα rules out the many other CR3 binding partners, including molecules expressed on platelet surfaces, as candidates for mediating chilled platelet clearance. Chilled platelets bind vWf and function normally *in vitro* and *ex vivo* after transfusion into CR3-deficient mice (Hoffmeister *et al.* 2003a).

During haemostasis, GPIbα on the surface of the resting discoid platelet functions to bind the activated form of vWF at sites of vascular injury. Cooling of platelets, however, causes GPIbα clustering rather than internalization. The observation that GPIbα interacts separately with vWF and with CR3 suggests that selective modification of GPIbα might inhibit cold-induced platelet clearance without impairing GPIbα's

619

haemostatically important reactivity with vWF. Hoffmeister and co-workers (2003b) have suggested that selective blockage of the exposed carbohydrate β-GlcNAc on the GPIbα clusters by UDP-galactose, a normal constituent of human cells, might neutralize the cold storage lesion and safely prolong the circulation of refrigerated platelets in humans.

Storage of platelets in the frozen state: not yet ready for prime time

Four methods of freezing platelets have been compared:
1 6% dimethylsulphoxide (DMSO) with a cooling rate of about 2–3°C/min (not controlled) and storage at –80°C (modification of a method described by Valeri (Valeri et al. 1974))
2 5% DMSO and 5% hydroxyethyl starch (HES) with the same cooling rate and storage temperature (Stiff et al. 1983)
3 3% glycerol with a cooling rate of 10°C/min from 15°C to –3°C followed by 35°C/min down to –140°C and storage in the vapour phase of liquid nitrogen (Dayian et al. 1974)
4 5% glycerol and 4% glucose with the same cooling programme and storage (Dayian et al. 1986).
The best results, obtained with method (1), showed mean platelet recovery and 24-h increment to be significantly better than with the other methods. Nevertheless, the post-transfusion increment was only about 30% of that of fresh platelets. In three out of eight patients receiving chemotherapy, episodes of epistaxis and moderately severe haemorrhage from the oral mucosa were arrested by transfusion of platelets frozen in 6% DMSO, and six of the eight patients were supported solely with such platelets until complete haematological recovery occurred (Angelini et al. 1992).

One strategy for managing immune refractory patients scheduled to receive repeated courses of chemotherapy is to collect autologous platelets during periods of haematopoietic recovery and freeze them for use during myeloablation. In a creative modification of this method Vadhan-Raj and co-workers (2002) administered recombinant human thrombopoietin at 2.4 g/kg to chemotherapy-naive patients with gynaecological malignancies, and cryopreserved the resulting autologous apheresis platelets in a mixture of ThromboSol and 2% DMSO. Subsequent transfusion of these autologous frozen platelets resulted in good increments in corrected counts, including in patients who were alloimmunized, allowing delivery of multiple cycles of intensive chemotherapy (Vadhan-Raj et al. 2002). Logistics, cost and potential side-effects of thrombopoietin make this approach impractical for all but a few particularly vexing alloimmunized platelet recipients.

Indications for platelet transfusions

Thrombocytopenia

Bleeding patients with severe thrombocytopenia and impaired platelet production require platelet transfusion support. However, most platelet transfusions are administered not to stem bleeding but to prevent it (McCullough et al. 1988). An autopsy study from the early years of leukaemia chemotherapy reported that 63% of leukaemia patients suffered haemorrhagic deaths in the year before prophylactic platelet transfusions were introduced (Han et al. 1966), a statistic that must seem incredible to those who trained in the era of platelet transfusion. Nevertheless, no controlled study has demonstrated that prophylactic platelet transfusions are superior to a strategy of timely transfusion when bleeding occurs.

A substantial body of evidence supports the value of prophylactic transfusions to prevent patients with a platelet count below $20 \times 10^9/l$ from bleeding. In a seminal publication, Gaydos and co-workers (1962) reported that serious bleeding on 92 children with acute leukaemia occurred on only 4% of hospital days when the child's platelet count exceeded $20 \times 10^9/l$, but on 10–30% when the count fell below $5 \times 10^9/l$. Too often forgotten is the absence of any obvious threshold effect for increased bleeding in their data analysis (Fig. 14.4).

Furthermore, during this period, the patients were administered aspirin as an antipyretic, which undoubtedly increased their bleeding tendency at higher platelet levels.

In a study of 62 leukaemic children, serious bleeding occurred in only 5% of patients with a platelet count between 20 and $40 \times 10^9/l$, but in 26% of those with counts $< 10 \times 10^9/l$. A double-blind randomized study of 21 patients with acute leukaemia confirmed the benefit of prophylaxis and observed that fever preceded haemorrhage in 10 out of 13 cases (Higby et al. 1974). Using the $20 \times 10^9/l$ trigger for prophylaxis,

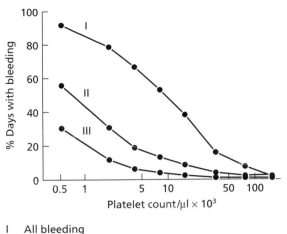

I   All bleeding
II Skin and epistaxis
III Melaena, haematuria, haematemesis

Fig 14.4 Relationship between platelet count and percentage of days with bleeding. Percentage of days with bleeding in 92 children with acute leukaemia: I, all bleeding; II, minor bleeding defined as skin and mucous membrane (purpura, epistaxis); III, significant bleeding (haematuria, haematemesis, melaena). Adapted from Gaydos *et al.* (1962).

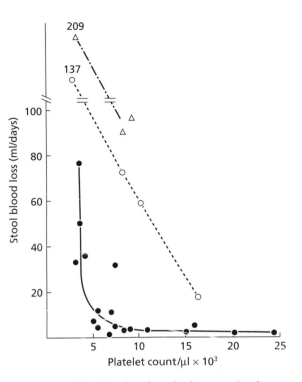

Fig 14.5 Stool blood loss based on platelet count. Stool blood loss (expressed as ml/day) was determined for 20 patients with stable aplastic thrombocytopenia and radiolabelled red cells. At a platelet count $> 10 \times 10^9$/l, blood loss averaged 9 ml/day, whereas at a count of $< 5 \times 10^9$/l, stool blood loss rose to 50 ml/day. Bleeding increased at every level when patients received prednisone (open circles) or semisynthetic penicillin (open triangles). Adapted from Slichter and Harker (1978).

Murphy and co-workers (1982) found a significant reduction in bleeding, but no reduction in mortality, when 28 acute leukaemia patients treated with prophylactic platelets were compared with control subjects. An earlier study, documented in letter form only, reported similar findings (Solomon *et al.* 1978).

Experimental and clinical data support a transfusion trigger well below 20×10^9/l for stable, non-infected, afebrile thrombocytopenic patients who have no additional anatomic or functional defects in haemostasis. Studies of patients with aplastic anaemia found that daily stool blood loss measured with radiolabelled red cells increased strikingly when the platelet count fell below 5×10^9/l (Fig. 14.5) (Slichter and Harker 1978).

Results of a 10-year experience in 103 patients with acute myeloid leukaemia indicate that for patients without other risk factors, such as bleeding or fever, a platelet count of 5×10^9/l is adequate to prevent bleeding; for patients with such risks the count was kept above 10×10^9/l and for those with an additional coagulation defect, or with anatomical lesions, the count was kept above 20×10^9/l (Gmur *et al.* 1991). Three fatal haemorrhages occurred. The serious episodes of

haemorrhage often occurred at relatively high platelet counts, emphasizing the importance of clinical factors as the cause of bleeding.

In 78 patients undergoing induction therapy for acute leukaemia who were randomized to receive prophylactic apheresis platelet concentrates, a 10×10^9/l threshold for prophylactic transfusion proved safe (Heckman *et al.* 1993). A subsequent large multicentre trial enrolled 255 assessable patients in 21 Italian centres (Rebulla *et al.* 1997). Adult acute leukaemia patients during the first remission induction were randomized to the traditional 20×10^9/l threshold or to a threshold of 10×10^9/l when in stable condition (but 20×10^9/l in the presence of fresh haemorrhage, fever greater than 38°C or invasive procedures). The lower threshold was associated with a 21.5% reduction in platelet requirements, yet no significant differences in the number of red cell transfusions, severe bleeding episodes or deaths during induction were detected. Overall, clinically significant haemorrhages occurred in 3.1% and 2% of the days in the lower and standard arms respectively.

The most contemporary evidence supporting the safety of the $10 \times 10^9/l$ threshold involved a multicentre trial in Germany that studied 105 leukaemia patients undergoing 216 remission–induction or consolidation treatment cycles in 17 centres (Wandt *et al.* 1998). Individual participating centres had previously chosen to adopt either a 20 or a $10 \times 10^9/l$ threshold level for their prophylactic transfusion policy. Twenty bleeding complications (18%) were recorded in 110 chemotherapy cycles in the lower threshold and 18 (17%) in 106 cycles in the higher one. Haemorrhagic deaths occurred in two patients at platelet counts of 36 and $50 \times 10^9/l$, treated in hospitals using the higher threshold. Similar data have been published for 159 patients undergoing haematopoietic stem cell transplant (Zumberg *et al.* 2002).

In summary, the venerated 'twenty-thousand' threshold represents a guideline to be modified based on the patient's diagnosis, clinical status and treatment. No algorithm replaces bedside evaluation. A threshold of $10 \times 10^9/l$ appears to be safe for prophylactic platelet transfusion in stable adult patients and children receiving therapy for acute leukaemia, although it is possible that this group of patients may not need prophylactic transfusions at all. Transfusion at higher levels may be advisable for newborns, for patients with signs of haemorrhage, high fever, mucositis, rapidly falling platelet count or other coagulation abnormalities (e.g. acute promyelocytic leukemia) and for those undergoing invasive procedures (Schiffer *et al.* 2001). The importance of a post-transfusion platelet count to confirm the expected efficacy of transfusion cannot be overemphasized.

Prophylactic platelet transfusions for invasive procedures

The generally accepted platelet threshold for patients undergoing invasive procedures is $50 \times 10^9/l$. A review of 95 patients with acute leukaemia who underwent 167 procedures, of which 70% were classified as major surgery, revealed no procedure-related deaths or excess bleeding when the platelet count exceeded

this level (Bishop *et al.* 1987). Platelet count was maintained at this level for three postoperative days in the case of surgery. No studies address either the safety of a threshold below $50 \times 10^9/l$ or delicate ophthalmological or neurosurgery in which a higher threshold may be prudent.

Few data serve to guide the use of platelet transfusions for other invasive procedures. Eight thrombocytopenic patients developed spinal subdural haematoma, an otherwise relatively uncommon complication, following lumbar puncture; five out of the eight had a platelet count below $50 \times 10^9/l$; no patient with a normal platelet count developed this complication during the same 4-year period (Edelson *et al.* 1974). A review of 5609 consecutive lumbar punctures in 956 children with acute leukaemia over a 15-year period reported no increased risk of neurological or haemorrhagic complications, even with platelet counts as low as $20 \times 10^9/l$ (Howard *et al.* 2002). However, all platelet counts of $100 \times 10^9/l$ or less were associated with an increased risk of traumatic and bloody lumbar puncture. In a review of 291 consecutive liver biopsies (155 standard, 22 fine needle) in thrombocytopenic patients, the frequency of bleeding was the same (3.4%) for patients at a platelet count between 50 and $99 \times 10^9/l$ as for patients with a mid-range normal count (McVay and Toy 1990). However, liver biopsy preceding a precipitous fall in platelet count has been associated with a lethal delayed haemorrhage (Reichert *et al.* 1983). Gastrointestinal endoscopy (Chu *et al.* 1983) and fibreoptic bronchoscopy in thrombocytopenic patients have not resulted in additional serious complications, although one life-threatening episode of severe epistaxis occurred during a transoral bronchoscopy in a patient who had prior epistaxis and a platelet count of $18 \times 10^9/l$ (Weiss *et al.* 1993).

Inherited qualitative defects in platelets

Patients with an inherited defect of platelet function (Wiskott–Aldrich syndrome, Bernard–Soulier syndrome and Glanzmann disease) should be treated with platelet transfusions when serious bleeding occurs, or before operation. In the last two disorders, alloimmunization, especially to GP IIb-IIIa in the case of Glanzmann disease, poses a particular problem, so that transfusions should be administered prudently (Kunicki *et al.* 1987). For alloimmunization related to other antigens, see Chapter 13.

Acquired qualitative defects in platelets

An acquired defect of platelet function, due apparently to damage by passage through a pump oxygenator, is sometimes observed in patients who have undergone cardiac bypass procedures. Troublesome bleeding may be observed even with a platelet count above $50 \times 10^9/l$. In these circumstances, transfusion of normal platelets may be effective (Moriau et al. 1977). Platelet transfusions may also have a role in managing patients receiving medications that interfere with platelet function, particularly those who are bleeding or require urgent surgery. Thioprenidines such as the antithrombotic agent clopidogrel (Plavix), specific inhibitors of ADP-stimulated platelet function, result in increased blood loss and red cell transfusion for coronary artery bypass graft surgery (Gansera et al. 2003). However, neither this drug nor its carboxylic acid metabolite inhibits platelets in vitro, suggesting that transfused platelets are unaffected (Bennett 2001). The monoclonal antibody Fab fragment abciximab (Reopro) blocks the platelet IIb/IIIa receptor and produces a Glanzmann-like effect. Unbound abciximab is rapidly cleared from circulation and little or no drug remains in serum or bound to tissues other than platelets. Subsequent platelet transfusion restores the platelet aggregation response, because previously bound abciximab redistributes to the new platelets, thus decreasing the overall percentage of blocked GPIIb/IIIa sites to fewer than the approximately 80% necessary to interfere with platelet aggregation and bleeding time (Coller 1997; Lemmer et al. 2000).

Thrombocytopenia due to immune destruction of platelets

Platelet transfusion in neonatal alloimmune thrombocytopenia and thrombotic thrombocytopenic purpura (TTP) is discussed in Chapter 13, and in post transfusion purpura in Chapter 15. Platelet transfusions are seldom indicated in autoimmune thrombocytopenia.

Thrombocytopenia due to consumption of platelets

In thrombotic thrombocytopenic purpura and in the haemolytic uraemic syndrome, the transfusion of platelets is rarely needed and tends to aggravate the condition (Chapter 13). The effects of platelet transfusion in DIC are less predictable but platelet transfusions are often given when serious bleeding is associated with thrombocytopenia.

Some other aspects of platelet transfusions

Expected rise in platelet count following transfusion: when it counts, it should be counted

Transfusion of one unit of fresh platelets (containing approximately 0.7×10^{11} platelets) to an adult weighing 70 kg produces an immediate post-transfusion increment of approximately $11 \times 10^9/l$ (Schiffer 1981). In order to make proper comparisons between different recipients, the number of platelets transfused and the approximate blood volume of the recipient must be taken into account. One formula defines the 'corrected count increment' as the rise in platelet count observed multiplied by the surface area (in metres squared) divided by the number of platelets transfused divided by 10^{11}. For example, for a 70-kg adult with a surface area of $1.7 \, m^2$ and the other figures given above, the corrected increment would be:

$$11 \times 10^9/l \times 1.7/0.7 = \text{approximately } 27 \times 10^9/l$$
$$\text{(Daly et al. 1980).} \qquad (14.2)$$

Calculation of the corrected increment at 1 h after transfusion is valuable in three circumstances: (1) when stored platelets are being used, as a check on their efficacy; (2) when platelet transfusions are being given to patients who may have formed alloantibodies; and (3) to check whether HLA-matched or crossmatch-compatible platelets are effective.

Two other methods for calculating platelet increment have been recommended. The percentage platelet recovery (PPR) also adjusts for the number of platelets transfused and for the blood volume, and a regression analysis method purports to separate the effects of dose and cell quality (Davis et al. 1999). Neither has been widely used.

Risks from red cell contamination

Platelet concentrates contain variable numbers of red cells and may induce Rh_0D sensitization in a D-negative subject. The risk is small, particularly in patients receiving immunosuppressive therapy for leukaemia or solid tumours (Goldfinger and McGinniss 1971; Lichtiger and Hester 1986; Lozano and Cid 2003). When platelet

623

concentrates from D-positive donors are transfused repeatedly to a D-negative woman who has not yet reached the menopause, provided that the recipient is not already immunized, a dose of anti-D immunoglobulin should be considered to suppress primary Rh_0D immunization. For further details, see Chapter 5.

Platelet concentrates from cytomegalovirus antibody-negative donors

The consequences of primary infection with cytomegalovirus (CMV) can be very serious in immunosuppressed patients. For those patients who are anti-CMV negative, platelet concentrates from anti-CMV-negative donors (see Chapters 13 and 16) should be made available; alternatively, the platelet concentrate should be depleted of white cells to reduce the risk of CMV transmission (Gilbert *et al.* 1989; Bowden *et al.* 1995).

The transfusion of leucocytes

A direct relationship between the number of circulating granulocytes and the risk of bacterial infection has been recognized for 40 years (Bodey *et al.* 1966). Early studies of granulocyte transfusions were limited by the short survival of circulating granulocytes, their poor viability when stored for more than a few hours and the difficulty in collecting sufficient numbers of cells to measure a post-transfusion increment. Freireich and co-workers (1964) elected to study the dose response of transfused granulocytes by collecting cells from adult donors (patients) with chronic myelocytic leukaemia (CML) and infusing them into granulocytopenic children. The initial 118 transfusions established several fundamental precepts: (1) the 1-h post-transfusion increment correlates directly with the number of granulocytes infused; (2) an estimated 10^{11} granulocytes per square metre of body surface area, more than the total number calculated to circulate in normal subjects, are needed to raise the recipient's circulating granulocytes by 1000/μl; (3) no increment is detected if fewer than 10^{10} cells are infused; and (4) clearance of circulating Gram-negative bacteria and resolution of fever occurred in most (10 out of 11) children who received more than 10^{10} granulocytes/m^2 (Frei *et al.* 1965). These studies established the basic principles of granulocyte transfusion. However, cells from patients with CML had two advantages over the mature gra-

nulocytes collected from normal volunteers during the following 30 years. First, these collections contained granulocyte precursors that circulated and matured for 24 h or more. Second, some of these cells clearly engrafted transiently in some of the immunosuppressed patients and proliferated for several days. Both factors probably contributed to the efficacy of the early treatments and made comparisons with these data difficult until methods to mobilize cells from normal subjects became available (Frei *et al.* 1965).

Labelling of granulocytes: distribution in the circulation

When labelled granulocytes are injected into the bloodstream, they equilibrate with the total blood granulocyte pool, consisting of cells that 'marginate' along, or adhere to, the walls of venules and others that circulate freely. Following intravenous injection of $DF^{32}P$-labelled granulocytes, the concentration in the bloodstream is only 45% of that expected if all the granulocytes circulated freely (Cartwright *et al.* 1964). This figure may slightly underestimate the true percentage of neutrophils that circulate freely, because some $DF^{32}P$ elutes rapidly from labelled granulocytes (Dancey *et al.* 1976). Moreover, when granulocytes were labelled *in vivo* with ^3H-thymidine and then transfused to another normal subject, the maximum recovery was 57%, suggesting that only 43% of the granulocytes (rather than 55%) were marginated (Dancey *et al.* 1976). However, using ^{111}In-labelled granulocytes, the marginating granulocyte pool was calculated to be 60% of the total blood granulocyte pool (Peters *et al.* 1985). Granulocytes labelled with ^3H-thymidine disappear from the bloodstream with a $T_{1/2}$ of 7.6 h. Based on this finding and other data, daily production of granulocytes was estimated to be 0.85×10^9/kg, about one-half of the previous estimate obtained with $DF^{32}P$. The total marrow metamyelocyte–granulocyte pool was estimated to be 6×10^9/kg (Dancey *et al.* 1976). In a 70-kg man the total pool of marrow granulocytes is thus about 4.2×10^{11}. Taking the granulocyte count in circulating blood at 4.0×10^9/l and assuming a blood volume of 5 l in a 70-kg man, total circulating granulocytes are estimated to be 2×10^{10} or about one-twentieth of the total marrow granulocyte pool. This estimate agrees well with data obtained following leucapheresis, which indicate an 'extracirculatory' reservoir of granulocytes of about

18 times the total number of granulocytes in the circulation (Bierman *et al.* 1962).

[111]In combined with a suitable chelating agent is the best label for granulocytes: little elution of the label occurs *in vivo* and labelled granulocytes can be detected readily by surface scanning. Following the injection of ^{111}In-labelled granulocytes, label accumulates immediately in the lungs, but granulocytes then redistribute to the liver and spleen. Granulocytes labelled with ^{111}In were cleared from the circulating blood with a $T_{1/2}$ of 7.5 h, confirming results obtained with ^{3}H-thymidine (Thakur *et al.* 1977a). ^{111}In-labelled granulocytes have been used successfully for the localization of abscesses (Thakur *et al.* 1977b; Dutcher *et al.* 1981) and, combined with imaging, have been used to study the distribution and sites of destruction of granulocytes in normal subjects (Saverymuttu *et al.* 1985).

Storage of granulocytes

Storage in the liquid state

Granulocytes do not store well. The effect of liquid storage on granulocyte function has been studied by measuring a variety of morphological markers, chemical changes in the supernatant, alterations in cell function *in vitro*, and cell recovery and circulation *in vivo*. Functional assays such as chemotaxis, phagocytosis, chemiluminescence and superoxide anion formation are not practical measurements for routine quality control. However, when the method of collection or of storage has been modified, granulocyte testing by a panel of functional assays should be undertaken. The definitive measure of efficacy is control of infection in the compromised host.

Of the *in vitro* assays, granulocyte chemotaxis is most often used as the surrogate measure of cell quality. Chemotaxis of neutrophils is maintained satisfactorily for about 8 h at 20–24°C, but is rapidly impaired by storage at 4°C (Lane and Windle 1979). The severe impairment of chemotaxis of granulocytes after prolonged storage is probably caused by a lesion of the cytoskeleton. After storage at 4°C, microfilaments are disorganized and few microtubes are visible (Palm *et al.* 1981). At room temperature, neutrophils consume glucose and maintenance of glucose concentration is essential for maintaining function (Glasser *et al.* 1985). The addition of bicarbonate to neutralize lactic acid formed as a result of glycolysis, and thus to maintain pH at acceptable levels, helps to maintain chemotactic function (Lane and Lamkin 1984). Granulocytes stored in the absence of protein deteriorate rapidly, but chemotaxis is maintained just as well in a synthetic medium supplemented with albumin as in autologous plasma (Glasser *et al.* 1985). Granulocytes stored for 24 h at either 1–6°C or 20–24°C have significantly reduced intravascular recovery and migration into skin windows. Granulocytes stored for only 8 h at 20–24°C have normal intravascular recovery and migration into skin windows (McCullough *et al.* 1983). Agitation of granulocytes during storage rapidly increases the rate at which their function deteriorates (McCullough *et al.* 1978).

Stimulating donors with granulocyte colony-stimulating factor (G-CSF), or G-CSF with dexamethasone, increases the yield of granulocytes compared with the yield from the traditional collection regimen of dexamethasone alone (Dale *et al.* 1998; Liles *et al.* 2000; Stroncek *et al.* 2001). When granulocytes are incubated with G-CSF or dexamethasone, apoptosis is delayed and *in vitro* survival prolonged. However, the effect does not appear to extend to cells collected from donors mobilized with these agents. The high cell counts in G-CSF- and G-CSF-plus-dexamethasone-mobilized concentrates cause a rapid decrease in pH, which limits component shelf-life. Dilutions of 1:8 to 1:16 with autologous plasma can maintain the pH of stored granulocyte concentrates, but the component volumes are impractical (Lightfoot *et al.* 2000). For the large number and high concentration of granulocytes in collections mobilized with G-CSF (see below), cell counts, viability and pH can be well maintained after 2, 24 and 48 h when cells are stored in the three cell culture media (Lightfoot *et al.* 2001). None of these media is approved for *in vivo* use. Standard infusible solutions are not buffered adequately and lack sufficient protein, but infusible solutions, such as lactated Ringer's solution or PlasmaLyte A supplemented with buffers and albumin, hold promise as effective and licensable solutions for granulocyte storage.

Storage in the frozen state

Critical granulocyte functions are impaired severely after freezing and subsequent thawing (Frim and Mazur 1980). Cryopreserved granulocytes are not satisfactory for transfusion purposes.

Irradiation of granulocyte concentrates

Granulocyte concentrates inevitably contain large numbers of immunocompetent T lymphocytes. Because many potential granulocyte recipients, especially those undergoing allogeneic transplantation procedures, are susceptible to transfusion-associated graft-versus-host disease, these cells are routinely exposed to 25-Gy gamma irradiation. Some early studies suggested that granulocytes collected by centrifugation are damaged by this irradiation dose (Buescher and Gallin 1987); however, studies of mobilized cells indicate that both phagocytosis and migration are preserved (Caspar et al. 1993).

Indications for granulocyte transfusions

Under normal circumstances, two and a half times the number of granulocytes present in the circulation at any given time is consumed each day. Granulocyte turnover can increase by an order of magnitude in the face of infection. Thus, for transfusions to be effective in neutropenic patients with life-threatening bacterial or fungal infections, large numbers of granulocytes must be administered repeatedly. If normal production in an adult is about 10^{11} granulocytes per day and if only 5–10% of the granulocyte pool is in the circulation, at least 2.1×10^{10} granulocytes should be transfused per day (Strauss 1993). To obtain such numbers without resorting to granulocytes from patients with chronic granulocyte leukaemia, the donor must be stimulated (mobilized) with cytokines, steroids or both, and blood cell separators must use an erythrocyte sedimenting agent such as hydroxyethyl starch during collection (Dale et al. 1998; Liles et al. 2000; Stroncek et al. 2001, 2002) (see also Chapter 17). Once granulocyte therapy has been started, transfusions should be continued for 4–7 days before reassessing patient status.

Therapeutic granulocyte transfusion in infected neutropenic patients

In adults and children. Several prospective, randomized, controlled clinical trials have shown an increased survival in neutropenic patients who are given leucocyte transfusions in addition to antibiotics (Higby et al. 1975; Alavi and Root 1977; Herzig et al. 1977; Vogler and Winton 1977). Seven controlled studies

have been reviewed in detail (Klein et al. 1996). Most of the patients studied suffered from Gram-negative septicaemia. Significant benefit from the transfusions was seen only when bone marrow recovery was delayed for more than 1 week, but did occur within 2 or 3 weeks when leucocyte transfusions were given daily for at least 4–7 days in patients with proven infections. However, the number of patients studied in these trials was small, the infections were heterogeneous, and the duration of granulocytopenia differed. In a later trial, no benefit was conferred by transfusion of granulocytes; patients treated with antibiotics alone survived just as well (Winston et al. 1982), but the number of granulocytes transfused (approximately 5×10^9 per transfusion) was totally inadequate (Schiffer 1990). Granulocyte transfusions have been reported to produce favourable results in patients with chronic granulomatous disease with pyogenic or fungal infections (Yomtovian et al. 1981). Several weeks of therapy may be required.

Although cytokine mobilization of donors has resulted in concentrates containing impressive numbers of granulocytes, evidence for clinical efficacy remains largely anecdotal. In patients with haematological malignancies, bacterial infections appear to respond well to a course of granulocyte therapy, even given the lack of controls and the difficulty in separating the effect of transfusion from that of antibiotics and systemic growth factor administration (Peters et al. 1999; Price et al. 2000). Although these infusions appear to be more effective against bacterial sepsis than against deep-seated fungal infections, case reports and uncontrolled small series are sufficiently promising that controlled studies with adequate numbers of compatible granulocytes should be carried out (Catalano et al. 1997; Dignani et al. 1997; Ozsahin et al. 1998).

Granulocyte transfusion should be considered only when the absolute neutrophil count falls below $0.5 \times 10^9/l$ and clinically significant infection persists despite 1–2 days of appropriate antibiotic therapy, or for patients with granulocyte dysfunction and progressive infection. Success for the former patients is unlikely unless haematopoiesis recovers (Higby and Burnett 1980; Klein et al. 1996).

Crossmatching of leucocytes

In the controlled studies, the best results were achieved when donors were selected to improve patient–donor leucocyte compatibility. Routine crossmatching for granulocytes is unnecessary. Although the presence of leucocyte antibodies does not invariably cause clinical problems (Adkins *et al.* 2000; Price *et al.* 2000), administration of granulocytes from random donors to alloimmunized patients is inadvisable. The effect of the transfusion will usually be negligible and the danger of severe transfusion reactions is substantial (see Chapter 15). In such cases, HLA-matched cells or granulocytes crossmatched against the recipient's serum should be used (Goldstein *et al.* 1971; Stroncek 1996; K Heim, personal communication). When lymphocytotoxicity alone was used as a 'compatibility test' in a study of 23 recipients of autologous haematopoietic transplants, the mean peak neutrophil increments of the last two out of four prophylactic transfusions were lower in the cohort with the positive assay, despite the transfusion of similar component cell doses. Although both cohorts received grafts with similar CD34(+) cell doses, the cohort with a positive assay had delayed neutrophil engraftment, a greater number of febrile days and more days of intravenous antibiotics and platelet transfusions (Adkins *et al.* 2000). A combination of the granulocyte immuno-fluorescence test, the most sensitive technique for the detection of granulocyte-specific antibodies (Verheugt *et al.* 1977), and the lymphocytotoxicity test, the assay of choice for detection of HLA antibodies, should be considered.

Granulocyte concentrates contain 30 ml or more red cells, so that red cell compatibility testing is advisable. When concentrates with incompatible red cells cannot be avoided, processing by sedimentation can reduce red cell contamination to about 2.5 ml with retention of 70% of the granulocytes. Such preparations have proved safe, although experience is limited. No clinical or laboratory signs of haemolysis occurred in a sensitized child (anti-c, -E, -Jka) during a course of 46 granulocyte transfusions, 37 of which were derived from c-, E- or Jka-positive donors (Depalma *et al.* 1989).

Newborn infants are more likely than adults to benefit from granulocyte transfusions because they have only a small reservoir of neutrophils (Christensen and Rothstein 1980) and have an impaired response to infection (Strauss 1986). In a large prospective, randomized study of infants who received granulocyte transfusions, 20 out of 21 survived, whereas of infants who received only supportive care, only 9 out of 14 survived (Cairo and Cairo 1987). In a further trial,

infected infants with neutrophil counts below $2.5 \times 10^9/l$ were randomized to receive either daily granulocyte transfusions for 3 days or IVIG, 1000 mg/kg per day for 3 days. All 10 who received granulocyte transfusions survived, but only two who received IVIG. Taking the two trials together, 30 out of 31 infants treated with granulocytes, but only 11 out of 21 who received other treatment survived ($P < 0.004$) (Cairo 1989).

Infants likely to benefit from granulocyte transfusions are those with bacterial sepsis, a neutrophil count below $3 \times 10^9/l$ and evidence of depletion of the neutrophil storage pool (< 10% of nucleated marrow cells being post-mitotic neutrophils) (Sacher *et al.* 1989). The daily dose should be $1–2 \times 10^9/kg$. To prevent CMV infection, anti-CMV-negative donors must be selected if the infant's mother is anti-CMV negative. Granulocyte concentrates given to newborn infants must be irradiated to prevent graft-versus-host disease (GvHD). No controlled studies of granulocyte therapy for infants have been reported since the introduction of G-CSF, and none using cells from donors mobilized with cytokines and steroids.

Prophylactic leucocyte transfusions in neutropenic patients

Twelve controlled trials of prophylactic granulocyte transfusion have been conducted before the introduction of cytokine mobilized cells; eight of these trials met the criteria for a formal meta-analysis (Vamvakas and Pineda 1997). The results of several of these trials suggest that leucocyte transfusions have temporary beneficial effects, but in none of them was survival improved. Interpretation is clouded by the small, variable numbers of leucocytes transfused, differing intervals of neutropenia and inconsistent compatibility testing. Prophylaxis of allogeneic bone marrow transplant patients with large numbers of G-CSF-mobilized HLA-matched granulocytes results in significant and sustained increments in the granulocyte and platelet count (Adkins *et al.* 1997). Benefit to clinical outcome has been less conclusive, although the four alternate-day transfusion regimen of the controlled trial may not be the ideal one (Adkins *et al.* 2000). However, in an era of meticulous surveillance and early administration of antiviral agents for CMV, it does appear that transplant recipients may receive at least two prophylactic granulocyte transfusions from CMV-seropositive mobilized donors (Vij *et al.* 2003).

Transfusion of haematopoietic cells

The object of transfusing allogeneic haematopoietic progenitor cells is to establish a permanent graft of transfused progenitor cells in the recipient. The fate of allogeneic progenitor cells infused into the venous circulation depends on their ability to traffic to sites of haematopoietic tolerance ('microenvironment') and on managing two immunological phenomena: (1) the rejection of donor progenitor cells by the host immunological response and (2) an immunological reaction of grafted immunologically competent cells against the host: GvHD. Both of these reactions depend on the degree of histocompatibility between donor and recipient and also on the immunological competence of the recipient. Engraftment and kinetics also depend on patient age, disease status, the preparative regimen, GvHD prophylaxis and the cellular content of the graft.

Bone marrow was the original source of progenitor cells for haematopoietic grafting, but mobilized peripheral blood and cord blood have gradually supplanted marrow as a source of PC. The engraftment potential of the component is commonly designated in terms of mononuclear cells that express the CD34 antigen, the cluster designation of a transmembrane glycoprotein present on haematopoietic progenitor cells (Krause et al. 1996), although accessory cells in the graft clearly play an important role (Ash et al. 1991). Cells that express CD34 include lineage-committed haematopoietic progenitors, multipotent progenitors and possibly pluripotent stem cells as well. Flow cytometric assays are used to quantify $CD34^+$ cells in both the donor and the component. However, problems with interlaboratory accuracy and reproducibility, especially of different PC sources, have been notorious, even with the adoption of a standardized technique (Sutherland et al. 1996; Keeney et al. 1998).

Peripheral blood-derived progenitor cells

Peripheral blood-derived progenitor cells (PBPCs) were reported to circulate in mammalian blood as early as 1909 (Maximow 1909), and the ability of circulating cells to repopulate a lethally irradiated animal was demonstrated in a parabiotic rat model in 1951 (Brecher and Cronkite 1951). However, circulating haematopoietic progenitor cells were not confirmed in human blood until the 1970s (McCredie et al. 1971). Collection of PBPCs obtained from peripheral blood

by leucapheresis (see Chapter 17) has now all but replaced infusion of bone marrow. PBPCs have the advantages of engrafting more rapidly and sparing the donor a general anaesthetic, which result in lower morbidity and cost (Kessinger et al. 1989; Azevedo et al. 1995; Bensinger et al. 1995; Korbling et al. 1995; Schmitz et al. 1995). Allogeneic PBPCs have a higher $CD34^+$ cell content than does marrow, which, independent of stem cell source, increases patient survival while reducing transplant-related mortality and relapse (Mavroudis et al. 1996; Bahceci et al. 2000; Zaucha et al. 2001). A theoretical argument against the use of PBPCs is the greater number of 'T' lymphocytes that contaminate these collections, compared with the number of T cells in bone marrow, suggesting the possibility of an increased risk of severe acute GvHD. Indeed, although the risk of acute GVHD after PBPCs is similar to that observed among historic bone marrow transplant (BMT) controls (Pavletic et al. 1997; Przepiorka et al. 1997), the probability and severity of chronic GVHD (cGVHD) appear to be increased (Bacigalupo et al. 1996; Flowers et al. 2002).

Liquid storage and cryopreservation

Collection of allogeneic PBPCs is ordinarily scheduled to coincide with the conclusion of the patient's preparatory regimen, so that the graft can be infused while fresh. Most centres opt to transfuse the cells as soon as possible. Refrigerated storage of unmanipulated mobilized collections at 2–6°C for 24 h and as long as 72 h results in little detectable loss of the in vitro functional properties (Beaujean et al. 1996; Moroff et al. 2004). PBPCs, like bone marrow, can be cryopreserved by slow cooling (1–3°C/min) in the presence of the cryprotectant dimethylsulphoxide (DMSO), variable amounts of plasma, with or without hydroxyethyl starch (Hubel 1997). Grafts can be stored at –80°C, but are usually placed in liquid nitrogen at –140°C or colder, at which engraftment potential is preserved for years.

Cryopreserved grafts are thawed in a waterbath at 37–40°C and infused through a 170-μ filter. Prolonged post-thaw storage is inadvisable, as prolonged exposure to 10% DMSO may harm the cells. Storage up to 1 h does not reduce viability or colony-forming activity (Rowley and Anderson 1993). Rapid infusion of DMSO has been associated with flushing, nausea, vomiting, diarrhoea and hypotension, probably the result of histamine release. Reversible encephalopathy has been reported when doses have approached 2 g/kg, so that caution is advisable when large volumes of PBSCs are thawed (Dhodapkar *et al.* 1994). The graft can be washed free of cryoprotectant, but progenitor cells may be lost in the process.

Cord blood progenitor cells

Umbilical cord blood is a rich source of progenitor cells (Knudtzon 1974; Broxmeyer *et al.* 1989a). The use of cord blood progenitor cells (CBPCs) has important real and potential advantages. The number of donors is unlimited, procurement is easy and inexpensive and the cells can be HLA typed and preserved in liquid nitrogen. Human CBPCs with high proliferative capacity and NOD/SCID mouse engrafting ability can be stored frozen for > 15 years, and probably remain effective for clinical transplantation (Broxmeyer *et al.* 2003). In addition, because many of the functions of the immunologically competent cells in cord blood are not fully developed, the chance of their inducing GvHD appears to be diminished (Szabolcs *et al.* 2003). Even after the transplantation of CBPCs from unrelated donors, mismatched for two, or as many as three, HLA antigens, the risk of severe GvHD seems to be low (Wagner 1995).

Umbilical cord blood banking

Umbilical cord blood is collected by either the obstetrician or the midwife *in utero* during the third stage of delivery or *ex utero* after delivery of the placenta by trained nurses or technologists (Wall *et al.* 1997; Fraser *et al.* 1998). Collection volume and cell yield appear to be similar with both methods (Lasky *et al.* 2002). A maternal blood specimen is screened for markers of transmissible disease, and a sample from the unit is cultured, HLA typed, analysed for cell count, viability and in many instances CD34+ cell number and colony count by culture. Suitable units are processed to remove red cells and plasma and are frozen at a controlled rate and stored in liquid nitrogen (Armitage *et al.* 1999).

Related donor transplants

The first successful transplantation of CBPCs from an HLA-identical sibling was given to a patient with Fanconi's anaemia (Broxmeyer *et al.* 1989a). In 44 paediatric transplantations of CBPCs from sibling donors, patients receiving HLA-identical or 1-antigen mismatched grafts showed an actuarial probability of engraftment of 85% at 50 days after transplantation; there were no instances of late graft failure (Wagner *et al.* 1995). The median total nucleated cells per kilogram (TNC/kg) was 5.2×10^7. The probability of GvHD at 100 days post transplant was 3% and of chronic GvHD at 1 year was 6%. The probability of survival with a median follow-up of 1.6 years was 72%. Among 102 children with acute leukaemia transplanted by the Eurocord collaborative investigators, 42 received a graft from a related cord blood donor; 12 of these were HLA mismatched (Locatelli *et al.* 1999). Nucleated cell dose (> 3.7×10^7/kg) correlated with engraftment; two-year survival was 41%. Rocha and co-workers (2000) compared 113 recipients of HLA-identical sibling CBPC transplants for malignant disease with records of 2052 siblings transplanted with bone marrow between 1990 and 1997. Although the umbilical cord blood (UCB) had a significantly longer delay in recovery of neutrophil and platelet reconstitution, no significant difference in survival and a significantly lower risk of GvHD and chronic GvHD was reported in the CBPC group. Bone marrow recipients received nearly 10-fold the total nucleated cells per kilogram body weight (TNC/kg). Of 44 children with non-malignant conditions (thalassaemia, sickle cell disease), two-year survivals were 79% and 90% respectively (Locatelli *et al.* 2003). One child with sickle cell disease and seven with thalassaemia failed to sustain engraftment. Four children suffered acute grade II GvHD.

Unrelated donor transplants

Several thousand CBPC transplants have been performed and more than 100 000 umbilical cord components are available worldwide. With the growth of public ('unrelated') CBPC banks, the number of CBPC transplants from unrelated donors now exceeds that from related donors. In one early series, a high rate of engraftment (23 out of 25 cases) was observed in children infused with allogeneic CBPC despite the donor–recipient pair discordance of 1–3 HLA antigens (Kurtzberg *et al.* 1996). A retrospective analysis of 562 unrelated CBPC transplants found that engraftment exceeded 80% and survival rate was 61%; pre-freeze cell count of the graft ranged from 0.7 to 10 TNC/kg (Rubinstein *et al.* 1998). The number of nucleated cord blood cells that were transfused per kilogram of the recipient's weight emerged as the main influence on engraftment. A retrospective analysis of 537 paediatric CBPC transplants from the Eurocord Registry, including 138 related transplants and 291 unrelated donors, reported similar results (Gluckman and Locatelli 2000). Laughlin and co-workers (2001) reported CBPC transplants in 68 adult recipients who received a median of 2.1×10^7 TNC/kg. TNC number per kilogram correlated with rapidity of engraftment and high CD34+ number was associated with event-free survival. Overall survival (22 months) was 28%. As expected from the experience with bone marrow transplantation, GvHD is significantly higher in the setting of grafts from unrelated donors and depends as well upon the age of the recipient, the degree of histocompatibility between donor and recipient, the nature of the preparatory regimen and a variety of other factors. In this series, grades III and IV GvHD occurred in 20% and chronic GvHD in 36%.

Reconstitution of adult recipients of cord blood

CBPCs have so far been used primarily for children and doubt has been expressed as to whether the number of progenitor cells in cord blood from a single donor will be sufficient to repopulate the majority of large adults who require a transplant. Most analyses indicate that the key clinical outcomes (days to neutrophil engraftment, platelet engraftment, severe GvHD and disease-free survival) are all superior in younger patients; age-related outcomes are widely attributed to the number of nucleated cells in a single unit of cord blood (Laughlin *et al.* 2001). There is, as yet, no quantitative assay for the progenitor cell subset that has the capacity for long-term bone marrow repopulation. On the other hand, the number of progenitor cells that can be assayed (CFU-GM, CFU-GEMM, etc.) is large enough, suggesting that the number of the more primitive progenitor cells may be sufficient (Broxmeyer 1995). There is evidence that the total cellular content of placental cord blood (PCB) grafts is related to the speed of engraftment, though the total nucleated cell (TNC) dose is not a precise predictor of the time of neutrophil or platelet engraftment. It is important to understand the reasons for the quantitative association and to improve the criteria for

selecting PCB grafts by using indices that are more precisely predictive of engraftment (Rubinstein *et al.* 1998). The post-transplant course of 204 patients who received grafts evaluated for haematopoietic colony-forming cell (CFC) content among 562 patients reported previously were analysed using univariate and multivariate life-table techniques to determine whether CFC doses predicted haematopoietic engraftment speed and risk for transplant-related events more accurately than the TNC dose. Actuarial times to neutrophil and platelet engraftment were shown to correlate with the cell dose, whether estimated as TNC or CFC per kilogram of recipient's weight. CFC association with the day of recovery of 500 neutrophils/µl was stronger than that of the TNC. In multivariate tests of speed of platelet and neutrophil engraftment and of probability of post-transplantation events, the inclusion of CFCs in the model displaced the significance of the high relative risks associated with TNC. The CFC content of PCB units is associated more rigorously with the major covariates of post-transplantation survival than is the TNC and is, therefore, a better index of the haematopoietic content of PCB grafts (Migliaccio *et al.* 2000). A positive correlation between CD34+ cells and circulating day-14 colony counts (CFU-GM) has been reported suggesting that with umbilical cord progenitor cells (UCPCs), as with PBPC, CD34 is a reliable measure of haematopoietic potential (Payne *et al.* 1995; Siena *et al.* 2000). Data from 102 patients identified CD34+ cell dose as the only factor that correlated with rate of engraftment (Wagner *et al.* 2002). Studies from Spain and Japan of small numbers of adults with haematological malignancies report promising rates of engraftment and disease-free survival (Sanz *et al.* 2001; Ooi *et al.* 2004).

Progenitor cell expansion

If the number of progenitor cells in cord blood proves to be scarcely sufficient for repopulation in many adults, the possibility of expanding the number by culture *in vitro* has been proposed (Apperley 1994; Broxmeyer *et al.* 1995) and several groups are developing methods to do so (Kogler *et al.* 1999; Pecora *et al.* 2000; Jaroscak *et al.* 2003). Whether the most important primitive progenitor cells are expanded by culture cannot be established *in vitro*. As yet, no evidence has confirmed that increase in engraftment kinetics or expansion of stem cells has been achieved, and the possibility of increased frequency of GvHD with some expansion methods has been raised (Shpall *et al.* 2002; Jaroscak *et al.* 2003).

Plasma from cord blood has been found to increase the self-renewal capacity of stem cells *in vitro* (Carow *et al.* 1993). Cord blood plasma, but not plasma from adults or fetal calf serum, had this effect and cord blood plasma also increased the expansion *in vitro* of the number of progenitor cells induced by growth factors (Bertolini *et al.* 1994). Furthermore, CBPCs fully retain this expansion potential after cryopreservation (Bertolini *et al.* 1994).

Use of multiple cord blood collections

Because limited cell dose compromises may comprom-ise the outcome of adult UCB transplants, multiple cord blood units have been combined to augment the dose. Zanjani and co-workers (2000) have trans-planted human UCB from multiple donors in a fetal sheep model. Short-term donor engraftment derived from both donors, but for long-term haematopoiesis, a single donor predominated.

Multidonor human UCB transplants using up to 12 units have been published (Ende and Ende 1972; Shen *et al.* 1994). Weinreb and co-workers (1998) reported that a unit that was partially HLA matched predominated in a recipient who received a combina-tion of 12 units. Another patient with advanced acute lymphocytic leukaemia received a mismatched, unre-lated UCB transplant using units from two donors and achieved a complete remission with double chimerism, which persisted until relapse (De Lima *et al.* 2002).

Barker and co-workers (2005) have augmented graft cell dose by combining two partially HLA-matched units. Twenty-three patients with high-risk haemato-logical malignancy received 2 UCB units (median infused dose, 3.5×10^7 NC/kg) and 21 evaluable patients engrafted at a median of 23 days. At day 21, engraftment was derived from both donors in 24% of patients and a single donor in 76% of patients. One unit predominated in all patients by day 100. Although neither nucleated or CD34$^+$ cell doses nor HLA match predicted which unit would predominate, the predominating unit had a significantly higher CD34$^+$ dose. The result is similar to the predominant lymphocyte chimerism that persists in trauma patients who receive multiple blood transfusions (Lee *et al.* 1999).

Law, ethics, related banks and genetic selection

Controversy continues regarding the propriety of related ('private') CBPCs for which the family pays to have the infant's cells cryopreserved for future use, as contrasted with unrelated ('public') banks, in which donated cords are stored for general use (Burgio *et al.* 2003). Both systems have their adherents and they should not be mutually exclusive. Although most related banks with commercial origins have sought participation from expectant mothers who agree to pay for storage of a cord from their newborn infant, others have been supported by federal grants (Reed *et al.* 2001). The infrequent utilization of a related cord blood unit does minimize its utility. The probabil-ity that the cord blood will be of use in a family with no history of blood or genetic disease is low (estimated at 1/200 000); moreover, one's own stem cells may be immunologically less potent than those of an unrelated donor for treating neoplastic diseases. However, several such transplants have been performed success-fully and prohibiting such storage despite appropriate informed consent seems curiously patronizing. The legal issues regarding property rights have been dis-cussed (Munzer 1999). *In vitro* fertilization and pre-natal genetic diagnosis to select an embryo donor on the basis of specific, desirable disease and HLA charac-teristics have been used successfully to treat a child with Fanconi's anaemia (Grewal *et al.* 2004).

Effect of ABO incompatibility of grafted cells

As ABO and HLA antigens are inherited independ-ently, ABO incompatibility may occur in 20–40% of HLA-matched allogeneic haematopoietic stem cell transplants. ABO incompatibility between donor pro-genitor cells and the recipient's plasma is not a barrier to successful transplantation (Storb *et al.* 1977; Buckner *et al.* 1978). In a series of 12 subjects who received major ABO-incompatible marrow, not one rejected the graft and the incidence of GvHD was no higher than in subjects who received ABO-compatible marrow (Hershko *et al.* 1980).

With major ABO-incompatible marrow grafts, defined as incompatibility of donor ABO antigens with the recipient's immune system, steps must be taken to prevent an acute haemolytic reaction due to lysis of incompatible red cells contained in the progenitor cell graft. To avoid haemolysis, grafts are purged of red cells. A satisfactory method has been described (Warkentin *et al.* 1985). An alternative method of removing red cells from marrow uses a cell separator (Blacklock *et al.* 1982). When PBPC or CBPC are used, the number of contaminating red cells is small.

Delayed donor red cell engraftment and pure red cell aplasia are well-recognized complications of major ABO-incompatible haematopoietic stem cell transplantation (Hows *et al.* 1983; Sniecinski *et al.* 1988; Stussi *et al.* 2002; Griffith *et al.* 2005). Donor red blood cell chimerism is delayed as long as three-fold (median 114 days) following reduced-intensity non-myeloablative compared with myeloablative conditioning for transplant and the delay correlates with the recipient anti-donor isohaemagglutinin titre (Bolan *et al.* 2001a). Late-onset red cell aplasia, most likely related to delayed lymphoid engraftment, may occur (Au *et al.* 2004). In some patients, thrombopoiesis may be delayed as well (Sniecinski *et al.* 1988).

After transplants of major ABO-incompatible grafts, the direct antiglobulin test (DAT) may turn positive after about 3 weeks. If substantial numbers of donor red cells enter the circulation, transient immune-mediated haemolysis may result (Sniecinski *et al.* 1987). Anti-A and anti-B may remain demonstrable in the recipient's plasma for some months and the DAT may remain positive during this time. In patients with minor ABO-incompatible transplants, defined as those in which the recipient antigens are incompatible with the donor's immune system, haemolysis may develop 1–2 weeks after transplantation owing to lysis of ABO-incompatible recipient cells as the donor immune lymphocytes engraft (Hows *et al.* 1986). This type of haemolysis has been seen only in patients receiving ciclosporin and prednisone GvHD prophylaxis, and may not develop in patients receiving methotrexate (Gajewski *et al.* 1992). Massive immune haemolysis may occur, and fatalities can be avoided by early, vigorous donor-compatible red cell transfusion until haemolysis subsides (Bolan *et al.* 2001a). Reactions are most common and severe when the donor is group O and the recipient group A, but neither blood group nor agglutinin titre reliably predict clinical severity. In some of the patients, haemolysis caused by anti-A or anti-B (or both) destroys transfused group O cells, probably as a result of activated complement components affixing the group O cells (*bystander haemolysis*). Haemolysis has also been observed when the donor lymphocytes produce anti-D, etc. (see Chapter 11).

Special consideration of the ABO group of components transfused to patients receiving ABO-incompatible grafts should begin with the initiation of the preparatory regimen to ensure that blood is compatible with both donor and recipient (Table 14.1). With bi-directional (major–minor) incompatibility, red cell transfusions should be limited to group O. Platelet concentrates administered to adults may be of any blood group, although plasma reduction may be prudent, especially for large-volume group O platelets. Plasma-compatible platelets should be used for infants and children. Some centres use the soluble antigens contained in plasma to neutralize isohaemagglutinins. As intravenous immunoglobulin contains variable titres of red cell antibodies, especially of anti-A, some centres screen for alloantibodies, whereas others avoid high-dose IVIG for group A recipients during the post-transplant period.

Donor lymphocyte infusion

Lymphocytes have been studied more often as blood component contaminants responsible for adverse effects than as therapeutic cells. However, some ostensibly adverse effects of mononuclear cell infusions can be exploited for therapeutic benefit. The mechanisms involved in TA-GvHD (see Chapters 13 and 15) are probably responsible for the graft-versus-malignancy effect in allogeneic stem cell transplantation. Studies in animal models are consistent with the observation by Barnes and Loutit (1957) that transplanted bone marrow has immune activity against residual leukaemia (Kloosterman *et al.* 1995). Clinical experience with haematopoietic transplantation has been consistent with the presence of antileukaemic activity also in humans, now commonly referred to as the graft-versus-leukaemia effect (GvL). The term 'adoptive immunotherapy' was coined by Mathé (1965) who used both marrow transplants and leucocyte infusions to treat acute leukaemia. Kolb and co-workers (1990) provided direct clinical evidence for GvL: the transfusion of donor lymphocytes in conjunction with the administration of alpha-interferon (IFN-α) induced cytogenetic remission in three patients with CML in relapse following allogeneic bone marrow transplantation. Numerous independent studies confirm the GvL effect in CML (Slavin *et al.* 1992; Bar *et al.* 1993; Porter *et al.* 1994). In both European and North American registries, more than 90% of the patients received original

Table 14.1 ABO and/or Rh-incompatible progenitor cell: transplant transfusion restrictions.

| Blood group | | Blood products | | |
Recipient	Donor	Red cells*	Platelets[†]	FFP*
A	B	O	Any	AB[‡]
A	O	O	Any	A[§]
A	AB	O,A	Any	AB[‡]
B	A	O	Any	AB[‡]
B	O	O	Any	B[§]
B	AB	O,B	Any	AB[‡]
O	A	O	Any	A[‡]
O	B	O	Any	B[‡]
O	AB	O	Any	AB[‡]
AB	A	O,A	Any	AB[§]
AB	B	O,B	Any	AB[§]
AB	O	O	Any	AB[§]
Rh pos	Rh neg	Rh neg[††]	Rh neg**	N/A
Rh neg	Rh pos	Rh pos[¶]	Rh pos	N/A

* Restrictions for ABO- and/or Rh-incompatible transplant recipients supported with blood components during pre-transplant conditioning and during the post-transplant period.

† Use *any* ABO group for platelet support for adults. Use plasma-compatible components for children.

‡ Plasma may be transfused to neutralize isohaemagglutinin(s).

§ Graft plasma depleted, no plasma neutralization required.

¶ Rh-positive components initiated on the day of transplant.

** Rh-negative platelets preferred.

†† Rh-negative red cells preferred during the pre-transplant conditioning regimen and post transplant.

grafts and subsequent donor lymphocyte infusion (DLI) from related donors, typically from an HLA-identical sibling. The results reported by the European Group for Blood and Marrow Transplantation (27 centres, 135 patients, 75 evaluable with CML) are similar to those reported by the North American Multicenter Bone Marrow Transplantation Registry (25 centres, 140 patients, 55 evaluable with CML): DLI-induced clinical remission at a rate approaching 80%, and molecular remission (inability to detect bcr-abl mRNA transcript using polymerase chain reaction) in nearly all patients entering clinical remission (Kolb et al. 1995; Collins et al. 1997).

Infusion of small numbers of lymphocytes (10^7) ('bulk dose') usually suffices, and excess cells collected by leucapheresis are often aliquoted and stored for repeated treatment if needed. The host's circulation, which often contains a mixture of both donor and host cells during chronic phase relapse, typically converts to cells of only donor origin. The time to remission ranges from 1 to 9 months, with a mean of about 3 months (Kolb et al. 1995; Collins et al. 1997). Nearly all responses are seen within 8 months after DLI, and the probability of remaining in remission at 2 and 3 years is 90% and 87% respectively (Kolb et al. 1995; Collins et al. 1997). Although late relapses occur and toxicity may be significant, DLI efficacy is durable in surviving patients with CML: 26 out of 39 (67%) patients were alive at follow-up with 25 (96% of survivors) remaining in complete remission (Porter et al. 1999).

Separating graft-versus-leukaemia from graft-versus-host-disease

GvHD occurring after DLI correlates strongly with antileukaemic response. However, the GvL effect and GvHD may be separable, and GvHD may not be required for durable disease remission (Weiss et al. 1994; Rocha et al. 1997; Slavin et al. 2002). Murine studies suggest that the rate of GvHD is inversely

633

proportional to the interval between transplant and DLI (Johnson *et al.* 1999). These considerations have popularized escalating dose DLI regimens (Dazzi *et al.* 2000). Although probability of achieving remission in relapsed CML does not differ, the escalating dose regimen is associated with a lower incidence of GvHD. DLI is typically initiated early in disease as soon as disease recurrence is anticipated, and a starting dose of 10^5 T cells/kg is escalated 10-fold at 2- to 4-week intervals (Weiss *et al.* 1994). Efforts to modify the composition of donor-derived lymphocytes (DDLs) have focused on selective CD8-positive T-cell depletion, which appears to be more effective than non-selective T-cell depletion in reducing GvHD while preserving GvL (Soiffer *et al.* 2002).

Target antigen as the primary determinant of efficacy and toxicity

Falkenburg and colleagues (1999) reported the first successful treatment of relapsed accelerated CML using *in vitro*-expanded leukaemia-specific lymphocytes. Presumably, cell selection and culture restored the anti-tumour activity and specificity against leukaemic cells that weakened with disease progression (Smit *et al.* 1998). Successful salvage therapy of a child with previously DLI-resistant CML by using DDL pulsed *in vitro* with a mixture of normal irradiated lymphocytes obtained from the child's parents has been reported.

Efficacy and toxicity in viral diseases

Walter and co-workers (1995) have used *in vitro*-stimulated, culture-expanded, CMV-specific donor-derived cytotoxic T cells to successfully reconstitute cellular immunity against CMV in 11 out of 14 allogeneic marrow transplant patients. The DLI therapy consisted of four escalating cell doses (0.33, 1.0, 3.3 and 10.0×10^8 cells) administered at weekly intervals beginning at days 30–40 after transplantation. DLI-associated toxicity, CMV disease and CMV viraemia were not observed. The results have been confirmed in similar studies (Einsele *et al.* 2002; Roback *et al.* 2003).

Epstein–Barr virus-related lymphoproliferative disorders

The incidence of Epstein–Barr virus-related lymphoproliferative disorders (EBV-LPDs) occurring in T cell-depleted transplants has been estimated at 6–12%, and secondary lymphomas occurring in this clinical setting respond readily to DLI at a dose approximately 10-fold smaller than that typically used for activity against the primary leukaemia. Sustained clinical remissions have been achieved with only mild GvHD, and patients have often required no additional maintenance therapy (Papadopoulos *et al.* 1994; Wagner *et al.* 2004). EBV-specific lymphocyte infusions have successfully treated EBV-LPD and EBV-positive Hodgkin disease (Rooney *et al.* 1998; Bollard *et al.* 2004).

The transfusion of plasma components

Fresh-frozen plasma

Fresh-frozen plasma (FFP) is plasma obtained from a single donor by normal donation or plasmapheresis and frozen within 6 h of collection to a temperature of −30°C or below. FFP contains all circulating coagulation factors in the concentration present in fresh plasma, and haemostatic activity is maintained for a year or longer, depending upon the storage temperature. Once thawed, FFP must be stored at $4 \pm 2°C$ for no longer than 24 h before infusion. FFP must not be refrozen, but once thawed (or after 1 year of storage and thaw), it can be used as single-donor plasma, i.e. not to replace labile coagulation factors, for as long as 5 weeks. The concentration of coagulation factor, the citrate concentration and the volume of each unit may vary depending on the characteristics of the donor and of the collection. In 51 units collected by apheresis from plasma donors, factor concentrations at the fifth and ninety-fifth percentile measured: V (690–1270 units/l); VII (830–1690 units/l); fibrinogen 1800–3700 µg/l; antithrombin (920–1290 units/l) (Beeck *et al.* 1999).

Risks of fresh-frozen plasma

Allergic reactions may occur after transfusion of FFP, of which the most serious is severe anaphylaxis, which may develop in IgA-deficient patients with class-specific anti-IgA (Chapter 15). Such reactions are rare. Transfusion-related acute lung injury (TRALI) may occur when the FFP contains strong leucocyte antibodies (see Chapter 15). The other main risk of treatment with FFP is the transmission of infectious agents, particularly viruses such as hepatitis B and C viruses, HIV, parvovirus and West Nile virus. Owing to donor selection and the availability of methods of inactivating viruses that are used to treat whole plasma in some countries, the risk of transmitting viruses has greatly decreased. However, the problem of inactivating non-lipid-enveloped viruses and the transmission of non-viral agents remains (Chapter 16). Therefore, FFP should still be used only when no safer alternative exists (Shimizu and Robinson 1996).

Precautions to be taken before infusion

FFP containing potent anti-A or anti-B agglutinins or haemolysins, or FFP that has not been tested for their presence, should not be given to recipients with corresponding red cell antigens. Fresh plasma, which is now rarely used, may contain red cells, so that appropriate measures should be taken to prevent immunization of D-negative women of childbearing age. There is no credible evidence that FFP presents such a risk.

Indications for fresh-frozen plasma: overused and abused

There is no justification for the use of FFP as a volume expander because safer alternatives (colloids and crystalloids) are available.

Factor V deficiency. No concentrate of factor V is available and FFP can be used as a source of factor V. Cryoprecipitate-poor plasma contains 80% of the amount of factor V in FFP and can be used as an alternative for FFP (Hellings 1981).

Severe liver disease. The liver is the major site of synthesis of coagulation factors II, V, VII, IX, X, XI, XII and fibrinogen as well as of factors with potential antithrombotic activity such as proteins C, S and antithrombin. Patients with severe liver disease may experience defects in factor synthesis and increased factor degradation that can result in generalized bleeding. Unfortunately, studies regarding the predictability of bleeding and its most effective management by transfusion in the presence of different degrees of hepatic impairment are old, poorly documented or both. Most recommendations rely upon expert opinion. What seems clear is that no single coagulation assay predicts bleeding (Spector and Corn 1967). Prolongations of the prothrombin time (PT) and activated partial thromboplastin time (aPTT) are the most fre-

quent abnormalities among the commonly performed clotting tests in patients with liver disease, and may reflect impaired protein synthesis, vitamin K deficiency or even disseminated intravascular coagulation (DIC). The presence of an abnormal test does not necessitate intervention, especially in the non-bleeding patient. Furthermore, in 30 patients with chronic liver disease, a moderate-dose plasma infusion (12 ml/kg or about 4 units) did not return the PT and aPTT to normal (Mannucci *et al.* 1982). In the bleeding patient, doses calculated to bring coagulation factor levels to the 20–30% range (20 ml/kg or 6–7 units) may be required as frequently as every 4–6 h to correct the abnormal coagulation tests (Spector *et al.* 1966). The routine use of FFP as prophylaxis for excessive surgical bleeding in patients with severe liver disease finds few supporters and less evidence of benefit (Oberman 1990).

Treatment of acquired deficiencies of factors II, VII, IX and X due to treatment with anticoagulants: warfarin reversal

The major risk of anticoagulant therapy is haemorrhage. For patients treated with the oral vitamin K antagonists, the annual risk of severe haemorrhage ranges from 1–5% (Levine *et al.* 2001). The intensity of anticoagulation (including poor control), its duration and, in some studies, advanced age and cerebrovascular disease all increase the bleeding risk (Landefeld and Goldman 1989). For the bleeding patient or the patient at extreme risk, urgent reversal of vitamin K antagonists can be achieved with plasma infusion to bring factor levels to 30–40%. The volume of plasma can be calculated easily based on the patient's body weight but as 6 units or more (1500 ml) may be required to reverse anticoagulation in an adult, volume considerations may make a prothrombin complex concentrate (PCC) the preferred infusion (Schulman 2003). Recombinant VIIa has also been used in this situation (Deveras and Kessler 2002) (see Chapter 18). Intravenous vitamin K_1, the specific warfarin antagonist, may require 12 h or more to be fully effective (Nee *et al.* 1999).

Disseminated intravascular coagulation: a vehicle on the road to multi-organ dysfunction syndrome

Disseminated intravascular coagulation is a condition in which the intravascular activation of the clotting cascade leads to the final common pathway of sustained and excessive thrombin generation. Liberated thrombin and proteolytic enzymes bring about the intravascular production of fibrin and deposition of platelets, with activation of the fibrinolytic system and an increased level of fibrin degradation products (FDPs) (Levi *et al.* 2001). In mild DIC the platelet count and the levels of clotting factors may be normal due to compensatory increases in production. As DIC becomes more severe, the levels of clotting factors and platelets fall, and a state that may be described as decompensated DIC may lead to multi-organ dysfunction syndrome (MODS).

DIC may be precipitated by a wide variety of stimuli, most related to the entry of tissue thromboplastins into the circulation, for example after abruptio placentae, crush injury, head trauma and snake envenomation. Other conditions associated with DIC include infections, malignancies, amniotic fluid embolism, giant haemangioma and intravascular lysis of incompatible red cells (Levi *et al.* 2004).

The cardinal principle of treatment of DIC remains elimination of the underlying cause as, once this has been accomplished, haemostasis usually returns to normal. When the underlying cause cannot be treated effectively, uncontrollable bleeding may result. The transfusion of blood may be essential and the replacement of clotting factors has to be considered. This replacement should be guided by coagulation assays and fibrinogen levels. If levels of clotting factors are severely reduced (< 25%), FFP may be given and if the fibrinogen concentration falls below 60 mg/dl, cryoprecipitate may be helpful. An initial dose of 10 bags, to provide 4–6 g of fibrinogen, has been suggested (Prentice 1985). Despite the theoretical objection of adding 'fuel to the fire', the administration of fibrinogen does not seem to be particularly dangerous.

Thrombotic thrombocytopenia purpura

Before the mechanisms involved in thrombotic thrombocytopenia purpura (TTP) were suspected, a plasma factor was postulated to correct the syndrome characterized by microangiopathic haemolysis and thrombocytopenia (Upshaw 1978). Relapses in chronic TTP were reversed or prevented by infusions of small volumes of FFP or cryoprecipitate-depleted FFP or by plasma infusion combined with plasmapheresis (Byrnes and Khurana 1977; Bukowski *et al.* 1981). The plasma

factor is not destroyed by the solvent detergent treatment of FFP used to inactivate lipid-encapsulated viruses (Moake *et al.* 1994). In the majority of cases, the plasma factor relates to the activity of a metallo-proteinase that cleaves unusually large multimers of vWF that are associated with the TTP thrombi (Asada *et al.* 1985; Tsai 1996) (see Chapter 17).

Cryoprecipitate-depleted fresh-frozen plasma (cryosupernatant)

Cryosupernatant is plasma from which about one-half of the fibrinogen, factor VIII and fibronectin has been removed as cryoprecipitate. The product is also depleted of the largest multimers of vWF, which sediment in the cryoprecipitate fraction and which may be partly responsible for platelet aggregation in TTP (Moake 2004). In some circumstances cryosupernatant may be more effective than FFP in the treatment of TTP. Seven patients with TTP who failed to respond to intensive plasma exchange with whole plasma responded to plasma exchange with cryosupernatant (Byrnes *et al.* 1990).

Cryoprecipitate

When plasma is fast frozen and then thawed slowly at 4–6°C, the small amount of protein precipitated is rich in fibrinogen, factor VIII, vWF and factor XIII. After decanting almost all of the supernatant plasma, the precipitated protein can be dissolved by warming to yield a small volume of solution. The introduction of cryoprecipitate revolutionized the treatment of haemophilia by providing a highly effective, convenient, readily available source of factor VIII. Modern treatment has moved away from cryoprecipitate to pathogen-inactivated factor VIII concentrate and to recombinant factor VIII. Cryoprecipitate is used now as a source of factor VIII and vWF only if safer concentrates are not available.

Cryoprecipitate, containing approximately 200–250 mg of fibrinogen in a volume of 10–15 ml, prepared from a single donor, is used primarily as a source of fibrinogen. The most common indication remains as a replacement for fibrinogen consumed in DIC, although it has been used as a topical haemostatic agent as well (fibrin glue) (Reiss and Oz 1996). Commercial fibrin sealants are safer, better standardized and more effective, and avoid the potential risk of immunization to contaminant factor V that has been reported when bovine thrombin is used to activate topical cryoprecipitate (Rousou *et al.* 1989; Rapaport *et al.* 1992; Atrah 1994) (see also Chapter 18). Thawing by microwave is rapid and preserves fibrinogen concentration (Bass *et al.* 1985).

Cryoprecipitate also contains about 60% of the vWF and 20–30% of the factor XIII of the original unit of FFP, but the component in not often used as a source of these proteins.

'Contaminants' in cryoprecipitate. Cryoprecipitates contain about 30–50% of the original fibrinogen and have about the same titre of anti-A and anti-B as that of the original plasma unit (Rizza and Biggs 1969; Pool 1970). Because of the risk of haemolysis, neonates should receive only ABO-compatible cryoprecipitate.

Plasma fractionation

The transfusion of whole plasma is unnecessary and usually inefficient if recipients require only a single protein, for example factor VIII. Plasma contains hundreds of different proteins, many of which are obvious candidates for replacement therapy, whereas others are well characterized physicochemically, but of unknown function. Commercial plasma fractionation uses dilution, pasteurization and nanofiltration to remove and inactivate most viruses, although no product can be guaranteed 'pathogen free'. The immunoglobulin (Ig) fraction (predominantly IgG) separated from whole plasma by alcohol fractionation was at first considered virtually free of the risk of transmitting viral hepatitis. However, HCV has been transmitted by both IVIG and anti-D Ig (Bjoro *et al.* 1994; Meisel *et al.* 1995; Power *et al.* 1995).

The most widely used method of fractionating plasma is still the cold alcohol precipitation technique described by Cohn and colleagues (1944) or modifications thereof (Kistler and Nitschmann 1962). Cohn fractionation relies on changes in ethanol concentration and pH for bulk precipitation of different protein fractions. An example of a fractionation scheme is shown in Fig. 14.6. Ethanol is removed by lyophilization or by ultrafiltration. Alcohol fractionation is now combined with glycine precipitation or polyethylene glycol, and with other separation methods such as chromatography to isolate specific proteins, such as coagulation factors and protease inhibitors.

Albumin

Albumin is available for clinical use either as human albumin in saline containing 4%, 4.5%, 5%, 20% or 25% protein, of which not less than 95% is albumin, or as plasma protein fraction (PPF), available only as a 5% solution, of which at least 83% is albumin. Compared with albumin, most preparations of PPF contain larger amounts of contaminating proteins. Hypotensive reactions attributed to pre-kallikrein activator and acetate have been observed with PPF, but not with albumin (Alving *et al.* 1978; Ng *et al.* 1981). For these reasons, most clinicians find little reason to select PPF when an albumin solution is indicated.

Albumin preparations are pasteurized by heat treatment at 60°C for 10 h and filtered. When prepared in this way, the fraction has proved free of transfusion-transmitted agents such as hepatitis viruses and HIV.

Although albumin contributes 75–80% of the colloid osmotic pressure of the plasma, subjects with a genetically determined total absence of plasma albumin, in whom the colloid osmotic pressure of plasma is between one-third and one-half of normal, may be completely asymptomatic (Bearn 1978). Such subjects show an increase in various plasma globulins and a slight decrease in blood pressure, changes that are regarded as compensatory. The indications for infusions of albumin in hypovolaemic patients are discussed in Chapter 2.

Recombinant albumin

Recombinant albumin has been synthesized in yeast, in *Saccharomyces cerevisiae* or *Pichia pastoris*, and appears to be similar to the plasma-derived protein (Dodsworth *et al.* 1996). A 20% solution (Recombumin 20%, Aventis Behring) prepared as a pharmaceutical excipient has been tested for safety in doses up to 65 mg in some 500 subjects. It is uncertain when, if ever, recombinant albumin might be commercially available as a product for transfusion.

Fibrinogen

The rate of disappearance of injected fibrinogen has been studied by giving infusions to patients with the very rare condition, hereditary afibrinogenaemia: in

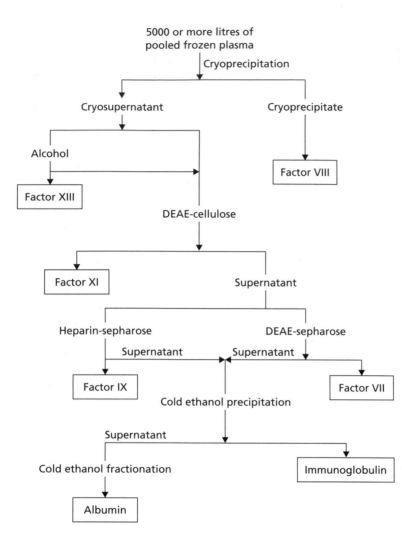

Fig 14.6 The various blood products (in squares) obtained by stepwise fractionation of large pools of fresh-frozen plasma using different cryoprecipitation, ethanol precipitation and adsorption procedures.

two cases, one-half of the injected fibrinogen disappeared during the first 24 h, presumably due to mixing with the protein 'pool'; thereafter the fibrinogen disappeared with a $T_{1/2}$ of 4 days (Gitlin and Borges 1953).

In clinical practice, hypofibrinogenaemia is most often encountered as one feature of the syndrome of DIC; in this condition the transfusion of fibrinogen is seldom indicated. Purified fibrinogen prepared by fractionation of pooled plasma, unless virally inactivated, carries a high risk of the transmission of viral diseases such as hepatitis and no commercial fractionation concentrate is licensed.

Factor VIII (anti-haemophilic factor)

Factor VIII levels in haemophiliacs

Severely affected patients with haemophilia A have no detectable factor VIII activity in their plasma and suffer from repeated episodes of spontaneous bleeding, particularly in the large joints and muscles. Patients whose factor VIII activity is 1–5% of normal, about 10% of affected individuals, are defined as 'moderate haemophilia' and have infrequent attacks of bleeding. Those with levels exceeding 5%, some 30–40% of patients, are mildly affected and seldom if ever suffer spontaneous bleeding. Intracranial haemorrhage is the most common cause of death from bleeding, is spontaneous in about 50% of cases and should always be considered in patients with haemophilia who complain of headache.

Treatment with factor VIII

In severe haemophilia A, treatment with factor VIII must be provided as soon as possible after bleeding has occurred. The dose depends on the kind of haemorrhage. The aim of initial 'episodic' therapy in the case of haemarthrosis or serious bruising is to raise the factor VIII level to 30–50% of normal; if a haematoma has developed, the level should be raised to 50%, and in case of gastrointestinal bleeding, to > 50%. The level should be raised to 100% if there is spontaneous intracerebral haemorrhage or head trauma (Furie *et al.* 1994). One unit of factor VIII is the amount of factor VIII activity in 1 ml of normal plasma. For example, as the plasma volume is about 50 ml/kg, 3500 units must be given to a recipient of 70 kg to increase the level to 100%. Regardless of the source of factor VIII, the plasma level reached after administration is only about 70% of the expected level and this must be taken into account in calculating the dose required. The half-life of factor VIII is 8–12 h. Thus if one-half of a dose is given at 12-h intervals after the initial dose, the level is kept relatively constant (Furie *et al.* 1994).

Prophylactic administration of factor VIII

The incidence of bleeding can be all but abolished and even arthropathy can be prevented if factor VIII is administered prophylactically from a very early age so as to maintain the factor VIII concentration above 1% of normal (Nilsson *et al.* 1994). Once joint damage has occurred, it cannot be reversed by prophylactic treatment (Manco-Johnson *et al.* 1994). The amount of factor VIII needed for universal application of prophylactic treatment is impractically large. Short-term prophylaxis (3 months of bi-weekly infusions calculated to keep trough values at 1–3%) should be considered for patients with frequent haemorrhages or with chronic synovitis, especially if active rehabilitation is considered (Kasper *et al.* 1989). With preoperative prophylaxis, surgical mortality from haemorrhage approaches zero for most procedures (Kitchens 1986). The initial infusion is routinely given several hours

prior to surgery and the factor VIII level confirmed before induction of anaesthesia. The duration of postoperative infusions depends on both the nature of the procedure and the clinical course (Kasper *et al.* 1985). Continuous postoperative factor infusion has become an increasingly popular strategy to maintain constant factor levels (> 50%) and consume less factor concentrate, although experience with this technique is still limited.

Factor VIII levels of healthy donors: maximizing collection potential

The factor VIII activity in group A donors is on average 8% higher than in group O donors, and the level in males is about 6% higher than in females (Preston and Barr 1964). Strenuous exercise produces an almost immediate increase in factor VIII levels, lasting for at least 6 h (Rizza 1961). These observations carried greater importance when cryoprecipitate was used as a source of factor VIII.

DDAVP (1-deamino-8-D arginine vasopressin, also known as desmopressin acetate), a synthetic derivative of vasopressin, injected intravenously, produces a rapid release of vWF into the circulation. Although vWF is a carrier protein for factor VIII, factor VIII and vWF may not increase concurrently (Cattaneo *et al.* 1994; Castaman *et al.* 1995). DDAVP is the treatment of choice in patients with mild haemophilia with factor VIII levels of > 10%, but should not be used in children under 1 year of age because of the risk of hyponatraemia (Weinstein *et al.* 1989; see also Chapter 18).

DDAVP is used primarily for therapeutic purposes. However, if DDAVP (0.2 µg/kg) is injected into blood donors 15 min before venepuncture, the yield of factor VIII in fractions prepared from the resulting plasma is increased two-fold (Nilsson *et al.* 1979; Mannucci 1986). DDAVP can also be administered intranasally and is effective within 1 h with minimal side-effects (Mikaelson *et al.* 1982).

Clotting factor concentrates: reducing the risk and allaying the fear

Treatment with clotting concentrates was revolutionized by methods to inactivate viruses in plasma fractions and by recombinant technology. The former advance all but eliminated the risks of the major transfusion-transmitted infections, whereas the latter added assurance that emerging agents would not evade inactivation technology.

Choice of factor VIII concentrate

Factor VIII can be administered as cryoprecipitate, as plasma-derived factor VIII concentrate or as recombinant factor VIII. Factor VIII activity is well maintained at −30°C to −40°C for cryoprecipitate or at 4°C for lyophilized products. Commercial plasma-derived factor VIII is now treated with at least two methods for inactivating transfusion-transmitted viruses, and no documented transmissions of the lipid-encapsulated viruses HIV, HBV or HCV have been reported since 1985. Non-enveloped viruses such as hepatitis A and parvovirus B19 may still be transmitted by plasma fractions (Mannucci 1992; Santagostino et al. 1997). Both plasma-derived and recombinant products are labelled for factor VIII potency and all preparations appear to be equally effective when assessed by post-administration factor levels. Patient age, susceptibility and product cost still largely determine the choice of treatment.

Purified factor VIII concentrates

Intermediate-/high-purity concentrate. Factor purity is commonly defined as specific activity (International Units of clotting activity per milligram of protein). Most fractionation centres use large pools of plasma (5000–30 000 donations) to prepare products of intermediate purity (< 50 units/mg) and high purity (> 50 units/mg). The primary procedure is cryoprecipitation, but additional fractionation steps are undertaken to give a higher potency, stability and solubility than are obtained with the freeze-dried cryoprecipitate.

Ultrapure concentrate. Concentrates purified by using affinity chromatography with monoclonal antibodies against factor VIII have a specific activity of factor VIIIC of > 3000 iu/mg protein. In a group of patients treated with this product for more than 24 months, clinical efficacy, $T_{1/2}$ and recovery were excellent (Brettler et al. 1989). One oft-stated advantage of purified high-potency concentrates is a less pronounced effect on the immune system of the patients, documented primarily in HIV-positive patients in whom the CD4+ cell count declines less rapidly after treatment with high- than after intermediate-purity

concentrates (de Biasi et al. 1991; Hilgartner et al. 1993; Seremetis et al. 1993). No increase in AIDS-associated infections or decrease in survival has been documented (Goedert et al. 1994). No difference in effect on the immune system in HIV-negative patients has been established. Suspicion that ultra high-purity concentrates (and recombinant concentrates) may more easily induce factor VIII inhibitors, particularly in children, have not been confirmed by prospective studies (Bray 1994; Peerlinck 1994). The relationship between mutation type and inhibitor development is probably far more important. As many as 35% of patients with 'severe molecular defects', intron 22 inversions, large deletions or stop mutations develop an inhibitor, whereas few with small insertions or deletions do so (Oldenburg et al. 2002).

Recombinant factor VIII. Recombinant clones encoding the complete 2351-amino-acid sequence for human factor VIII have been isolated and used to produce factor VIII in cultured mammalian cells. The recombinant protein corrects the clotting time of plasma from haemophiliacs and is virtually indistinguishable from plasma-derived factor VIII (Wood et al. 1984).

Clinical trials have shown that *in vivo* recovery and $T_{1/2}$ of recombinant factor VIII (r-factor VIII) are not significantly different from those of plasma-derived factor VIII. The r-factor VIII Recombinate (Baxter Bioscience) and Koginate (Cutter Biological/Miles) have now been used successfully in the treatment of bleeding episodes and for prophylaxis. The observed incidence of inhibitor formation is similar to studies of previously untreated patients (PUPs) receiving plasma-derived FVIII. Long-term trials demonstrate the safety and efficacy of r-FVIII in chronic treatment of haemophilia A (Lusher 1994; White et al. 1997). Preparations of the early recombinant proteins used plasma-derived reagents during manufacture. However the most recent generation is processed and formulated without the addition of human or animal plasma additives.

Animal factor VIII concentrates. Concentrates prepared from bovine or porcine plasma have 100 times more factor VIII activity per milligram of protein than normal human plasma. The original preparations were immunogenic and could as a rule be used effectively for only 7–10 days, following which antibodies against the animal protein developed. Polyelectrolyte-fractionated porcine factor VIII concentrate (PE porcine VIII) appears to be considerably less antigenic and contains negligible amounts of platelet-aggregating factor (Kernoff *et al.* 1984).

Factor VIII inhibitors (antibodies)

Factor VIII inhibitors are found either as isoantibodies in 15–35% of haemophilia A patients following treatment with factor VIII-containing materials or, more rarely, as autoantibodies in non-haemophiliacs. The titre of the antibody measured in Bethesda units (Bu) determines both risk and management. About one-half of the antibodies in haemophiliacs are of low titre and transient. Patients with factor VIII inhibitors are relatively refractory to treatment with factor VIII and must be given very high doses to secure a response. Concentrates of factor VIII are effective if the inhibitor titre is less than 20 Bu/ml; with higher titres, factor VIII concentrates alone are ineffective. Haemophiliacs with factor VIII inhibitors may show a rise in inhibitor titre following the infusion of factor VIII; in such patients factor VIII concentrates are not effective after 5–7 days of treatment (Blatt 1982).

In treating major haemorrhage in haemophiliacs with inhibitors, provided that the inhibitor titre does not exceed 20 Bu/ml, human factor VIII concentrate can be used initially. In average-sized adults (70 kg), 5000 units of factor VIII are given initially, followed by 500–1000 units per hour. Thereafter, the dose is adjusted according to the factor VIII level (Blatt 1982). In patients with inhibitor titres exceeding 20 Bu/ml, activated prothrombin complex concentrates appear to be effective, but have an increased risk of thromboembolic complications (Hilgartner *et al.* 1990; Tjonnfjord *et al.* 2004). These concentrates bypass the need for factor VIII in a manner not thoroughly understood. Recombinant activated factor VII (rFVIIa) has been found effective in patients with antibodies against factor VIII (see also Chapter 18) (Hedner and Kisiel 1983; Abshire and Kenet 2004). Standard dosing of rFVIIa (90 µg/kg) allows binding of FVIIa to the surface of activated platelets and can directly activate factor X in the absence of tissue factor. Experience with bolus dosing suggests that higher dosing (> 200 µg/kg) may be more efficacious in treating haemophilia patients.

In patients who require very large amounts of factor VIII, animal factor concentrates have been used successfully (Kernoff *et al.* 1984). Four haemophiliacs with factor VIII inhibitors received repeated infusions of porcine VIII for periods up to 27 days with satisfactory results. An antibody response was detected in only one out of the four patients. Equally good results were obtained in a later trial (Hay *et al.* 1990). The newer treatments should render animal factor concentrates a historical curiosity.

In about 50% of patients with high-titre inhibitors and up to 90% of those with titre < 5, immune tolerance can be induced by desensitization regimens that involve daily factor VIII infusions (Ewing *et al.* 1988). Treatment may be required for weeks or months and infusions of factor VIII are sometimes combined with short courses of immunosuppressive agents such as corticosteroids, cyclophosphamide and IVIG (Kasper *et al.* 1989; Mariani *et al.* 1994).

Treatment with IVIG is beneficial in some patients with haemophilia A and inhibitors and particularly in patients with factor VIII autoantibodies. The effect may be due to anti-idiotype antibodies (Sultan *et al.* 1994; Schwartz *et al.* 1995).

Transfusion in patients with von Willebrand disease

Von Willebrand disease is a common inherited autosomal dominant bleeding disorder characterized by easy bruising, epistaxis, bleeding with dental procedures and gastrointestinal haemorrhage. In the majority of patients, bleeding results from decreased von Willebrand factor (vWF), a protein carrier of factor VIII that mediates platelet–platelet interaction and platelet binding to vascular subendothelium (Ruggeri and Ware 1993). The vWF gene is located on chromosome 12, and numerous polymorphisms and mutations have been reported; the von Willebrand syndromes are now classified by molecular, functional and clinical criteria (Sadler 1998).

Appropriate treatment depends on the specific type of vWD. Type 1 vWD, the most common form, usually presents with mild or moderate bleeding. Laboratory diagnosis shows low vWF antigen, activity (ristocetin cofactor) and factor VIII levels, as well as a prolonged bleeding time. Such patients usually respond well to an infusion of DDAVP (0.3 µg/kg) with release of sufficient vWF and factor VIII from tissue stores within 30 min to elevate these levels several fold for about 4 h (Scott and Montgomery 1993). Some of the less common vWD variants do not respond well to

DDAVP (Ruggeri *et al.* 1980; Sutor 2000). For the 10–20% of patients with vWD who do not respond to DDAVP and for patients who become refractory ('tachyphylactic') with repeated treatment given over a long period of time (Rodeghiero *et al.* 1992), replacement therapy is available in several forms. Patients who require treatment with vWF should be given high-purity, solvent detergent-treated vWF concentrate (Pasi *et al.* 1990; Burnouf-Radosevich and Burnouf 1992). If this is not available, factor VIII concentrate which contains vWF should be used instead (Cohen and Kernoff 1990). Cryoprecipitate, although rich in vWF, has generally not been treated to reduce the risk of viral transmission, and is therefore the least desirable of the available components. For planned surgery, the products should be given a few hours before operation and, if factor VIII or ristocetin cofactor is used to estimate effectiveness, the level should be measured immediately before the operation is started; if the level is not high enough (50–100%), more concentrate should be given. Repeated infusions every 12 h may be necessary for a week or more.

Treatment of factor IX deficiency (haemophilia B or Christmas disease)

Patients with haemophilia B are treated with factor IX concentrate. The administration of crude factor IX concentrates derived from cryoprecipitate supernatant ('prothrombin complex concentrate') was associated with thrombotic complications (Kohler 1999), but highly purified, virus-inactivated factor IX concentrates, based either on a combination of three conventional chromatographic steps (Burnouf *et al.* 1989) or on immune-affinity chromatography with monoclonal antibodies against factor IX, are now available (Kim *et al.* 1990; Tharakan *et al.* 1990). Recombinant factor IX is also available. Some patients achieve only 80% of the predicted plasma level and interpatient variability is wide when this product is used, so that baseline recovery measurements are important to ensure adequate treatment. Treatment with highly purified or recombinant product avoids the side-effects mentioned above (Kim *et al.* 1990). Each unit of factor IX administered raises the plasma concentration by 1%. The $T_{1/2}$ of plasma factor IX is 20 h. As in haemophilia A, the dose needed is determined by the kind of bleeding (see above) (Furie *et al.* 1994). If no factor IX concentrate is available, PCC (see below) can be used instead. Treatment with PCC may lead to thrombotic disorders and DIC (Aronson and Menache 1987).

Treatment with factor IX concentrate may induce inhibitor formation, although this is less frequent than the formation of factor VIII inhibitors in patients with haemophilia A (Knobel *et al.* 2002). The treatment of patients with factor IX inhibitors is essentially the same as that of patients with factor VIII inhibitors (see below).

Prothrombin complex concentrates (concentrates containing factors II, VII, IX and X)

Concentrates containing these vitamin K-dependent factors were originally produced for the treatment of inherited factor IX deficiency but are also used for acquired deficiencies of factors II, VII, IX and X, for example in patients with liver disease or warfarin overdose. As described above, PCCs have also been used for treating minor bleeding episodes in haemophiliacs with inhibitors. The concentrates should be administered rapidly, and immediately after reconstitution.

PCCs are thrombogenic and their use remains controversial except in the treatment of haemophilia B, although, even here, purified factor IX concentrate has largely replaced them (see above).

Use of some other coagulation factors

Factor VII

Fresh-frozen plasma can be used to treat factor VII deficiency; however, the need for frequent infusions and the risk of viral transmission have all but eliminated its use for this indication. Plasma-derived factor VII concentrate has been used successfully to treat patients with hereditary factor VII deficiency (Dike *et al.* 1980). Long-term prophylaxis in children has also been successful (Cohen *et al.* 1995). Because of its short half-life (3–4 h), frequent infusions are necessary, especially for surgery, although levels of 15–25% of normal are sufficient for this indication. Recombinant factor VIIa has been found to be effective in haemophiliacs with antibodies to factor VIII and in some subjects with poorly controlled massive or life-threatening haemorrhage (see above and Chapter 18) (Hedner *et al.* 1988; Schmidt *et al.* 1994). rFactor VIIa is the treatment of choice when no pathogen-reduced VII concentrate is available (Lusher *et al.* 1998).

Factor XIII

Pasteurized factor XIII concentrates prepared from either plasma or placenta are used to treat patients with factor XIII deficiency, a condition that can be as dangerous as haemophilia A or B (Smith 1990). Levels as low as 5% are sufficient to control bleeding. Because the half-life of factor XIII is measured in weeks, infusions may be given every 14–21 days. In the USA, where no factor XIII concentrate is licensed, FFP and cryoprecipitate are the components of choice.

Protein C

Protein C is a serine protease zymogen, which is activated by thrombin. Activated protein C interferes with the activated forms of factors V and VIII; it requires a cofactor, protein S. Activated protein C also stimulates fibrinolysis by neutralizing the inhibitor of tissue plasminogen activator. Protein C deficiency, whether hereditary or acquired as, for example, in severe liver disease, leads to venous thrombosis. Protein C concentrates are now available: a vapour-treated protein C concentrate that has been shown to be effective for long-term therapy in an infant with severe protein C deficiency (Dreyfus et al. 1995) and an immunoaffinity-purified, activated protein C concentrate, virus inactivated by chemical treatment (Orthner et al. 1995). Recombinant human activated protein C has anti-inflammatory and profibrinolytic properties in addition to its antithrombotic activity. One recombinant formulation, drotrecogin alpha, produced dose-dependent reductions in the levels of markers of coagulation and inflammation in patients with severe sepsis. In a randomized trial, treatment with drotrecogin alfa activated significantly reduced mortality in patients with severe sepsis, but seemed to be associated with an increased risk of bleeding (Bernard et al. 2001). The mechanism of the anti-inflammatory effect is poorly understood, but may involve inhibition of tumour necrosis factor production by blockade of leucocyte adhesion or interference with thrombin-induced inflammation.

C1 esterase inhibitor (C1 inh.)

Hereditary functional deficiency of C1 inh. is due to either a deficiency or a dysfunction of the protein. Acquired deficiencies of C1 inh. also occur. This pro- tease inhibitor is involved in the regulation of several proteolytic systems in plasma, including the complement system, the contact system of intrinsic coagulation and kinin release and the fibrinolytic system (Cugno et al. 1990). Functional deficiency of C1 inh. permits production of vasoactive peptides that alter vascular permeability and cause angioneurotic oedema, a serious, potentially fatal syndrome characterized by attacks of swelling of the subcutaneous tissues and mucous membranes of the face, bowel and upper airway. Mortality rate in affected kindred approaches 30%. The pathogenesis of angioedema is not completely understood (Baldwin et al. 1991).

Pasteurized C1 inh. concentrates are now available and acute attacks of angioedema respond within hours of treatment (Brummelhuis 1980; Gadek et al. 1980; Bork and Barnstedt 2001). Long-term prophylaxis with C1 inh. concentrate in hereditary as well as acquired C1 inh. deficiency has also been successful (Bork and Witzke 1989; Waytes et al. 1996). Activation of the complement and contact systems occurs in septic shock, together with a decrease of plasma C1 inh. levels. Preliminary results show that complement and contact activation can be diminished by treatment with high-dose C1 inh. concentrate (Hack et al. 1992).

Immunoglobulins

IgG

Following i.v. injection, IgG distributes between the intravascular and extravascular compartments; equilibrium is reached in about 5 days (Cohen and Freeman 1960). The daily movement of IgG from the intravascular to the extravascular compartment is equivalent to about 25–30% of the plasma IgG and is balanced by a similar transfer in the opposite direction.

When equilibrium has been attained, the plasma level declines with a $T_{1/2}$ of 21 days. The fractional rate of catabolism is largely independent of plasma IgG concentration so that the total IgG turnover varies directly with the plasma IgG level. The rate of IgG synthesis is the primary factor determining the serum IgG level (Schultze 1966). The catabolism of IgG has also been studied by injecting HBs antibody in high titre, with disappearance of antibody followed with a very sensitive radio-immunoassay. The $T_{1/2}$ of these IgG antibodies was calculated to be 19.7 days (Shibata et al. 1983). Catabolism may be enhanced by fever,

643

burns and infection. For further information, including the turnover rates of IgG subclasses, see Chapter 3.

Intravenous infusion of the 'standard' 16% Ig preparations prepared for intramuscular injection may produce severe reactions (see Chapter 15). This preparation should not be administered intravenously.

Following i.m. injection of IgG, the protein passes via the lymphatics into the bloodstream. Analysis of plasma concentration curves is relatively complex as the influx into the plasma from the site of injection is offset by efflux from the plasma into the extravascular space and also by catabolism. In a study in which ^{125}I-labelled IgG was used, the average fraction of the dose cleared per day from the site of i.m. injection, after injecting 2 ml of solution into the deltoid muscle, was estimated to be about 0.37. Plasma levels were almost maximal at 2 days, and corresponded to about 40% of the values that would have been attained immediately after i.v. injection of the same doses (Smith *et al.* 1972; see also Table 10.1). In a single case, surface counting over the site of injection showed that approximately 45% of the total injected dose was cleared per day (Jouvenceaux 1971). In two normal subjects following the injection of 10 ml of 16% Ig into the gluteal region, plasma levels corresponded to 32% of the injected dose on day 5 in one case and 20% on day 7 in the other (Morell *et al.* 1980). In retrospect, uptake may have been poor in these two cases because the injections were made into fatty tissue rather than into muscle. One survey indicated that when injections are given into the gluteal region, few female patients and fewer than 15% of male patients receive an i.m. injection (Cockshott *et al.* 1982).

Following subcutaneous injection of IgG into the buttock, the rate of uptake is distinctly slower than after i.m. injection and maximum plasma levels have still not been attained 5 days after injection (Smith *et al.* 1972).

Composition of IVIG preparations: not all are created equal

Several Ig preparations containing fully functional immunoglobulins are now available for i.v. use. These are generally 5% or 10% solutions but concentrations range from 3% to 12%. One product is prepared by DEAE fractionation, followed by treatment of the IgG-containing fraction at pH 4 with a low concentration of pepsin; the IgG molecule is not cleaved, but high-molecular-weight aggregates responsible for anaphylaxis and some of the other adverse reactions are dispersed (Jungi and Barandun 1985). If Ig for i.v. use is to be stored in the liquid state, pH must be kept low to maintain purity and stability. The low pH of the product may be responsible for pain, erythema and even phlebitis sometimes experienced at the injection site. Freeze-dried preparations can be reconstituted immediately before use at a pH of 6.6, thus avoiding the above side-effects.

Stringent requirements for IVIG have been set by the Committee for Proprietary and Medicinal Products (http://pharmacos.eudra.org). Human Ig preparations contain very little IgM, but variable amounts of IgA. Some two dozen commercial preparations are available and vary in physicochemical characteristics including concentration, volume, osmolality, sodium and sugar content (Lemm 2002).

Changes in immunoglobulin preparations on storage

Although most IgG antibodies show no obvious change in potency over a period of several years in Ig preparations kept at 4°C, the concentration of anti-D diminished at about 8% a year over 2–4.5 years in 28 preparations tested (Hughes-Jones *et al.* 1978). There was no evidence of appreciable breakdown of IgG molecules in the preparations in the same period. Low levels of immune complexes and variable amounts of IgG dimer are found in commercial preparations derived from large numbers of donor plasma collections. The proportion of dimer increases over months of storage and is enhanced by low temperature (Tankersley *et al.* 1988).

Use of human immunoglobulin

Prophylaxis of infectious disease. Standard human Ig, prepared for i.m. injection from unselected plasma, is used in protection against hepatitis A, rubella, measles and other disorders. The immunity conferred by an injection of Ig is, of course, temporary and depends upon the amount of antibody injected. Ordman and co-workers (1944) found that a dose of Ig that would protect children from measles for periods up to 14 days would not protect them for as long as 7–10 weeks (Ordman *et al.* 1944). A relatively large dose (450 mg) of Ig provides some protection for periods up to 6 weeks

(Kekwick and Mackay 1954, p. 58). In the prophylaxis of hepatitis A, a single dose of Ig (750 mg) may protect for about 5 months (Pollock and Reid 1969).

Hyperimmune Igs prepared from selected donors with high titres of the relevant antibodies are used in the prophylaxis of hepatitis B, diphtheria, tetanus, rubella, herpes zoster, rabies, measles and infection with CMV, pseudomonas and other agents. Anti-D Ig is used in the prevention of primary Rh D immunization (see Chapter 10).

Anti-HBs Ig in very high doses can prevent reactivation of hepatitis in 65–80% of HbsAg-positive patients receiving liver transplant grafts (Terrault and Vyas 2003). Monoclonal anti-HBs is available. Specific anti-pertussis toxoid Ig in high titre has been shown in a randomized trial to reduce significantly the number of 'whoops' in 47 children with less than 14 days of disease before therapy. Duration of whoops post treatment was 8.7 days for patients with whooping cough (Granstrom et al. 1991).

AIDS. A decreased incidence of bacterial infections and sepsis and an improved survival rate have been observed in infants with congenital AIDS receiving monthly IVIG (Calvelli and Rubinstein 1986). The beneficial effect of IVIG has been confirmed in children with advanced AIDS receiving zidovudine. The benefit, however, was only apparent in children who were not receiving trimethoprim-sulphamethoxazole as prophylaxis (Spector et al. 1994). In one study, prophylactic administration of IVIG to premature infants significantly reduced the risk of infections (Baker et al. 1992), but in another similar study, in which a different preparation was used, IVIG had no effect (Fanaroff et al. 1992). No recent study has evaluated IVIG therapy in children with AIDS receiving highly active antiretroviral agents (HAARTs), and the use of IVIG should probably be restricted to children who develop recurrent infections despite the administration of HAARTs and prophylactic cotrimoxazole.

Replacement therapy for immunodeficiency syndromes. Patients with either congenital or acquired hypogammaglobulinaemia with IgG levels of less than 2 g/l are candidates for treatment. Intravenous infusion is usually preferred, because large amounts of Ig have to be given that are poorly tolerated when given by repeated i.m. injection. Although subcutaneous injection of Ig preparations for i.m. use has also been satisfactory (Roord et al. 1982), the ease and ready acceptance of intravenous administration has largely replaced all other regimens. Patients with X-linked agammaglobulinaemia, severe combined immunodeficiency (SCID), Wiskott–Aldrich syndrome among others have benefited. Dosage has been determined empirically, although prospective unblinded studies confirm their effectiveness (Buckley and Schiff 1991). The recommended intravenous dose is 300–400 mg/kg body weight once per month. If the response is unsatisfactory, the dose can be increased to attain a trough level of 400–500 mg/dl.

Neonatal sepsis. Promising results in treating neonatal sepsis, particularly in premature infants, led to the recommendation that infants weighing less than 1500 g at birth should be given 0.5 g of Ig daily for 6 days, as a routine measure (Sidiropoulos et al. 1981). In a randomized study, 133 newborn infants were divided into two groups based on whether the duration of gestation was shorter or longer than 34 weeks. The infants were assigned to receive either 500 mg/kg IVIG weekly for 4 weeks or no therapy. Septicaemia and infection-related deaths were significantly less frequent in the group of infants born before 34 weeks who had received IVIG (Chiroco et al. 1987). In another prospective randomized study, 753 premature infants with early onset sepsis were randomly assigned to receive a single injection of IVIG (500 mg/kg) or albumin (5 mg/kg). At 7 days, none of the infants who received IVIG but five of the control subjects had died ($P < 0.05$). However, at 56 days, there was no difference in death rate. A single infusion may be insufficient to reduce infection-related mortality for more than a few weeks. No serious side-effects occurred in any of the treated infants (Weisman et al. 1992).

Infection in adults. Selected Ig preparations containing antibodies in high titre may have a role in severe viral and bacterial infection (Sawyer 2000). Trials with anti-*Pseudomonas* Ig prepared from plasma from vaccinated volunteers reduced the number of *Pseudomonas* infections and mortality in children and adults with severe burns (Jones et al. 1980). The protective effect of human IVIG preparations in bacterial infection has been shown clearly in mice (Imaizumi et al. 1985). However, results of other trials in patients with severe burns or multiple injuries have been less convincing (Berkman et al. 1990).

645

Chronic lymphocytic leukaemia

Hypogammaglobulinaemia is common in patients with chronic lymphocytic leukaemia (CLL) and response to immunization is impaired. The incidence of infections was reduced by 50% in 42 patients with CLL who received IVIG (400 mg/kg every 3 weeks) compared with 42 patients receiving a placebo (Cooperative Group for the Study of Immunoglobulin in Chronic Lymphocytic Leukemia 1988). This result has been confirmed (Griffiths *et al.* 1989). A dose of 250 mg per kilogram appears to be equally effective (Gamm *et al.* 1994).

Multiple myeloma. In two prospective studies, a substantial reduction in bacterial infections has been observed in patients treated with IVIG (Schedel 1986; Lee *et al.* 1994).

Kawasaki syndrome. Kawasaki syndrome, a childhood vasculitis thought by some to be associated with infection by a retrovirus, responds to treatment with high-dose IVIG (400 mg/kg per day for 3 days) combined with aspirin (Nagashima *et al.* 1987). Fever resolves in more than 85% of patients within 48 h and coronary aneurysm formation is prevented (Burns *et al.* 1998). Although the mechanism of action is unknown, IVIG reduces nitric oxide production and the expression of inducible nitric oxide synthase, factors associated both with vascular smooth muscle relaxation and with aneurysm formation (Fukunishi *et al.* 2000).

Immune thrombocytopenic purpura. The chance observation that IVIG raised the platelet count in immunodeficient children with severe thrombocytopenia has led to its widespread use in the treatment of immune thrombocytopenic purpura (ITP), first in children and subsequently in adults (Imbach *et al.* 1981; Fehr *et al.* 1982). The mechanism of action in this and in other autoimmune disorders is unknown, but may involve anti-idiotype antibodies, regulatory effects on lymphocytes and macrophages or interference with the effects of complement activation (Tankersley *et al.* 1988; Mollnes *et al.* 1997; Hansen and Balthasar 2004). Because children with acute thrombocytopenic purpura are at risk for life-threatening haemorrhages, treatment with IVIG has been advised when the platelet count falls below $10 \times 10^9/l$ (Blanchette and Turner 1986). In adults, treatment with IVIG has been recommended for patients who are bleeding or as prophylaxis for surgery, because infusions usually induce a significant, albeit short-term rise in the platelet count (Oral *et al.* 1984). The recommended dose is the original empirical schedule of 400 mg/kg per day for 4 days or 1 g per kilogram per day. The injection of relatively small amounts of anti-Rh D Ig has also been successful in inducing remissions in ITP. In D-positive adults, 750–4500 µg of anti-D was given in one series (Salama *et al.* 1986); in another, all of 13 D-positive patients given 2500 µg responded, and a single D-negative patient failed to respond (Boughton *et al.* 1988). Success has also been achieved by giving a single dose of 4 ml of D-positive red cells coated *in vitro* with 100 µg of anti-D (Ambriz *et al.* 1987). These observations suggest that anti-D produces its beneficial effects by causing D-positive red cells to bind to, and thus block, Fc receptors on macrophages. Remission has been reported in one D-negative pregnant woman who had failed to respond to steroids and who was given 120 µg of anti-D intravenously (Moise *et al.* 1990). The effective agent in anti-D Ig may be HMW IgG polymers rather than anti-D. Preparations of anti-D Ig contain a substantially higher proportion of HMW IgG polymers than non-specific Ig preparations and these polymers are more effective in blocking Fc receptors (Boughton *et al.* 1990). In a randomized study, the effect of intravenous anti-D on the platelet count in childhood acute ITP has been found to be inferior to that of IVIG (McMillan *et al.* 1994); however, one treatment occasionally proves effective after the other has failed. IVIG and anti-D may work through different mechanisms (Cooper *et al.* 2004).

Other autoimmune diseases

IVIG has been used successfully in treating patients with autoimmune neutropenia (Pollack *et al.* 1982; Bussel and Lalezari 1983). For the effect of IVIG in autoimmune haemolytic anaemia, see Chapter 7.

IVIG has also been used in treating patients with other autoimmune diseases, among them myasthenia gravis, the Guillain–Barré syndrome, multiple sclerosis and chronic demyelinating polyneuropathy (Knezevic-Maramica and Kruskall 2003). In patients with factor VIII or factor IX inhibitors, the antibody titre decreases following the administration of IVIG (Nilsson and Sundqvist 1984; Sultan *et al.* 1994).

Alloimmune diseases. High-dose IVIG has been used in Rh D haemolytic disease (see Chapter 12), in neonatal alloimmune thrombocytopenia (see Chapter 13) and in post-transfusion purpura (see Chapter 15).

Bone marrow transplantation

IVIG has been shown to reduce the incidence of septicaemia, interstitial pneumonia, fatal CMV disease, acute GvHD and transplant-related mortality in adult recipients of related marrow transplants (Siadak *et al.* 1994). The mechanism responsible for this effect is not known (Gale and Winston 1991; Sullivan *et al.* 1991). A meta-analysis of 12 randomized, controlled trials of prophylaxis in bone marrow transplantation revealed a significant reduction in fatal CMV infection; CMV-interstitial pneumonia, non-CMV pneumonia and transplant-related mortality (Bass *et al.* 1993). Continued administration after day 90 does not appear to reduce late-occurring infections or chronic GvHD (Sullivan *et al.* 1996).

Adverse reactions

Adverse reactions occur in as many as 15% of administrations (Boshkov and Kelton 1989). A commonly recognized complex of symptoms including flushing, headache, nausea and fever has been attributed to the presence of IgG aggregates and complement fixation by IgG dimers. The syndrome was first reported with i.m. administration, but clearly occurs with IVIG, especially when infusion is rapid (Nydegger and Sturzenegger 1999). An anaphylaxis-like syndrome that includes chills, arthralgias, flank pain, urticaria and circulatory collapse was reported with the first IVIG preparations, but occurs less commonly with the low pH pepsin treatment described above (Barandun and Isliker 1986; Tankersley 1994).

Passive antibody transfer is the intended consequence of treatment with immunoglobulin preparations; however, some passive antibodies cause diagnostic uncertainty, whereas others such as red cell alloantibodies may cause haemolysis. Persistent measurable titres of anti-HBs and anti-CMV in particular may persist for months, although the titre will fall over time and evidence of virus by other assays will be lacking (Lichtiger and Rogge 1991). Antibodies to numerous red cell antigens have been reported in up to one-half of commercial Ig preparations in the past,

although this is a less common fining in the newer preparations (Niosi *et al.* 1971; Nydegger and Sturzenegger 1999). Both passively acquired DAT and haemolysis occur after infusion of passive antibody (Copelan *et al.* 1986; Moscow *et al.* 1987). In a series of 47 patients who received high-dose IVIG as prophylaxis for cytomegalovirus infection following bone marrow transplantation, almost one-half were found to have an acquired DAT, and a quarter a positive indirect antiglobulin test (IAT) caused by passive anti-A, -B, -D and -K (Robertson *et al.* 1987). Most findings appeared within 1 week of initiation of IVIG therapy. Transient neutropenia, presumably as a result of passive neutrophil antibody, has been reported as well (Tam *et al.* 1996).

Thromboembolism, including venous thrombosis, pulmonary embolism, myocardial infarction, stroke and hepatic veno-occlusive disease, has been associated with IVIG infusion (Go and Call 2000). The mechanism is unclear; however, changes in viscosity, procoagulant contaminants and platelet activation have all been implicated. Manufacturers and regulatory agencies have called specific attention to this complication (Dalakas and Clark 2003).

Renal dysfunction, including acute renal failure and 17 fatalities, has been reported to the FDA (Epstein and Zoon 2000). The pathological appearance of the proximal renal tubules of the kidney has suggested 'sucrose nephropathy', so that sucrose added to some IVIG preparations has been implicated as the cause (Cayco *et al.* 1997). Patients with underlying renal disease, especially the elderly and those with diabetes mellitus sepsis, monoclonal gammopathies and volume depletion seem particularly susceptible to renal failure.

Aseptic meningitis has been reported as a dose-related complication of IVIG infusion, particularly in patients with pre-existing migraine (Sekul *et al.* 1994). Case reports of recurrent migraine and seizures have been published and may be causally related, but the most intriguing is that of a patient who suffered recurrent episodes of hypothermia with IVIG infusion (Duhem *et al.* 1996).

Transmission of HCV through IVIG has been referred to above (Bresee *et al.* 1996).

Novel intravenous immunoglobulins

By hybridoma technology, genetic engineering and chemical methods, novel specific monoclonal antibody preparations now constitute a significant proportion of biopharmaceutical products in development. Several chimeric and humanized monoclonal antibodies are now licenced therapeutics (Roque *et al.* 2004).

Antithrombin

Hereditary AT deficiency occurs in at least two forms: in one, the level of antithrombin is low (about 50% of normal), and in the second, antithrombin is functionally deficient. In both cases the deficiency of this natural anticoagulant is associated with a high risk of venous thrombosis. The first event often presents in adolescence or young adulthood (Demers *et al.* 1992). Antithrombin inactivates five of the activated coagulation factors. This function of antithrombin at several levels of the coagulation pathway probably explains why an apparently modest decrease in antithrombin activity, as in patients with familial low antithrombin levels, leads to a thrombotic tendency (Abilgaard 1984).

Heat-treated antithrombin concentrates are available with an initial 50% disappearance time of 22 h and a biological half-life of 3.8 days, and are indicated for the prevention or treatment of thromboembolic disorders in patients with hereditary antithrombin deficiency (Lechner *et al.* 1983; Menache *et al.* 1990; Lebing *et al.* 1994). A recombinant human antithrombin has been used in congenitally deficient patients who require surgery; the optimal dosing regimen remains to be defined (Konkle *et al.* 2003).

Acquired AT deficiency has several causes. Administration of antithrombin may benefit patients with cirrhosis who are to undergo surgery and patients in hepatic coma or pre-coma (Lechner *et al.* 1983). In DIC, in which antithrombin levels are often low, treatment with antithrombin concentrate may help, particularly when treatment is started early and enough concentrate is given to maintain a plasma level of at least 100% of normal (Lammle *et al.* 1984; Gabriel 1994; Schwartz 1994).

Fibronectin

Plasma fibronectin, an opsonic glycoprotein that may play a role in wound healing, infection and vascular integrity, enjoyed a short but enthusiastic vogue as a therapeutic agent when administered in the form of cryoprecipitate (Saba *et al.* 1978; Saba and Jaffe 1980). Treatment of trauma and burn patients deficient in plasma fibronectin with cryoprecipitate purportedly resulted in clinical improvement (Saba *et al.* 1986). However, a controlled trial of fibronectin found no benefit for patients with severe abdominal infections (Lundsgaard-Hansen *et al.* 1985). Similarly, patients with septic shock or severe injury showed no evidence of improvement after treatment with fibronectin (Rubli *et al.* 1983; Hesselvik *et al.* 1987; Mansberger *et al.* 1989).

α_1-Antitrypsin

α_1-Antitrypsin (α_1-AT) is a major serine endopeptidase inhibitor in human plasma, which inhibits neutrophil elastase, an enzyme involved in the proteolysis of connective tissue, especially in the lung. Hereditary deficiency of α_1-AT may lead to progressive emphysema. Clinical trials have suggested that replacement therapy in deficient patients may restore the concentration of α_1-AT in plasma and thereby limit the development of emphysema (Gadek *et al.* 1981). Concentrates of α_1-AT, which can be treated at 60°C for 10 h, are available. Weekly injections of 4 g for 6 months were given to 21 patients homozygous for the deficiency allele P1Z (Wewers *et al.* 1987). Peak levels in plasma were above the normal upper range. After a rapid decline during the first 2 days after infusion, corresponding to redistribution of α_1-AT into the intravascular space, there was a slower rate of decline consistent with the normal 4- to 5-day half-life of plasma α_1-AT. The lowest levels before the next injection were always above the threshold level. Diffusion of the infused material across the alveolus and a significant increase in elastase activity in epithelial lining fluid could be demonstrated. Similar results were obtained in another study (Konietzko *et al.* 1988). There are, however, still unanswered questions with regard to replacement therapy with α_1-AT. Whether such therapy actually prevents the development or the further progress of emphysema remains unknown and would require a large randomized trial (Dirksen *et al.* 1999). Neither has the question as to which deficient patients should be treated been answered. Considering the number of deficient patients (estimated at 70 000 in the USA), long-term demand cannot be met by α_1-AT produced from plasma. Recombinant α_1-AT would surely be needed and such products are in development. The American Thoracic Society and European Respiratory Society have reviewed this subject (2003).

References

Aas KA, Gardner FH (1958) Survival of blood platelets labeled with chromium 51. J Clin Invest 37: 1257

Abilgaard U (1984) Biological action and clinical significance of antithrombin III. Haematologia 17: 77–79

Abrahamsen AF (1970) Survival of 51Cr-labelled autologous and isologous platelets as differential diagnostic aid in thrombocytopenic states. Scand J Haematol 7: 525

Abshire T, Kenet G (2004) Recombinant factor VIIa: review of efficacy, dosing regimens and safety in patients with congenital and acquired factor VIII or IX inhibitors. J Thromb Haemost 2: 899–909

Adkins D, Spitzer G, Johnston M et al. (1997) Transfusions of granulocyte-colony-stimulating factor-mobilized granulocyte components to allogeneic transplant recipients: analysis of kinetics and factors determining posttransfusion neutrophil and platelet counts. Transfusion 37: 737–748

Adkins DR, Goodnough LT, Shenoy S et al. (2000) Effect of leukocyte compatibility on neutrophil increment after transfusion of granulocyte colony-stimulating factor-mobilized prophylactic granulocyte transfusions and on clinical outcomes after stem cell transplantation. Blood 95: 3605–3612

Alavi JB, Root RK (1977) A randomized clinical trial of granulocyte transfusions for infection in acute leukemia. N Engl J Med 296: 706

Alving BM, Hojima Y, Pisano JJ (1978) Hypotension associated with prekallikrein activator (Hageman-factor fragments) in plasma protein fraction. N Engl J Med 299: 66

Ambriz R, Munoz, R, Pizzuto J (1987) Low-dose autologous in vitro opsonised erythrocytes. Arch Intern Med 147: 105–108

American Thoracic Society/European Respiratory Society Statement: Standards for the Diagnosis and Management of Individuals with Alpha-1 Antitrypsin Deficiency. (2003). Am J Respir Crit Care Med 168: 818–900

Angelini A, Dragani A, Berardi A (1992) Evaluation of four different methods of freezing platelets. In vitro and in vivo studies. Vox Sang 62: 146–151

Apperley JF (1994) Umbilical cord blood progenitor cell transplantation. The International Conference Workshop on Cord Blood Transplantation, Indianapolis, November 1993. Bone Marrow Transplant 14: 187–196

Armitage S, Warwick R, Fehily D et al. (1999) Cord blood banking in London: the first 1000 collections. Bone Marrow Transplant 24: 139–145

Aronson DL, Menache D (1987) Thrombogenicity of Factor IX complex: in vivo investigation. Joint IABS CSL Symposium on Standardization in Blood Fractionation including Coagulation Factors, Melbourne 1986. Div Biol Standard. Basel: S Karger

Asada Y, Sumiyoshi A, Hayashi T et al. (1985) Immunohistochemistry of vascular lesion in thrombotic thrombocytopenic purpura, with special reference to factor VIII related antigen. Thromb Res 38: 469–479

Ash RC, Horowitz MM, Gale RP et al. (1991) Bone marrow transplantation from related donors other than HLA-identical siblings: effect of T cell depletion. Bone Marrow Transplant 7: 443–452

Aster RH (1965) Effect of anticoagulant and ABO incompatibility on recovery of transfused human platelets. Blood 26: 732

Aster RH (1966) Pooling of platelets in the spleen: role in the pathogenesis of 'hypersplenic' thrombocytopenia. J Clin Pathol 45: 645

Aster RH, Jandl JH (1964) Platelet sequestration in man. I. Methods. J Clin Invest 43: 843–855

Atrah HI (1994) Fibrin glue topical haemostasis for areas of bleeding large and small. BMJ 308: 933–934

Au WY, Lie AK, Ma ES et al. (2004) Late-onset pure red blood cell aplasia owing to delayed lymphoid engraftment complicating ABO-mismatched hematopoietic stem cell transplantation. Transfusion 44: 946–947

AuBuchon JP, Herschel L, Roger J et al. (2004) Preliminary validation of a new standard of efficacy for stored platelets. Transfusion 44: 36–41

Azevedo WM, Aranka FJP, Gonvea JV et al. (1995) Allogeneic transplantation with blood stem cells mobilized by rc-CSF for hematological malignancies. Bone Marrow Transplant 16: 647–653

Bacigalupo A, Van Lint MT, Valbonesi M et al. (1996) Thiotepa cyclophosphamide followed by granulocyte colony-stimulating factor mobilized allogeneic peripheral blood cells in adults with advanced leukemia. Blood 88: 353–357

Bahceci E, Read EJ, Leitman S et al. (2000) CD34+ cell dose predicts relapse and survival after T-cell-depleted HLA-identical haematopoietic stem cell transplantation (HSCT) for haematological malignancies. Br J Haematol 108: 408–414

Baker CJ, Melish ME, Hall RT (1992) Intravenous immunoglobulin for the prevention of nosocomial infection in low-birth-weight neonates. N Engl J Med 327: 213–219

Baldwin J, Pence HL, Karibo JM (1991) C1 esterase inhibitor deficiency: three presentations. Ann Allergy 67: 107

Bar BM, Schattenberg A, Mensink EJ et al. (1993) Donor leukocyte infusions for chronic myeloid leukemia relapsed after allogeneic bone marrow transplantation. J Clin Oncol 11: 513–519

Barandun S, Isliker H (1986) Development of immunoglobulin preparations for intravenous use. Vox Sang 51: 157–160

Barker JN, Weisdorf DJ, DeFor TE et al. (2005) Transplantation of 2 partially HLA-matched umbilical cord blood units to enhance engraftment in adults with hematologic malignancy. Blood 105: 1343–1347

Barnes DW, Loutit JF (1957) Treatment of murine leukaemia with x-rays and homologous bone marrow. II. Br J Haematol 3: 241–252

Bass EB, Powe NR, Goodman SN (1993) Efficacy of immunoglobulin in preventing complications of bone marrow transplantation: a meta analysis. Bone Marrow Transplant 12: 273–282

Bass H, Trenchard PM, Mustow MJ (1985) Microwave-thawed plasma for cryoprecipitate production. Vox Sang 48: 65–71

Bautista AP, Buckler PW, Towler HMA (1984) Measurement of platelet life-span in normal subjects and patients with myeloproliferative disease with indium oxine labelled platelets. Br J Haematol 58: 679–687

Bearn AG, Litwin S (1978) Deficiencies of circulating enzymes and plasma proteins. In: The Metabolic Basis of Inherited Disease, 4th edn. SB Stanbury, JB Wyngaarden, DS Fredrickson (eds). New York: McGraw Hill

Beaujean F, Pico J, Norol F et al. (1996) Characteristics of peripheral blood progenitor cells frozen after 24 hours of liquid storage. J Hematother 5: 681–686

Becker GA, Tuccelli M, Kunicki T et al. (1973) Studies of platelet concentrates stored at 22°C and 4°C. Transfusion 13: 61–68

Beeck H, Becker T, Kiessig ST et al. (1999) The influence of citrate concentration on the quality of plasma obtained by automated plasmapheresis: a prospective study. Transfusion 39: 1266–1270

Bennett JS (2001) Novel platelet inhibitors. Annu Rev Med 52: 161–184

Bensinger WJ, Weaver CH, Appelbaum FR et al. (1995) Transplantation of allogeneic peripheral blood stem cells mobilized by recombinant human granulocyte colony stimulating factor. Blood 85: 1655–1658

Berger G, Hartwell DW, Wagner DD (1998) P-Selectin and platelet clearance. Blood 92: 4446–4452

Berkman SA, Lee ML, Gale RPG (1990) Clinical uses of intravenous immunoglobulins. Ann Intern Med 112: 278–292

Bernard GR, Vincent JL, Laterre PF et al. (2001) Efficacy and safety of recombinant human activated protein C for severe sepsis. N Engl J Med 344: 699–709

Bertolini F, Murphy S, Rebulla P (1992) Role of acetate during storage of platelet concentrates in a synthetic medium. Transfusion 32: 152–156

Bertolini F, Lazzari L, Lauri E et al. (1994) Cord blood plasma-mediated ex vivo expansion of hematopoietic progenitor cells. Bone Marrow Transplant 14: 347–353

de Biasi R, Rocino A, Miraglia E et al. (1991) The impact of a very high purity factor VIII concentrate on the immune system of human immunodeficiency virus-infected hemophiliacs: a randomized, prospective, two-year comparison with an intermediate purity concentrate. Blood 78: 1919–1922

Bierman HR, Marshall GJ, Kelly KH (1962) Leucopheresis in man. II. Changes in circulating granulocytes, lymphocytes and platelets in the blood. Br J Haematol 8: 77

Bishop JF, Schiffer CA, Aisner J et al. (1987) Surgery in acute leukemia: a review of 167 operations in thrombocytopenic patients. Am J Hematol 26: 147–155

Bjoro K, Froland SS, Yun Z (1994) Hepatitis C infection in patients with primary hypogammaglobulinemia after treatment with contaminated immunoglobulin. N Engl J Med 331: 1607–1611

Blacklock HA, Prentice HG, Evans JPM (1982) ABO incompatible bone-marrow transplantation; removal of red blood cells from donor marrow avoiding recipient antibody depletion. Lancet ii: 1061–1064

Blanchette VS, Turner C (1986) Treatment of acute idiopathic thrombocytopenic purpura. J Pediatr 108: 326–327

Blatt PM , White GC 2nd, McMillan CW (1982) The treatment of hemorrhage in hemophiliacs with anti-Factor VIII antibodies. In: Safety in Transfusion Practices. Skokie, IL: College of American Pathologists

Bode AP, Miller DT (1988) Preservation of in vitro function of platelets stored in the presence of inhibitors of platelet activation and a specific inhibitor of thrombin. J Lab Clin Med 111: 118–124

Bode AP, Miller DT (1989) The use of thrombin inhibitors and aprotinin in the preservation of platelets stored for transfusion. J Lab Clin Med 113: 753–758

Bodey GP, Buckley M, Sathe YS et al. (1966) Quantitative relationships between circulating leukocytes and infection in patients with acute leukemia. Ann Intern Med 64: 328–340

Bolan CD, Childs RW, Procter JL et al. (2001a) Massive immune haemolysis after allogeneic peripheral blood stem cell transplantation with minor ABO incompatibility. Br J Haematol 112: 787–795

Bolan CD, Leitman SF, Griffith LM et al. (2001b) Delayed donor red cell chimerism and pure red cell aplasia following major ABO-incompatible nonmyeloablative hematopoietic stem cell transplantation. Blood 98: 1687–1694

Bollard CM, Aguilar L, Straathof KC et al. (2004) Cytotoxic T lymphocyte therapy for Epstein–Barr virus and Hodgkin's disease. J Exp Med 200: 1623–1633

Bork K, Barnstedt SE (2001) Treatment of 193 episodes of laryngeal edema with C1 inhibitor concentrate in patients with hereditary angioedema. Arch Intern Med 161: 714–718

Bork K, Witzke G (1989) Long-term prophylaxis with C1-inhibitor (C1 INH) concentrate in patients with recurrent angioedema caused by hereditary and acquired C1-inhibitor deficiency. J Allergy Clin Immunol 83: 677–682

Boshkov LK, Kelton JG (1989) Use of intravenous gamma-globulin as an immune replacement and an immune suppressant. Transfusion Med Rev 3: 82–120

Boughton BJ, Chaskraverty R, Baglin TP (1988) The treatment of chronic idiopathic thrombocytopenia with anti-D (RhD) immunoglobulin; its effectiveness, safety and mechanism of action. Clin Lab Haematol 10: 275–284

Boughton BJ, Chakravertyy RK, Simpson A (1990) The effect of anti-RhD and non-specific immunoglobulins on monocyte Fc receptor function: the role of high molecular weight IgG polymers and IgG subclasses. Clin Lab Haematol 12: 17–23

Bowden RA, Slichter SJ, Sayers M et al. (1995) A comparison of filtered leukocyte-reduced and cytomegalovirus (CMV) seronegative blood products for the prevention of transfusion-associated CMV infection after marrow transplant. Blood 86: 3598–3603

Bray G (1994) Inhibitor questions: plasma-derived factor VIII and recombinant factor VIII. Semin Hematol 68 Suppl. 3: 529–534

Brecher G, Cronkite EP (1951) Post-radiation parabiosis and survival in rats. Proc Soc Exp Biol Med 77: 292–294

Bresee JS, Mast EE, Coleman PJ et al. (1996) Hepatitis C virus infection associated with administration of intravenous immune globulin. A cohort study. JAMA 276: 1563–1567

Brettler DB, Forsberg AD, Levine PH (1989) Factor VIII: concentrate purified from plasma using monoclonal antibodies: human studies. Blood 73: 1859–1863

Broxmeyer HE (1995) Questions to be answered regarding umbilical cord blood hematopoietic stem and progenitor cells and their use in transplantation. Transfusion 35: 694–702

Broxmeyer HE, Douglas GW, Hangoc G (1989) Human umbilical cord blood as a potential source of transplantable hematopoietic stem/progenitor cells. Proc Natl Acad Sci USA 86: 3828–3832

Broxmeyer HE, Lu L, Cooper S et al. (1995) Flt3 ligand stimulates/costimulates the growth of myeloid stem/progenitor cells. Exp Hematol 23: 1121–1129

Broxmeyer HE, Srour EF, Hangoc G et al. (2003) High-efficiency recovery of functional hematopoietic progenitor and stem cells from human cord blood cryopreserved for 15 years. Proc Natl Acad Sci USA 100: 645–650

Brummelhuis HGJ (1980) Preparation of C1 esterase inhibitor and its clinical use. Proc Joint Meeting of the 18th Congr Int Soc Hemat and 16th Congr Int Soc Blood Transfus, Montreal, Canada

Buckley RH, Schiff RI (1991) The use of intravenous immune globulin in immunodeficiency diseases. N Engl J Med 325: 110–117

Buckner CD, Clift RA, Sanders JE et al. (1978) ABO-incompatible marrow transplants. Transplantation 26: 233–238

Buescher ES, Gallin JI (1987) Effects of storage and radiation on human neutrophil function in vitro. Inflammation 11: 401–416

Bukowski RM, Hewlett JS, Reimer RR et al. (1981) Therapy of thrombotic thrombocytopenic purpura: an overview. Semin Thromb Hemost 7: 1–8

Burgio GR, Gluckman E, Locatelli F (2003) Ethical reappraisal of 15 years of cord-blood transplantation. Lancet 361: 250–252

Burnouf T, Michalski C, Coudemand M (1989) Properties of a highly purified human plasma factor IX:c therapeutic concentrate prepared by conventional chromatography. Vox Sang 57: 225–232

Burnouf-Radosevich M, Burnouf T (1992) Chromatographic preparation of a therapeutic highly purified von Willebrand Factor concentrate from human cryoprecipitate. Vox Sang 62: 1–11

Burns JC, Capparelli EV, Brown JA et al. (1998) Intravenous gamma-globulin treatment and retreatment in Kawasaki disease. US/Canadian Kawasaki Syndrome Study Group. Pediatr Infect Dis J 17: 1144–1148

Bussel J, Lalezari PH (1983) Reversal of neutropenia with intravenous gammaglobulin in autoimmune neutropenia of infancy. Blood 62: 398–400

Byrnes JJ, Khurana M (1977) Treatment of thrombotic thrombocytopenic purpura with plasma. N Engl J Med 297: 1386–1389

Byrnes JJ, Moake JL, Klug P (1990) Effectiveness of the cryosupernatant fraction of plasma in the treatment of refractory thrombotic thrombocytopenic purpura. Am J Hematol 34: 169–174

Cairo MS (1989) Neutrophil transfusions in the treatment of neonatal sepsis. Am J Pediatr Hematol Oncol 11: 227–234

Cairo MS, Cairo MS (1987) Role of circulating complement and polymorphonuclear leukocyte transfusion in treatment and outcome in critically ill neonates with sepsis. J Pediatr 110: 935–941

Calvelli TA, Rubinstein A (1986) Intravenous gammaglobulin in infants with acquired immunodeficiency syndrome. Pediatr Infect Dis 5: 207–210

Carow CE, Hangoc G, Broxmeyer HE (1993) Human multipotential progenitor cells (CFU-GEMM) have extensive replating capacity for secondary CFU-GEMM: an effect enhanced by cord blood plasma. Blood 81: 942–949

Cartwright GE, Athens JW, Wintrobe MM (1964) The kinetics of granulopoiesis in normal man. Blood 24: 780

Caspar CB, Seger RA, Burger J et al. (1993) Effective stimulation of donors for granulocyte transfusions with recombinant methionyl granulocyte colony-stimulating factor. Blood 81: 2866–2871

Castaman G, Lattezada A, Mannucci PM (1995) Factor VIII: C increases after desmopressin in a subgroup of patients with von Willebrand disease. Br J Haematol 89: 147–151

651

Catalano L, Fontana R, Scarpato N *et al.* (1997) Combined treatment with amphotericin-B and granulocyte transfusion from G-CSF-stimulated donors in an aplastic patient with invasive aspergillosis undergoing bone marrow transplantation. Haematologia 82: 71–72

Cattaneo M, Simoni L, Gringeri A (1994) Patients with severe von Willebrand disease are insensitive to the releasing effect of DDAVP: evidence that the DDAVP-induced increase in plasma factor VIII is not secondary to the increase in plasma von Willebrand factor. Br J Haematol 86: 333–337

Cayco AV, Perazella MA, Hayslett JP (1997) Renal insufficiency after intravenous immune globulin therapy: a report of two cases and an analysis of the literature. J Am Soc Nephrol 8: 1788–1794

Chiroco G, Rondini G, Plenbani A (1987) Intravenous gammaglobulin therapy for prophylaxis of infection in high-risk neonates. J Pediatr 110: 437–442

Christensen RD, Rothstein G (1980) Exhaustion of mature marrow neutrophils in neonates. J Pediatr 96: 316–318

Chu DZ, Shivshanker K, Stroehlein JR *et al.* (1983) Thrombocytopenia and gastrointestinal hemorrhage in the cancer patient: prevalence of unmasked lesions. Gastrointest Endosc 29: 269–272

Cockshott WP, Thompson GT, Howlett LJ (1982) Intramuscular or intralipomatous injections. N Engl J Med 307: 356–368

Cohen H, Kernoff PBA (1990) Plasma, plasma products, and indications for their use. BMJ 300: 803–806

Cohen LJ, McWilliams NB, Neuberg R *et al.* (1995) Prophylaxis and therapy with factor VII concentrate (human) immuno, vapor heated in patients with congenital factor VII deficiency: a summary of case reports. Am J Hematol 50: 269–276

Cohen S, Freeman T (1960) Metabolic heterogeneity of human gamma-globulin. Biochem J 76: 475

Cohn EJ, Oncley JL, Strong LE (1944) Chemical, clinical and immunological studies on the products of human plasma fractionation. I. The characterization of the protein fractions in human plasma. J Clin Invest 23: 417

Coller BS (1997) GPIIb/IIIa antagonists: pathophysiologic and therapeutic insights from studies of c7E3 Fab. Thromb Haemost 78: 730–735

Collins RH Jr, Shpilberg O, Drobyski WR *et al.* (1997) Donor leukocyte infusions in 140 patients with relapsed malignancy after allogeneic bone marrow transplantation. J Clin Oncol 15: 433–444

Cooper N, Heddle NM, Haas M *et al.* (2004) Intravenous (IV) anti-D and IV immunoglobulin achieve acute platelet increases by different mechanisms: modulation of cytokine and platelet responses to IV anti-D by FcgammaRIIa and FcgammaRIIIa polymorphisms. Br J Haematol 124: 511–518

Cooperative Group for the Study of Immunoglobulin in Chronic Lymphocytic Leukemia (1988) Intravenous immunoglobulin for the prevention of infection in chronic lymphocytic leukemia. A randomized, controlled clinical trial. N Engl J Med 319: 902–907

Copelan EA, Strohm PL, Kennedy MS *et al.* (1986) Hemolysis following intravenous immune globulin therapy. Transfusion 26: 410–412

Corash LM (1978) Platelet heterogeneity: relationship between density and age. In: The Blood Platelet in Transfusion Therapy. TJ Greenwalt, CA Jamieson (eds). New York: Alan R Liss

Cugno M, Nuijens J, Hack E (1990) Plasma levels of C1 inhibitor complexes and cleaved C1 inhibitor in patients with hereditary angioneurotic edema. J Clin Invest 85: 1215–1220

Dalakas MC, Clark WM (2003) Strokes, thromboembolic events, and IVIg: rare incidents blemish an excellent safety record. Neurology 60: 1736–1737

Dale DC, Liles WC, Llewellyn C *et al.* (1998) Neutrophil transfusions: kinetics and functions of neutrophils mobilized with granulocyte-colony-stimulating factor and dexamethasone. Transfusion 38: 713–721

Daly PA, Schiffer CA, Aisner J (1980) Platelet transfusion therapy. One-hour posttransfusion increments are valuable in predicting the need for HLA-matched preparations. JAMA 243: 435–438

Dancey IT, Deubelbeiss KA, Harker LA (1976) Neutrophil kinetics in man. J Clin Invest 58: 705

Danpure HJ, Osman S, Peters AM (1990) Labelling autologous platelets with 111In tropolonate for platelet kinetic studies: limitations imposed by thrombocytopenia. Eur J Haematol 45: 223–230

Davis KB, Slichter SJ, Corash L (1999) Corrected count increment and percent platelet recovery as measures of posttransfusion platelet response: problems and a solution. Transfusion 39: 586–592

Dayian G, Reich LM, Mayer K (1974) Use of glycerol to preserve platelets suitable for transfusion. Cryobiology II: 563–571

Dayian G, Harris HL, Vlahides GD (1986) Improved procedure for platelet freezing. Vox Sang 51: 292–298

Dazzi F, Szydlo RM, Craddock C *et al.* (2000) Comparison of single-dose and escalating-dose regimens of donor lymphocyte infusion for relapse after allografting for chronic myeloid leukemia. Blood 95: 67–71

De Lima M, St John LS, Wieder ED *et al.* (2002) Double-chimaerism after transplantation of two human leucocyte antigen mismatched, unrelated cord blood units. Br J Haematol 119: 773–776

Demers C, Ginsberg JS, Hirsh J *et al.* (1992) Thrombosis in antithrombin-III-deficient persons. Report of a large kindred and literature review. Ann Intern Med 116: 754–761

Depalma L, Leitman SF, Carter CS et al. (1989) Granulocyte transfusion therapy in a child with chronic granulomatous disease and multiple red cell alloantibodies. Transfusion 29: 421–423

Deveras RA, Kessler CM (2002) Reversal of warfarin-induced excessive anticoagulation with recombinant human factor VIIa concentrate. Ann Intern Med 137: 884–888

Dhodapkar M, Goldberg SL, Tefferi A et al. (1994) Reversible encephalopathy after cryopreserved peripheral blood stem cell infusion. Am J Hematol 45: 187–188

Dignani MC, Anaissie EJ, Hester JP et al. (1997) Treatment of neutropenia-related fungal infections with granulocyte colony-stimulating factor-elicited white blood cell transfusions: a pilot study. Leukemia 11: 1621–1630

Dike GWR, Griffiths D, Bidwell E (1980) A Factor VII concentrate for therapeutic use. Br J Haematol 45: 107–118

Dirksen A, Dijkman JH, Madsen F et al. (1999) A randomized clinical trial of alpha(1)-antitrypsin augmentation therapy. Am J Respir Crit Care Med 160: 1468–1472

Divers SG, Kaunan K, Stewart RM (1995) Quantitation of CD62, soluble CD62, and lysome-associated membrane proteins 1 and 2 for evaluation of the quality of stored platelet concentrates. Transfusion 35: 292–297

Dodsworth N, Harris R, Denton K et al. (1996) Comparative studies of recombinant human albumin and human serum albumin derived by blood fractionation. Biotechnol Appl Biochem 24 (Pt 2): 171–176

Dreyfus M, Masterson M, David M et al. (1995) Replacement therapy with a monoclonal antibody purified protein C concentrate in newborns with severe congenital protein C deficiency. Semin Thromb Hemost 21: 371–381

Duhem C, Ries F, Dicato M (1996) Intravenous immune globulins and hypothermia. Am J Hematol 51: 172–173

Dumont LJ, AuBuchon JP, Whitley P et al. (2002) Seven-day storage of single-donor platelets: recovery and survival in an autologous transfusion study. Transfusion 42: 847–854

Dutcher JP, Schiffer CA, Johnston GS (1981) Rapid migration of 111indium-labeled granulocytes to sites of infection. N Engl J Med 304: 586–589

Edelson RN, Chernik NL, Posner JB (1974) Spinal subdural hematomas complicating lumbar puncture. Arch Neurol 31: 134–137

Einsele H, Roosnek E, Rufer N et al. (2002) Infusion of cytomegalovirus (CMV)-specific T cells for the treatment of CMV infection not responding to antiviral chemotherapy. Blood 99: 3916–3922

Ende M, Ende N (1972) Hematopoietic transplantation by means of fetal (cord) blood. A new method. V Med 99: 276–280

Epstein JS, Zoon KC (2000) Important drug warning: Immune Globulin Intravenous (human) (IGIV) products. Neonatal Netw 19: 60–62, No. 286

Ewing NP, Sanders NL, Dietrich SL et al. (1988) Induction of immune tolerance to factor VIII in hemophiliacs with inhibitors. JAMA 259: 65–68

Falkenburg JH, Wafelman AR, Joosten P et al. (1999) Complete remission of accelerated phase chronic myeloid leukemia by treatment with leukemia-reactive cytotoxic T lymphocytes. Blood 94: 1201–1208

Fanaroff A, Wright E, Korones S (1992) A controlled trial of prophylactic intravenous immunoglobulin (IVIG) to reduce nosocomial infections in VLBW infants. Pediatr Res 31: 202A (Abstract)

Fantl P (1968) Osmotic stability of blood platelets. J Physiol 198: 1–16

Fehr J, Hofman V, Kappeler U (1982) Transient reversal of thrombocytopenia in idiopathic thrombocytopenic purpura by high-dose intravenous gamma globulin. N Engl J Med 306: 1254–1258

Fijnheer R (1991) Survival of activated platelets after transfusion. In: Biochemical and Clinical Aspects of Platelet Transfusion, pp. 121–130. Amsterdam: University of Amsterdam

Fijnheer R, Pietersz RNI, de Korte D (1989) Monitoring of platelet morphology during storage of platelet concentrates. Transfusion 29: 36–40

Fijnheer R, Modderman PW, Veldman WH (1990) Detection of platelet activation with monoclonal antibodies and flow cytometry: changes during platelet storage. Transfusion 30: 20–25

Flowers ME, Parker PM, Johnston LJ et al. (2002) Comparison of chronic graft-versus-host disease after transplantation of peripheral blood stem cells versus bone marrow in allogeneic recipients: long-term follow-up of a randomized trial. Blood 100: 415–419

Franco RS, Lee KN, Bakker-Gear R (1994) Use of bi-level biotinylation for concurrent measurement of in vivo recovery and survival in two rabbit platelet populations. Transfusion 34: 784–789

Fraser JK, Cairo MS, Wagner EL et al. (1998) Cord Blood Transplantation Study (COBLT): cord blood bank standard operating procedures. J Hematother 7: 521–561

Fratantoni JC, Poindexter BJ, Bonner RF (1984) Quantitative assessment of platelet morphology by light scattering: a potential method for the evaluation of platelets for transfusion. J Lab Clin Med 103: 620–631

Frei E III, Levin RH, Bodey GP et al. (1965) The nature and control of infections in patients with acute leukemia. Cancer Res 25: 1511–1515

Freireich EJ, Kliman A, Lawrence AG et al. (1963) Response to repeated platelet transfusion from the same donor. Ann Intern Med 59: 277–287

Freireich EJ, Levin RH, Whang J et al. (1964) The function and fate of transfused leukocytes from donors with chronic myelocytic leukemia in leukopenic recipients. Ann NY Acad Sci 113: 1081–1089

Frim J, Mazur P (1980) Approaches to the cryopreservation of human granulocytes. Cryobiology 17: 282–286

Fukunishi M, Kikkawa M, Hamana K *et al.* (2000) Prediction of non-responsiveness to intravenous high-dose gamma-globulin therapy in patients with Kawasaki disease at onset. J Pediatr 137: 172–176

Furie B, Limentani SA, Rosenfield CG (1994) A practical guide to the evaluation and treatment of hemophilia. Blood 84: 3–9

Gabriel DA (1994) The use of antithrombin III in treatment of disseminated intravascular coagulation. Semin Hematol 31 (Suppl. 1): 60–64

Gadek JE, Hosea SW, Gelfand MA (1980) Replacement therapy in hereditary angioedema. Successful treatment of acute episodes of angioedema with partly purified C1 inhibitor. N Engl J Med 302: 542–546

Gadek JE, Klein HG, Holland PV (1981) Replacement therapy of alpha 1-antitrypsin deficiency. Reversal of pro-tease-antiprotease imbalance within the alveolar structures of PiZ subjects. J Clin Invest 68: 1158–1165

Gajewski JL, Petz LD, Calhoun L *et al.* (1992) Hemolysis of transfused group O red blood cells in minor ABO-incompatible unrelated-donor bone marrow transplants in patients receiving cyclosporine without posttransplant methotrexate. Blood 79: 3076–3085

Gale RP, Winston D (1991) Intravenous immunoglobulin in bone marrow transplantation. Cancer 68: 1451–1453

Gamm H, Huber C, Chapel H *et al.* (1994) Intravenous immune globulin in chronic lymphocytic leukaemia. Clin Exp Immunol 97 (Suppl. 1): 17–20

Gansera B, Schmidtler F, Spiliopoulos K *et al.* (2003) Urgent or emergent coronary revascularization using bilateral inter-nal thoracic artery after previous clopidogrel antiplatelet therapy. Thorac Cardiovasc Surg 51: 185–189

Gaydos LA, Freireich EJ, Mantel N (1962) The quantitat-ive relation between platelet count and hemorrhage in patients with acute leukemia. N Engl J Med 266: 905–909

George VM, Holme S, Moroff G (1989) Evaluation of two instruments for non invasive platelet concentrate quality assessment. Transfusion 29: 273–275

Gilbert GL, Hayes K, Hudson IL *et al.* (1989) Prevention of transfusion-acquired cytomegalovirus infection in infants by blood filtration to remove leucocytes. Neonatal Cytomegalovirus Infection Study Group. Lancet 1: 1228–1231

Gitlin D, Borges WH (1953) Studies on the metabolism of fibrinogen in two patients with congenital afibrinogene-mia. Blood 8: 679

Glasser L, Fiederlein RL, Huestis DW (1985) Liquid preserva-tion of human neutrophils stored in synthetic media at 22°C: controlled observations on storage variables. Blood 66: 267–272

Gluckman E, Locatelli F (2000) Umbilical cord blood trans-plants. Curr Opin Hematol 7: 353–357

Gmur J, Burger J, Schanz U (1991) Safety of stringent prophy-lactic platelet transfusion policy for patients with acute leukaemia. Lancet ii: 1223–1226

Go RS, Call TG (2000) Deep venous thrombosis of the arm after intravenous immunoglobulin infusion: case report and literature review of intravenous immunoglobulin-related thrombotic complications. Mayo Clin Proc 75: 83–85

Goedert JJ, Cohen AR, Kessler CM *et al.* (1994) Risks of immunodeficiency, AIDS, and death related to purity of factor VIII concentrate. Multicenter Hemophilia Cohort Study. Lancet 344: 791–792

Goldfinger D, McGinniss MH (1971) Rh-incompatible platelet transfusions: risks and consequences of sensitizing immunosuppressed patients. N Engl J Med 284: 942

Goldstein IM, Eyre HJ, Terasaki PI (1971) Leukocyte trans-fusions: role of leukocyte alloantibodies in determining transfusion response. Transfusion 11: 19

Gottschall JL, Johnston VL, Azod L (1984) Importance of white blood cells in platelet storage. Vox Sang 47: 101–107

Gottschall JL, Rzad L, Aster RH (1986) Studies of the minimum temperature at which human platelets can be stored with full maintenance of viability. Transfusion 26: 460–462

Granstrom M, Olinder-Nielsen AM, Holmblad P *et al.* (1991) Specific immunoglobulin for treatment of whoop-ing cough. Lancet 338: 1230–1233

Grewal SS, Kahn JP, MacMillan ML *et al.* (2004) Successful hematopoietic stem cell transplantation for Fanconi ane-mia from an unaffected HLA-genotype-identical sibling selected using preimplantation genetic diagnosis. Blood 103: 1147–1151

Griffith LM, McCoy JP, Bolan CD *et al.* (2005) Persistence of recipient plasma cells and anti-donor isohaemagglutinins in patients with delayed donor erythropoiesis after major ABO incompatible non-myeloablative haematopoietic cell transplantation. Br J Haematol 128: 668–675

Griffiths H, Brennan V, Lea J (1989) Crossover study of immunoglobulin replacement therapy in patients with low-grade B-cell tumors. Blood 73: 366–368

Gullikson H, Shanwell A, Wikman A (1991) Storage of platelets in a new plastic container. Vox Sang 61: 165–170

Gunson HH, Merry AH, Makar Y (1983) Five day storage of platelet concentrates. II. *In vivo*-studies. Clin Lab Haematol 5: 287–294

Guppy M, Whisson ME, Sabaratuam R (1990) Alternative fuels for platelet storage: a metabolic study. Vox Sang 59: 146–152

Hack EC, Voerman J, Eiselo B (1992) C1-esterase inhibitor substitution therapy in sepsis (Letter). Lancet 339: 378

Han T, Stutzman L, Cohen E *et al.* (1966) Effect of platelet transfusion on hemorrhage in patients with acute leukemia. An autopsy study. Cancer 19: 1937–1942

Hansen RJ, Balthasar JP (2004) Mechanisms of IVIG action in immune thrombocytopenic purpura. Clin Lab 50: 133–140

Hanson SR, Slichter SJ (1985) Platelet kinetics in patients with bone marrow hypoplasia: evidence for a fixed platelet requirement. Blood 66: 1105–1109

Harker LA (1977) The kinetics of platelet production and destruction in man. Clin Haematol 6: 671

Harker LA, Finch CA (1969) Thrombokinetics in man. J Clin Invest 48: 963

Harker LA, Slichter SJ (1972a) Platelet and fibrinogen consumption in man. N Engl J Med 287: 999–1005

Harker LA, Slichter SJ (1972b) The bleeding time as a screening test for evaluating platelet function. N Engl J Med 287: 155

Hay CRM, Laurian Y, Verroust F (1990) Induction of immune tolerance in patients with hemophilia A and inhibitors treated with porcine VIIIC by home therapy. Blood 76: 882–886

Heaton WA, Davis HH, Welch MJ (1979) Indium-111: a new radionuclide label for studying human platelet kinetics. Br J Haematol 42: 613–622

Heckman K, Weiner GJ, Strauss RC (1993) Randomized evaluation of the optimal platelet count for prophylactic platelet transfusion in patients undergoing induction therapy for acute leukemia (Abstract). Blood 82 (Suppl. 1): 192a

Hedner U, Kisiel W (1983) Use of human Factor VIIa in the treatment of two haemophilia A patients with high titre inhibitors. J Clin Invest 71: 1836–1841

Hedner U, Glazer S, Pingel K (1988) Successful use of recombinant Factor VIIa in a patient with severe haemophilia A during synovectomy. Lancet ii: 1193

Hellings JA (1981) On the structure and function of Factor VIII: von Willebrand factor. Thesis, University of Amsterdam, Amsterdam

Hershko C, Gale RP, Ho W (1980) ABH antigens and bone marrow transplantation. Br J Haematol 44: 65–73

Herzig RH, Herzig GP, Graw R Jr (1977) Successful granulocyte transfusion therapy for gram-negative septicemia. N Engl J Med 296: 701

Hesselvik R, Brodin B, Carlsson C (1987) Cryoprecipitate infusion fails to improve organ function in septic shock. Crit Care Med 15: 594–597

Heyns AD, Lotter MG, Badenhorst PN *et al.* (1980) Kinetics, distribution and sites of destruction of 111indium-labelled human platelets. Br J Haematol 44: 269–280

Higby DJ, Burnett D (1980) Granulocyte transfusions: current status. Blood 55: 2–8

Higby DJ, Cohen E, Holland JF (1974) The prophylactic treatment of thrombocytopenic leukemic patients with platelets: a double blind study. Transfusion 14: 440

Higby DL, Yates JW, Henderson ES (1975) Filtration leukapheresis for granulocyte transfusion therapy: clinical and laboratory studies. N Engl J Med 292: 761

Hilgartner M, Aledort L, Andes A *et al.* (1990) Efficacy and safety of vapor-heated anti-inhibitor coagulant complex in hemophilia patients. FEIBA Study Group. Transfusion 30: 626–630

Hilgartner MW, Buckley JD, Operskalski EA *et al.* (1993) Purity of factor VIII concentrates and serial CD4 counts. The Transfusion Safety Study Group. Lancet 341: 1373–1374

Hirosue A, Yamamoto K, Shiraki H (1988) Preparation of white-cell poor blood components using a quadruple bag system. Transfusion 28: 261–264

Hoffmeister KM, Falet H, Toker A *et al.* (2001) Mechanisms of cold-induced platelet actin assembly. J Biol Chem 276: 24751–24759

Hoffmeister KM, Felbinger TW, Falet H *et al.* (2003a) The clearance mechanism of chilled blood platelets. Cell 112: 87–97

Hoffmeister KM, Josefsson EC, Isaac NA *et al.* (2003b) Glycosylation restores survival of chilled blood platelets. Science 301: 1531–1534

Hogge DE, Thompson BW, Schiffer CA (1986) Platelet storage for 7 days in second-generation blood bags. Transfusion 26: 131–135

Högman CF, Eriksson L, Tapper K (1989) The Opti system. A new technique for automated separation of whole blood into red cells, plasma and buffy coat. Transfusion 29 (Suppl.): 40S

Högman CF, Eriksson L, Ericson A (1991a) Storage of saline-adenine-glucose-mannitol-suspended red cells in a new plastic container: polyvinylchloride plasticized with butyryl-n-trihexyl-citrate. Transfusion 31: 26–29

Högman CF, Gong J, Eriksson L *et al.* (1991b) White cells protect donor blood against bacterial contamination. Transfusion 31: 620–626

Holme S, Heaton A, Momoda G (1989) Evaluation of a new, more oxygen-permeable, polyvinylchloride container. Transfusion 29: 159–164

Holme S, Heaton WAL, Courtright WL (1987) Improved *in vivo* and *in vitro* viability of platelet concentrates stored for seven days in a platelet additive solution. Br J Haematol 66: 233–238

Howard SC, Gajjar AJ, Cheng C *et al.* (2002) Risk factors for traumatic and bloody lumbar puncture in children with acute lymphoblastic leukemia. JAMA 288: 2001–2007

Hows J, Beddow K, Gordon-Smith E (1986) Donor derived red blood cell antibodies and immune hemolysis after allogeneic bone marrow transplantation. Blood 67: 177–181

655

Hows JM, Chipping PM, Palmer S (1983) Regeneration of peripheral blood cells following ABO-incompatible allogeneic BMT for severe aplastic anaemia. Br J Haematol 53: 145–151

Hubel A (1997) Parameters of cell freezing: implications for the cryopreservation of stem cells. Transfusion Med Rev 11: 224–233

Hughes-Jones NC, Hunt VA, Maycock W (1978) Anti-D immunoglobulin preparations: the stability of anti-D concentrations and the error of the assay of anti-D. Vox Sang 35: 100

Hunter S, Nixon J, Murphy S (2001) The effect of the interruption of agitation on platelet quality during storage for transfusion. Transfusion 41: 809–814

Imaizumi A, Suzuki Y, Sato H (1985) Protective effects of human gamma-globulin preparation against experimental aerosol infections of mice with *Bordetella pertussis*. Vox Sang 48: 18–25

Imbach P, Barandun S, d'Apuzzo V et al. (1981) High-dose intravenous gammaglobulin for idiopathic thrombocytopenic purpura in childhood. Lancet 1: 1228–1231

Jaroscak J, Goltry K, Smith A et al. (2003) Augmentation of umbilical cord blood (UCB) transplantation with *ex vivo*-expanded UCB cells: results of a phase 1 trial using the AastromReplicell System. Blood 101: 5061–5067

Johnson BD, Becker EE, Truitt RL (1999) Graft-vs.-host and graft-vs.-leukemia reactions after delayed infusions of donor T-subsets. Biol Blood Marrow Transplant 5: 123–132

Jones RJ, Roe EA, Gupta JC (1980) Controlled trial of pseudomonas immunoglobulin and vaccine in burn patients. Lancet ii: 1263–1265

Jouvenceaux A (1971) Prévention de l'immunisation anti-Rh. Rév Fr Transfusion 14: 39

Jungi TW, Barandun S (1985) Estimation of the degree of opsonization of homologous erythrocytes by IgG for intravenous and intramuscular use. Vox Sang 49: 9–20

Kasper CK, Boylen AL, Ewing NP et al. (1985) Hematologic management of hemophilia A for surgery. JAMA 253: 1279–1283

Kasper CK, Graham JB, Kernoff P (1989) Hemophilia: state of the art of haematologic care 1988. Vox Sang 56: 141–144

Keegan T, Heaton A, Holme S (1992) Paired comparison of platelet concentrates prepared from platelet-rich plasma and buffy coats using a new technique with 111In and 51Cr. Transfusion 32: 113–120

Keeney M, Chin-Yee I, Weir K et al. (1998) Single platform flow cytometric absolute CD34+ cell counts based on the ISHAGE guidelines. International Society of Hematotherapy and Graft Engineering. Cytometry 34: 61–70

Kekwick RA, Mackay ME (1954) The separation of protein fractions from human plasma with ether. Spec Rep Ser Med Res Coun (Lond) No. 286

Kernoff PB, Thomas ND, Lilley PA et al. (1984) Clinical experience with polyelectrolyte-fractionated porcine factor VIII concentrate in the treatment of hemophiliacs with antibodies to factor VIII. Blood 63: 31–41

Kessinger A, Smith CM, Standford SE (1989) Allogeneic transplantation of blood-derived T-cell depleted hemopoietic stem cells after myeloablative treatment in a patient with acute lymphoblastic leukemia. Bone Marrow Transplant 4: 643–646

Kilkson H, Holme S, Murphy S (1984) Platelet metabolism during storage of platelet concentrates at 22 degrees C. Blood 64: 406–414

Kim HC, McMillan CW, White GC (1990) Clinical experience of a new monoclonal antibody purified Factor IX: half-life, recovery, safety in patients with hemophilia B. Semin Haematol 27: 30–35

Kistler P, Nitschmann H (1962) Large scale production of human plasma fractions. Eight years experience with the alcohol fractionation procedure of Nitschmann, Kistler and Lergies. Vox Sang 7: 414–424

Kitchens CS (1986) Surgery in hemophilia and related disorders. A prospective study of 100 consecutive procedures. Medicine (Baltimore) 65: 34–45

Klein HG, Strauss RG, Schiffer CA (1996) Granulocyte transfusion therapy. Semin Hematol 33: 359–368

Kloosterman TC, Martens AC, van Bekkum DW et al. (1995) Graft-versus-leukemia in rat MHC-mismatched bone marrow transplantation is merely an allogeneic effect. Bone Marrow Transplant 15: 583–590

Knezevic-Maramica I, Kruskall MS (2003) Intravenous immune globulins: an update for clinicians. Transfusion 43: 1460–1480

Knobel KE, Sjorin E, Tengborn LI et al. (2002) Inhibitors in the Swedish population with severe haemophilia A and B: a 20-year survey. Acta Paediatr 91: 910–914

Knudtzon S (1974) *In vitro* growth of granulocytic colonies from circulating cells in human cord blood. Blood 43: 357–361

Koerner K (1984) Platelet function of room temperature platelet concentrates stored in a new plastic material with high gas permeability. Vox Sang 47: 406–411

Kogler G, Nurnberger W, Fischer J et al. (1999) Simultaneous cord blood transplantation of *ex vivo* expanded together with non-expanded cells for high risk leukemia. Bone Marrow Transplant 24: 397–403

Kohler M (1999) Thrombogenicity of prothrombin complex concentrates. Thromb Res 95: S13–S17

Kolb HJ, Mittermuller J, Clemm C et al. (1990) Donor leukocyte transfusions for treatment of recurrent chronic myelogenous leukemia in marrow transplant patients. Blood 76: 2462–2465

Kolb HJ, Schattenberg A, Goldman JM et al. (1995) Graft-versus-leukemia effect of donor lymphocyte transfusions in marrow grafted patients. European Group for Blood and Marrow Transplantation Working Party Chronic Leukemia. Blood 86: 2041–2050

Konietzko N, Becker M, Schmidt EW (1988) Substitution therapy with alpha-1-Pi in patients with alpha-1-Pi deficiency and progressive pulmonary emphysema. Dtsch Med Wschr 113: 369–373

Konkle BA, Bauer KA, Weinstein R et al. (2003) Use of recombinant human antithrombin in patients with congenital antithrombin deficiency undergoing surgical procedures. Transfusion 43: 390–394

Korbling M, Przepiorka D, Huh YO et al. (1995) Allogeneic blood stem cell transplantation for refractory leukemia and lymphoma: potential advantage of blood over marrow allografts. Blood 85: 1659–1665

de Korte D, Gouwerok CWN, Fijnheer R (1990) Depletion of dense granule nucleotides during storage of human platelets. Thromb Haemost 63: 275–278

Kotilainen M (1969) Platelet kinetics in normal subjects and in haematological disorders. Scand J Haematol Suppl 5: 5–97

Kotze HF, Heyns AD, Lotter MG et al. (1991) Comparison of oxine and tropolone methods for labeling human platelets with indium-111. J Nucl Med 32: 62–66

Krause DS, Fackler MJ, Civin CI et al. (1996) CD34: structure, biology, and clinical utility. Blood 87: 1–13

Kunicki TJ, Tuccelli M, Becker GA et al. (1975) A study of variables affecting the quality of platelets stored at room temperature. Transfusion 15: 414

Kunicki TJ, Furihata K, Bull B et al. (1987) The immunogenicity of platelet membrane glycoproteins. Transfusion Med Rev 1: 21–33

Kurtzberg J, Laughlin M, Graham ML (1996) Placental blood as a source of hematopoietic stem cells for transplantation into unrelated recipients. N Engl J Med 335: 157–166

Lammle B, Tran TH, Ritz R (1984) Plasma prekallikrein factor XII, antithrombin III, protein C, C1-inhibitor and α2 macroblobulin in critically ill patients with suspected disseminated intravascular coagulation (DIC). Am J Clin Pathol 82: 396–404

Landefeld CS, Goldman L (1989) Major bleeding in outpatients treated with warfarin: incidence and prediction by factors known at the start of outpatient therapy. Am J Med 87: 144–152

Lane TA, Lamkin GE (1984) Hydrogen ion maintenance improves the chemotaxis of stored granulocytes. Transfusion 24: 231–237

Lane TA, Windle BE (1979) Granulocyte concentrate preservation: effect of temperature on granulocyte preservation. Blood 54: 216–255

Lasky LC, Lane TA, Miller JP et al. (2002) In utero or ex utero cord blood collection: which is better? Transfusion 42: 1261–1267

Laughlin MJ, Barker J, Bambach B et al. (2001) Hematopoietic engraftment and survival in adult recipients of umbilical-cord blood from unrelated donors. N Engl J Med 344: 1815–1822

Lebing WR, Hammond DJ, Wydick JE (1994) A highly purified antithrombin III concentrate prepared from human plasma fraction IV-1 by affinity chromatography. Vox Sang 67: 117–124

Lechner K, Thaler E, Niessner H (1983) Ursache, klinische Bedeutung and Therapie von Antithrombin III-Mangelzustanden. Acta Med Austriaca 10: 129–135

Lee M, Hargreaves R, Pamphilon DH (1994) Randomised trial of intravenous immunoglobulin as prophylaxis against infection in plateau-phase multiple myeloma. Lancet 343: 1059–1064

Lee TH, Paglieroni T, Ohto H et al. (1999) Survival of donor leukocyte subpopulations in immunocompetent transfusion recipients: frequent long-term microchimerism in severe trauma patients. Blood 93: 3127–3139

Lemm G (2002) Composition and properties of IVIg preparations that affect tolerability and therapeutic efficacy. Neurology 59: S28–S32

Lemmer JH Jr, Metzdorff MT, Krause AH Jr et al. (2000) Emergency coronary artery bypass graft surgery in abciximab-treated patients. Ann Thorac Surg 69: 90–95

Levi M, de Jonge E, van der PT (2001) Advances in the understanding of the pathogenetic pathways of disseminated intravascular coagulation result in more insight in the clinical picture and better management strategies. Semin Thromb Hemost 27: 569–575

Levi M, de Jonge E, van der Poll T (2004) New treatment strategies for disseminated intravascular coagulation based on current understanding of the pathophysiology. Ann Med 36: 41–49

Levine MN, Raskob G, Landefeld S et al. (2001) Hemorrhagic complications of anticoagulant treatment. Chest 119: 108S–121S

Lichtiger B, Hester JP (1986) Transfusion of Rh-incompatible blood components to cancer patients. Haematologia 19: 81–88

Lichtiger B, Rogge K (1991) Spurious serologic test results in patients receiving infusions of intravenous immune gammaglobulin. Arch Pathol Lab Med 115: 467–469

Lightfoot T, Leitman SF, Stroncek DF (2000) Storage of G-CSF-mobilized granulocyte concentrates. Transfusion 40: 1104–1110

Lightfoot T, Gallelli J, Matsuo K et al. (2001) Evaluation of solutions for the storage of granulocyte colony-stimulating factor-mobilized granulocyte concentrates. Vox Sang 80: 106–111

Liles WC, Rodger E, Dale DC (2000) Combined administration of G-CSF and dexamethasone for the mobilization of granulocytes in normal donors: optimization of dosing. Transfusion 40: 642–644

Locatelli F, Rocha V, Chastang C et al. (1999) Factors associated with outcome after cord blood transplantation in children with acute leukemia. Eurocord-Cord Blood Transplant Group. Blood 93: 3662–3671

Locatelli F, Rocha V, Reed W et al. (2003) Related umbilical cord blood transplantation in patients with thalassemia and sickle cell disease. Blood 101: 2137–2143

Lotter MG, Heyns AD, Badenhorst PN et al. (1986) Evaluation of mathematic models to assess platelet kinetics. J Nucl Med 27: 1192–1201

Lozano M, Cid J (2003) The clinical implications of platelet transfusions associated with ABO or Rh(D) incompatability. Transfus Med Rev 17: 57–68

Lundsgaard-Hansen P, Doran JE, Rubli E (1985) Purified fibronectin administration to patients with severe abdominal infections. Ann Surg 202: 745–758

Lusher J, Ingerslev J, Roberts H et al. (1998) Clinical experience with recombinant factor VIIa. Blood Coagul Fibrinolysis 9: 119–128

Lusher JM (1994) Summary of clinical experience with recombinant Factor VIII product-Kogenate. Am J Hematol 68, Suppl 3: 53–57

McCredie KB, Hersh EM, Freireich EJ (1971) Cells capable of colony formation in the peripheral blood of man. Science 171: 293–294

McCullough J, Weiblen BJ, Peterson PK (1978) Effect of temperature on granulocyte preservation. Blood 52: 301–310

McCullough J, Weiblen BJ, Fine D (1983) Effects of storage of granulocytes on their fate in vivo. Transfusion 23: 20–24

McCullough J, Steeper TA, Connelly DP et al. (1988) Platelet utilization in a university hospital. JAMA 259: 2414–2418

McMillan J, Wang E, Milner R (1994) Randomized trial of intravenous immunoglobulin S, intravenous anti-D and oral prednisone in childhood acute immune thrombocytopenic purpura. Lancet 344: 703–707

McVay PA, Toy PT (1990) Lack of increased bleeding after liver biopsy in patients with mild hemostatic abnormalities. Am J Clin Pathol 94: 747–753

Manco-Johnson MJ, Nuss R, Ceraghty S (1994) A prophylactic program in the United States: experience and issues. Semin Hematol 31 (Suppl. 2): 10–13

Mannucci PM (1986) Desmopressin (DDAVP) for treatment of disorders of hemostasis. Prog Hemost Thromb 8: 19–45

Mannucci PM (1992) Outbreak of hepatitis A among Italian patients with haemophilia. Lancet 339: 819

Mannucci PM, Federici AB, Sirchia G (1982) Hemostasis testing during massive blood replacement. Vox Sang 42: 113–123

Mansberger AR, Doran JE, Treat R (1989) The influence of fibronectin administration on the incidence of sepsis and septic mortality in severely injured patients. Ann Surg 210: 297

Mariani G, Scheibel E, Nogao T (1994) Immune tolerance as treatment of alloantibodies to Factor VIII in hemophilia. Semin Hematol 31 (Suppl. 4): 62–64

Mathé G, Amiel JL, Schwarzenberg L et al. (1965) Adoptive immunotherapy of acute leukemia: experimental and clinical results. Cancer Res 25: 1525–1531

Mavroudis D, Read E, Cottler-Fox M et al. (1996) CD34+ cell dose predicts survival, posttransplant morbidity, and rate of hematologic recovery after allogeneic marrow transplants for hematologic malignancies. Blood 88: 3223–3229

Maximow A (1909) Der Lymphozyt als gemeinsame Stamzelle der verschieden Blutelemente in der embryonalen Entwicklung und in post fetalen Leiben der Saugetiere. Folia Haematol (Leipzig) 8: 125–141

Meisel H, Reip A, Faltus B (1995) Transmission of hepatitis C virus to children and husbands by women infected with contaminated anti-D immunoglobulin. Lancet 345: 1209–1211

Menache D, O'Malley JP, Schorr JB (1990) Evaluation of the safety, recovery, half-life, and clinical efficacy of antithrombin III (human) in patients with hereditary antithrombin III deficiency. Blood 75: 33–39

Michelson AD, Barnard MR, Hechtman HB et al. (1996) In vivo tracking of platelets: circulating degranulated platelets rapidly lose surface P-selectin but continue to circulate and function. Proc Natl Acad Sci USA 93: 11877–11882

Mielke CH, Kaneshiro MM, Maher IA (1969) The standardized normal Ivy bleeding time and its prolongation by aspirin. Blood 34: 204

Migliaccio AR, Adamson JW, Stevens CE et al. (2000) Cell dose and speed of engraftment in placental/umbilical cord blood transplantation: graft progenitor cell content is a better predictor than nucleated cell quantity. Blood 96: 2717–2722

Mikaelson M, Nilsson IM, Vilhardt H (1982) Factor VIII concentrate prepared from blood donors stimulated with intranasal DDAVP. Transfusion 22: 229–233

Moake JL (2004) von Willebrand factor, ADAMTS-13, and thrombotic thrombocytopenic purpura. Semin Hematol 41: 4–14

Moake J, Chintagumpala M, Turner N (1994) Solvent/detergent-treated plasma suppresses shear induced platelet aggregation and prevents episodes of thrombotic thrombocytopenic purpura. Blood 84: 490–497

Moise KJ Jr, Cano LE, Sala D (1990) Resolution of severe thrombocytopenia in a pregnant patient with rhesus-negative blood with autoimmune thrombocytopenic purpura after intravenous rhesus immune globulin. Am J Obstet Gynecol 162: 1237–1238

Mollnes TE, Andreassen IH, Hogasen K et al. (1997) Effect of whole and fractionated intravenous immunoglobulin on complement in vitro. Mol Immunol 34: 719–729

Morell A, Schurch B, Ryser D (1980) In vivo behaviour of gamma globulin preparations. Vox Sang 38: 272–283

Moriau M, Masure R, Hurler A (1977) Haemostasis disorders in open heart surgery with extracorporeal circulation. Importance of the platelet function and the heparin neutralization. Vox Sang 32: 41

Moroff G, George VM (1990) The maintenance of platelet properties upon limited discontinuation of agitation during storage. Transfusion 30: 427–430

Moroff GH, George VM (1994) Effect on platelet properties of exposure to temperatures below 20° for short periods during storage at 20 to 24°C. Transfusion 34: 317–321

Moroff G, Holme S (1991) Concepts about current conditions for the preparation and storage of platelets. Transfusion Med Rev 5: 48–59

Moroff G, Holme S, Heaton WAL (1990) Effect of an 8-hour holding period on in vivo and in vitro properties of red cells and Factor VIII content of plasma after collection in a red cell additive system. Transfusion 30: 828–830

Moroff G, Holme S, Dabay MH et al. (1993) Storage of pools of six and eight platelet concentrates. Transfusion 33: 374–378

Moroff G, Seetharaman S, Kurtz JW et al. (2004) Retention of cellular properties of PBPCs following liquid storage and cryopreservation. Transfusion 44: 245–252

Moscow JA, Casper AJ, Kodis C et al. (1987) Positive direct antiglobulin test results after intravenous immune globulin administration. Transfusion 27: 248–249

Mourad N (1968) A simple method for obtaining platelet concentrates free of aggregates. Transfusion 8: 48

Munzer SR (1999) The special case of property rights in umbilical cord blood for transplantation. Rutgers Law Rev 51: 493–568

Murphy S (1985) Platelet storage for transfusion. Semin Hematol 22: 165–177

Murphy S (2002) What's so bad about old platelets? Transfusion 42: 809–811

Murphy S (2004) Radiolabeling of PLTs to assess viability: a proposal for a standard. Transfusion 44: 131–133

Murphy S, Gardner FH (1969) Effect of storage temperature on maintenance of platelet viability: deleterious effect of refrigerated storage. N Engl J Med 280: 1094–1098

Murphy S, Gardner FH (1971) Platelet storage at 22 degrees C; metabolic, morphologic, and functional studies. J Clin Invest 50: 370–377

Murphy S, Gardner FH (1976) Room temperature storage of platelets. Transfusion 16: 2

Murphy S, Sayar SN, Gardner FH (1970) Storage of platelet concentrates at 22°C. Blood 35: 549

Murphy S, Kahn RA, Holme S (1982) Improved storage of platelets for transfusion in a new container. Blood 60: 194–200

Murphy S, Kogen L, Holme S (1991) Platelet storage in synthetic media lacking glucose and bicarbonate. Transfusion 31: 16–20

Murphy S, Rebulla P, Bertolini F (1994) In vitro assessment of the quality of stored platelet concentrates. Transfusion Med Rev 8: 29–36

Murphy S, Shimizu T, Miripol J (1995) Platelet storage for transfusion in synthetic media: further optimization of ingredients and definition of their roles. Blood 86: 3951–3960

Nagashima M, Matsushima M, Massuoko H (1987) High-dose gammaglobulin therapy for Kawasaki disease. J Pediatr 110: 710–712

Nee R, Doppenschmidt D, Donovan DJ et al. (1999) Intravenous versus subcutaneous vitamin K1 in reversing excessive oral anticoagulation. Am J Cardiol 83: 286–287

Ng PK, Fournel MH, Lundblad JL (1981) PPF: product improvement studies. Transfusion 21: 682–685

Nilsson IM, Sundqvist SB (1984) Suppression of secondary antibody response by intravenous immunoglobulin and development of tolerance in a patient with haemophilia B and antibodies. Scand J Haematol 40 (Suppl.): 203–206

Nilsson IM, Walter H, Mikaelsson M (1979) Factor VIII concentrate prepared from DDAVP stimulated blood donor plasma. Scand J Haematol 22: 42–46

Nilsson IM, Berntorp E, Ljung R (1994) Prophylactic treatment of severe hemophilia A and B can prevent joint disability. Semin Haematol 31 (Suppl. 2): 5–10

Niosi P, Lundberg J, McCullough J et al. (1971) Blood group antibodies in human immune serum globulin. N Engl J Med 285: 1435–1436

Nydegger UE, Sturzenegger M (1999) Adverse effects of intravenous immunoglobulin therapy. Drug Safety 21: 171–185

Oberman HA (1990) Appropriate use of plasma and plasma derivatives. In: Transfusion Therapy: Guidelines for Practice. SH Summers, DM Smith, DM Agranenko (eds). Arlington, VA: Am Assoc Blood Banks

Oldenburg J, El Maarri O, Schwaab R (2002) Inhibitor development in correlation to factor VIII genotypes. Haemophilia 8 (Suppl. 2): 23–29

Ooi J, Iseki T, Takahashi S et al. (2004) Unrelated cord blood transplantation after myeloablative conditioning in patients over the age of 45 years. Br J Haematol 126: 711–714

Oral A, Nusbacher J, Hill JB et al. (1984) Intravenous gammaglobulin in the treatment of chronic idiopathic thrombocytopenic purpura in adults. Am J Med 76 (3a): 187–192

Ordman CW, Jennings CG, Janeway CA (1944) Chemical, clinical and immunological studies on the products of human plasma fractionation. XII. The use of concentrated normal human serum gamma globulin (human immune serum globulin) in the prevention and attenuation of measles. J Clin Invest 23: 541

Orthner CL, Ralston AH, Gee D (1995) The large scale production and properties of immunoaffinity-purified human activated protein C concentrate. Vox Sang 69: 309–319

Ozsahin H, von Planta M, Muller I et al. (1998) Successful treatment of invasive aspergillosis in chronic granulomatous disease by bone marrow transplantation, granulocyte colony-stimulating factor-mobilized granulocytes, and liposomal amphotericin-B. Blood 92: 2719–2724

Palm SL, Furcht LT, McCullough J (1981) Effects of temperature and duration of storage on granulocyte adhesion, spreading and ultrastructure. Lab Invest 45: 82–88

Papadopoulos EB, Ladanyi M, Emanuel D et al. (1994) Infusions of donor leukocytes to treat Epstein-Barr virus-associated lymphoproliferative disorders after allogeneic bone marrow transplantation. N Engl J Med 330: 1185–1191

Pasi KJ, Williams MD, Enayat MS et al. (1990) Clinical and laboratory evaluation of the treatment of von Willebrand's disease patients with heat-treated factor VIII concentrate (BPL 8Y). Br J Haematol 75: 228–233

Pavletic ZS, Bishop MR, Tarantolo SR et al. (1997) Hematopoietic recovery after allogeneic blood stem-cell transplantation compared with bone marrow transplantation in patients with hematologic malignancies. J Clin Oncol 15: 1608–1616

Payne TA, Traycoff CM, Laver J et al. (1995) Phenotypic analysis of early hematopoietic progenitors in cord blood and determination of their correlation with clonogenic progenitors: relevance to cord blood stem cell transplantation. Bone Marrow Transplant 15: 187–192

Pecora AL, Stiff P, Jennis A et al. (2000) Prompt and durable engraftment in two older adult patients with high risk chronic myelogenous leukemia (CML) using ex vivo expanded and unmanipulated unrelated umbilical cord blood. Bone Marrow Transplant 25: 797–799

Peerlinck K (1994) Haemophilia A: inhibitors. In: Haemorrhagic Disorders and Transfusion Medicine. European School of Medicine. SJ Machin, L Donet, PM Mannuci (eds). Bilirigate, Italy, pp. 57–60

Penny R, Rozenberg MC, Firkin BG (1966) The splenic platelet pool. Blood 27: 1

Peters AM, Klonizakis I, Lavender JP (1980) Use of 111Indium-labelled platelets to measure spleen function. Br J Haematol 46: 587–593

Peters AM, Saverymuttu SH, Wonke B (1984) The interpretation of sites of abnormal platelet destruction. Br J Haematol 57: 637–649

Peters AM, Saverymuttu SH, Bell RN (1985) Quantification of the distribution of the marginating granulocyte pool in man. Scand J Haematol 34: 111–120

Peters C, Minkov M, Matthes-Martin S et al. (1999) Leucocyte transfusions from rhG-CSF or prednisolone stimulated donors for treatment of severe infections in immunocompromised neutropenic patients. Br J Haematol 106: 689–696

Pietersz RN, Loos JA, Reesink HW (1985) Platelet concentrates stored in plasma for 72 hours at 22 degrees C prepared from buffycoats of citrate-phosphate-dextrose blood collected in a quadruple-bag saline-adenine-glucose-mannitol system. Vox Sang 49: 81–85

Pietersz RNI, Reesink HW, Dekker WJA (1987) Preparation of leukocyte-poor platelet concentrates from buffy coats. I. Special inserts for centrifuge cups. Vox Sang 53: 203–208

Pietersz RNI, Dekker WJA, Reesink HW (1989) Comparison of a conventional quadruple-bag system with a 'top and bottom' system for blood processing. Transfusion 29 (Suppl.): 8S

Pollack S, Cunningham-Rundles C, Smithwick EM (1982) High dose intravenous gamma globulin in autoimmune neutropenia. N Engl J Med 307: 253

Pollock TM, Reid D (1969) Immunoglobulin for the prevention of infectious hepatitis in persons working overseas. Lancet i: 281

Pool JG (1970) Cryoprecipitated Factor VIII concentrate. Bibl Haematol (Basel) 34: 23

Porter DL, Roth MS, McGarigle C et al. (1994) Induction of graft-versus-host disease as immunotherapy for relapsed chronic myeloid leukemia. N Engl J Med 330: 100–106

Porter DL, Collins RH Jr, Shpilberg O et al. (1999) Long-term follow-up of patients who achieved complete remission after donor leukocyte infusions. Biol Blood Marrow Transplant 5: 253–261

Power JP, Lawlor E, Davidson F (1995) Molecular epidemiology of an outbreak of infection with hepatitis C virus in recipients of anti-D immunoglobulin. Lancet 345: 1211–1213

Prentice CRM (1985) Acquired coagulation disorders. In: Coagulation Disorders. AN Ruggeri (ed.) Clinics in Haematol 14: 413–442

Preston AE, Barr A (1964) The plasma concentration of Factor VIII in the normal population. II. The effects of age, sex and blood group. Br J Haematol 10: 238

Price TH, Bowden RA, Boeckh M et al. (2000) Phase I/II trial of neutrophil transfusions from donors stimulated with G-CSF and dexamethasone for treatment of patients with infections in hematopoietic stem cell transplantation. Blood 95: 3302–3309

Przepiorka D, Anderlini P, Ippoliti C et al. (1997) Allogeneic blood stem cell transplantation in advanced hematologic cancers. Bone Marrow Transplant 19: 455–460

Rapaport SI, Zivelin A, Minow RA et al. (1992) Clinical significance of antibodies to bovine and human thrombin and factor V after surgical use of bovine thrombin. Am J Clin Pathol 97: 84–91

Rebulla P, Finazzi G, Marangoni F et al. (1997) The threshold for prophylactic platelet transfusions in adults with acute myeloid leukemia. Gruppo Italiano Malattie Ematologiche Maligne dell'Adulto. N Engl J Med 337: 1870–1875

Reed W, Walters M, Trachtenberg E et al. (2001) Sibling donor cord blood banking for children with sickle cell disease. Pediatr Pathol Mol Med 20: 167–174

Reichert CM, Weisenthal LM, Klein HG (1983) Delayed hemorrhage after percutaneous liver biopsy. J Clin Gastroenterol 5: 263–266

Reiss RF, Oz MC (1996) Autologous fibrin glue: production and clinical use. Transfusion Med Rev 10: 85–92

Rizza CR (1961) Effect of exercise on the level of anti-haemophilic globulin in human blood. J Physiol (Lond) 156: 128

Rizza CR, Biggs R (1969) Blood products in the management of haemophilia and Christmas disease. In: Recent Advances in Blood Coagulation. L Poller (ed.). London: J & A Churchill

Roback JD, Hossain MS, Lezhava L et al. (2003) Allogeneic T cells treated with amotosalen prevent lethal cytomegalovirus disease without producing graft-versus-host disease following bone marrow transplantation. J Immunol 171: 6023–6031

Robertson VM, Dickson LG, Romond EH et al. (1987) Positive antiglobulin tests due to intravenous immunoglobulin in patients who received bone marrow transplant. Transfusion 27: 28–31

Rocha M, Umansky V, Lee KH et al. (1997) Differences between graft-versus-leukemia and graft-versus-host reactivity. I. Interaction of donor immune T cells with tumor and/or host cells. Blood 89: 2189–2202

Rocha V, Wagner JE Jr, Sobocinski KA et al. (2000) Graft-versus-host disease in children who have received a cord-blood or bone marrow transplant from an HLA-identical sibling. Eurocord and International Bone Marrow Transplant Registry Working Committee on Alternative Donor and Stem Cell Sources. N Engl J Med 342: 1846–1854

Rock C, Tittley P (1990) A comparison of results obtained by two different chromium-51 methods of determining platelet survival and recovery. Transfusion 30: 407–410

Rock G, Figueredo A (1976) Metabolic changes during platelet storage. Transfusion 16: 571–579

Rodeghiero F, Castaman G, Meijer D (1992) Replacement therapy with virus-inactivated plasma concentrate in Von Willebrand's disease. Vox Sang 62: 193–200

Rooney CM, Smith CA, Ng CY et al. (1998) Infusion of cytotoxic T cells for the prevention and treatment of Epstein–Barr virus-induced lymphoma in allogeneic transplant recipients. Blood 92: 1549–1555

Roord JJ, van der Meer JWM, Kuis W (1982) Home treatment in patients with antibody deficiency by slow subcutaneous infusion of gammaglobulin. Lancet i: 689–690

Roque AC, Lowe CR, Taipa MA (2004) Antibodies and genetically engineered related molecules: production and purification. Biotechnol Prog 20: 639–654

Rousou J, Levitsky S, Gonzalez-Lavin L et al. (1989) Randomized clinical trial of fibrin sealant in patients undergoing resternotomy or reoperation after cardiac operations. A multicenter study. J Thorac Cardiovasc Surg 97: 194–203

Rowley SD, Anderson GL (1993) Effect of DMSO exposure without cryopreservation on hematopoietic progenitor cells. Bone Marrow Transplant 11: 389–393

Rubinstein P, Carrier C, Scaradavou A et al. (1998) Outcomes among 562 recipients of placental-blood transplants from unrelated donors. N Engl J Med 339: 1565–1577

Rubli E, Buessard S, Frei E (1983) Plasma fibronectin and associated variables in surgical intensive care patients. Ann Surg 197: 310

Ruggeri ZM, Ware J (1993) von Willebrand factor. FASEB J 7: 308–316

Ruggeri ZM, Pareti FI, Mannucci PM et al. (1980) Heightened interaction between platelets and factor VIII/von Willebrand factor in a new subtype of von Willebrand's disease. N Engl J Med 302: 1047–1051

Saba TM, Jaffe E (1980) Plasma fibronectin (opsonic glycoprotein), its synthesis by vascular endothelial cells and role in cardiopulmonary integrity after trauma is related to reticulo-endothelial function. Am J Med 68: 577–594

Saba TM, Blumenstock FA, Scovill WA (1978) Cryoprecipitate reversal of opsonic alpha 2 surface binding glycoprotein deficiency in septic surgical and trauma patients. Science 201: 622

Saba TM, Blumenstock FA, Shah DM (1986) Reversal of opsonic deficiency in surgical, trauma and burn patients by infusion of purified human plasma fibronectin. Am J Med 80: 229

Sacher RA, Luban NL, Strauss RG (1989) Current practice and guidelines for the transfusion of cellular blood components in the newborn. Transfusion Med Rev 3: 39–54

Sadler JE (1998) Biochemistry and genetics of von Willebrand factor. Annu Rev Biochem 67: 395–424

Salama A, Kiefel V, Mueller-Eckhardt C (1986) Effect of IgG anti-Rho(D) in adult patients with chronic autoimmune thrombocytopenia. Am J Haematol 22: 241–250

Santagostino E, Mannucci PM, Gringeri A et al. (1997) Transmission of parvovirus B19 by coagulation factor concentrates exposed to 100 degrees C heat after lyophilization. Transfusion 37: 517–522

Sanz GF, Saavedra S, Planelles D et al. (2001) Standardized, unrelated donor cord blood transplantation in adults with hematologic malignancies. Blood 98: 2332–2338

661

Saverymuttu SH, Peters AM, Keshavarzian A (1985) The kinetics of 111 Indium distribution following injection of 111 Indium labelled autologous granulocytes in man. Br J Haematol 61: 675–685

Sawyer L (2000) Antibodies for the prevention and treatment of viral diseases. Antiviral Res 47: 57–77

Schedel L (1986) Application of immunoglobulin preparations in multiple myeloma. In: Clinical Uses of Intravenous Immunoglobulins. London: Academic Press, pp. 123–132

Schiffer CA (1981) In International Forum: Which are the parameters to be controlled in platelet concentrates in order that they may be offered to the medical profession as a standardised product with specific properties? Vox Sang 40: 122–124

Schiffer CA (1990) Granulocyte transfusions: an overlooked therapeutic modality. Transfusion Med Rev 4: 2–7

Schiffer CA, Anderson KC, Bennett CL et al. (2001) Platelet transfusion for patients with cancer: clinical practice guidelines of the American Society of Clinical Oncology. J Clin Oncol 19: 1519–1538

Schmidt ML, Gamerman S, Smith HE (1994) Recombinant activated Factor VII (= FVIIa) therapy for intracranial hemorrhage in hemophilia A patients with inhibitors. Am J Hematol 47: 36–40

Schmitz N, Dreger P, Suttorp M (1995) Primary transplantation of allogeneic peripheral blood progenitor cells mobilized by filgrastin (granulocyte-colony-stimulating factor). Blood 85: 1666

Schulman S (2003) Clinical practice. Care of patients receiving long-term anticoagulant therapy. N Engl J Med 349: 675–683

Schultze HE, Heremans JF (1966) Molecular Biology of Human Proteins with Special Reference to Plasma Proteins, vol 1. Amsterdam: Elsevier

Schwartz RS (1994) Clinical studies using antithrombin III in patients with acquired antithrombin III deficiency. Semin Hematol 31 (Suppl. 1): 52–59

Schwartz RS, Gabriel DA, Aledort LM et al. (1995) A prospective study of treatment of acquired (autoimmune) Factor VIII inhibitors with high-dose intravenous gamma-globulin. Blood 86: 797–804

Scott EP, Slichter SJ (1980) Viability and function of platelet concentrates stored in CPD-adenine (CPDA1). Transfusion 20: 489–497

Scott JP, Montgomery RR (1993) Therapy of von Willebrand disease. Semin Thromb Hemost 19: 37–47

Sekul EA, Cupler EJ, Dalakas MC (1994) Aseptic meningitis associated with high-dose intravenous immunoglobulin therapy: frequency and risk factors. Ann Intern Med 121: 259–262

Seremetis SV, Aledort LM, Bergman GE et al. (1993) Three-year randomised study of high-purity or intermediate-purity factor VIII concentrates in symptom-free HIV-seropositive haemophiliacs: effects on immune status. Lancet 342: 700–703

Shen BJ, Hou HS, Zhang HQ et al. (1994) Unrelated, HLA-mismatched multiple human umbilical cord blood transfusion in four cases with advanced solid tumors: initial studies. Blood Cells 20: 285–292

Shibata Y, Baba M, Kaniyoki M (1983) Studies on the retention of passively transferred antibodies in man. II. Antibody activity in the blood after intravenous or intramuscular administration of anti-HBs human immunoglobulin. Vox Sang 45: 77–82

Shimizu M, Robinson EAE (1996) Clinical indications for FFP (Abstract). Vox Sang 70 (Suppl. 2): 59

Shimizu T, Murphy S (1993) Roles of acetate and phosphate in the successful storage of platelet concentrates prepared with the Seto additive solution. Transfusion 33: 304–310

Shively JA, Gott CL, De Jongh DS (1970) The effect of storage on adhesion and aggregation of platelets. Vox Sang 18: 204–215

Shpall EJ, Quinones R, Giller R et al. (2002) Transplantation of ex vivo expanded cord blood. Biol Blood Marrow Transplant 8: 368–376

Siadak MF, Kopecky K, Sullivan KM (1994) Reduction in transplant-related complications in patients given intravenous immuno globulin after allogeneic marrow transplantation. Clin Exp Immunol 97 (Suppl. 1): 53–57

Siena S, Schiavo R, Pedrazzoli P et al. (2000) Therapeutic relevance of CD34 cell dose in blood cell transplantation for cancer therapy. J Clin Oncol 18: 1360–1377

Simon DI, Chen Z, Xu H et al. (2000) Platelet glycoprotein ibalpha is a counterreceptor for the leukocyte integrin Mac-1 (CD11b/CD18). J Exp Med 192: 193–204

Simon TL, Sierra ER (1982) Lack of adverse effect of transportation on room temperature stored platelet concentrates. Transfusion 22: 496–497

Simon TL, Sierra E (1989) Platelet viability after extensive transportation (Abstract). Transfusion 29: S186

Simon TL, Marcus CS, Myhre BA (1987) Effects of AS-3 nutrient additive solution on 42 and 49 days of storage of red cells. Transfusion 27: 178–182

Slavin S, Ackerstein A, Weiss L et al. (1992) Immunotherapy of minimal residual disease by immunocompetent lymphocytes and their activation by cytokines. Cancer Invest 10: 221–227

Slavin S, Morecki S, Weiss L et al. (2002) Donor lymphocyte infusion: the use of alloreactive and tumor-reactive lymphocytes for immunotherapy of malignant and nonmalignant diseases in conjunction with allogeneic stem cell transplantation. J Hematother Stem Cell Res 11: 265–276

Slichter SJ (1985) Optimum platelet concentrate preparation and storage. In: Current Concepts in Transfusion Therapy. G Garratty (ed.) Arlington, VA: Am Assoc Blood Banks

Slichter SJ, Harker LA (1976a) Preparation and storage of platelet concentrates. Transfusion 16: 8–12

Slichter SJ, Harker LA (1976b) Preparation and storage of platelet concentrates. I. Factors influencing the harvest of viable platelets from whole blood. Br J Haematol 34: 395–402

Slichter SJ, Harker LA (1976c) Preparation and storage of platelet concentrates. II. Storage variables influencing platelet viability and function. Br J Haematol 34: 403–419

Slichter SJ, Harker LA (1978) Thrombocytopenia: mechanisms and management of defects in platelet production. Clin Haematol 7: 523–539

Sloand EM, Klein HG (1990) Effect of white cells on platelets during storage. Transfusion 30: 333–338

Smit WM, Rijnbeek M, van Bergen CA et al. (1998) T cells recognizing leukemic CD34(+) progenitor cells mediate the antileukemic effect of donor lymphocyte infusions for relapsed chronic myeloid leukemia after allogeneic stem cell transplantation. Proc Natl Acad Sci USA 95: 10152–10157

Smith GN, Griffiths B, Mollison DP (1972) Uptake of IgG following intramuscular and subcutaneous injection. Lancet i: 1208

Smith JK (1990) Trends in the production and use of coagulation factor concentrates. In: Developments in Hematology and Immunology, Vol 26. JK Smith (ed.) Dordrecht: Kluwer Academic Publishers

Sniecinski IJ, Petz LD, Orien L (1987) Immunohematologic problems arising from ABO incompatible bone marrow transplantation. Transplant Proc 19: 4609–4611

Sniecinski IJ, Orien L, Petz LP (1988) Immunohematologic consequences of major ABO-mismatched bone marrow transplantation. Transplantation 45: 530–534

Snyder EL, Ferri P, Brown R (1985) Evaluation of flatbed reciprocal motion agitators for resuspension of stored platelet concentrates. Vox Sang 48: 269–275

Snyder EL, Moroff T, Simon A et al. (1986) Recommended methods for conducting radiolabelled platelet survival studies. Transfusion 26: 37–42

Snyder EL, Stack G, Napychank P et al. (1989a) Storage of pooled platelet concentrates. In vitro and in vivo analysis. Transfusion 29: 390–395

Snyder EL, Horne WC, Napychank P et al. (1989b) Calcium-dependent proteolysis of actin during storage of platelet concentrates. Blood 73: 1380–1385

Soiffer RJ, Alyea EP, Hochberg E et al. (2002) Randomized trial of CD8+ T-cell depletion in the prevention of graft-versus-host disease associated with donor lymphocyte infusion. Biol Blood Marrow Transplant 8: 625–632

Solomon J, Bofenkamp T, Fahey JL et al. (1978) Platelet prophylaxis in acute non-lymphoblastic leukaemia. Lancet 1: 267

Spector I, Corn M (1967) Laboratory tests of hemostasis. The relation to hemorrhage in liver disease. Arch Intern Med 119: 577–582

Spector I, Corn M, Ticktin HE (1966) Effect of plasma transfusions on the prothrombin time and clotting factors in liver disease. N Engl J Med 275: 1032–1037

Spector SA, Gelber RD, McGrath N (1994) A controlled trial of intravenous immunoglobulin for the prevention of serious bacterial infections in children receiving zidovudine for advanced human immunodeficiency virus infection. N Engl J Med 331: 1181–1187

Stiff PJ, Murgo AJ, Zaroulis CG (1983) Unfractionated human marrow cell cryopreservation using dimethylsulfoxide and hydroxylethyl starch. Cryobiology 20: 17–24

Storb R, Prentice RL, Thomas ED (1977) Treatment of aplastic anemia by marrow transplantation from HLA identical siblings. Prognostic factors associated with graft versus host disease and survival. J Clin Invest 59: 625–632

Strauss RG (1986) Current issues in neonatal transfusions. Vox Sang 51: 1–9

Strauss RG (1993) Therapeutic granulocyte transfusions in 1993. Blood 81: 1675–1678

Stroncek DF, Leonard K, Eiber G et al. (1996) Alloimmunization after granulocyte transfusions. Transfusion 36: 1009–1015

Stroncek DF, Yau YY, Oblitas J et al. (2001) Administration of G-CSF plus dexamethasone produces greater granulocyte concentrate yields while causing no more donor toxicity than G-CSF alone. Transfusion 41: 1037–1044

Stroncek DF, Matthews CL, Follmann D et al. (2002) Kinetics of G-CSF-induced granulocyte mobilization in healthy subjects: effects of route of administration and addition of dexamethasone. Transfusion 42: 597–602

Stussi G, Muntwyler J, Passweg JR et al. (2002) Consequences of ABO incompatibility in allogeneic hematopoietic stem cell transplantation. Bone Marrow Transplant 30: 87–93

Sullivan KM, Kopecky KJ, Buckner CD (1991) Intravenous immunoglobulin to prevent graft-versus-host disease after bone marrow transplantation. N Engl J Med 324: 631–633

Sullivan KM, Storek J, Kopecky KJ et al. (1996) A controlled trial of long-term administration of intravenous immunoglobulin to prevent late infection and chronic graft-vs.-host disease after marrow transplantation: clinical outcome and effect on subsequent immune recovery. Biol Blood Marrow Transplant 2: 44–53

Sultan Y, Kazatchkine MD, Algiman M (1994) The use of intravenous immunoglobulin in the treatment of Factor VIII inhibitors. Semin Hematol 31 (Suppl.) 4: 65–66

Sutherland DR, Anderson L, Keeney M et al. (1996) The ISHAGE guidelines for CD34+ cell determination by flow cytometry. International Society of Hematotherapy and Graft Engineering. J Hematother 5: 213–226

663

Sutor AH (2000) DDAVP is not a panacea for children with bleeding disorders. Br J Haematol 108: 217–227

Sweeney JD, Holme SH, Heaton A (1995) Quality of platelet concentrates. Immunol Invest 24: 353–370

Sweeney JD, Kouttab NM, Holme S *et al.* (2004) Prestorage pooled whole-blood-derived leukoreduced platelets stored for seven days, preserve acceptable quality and do not show evidence of a mixed lymphocyte reaction. Transfusion 44: 1212–1219

Szabolcs P, Park KD, Reese M *et al.* (2003) Coexistent naive phenotype and higher cycling rate of cord blood T cells as compared to adult peripheral blood. Exp Hematol 31: 708–714

Tam DA, Morton LD, Stroncek DF *et al.* (1996) Neutropenia in a patient receiving intravenous immune globulin. J Neuroimmunol 64: 175–178

Tankersley DL (1994) Dimer formation in immunoglobulin preparations and speculations on the mechanism of action of intravenous immune globulin in autoimmune diseases. Immunol Rev 139: 159–172

Tankersley DL, Preston MS, Finlayson JS (1988) Immunoglobulin G dimer: an idiotype-anti-idiotype complex. Mol Immunol 25: 41–48

Terrault NA, Vyas G (2003) Hepatitis B immune globulin preparations and use in liver transplantation. Clin Liver Dis 7: 537–550

Thakur ML, Welch MJ, Joist JH (1976) Indium-111 labelled platelets: studies on preparation and evaluation of *in vitro* and *in vivo* functions. Thromb Res 9: 345–357

Thakur ML, Lavender JP, Arnot RN (1977a) Indium-111-labeled autologous leukocytes in man. J Nucl Med 18: 1014

Thakur ML, Coleman RE, Welch MJ (1977b) Indium-111-labeled leukocytes for the localization of abscesses: preparation, analysis, tissue distribution, and comparison with gallium-67 citrate in dogs. J Lab Clin Med 89: 217

Tharakan J, Strickland D, Burgess W (1990) Development of an immunoaffinity process for Factor IX purification. Vox Sang 58: 21–29

Tjonnfjord GE, Brinch L, Gedde-Dahl T *et al.* (2004) Activated prothrombin complex concentrate (FEIBA) treatment during surgery in patients with inhibitors to FVIII/IX. Haemophilia 10: 174–178

Tsai HM (1996) Physiologic cleavage of von Willebrand factor by a plasma protease is dependent on its conformation and requires calcium ion. Blood 87: 4235–4244

Upshaw JD Jr (1978) Congenital deficiency of a factor in normal plasma that reverses microangiopathic hemolysis and thrombocytopenia. N Engl J Med 298: 1350–1352

Vadhan-Raj S, Kavanagh JJ, Freedman RS *et al.* (2002) Safety and efficacy of transfusions of autologous cryopreserved platelets derived from recombinant human thrombopoietin to support chemotherapy-associated severe thrombocyto-penia: a randomised cross-over study. Lancet 359: 2145–2152

Valeri CR (1976) Circulation and hemostatic effectiveness of platelets stored at 4°C or 22°C: studies in aspirin-treated normal volunteers. Transfusion 16: 20–23

Valeri CR, Feingold H, Marchionni CD (1974) A simple method for freezing human platelets using 6% dimethyl sulfoxide and storage at –80°C. Blood 43: 131–136

Vamvakas EC, Pineda AA (1997) Determinants of the efficacy of prophylactic granulocyte transfusions: a meta-analysis. J Clin Apheresis 12: 74–81

Verheugt FWA, dem Borne AEGK, Décary F (1977) The detection of granulocyte alloantibodies with an indirect immunofluorescence test. Br J Haematol 36: 533

Vij R, DiPersio JF, Venkatraman P *et al.* (2003) Donor CMV serostatus has no impact on CMV viremia or disease when prophylactic granulocyte transfusions are given following allogeneic peripheral blood stem cell transplantation. Blood 101: 2067–2069

Vogler WR, Winton EF (1977) A controlled study of the efficacy of granulocyte transfusions in patients with neutropenia. Am J Med 63: 548

Wadenvik H, Kutti J (1991) The *in vivo* kinetics of 111 In and 51Cr-labelled platelets: a comparative study using both stored and fresh platelets. Br J Haematol 78: 523–528

Wagner HJ, Cheng YC, Huls MH *et al.* (2004) Prompt versus pre-emptive intervention for EBV-lymphoproliferative disease. Blood 103: 3979–3981

Wagner JE (1995) Umbilical cord blood transplantation. Transfusion 35: 619–621

Wagner JE, Kirnan NA, Steinbuch M (1995) Allogeneic sibling cord blood transplantation in 44 children with malignant and non-malignant disease. Lancet 356: 214–219

Wagner JE, Barker JN, DeFor TE *et al.* (2002) Transplantation of unrelated donor umbilical cord blood in 102 patients with malignant and nonmalignant diseases: influence of CD34 cell dose and HLA disparity on treatment-related mortality and survival. Blood 100: 1611–1618

Wall DA, Noffsinger JM, Mueckl KA *et al.* (1997) Feasibility of an obstetrician-based cord blood collection network for unrelated donor umbilical cord blood banking. J Matern Fetal Med 6: 320–323

Walter EA, Greenberg PD, Gilbert MJ *et al.* (1995) Reconstitution of cellular immunity against cytomegalovirus in recipients of allogeneic bone marrow by transfer of T-cell clones from the donor. N Engl J Med 333: 1038–1044

Wandt H, Frank M, Ehninger G *et al.* (1998) Safety and cost effectiveness of a $10 \times 10(9)$/L trigger for prophylactic platelet transfusions compared with the traditional $20 \times 10(9)$/L trigger: a prospective comparative trial in

105 patients with acute myeloid leukemia. Blood 91: 3601–3606

Warkentin PI, Hilden JM, Kersey JH (1985) Transplantation of major ABO-incompatible bone marrow depleted of red cells by hydroxyethyl starch. Vox Sang 48: 89–104

Waytes AT, Rosen FS, Frank MM (1996) Treatment of hereditary angioedema with a vapor-heated C1 inhibitor concentrate. N Engl J Med 334: 1630–1634

Weinreb S, Delgado JC, Clavijo OP et al. (1998) Transplantation of unrelated cord blood cells. Bone Marrow Transplant 22: 193–196

Weinstein RE, Bona RD, Altman AJ (1989) Severe hyponatremia after repeated intravenous administration of desmopressin. Am J Hematol 32: 258–261

Weisman LE, Stoll BJ, Kneser TJ (1992) Intravenous immunoglobulin therapy for early-onset sepsis in premature neonates. J Pediatr 121: 434–443

Weiss L, Lubin I, Factorowich I et al. (1994) Effective graft-versus-leukemia effects independent of graft-versus-host disease after T cell-depleted allogeneic bone marrow transplantation in a murine model of B cell leukemia/lymphoma. Role of cell therapy and recombinant IL-2. J Immunol 153: 2562–2567

Weiss SM, Hert RC, Gianola FJ et al. (1993) Complications of fiberoptic bronchoscopy in thrombocytopenic patients. Chest 104: 1025–1028

Whisson ME, Wakhoul A, Howman P (1993) Quantitative study of starving platelets in a minimal medium: maintenance by acetate or plasma but not by glucose. Transfusion Med 3: 103–113

White GC, Courter S, Bray GL et al. (1997) A multicenter study of recombinant factor VIII (Recombinate) in previously treated patients with hemophilia A. The Recombinate Previously Treated Patient Study Group. Thromb Haemost 77: 660–667

White JG, Krivit W (1967) An ultrastructural basis for the shape changes induced in platelets by chilling. Blood 30: 625–635

Wildt-Eggen J, Bins M, van Prooijen HC (1996) Evaluation of storage conditions of platelet concentrates prepared from pooled buffy coats. Vox Sang 70: 11–15

Wildt-Eggen J, Schrijver JG, Bins M (2001) WBC content of platelet concentrates prepared by the buffy coat method using different processing procedures and storage solutions. Transfusion 41: 1378–1383

Winston DJ, Ho WG, Gale RP (1982) Therapeutic granulocyte transfusions for documented infections. A controlled trial in ninety-five infectious granulocytopenic episodes. Ann Intern Med 97: 509–515

Wood WI, Capon DJ, Simonsen CC (1984) Expression of active human factor VIII from recombinant DNA clones. Nature (Lond) 312: 330–337

Yomtovian R, Abramson J, Quie P (1981) Granulocyte transfusion therapy in chronic granulomatous disease. Transfusion 21: 739–743

Zanjani E, Almeida-Porada G, Hangoc G et al. (2000) Enhanced short term engraftment of human cells in sheep transplanted with multiple cord bloods: implications for transplantation of adults (Abstract). Blood 96: 552a

Zaucha JM, Gooley T, Bensinger WI et al. (2001) CD34 cell dose in granulocyte colony-stimulating factor-mobilized peripheral blood mononuclear cell grafts affects engraftment kinetics and development of extensive chronic graft-versus-host disease after human leukocyte antigen-identical sibling transplantation. Blood 98: 3221–3227

Zumberg MS, del Rosario ML, Nejame CF et al. (2002) A prospective randomized trial of prophylactic platelet transfusion and bleeding incidence in hematopoietic stem cell transplant recipients: 10 000/L versus 20 000/microL trigger. Biol Blood Marrow Transplant 8: 569–576

15 Some unfavourable effects of transfusion

Adverse effects due to overloading the circulation are discussed in Chapter 2, reactions caused by red cell incompatibility in Chapter 11, and transmission of infectious agents in Chapter 16. The present chapter includes reactions due to incompatibility of white cells, platelets or plasma components. Cases in which the incompatible antibody is present in transfused plasma, or is made by grafted lymphocytes, are discussed, as well as those in which the antibody concerned is made by the recipient. Non-immunological reactions, such as those due to the presence of cytokines in stored blood components and those due to citrate anticoagulant and iron overload, are also described.

Reactions due to leucocyte antibodies

Febrile reactions due to antibodies in the recipient

Frequency of febrile reactions

The frequency of febrile reactions to transfusion depends on the type of blood component, its storage conditions and a variety of factors specific to the recipient. Of nearly 100 000 units of whole blood and red cells transfused from one blood centre in 1980, less than 1% was reported to result in a febrile reaction, and only 15% of recipients who were subsequently transfused experienced a second episode of fever (Menitove *et al.* 1982). This oft-cited statistic is undoubtedly too conservative because of an under-reporting bias in the study design. A prospective study of 531 HIV-infected and AIDS patients who received 3864 red cell units during 1745 transfusion episodes documented the frequency of fever as 16.8%, 12.4% if patients with fever in the week prior to transfusion were excluded (Lane *et al.* 2002). The study investigators found that fever associated with transfusion was recorded about four times as often as the hospital attending staff reported it using a voluntary transfusion reaction form. Fever exceeding 2°C occurred in 3.1% of transfusions. Because patients with AIDS are particularly susceptible to infection and possibly more likely to develop fever during the course of transfusion, the true rate of febrile reactions following red cell transfusion probably lies between these two values. In contrast, fever occurs in as many as 30% of platelet transfusions, a striking disparity that may reflect platelet-specific factors as well as the effects of inflammatory cytokines, chemokines and bacterial pyrogens (Chapter 16) that accumulate in platelet concentrates over the course of room temperature storage (Mangano *et al.* 1991; Heddle 1999). In a study of 598 leukaemia patients who received 8769 transfusions, fever occurred in 4.4% of patients, but rose to more than 22% if chills with rigors were included in the definition of these reactions (Enright *et al.* 2003). Only 2.2% of platelet transfusions resulted in a moderate or severe reaction of any kind.

Leucocyte antibodies in febrile reactions

The possibility that leucocyte antibodies might cause transfusion reactions was suggested by the association of potent leucoagglutinins in the serum of patients who had received multiple transfusions and who suffered febrile reactions (Brittingham and Chaplin 1957; Payne 1957). Evidence confirming this association was

Fig 15.1 Effect of transfusing the buffy coat to a patient whose serum contained leucoagglutinins. Two fractions were prepared from fresh blood: fraction I, containing many red cells with very few white cells and platelets and fraction II, containing a few red cells and most of the plasma, platelets and white cells. Transfusion of this second fraction produced a very severe febrile reaction whereas transfusion of the first 'buffy-poor' fraction produced no fever. From Brittingham and Chaplin (1957) with permission.

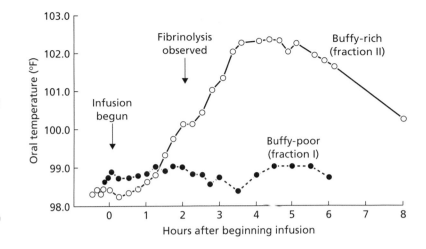

published subsequently (van Loghem *et al.* 1958). The role of leucocytes in causing transfusion reactions was shown clearly in a study of five patients who had a history of severe febrile reactions following blood transfusion and whose serum contained leucoagglutinins; transfusion of a fraction of blood containing more than 90% of the buffy coat produced a severe febrile reaction, but transfusion from the same unit of red cells and plasma with less than 10% of the buffy coat caused no reaction (Fig. 15.1). The severe reactions were characterized by flushing within 5 min of the start of transfusion and a sensation of warmth. The patient then felt well for 45 min; about 60 min after the start of the transfusion, temperature spiked and a severe febrile reaction began (Brittingham and Chaplin 1957). In complementary observations, Payne (1957) found leucoagglutinins in the serum of 32 out of 49 patients with a history of febrile transfusion reactions. Moreover, in 13 out of 15 patients receiving repeated transfusions, leucoagglutinins appeared at about the time the patients developed the first transfusion reactions. Blood containing less than 0.2×10^9 leucocytes per litre provoked no reaction in these patients.

In a detailed study of a single subject 0.4×10^9 leucocytes (the number present in 50 ml of normal blood) would not produce a reaction whereas the injection of 1.5×10^9 or more would do so regularly. The reactions produced by 1.5×10^9 leucocytes were mild when the titre of the leucoagglutinins was low, but severe at a time when the titre was high (Brittingham and Chaplin 1961). From another study of eight patients, the least number of leucocytes required to produce a reaction

varied from 0.25×10^9 to more than 25×10^9. The degree of temperature elevation was related to the number of incompatible leucocytes transfused (Perkins *et al.* 1966).

These early studies indicate that leucocyte-poor blood prepared for transfusion to patients who have had febrile reactions due to leucoagglutinins should contain fewer than 0.5×10^9 leucocytes or about 10% of the number contained in a fresh unit of whole blood. Current component filtration technology achieves leucocyte levels that are lower by several orders of magnitude.

Features of febrile reaction

By convention, an increase in body temperature of 1°C or more (body temperature > 38°C) that occurs during or within several hours of transfusion merits evaluation as a transfusion-related event. In practice, transfusion reactions related to leucocyte antibodies may include an array of signs and symptoms in addition to fever, including dyspnoea, hypotension, hypertension and rigors; placing them in the 'febrile' reaction category is convenient, but somewhat arbitrary. Patients who develop febrile reactions related to leucoagglutinins usually do not start to feel cold for at least 30 min after the transfusion has started, and signs may not develop for 60–80 min (see Fig. 15.2). However, non-specific symptoms such as chilliness, nausea and headache may precede the onset of chills and fever. Antibodies bind to the transfused leucocytes and the resulting complexes bind to and activate monocytes,

667

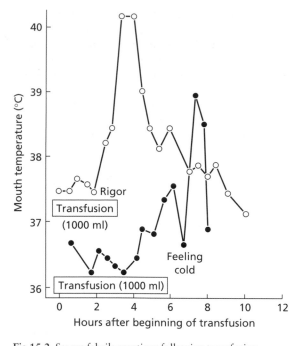

Fig 15.2 Severe febrile reactions following transfusion.
○–○, transfusion completed in 2 h; rigor (chill) began before
the transfusion was finished; ●–●, transfusion of the same
amount of blood in 5.5 h. The temperature started to rise at
the end of about 5 h. About 1 h later the patient felt cold but
did not shiver; the temperature then rose and reached its
maximum about 2 h after the end of the transfusion.

which release cytokines with pyrogenic properties
(Dzik 1992). The flushing that commonly develops
within minutes of the start of transfusion is probably
related to complement activation with the release
of vasoactive substances, while cytokine release by
monocytes may be somewhat delayed. Fever may last
for several hours, but if fever persists more than 8 h,
causes other than transfusion should be suspected.

The high fever that regularly follows transfusion
of some multiparous women and patients who have
received many transfusions is often associated with
serum leucocyte antibodies; mild febrile reactions,
observed after only one of a series of transfusions,
commonly are not (Kevy et al. 1962). Such reactions
may be mediated by antibodies undetected in standard
screening techniques or by passive transfer of cytokines
and other pyrogens (see below).

Granulocytes react with anti-HLA-A, -B and -C, as
well as with granulocyte-specific antibodies. Monocytes

react with the same HLA antibodies, with antibodies
against HLA class II antigens and with monocyte-
specific antibodies as well. Several studies support the
conclusion that HLA antibodies play a leading role in
causing febrile transfusion reactions. First, sera from
101 patients with a history of non-haemolytic transfusion reactions were tested against granulocytes
and lymphocytes using several different methods. The
highest percentage of positives was obtained with a
modified cytotoxicity test against B lymphocytes;
32% of these positive reactions, probably due to weak
HLA-A, -B or -C antibodies, were missed by the standard cytotoxicity test (Décary et al. 1984). Second, in a
study in which leucocyte agglutination, lymphocytotoxicity and immunofluorescence tests using granulocytes, lymphocytes and platelets were applied, HLA
alloantibodies were found far more frequently than
were granulocyte-specific antibodies; alloantibodies
of one kind or another were found in every case of a
reaction; in 36 out of 40 patients, leucocyte antibodies
were found, but antibodies directed against platelet-
specific antigens were detected in the remaining four
(De Rie et al. 1985). Finally, Mangano and co-workers
(1991) found a reaction rate of 14% after single-donor
platelet transfusions that fell to 6.5% when HLA-
matched platelets were used, whereas previously
Chambers and co-workers (1990) found the rate of
unmatched platelets to be almost twice that of matched
platelets. In both studies, unmatched pools of platelets
resulted in the highest reaction rates. The reduction of
febrile reactions with HLA-matched platelets has been
confirmed in other studies (Williamson et al. 1994).

Two caveats bear repeating: (1) In patients who
have had febrile reactions following transfusions, the
presence of serum alloantibodies cannot be excluded
with any confidence unless several different assay
methods and an extensive panel of cells are used.
(2) Antibodies directed against leucocyte antigens,
particularly anti-HLA, are common in multiparous
women and repeatedly transfused patients. Their presence in patients with fever does imply cause and effect.

Febrile reactions in infants

Infants seem incapable of shivering. Perhaps this
explains an apparent lack of interest in the infant's
reaction to transfusion. If an infant's temperature
is recorded at intervals after transfusion, it is not
unusual to observe rises in temperature up to 38.5°C

or thereabouts. Sometimes a temporary refusal to feed and diarrhoea accompany the rise in temperature.

Although an infant does not shiver in the early phase of a febrile reaction, the infant may look pale and its skin may feel cold. The following is an example:

Baby R, aged 5 weeks, was recovering from haemolytic disease of the newborn. Although the Hb concentration was 100 g/l, a transfusion was administered as the infant was shortly going on a journey by air and would not be under medical supervision for a long period thereafter.

Seventy-five millilitres of fresh Rh D-negative blood were injected into a scalp vein in 20 min. The infant appeared to have tolerated the transfusion well but, 75 min later, turned pale and refused to feed. During the next 2 h it was restless, and 3 h after the transfusion, its pulse rate reached 200/min. Four hours after transfusion the temperature was 39.1°C and the pulse rate 180 per minute. The temperature remained above 39°C for a further 3 h and then fell gradually. By the following day the baby appeared perfectly well.

Reactions following granulocyte transfusion

Reactions to transfused granulocytes may be severe and even life threatening. The majority of these reactions occur in patients who have pre-existing leucoagglutinins, most often HLA antibodies. Reactions have also been associated with isolated granulocyte-specific antibodies. Although fever is the most common sign, additional signs and symptoms include anxiety, sudden hypotension, hypertension, dyspnoea and cyanosis with moderate oxygen desaturation. In a study of 18 patients with chronic granulomatous disease (CGD) and frequent courses of granulocyte transfusions, 14 patients had evidence of leucocyte antibodies measured by lymphocytotoxicity, granulocyte immunofluorescence or granulocyte agglutination assays. Febrile reactions occurred in 11 out of the 14 sensitized patients; seven suffered pulmonary reactions. None of the four patients who lacked antibodies reacted to granulocyte transfusion (Stroncek 1996). A similar case with repeated severe pulmonary compromise was reported when granulocytes were transfused to a patient who was found to have a strongly positive granulocyte cross-match. That reaction has been categorized as transfusion-related acute lung injury (TRALI) (see below) (Sachs and Bux 2003). Cell labelling studies provide further evidence that these reactions are caused by granulocyte–antibody interaction. The fluorescent label, dihydrorhodamine-123, can distinguish normal granulocytes from those that lack the oxidative burst, such as granulocytes from patients with CGD. Less than 1% of transfused granulocytes could be detected by dihydrorhodamine-labelling in alloimmunized CGD patients who developed reactions during granulocyte transfusion; in contrast, measurable increments were found in patients who sustained no reaction (Heim et al. in press). Granulocyte circulation, severe febrile and pulmonary reactions may correlate less well with the presence of alloantibodies in patients with acute leukaemia and haematopoietic transplant than in those with CGD and aplastic anaemia (T Price, personal communication). Patients who develop fever with granulocyte transfusions are unlikely to derive benefit from this treatment, may become seriously ill as a result of further granulocyte transfusion and should receive only serologically compatible transfusions in the future.

Febrile reactions induced by other soluble factors in stored blood

Plasma factors have been associated with febrile transfusion reactions for more than 50 years (Dameshek and Neber 1950). As these observations occurred before the era of sterile, interconnected plastic storage bags, the plasma factor(s) may have been bacterial pyrogens, leucoagglutinins or, less likely, cytokines derived from the cellular components. Patients still develop fever after platelet transfusion even if platelet concentrates have been depleted of leucocytes immediately before the transfusion (Mangano et al. 1991; Muylle and Peetermans 1994). Heddle and co-workers (1993) demonstrated that infusion of the plasma supernatant removed from stored platelets is associated with these febrile reactions. Evidence is mounting that many febrile reactions, particularly those related to platelet concentrates, are caused by cytokines, chemokines and possibly other cell-derived soluble factors that accumulate during component storage (Heddle 1999). Viable leucocytes are the prime suspects. Leucocyte removal prior to platelet storage (and prior to cytokine elaboration) appears to reduce the number of reactions. In a randomized study of 1190 transfusions of 129 patients, the frequency of reactions was 13.6% when platelets were leucoreduced prior to storage (Heddle et al. 2002). Severe reactions declined to 1–2%. As might be expected, the frequency of febrile reactions induced by platelet concentrates increases with the length of platelet storage (Muylle *et al.* 1992; Heddle *et al.* 1993). Chills, rigors and flushing have also been associated with elevated concentrations of these soluble factors, although these symptoms alone are usually not reported as 'febrile' reactions.

The concentration of various cytokines (TNF-α, IL-1α and -β, IL-6) increases during platelet storage and correlates with the number of leucocytes in the concentrate (Muylle *et al.* 1993; Enright *et al.* 2003). IL-8 has also been found to increase during storage (Stack and Snyder 1994). Not unexpectedly, stored platelet concentrates prepared by the platelet-rich plasma (PRP) method induce febrile reactions more frequently than do concentrates prepared by the buffy coat method, which contain fewer leucocytes (Flegel *et al.* 1995; Muylle *et al.* 1996). The frequency of febrile reactions induced by plasma separated from stored platelet concentrates correlates strongly with the concentration of IL-1 and IL-6 in the plasma (Heddle *et al.* 1994).

As the leucocytes in a platelet concentrate do not contain detectable amounts of IL-1 or IL-6 immediately after preparation, the released cytokines that result must be synthesized by activated cells (probably monocytes), although no cause of the activation has been established (Gottschall *et al.* 1984). Prestorage removal of leucocytes from platelet concentrates prevents the accumulation of cytokines (Muylle and Peetermans 1994; Stack and Snyder 1994). However, the platelet has not yet been exonerated. Soluble factors associated with the platelets may play a role as well (Phipps *et al.* 2001).

Refrigerated storage almost certainly accounts for the lower frequency of fever observed after RBC transfusion compared with platelet transfusion. Even after refrigerated storage for 42 days, red blood cell (RBC) concentrates contain levels of IL-1 and IL-6 only slightly greater than at the time of collection, as cellular metabolism all but ceases at 4°C (Smith *et al.* 1993).

Effect of rate of infusion

It seems intuitive that when pyrogenic substances are being infused, the rate of infusion will affect the severity of the reactions. The recommendation for initiating transfusion slowly and for increasing the rate gradually to about 500 ml in 1 h in non-urgent cases rests in part on this reasoning. Clinical experience certainly supports an impression that febrile reactions are more severe when transfusions are given rapidly; however, surprisingly few data address this issue (see Grant and Reeve 1951).

Removal of leucocytes from red cell and platelet concentrates

The majority of febrile non-haemolytic transfusion reactions can be attenuated if not prevented entirely by ensuring that red cell concentrates contain fewer than 0.5×10^9 leucocytes (Perkins *et al.* 1966). These levels can be achieved by centrifugation and removal of the buffy coat. Red cells that have been frozen in glycerol, thawed and washed contain only 2% of the original number of leucocytes and are unlikely to cause febrile transfusion reactions (Chaplin *et al.* 1956). However, highly sensitized patients may require more rigorous treatment of red cells. In a cohort of 82 thalassaemic patients receiving chronic transfusion therapy, more than one-half experienced febrile reactions following treatment with buffy coat-reduced red cells and more than one-half of all transfusions resulted in fever. Adoption of filtration methods to remove additional leucocytes (to $< 5 \times 10^6$ per unit) reduced both figures below 5% (Sirchia 1994). Yet even leucocyte reduction to these levels does not reduce the number of febrile reactions for certain patients. In a multicentre randomized study of 531 patients with HIV infection and AIDS, 3864 red cell units were administered during 1745 transfusion episodes. Fever occurred in 16.8% of transfusions and prestorage leucocyte reduction had no effect on overall rates of elevated temperature (Lane *et al.* 2002). No explanation has been offered for the apparent heightened sensitivity of these patients to transfusion.

Removal of leucocytes from platelets reduces febrile reactions, but this technique is most effective when performed immediately following collection (see above). Although bedside filtration effectively removes leucocytes from platelet concentrates, controlled studies fail to demonstrate a reduction in either febrile reactions or severe reactions in the recipients (Williamson *et al.* 1994). Significant reductions in both febrile reactions and all categories of moderate and severe reactions have been documented when fresh platelets and platelets that are leucocyte reduced before issue are used (Enright *et al.* 2003).

The various filters used to remove leucocytes from red cell or platelet concentrates are discussed in Chapter 13.

In summary, for patients who have had previous transfusion reactions and in whom leucocyte-poor red cells are indicated, blood depleted of white cells by most methods will generally be effective. If the patient still experiences febrile reactions, blood passed through a white cell depletion filter should be used. As febrile reactions increase the patient's oxygen requirement, complicate diagnosis and cause the patient distress, and as many patients will suffer repeated reactions (Kevy et al. 1962), the common practice of delaying the use of leucocyte-reduced components until several reactions have been experienced should be abandoned.

The effect of drugs in suppressing febrile reactions

Antipyretics are used widely for treatment and prophylaxis of febrile transfusion reactions. Although generations of clinicians have endorsed their use, primarily for fever related to red cell transfusion, the effectiveness of antipyretics may vary depending upon the specific blood component transfused and the mechanism of fever production. Pre-medication for platelet concentrate transfusion has not been particularly successful in preventing chills and fever, whether related to cytokine accumulation, bacterial contamination or leucocyte antibodies (Heddle et al. 1993; Morrow et al. 1993; Wang et al. 2002). However, when volunteers were given intravenous pyrogens and aspirin (1 g) was administered at the onset of shivering, symptoms were suppressed within 20 min in all but the most severe cases; moreover, there was no subsequent rise in temperature (Dare and Mogey 1954). In a single case in which a subject was given 1 g of aspirin 1 h before the injection of 10 ml of anti-D sensitized red cells, followed by three doses of 1 g at 2-h intervals, the expected febrile reactions failed to occur (Jandl and Tomlinson 1958). For severe rigors, especially with granulocyte transfusions, intravenous meperidine 25–50 mg is remarkably effective. The mechanism of action is unknown. For less threatening reactions, paracetamol is the drug of choice in the treatment and prophylaxis of febrile reactions. Compared with aspirin, corticosteroids and non-steroidal anti-inflammatory agents, paracetamol is equally effective, does not interfere with platelet function and has a more benign adverse event profile.

No compelling evidence suggests that antihistamines prevent febrile reactions, although the use is widespread. A randomized, placebo-controlled study of highly selected oncology patients could not show that oral paracetamol 650 mg and intravenous diphen-hydramine 25 mg prevented any of an assortment of non-haemolytic transfusion reactions in recipients of leucoreduced single-donor platelets (Wang et al. 2002). In separate studies, when 5 mg of diphenhydramine hydrochloride, or 10 mg of chlorpheniramine maleate, were added to 500 ml of blood at the time of transfusion, the recipients were as likely to develop febrile reactions as those receiving untreated blood (Wilhelm et al. 1955; Hobsley 1958).

Transfusion-related acute lung injury

A severe transfusion reaction, originally termed *non-cardiogenic pulmonary oedema*, has been associated with leucocyte antibodies in donor plasma. The typical reaction is characterized by chills, fever, a non-productive cough, dyspnoea, cyanosis and hypotension or hypertension occurring within an hour or two of transfusion (Popovsky and Moore 1985). Characteristic chest radiograph findings include bilateral fluffy pulmonary infiltrates, numerous, predominantly perihilar opacities and infiltration of the lower lung fields without cardiac enlargement or engorgement of the vessels (Ward 1970). Unlike pulmonary oedema associated with circulatory overload, central venous pressure and pulmonary wedge pressure are not elevated with transfusion related acute lung injury (TRALI). Brittingham and Chaplin (1957) first described the syndrome and the ability to provoke it by injecting leucoagglutinins into a recipient. Fifty millilitres of blood containing leucoagglutinins with a titre of 256 were transfused to one of the two authors, who developed several of the above-mentioned signs and symptoms. Almost half a century later, an unusual opportunity to confirm the role of antibody specificity arose when a 34-year-old woman who underwent a single lung transplant developed pulmonary infiltrates in the transplanted lung following transfusion of leucocyte-reduced red cells containing anti-HLA-B44 in the plasma (Fig. 15.3). The donor lung expressed the HLA-B44 antigen, but the native lung did not (Dykes et al. 2000).

Several hundred cases of the classic 'pulmonary' reaction, now called TRALI, have been reported; the condition is clearly underdiagnosed and infrequently considered, especially in the intensive care setting. Severe lung injury following transfusion represents only the tip of a respiratory iceberg. Many patients with unexplained pulmonary insufficiency and severe hypoxaemia, as well as others who present with few of

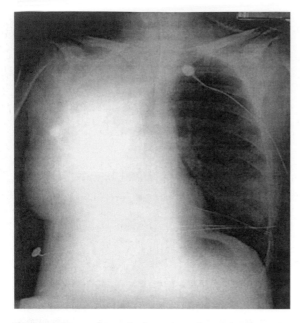

Fig 15.3 Chest radiograph of a patient who received a single lung transplant and developed TRALI in the transplanted lung following red cell transfusion. The native lung is clear on the radiograph. From Dykes *et al.* (2000) with permission.

the characteristic signs and symptoms suffer from TRALI. Some 15% of cases present with mild to moderate hypotension, typically unresponsive to fluid challenge, whereas another 15% present with hypertension (Popovsky and Haley 2000; Silliman *et al.* 2003). Mortality is estimated at 6–10% (Silliman *et al.* 1997; Wallis 2003).

In the USA, TRALI has been estimated to occur after about 1:5000 blood component transfusions (Popovsky and Moore 1985). A review of the charts of 36 evaluable recipients of plasma from one donor whose plasma containing anti-5b (anti-HNA-3a) was implicated in a fatal pulmonary reaction, found evidence of seven mild-to-moderate and eight severe pulmonary reactions (Kopko *et al.* 2002; Silliman *et al.* 2003). Only two of the eight severe reactions had been reported to the hospital transfusion service, and only 2 out of the 15 reactions were known to the blood collector. European haemovigilance studies report a lower incidence (Andreu *et al.* 2002).

TRALI has been observed following transfusion of most plasma-containing blood components. The single exception appears to be solvent detergent-treated plasma where pooling of 12 000 units during manufacture may dilute even high-titre antibody present in any single unit. As little as 2 ml of plasma seems to be sufficient to cause respiratory distress. In most cases the responsible antibodies are found in the donor. However, TRALI may also occur when the antibodies are present in the recipient and granulocytes are transfused (Ward 1970; Gans *et al.* 1988; Stroncek 1996). The pulmonary infiltrates and respiratory compromise may persist for 24 to 48 h.

Antibodies directed against numerous leucocyte antigens have been implicated in TRALI, including HLA antibodies (Andrews *et al.* 1976; Popovsky and Moore 1985; Gans *et al.* 1988; Eastlund *et al.* 1989; Kao *et al.* 2003), granulocyte-specific antibodies [anti-NA2, (Yomtovian *et al.* 1984); anti-NB2 (van Buren *et al.* 1990) and anti-5b (Nordhagen *et al.* 1986; Kopko *et al.* 2002)]. Dooren and co-workers (1998) reported a 31-year-old previously healthy man who suffered a severe pulmonary reaction after a 10-ml infusion of an experimental intravenous gamma globulin concentrate containing monocyte-reactive IgG antibodies. An intradonor leucocyte–antibody reaction in a patient receiving multiple platelet units has also been associated with TRALI (Virchis *et al.* 1997). In 20–30% of TRALI cases, no leucocyte antibody is detected. Absence of antibody may mean that the syndrome has an alternative cause (see below) or that the culprit is an antibody not detected by current methods, an important consideration as therapeutic monoclonal antibodies are used increasingly in the clinic.

Pathogenesis of TRALI

The exact mechanism of TRALI, and therefore the essential characteristics of the antibodies responsible for it, remains uncertain. However, in an *in vitro* model in which isolated rabbit lungs and 5b antibodies were used, severe vascular leakage could be induced, but only in the presence of rabbit complement (Seeger *et al.* 1990). This finding implies that activation of complement is essential for inducing TRALI. Fragments of activated C5 injected into rabbits have been shown to produce pulmonary inflammation, characterized by accumulation of neutrophils and oedema (Larsen *et al.* 1980; Henson *et al.* 1982). An alternative mechanism that implicates bioactive lipids capable of priming neutrophil degranulation has been proposed (Silliman *et al.* 1997). In a prospective study of TRALI, Silliman and co-workers (2003) observed 90 instances of TRALI in 81 patients, a frequency of 1 in 1120 components transfused. HLA antibodies were detected in only 3.6%. Significant associations were found with increasing length of platelet storage, increased leucocyte priming activity, lipid priming activity and IL-6 concentration. In a retrospective analysis of 10 patients with TRALI, each had an antecedent 'first event' such as surgery, sepsis cytokine administration or massive transfusion (Silliman *et al.* 1997). These authors propose a 'two-hit model' that might explain antibody-negative cases of TRALI as well as the absence of clinical reactions in some susceptible patients who receive passively transfused antibody. However, it is clear that antibody alone can effect TRALI in an otherwise healthy subject (Dooren *et al.* 1998).

Prevention and treatment of TRALI

Several strategies have been proposed to prevent TRALI. Many investigators recommend disqualification of donors associated with a case of TRALI, although most will reinstate such donors if further study detects no evidence of an antibody to a leucocyte antigen. In the Netherlands, plasma that tests positive for HLA antibodies is discarded. Few cases of TRALI have been reported since the initiation of this policy. In a randomized study, Palfi and co-workers (2001) report that plasma from multiparous women is more likely to impair pulmonary function in intensive care patients. The UK has disqualified all multiparous females from plasma donation, a policy that seems somewhat extreme in the absence of evidence that such plasma infusions are implicated disproportionately in transfusion reactions. Washing red cell components will remove both antibody and lipid priming activity; however, such a recommendation, even for major surgical procedures, seems premature.

The treatment of TRALI requires prompt and vigorous respiratory support. Oxygenation and mechanical ventilatory assistance are often necessary (Popovsky *et al.* 1992). Plasmapheresis to remove the offending antibody and corticosteroids to reduce the inflammatory response have been recommended on occasion; however, little evidence supports their routine use. Patients who recover appear to suffer no residual pulmonary impairment.

Graft-versus-host disease

Transfusion-associated graft-versus-host disease (TA-GvHD) occurs when immunocompetent allogeneic lymphocytes in a blood component engraft in the recipient, proliferate and mount an attack against the host tissues. The earliest reports of what was once thought to be a rare and invariably fatal disease involved children with immunodeficiency syndromes. The clinical picture evoked comparison with the runt syndrome developed by newborn mice that were challenged with adult splenocyte infusion (Hathaway *et al.* 1965). TA-GvH disease is probably underdiagnosed because the syndrome often affects patients who are already severely ill. The combination of symptoms may be wrongly attributed to the underlying disease, intercurrent infection or a severe reaction to a drug. Although baseline prospective studies are lacking, the frequency of TA-GvHD appears to be increasing as a result of increases in the surgical procedures, immunosuppressive therapies and transfusion strategies that predispose to allogeneic cell engraftment.

Circulating lymphocyte chimerism

Lymphocyte chimerism in fraternal twins, in transplant recipients and (bidirectional) in maternal–child pairs has long been recognized, but only relatively recently has the extent of chimerism following blood transfusion been appreciated (Schechter *et al.* 1972; Lee *et al.* 1999). Although the detailed fate of transfused lymphocytes is unknown, Lee and co-workers (1999) followed the kinetics of transfused lymphocytes in 10 otherwise immunocompetent trauma victims who received multiple units of red cells stored for two weeks or less. Seven of the 10 patients had evidence of multilineage (CD4, CD8, CD15, CD19) cell proliferation and circulation for up to 1.5 years; none developed GvHD.

Features of TA-GvHD

The main features of TA-GvHD involve a complex of fever and rash, nausea, vomiting and watery or bloody diarrhoea, hepatitis, lymphadenopathy and pancytopenia. Bone marrow aplasia differentiates TA-GvHD from the GvHD that follows allogeneic bone marrow transplantation. The dermatological features usually begin as a central erythematous, maculopapular eruption, which spreads to the extremities and may progress to generalized erythroderma and the formation of bullae. The histological features of most affected tissues, although not pathognomonic, are sufficiently typical, so that skin biopsy, once considered, proves an easy, sensitive and relatively benign course to early diagnosis.

TA-GvHD disease occurs between 4 and 30 days after transfusion. When the full-blown syndrome is observed and multiple organ systems are involved, mortality is high, approaching 90% (von Fliedner *et al.* 1983; Juji *et al.* 1989). However, less severe disease, especially if transient, may not be recognized, much less reported. The postoperative erythroderma syndrome reported primarily in Japan is one such example (Ito *et al.* 1988). TA-GvHD has been observed after transfusion of whole blood, packed red cells, platelet concentrates, granulocyte concentrates and fresh plasma, but not after fresh-frozen plasma or cryoprecipitate (Anderson and Weinstein 1990). Fresh blood may predispose to lymphocyte engraftment, although 'freshness' may be no more than a surrogate marker for the number of immunocompetent lymphocytes in the component.

Factors that predispose to TA-GvHD

TA-GvH disease has been reported in six clinical circumstances:

1 *In subjects with an immature immunological system, such as fetuses following intrauterine transfusion, premature infants after exchange transfusion and full-term infants after transfusion and exchange.* Two cases of fatal GvHD in immunologically normal infants who had been given intrauterine transfusions at 30 and 32 weeks, with blood that had been stored for not more than 48 h before transfusion, were reported by Parkman and co-workers (1974). Both infants, born at 36 weeks, were treated by exchange transfusion, but died 2–3 weeks after birth. The cells causing the GvH reaction came from the donors used for the exchange transfusion. TA-GvHD following exchange transfusion in premature infants has also been observed (Seemayer and Bolande 1980). Of the 27 cases of TA-GvHD reported in Japanese newborns over a 10-year interval, 20 were in premature infants and seven in full-term infants. Seventeen infants received red cell transfusion. Twenty-three infants received

blood less than 72 h old, often from relatives (Ohto and Anderson 1996a).

2 *In subjects with an impaired immunological system, for example thymic alymphoplasia, severe combined immunodeficiency disease and Wiskott–Aldrich syndrome.* In these cases, GvHD, which may occur following a single transfusion, is usually fatal. However, no cases of TA-GvHD have been reported in patients with AIDS, despite *in vitro* evidence of profound immunodeficiency (Kaslow *et al.* 1987). Perhaps HIV destroys or incapacitates the transfused lymphocytes. Lymphocyte microchimerism is rarely detected in multitransfused patients with HIV/AIDS (Kruskall *et al.* 2001).

3 *In patients with an immunological system impaired by immunosuppressive medications, for example patients treated for acute leukaemia (Ford et al. 1976) or Hodgkin's disease (Burns et al. 1984), and patients with stem cell and organ transplants (Wisecarver et al. 1994).* The increasing use of purine analogues with potent immunosuppressive properties, such as fludarabine and cladribine, for both malignant conditions and autoimmune disorders presents a singular challenge for clinicians. During the evaluation of fludarabine, three out of eight treated patients with B-cell chronic lymphocytic leukaemia developed TA-GvHD (Maung *et al.* 1994). Subsequent experience led to the recommendation to transfuse only gamma-irradiated blood components. However, evidence of immune dysregulation after treatment with this powerfully immunosuppressive class of drug may persistent for a year or more. Widespread use of these agents among patients who do not traditionally require transfusion increases the chance of overlooking patients at risk for TA-GvHD when transfusion is administered:

A 42-year-old woman was treated on an experimental protocol with three courses of fludarabine and cyclophosphamide for systemic lupus erythematosis. Ninety days later, she was treated at an institution in a distant state where she required transfusion of 2 units of red cells and 6 units of pooled platelets. The implications of her earlier immunosuppressive treatment were not appreciated. Two weeks later she developed fever, rash, hyperbilirubinaemia and marrow aplasia, which proved to herald fatal TA-GvHD. Molecular testing of her lymphocytes detected her two native HLA haplotypes as well as two haplotypes identical to those from one of the platelet donors (Leitman *et al.* 2003).

4 *In immunocompetent patients TA-GvH disease may occur when a blood donor who is homozygous at*

the HLA loci shares one of the patient's HLA haplotypes. In this situation the patient is incapable of rejecting the donor's T lymphocytes; however, donor cells can react against the HLA antigens encoded by the patient's non-shared haplotype (Sakatibara and Juji 1986; Ito *et al*. 1988; Otsuka *et al*. 1989, 1991; Thaler *et al*. 1989). This situation occurs increasingly as relatives of patients 'direct' their blood donations. Otherwise, the chance that a donor is homozygous for one of the patient's haplotypes is very small in the ethnically diverse populations of most North American and European countries. The risk of TA-GvHD estimated by one model lies between 1:17 700 and 1:39 000 in white people in the USA, but is far greater among first-degree relatives and in populations such as Japan (estimated risk 1:600–1:7900) in which homozygosity for HLA haplotypes is common (Wagner and Flegel 1995).

5 *In patients with certain malignancies, particularly acute lymphocytic leukaemia, Hodgkin's disease, lymphoma and neuroblastoma, but also with glioblastoma, rhabdomyosarcoma and other solid tumours*. The malignancy itself may represent an independent risk factor for TA-GvHD (Anderson and Weinstein 1990; Ohto and Anderson 1996b). The respective roles of the chemotherapy and HLA homozygosity are often difficult to dissect out of the various case reports.

6 *In patients undergoing cardiac surgery in Japan*. The prevalence of TA-GvHD, most often presenting with postoperative erythroderma, has been calculated to be as high as 0.47% (Juji *et al*. 1989; Ohto and Anderson 1996b). Whether this high frequency results from the surgical procedure and drug administration, the use of fresh blood, the use of directed donations, a donor population with unusually high HLA homology or a combination of factors cannot be determined easily.

Diagnosis and prevention of TA-GvHD

The diagnosis of post-transfusion GvH disease can be made when the appropriate clinical picture is supported by skin biopsy; diagnosis is confirmed by detection of donor DNA. A technique based on the analysis of polymorphisms associated with variations in the length of dinucleotide or trinucleotide microsatellite repeats has been described (Wang *et al*. 1994).

In order to avoid the risk of GvHD from blood transfusion, the transfused components must be irradiated to inactivate donor T lymphocytes. T-cell responses become undetectable only after exposure to at least 25 Gy (Pelszynski *et al*. 1994). Prevention has been approached by both targeted and global irradiation strategies. Irradiation of cellular components has been advised for patients (1) with congenital immune deficiencies; (2) undergoing high-dose chemotherapy; (3) with Hodgkin's disease and for (4) intrauterine transfusions; (5) transfusions for premature infants; and (6) HLA-matched platelet transfusions (Petz *et al*. 1993; Benson *et al*. 1994; Pelszynski *et al*. 1994) and for 'fresh' components (stored for 3 days or less). However, some oncology units and paediatric hospitals have elected to irradiate all blood components, and in Japan, blood component irradiation is universal. Photochemical treatment of blood components to reduce transmission of infectious agents may have the added benefit of protection against TA-GvHD (Grass *et al*. 1999).

Data from a mouse model suggest that as few as 10^7 lymphocytes per kilogram can induce the syndrome. Although methods are available to prepare blood components with such low levels of leucocyte contamination, removal of leucocytes from blood components by centrifugation or filtration has not been proven to prevent TA-GvHD. Leucocyte reduction alone is therefore not recommended as a measure to prevent TA-GvHD (see Anderson 1995).

Treatment for TA-GvHD ranges from difficult to singularly unsuccessful. A variety of new approaches based on recent information regarding pathogenesis have been reviewed (Williamson 1998).

Reactions due to platelet antibodies

Febrile reactions

The role of platelet antibodies in causing transfusion reactions is difficult to assess, first because suspensions of platelets are always contaminated to some extent with leucocytes, and second because platelet alloantibodies are usually accompanied by leucocyte antibodies. Fever resulting from reactions to platelet-specific antibodies must be uncommon; however, Kroll and coworkers (1993) reported six cases of fever in patients with antibodies and post-transfusion purpura, who were unsuccessfully transfused with platelets. Fever, rash and thrombocytopenia were also observed in patients who were infused with plasma containing platelet-specific antibodies (Ballem *et al*. 1987). There is no doubt that the destruction of platelets by other alloantibodies can cause adverse reactions. The association was shown convincingly by Aster and Jandl (1964). HLA-A2-negative recipients were transfused with HLA-A2-positive platelets and, a day or two later, with serum containing anti-HLA-A2. In three out of the four recipients, frontal headache developed at 30 min and rigors at 45–50 min (lasting 15–30 min), followed by fever.

As mentioned above, only platelet-specific antibodies were detectable in the serum of four of 40 patients who developed a typical febrile reaction after transfusion (De Rie *et al.* 1985). However, the observation that febrile reactions may be associated with the accumulation of cytokines in stored platelets complicates interpretation of these findings.

Post-transfusion purpura

In this uncommon syndrome, some patients with platelet-specific alloantibodies develop profound thrombocytopenia between 2 days and 2 weeks after a transfusion. The clinical syndrome is characterized by purpura, epistaxis, gastrointestinal bleeding and haematuria. If untreated, the course may be mild and self-limited, lasting as little as a few days or as long as several months. However, haemorrhage can be dramatic, and even when treated, mortality is reported as 5–10% (Kroll *et al.* 1993). It is important to distinguish this disorder from the more common syndrome of heparin-induced thrombocytopenia and thrombosis (HITT), as the clinical course, management and outcome are quite different (Lubenow *et al.* 2000).

In the first recorded example of post-transfusion purpura (PTP), a platelet-specific antibody was detected and named anti-Zw^a (van Loghem *et al.* 1959), but only later was the antibody recognized as the cause of thrombocytopenia. Shulman and co-workers (1961) described two women who developed severe generalized purpura with thrombocytopenia 6–7 days after transfusion; in both, a platelet antibody termed anti-Pl^{A1} (later shown to be identical with anti-Zw^a) was present. The investigators postulated that these two patients had been immunized to Pl^{A1} previously during pregnancy, and that the subsequent transfusion of Pl^{A1+} platelets had stimulated an anamnestic response. The mechanism by which the patient's native Pl^{A1-} platelets were destroyed was (and remains) more problematic. The authors suggested that sufficient

Pl^{A1} antigen from transfused platelets circulated at least 1 week after transfusion, interacted with anti-Pl^{A1} and somehow caused the non-specific destruction of the patient's own Pl^{A1}-negative platelets (Shulman *et al.* 1961) (see below). However, the authors did not succeed in demonstrating residual Pl^{A1} antigen in their patients. (Pl^{A1}/Zwa has now been renamed HPA-1a; see Chapter 13).

Almost all PTP patients are women; most appear to have been immunized by previous pregnancies. In a few cases, men, or women who have either never been pregnant or who had only HPA-1a-negative children, have been immunized by a previous transfusion; one case has been described in a woman without a recognized previous pregnancy or transfusion (Nicholls *et al.* 1970). Of the several hundred reported cases, only five were men, four of whom had been transfused many years before the transfusion implicated in PTP (Shulman 1991).

In almost all cases, the platelet-specific antibodies responsible for PTP are directed against antigens located on the GPIIb–IIIa complex. In a Joint European Study comprising 104 cases, anti-HPA-1a was found in 88, anti-HPA-1b in five, anti-HPA-3a in six and anti-HPA-3b in one case (Mueller-Eckhardt 1991). Antibodies against an antigen on GPI^a–IIa (anti-HPA-5b) were found in one case (Christie *et al.* 1991). In another case the alloantibody anti-Nak^a (GPIV) was detected, but thrombocytopenia in this case may not have represented PTP (Bierling *et al.* 1995).

Anti-HPA-1a has usually been found in its highest titre on about the seventh day after transfusion and in many cases has disappeared completely within the following month. However, in one case the antibody persisted at 50% of its peak level after 12 months (Lau *et al.* 1980) and, in another, remained detectable for 18 months. The antibody was IgG alone in six out of eight cases and a combination of IgM and IgG in the remaining two. The IgG antibody was IgG1 alone in five cases and IgG1/IgG3 combined in three others. In most cases, the antibody activated complement (Pegels *et al.* 1981).

Pathogenesis of post-transfusion purpura

The mechanism of destruction of the patient's own platelets in PTP remains unknown. The following hypotheses have been proposed:

Immune complex absorption. Shulman and co-workers (1961) suggested that HPA-1a antigens present in the donor blood form immune complexes with anti-HPA-1a in the patient or that such complexes might be released after destruction of donor platelets. In either case, the complexes might adhere to the patient's platelets, which would subsequently be sequestered. Particulate HPA-1a antigen has been detected in stored blood from HPA-1a+ donors (Shulman *et al.* 1961) and an increased amount of IgG has been demonstrated on the recipient's platelets in several cases – up to 10 times the normal amount in one case on the fourth day after the onset of thrombocytopenia (Cines and Schreiber 1979). Increased antibody was demonstrable by immunofluorescence in two cases during the acute phase of the illness (Pegels *et al.* 1981) and, together with IgA and IgM, in five cases, in three of which anti-HPA-1a could be eluted from the patient's HPA-1a– platelets (von dem Borne and van der Plas-van Dalen 1985). In two cases anti-HPA-1a could be eluted from the patient's platelets even after the platelet count had returned to normal (Taaning and Skov 1991). An argument against the immune complex theory is a lack of correlation between the titre of anti-HPA-1a and the severity of thrombocytopenia (Hamblin *et al.* 1985; Chong *et al.* 1986). However, this may be due to differences in the immunochemical characteristics of the antibodies.

One possible explanation for the adherence of immune complexes to platelets in PTP involves the interaction of specific glycoproteins on the platelet membrane. In almost all cases of PTP, the platelet antigens involved are found either on glycoprotein GPIIb (HPA-3a, HPA-3b) or on GPIIIa (HPA-1a, HPA-1b; HPA-4a). GPIIb and GPIIIa associate readily to form the complex GPIIb–IIIa; in fact, under experimental conditions, these proteins can be kept apart only in the absence of Ca^{2+} (Kunicki *et al.* 1981; Hagen *et al.* 1982; Howard *et al.* 1982). It is possible that fragments of HPA-1a+ platelets, if they contain GPIIb–IIIa, adhere to GPIIb–IIIa on intact HPA-1a– platelets. When the platelet fragments are bound to IgG (i.e. anti-HPA-1a), the intact HPA-1a– platelets with the adherent immune complexes undergo destruction by the mononuclear phagocyte system (MPS). In support of this theory is the observation that patients with Glanzmann's disease, whose platelets lack GPIIb–IIIa, and who have antibodies

against determinants on GPIIb–IIIa, have not developed PTP. In addition, two cases in which anti-HPA-5b was involved have been described; in one instance, HPA-5b was the sole antibody (Christie *et al.* 1991) and in the other, anti-HPA-1b was present as well (Walker *et al.* 1988). HPA-5b is located on GPI[a], which forms a complex with GPIIa, so that the mechanism described above may be the same in these cases.

Binding of HPA-1a antigen to recipient's platelets. *In vitro*, HPA-1a antigen in plasma from HPA-1a+ subjects is bound by HPA-1a– platelets (Kickler *et al.* 1986). If plasma containing HPA-1a antigen is transfused to HPA-1a– subjects, the antigen may bind to the recipient's platelets and thus render them susceptible to destruction by anti-HPA-1a.

Formation of crossreacting antibodies. It has been proposed that in the secondary immune response, in addition to anti-HPA-1a, crossreactive antibodies are formed against an epitope common to HPA-1a and -1b (Morrison and Mollison 1966). Crossreactive antibodies could not be detected, but the techniques used at that time were insensitive (see below).

Formation of autoantibodies. Another explanation for PTP proposes the formation of autoantibodies during the secondary immune response to the alloantigen; the difference between crossreactive antibodies (see above) and autoantibodies may be more one of definition than of biology.

In animals, alloimmunization against platelets may induce the formation of autoantibodies and thrombocytopenia (Gengozian and McLaughlin 1978). In some cases, when sensitive techniques were used, serum taken during the acute phase was found to react with HPA-1a– platelets including the patient's own platelets taken after recovery (Pegels *et al.* 1981; Minchinton *et al.* 1990). Furthermore, eluates from patients' platelets in the acute phase reacted weakly with HPA-1a– platelets although much more strongly with HPA-1a+ platelets (von dem Borne and van der Plas-van Dalen 1985). Such reactions with HPA-1a– platelets probably result from auto-antibodies, or from crossreactive antibodies. However, in most cases acute phase serum does not react with HPA-1a– platelets and the role of autoantibodies in PTP remains unclear.

Post-transfusion purpura: persisting puzzles

One of the many perplexing features of PTP is the unpredictability of disease recurrence. No untoward episode occurred in two cases in which HPA-1a+ blood was transfused to patients who had previously suffered from PTP, even although anti-HPA-1a was still detectable in the serum. The explanation may be that some special characteristic of the antibody is required for inducing PTP. Shulman and co-workers (1961) noticed that the anti-HPA-1a antibodies in their first two patients with PTP were complement fixing in the acute phase but not in the recovery phase. Perhaps a sufficient number of immune complexes to induce PTP is released only with intravascular destruction of platelets.

PTP may recur with re-exposure years after the initial episode. An HPA-1a-negative patient who had two relatively mild episodes of thrombocytopenia separated by an interval of 3 years, both occurring a week or two after transfusion, was found to have potent anti-HPA-1a in her plasma (Soulier et al. 1979). Shulman's original patient, who failed to develop thrombocytopenia after repeated exposure to HPA-1a+ in the months after her first episode, sustained a second, dramatic episode of thrombocytopenia following transfusion for cardiac surgery more than a decade later (NR Shulman, personal communication). Another patient had three episodes of PTP due to anti-HPA-1a (Budd et al. 1985).

A curious relationship is worth noting between PTP and neonatal alloimmune thrombocytopenia (NAIT), two different manifestations of sensitization to HPA-1a. Although 2% of the USA population lacks HPA-1a, PTP and NAIT occur less frequently than might be expected. A 'two-hit' mechanism has been proposed to explain this discrepancy (de Waal et al. 1986). The majority of PTP and NAIT patients express the HLA-DR3 allele, and all have the supertypic determinant DRw52. DRw52a may be the class II chain that presents the HPA-1a immunogenic peptide to antigen-specific T cells to initiate the immune response. According to this hypothesis, the majority of patients must inherit at least two specific gene loci (DRw52a and homozygous HPA-1b) to develop anti-HPA-1a and be rendered 'at risk' for PTP and NAIT. It is equally puzzling that among the multiparous women who have developed anti-HPA-1a and subsequent PTP, none has been reported with NAIT.

Management of post-transfusion purpura

Many patients have been treated with corticosteroids, usually without benefit. Administration of prednisone in doses of approximately 1–2 mg/kg per day has produced a prompt rise in platelet count in a few instances (Vaughan-Neil et al. 1975; Slichter 1982).

Exchange transfusion produced excellent responses in two of the original cases (Shulman et al. 1961; Cimo and Aster 1972) and, subsequently, many examples of rapid response to plasma exchange have been recorded. However, in at least one case the exchange of 5 l of plasma in 3 days produced no improvement (Erichson et al. 1978).

Until recently, transfusion of HPA-1a-negative platelets to patients with established PTP due to anti-HPA-1a had been considered fruitless (Vogelsang et al. 1986; Mueller-Eckhardt and Kiefel 1988). This experience contrasts with the successful practice of transfusing antigen-negative platelets to neonates with NAIT. However, infusions of large numbers of antigen-negative platelets can effect transient increases in the patient's platelet count and clinical haemostasis in PTP (Brecher et al. 1990; Win et al. 1995). Antigen-negative platelets, when available – usually from the patient's relatives – can be a critical temporizing measure in emergencies. The combination of antigen-negative platelets and IVIG (see below) can reverse the course of the disease within 24 h.

Treatment with high-dose IVIG has altered the management of PTP and has become the initial treatment of choice. Following IVIG infusion, 16 out of 17 patients achieved normal platelet counts within a few days. Relapse occurred in five patients, but platelet counts returned to normal after a second dose of IVIG (Mueller-Eckhardt and Kiefel 1988). In one patient with massive bleeding, PTP was refractory to corticosteroids, IVIG and plasma exchange. An immediate and sustained rise in the platelet count followed splenectomy (Cunningham and Lind 1989).

Effect of transfusing platelet alloantibodies

Experimental studies

The effect of transfusing plasma containing platelet alloantibodies to a normal subject was described by Harrington (1954). The donor was a subject who had received many transfusions previously. Potent platelet agglutinins were found in his plasma and an injection of 10 ml into a normal subject produced profound thrombocytopenia.

Similarly, Shulman and co-workers (1961) showed that a transfusion of as little as 5–10 ml of plasma containing potent complement-fixing anti-HPA-1a would produce thrombocytopenia in normal HPA-1a+ subjects. In a subsequent review, Shulman and co-workers (1964) concluded that the concentration of alloantibody capable of producing effects *in vivo* was about 10 times less than the minimum concentration detectable by the most sensitive tests *in vitro*.

Further studies. ^{51}Cr-labelled HLA-A2 platelets were transfused to four recipients whose own platelets lacked the antigen; 1–2 days later various amounts of serum containing anti-HLA-A2 were injected. This serum, in the presence of positive platelets, fixed complement *in vitro* at a dilution of 1 in 300. In the first recipient the injection of 0.25 ml of serum produced clearance of the labelled platelets with a $T_{1/2}$ of 160 min and sequestration only in the spleen. In the second recipient the injection of 0.5 ml of serum produced clearance with a $T_{1/2}$ of 80 min with sequestration in both liver and spleen, and the injection of 2.0 ml of serum brought about clearance with a $T_{1/2}$ of 15 min and sequestration in the liver. Three of the four subjects developed febrile reactions (Aster and Jandl 1964).

Clinical reactions

Following the transfusion of 80 ml of blood, a patient developed a severe reaction characterized by dyspnoea, rash and fever; there was marked oozing of blood and the platelet count fell from $193 \times 10^9/l$ to $11 \times 10^9/l$. The donor plasma was found to contain anti-HPA-1a with a titre of 1000; the patient was HPA-1a+. Three previous recipients of blood from the same donor had developed unexplained thrombocytopenia (Scott *et al.* 1988). In a similar case, a patient developed severe thrombocytopenia immediately after receiving a unit of red blood cells that contained strong anti-HPA-1a (Ballem *et al.* 1987). Compared with six reported cases involving passive transfer of anti-HPA-1, milder thrombocytopenia has been reported following infusion of a unit of FFP that contained anti-HPA-5b; this observation may be related to the lower number of GPIa–IIa molecules on the platelet surface (2000) than with GP IIb/IIIa (60 000) (Warkentin *et al.* 1992).

Granulocytopenia following transfusion of incompatible platelets

In two patients with aplastic anaemia, the transfusion of HLA-incompatible platelets was followed by a prolonged decrease in the number of circulating granulocytes. At 20 h, the count was still only 30% of the pre-transfusion value and remained depressed at 48 h. No rebound granulocytosis, as noted after the transfusion of incompatible red cells, was found. HLA-matched platelets did not cause granulocytopenia (Herzig *et al.* 1974). The authors discussed the possibility that the transfusion of incompatible platelets may increase the risk of infection.

Reactions due to transfused proteins

Immediate-type hypersensitivity reactions following plasma transfusion

Following the transfusion of plasma-containing blood components, the recipient may develop an anaphylactic-type reaction; the severest form (anaphylactic shock) is characterized by flushing, hypotension, substernal pain, laryngospasm and dyspnoea, and the mildest simply by urticaria (hives). Common skin hypersensitivity reactions are IgE mediated. Symptoms and signs, usually pruritus, urticaria and angioedema but including a wide range of cutaneous eruptions, have been attributed to histamine release. Severe reactions also appear to be IgE mediated, but involve a variety of chemical mediators including fragments of complement components, C3a, C4a and C5a, tryptase, cytokines, leukotrienes and platelet activating factor (Kemp and Lockey 2002).

Many cases of anaphylactic shock are attributed to an interaction between transfused IgA and class-specific anti-IgA (Chapter 14) in the recipient's plasma, but often the cause of the reaction is unknown.

The frequency of severe anaphylactic reactions following transfusion is very low, one case per 20 000 transfusions in one series (Bjerrum and Jersild 1971). In contrast, urticaria during transfusion is relatively common. Kevy and co-workers (1962) report the incidence at 1.1%; in another series in which even the occasional weal was counted, the incidence was approximately 3% (Stephen *et al.* 1955). In a retrospective analysis of 1613 transfusion reactions during a 9-year period at a single institution, allergic reactions accounted for 17%, but of these only 7% were severe, accounting for 1.7% of all transfusion reactions. In a prospective study of platelet transfusion, 8679 transfusions in 598 patients, extensive urticaria occurred during 0.4% of transfusions and in 4.4% of patients (Enright *et al.* 2003). Allergic reactions occurred with a frequency of 1 in 4124 blood components and 1 in 2338 transfusion episodes (Domen and Hoeltge 2003).

IgA

Reactions due to class-specific anti-IgA

Several cases have been described in which the transfusion of only a few millilitres of blood has caused such symptoms as dyspnoea, substernal pain, laryngeal oedema and circulatory collapse. These patients usually have undetectable IgA and high-titre, naturally occurring class-specific anti-IgA.

In a woman aged 60 years who denied previous pregnancies and had no previous history of exposure to blood antigens, the transfusion of as little as 10 ml of blood was followed by severe hypotension and cyanosis. The reaction was at first ascribed to a coincidental pulmonary embolism and a second transfusion, of packed red cells, was begun a few days later. Almost immediately the patient developed light-headedness, sternal pain, nausea and flushing of the face and upper part of the chest, with hypotension. The symptoms lasted 10 min and were followed by chills and fever. On several further occasions, the transfusion of a few millilitres of blood produced very severe anaphylactic reactions. The patient was eventually found to lack IgA and to have a potent IgG, complement-fixing anti-IgA: the titre of a sample taken before the first transfusion was 1750; after the second transfusion it rose to 17 500 (Schmidt *et al.* 1969).

In a man who had received a transfusion of plasma some years previously, a transfusion of plasma resulted in severe symptoms, including shortness of breath and substernal pain after only 10–15 ml had been given. The symptoms subsided rapidly after the transfusion was discontinued and hydrocortisone was administered (Vyas 1970). In a similar case, intense malaise, laryngeal oedema, sweating and collapse followed the transfusion of only a few millilitres of whole blood. The patient gave a history of a similar reaction after receiving an injection of intramuscular Ig a year earlier. The very slow transfusion of washed red cells produced only slight malaise. The patient's

serum contained a potent anti-IgA (titre varying from 64 to 1000) (Ropars *et al.* 1973).

In another case, red cells that had been frozen and deglycerolized could be transfused without incident, provided that the rate was slow enough; rapid infusion produced a mild reaction. The transfusion of twice-washed red cells, cell-free plasma or plasma protein fraction (PPF) all produced a reaction. The patient's own stored blood and blood from donors known to lack IgA was well tolerated (Miller *et al.* 1970). Subsequently, the same patient received RBC transfusions washed with 2 l of saline without incident.

In yet another patient, twice-washed red cells gave only a mild reaction and five-times-washed red cells no reaction. In this patient, and in three others, anaphylactic reactions developed after giving a small amount of whole blood. In one case, symptoms developed within a few seconds. All four patients had anti-IgA titres in the range 500–16 000 (Leikola *et al.* 1973).

The frequency of IgA deficiency and of anti-IgA depends on the assay used. Rate nephelometry is a relatively insensitive assay and will not detect IgA levels of < 7 mg/dl. Absent IgA by this assay requires further testing with a haemagglutination or ELISA assay that is sensitive to 0.05 mg/dl. Patients with IgA levels above this do not often have clinically important anti-IgA or anaphylaxis from transfusion.

Class-specific anti-IgA has been detected in 76.3% of 80 IgA-deficient patients with a history of anaphylactic transfusion reaction. Of these patients, 48 received 525 components drawn from IgA-deficient donors without clinical reaction (Sandler *et al.* 1994). However, the same study confirmed that sera of 1 in 1200 of 32 376 random blood donors tested negative for IgA and positive for class-specific anti-IgA. As the incidence of anaphylaxis is estimated at between 1 in 20 000 and 1 in 47 000 transfusions (Pineda and Taswell 1975), screening for class-specific anti-IgA by current methodology probably overestimates the risk to current transfusion recipients.

Reaction to IgA following injected immunoglobulin

Although Ig preparations usually contain about 95% IgG, all of them contain some IgA. One serious reaction following the intramuscular administration of Ig was shown to be associated with the presence in the recipient's serum of potent anti-IgA; other patients with weaker anti-IgA suffered no reactions (Vyas *et al.* 1968). Anaphylactic reactions due to anti-IgA occur more frequently after intravenous administration of Ig. Reactions have been shown to be particularly severe in patients with IgE anti-IgA (Burks *et al.* 1986; Ferreira *et al.* 1988). The routine screening for anti-IgA in patients to be treated with IVIG has been advocated (McCluskey and Boyd 1990). Simple methods for screening for anti-IgA have been described (Hunt and Reed 1990; Mohabir and Rees 1995).

Reactions due to anti-IgA of limited specificity

The term 'limited specificity' applies to antibodies against Am factors and subclass antibodies (i.e. anti-α1 and anti-α2). Only a few cases have been described in which anti-IgA of limited specificity seems to have been responsible for anaphylactic reactions.

In one case the patient, who had a severe erythematous rash, abdominal pain and difficulty in breathing following the transfusion of 100 ml of packed red cells from one donor, showed a rise in anti-IgA titre from 8 to 32. Subsequently, she was given 60 ml of plasma from the same donor, developed a severe hypersensitivity reaction and lost consciousness. Previously, she had been transfused with IgA-deficient plasma without reaction (Vyas *et al.* 1968).

Details of two further cases were as follows: The first patient was a woman whose second transfusion, given 2 years after the first, was followed by severe urticaria, hypotension and oliguria. A third transfusion given 2 years later produced a similar clinical picture accompanied by apprehension and respiratory distress. The patient's serum contained anti-IgA of limited specificity with a titre of 256. In the second case a man, who may have been transfused previously, was given 2 units blood during operation and a third unit on the following day. After 25–30 ml had been transfused, he developed apprehension and restlessness and died 45 min later. The only abnormal finding in his serum was anti-IgA of limited specificity with a titre of 64 before transfusion and of 16 immediately afterwards (Pineda and Taswell 1975). In four patients of the phenotype A2m(–1), with normal levels of IgM in their serum, anaphylactoid reactions following transfusion were due to anti-A2m(1) in the recipient's plasma and could be avoided by transfusion of

A2m(–1) or IgA-deficient plasma (Vyas and Perkins 1976). In one of these patients the antibody had a titre of 256 and the patient twice had a serious anaphylactic reaction following transfusion of only small amounts of A2m(1) blood (Vyas and Fudenberg 1970).

Finally, in a patient who developed a life-threatening reaction with shortness of breath, itching, hot flushes, substernal pain, marked hypotension and cardiorespiratory arrest after the transfusion of 50 ml of pooled platelet concentrate, the serum contained an antibody reactive only with red cells coated with an A2m(1) protein from one particular subject; the patient subsequently received platelet concentrates from an A2m(1)-negative relative without incident (Strauss *et al.* 1983).

Prevention of anaphylaxis in patients who lack IgA. Patients who have suffered anaphylactic transfusion reactions related to plasma proteins may be transfused safely with frozen deglycerolyzed red cells or cellular components that have been washed extensively to remove contaminant plasma (Silvergleid *et al.* 1977; Yap *et al.* 1982; Sloand *et al.* 1990; Toth *et al.* 1998). Blood services have established a registry of IgA-deficient donors. Some transfusion centres now stock fresh-frozen plasma (FFP) made from such donors.

Subjects who have sustained anaphylactic reactions with transfusion and those found to have potent, class-specific anti-IgA should be given some means of emergency identification, such as a card with the information on it or a Medic Alert bracelet (Morton *et al.* 2002).

Other immunoglobulins

Antibodies to haptoglobin

Patients with haptoglobin deficiency associated with haptoglobin IgG and IgE antibodies, and who experienced severe non-haemolytic transfusion reactions have been identified in Japan (Shimada *et al.* 2002). The incidence of individuals homozygous for the haptoglobin deletion has been calculated at 1 in 4000 in Japanese, 1 in 1500 in Koreans and 1 in 1000 in Chinese (Koda *et al.* 2000). This incidence is higher than that of IgA deficiency in Japanese, so that more attention should be paid to haptoglobin deficiency and haptoglobin antibody as the cause of transfusion-related anaphylactic reactions in Asian populations.

IgG

Immediate reactions. Injection of early preparations of Ig modified for intravenous use commonly resulted in adverse reactions, due to the presence of either substantial amounts of aggregates or prekallikrein activator in the preparations (see below). With current IVIG preparations, such reactions are rare. However, patients with hypogammaglobulinaemia, who are especially prone to anaphylactic reactions following the administration of IgG, may develop reactions with intramuscular Ig. This hypersensitivity may be related to the paucity of tissue-bound Ig in these patients (Barandun and Isliker 1986).

The intravenous injection of relatively small amounts of IgG, as in vials containing anti-Rh D Ig prepared by fractionation on DEAE Sephadex, seldom causes reactions; see Chapter 12. Similarly, the commercial preparation of anti-D Ig 'Rho-GAM', which contains 300 µg of anti-D and, presumably, about 300 mg of IgG per 2-ml vial, although intended for intramuscular use, has been given intravenously on many occasions without producing any obvious untoward effects (W Pollack, personal communication).

Reactions associated with repeated intramuscular injections of immunoglobulin. Among 43 normal adults (the staff of a dialysis unit) receiving 5 ml of a 165-g/l solution of Ig as a source of anti-HBs every 8 weeks, four developed either chills or local oedema or generalized urticaria. Of the 43 subjects, about 80% developed IgE antibodies against other Ig classes and about 60% showed a decrease in IgE levels that lasted for several months (Ropars *et al.* 1979).

Possible role of anti-Gm. Two cases in which anti-G1m(a) appeared to be responsible for a transfusion reaction have been described (Fischer 1964; Fudenberg *et al.* 1964), but these cases were reported before the role of anti-IgA was appreciated, and no investigations were made to exclude anti-IgA as a possible cause. In a more recent case, in which the role of anti-IgA was excluded, following a febrile reaction the only protein antibody demonstrable in the patient's serum was anti-G1m(z). The antibody was remarkable in that it was IgG (unlike most Gm antibodies, which are IgM) and that it had a titre of 10 000. No tests were conducted to determine the subclass of the antibody or whether it bound complement (van Loghem and de Lange 1975).

Serum sickness-like syndromes due to anti-IgG seem to be rare. One case followed an intramuscular injection of IgG (see sixth edition, p. 631).

The subject was a male volunteer who was given an i.m. injection of a standard preparation of anti-Rh D Ig (100 µg). Three days later he developed polyarthritis, affecting particularly the hands. Two days after this he was a little worse but after a further 2 days he had started to improve and within 2–3 weeks of the injection he was completely free of symptoms. He never developed a rash or fever. Ten days after the injection the level of haemolytic complement in his serum was reduced (6 units compared with the normal level of 22–27) and significant amounts of C1q and IgG could be precipitated from the serum.

Results on a further sample taken on the following day were similar but 16 days after the injection the level of haemolytic complement was almost normal (20 units) and only trace amounts of C1q and IgG were precipitated in the polyethylene glycol (PEG) test. The results were interpreted as typical of the development of immune complexes and their subsequent removal from the circulation within a few days (JF Mowbray, personal communication). The subject had had one previous injection of Ig 18 months earlier and it may be significant that the preparation, an experimental one, was known to have contained 15% denatured material.

A case in which serum sickness-like reactions developed 2 days or more after transfusions of materials containing plasma (red cells) was described by Avoy (1981); the patient's plasma was found to contain 'autoantibodies directed against IgG'. A clinical case of serum sickness has been reported during repeated plasma exchange used to treat a patient with thrombotic thrombocytopenic purpura (TTP) (Rizvi *et al.* 2000).

For additional adverse reaction associated with administration of IVIG see Chapter 14.

Atopens

In a series of atopic subjects, those known to be sensitive to such common atopens as pollen, dust, milk and egg protein, the transfusion of pooled serum was almost always followed by moderate or severe urticaria, whereas in normal subjects no more than an occasional weal developed (Maunsell 1944). Presumably, these reactions were due to IgE anti-atopens.

Hypersensitivity reactions due to passively acquired antibodies

In a classical case, a patient, who had received a transfusion 2 weeks previously, went for a carriage drive and promptly developed a severe attack of asthma, something that had never happened to him before. It was subsequently discovered that the blood donor had long known that he suffered asthma attacks when exposed to horses and his skin tests to horse dander were strongly positive (Ramirez 1919). Those occasional donors who give a really striking history of hypersensitivity should best be deferred.

Reactions due to passively acquired penicillin antibody

In a patient who developed a generalized maculopapular rash 1 h after receiving 4 units of blood, highly suggestive evidence was obtained that the reaction was due to the presence of penicillin antibody in the plasma of one of the transfused units. The recipient had been receiving ampicillin until the day before transfusion and red cells in a pre-transfusion sample were found to be coated with penicillin; another similar case has been mentioned (McGinniss and Goldfinger 1971).

Reaction due to passively acquired penicillin

In a patient known to be allergic to penicillin, transfusion was followed by the development of a maculopapular eruption with pruritus and fever; the donor unit was shown to contain penicillin (Michel and Sharon 1980).

Sensitivity to nickel

Two patients who, within 24 h of receiving transfusions of blood or plasma, developed an urticarial rash (generalized in one case, around the site of infusion in the other) had a history of sensitivity to nickel. It was presumed that the nickel steel shafts of the needles used for transfusion were responsible (Stoddart 1960).

Sensitivity to latex

A 27-year-old transfusion-dependent patient with thalassaemia major developed progressively severe transfusion reactions characterized by swollen lips, bone pain and vomiting that appeared at least initially to respond in part to antihistamine and corticosteroid administration. During a 4-year interval the reaction complex expanded to include facial oedema, laryngeal spasm, numbness of the tongue, back pain, chest pain and frank anaphylactic shock. Skin testing and IgE radio allergosorbent test (RAST) testing were strongly positive for latex allergy. No benefit was derived from pre-storage leucocyte filtration, extensive cell washing or prophylaxis with high doses of corticosteroids. However, blood collected into latex-free containers and infused through latex-free administration sets was tolerated without incident. Special precautions were necessary to avoid solutions and medications with latex seals and stoppers and latex-containing cannulas (JB Porter, personal communication).

Prophylaxis and treatment of allergic reactions

Antihistamines

After slowing or discontinuing the transfusion, clinicians have traditionally administered antihistamines to ameliorate mild allergic reactions, such as urticaria, and have premedicated patients prior to subsequent transfusion. Based on extensive clinical experience, an H_1-blocking antihistamine such as diphenhydramine (25–50 mg i.v. or p.o.) has become the drug of choice. A variety of similar agents is available and probably equally effective. Little scientific evidence supports any specific medication, dose or dose schedule in the transfusion setting. Combined H_1 and H_2 blockade is sometimes used when urticaria is difficult to control. As prophylaxis, combinations appear to be superior to either agent alone, at least for urticarial reactions that do not involve transfusion (Runge et al. 1992). There is no evidence to support the use of glucocorticoids in these situations. When antihistamines are indicated they should not be added to the blood to be transfused.

For recurrent reactions, cellular components washed free of plasma may ameliorate or eliminate subsequent reactions (Silvergleid et al. 1977).

The above discussion refers predominantly to the suppression of dermatological reactions. For severe allergic reactions involving circulatory or respiratory distress, and certainly for anaphylactic shock, adrenaline should be given intramuscularly (1:1000 solution, 0.5 ml/kg for adults, 0.01 ml/kg for children) or, slowly, intravenously (1:10 000 solution, 0.1 ml/kg)

(Kemp and Lockey 2002), and supportive care should be initiated in an intensive care setting.

Some non-immunological reactions

Effects of vasoactive substances

Prekallikrein activator and angiotensin

Hypotension, vasodilatation, nausea, sweating and chest pain have been noted after the rapid administration of certain batches of plasma protein fraction (PPF), and were found to be related to prekallikrein activator (PKA) generated during the fractionation process (Alving *et al.* 1978; Bleeker *et al.* 1982). Now that tests for PKA are part of the quality control release criteria of plasma fractions, adverse reactions due to PKA are rare except when the patient is receiving angiotensin-converting enzyme (ACE) inhibitors, drugs that block normal bradykinin metabolism (Perseghin *et al.* 2001; see below).

Angiotensin may be generated in plasma pools kept at room temperature. The amounts present are sufficient to affect blood pressure and aldosterone secretion when infused rapidly. In nine different pools the mean level was found to vary between 320 and 830 ng/ml (Vandongen and Gordon 1969).

Hypotensive reactions with bedside filtration and haemapheresis. Hypotensive reactions, occasionally severe enough to require circulatory support, have been encountered when bradykinin components and angiotensin are generated as plasma is exposed to charged synthetic surfaces, or when small amounts of PKA (e.g. residual in albumin fractions) are administered to patients medicated with ACE inhibitors. These reactions have been well documented in patients with ACE inhibitors who undergo haemodialysis or haemapheresis with albumin replacement (Owen and Brecher 1994). A mild reduction in systolic blood pressure and accumulation of bradykin occurs in plasmapheresis subjects who ingested ACE inhibitors. After a series of reports of hypotensive reactions following platelet transfusion in 1993, an American Association of Blood Banks survey reported 17 hypotensive reactions, the vast majority of which began within an hour of transfusion and were associated with blood administration through a filter used to remove leucocytes (Hume *et al.* 1996). Subsequent reports implicated filters from several different manufacturers; all of the different blood components passed through these filters at the bedside may result in hypotension; the mechanism appears to be generation of labile vasoactive proteins such as bradykinin (Shiba *et al.* 1997; Mair and Leparc 1998). In a study of patients undergoing orthotopic heart transplantation, Lavee and Paz (2001) reported 24 episodes of hypotension in their 30 patients (47% of patients) who received components filtered at the bedside. Eleven of these patients (79%) were receiving ACE inhibitors. Filtering blood with these filters immediately prior to transfusion poses an unnecessary risk to the recipient, and filtration prior to storage of blood is clearly preferable. Patients who are being treated with ACE inhibitors at the time of transfusion appear to be particularly susceptible to these reactions and deaths have been reported.

Bacterial pyrogens

Lipopolysaccharides of bacterial origin are the most potent pyrogens known; as little as 0.001 μg/kg of *E. coli* 08 lipopolysaccharide will produce a rise in body temperature when injected intravenously into rabbits; doses of 1 μg/kg regularly produce leucopenia, and doses of 20–30 μg/kg are fatal. In an adult human, 0.1 μg of the same pyrogen may produce fever with leucopenia, followed by leucocytosis (Westphal 1957).

Many bacteria produce pyrogens (Tui and Schrift 1942), but pyrogen testing of solutions for parenteral use is now routine. However, endotoxin and other pyrogens may be responsible for the severe, sometimes fatal reactions seen with bacterial contamination of blood components (Chapter 16). Bottles of commercially prepared protein fractions have been cracked and contaminated during transportation and handling.

Effects of transfusing ice-cold blood

In patients transfused with large amounts of cold (stored) blood, oesophageal temperatures as low as 27.5–29°C have been recorded (MacLean and van Tyn 1961; Boyan and Howland 1963).

Rapid transfusion of large volumes (3000 ml of citrated blood at 50 ml or more/min) of cold blood can be dangerous. In 25 patients transfused with cold blood at 50–100 ml/min, 12 episodes of cardiac arrest occurred; 11 other patients transfused with more than

6000 ml of cold blood at more than 100 ml/min suffered nine episodes of arrest. By contrast, in 105 patients transfused with warm blood at 50–110 ml/min there were only three episodes of cardiac arrest, although in 13 further patients transfused with warm blood at the rate of more than 100 ml/min five episodes were reported (Boyan 1964). The patients in this series were undergoing extensive operations for terminal cancer and the high incidence of cardiac arrest may not indicate the level of risk for other patient groups.

In another series, several episodes of ventricular arrhythmia were observed during neurological operations in which a large amount of blood had been transfused. There were 13 cases of cardiac arrest, 11 of which were fatal. It seemed doubtful that either citrate or potassium toxicity caused the deaths because supplemental calcium had been infused, and blood less than 1 week old had been used. The authors concluded that the administration of cold blood might be responsible and when for a further 2-year period warmed blood was used, no deaths occurred (Dybkjaer and Elkjaer 1964). The same authors showed that when warm blood was given, body temperature fell very slightly during operations lasting 3–4 h, whereas with cold blood, body temperature sometimes fell by 3°C or more. One patient whose temperature fell from 37°C to 34.8°C developed frequent extrasystoles; administration of calcium was without effect, but the transfusion of warmed blood reversed the signs.

Experiments in rabbits indicate that in some circumstances the transfusion of ice-cold blood may be relatively safe. In exchange transfusions, blood at 1°C was injected rapidly (10-ml amounts in about 30 s) into a catheter whose tip lay in the external jugular vein near the right atrium. In a series of experiments designed to test the toxicity of citrate and potassium, blood transfused at 1°C seemed to be no more dangerous than blood injected at 21°C. Indeed there was some evidence that the animal could tolerate larger amounts of citrated, high-potassium blood when this was injected at 1°C (Taylor et al. 1961).

Hypothermia as a result of rapid infusion of cold blood has been implicated as a factor contributing to the coagulopathy reported with massive transfusion (Chapter 2). Hypothermia interferes with platelet function, clotting factor interaction and bleeding time, and slows clotting in a porcine haemorrhagic shock model (Valeri et al. 1995; Heinius et al. 2002).

Methods of warming blood

The simplest method is to pass the blood (on its way from the container to the patient) through a coil of tubing in a waterbath at approximately 40°C (e.g. Dybkjaer and Elkjaer 1964). This method is rarely used today because a relatively long piece of tubing is required to achieve the necessary warming, temperature is poorly monitored, the blood may be exposed to waterbath temperatures for relatively long periods and considerable pressure may be required to force blood through the tubing. A better method is to use a disposable heat exchanger in which the coils of tubing are warmed by electric heating plates. Several devices that use microwave technology for rapid warming of red cells, plasma and other resuscitation fluids are commercially available (Iserson and Huestis 1991; Pappas et al. 1995; Hirsch et al. 2003). In any case, blood should be warmed for transfusion only in a few special circumstances such as when massive amounts are being transfused (see above), or in occasional patients who develop pain at the site of transfusion due to venous spasm. Blood should never be warmed with instruments not designed specifically for this purpose (e.g. a sink filled with hot water, a microwave oven, the top of a television set), as damage to blood cells and proteins may result, and thermal haemolysis of RBC units can prove lethal to the recipient.

Metabolic complications of transfusion

Citrate toxicity

Citrate toxicity may become a hazard under special circumstances: following massive transfusion, especially in subjects with impaired liver function; after exchange transfusion in newborn infants; and during haemapheresis procedures when citrate-containing anticoagulants are infused. In the former cases, the use of packed red cells or red cells in additive solution, rather than whole blood, greatly reduces the hazard. During haemapheresis, reduction in the rate of blood flow and the use of either oral or intravenous calcium preparations ameliorate symptoms (Bolan et al. 2002).

Plasma contains approximately 10 mg of citrate/l expressed as citric acid (Howland et al. 1957). During the infusion of citrate, the plasma level rises and may reach approximately 1 g/l (5 mmol/l). At such levels serious toxic effects may be observed as ionized calcium falls.

In dogs, the administration of 0.06 mmol citrate/kg/min for 20 min was lethal, although 0.04 mmol/kg/min was tolerated (Adams *et al.* 1944). In other canine experiments, an inverse relationship was found between the rate of intravenous infusion of acid-citrate-dextrose (ACD) solution and the cumulative amount of citrate required to produce equivalent electrocardiogram (ECG) changes. The signs observed on the ECG included prolongation of the QT interval, pulsus alternans, depression of P and T waves and development of muscle tremor. With higher doses, the arterial pressure declined to zero and the animal died unless calcium was injected promptly. By keeping the rate of administration at 0.02 mmol/kg/min, it was possible to inject a total dose of approximately 1.8 mmol citrate/kg in 90 min (Nakasone *et al.* 1954), corresponding to the administration of almost 7 l of citrated blood to an adult. In another study in dogs, arrhythmias developed when the blood citrate level reached 0.6 g/l and, unless remedial measures were taken, ventricular fibrillation followed. The administration of sodium citrate at rates of 2.5–12 mg/kg/min led to a significant decrease in cardiac output, stroke volume, left ventricular work, mean and systolic aortic pressures and left ventricular pressure (Corbascio and Smith 1967).

Observations in man are in general agreement with those in experimental animals. For example, following the infusion of 40 ml of ACD/min for 20–30 min to three anaesthetized patients, a rate corresponding to 6–8 mg of citric acid/kg/min, i.e. almost 0.04 mmol/kg/min, the plasma citrate level rose to about 800 mg/l and the QT segment of the ECG was prolonged (Howland *et al.* 1957). In a later report, two series were compared retrospectively: among 152 patients transfused without additional calcium there were three deaths and among 114 patients who had been given calcium there were 13 deaths (Howland *et al.* 1960). However, valid comparison between the two series is impossible, as, of patients receiving 20 or more units of blood, 13 out of 14 were in the series treated with calcium and there were eight deaths among these. As the authors pointed out, the apparent association of death with the administration of calcium may reflect the extreme circumstances that led to calcium administration as a last resort.

Rather surprisingly, the papers just referred to (Howland *et al.* 1957, 1960) are sometimes quoted to support the contention that citrate intoxication is not a significant problem. As mentioned above, a rate of 0.04 mmol citrate/kg/min is tolerated only if it is not maintained very long.

In the era when exchange transfusion of newborn infants was carried out with citrated whole blood, several reports of citrate toxicity and of reversal of signs after injecting calcium were published (Wexler *et al.* 1949; Furman *et al.* 1951; Gustafson 1951). In a review of 140 exchange transfusions among 106 neonates, hypocalcaemia was found in more than one-third; 1 in 20 demonstrated ECG changes; and one sustained cardiac arrest (Jackson 1997). Among the subset of ill neonates, 12% developed severe complications including two deaths attributed to transfusion.

Although the injection of calcium reverses the toxic effects of citrate, and correlation between symptoms and ionized calcium is generally good (Bolan *et al.* 2001), the concentration of calcium below which any patient may become symptomatic is variable (Ladenson *et al.* 1978). The signs and symptoms observed are not due solely to the decrease of ionized calcium, but may be due in part to other effects of citrate, or of the accompanying potassium, glucose or magnesium concentration. Thus the administration of blood rendered hypocalcaemic by passage across an anion-exchange resin does not produce circulatory derangements as severe as those caused by citrated blood (Nakasone *et al.* 1954). As described below, the low pH and raised plasma potassium concentration of citrated blood may contribute to its toxicity.

From data described above, it is safe to conclude that, in adults, signs of citrate toxicity are likely to develop when blood is transfused at the rate of 1 l in 10 min and that the toxic effects can be minimized by giving calcium, for example 10 ml of 10% calcium gluconate for every litre of citrated blood. When even higher rates of transfusion have to be used, even more aggressive calcium restoration has been recommended. For example, when citrated blood is going to be given at rates up to 500 ml/min, one protocol specifies that 10 ml of 10% calcium gluconate be given immediately before transfusion, a further 15 ml intravenously (into another vein) after the first 100 ml and a further 10 ml after each subsequent 500 ml (Firt and Hejhal 1957).

When calcium gluconate is used the dose must be almost four times greater than when calcium chloride is used. The molecular weight of calcium gluconate is

448 and that of calcium chloride 111; each of the molecules contains one atom of calcium (atomic weight 40) so that the amount of calcium (by weight) in calcium gluconate is 9% but in calcium chloride 37%.

Fatal cardiac arrest, apparently due to calcium overdosage, was reported by Wolf and co-workers (1970). A child who had been transfused with 1250 ml of citrated blood in 20 h following cardiac surgery received a total of about 2 g of calcium (2 ml of 10% $CaCl_2$ with each 50 ml of blood). Serum calcium was approximately 50 mg/dl at the end of the transfusion. Excessive amounts of calcium have also been administered by error during haemapheresis, on one occasion related to erroneous dilution of calcium chloride and on another because of poorly monitored gravity infusion (C. Bolan, personal communication); rapid recognition and reversal prevented clinical problems. Calcium solutions must not be administered intravenously unless accompanied by careful monitoring and control of the infusion rate

Factors that increase citrate toxicity

Impaired liver function. In patients with liver disease or with mechanical obstruction to the hepatic circulation, the rapid administration of citrate is more likely to produce toxic effects. When citrated blood was infused at a rate of 500 ml in 15 min, the plasma citrate concentration rose above 0.5 mmol/l in almost all patients with liver disease, but in only 50% of normal subjects. In five patients with severe liver disease or with mechanical obstruction to the hepatic circulation, the calculated concentration of ionized calcium was 0.6 mmol/l or less, compared with the normal value of 1.0 mmol/l (Bunker *et al.* 1955). A concentration of 0.6 mmol/l must be regarded as dangerous in view of the fact that at a concentration of 0.5 mmol/l the isolated frog's heart stops beating (McLean and Hastings 1934) and the clotting time of blood is prolonged (Stefanini 1950).

Acid load in massive blood transfusion

Citrated blood becomes progressively more acid on storage. Nevertheless, in war casualties who were initially profoundly hypotensive and severely acidotic following massive transfusions of 3-week-old blood, acid–base status returned almost to normal during transfusion provided that blood loss was arrested, even although no alkali was administered (Collins *et al.* 1971).

Potassium toxicity

As most transfusions are given with citrate, it is more realistic to consider the combined effects of potassium and citrate rather than of potassium alone.

When red cells are stored in the cold, the potassium content of the red cells decreases and that of the supernatant plasma increases. Normally, red cells contain approximately 100 mmol K/l (of packed cells) and plasma contains 4–5 mmol/l.

In whole blood mixed with CPDA-1 solution, extracellular potassium increases from an initial level of 4.2 mmol/l to 27.3 mmol/l after 35 days; in red cell concentrates prepared from CPDA-1 blood, extracellular potassium increases from 5.1 to 78.5 mmol/l in the same period. The amount of plasma in a unit of CPDA-1 blood is approximately 300 ml and in the corresponding red cell concentrate, 70 ml. Thus, the total potassium load (extracellular) of a unit of whole blood stored for 35 days is 8.2 mmol and that of a red cell concentrate is 5.5 mmol (Moore *et al.* 1981). The rate of increase in plasma potassium in blood stored with ACD is slightly greater; for example, the total extracellular potassium in a unit stored for 28 days was 10.2 mmol (Loutit *et al.* 1943).

In blood that has been irradiated, the level of extracellular potassium is increased; see Chapter 9.

Marked ECG changes occur when a patient's plasma potassium concentration reaches about 8 mmol/l and, in conditions in which the plasma potassium level is thought to be the immediate cause of death, levels of approximately 10 mmol/l are found (Hoff *et al.* 1941; Stewart *et al.* 1948). When the plasma potassium concentration is found to be raised after circulatory collapse has occurred, the rise in potassium concentration is likely to be a consequence rather than a cause of the collapse; immediately after respiratory arrest, dogs sustain a rapid agonal rise in serum potassium (Winkler and Hoff 1943).

In subjects treated with citrated blood, the toxic effects of potassium and citrate should be considered jointly. The addictive effect has been demonstrated on the isolated heart (Baker *et al.* 1957) and during exchange transfusions in rabbits (Taylor *et al.* 1961). In the latter experiments, 10-ml volumes of blood were withdrawn and replaced within 1 min, to a total of 60 or even 100 ml/kg. The blood used had a slightly higher citrate concentration than citrated blood used in normal transfusion practice. Fresh blood was used, but in some experiments potassium was added to bring the plasma potassium concentration to about 25 mmol/l (equivalent to 3- or 4-week-old stored blood). When citrated blood without added potassium was exchanged, there was only one death among 10 rabbits, but when blood with added potassium was used 15 out of 19 rabbits died. The figures for heparinized blood were: without added potassium, none out of 13 died and with added potassium, two out of 15 died. The common mode of death was ventricular fibrillation. These figures show that the combination of citrate and a raised potassium concentration is more dangerous than moderate elevation of potassium alone. It should be emphasized that the rate of exchange transfusion in these experiments was considerably greater than the rate employed in exchange transfusion in infants, that the amounts of citrate and, even more, of potassium that were injected were considerably greater than the amounts involved in exchange transfusion in infants, and that rabbits are more susceptible to citrate toxicity than are humans.

Apart from the special circumstances in which large amounts of blood are rapidly infused, potassium toxicity need be considered only when transfusing patients whose plasma potassium concentration is already raised, for example anuric patients with extensive wounds involving muscle.

Premature and very low birthweight (immature) infants are at particular risk of developing metabolic complications. Based on their observation of 14 episodes of severe hypoglycaemia in six infants receiving transfusion, Mahon and co-workers (1985) suggest that hypoglycaemia may go unrecognized during neonatal transfusion. Hypoglycaemia as a consequence of replacement transfusion in very premature infants occurs as a result of decreased glucose infusion as red cell transfusion with small volumes of CPDA-1 or AS-1 is substituted for dextrose infusion for 3–4 h (Luban 2002). During the transfusion interval, glucose infusion rates drop to 0.2–0.5 mg/kg/min, far below the normal glucose requirement. Two-thirds of premature infants who received red cell concentrates at 17 ml/kg required supplemental glucose within the first 2 h of transfusion as blood glucose fell below 40 mg/dl or clinical evidence of hypoglycaemia developed (Goodstein et al. 1993). The higher dextrose content of red cells preserved in additive solutions may improve glucose homeostasis during transfusion.

In infants transfused with blood stored for less than a week, serum potassium did not change significantly but in those transfused with blood stored for 9–21 days, with a plasma citrate potassium concentration of approximately 15 mEq/l, serum potassium rose to 8 mEq/l in two cases; no ECG changes were observed (Miller et al. 1954). In 36 infants undergoing exchange transfusion with donor blood having a plasma potassium concentration of approximately 7.5 mEq/l, mean potassium values rose from initial values of 4.0–4.5 mEq/l to 5.5–6.0 mEq/l after the exchange of 500 ml. A few samples, mostly from infants who showed signs of circulatory collapse or who actually died shortly after the samples were taken, had concentrations of 8 or 9 mmol/l. When infants require rapid infusion of red cells, it seems prudent to use either blood stored for less than one week or cells saline-washed free of plasma, although blood stored for longer period seems safe when small volumes (10–20 ml/kg) are transfused slowly (Liu et al. 1994).

Ammonia in stored blood

Fresh blood contains only about 100 µg/dl of ammonia but this may increase in blood stored for 3 weeks to about 900 µg/dl; this amount of ammonia may make it undesirable to give large amounts of stored blood to patients with liver failure (Spear et al. 1956).

Transfusion of extraneous matter

Air embolism

When blood was commonly drawn into glass bottles, pumping air into the bottle was a commonly accepted means of accelerating the flow of blood. As rubber tubing and glass drip chambers provided possibilities of air leaks, air embolism was a very real hazard of transfusion. Schmidt and Kevy (1958) described an episode in which a blood donor became severely ill after receiving 60–80 ml of air intravenously.

The introduction of interconnected plastic bags that contain no air has all but eliminated the possibility of introducing air during transfusion. Nevertheless, there are still a few ways in which at least small amounts of air can be introduced into patients' veins during transfusion. For example, air can be introduced at the beginning of the transfusion by failing to expel air from the transfusion tubing or can be introduced into the infusion line when changing from one bag to another. Although the introduction of a few bubbles of air into a patient is harmless, the introduction of large amounts should be avoided.

The most hazardous setting for fatal air embolism from transfusion is now the operating room where recovered ('salvaged') blood in air-containing recovery containers may be infused under pressure. In a review of all perioperative procedures and conventional transfusions in the state of New York between 1990 and 1995, five fatal cases of air embolism were reported, all involving recovered blood infused under pressure (Linden *et al.* 1997). In all cases, insufficient knowledge, vigilance or adherence to standard operating procedures by technical staff were implicated as causes. The fatality rate, approximately 1:38 000, far exceeded the rate of fatal haemolytic transfusion reactions or fatal infectious disease transmission.

Particulate matter

Aggregates in stored blood

In blood mixed with either ACD or heparin, aggregates of leucocytes and platelets up to 200 μm in diameter form during storage (Swank 1961). In ACD, the formation of these aggregates begins within 24 h of drawing the blood and the aggregates are always very marked by 8–10 days. In heparin, formation begins within 2 h and the changes are marked by 8 h. The presence of these particles was demonstrated by measuring the screen filtration pressure (SFP), the pressure needed to force blood at a constant rate through a microfilter with a pore size of 20 μm. The aggregates could be removed by passing stored blood through Pyrex glass wool, although not by passing it through a nylon filter of pore size 200 μm.

In blood stored at 4–6°C with ACD, the microaggregates formed during the first week consist almost entirely of platelets; only subsequently do leucocytes begin to disintegrate and contribute to the particulates (Solis *et al.* 1974).

In the studies of the formation of aggregates in stored blood, the most commonly used method has been to measure the SFP; it has often been assumed that the formation of aggregates of platelets and leucocytes is the most important determinant of SFP. On the other hand, the formation of fibrin is an important determinant of SFP. The source of fibrin in aggregates is predominantly platelet fibrinogen rather than plasma fibrinogen. In experiments in which platelet-rich serum was stored, fibrin formation was observed in the absence of plasma fibrinogen (Marshall *et al.* 1975).

In blood stored with ACD or CPD, little increase in SFP develops during the first 5 days but then a sharp increase occurs, coinciding with the onset of fibrin formation as seen by scanning electron microscopy (Marshall *et al.* 1975). After 4–8 days' storage, SFP was found to be substantially higher in CPD blood than in ACD blood (Wright and Sanderson 1974). Similarly, during the first week of storage greater formation of microaggregates was found with CPD than with ACD, although at 14 and 21 days there were no differences (Marshall *et al.* 1975).

In standard administration sets the nylon filter has a pore size of 170 μm. There is some evidence that debris that can pass through such a filter is harmful to recipients (see below). Macroaggregates weighing up to 9 g have been observed in red cell concentrates stored with saline–adenine–glucose–mannitol solution (Robertson *et al.* 1985). The aggregates were composed of leucocytes and platelet debris, together with some fibrin. Macroaggregate formation was halved by using less centrifugal force during the preparation of the concentrates and was further reduced by the use of an additive solution containing citrate. The separation of the buffy coat from red cell concentrates, which results in removal of more than 80% of the platelets and more than 60% of the leucocytes, as expected reduces aggregate formation (Prins *et al.* 1980).

Macroaggregates, described as 'white particulate matter' in red cells removed from refrigerated storage for issue, resulted in a massive recall of blood components in the USA in 2002. Extensive studies of anticoagulant containers and processing procedures failed to identify impurities or exotic elements; the particulate matter consisted of the same biological debris as found in previous studies. Particulate matter was reduced when soft-spin centrifugation was used or after components were processed with the current generation of leucocyte reduction filters.

Clinical importance of microaggregates in stored blood

In patients who have received a massive transfusion of blood, hypoxia commonly develops and the degree of hypoxia appears to be related to the volume of blood transfused. One possible cause is pulmonary micro-embolism due to debris in stored blood (McNamara et al. 1970). A study by Reul and co-workers (1974) appeared to support this conclusion. In a series of severely traumatized patients who were given massive transfusions, some degree of pulmonary insufficiency developed in 7 out of 17 patients transfused with an average of about 19 units through standard filters (pore size 170 μm) compared with only 2 out of 27 subjects who received an average of 18 units through filters with a pore size of 40 μm. This evidence is suggestive of a causal relationship; the patients in the two series were not strictly comparable, and other evidence casts doubt on the role of microaggregates in causing pulmonary insufficiency. For example, in an experimental study in baboons, oligaemic shock was induced and the animals were then resuscitated with large amounts of blood stored for 16–21 days, after which they were given an exchange transfusion with stored blood equivalent to twice their blood volume. The stored blood used contained aggregates similar to those found in human stored blood. Blood was administered through standard filters of pore size 170 μm. No detectable changes in lung function and no rise in pulmonary arterial pressure were observed. Sections of lungs examined by electron microscopy showed no evidence of pulmonary emboli (Tobey et al. 1974).

In patients dying from respiratory failure following wounding and massive transfusion (65 units and more than 100 units in two cases) it may be impossible to demonstrate pulmonary microemboli. Although particulate emboli from stored blood may contribute to pulmonary impairment following traumatic shock and transfusion, their role is probably a minor one (Bredenberg 1977). A study of combat casualties in Vietnam led to a similar conclusion: differences in pulmonary function related to the type of injury far exceeded differences associated with transfusion (Collins et al. 1978). Furthermore, in a randomized prospective study, results in two groups each of 20 patients undergoing abdominal aortic surgery were compared. Patients were transfused with 6–7 units of blood stored for 10–11 days, either through a standard filter (170 μm) or through a microaggregate filter (40 μm). No difference in postoperative lung function was found between the two groups (Virgilio et al. 1977).

The passage of blood through microaggregate filters may actually induce particle formation. With fresh blood or with blood stored for not more than 10 days, the number of particles was found to be greater after than before filtration (Eisert and Eckert 1979).

There is now little support for the practice of using microaggregate filters. However, removal of particulates may provide an additional benefit for patients who receive components processed with leucocyte depletion filters (see Chapter 13).

Accidental loss of plastic tubes into veins

Many instances of catheter embolism have been recorded. In one case, part of a plastic tube was lost into an arm vein and observed in the right atrium where it caused no symptoms (Taylor and Rutherford 1963). In another case, 10 cm of plastic catheter disappeared into a vein without apparent ill effect (Bennett 1963); the author referred to six previous publications with eight recorded cases; in one, the catheter was found in the pulmonary artery of a patient who had died from pulmonary embolism. In two cases a 'lost catheter' was successfully recovered – in one instance from the right atrium.

In many of the reported accidents the catheter has been severed during attempts to withdraw it through a needle; the bevel of the needle has cut it in two. This accident can be avoided by using the type of catheter that fits over the outside of the needle.

Fragments of skin

Small fragments of skin (visible to the naked eye) are commonly taken into the lumen of the needle when the skin is punctured; using needles with an internal diameter of 0.30–0.75 mm (SWG 18–24), fragments are found after about two-thirds of punctures (Gibson and Norris 1958). If skin fragments are injected into animals, they can sometimes be found in pulmonary vessels and, if injected subcutaneously, dermoid cysts may result. Nevertheless, no ill effects from this cause have yet been reported in humans. Non-coring needles that reduce (but do not eliminate) skin fragmenting are in general use for blood collection.

Toxic substances in plastic

Polyvinyl chloride (PVC) plastic as used in blood transfusion equipment contains plasticizers and stabilizers. According to Gullbring and co-workers (1964), the common plasticizers are: dioctyl phthalate (most commonly added to soft polyvinyl chloride), trioctyl phthalate, and dioctyl sebacate and adipate (used with soft vinyl polymers). The 'stabilizers' used are: mild alkalis, fatty acid salts, ethylene oxide compounds and organic compounds of lead, barium, cadmium and tin.

Animal experiments have shown that some batches of PVC tubing liberate a substance or substances capable of: (1) arresting the isolated rat's heart (Meijler and Durrer 1959); (2) killing minnows (Roggen et al. 1964); and (3) damaging mammalian cells cultured in vitro (Gullbring et al. 1964; Roggen et al. 1964).

Phthalates

The plasticizer di (2-ethylhexyl) phthalate (DEHP) dissolves readily in lipids and can be found in lipid extracts of plasma that has been stored (as blood) in ordinary plastic packs (Marcel and Noel 1970). In vitro studies have shown that DEHP inhibits the deterioration of RBCs during refrigerated storage in containers that use this compound as a plasticizer (AuBuchon et al. 1988). The level of DEHP in the plasma increases with time, reaching 5–7 mg/dl at 21 days; moreover, in transfused patients significant amounts of plasticizer are found in the tissues, the largest amounts being in abdominal fat (Jaeger and Rubin 1970). In a study carried out in infants, those who had died from necrotizing enterocolitis following umbilical catheterization with PVC tubes were found to have significantly higher amounts of DEHP in their tissues than those who had not been catheterized (Hillman et al. 1975).

Monoethylhexylphthalate (MEHP) is at least as toxic as DEHP and should be measured as well as DEHP in assessing the potential toxicity of phthalates in extracts (Vessman and Rietz 1978). One potential advantage of fractionating fresh plasma rather than outdated plasma is that the former contains far smaller amounts of phthalates. MEHP (as contrasted with DEHP) has a particular affinity for albumin and, as the conversion of DEHP to MEHP may continue even in frozen plasma, it is desirable to prepare albumin from fresh rather than stored plasma (Cole et al. 1981).

DEHP, at a concentration of 0.4 mg/dl, was found to be lethal to chick embryo beating hearts in tissue culture (Jaeger and Rubin 1970). Although DEHP seems to be only mildly toxic in animals (including humans), it is highly toxic in plants (Hardwick and Cole 1986). Neither DEHP nor its two major metabolites MEHP and ethylhexanol are mitogenic in rats (De Angelo and Garrett 1983; Kornbrust et al. 1984).

Butyryl-n-trihexyl citrate (BTHC), which is now used in the filter PL-2209 (Fenwal), does not leach into blood components during storage (Gullikson et al. 1991; Högman et al. 1991).

Ethylene oxide

Sensitization to ethylene oxide gas (used for sterilizing plastic equipment), associated with the formation of IgE antibodies, has been demonstrated in patients developing acute hypersensitivity reactions during haemodialysis (Nicholls 1986) and in donors during plateletpheresis (Leitman et al. 1986). Signs, although predominantly ocular in the latter patients, were clear manifestations of mild anaphylaxis as confirmed by skin test reactivity and the presence of anti-IgE. Cutaneous reactions (including fiery red ears), nausea, diarrhoea, wheezing, coughing and sneezing have been noted as well.

Transfusion haemosiderosis

One litre of blood contains about 500 mg of iron, whereas the daily excretion of iron from the body is only about 1 mg. Thus if numerous transfusions are given to a patient who is not bleeding, the amount of iron in the body increases progressively with toxic accumulation in the heart, liver and endocrine organs. The association of multiple blood transfusions with haemosiderosis was first recognized in a patient who had received more than 290 transfusions over a period of 9 years (Kark 1937).

In patients who have received relatively few transfusions and in whom serum transferrin is not fully saturated, iron liberated from senescent red cells is taken up by the reticuloendothelial system, where it is relatively harmless. However, even after the transfusion of as few as 10–15 units of blood, transferrin is almost saturated (Ley et al. 1982). Following further transfusions, iron is deposited in parenchymal cells, causing widespread tissue damage (Marcus and Huehns 1985).

691

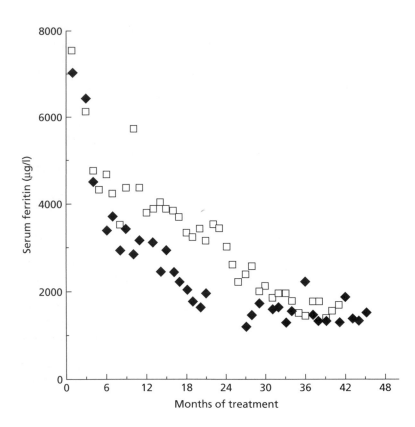

Fig 15.4 Decline of serum ferritin levels in response to continuous intravenous 24-h desferrioxamine infusion in two iron-overloaded patients with homozygous beta thalassaemia. Biphasic kinetics are characterized by an early rapid fall in serum ferritin, followed by a slower rate of decline in patients with ferritin elevations exceeding 3000 ug/l (Davis and Porter 2000).

Moreover, in chronic dyshaemopoietic anaemias for which patients receive regular transfusions, excess iron is absorbed from the gut and transported via the portal vein to hepatocytes with resultant interference with hepatic function.

Iron can be removed from the body by giving injections of desferrioxamine (DFO), but even when 500 mg is given by daily intramuscular injection, serious iron overload is not prevented and retardation of growth and sexual development ensues (Modell 1975). When given by constant subcutaneous or intravenous injection, DFO is much more effective, so that it is actually possible to obtain a net excretion of iron (Fig. 15.4), increased survival and decreased cardiac complications in patients receiving regular transfusion therapy (Brittenham *et al.* 1994; Davis and Porter 2000). Chelation efficiency is related to the total body burden of iron. Endocrine dysfunction is not reversible; however, aggressive chelation can prevent further decline. Cardiac accumulation is reversible and determined chelation can postpone or prevent the primary

cause of death in these patients (Anderson *et al.* 2004; Davis *et al.* 2004). The disadvantages of DFO therapy include reversible retinal toxicity and catheter complications such as infection and thrombosis with continuous intravenous infusion. Lack of patient compliance is a particular problem during the social sufferings of adolescence.

An oral iron chelator, L1 (deferiprone), has been shown to be effective in causing negative iron balance in long-term trials in thalassaemia major and other transfusion-dependent refractory anaemias and at present is licensed in Europe. Widespread use of L1 has been limited by inconsistency of effect and concerns about toxicity, primarily agranulocytosis. Treatment with L1 should be carefully considered for patients unable or unwilling to use DFO or for patients with an unsatisfactory response to DFO as judged by liver iron and serum ferritin measurements or evidence of cardiac iron overload or iron-induced cardiac dysfunction (Hoffbrand *et al.* 2003). All patients receiving the drug should be closely monitored.

References

Adams WE, Thornton TF, Allen JG (1944) Danger and prevention of citrate intoxication in massive transfusions of whole blood. Ann Surg 120: 656

Alving BM, Hojima Y, Pisano JJ (1978) Hypotension associated with prekallikrein activator (Hageman-factor fragments) in plasma protein fraction. N Engl J Med 299: 66

Anderson KC (1995) Current trends: evolving concepts in transfusion medicine. Leukodepleted cellular blood components for prevention of transfusion-associated graft-versus-host disease. Transfusion Sci 16: 265–268

Anderson KC, Weinstein HJ (1990) Transfusion-associated graft-versus-host disease. N Engl J Med 323: 315–319

Anderson LJ, Westwood MA, Holden S et al. (2004) Myocardial iron clearance during reversal of siderotic cardiomyopathy with intravenous desferrioxamine: a prospective study using T2* cardiovascular magnetic resonance. Br J Haematol 127: 348–355

Andreu G, Morel P, Forestier F et al. (2002) Hemovigilance network in France: organization and analysis of immediate transfusion incident reports from 1994 to 1998. Transfusion 42: 1356–1364

Andrews AT, Zinigewski CM, Bowman HS (1976) Transfusion reaction with pulmonary infiltration associated with HLA-specific leukocyte antibodies. Am J Clin Pathol 66: 483

Aster RH, Jandl JH (1964) Platelet sequestration in man. I. Immunological and clinical studies. J Clin Invest 43: 856

AuBuchon JP, Estep TN, Davey RJ (1988) The effect of the plasticizer di-2-ethylhexyl phthalate on the survival of stored RBCs. Blood 71: 448–452

Avoy DR (1981) Delayed serum sickness-like transfusion reactions in a multiply transfused patient. Vox Sang 41: 239–244

Baker JBE, Bentall HH, Dreyer B (1957) Arrest of isolated heart with potassium citrate. Lancet ii: 555

Ballem PJ, Buskard NA, Decary F et al. (1987) Post-transfusion purpura secondary to passive transfer of anti-PlA1 by blood transfusion. Br J Haematol 66: 113–114

Barandun S, Isliker H (1986) Development of immunoglobulin preparations for intravenous use. Vox Sang 51: 157–160

Bennett PJ (1963) The use of intravenous plastic catheters. BMJ ii: 1252

Benson K, Marks AR, Marshall MJ et al. (1994) Fatal graft-versus-host disease associated with transfusions of HLA-matched, HLA-homozygous platelets from unrelated donors. Transfusion 34: 432–437

Bierling PM, Godeau B, Fromont P (1995) Post-transfusion purpura-like syndrome associated with CD36 (Nak^a) isoimmunisation. Transfusion 35: 777–782

Bjerrum OJ, Jersild C (1971) Class-specific anti-IgA associated with severe anaphylactic transfusion reactions in a patient with pernicious anaemia. Vox Sang 21: 411

Bleeker WK, van Rosevelt RF, Ufkes JGR (1982) Hypotensive effects of plasma protein fraction. J Lab Clin Med 100: 540–547

Bolan CD, Greer SE, Cecco SA et al. (2001) Comprehensive analysis of citrate effects during plateletpheresis in normal donors. Transfusion 41: 1165–1171

Bolan CD, Cecco SA, Wesley RA et al. (2002) Controlled study of citrate effects and response to i.v. calcium administration during allogeneic peripheral blood progenitor cell donation. Transfusion 42: 935–946

Boyan CP (1964) Cold or warmed blood for massive transfusions. Ann Surg 160: 282

Boyan CP, Howland WS (1963) Cardiac arrest and temperature of bank blood. JAMA 183: 58

Brecher ME, Moore SB, Letendre L (1990) Posttransfusion purpura: the therapeutic value of Pl^{A1}-negative platelets. Transfusion 30: 433–435

Bredenberg CE (1977) In International Forum. Does a relationship exist between massive blood transfusions and the adult respiratory distress syndrome? Vox Sang 32: 311

Brittenham GM, Griffith PM, Nienhuis AW et al. (1994) Efficacy of deferoxamine in preventing complications of iron overload in patients with thalassemia major. N Engl J Med 331: 567–573

Brittingham TE, Chaplin H Jr (1957) Febrile transfusion reactions caused by sensitivity to donor leukocytes and platelets. JAMA 165: 819

Brittingham TE, Chaplin H Jr (1961) The antigenicity of normal and leukemic human leukocytes. Blood 17: 139

Budd JL, Wiegers SE, O'Hara JM (1985) Relapsing post-transfusion purpura. A preventable disease. Am J Med 78: 361–362

Bunker JP, Stetson JB, Coe RC (1955) Citric acid intoxication. JAMA 157: 1361

van Buren NL, Stroncek DF, Clay ME (1990) Transfusion-related acute lung injury caused by an NB2 granulocyte-specific antibody in a patient with thrombotic thrombocytopenic purpura. Transfusion 30: 42–45

Burks AW, Sampson HA, Buckley RH (1986) Anaphylactic reactions after gamma globulin administration in patients with hypogammaglobulinemia. N Engl J Med 314: 560–564

Burns LJ, Westberg MW, Burn CF (1984) Acute graft-versus-host disease resulting from normal donor blood transfusion. Acta Haematol 71: 270–276

Chambers LA, Kruskall MS, Pacini DG et al. (1990) Febrile reactions after platelet transfusion: the effect of single versus multiple donors. Transfusion 30: 219–221

Chaplin H Jr, Crawford H, Cutbush M (1956) The preservation of red cells at −79°C. Clin Sci 15: 27

Chong BH, Cade J, Smith JA (1986) An unusual case of post-transfusion purpura: good transient response to high-dose immunoglobulin. Vox Sang 51: 182–184

Christie DJ, Pulkrabek S, Putman JL (1991) Post-transfusion purpura due to an alloantibody reactive with glycoprotein Ia/IIa (anti-HPA-5b). Blood 12: 2785–2789

Cimo PL, Aster RH (1972) Post-transfusion purpura. Successful treatment by exchange transfusion. N Engl J Med 287: 290

Cines DB, Schreiber AD (1979) Immune thrombocytopenia. Use of a Coombs antiglobulin test to detect IgG and C3 on platelets. N Engl J Med 300: 106–111

Cole RS, Tocchi M, Wye E (1981) Contamination of commercial blood products by di-2-ethylhexyl phthalate and mono-2-ethylhexyl phthalate. Vox Sang 40: 317–322

Collins JA, Simmons RL, James PM (1971) Acid-base status of seriously wounded combat casualties. II. Resuscitation with stored blood. Ann Surg 173: 6

Collins JA, James PM, Bredenberg CE (1978) The relationship between transfusion and hypoxemia in combat casualties. Ann Surg 188: 513

Corbascio AN, Smith NT (1967) Hemodynamic effects of experimental hypercitremia. Anesthesiology 28: 510

Cunningham CC, Lind SE (1989) Apparent response of refractory post-transfusion purpura to splenectomy. Am J Hematol 30: 112–113

Dameshek W, Neber J (1950) Transfusion reactions to plasma constituent of whole blood: their pathogenesis and treatment by washed red blood cell transfusions. Blood 5: 129–147

Dare JG, Mogey GA (1954) Rabbit responses to human threshold doses of a bacterial pyrogen. J Pharm Pharmacol 6: 325–332

Davis BA, Porter JB (2000) Long-term outcome of continuous 24 h deferoxamine infusion via indwelling intravenous catheters in high-risk beta-thalassemia. Blood 95: 1229–1236

Davis BA, O'Sullivan C, Jarritt PH et al. (2004) Value of sequential monitoring of left ventricular ejection fraction in the management of thalassemia major. Blood 104: 263–269

De Angelo AB, Garrett CT (1983) Inhibition of development of preneoplastic lesions in the livers of rats fed a weakly carcinogenic environmental contaminant. Cancer Lett 20: 199–205

Décary F, Ferner P, Giavedoni L (1984) An investigation of nonhemolytic transfusion reactions. Vox Sang 46: 277–285

De Rie MA, van der Plas-van Dalen CM, Engelfriet CP (1985) The serology of febrile transfusion reactions. Vox Sang 49: 126–134

Domen RE, Hoeltge GA (2003) Allergic transfusion reactions: an evaluation of 273 consecutive reactions. Arch Pathol Lab Med 127: 316–320

Dooren MC, Ouwehand WH, Verhoeven AJ et al. (1998) Adult respiratory distress syndrome after experimental intravenous gamma-globulin concentrate, monocyte-reactive IgG antibodies. Lancet 352: 1601–1602

Dybkjaer E, Elkjaer P (1964) The use of heated blood in massive blood replacement. Acta Anaesth Scand 8: 271

Dykes A, Smallwood D, Kotsimbos T et al. (2000) Transfusion-related acute lung injury (Trali) in a patient with a single lung transplant. Br J Haematol 109: 674–676

Dzik WH (1992) Is the febrile response to transfusion due to donor or recipient cytokines. Transfusion 32: 594

Eastlund T, McGrath PC, Britten A (1989) Fatal pulmonary transfusion reaction to plasma containing donor HLA antibody. Vox Sang 57: 63–66

Eisert WG, Eckert G (1979) Current problems and results in testing microaggregate filters. Vox Sang 37: 310–320

Enright H, Davis K, Gernsheimer T et al. (2003) Factors influencing moderate to severe reactions to PLT transfusions: experience of the TRAP multicenter clinical trial. Transfusion 43: 1545–1552

Erichson RB, Viles H, Grann V (1978) Posttransfusion purpura. Arch Intern Med 138: 998

Ferreira A, Rodriguez MCC, Lopz-Trascasa M (1988) Anti-IgA antibodies in selective IgA deficiency and in primary immunodeficient patients treated with globulin. Clin Immunol Immunopathol 47: 199–207

Firt P, Hejhal L (1957) Treatment of severe haemorrhage. Lancet ii: 1132

Fischer K (1964) Immunhaematologische und klinische Befunde bei einem Transfusions-Zwischen-fall infolge Gm (a)-Antikoerperbildung. Commun 10th Congr Int Soc Blood Transf, Stockholm

Flegel WA, Wiesneth M, Stampe D (1995) Low cytokine contamination in buffy coat-derived platelet concentrates without filtration. Transfusion 35: 917–920

von Fliedner VE, Grob JP, Barrelet L (1983) Clinical characteristics and evaluation of risk in the graft versus host reaction following transfusion. Schweiz Med Wochenschr 113: 1521–1523

Ford JM, Lucey JJ, Cullen MH (1976) Fatal graft-versus-host disease following transfusion of granulocytes from normal donors. Lancet ii: 1167

Fudenberg HH, Franklin EC, Meltzer M et al. (1964) Antigenicity of hereditary human gamma-globulin (Gm) factors – biological and chemical aspects. Cold Spring Harb Symp Quart Biol 29: 463

Furman RA, Hellerstein HK, Startzman (1951) ECG changes occurring during the course of replacement transfusions. J Pediatr 38: 45

Gans ROB, Duurkens VAM, van Zundert AA (1988) Transfusion-related acute lung injury. Intens Care Med 14: 654–659

Gengozian N, McLaughlin CL (1978) Activity induced platelet-bound IgG associated with thrombocytopenia in the marmoset. Blood 51: 1197–1210

Gibson T, Norris W (1958) Skin fragments removed by injection needles. Lancet ii: 983

Goodstein MH, Locke RG, Wlodarczyk D et al. (1993) Comparison of two preservation solutions for erythrocyte transfusions in newborn infants. J Pediatr 123: 783–788

Gottschall IL, Johnston VL, Azod L (1984) Importance of white blood cells in platelet storage. Vox Sang 47: 101–107

Grant RT, Reeve EB (1951) Observations on the general effects of injury in man, with special reference to wound shock. Spec Rep Ser Med Res Coun (Lond) 277

Grass JA, Wafa T, Reames A et al. (1999) Prevention of transfusion-associated graft-versus-host disease by photochemical treatment. Blood 93: 3140–3147

Gullbring B, Eklund LH, Svartz-Malmberg G (1964) Chemical and biological test-methods applied to plastic products used in transfusion equipment. Vox Sang 9: 530

Gullikson H, Shanwell A, Wikman A (1991) Storage of platelets in a new plastic container. Vox Sang 61: 165–170

Gustafson JE (1951) Electrocardiographic changes in exchange transfusion. J Pediatr 39: 593

Hagen J, Bierrum OJ, Gogstad G (1982) Involvement of divalent cations in the complex between the platelet glycoproteins IIb and IIIa. Biochim Biophys Acta 701: 1–6

Hamblin TJ, Naoroase Abide SM, Nee PA (1985) Successful treatment of post-transfusion purpura with high dose immunoglobulin after lack of response to plasma exchange. Vox Sang 49: 164–167

Hardwick R, Cole R (1986) Plastics that kill plants. The Garden 111: 264–267

Harrington WJ (1954) The clinical significance of antibodies for platelets. Commun 5th Congr Int Soc Haematol (Paris)

Hathaway WE, Githens JH, Blackburn WR et al. (1965) Aplastic anemia, histiocytosis and erythrodermia in immunologically deficient children. Probable human runt disease. N Engl J Med 273: 953–958

Heddle NM (1999) Pathophysiology of febrile nonhemolytic transfusion reactions. Curr Opin Hematol 6: 420–426

Heddle NM, Klama LN, Griffits L (1993) A prospective study to identify the risk factors associated with acute reactions to platelet and red cell transfusions. Transfusion 33: 794–797

Heddle NM, Klama L, Singer J (1994) The role for the plasma from platelet concentrates in transfusion reactions. N Engl J Med 331: 625–628

Heddle NM, Blajchman MA, Meyer RM et al. (2002) A randomized controlled trial comparing the frequency of acute reactions to plasma-removed platelets and prestorage WBC-reduced platelets. Transfusion 42: 556–566

Heim KF, Stroncek DF, Fleisher TA et al. Use of flow cytometry to evaluate the clinical efficacy of granulocyte transfusions in alloimmunized patients: experience in a chronic granulomatous disease cohort. Transfusion (in press)

Heinius G, Wladis A, Hahn RG et al. (2002) Induced hypothermia and rewarming after hemorrhagic shock. J Surg Res 108: 7–13

Henson PM, Larsen CL, Webster RO (1982) Pulmonary microvascular alterations and injury induced by complement fragments: synergistic effect of complement activation, neutrophil sequestration and prostaglandins. Ann NY Acad Sci 384: 300

Herzig RH, Poplack DG, Yankee RA (1974) Prolonged granulocytopenia from incompatible platelet transfusions. N Engl J Med 290: 1220

Hillman LS, Goodwin SL, Sherman WR (1975) Identification and measurement of plasticizer in neonatal tissues after umbilical catheters and blood products. N Engl J Med 292: 381

Hirsch J, Bach R, Menzebach A et al. (2003) Temperature course and distribution during plasma heating with a microwave device. Anaesthesia 58: 444–447

Hobsley M (1958) Chlorpheniramine maleate in prophylaxis of pyrexial reactions during blood-transfusions. Lancet i: 497

Hoff HE, Smith PK, Winkler AW (1941) The cause of death in experimental anuria. J Clin Invest 20: 607

Hoffbrand AV, Cohen A, Hershko C (2003) Role of deferiprone in chelation therapy for transfusional iron overload. Blood 102: 17–24

Högman CF, Eriksson L, Ericson A et al. (1991) Storage of saline-adenine-glucose-mannitol-suspended red cells in a new plastic container: polyvinylchloride plasticized with butyryl-n-trihexyl-citrate. Transfusion 31: 26–29

Howard L, Shulman S, Sadanandan S (1982) Crossed immunoelectrophoresis of human platelet membranes. The major antigen consists of a complex of glycoproteins GPIIb and GPIIIa held together by Ca^{2+} and missing in Glanzmann's thrombasthenia. J Biol Chem 257: 8331–8336

Howland WS, Bellville JW, Zucker MB (1957) Massive blood replacement. V. Failure to observe citrate intoxication. Surg Gynecol Obstet 105: 529

Howland WS, Jacobs R, Goulet AG (1960) An evaluation of calcium administration during rapid replacement. Anaesth Analg 39: 557

Hume HA, Popovsky MA, Benson K et al. (1996) Hypotensive reactions: a previously uncharacterized complication of platelet transfusion? Transfusion 36: 904–909

Hunt AF, Reed MI (1990) Anti-IgA screening and use of IVIG. Lancet 336: 1197

Iserson KV, Huestis DW (1991) Blood warming: current applications and techniques. Transfusion 31: 558–571

Ito K, Yoshida H, Yanagibashi K (1988) Change of HLA phenotype in postoperative erythroderma. Lancet i: 413–414

Jackson JC (1997) Adverse events associated with exchange transfusion in healthy and ill newborns. Pediatrics 99: E7

Jaeger RJ, Rubin RJ (1970) Plasticizers from plastic devices; extraction, metabolism, and accumulation by biological systems. Science 170: 460

Jandl JH, Tomlinson AS (1958) The destruction of red cells by antibodies in man. II. Pyrogenic, leukocytic and dermal responses to immune hemolysis. J Clin Invest 37: 1202

Juji T, Shibata Y, Ide H (1989) Post-transfusion graft-versus-host disease in immunocompetent patients after cardiac surgery in Japan (Letter). N Engl J Med 321: 56

Kao GS, Wood IG, Dorfman DM et al. (2003) Investigations into the role of anti-HLA class II antibodies in TRALI. Transfusion 43: 185–191

Kark RM (1937) Two cases of aplastic anaemia. One with secondary haemochromatosis following 290 transfusions in nine years, the other with secondary carcinoma of the stomach. Guy's Hosp Rep 87: 343

Kaslow RA, Phair JP, Friedman HB (1987) Infection with the human immunodeficiency virus: clinical manifestations and their relationship to immune deficiency: a report from the multicenter AIDS Cohort Study. Ann Intern Med 107: 474–480

Kemp SF, Lockey RF (2002) Anaphylaxis: a review of causes and mechanisms. J Allergy Clin Immunol 110: 341–348

Kevy SV, Schmidt PJ, McGinniss MH et al. (1962) Febrile, nonhemolytic transfusion reactions and the limited role of leukoagglutinins in their etiology. Transfusion 2: 7–16.

Kickler TS, Ness PM, Herman JH (1986) Studies on the pathophysiology of posttransfusion purpura. Blood 68: 347–350

Koda Y, Watanabe Y, Soejima M et al. (2000) Simple PCR detection of haptoglobin gene deletion in anhaptoglobinemic patients with antihaptoglobin antibody that causes anaphylactic transfusion reactions. Blood 95: 1138–1143

Kopko PM, Marshall CS, MacKenzie MR et al. (2002) Transfusion-related acute lung injury: report of a clinical look-back investigation. JAMA 287: 1968–1971

Kornbrust OJ, Barfknecht TR, Ingram P (1984) Effect of di(2-ethylhexyl) phthalate on DNA repair and lipid peroxidation in rat hepatocytes and on metabolic cooperation in chinese hamster V-79 cells. J Toxicol Environ Health 13: 99–116

Kroll H, Kiefel V, Mueller-Eckhardt C (1993) Post-transfusion purpura: clinical and immunologic studies in 38 patients. Infusionsther Transfusionsmed 20: 198–204

Kruskall MS, Lee TH, Assmann SF et al. (2001) Survival of transfused donor white blood cells in HIV-infected recipients. Blood 98: 272–279

Kunicki TJ, Pidard D, Rosa JP (1981) The formation of Ca^{2+}-dependent complexes of platelet membrane glycoproteins IIb and IIIa in solution, as determined by crossed immuno-electrophoresis. Blood 58: 268–278

Ladenson JH, Miller WV, Sherman LA (1978) Relationship of physical symptoms, ECG, free calcium, and other blood chemistries in reinfusion with citrated blood. Transfusion 18: 670–679

Lane TA, Gernsheimer T, Mohandas K et al. (2002) Signs and symptoms associated with the transfusion of WBC-reduced RBCs and non-WBC-reduced RBCs in patients with anemia and HIV infection: results from the Viral Activation Transfusion Study. Transfusion 42: 265–274

Larsen GL, McCarthy K, Webster RV (1980) A differential effect of C5a and C5a des Arg. in induction of pulmonary inflammation. Am J Pathol 100: 179–192

Lau P, Sholtis CM, Aster RH (1980) Post-transfusion purpura: an enigma of alloimmunization. Am J Hematol 9: 331–336

Lavee J, Paz Y (2001) Hypotensive reactions associated with transfusion of bedside leukocyte-reduction filtered blood products in heart transplanted patients. J Heart Lung Transplant 20: 759–761

Lee TH, Paglieroni T, Ohto H et al. (1999) Survival of donor leukocyte subpopulations in immunocompetent transfusion recipients: frequent long-term microchimerism in severe trauma patients. Blood 93: 3127–3139

Leikola J, Koistinen J, Lehtinen M (1973) IgA-induced anaphylactic transfusion reactions: a report of four cases. Blood 42: 111

Leitman SF, Boltansky H, Alter HJ (1986) Allergic reactions in healthy plateletpheresis donors caused by sensitization to ethylene oxide gas. N Engl J Med 315: 1192–1196

Leitman SF, Tisdale JF, Bolan CD et al. (2003) Transfusion-associated GVHD after fludarabine therapy in a patient with systemic lupus erythematosus. Transfusion 43: 1667–1671

Ley TJ, Griffith P, Nienhuis AW (1982) Transfusion haemosiderosis and chelation therapy. Clin Haematol 11: 437–464

Linden JV, Kaplan HS, Murphy MT (1997) Fatal air embolism due to perioperative blood recovery. Anesth Analg 84: 422–426

Liu EA, Mannino FL, Lane TA (1994) Prospective, randomized trial of the safety and efficacy of a limited donor exposure transfusion program for premature neonates. J Pediatr 125: 92–96

van Loghem E, de Lange G (1975) Transfusion reactions caused by antibodies against immunoglobulins. Dr Karl Landsteiner Foundation Annual Report, Central Laboratory of the Netherlands Red Cross Blood Transfusion Service

van Loghem JJ, van der Hart M, Hijmans W (1958) The incidence and significance of complete and incomplete white cell antibodies with special reference to the use of the Coombs consumption test. Vox Sang 3: 203

van Loghem JJ, Dorfmeier H, van der Hart M (1959) Serological and genetical studies on a platelet antigen (Zw). Vox Sang 4: 161

Loutit JF, Mollison PL, Young IM (1943) Citric acid-sodium-citrate-glucose mixtures for blood storage. Quart J Exp Physiol 32: 183

Luban NL (2002) Neonatal red blood cell transfusions. Curr Opin Hematol 9: 533–536

Lubenow N, Eichler P, Albrecht D et al. (2000) Very low platelet counts in post-transfusion purpura falsely diagnosed as heparin-induced thrombocytopenia. Report of four cases and review of literature. Thromb Res 100: 115–125

McCluskey DR, Boyd NAM (1990) Anaphylaxis with intravenous gamma-globulin. Lancet i: 874

McGinniss MH, Goldfinger D (1971) Drug reactions due to passively transfused penicillin antibody. Commun Am Assoc Blood Banks, Chicago

McLean FC, Hastings AB (1934) A biological method for the estimation of calcium ion concentration. J Biol Chem 107: 337

MacLean LD, van Tyn RA (1961) Ventricular defibrillation. JAMA 175: 471

McNamara JJ, Molot MD, Stremple JF (1970) Screen filtration pressure in combat casualties. Ann Surg 172: 334

Mahon PM, Jones ST, Kovar IZ (1985) Hypoglycaemia and blood transfusions in the newborn. Lancet 2: 388

Mair B, Leparc GF (1998) Hypotensive reactions associated with platelet transfusions and angiotensin-converting enzyme inhibitors. Vox Sang 74: 27–30

Mangano MM, Chambers LA, Kruskall MS (1991) Limited efficacy of leukopoor platelets for prevention of febrile transfusion reactions. Am J Clin Pathol 95: 733–738

Marcel YL, Noel SP (1970) Contamination of blood stored in plastic packs. Lancet i: 35

Marcus RE, Huehns ER (1985) Transfusional iron overload. Clin Lab Haematol 7: 195–212

Marshall BE, Ellison N, Wurzel HA (1975) Microaggregate formation in stored blood. II. Influence of anticoagulants and blood components. Circ Shock 2: 185

Maung ZT, Wood AC, Jackson GH et al. (1994) Transfusion-associated graft-versus-host disease in fludarabine-treated B-chronic lymphocytic leukaemia. Br J Haematol 88: 649–652

Maunsell K (1944) Urticarial reactions and desensitization in allergic recipients after serum transfusions. BMJ ii: 236

Meijler FL, Durrer D (1959) The influence of polyvinylchloride tubing on the isolated perfused rat's heart. Vox Sang 4: 239

Menitove JE, McElligott MC, Aster RH (1982) Febrile transfusion reaction: what blood component should be given next? Vox Sang 42: 318–321

Michel J, Sharon R (1980) Non-haemolytic adverse reaction after transfusion of a blood unit containing penicillin. BMJ i: 152–153

Miller G, McCoord AB, Joos HA (1954) Studies of serum electrolyte changes during exchange transfusion. Pediatrics 13: 412

Miller WV, Holland PV, Sugarbaker E (1970) Anaphylactic reactions to IgA: a difficult transfusion problem. Am J Clin Pathol 54: 618

Minchinton RM, Cunningham J, Cole-Sinclair M (1990) Autoreactive platelet antibody in post transfusion purpura. Aust NZ J Med 20: 111–115

Modell CB (1975) Transfusion and haemochromatosis. In: Iron Metabolism and its Disorders. H Kiel (ed.). Amsterdam: Excerpta Medica

Mohabir LA, Rees TJ (1995) Screening for IgA deficiency on the Olympus PK7100 by haemagglutination inhibition. Transfusion Med 5: 275–279

Mollison PL (1979) Blood Transfusion in Clinical Medicine, 6th edition. Oxford: Blackwell Scientific Publications

Moore GL, Peck CC, Sohmer PR (1981) Some properties of blood stored in anticoagulant CPDA-1 solution. A brief summary. Transfusion 21: 135–137

Morrison FS, Mollison PL (1966) Post-transfusion purpura. N Engl J Med 275: 243–248

Morrow JF, Braine HG, Kickler TS et al. (1993) Septic reactions to platelet transfusions. A persistent problem. JAMA 266: 555–558

Morton L, Murad S, Omar RZ et al. (2002) Importance of emergency identification schemes. Emerg Med J 19: 584–586

Mueller-Eckhardt C (1991) Posttransfusion purpura. In: Platelet Immunology; Fundamental and Clinical Aspects. C Kaplan-Gouet (ed.). Paris: Eurotext, pp. 249–255

Mueller-Eckhardt C, Kiefel V (1988) High-dose IgG for post-transfusion purpura – revisited. Blut 57: 163–167

Muylle L, Peetermans ME (1994) Effect of prestorage leucocyte removal on the cytokine levels in stored platelet concentrates. Vox Sang 66: 14–17

Muylle L, Wouters E, de Bock R (1992) Transfusion reactions to platelet concentrates: the effect of the storage time of the concentrate. Transfusion Med 2: 289–293

Muylle L, Joos M, Wouters E (1993) Increased tumor necrosis factor a (TNF-α) interleukin 1 and interleukin 6 (IL-6) levels in plasma of stored platelet concentrates: relationship between TNF-α and IL-6 and febrile transfusion reactions. Transfusion 33: 195–199

Muylle L, Wouters E, Peetermans ME (1996) Febrile reactions to platelet transfusion: the effect of increased interleukin 6 levels in concentrates prepared by the platelet-rich plasma method. Transfusion 36: 886–890

Nakasone N, Watkins E Jr, Janeway CA (1954) Experimental studies of circulatory derangement following the massive transfusion of citrated blood. Comparison of blood treated with ACD solution and blood decalcified by ion exchange resin. J Lab Clin Med 43: 184

Nicholls A (1986) Ethylene oxide and anaphylaxis during haemodialysis. BMJ 292: 1221–1222

Nicholls RJ, Davies P, Kenwright MG (1970) Thrombocytopenic purpura after blood transfusion. BMJ ii: 581

Nordhagen R, Conradi M, Dromtorp SM (1986) Pulmonary reaction associated with transfusion of plasma containing anti-5b. Vox Sang 51: 102–108

Ohto H, Anderson KC (1996a) Posttransfusion graft-versus-host disease in Japanese newborns. Transfusion 36: 117–123

Ohto H, Anderson KC (1996b) Survey of transfusion-associated graft-versus-host disease in immunocompetent recipients. Transfusion Med Rev 10: 31–43

Otsuka S, Kunieda K, Hirose M (1989) Fatal erythroderma (suspected graft-versus-host disease) after cholecystectomy. Transfusion 29: 544

Otsuka S, Kunieda K, Kitamura F (1991) The critical role of blood from HLA-homozygous donors in fatal transfusion-associated graft-versus-host disease in immunocompetent patients. Transfusion 31: 260–264

Owen HG, Brecher ME (1994) Atypical reactions associated with use of angiotensin-converting enzyme inhibitors and apheresis. Transfusion 34: 891–894

Palfi M, Berg S, Ernerudh J et al. (2001) A randomized controlled trial of transfusion-related acute lung injury: is plasma from multiparous blood donors dangerous? Transfusion 41: 317–322

Pappas CG, Paddock H, Goyette P et al. (1995) In-line microwave blood warming of in-date human packed red blood cells. Crit Care Med 23: 1243–1250

Parkman R, Mosier D, Umansky I (1974) Graft-versus-host disease after intrauterine and exchange transfusions for hemolytic disease of the newborn. N Engl J Med 290: 359

Payne R (1957) The association of febrile transfusion reactions with leukoagglutinins. Vox Sang 2: 233

Pegels JG, Bruynes ECE, Engelfriet CP (1981) Post-transfusion purpura: a serological and immunochemical study. Br J Haematol 49: 521–530

Pelszynski MM, Moroff G, Luban NL et al.(1994) Effect of gamma irradiation of red blood cell units on T-cell inactivation as assessed by limiting dilution analysis: implications for preventing transfusion-associated graft-versus-host disease. Blood 83: 1683–1689

Perkins HA, Payne R, Ferguson J (1966) Nonhemolytic febrile transfusion reactions. Quantitative effects of blood components with emphasis on isoantigenic incompatibility of leukocytes. Vox Sang 11: 578

Perseghin P, Capra M, Baldini V et al. (2001) Bradykinin production during donor plasmapheresis procedures. Vox Sang 81: 24–28

Petz LD, Calhoun L, Yam P (1993) Transfusion-associated graft-versus-host disease in immunocompetent patients: report of a fatal case associated with transfusion of blood from a second-degree relative and survey of predisposing factors. Transfusion 33: 742–750

Phipps RP, Kaufman J, Blumberg N (2001) Platelet derived CD154 (CD40 ligand) and febrile responses to transfusion. Lancet 357: 2023–2024

Pineda AA, Taswell HF (1975) Transfusion reactions associated with anti-IgA antibodies: report of four cases and review of the literature. Transfusion 15: 10

Popovsky MA, Haley NR (2000) Further characterization of transfusion-related acute lung injury: Demographics, clinical and laboratory features and morbidity. Immuno-hematology 16, 157–159.

Popovsky MA, Moore SB (1985) Diagnostic and pathogenetic considerations in transfusion-related acute lung injury. Transfusion 25: 573–577

Popovsky MA, Chaplin HC, Moore SB (1992) Transfusion related acute lung injury: a neglected, serious complication of hemotherapy. Transfusion 32: 589–592

Prins HK, De Bruyn JCGH, Henrichs HPJ (1980) Prevention of microaggregate formation by removal of 'buffycoats'. Vox Sang 39: 48–51

Ramirez MA (1919) Horse asthma following blood transfusion: report of a case. JAMA 73: 985

Reul GJ Jr, Beall A Jr, Greenberg SD (1974) Protection of the pulmonary microvasculature by fine screen blood filtration. Chest 66: 4

Rizvi MA, Vesely SK, George JN et al. (2000) Complications of plasma exchange in 71 consecutive patients treated for clinically suspected thrombotic thrombocytopenic purpura-hemolytic-uremic syndrome. Transfusion 40: 896–901

Roggen G, Bertschmann M, Berchtold H (1964) A contribution to the comparative chemical and biological assay procedures for plastic containers used for blood preservation. Vox Sang 9: 546

Ropars C, Whylie S, Cartron JP (1973) Anticorps chez les polytransfusés dirigés contres certaines immunoglobulines IgM. Nouv Rév Fr Hematol 13: 459

Ropars C, Geay-Chicot D, Cartron JP (1979) Human IgE response to the administration of blood components. II. Repeated gammaglobulin injections. Vox Sang 37: 149–157

Runge JW, Martinez JC, Caravati EM et al. (1992) Histamine antagonists in the treatment of acute allergic reactions. Ann Emerg Med 21: 237–242

Sachs UJ, Bux J (2003) TRALI after the transfusion of cross-match-positive granulocytes. Transfusion 43: 1683–1686

Sakatibara T, Juji T (1986) Post-transfusion graft-versus host disease after open heart surgery. Lancet ii: 1099

Sandler SG, Eckrich R, Malamut D et al. (1994) Hemagglutination assays for the diagnosis and prevention of IgA anaphylactic transfusion reactions. Blood 84: 2031–2035

Schechter GP, Soehlen F, McFarland W (1972) Lymphocyte response to blood transfusion in man. N Engl J Med 28: 1169

Schmidt PJ, Kevy SV (1958) Air embolism. N Engl J Med 258: 424

Schmidt AP, Taswell F, Gleich GJ (1969) Anaphylactic transfusion reactions associated with anti-IgA antibody. N Engl J Med 280: 188

Scott EP, Moilan-Bergeland J, Dalmasso AP (1988) Post-transfusion thrombocytopenia associated with passive transfusion of a platelet-specific antibody. Transfusion 28: 73–76

Seeger W, Schneider U, Kreusler B (1990) Reproduction of transfusion-related acute lung injury in an *ex-vivo* lung model. Blood 76: 1438–1444

Seemayer TA, Bolande RP (1980) Thymic involution mimicking thymic dysplasia. A consequence of transfusion induced graft versus-host disease in a premature infant. Arch Pathol Lab Med 104: 141–144

Shiba M, Tadokoro K, Sawanobori M *et al.* (1997) Activation of the contact system by filtration of platelet concentrates with a negatively charged white cell-removal filter and measurement of venous blood bradykinin level in patients who received filtered platelets. Transfusion 37: 457–462

Shimada E, Tadokoro K, Watanabe Y *et al.* (2002) Anaphylactic transfusion reactions in haptoglobin-deficient patients with IgE and IgG haptoglobin antibodies. Transfusion 42: 766–773

Shulman NR (1991) Posttransfusion purpura: clinical features and the mechanism of platelet destruction. In: Clinical and Basic Science Aspects of Immunohematology. ST Nance (ed.). Arlington, VA: Am Assoc of Blood Banks

Shulman NR, Aster RH, Leitner A (1961) Immunoreactions involving platelets. V. Post-transfusion purpura due to a complement-fixing antibody against a genetically controlled platelet antigen. A proposed mechanism for thrombocytopenia and its relevance in 'autoimmunity'. J Clin Invest 40: 1597

Shulman NR, Marder VJ, Hiller MC (1964) Platelet and leukocyte isoantigens and their antibodies: serologic, physiologic and clinical studies. Progr Hematol 4: 222

Silliman CC, Paterson AJ, Dickey WO *et al.* (1997) The association of biologically active lipids with the development of transfusion-related acute lung injury: a retrospective study. Transfusion 37: 719–726

Silliman CC, Boshkov LK, Mehdizadehkashi Z *et al.* (2003) Transfusion-related acute lung injury: epidemiology and a prospective analysis of etiologic factors. Blood 101: 454–462

Silvergleid AJ, Hafleigh EB, Harabin MA (1977) Clinical value of washed-platelet concentrates in patients with non-hemolytic transfusion reactions. Transfusion 17: 33

Sirchia G, Rebulla P, Patayaccini A (1994) Leukocyte depletion of red cells. In: Leukocyte-depleted Blood Products: Current Studies in Hematology and Blood Transfusion. Lane TT (ed.). Basel: Karger, p. 60

Slichter S (1982) Post-transfusion purpura: response to steroids and association with red blood cell and lymphocytotoxic antibodies. Br J Haematol 50: 599–605

Sloand EM, Fox SM, Banks SM *et al.* (1990) Preparation of IgA-deficient platelets. Transfusion 30: 322–326

Smith KJ, Sierra ER, Nelson EJ (1993) Histamine, IL-1α and IL-8 increase in packed RBCs stored for 42 days but not in RBCs leukodepleted prestorage. Transfusion 33 (Suppl.): S202

Solis RT, Goldfinger D, Gibbs MB (1974) Physical characteristics of microaggregates in stored blood. Transfusion 14: 538

Soulier J-P, Patereau C, Gobert N (1979) Posttransfusional immunologic thrombocytopenia. A case report. Vox Sang 37: 21–29

Spear PW, Sass M, Cincotti JJ (1956) Ammonia levels in transfused blood. J Lab Clin Med 48: 702

Stack G, Snyder EL (1994) Cytokine generation in stored platelet concentrates. Transfusion 34: 20–25

Stefanini M (1950) Studies on the role of calcium in the coagulation of blood. Acta Med Scand 136: 250

Stephen CR, Martin RC, Bourgeois-Gavardin M (1955) Antihistaminic drugs in treatment of nonhemolytic transfusion reactions. JAMA 158: 525

Stewart HJ, Shepard EM, Horger EL (1948) Electrocardiograph manifestations of potassium intoxication. Am J Med 5: 821

Stoddart JC (1960) Nickel sensitivity as a cause of infusion reactions. Lancet ii: 741

Strauss RA, Gloster E, Shanfield MS (1983) Anaphylactic transfusion reaction associated with a possible anti-A2m(1). Clin Lab Haematol 5: 371–377

Stroncek DF, Leonard K, Eiber G *et al.* (1996) Alloimmunization after granulocyte transfusions. Transfusion 36: 1009–1015

Swank RL (1961) Alteration of blood on storage: measurement of adhesiveness of 'aging' platelets and leucocytes and their removal by filtration. N Engl J Med 265: 728

Taaning E, Skov F (1991) Elution of anti-Zwᵃ (-Plᴬ¹) from autologous platelets after normalization of platelet count in post-transfusion purpura. Vox Sang 60: 40–44

Taylor IW, Rutherford CE (1963) Accidental loss of plastic tube into venous system. Arch Surg 86: 177

Taylor WC, Gillis CN, Nash CW (1961) Experimental observations on cardiac arrhythmia during exchange transfusion in rabbits. J Pediatr 58: 470

Thaler M, Shamis A, Orgad S (1989) The role of blood from HLA-homozygous donors in fatal transfusion-associated graft-versus-host disease after open-heart surgery. N Engl J Med 321: 25–28

Tobey RE, Kopriva CJ, Homer LD (1974) Pulmonary gas exchange following hemorrhagic shock and massive transfusion in the baboon. Ann Surg 179: 316

Toth CB, Kramer J, Pinter J *et al.* (1998) IgA content of washed red blood cell concentrates. Vox Sang 74: 13–14

Tui C, Schrift MN (1942) Production of pyrogen by some bacteria. J Lab Clin Med 27: 569

Valeri CR, MacGregor H, Cassidy G *et al.* (1995) Effects of temperature on bleeding time and clotting time in normal male and female volunteers. Crit Care Med 23: 698–704

Vandongen R, Gordon RD (1969) Generation and survival of angiotensin in non-refrigerated plasma: an explanation for presence of pressor material in human plasma protein solutions used clinically. Transfusion 9: 205

Vaughan-Neil EF, Ardeman S, Bevan G (1975) Post-transfusion purpura associated with unusual platelet antibody (anti-PlBl). BMJ i: 436

Vessman J, Rietz G (1978) Formation of mono(ethylhexyl)phthalate from di(ethylhexyl)phthalate in human plasma stored in PVC bags and its presence in fractionated plasma proteins. Vox Sang 35: 75

Virchis AE, Patel RK, Contreras M et al. (1997) Lesson of the week. Acute non-cardiogenic lung oedema after platelet transfusion. BMJ 314: 880–882

Virgilio RW, Smith DE, Rice CL (1977) To filter or not to filter? (Abstract). Intens Care Med 3: 144

Vogelsang GB, Kickler TS, Bell WR (1986) Post-transfusion purpura: a report of five patients and a review of the pathogenesis and management. Am J Hematol 21: 259–267

Von dem Borne AEK, van der Plas-van Dalen CM (1985) Further observations on posttransfusion purpura (Letter). Br J Haematol 61: 374–375

Vyas GN (1970) Antibodies to IgA causing anaphylactic reactions to small transfusions. Am Assoc Blood Banks Workshop on Transfusion Problems 2: 21

Vyas GN, Fudenberg HH (1970) Immunobiology of human anti-IgA: a serologic and immunogenetic study of immunization to IgA in transfusion and pregnancy. Clin Genet 1: 45

Vyas GN, Perkins HA (1976) Anti-IgA in blood donors (Letter). Transfusion 16: 289

Vyas GN, Perkins HA, Fudenberg HH (1968) Anaphylactoid transfusion reactions associated with anti-IgA. Lancet ii: 312

de Waal LP, van Dalen CM, Engelfriet CP et al. (1986) Alloimmunization against the platelet-specific Zwa antigen, resulting in neonatal alloimmune thrombocytopenia or posttransfusion purpura, is associated with the supertypic DRw52 antigen including DR3 and DRw6. Hum Immunol 17: 45–53

Wagner FF, Flegel WA (1995) Transfusion-associated graft-versus-host disease: risk due to homozygous HLA haplotypes. Transfusion 35: 284–291

Walker WS, Yap PL, Kilpatrick DC (1988) Post transfusion purpura following open heart surgery: management by high dose intravenous immunoglobulin transfusion. Blut 57: 323–325

Wallis JP (2003) Transfusion-related acute lung injury (TRALI): under-diagnosed and under-reported. Br J Anaesth 90: 573–576

Wang L, Juji T, Tokunaga K (1994) Polymorphic microsatellite markers for the diagnosis of graft-versus-host disease. N Engl J Med 330: 398–401

Wang SE, Lara PN Jr, Lee-Ow A et al. (2002) Acetaminophen and diphenhydramine as premedication for platelet transfusions: a prospective randomized double-blind placebo-controlled trial. Am J Hematol 70: 191–194

Ward HN (1970) Pulmonary infiltrates associated with leukoagglutinin transfusion reactions. Ann Intern Med 73: 689

Warkentin TE, Smith JW, Hayward CP et al. (1992) Thrombocytopenia caused by passive transfusion of anti-glycoprotein Ia/IIa alloantibody (anti-HPA-5b). Blood 79: 2480–2484

Westphal O (1957) Pyrogens. In: Polysaccharides in Biology. New York: Transactions 2nd Conf 1956 Josiah Macy Jr Foundation, p. 115

Wexler LB, Pincus JB, Matelson S (1949) The fate of citrate in erythroblastic infants treated with exchange transfusion. J Clin Invest 28: 474

Wilhelm RE, Nutting HM, Devlin HB (1955) Antihistaminics for allergic and pyrogenic transfusion reactions. JAMA 158: 529

Williamson LM (1998) Transfusion associated graft versus host disease and its prevention. Heart 80: 211–212

Williamson LM, Wimperis JZ, Williamson P et al. (1994) Bedside filtration of blood products in the prevention of HLA alloimmunization – a prospective randomized study. Alloimmunisation Study Group. Blood 83: 3028–3035

Win N, Peterkin MA, Watson WH (1995) The therapeutic value of HPA-1a-negative platelet transfusion in post-transfusion purpura complicated by life-threatening haemorrhage. Vox Sang 69: 138–139

Winkler AW, Hoff HE (1943) Potassium and the cause of death in traumatic shock. Am J Physiol 139: 686

Wisecarver JL, Cattral MS, Langnas AN et al. (1994) Transfusion-induced graft-versus-host disease after liver transplantation. Documentation using polymerase chain reaction with HLA-DR sequence-specific primers. Transplantation 58: 269–271

Wolf PL, McCarthy LJ, Hafleigh B (1970) Extreme hypercalcemia following blood transfusion combined with intravenous calcium. Vox Sang 19: 544

Wright G, Sanderson JM (1974) ACD and CPD blood preservation. Lancet ii: 173

Yap PL, Pryde EA, McClelland DB (1982) IgA content of frozen-thawed-washed red blood cells and blood products measured by radioimmunoassay. Transfusion 22: 36–38

Yomtovian R, Kline W, Press C (1984) Severe pulmonary hypersensitivity associated with passive transfusion of a neutrophil-specific antibody. Lancet i: 244–246

16 Infectious agents transmitted by transfusion

Most deaths caused by blood transfusion worldwide are due to the transmission of infectious agents: viruses, bacteria or protozoa. As civilization encroaches upon undeveloped forest and jungle, the evolving suburban wilderness and global travel ensure the emergence and spread of 'new' blood-borne pathogens. Microbial adaptation, climate and weather changes, war and famine, and the spectre of bioterrorism all raise the concern of emerging infectious threats to the blood supply. The agents responsible share the following characteristics: persistence in the donor's bloodstream, giving rise to carrier or latent states; a susceptible recipient population; the ability to cause asymptomatic infections; stability in stored blood and, in many cases, in plasma fractions. Ideally, blood for transfusion should be either tested for all pathogens that are prevalent in a given population and can cause serious disease or treated to inactivate all such agents. In practice, neither is possible. Furthermore, some agents are pathogens primarily for certain susceptible patients, such as premature infants or patients immunosuppressed for organ transplantation. Testing is an effective reactive strategy but it cannot interdict an emerging agent such as HIV in the early 1980s or West Nile virus (WNV) at the beginning of this century.

Tests suitable for mass screening of blood donations are available for many of the infectious agents capable of causing significant morbidity in recipients. However, even the most sensitive tests do not detect all infectious donors. The chance of becoming a carrier of a particular agent varies widely in different populations and the risk of transmitting the agent can be reduced by appropriate selection of donors. For example, the risk of transmitting malaria in non-endemic areas can be minimized by excluding donors from areas in which the disease is endemic, and the risk of transmitting human immunodeficiency virus (HIV) can be greatly reduced by excluding donors with high-risk activity.

Infectious agents that are present only in blood cells, for example malarial parasites, can be transmitted by all blood components except cell-free plasma. On the other hand, those viruses that are present in plasma (e.g. hepatitis B virus (HBV)) can be transmitted by cell-free plasma and plasma fractions, as well as by cellular components. HIV is found in both mononuclear cells and free in plasma.

Some infectious agents, e.g. cytomegalovirus, CMV, human T-lymphotropic virus (HTLV), *Treponema pallidum* are transmitted more readily by relatively fresh blood components, whereas other agents (HBV, HIV) are stable in stored, and even in frozen, red cells or plasma.

Screening assays for microbiological agents (Fig. 16.1)

In most countries, blood donations are routinely screened by serology for HBsAg (and in some for anti-HBc) as well as for hepatitis C virus (HCV), HIV and syphilis. In several countries, for example Japan, the USA, France, some Caribbean countries and the Netherlands, donations are screened for HTLV antibodies. In most Central and South American countries, donations are also screened for *Treponema cruzi* antibodies and in some South American countries,

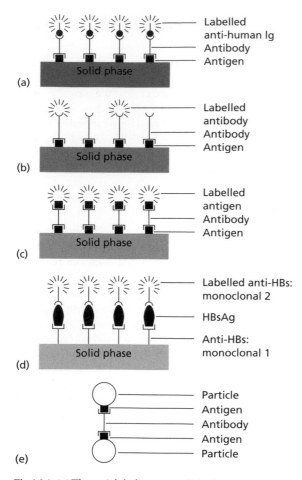

(a)

(b)

(c)

(d)

(e)

Labelled
anti-human Ig
Antibody
Antigen
Solid phase

Labelled
antibody
Antibody
Antigen
Solid phase

Labelled
antigen
Antibody
Antigen
Solid phase

Labelled anti-HBs:
monoclonal 2

HBsAg

Anti-HBs:
monoclonal 1
Solid phase

Particle
Antigen
Antibody
Antigen
Particle

Fig 16.1 (a) The antiglobulin enzyme-linked immunosorbent assay (ELISA); (b) the competitive ELISA; (c) the sandwich ELISA (d); the monoclonal sandwich ELISA; and (e) the sandwich particle assay. For an explanation of these assays, see text.

such as Colombia, for brucellosis. In several countries a proportion of blood units are tested for CMV antibodies to supply CMV seronegative blood to selected recipients. Increasingly, direct detection of virus is performed by molecular assays (nucleic acid testing, NAT). Most countries use NAT for HIV and HCV; some European countries have added HBV, and in the USA and Canada, NAT testing is performed for West Nile virus. Screening tests for malaria antibodies are being developed for use in countries where the disease is not endemic.

The need to develop sensitive and specific assays amenable to mass screening and automation has become apparent. Transfusion services are faced with the conflict between increasing test sensitivity to protect recipients from the risk of acquiring infections by transfusion and, at the same time, increasing the specificity of assays to reduce the number of false-positive results. This is a difficult balance to achieve. More than 10–15% of blood donations are discarded in many countries in addition to the rejection of a similar number of donors before they are bled (Sarkodie *et al.* 2001). These losses have a major impact on blood transfusion services, many of which are struggling to meet demand. An added complication is the number of blood components that must be held in quarantine while initially positive screening tests are repeated; even in fully computerized transfusion services, the possibility of mistakes with the consequent release of the incompletely tested units increases with the number of units held.

The first screening tests were developed to detect viral antigen (HBsAg) and antibody (HIV, HCV). The confirmation of antigen assays by neutralization of reactivity using specific antibody is more reliable than the open 'confirmatory' techniques available for antibody assays. In an effort to reduce the risk of transmitting infection to the lowest possible level, molecular techniques to detect the microbial genomes are used widely for HBV, HCV, HIV and WNV. For ease and cost, pools of 16–90 specimens are screened, but as combination tests evolve, testing of individual donations for each agent will certainly become standard practice. The principles for most of the commonly used screening assays are described below.

Passive haemagglutination or particle agglutination

Standardized antigen or antibody is used to coat tanned red cells or particles such as gelatin or latex. If the specific, complementary antibody or antigen is present in the serum under investigation, the red cells or particles are agglutinated. This type of assay is usually performed in U- or V-well microplates that can be centrifuged to enhance agglutination. The assay is also amenable to automation in blood grouping machines. If antibodies are used to coat the cells for agglutination by antigen in the serum under investigation, the term 'reverse passive agglutination' is used.

Enzyme-linked immunosorbent assay

Standardized antigen (e.g. HIV antigen) is linked to a solid phase in the form of beads, the wells of microplates or dipsticks, etc. If antibody (e.g. anti-HIV) is present in the test sample (donor's serum), which is generally diluted according to the manufacturer's instructions, it will adhere to the solid phase. The coated wells or beads are then washed; if antibodies are present, they will be detected with an enzyme-linked human antiglobulin reagent, which will, in turn, be detected by the appropriate chromogenic substrate (Fig. 16.1a). The antigens can be: (1) disrupted microbial agents with different grades of purity and of contamination with cells in which they are cultured; (2) recombinant polypeptides obtained by molecular genetic methods; or (3) synthetic antigens. The enzymes most widely used are horseradish peroxidase and alkaline phosphatase. The sensitivity of the enzyme-linked immunosorbent assay (ELISA) can be enhanced with biotin–avidin or biotin–streptavidin, or by amplification through the addition of NADP, alcohol dehydrogenase and diaphorase.

Radioimmunoassay

The basic principles are the same as for ELISA, but the label for the antiglobulin is a radioisotope, such as ^{125}I.

Chemiluminescence assays

The assay is similar to an ELISA but the horseradish peroxidase reacts with luminol in the presence of an enhancer to produce light emission.

Competitive enzyme-linked immunosorbent assay or radioimmunoassay

Known antigen (for example HIV-1) is linked to the solid phase and any antibody in the serum will compete for binding with enzyme-labelled or radiolabelled antibody (Fig. 16.1b). The more antibody in the sample, the weaker the enzyme reaction available to colour the substrate, or the weaker the radioactive signal. In a competitive assay, the weaker the reaction, the larger is the amount of antibody present, whereas in the antiglobulin assay, the stronger the reaction, the larger is the amount of antibody present.

Sandwich enzyme-linked immunosorbent assay or radioimmunoassay

Antigen molecules coat the solid phase as in the antiglobulin ELISA and any antibody present in the test sample will be detected by the reaction with labelled antigen (Fig. 16.1c). For the detection of viral antigen, two types of monoclonal antibodies can be used in 'one-step' assays, reacting with different epitopes of the antigen to avoid blocking the sites which attach the antibody onto the solid phase (Fig. 16.1d).

Sandwich particle assay

Particles in suspension are coated with several molecules of antigen. When antibody is present in the test sample, the particles agglutinate (Fig. 16.1e).

Screening assays: testing strategy

If donor serum or plasma reacts with a screening assay, most tests are repeated in duplicate. If at least one of the repeat tests reacts, the specimen is considered 'reactive'. The original sample should then be tested with a 'supplementary' or with a 'confirmatory' assay using a methodology different from that used in the screening assay. The most definitive type of confirmation is that used for viral antigen and consists of neutralization or inhibition of the antigen–antibody reaction by a well-authenticated antibody.

Western blot

Lysed viral or recombinant antigens, for example of HIV, are subjected to electrophoresis in sodium dodecyl sulphate (SDS) polyacrylamide gel. The viral polypeptides are separated by migration on the gel, according to their molecular weight. The polypeptide pattern on the gel is transferred ('blotted') on to nitrocellulose paper, which is dried and cut into strips. Dilutions of the serum samples found to be positive in screening assays are incubated with the strips; if antibodies to HIV antigens are present, they will combine with different and precise sections of the strip carrying the specific polypeptides. As in any other antiglobulin assay, the strips are washed and antigen–antibody reactions are detected by an appropriately labelled antiglobulin reagent. Antiglobulin is usually labelled with enzyme and a positive reaction is detected by the reaction of the enzyme with its substrate. Antibodies to defined polypeptides can be detected according to the position of the bands on the strip. Criteria of a positive reaction should be well defined for each agent for which Western blot is used as the confirmatory test. Unfortunately, contaminating proteins from viral lysates may travel to positions that are the same as those of specific viral antigens and may sometimes bind to crossreacting antibodies, leading to false-positive reactions.

Recombinant immunoblot assay(RIBA)

This assay is used for confirmation of the presence of HCV antibodies. Recombinant and synthetic antigens on a nitrocellulose strip are incubated with the test serum; specific antibodies react when present in the serum and the reactions are visualized as bands.

Nucleic acid testing technology

The principle underlying nucleic acid testing (NAT) is the polymerase chain reaction (PCR), a technique that makes it possible to amplify a short specific sequence of viral deoxyribonucleic acid (DNA) in a sample (see Plate 16.1 shown in colour between pages 528 and 529) (Mullis and Faloona 1987). Ribonucleic acid (RNA) viruses can also be used after treatment with reverse transcriptase. For PCR it is essential to know the sequence of bases flanking the target DNA region. Two specific short fragments of synthetic DNA (oligonucleotide primers) are then synthesized to match (hybridize) the sequences at either end of the target from the 5′-end (see Plate 16.1). The first primer is a copy of the end of the coding strand and the second primer is a copy of the end of the non-coding homologous strand. DNA polymerase is essential in PCR for the synthesis of the complementary strand of a DNA sequence in the presence of the appropriate primers and deoxyribonucleotide triphosphates (dNTPs). A thermostable polymerase enzyme from the bacillus *Thermus aquaticus* (*Taq*) has simplified the procedure considerably, as it is relatively unaffected at the denaturation temperature of 94°C and does not need to be replenished at each cycle. The PCR mixture contains the specimen under study, excess oligonucleotide primers, *Taq* polymerase and abundant dNTPs as well as electrolytes such as Mg^{2+}. The binding of the

primers to the flanking sequences of the target DNA (annealing) is possible after separation of the two strands of DNA by melting at 94°C and cooling at 40–55°C. At its optimal temperature of 70–75°C, the *Taq* polymerase will stimulate the synthesis of complementary DNAs (extension) to the coding and non-coding strands starting from the annealed primers in the 5′ to 3′ direction. The whole process of melting, cooling, reassociation or annealing and synthesis takes 2–3 min and is repeated cyclically. As more than 30 cycles are undertaken per procedure, the target DNA becomes amplified exponentially because the new strands, as well as the old ones, become templates for the excess primers (Plate 16.1). The end result is that the target DNA sequence is amplified 10^5–10^6 times in just a few hours. The amplified sequences are detected by electrophoretic separation or by hybrididization to radiolabelled or enzyme-tagged probes. PCR cycling has been automated using microprocessor-controlled heating blocks. Commercial systems can detect fewer than 100 viral copies in plasma or cell samples (Hawkins *et al.* 1997; Nolte *et al.* 2001). The major problems with PCR relate to the specificity of the oligonucleotide primers and to the possibility of amplification of non-target sequences that can occur, especially in contaminated samples. Crosscontamination with foreign DNA during PCR assays is by far the greatest problem because the contaminating DNA can also be amplified.

NAT involves more than one kind of assay, but the general principles are similar. The NASBA technique amplifies RNA, based on the principles of bacteriophage replication, with no requirement for thermal cycling; the amplified RNA is detected either by an enzyme-linked assay or by luminometry (Romano *et al.* 1996). Other amplification techniques include transcription-mediated amplification (Sarrazin *et al.* 2000), the ligase chain reaction for amplification of DNA and the branched DNA signal amplification assay (Allain 2000). Equipment providing varying degrees of automation has been applied to these techniques, and full automation is close to licensure.

Current practice involves two different approaches to NAT screening: plasma pool and single-donation testing. Pool testing costs less, but suffers some loss of sensitivity. Single-unit testing is not yet fully automated and will be more costly unless multiplex testing can be used (Allain 2000).

Hepatitis B virus

Despite the dramatic reduction in risk of viral transmission during the past three decades, viral hepatitis remains a serious complication of transfusion worldwide. The discovery in 1968 that the viraemic phase of serum hepatitis (hepatitis B) could be recognized serologically (Blumberg et al. 1968; Prince 1968) sparked the hope that all infectious donors could be identified and that post-transfusion hepatitis could be eliminated. However, most transfusion-transmitted cases of hepatitis proved to be associated with viruses other than B (or A), and several other viruses, most importantly HCV, were eventually discovered.

HBV remains a major human pathogen that causes acute and chronic hepatitis, cirrhosis and hepatocellular carcinoma (Ganem and Prince 2004). However, the risk of HBV infection in transfusion recipients is extremely low when sensitive tests for HBsAg, capable of detecting less than 1 ng/ml, and tests for anti-HBc (see below) are used routinely (Biswas et al. 2003). Nevertheless, cases in which HBV is transmitted by HBsAg and anti-HBc-negative donations still occur (Allain 2004). The risk has been estimated to be 1 in 205 000 per unit in the USA (Dodd et al. 2002).

HBV-associated antigens and antibodies: the 'B-markers'

Hepatitis B surface antigen (HBsAg, formerly Australia antigen) is unassembled viral coat. Electron microscopy of concentrated serum containing HBsAg reveals the presence of so-called Dane particles, diameter 42 nm, which are known to be the complete virus (Dane et al. 1970). The particles are made up of an inner protein core (HBc) containing partially double-stranded DNA with a single-stranded region of variable length, protein kinases and DNA polymerase, surrounded by an outer coat of HBsAg (see Plate 16.2 shown in colour between pages 528 and 529). HBsAg is shed into the plasma in large quantities in the form of spheres and rods (diameter 18–22 nm). Antibodies to the surface antigen and the core antigen are known, respectively, as anti-HBs and anti-HBc. The major polypeptide in the core of HBV, p19, carries the antigenic determinants of HBcAg and HBeAg (Takahashi et al. 1981). HBseAg is a soluble protein (although also particle associated), found only in some sera containing HBsAg and thought to be a cleavage product of HBcAg. HBeAg in serum reflects viral replication and its presence is associated with infectivity.

In the partially double-stranded DNA, the long (L–) strand is of fixed length, whereas the length of the short strand (S+) is variable. The circular HBV genome is about 3200 nucleotides long. The L– strand carries virtually all the protein capacity of HBV in four open reading frames (ORFs) termed S/pre-S, C, P and X, which overlap one another. The S/pre-S region codes for the envelope proteins and is divided into: (1) the S gene coding for the major protein, HBsAg, 226 amino acids long, carrying the 'a' immunodominant determinant, with allelic variations for d/y and w/r (see below); (2) the pre-S2 region, coding for the pre-S2 antigen, a very immunogenic sequence of 55 amino acids, resistant to denaturation, which elicits neutralizing antibodies and, together with the major protein, codes for the middle protein, a glycoprotein 281 amino acids long; and (3) the pre-S1 region coding for a variable sequence of 108–119 amino acids, depending on the subtype, which is essential for recognition of hepatocyte receptors and, together with the S gene and the pre-S2 region, codes for the large envelope protein of HBV. The C region codes for the core protein and the P region for the DNA polymerase; the function of the X gene is still unknown (Tiollais 1988).

Subtypes and genotypes of HBV

All HBV strains have one antigenic determinant (a) in common, which may be of d or y subtypes: the subtypes (ad and ay) have a further determinant that may be either w or r. The subtypes are useful in epidemiological studies, as their distribution varies geographically.

Eight distinct genotypes, A–H, which vary in geographic distribution have been identified. Pathogenicity and response to therapy vary according to genotype. Genotype A is most common in the USA, whereas genotypes B and C are widespread in Asia (Kao et al. 2000; Kato et al. 2004).

HBsAg carriers

The prevalence of HBsAg varies considerably in different parts of the world and exceeds 15% in some populations in Africa, South-East Asia, China and Latin America. In some countries, such as the USA, in which the disease is not endemic, donors with a history of hepatitis after the age of 11 years are permanently deferred from donation. Soon after the introduction of testing for HBsAg, the frequency of positive results in volunteer donors giving blood for the first time was about 0.1%, both in the UK (Wallace *et al.* 1972) and in the USA (Cherubin and Prince 1971). In paid donors the frequency of HBsAg-positive donors was about 10 times greater than in volunteer donors (Walsh *et al.* 1970; Cherubin and Prince 1971). In donors with previously negative tests who give blood on subsequent occasions, the frequency of a positive test for HBsAg is very low: one in 60 000 in one series in north London. Almost all of the positive tests were due to acute infections in young men (Barbara and Briggs 1981). In north London, up to 1983, about 85% of the HBsAg-positive donations detected by screening were from long-term HBsAg carriers; the remainder came from donors with acute HBV infections (Barbara 1983). In a 6-year study of 1.9 million blood donors at five USA collection centres between the years 1991 and 1996, no reduction in the frequency (0.2%) of HBsAg in first-time blood donors could be documented (Glynn *et al.* 2000). A donor can transmit HBV for as long as 19 years after a positive test for HBsAg has been detected (Zuckerman and Taylor 1969). Carriers clear their HBsAg at a rate of about 1.7% per annum (Sampliner *et al.* 1979; Barbara 1983). When HBsAg is eventually lost, it is replaced ordinarily by anti-HBs as a marker of immunity.

More than 70% of apparently healthy British blood donors who are found to be HBsAg positive have normal liver function, as judged by serum aspartate transaminase (AST) and aminotransferase (ALT) levels (Barbara and Mijovic 1978). In a Dutch series a similar figure was observed: in the 30% with abnormal liver function tests (LFTs), when the tests remained abnormal over a period of time, moderate to severe liver disease, as judged histologically, was present in eight out of nine cases. All carriers of HBV were found to be either HBeAg positive (21%) or anti-HBe positive (79%). Abnormal LFTs were found significantly more often in HBeAg-positive carriers than in anti-HBe-positive carriers (Reesink *et al.* 1980). In countries where HBV is endemic, the proportion of HBsAg carriers who are HBeAg positive is higher.

Immunosuppression may cause recrudescence of latent HBV. In patients in whom anti-HBc is the only detectable HBV marker before immunosuppression, HBsAg may appear after immunosuppressive therapy (Nagington *et al.* 1977). Activation of latent HBV may be mistaken for post-transfusion hepatitis (PTH) in leukaemic patients or in patients with AIDS who receive blood component therapy. Haemophilia patients infected with HBV are more likely to progress to end-stage liver disease when they are co-infected with HCV and HIV (Goedert *et al.* 2002).

Anti-HBs

Anti-HBs develop in most people who recover from hepatitis B infection. The presence of the antibody in the plasma marks the end of acute infection and prevents re-infection with HBV.

Anti-HBc

Anti-HBc is found lifelong in persons who have been infected with HBV and is a marker of past or current viral replication. In acute infection, high levels of IgM anti-HBc appear during the incubation period after the appearance of HBsAg, persist for 3–4 months and are then replaced by IgG anti-HBc. High titres of IgG anti-HBc can be found in carriers who may sometimes also have low levels of IgM anti-HBc (see below). During the recovery phase of acute hepatitis B, anti-HBc may be present in the absence of HBsAg and anti-HBs. Donations taken at this time ('window' period) can transmit HBV (Hoofnagle *et al.* 1978). In a small proportion of carriers, only anti-HBc can be detected in the plasma. Such subjects may transmit HBV by transfusion (Larsen *et al.* 1990). In countries such as the USA, where screening of blood donations for anti-HBc has been introduced, the incidence of PTH due to HBV may have decreased considerably compared with that in countries such as the UK where routine screening for anti-HBc is not mandatory. The presence of both anti-HBc and anti-HBs confirms immunity to HBV, whereas their absence suggests susceptibility. However, passive transfer of these antibodies may follow transfusion or childbirth.

HBeAg and anti-HBe

HBeAg is a marker of infectivity associated with the presence of large numbers of Dane particles, found during the incubation period and the acute phase of clinical hepatitis B. Anti-HBe develops during recovery. HBsAg carriers initially have HBeAg in their blood, together with a high level of HBsAg. This phase may last for a variable period, sometimes measured in years. Approximately 20% of HBsAg-positive blood donors in the UK have HBeAg (Dow *et al.* 1980; Harrison *et al.* 1985), compared with 50% in Mediterranean countries (Lieberman *et al.* 1983). The HBeAg-positive phase is followed by a second phase in which anti-HBe replaces HBeAg, with HbsAg often falling to lower levels. Although infectivity is greatly reduced during this second phase, blood transfusion can still transmit HBV. Some HBV mutants that are incapable of synthesizing HBeAg have been shown to induce fulminant hepatitis (see section on HBV variants, below).

DNA polymerase

DNA polymerase is a marker of viraemia. Biochemical assays for the detection of DNA polymerase have been developed, but the assay is not as sensitive as that for detecting HBV-DNA and therefore not useful for mass screening of blood donors.

Serum HBV-DNA

HBV-DNA can be detected in serum by molecular hybridization techniques and PCR; however, PCR is more sensitive by several orders of magnitude than direct hybridization. A low level of HBV-DNA appears before HBsAg at the time of infection and remains detectable in serum and liver tissue in some patients who clear HBsAg from either acute self-limited or chronic HBV infection, or even after a successful anti-HBV treatment (Hu 2002). Occult, silent or latent HBV infection, defined as the presence of HBV infection with undetectable HBsAg, is well documented, although the prevalence of this clinical entity is unknown (Thiers *et al.* 1988; Allain 2004). HBV-DNA was detected in 8–12% of healthy Chinese people who were positive only for anti-HBc or anti-HBs, and in some healthy Chinese people without any serological HBV markers. On the other hand HBV-DNA was detected in only one-third of HBsAg positives (Pao *et al.* 1991). The viral load in occult infections is < 1000 IU/ml, so that pooled testing would improve blood safety minimally. If blood donors were to be screened for HBV-DNA in addition to HBsAg, the number of extra infectious donors detected would be small in countries with a low prevalence of HBsAg,

and increasing immunization together with effective treatment minimize the public health benefit of such screening. In a study of 600 000 volunteer blood donations in the USA, HBV 24-sample minipool NAT detected only two additional positive donors, which extrapolates to about 50 interdicted infectious donations transmitted to about 85 blood component recipients per year. Whether screening blood donors in populations with a very high prevalence of HbsAg, such as the Chinese (25%), would be of value, is another matter.

Screening tests for HBsAg in blood donations

The first tests used, such as immunodiffusion and counterimmunoelectrophoresis, were soon replaced by the more sensitive immunoradiometric assay (RIA) and the ELISA, which detect less than 0.5 ng of HBsAg/ml. However, taking the molecular weight of HBsAg as 3×10^6, 0.5 ng is equivalent to 1×10^7 particles. Thus, with a negative result of these tests, as many as $4-10 \times 10^7$ antigen molecules may be present per millilitre. Complete prevention of post-transfusion hepatitis B probably cannot be achieved by screening for HBsAg.

Immunoassays are available for the simultaneous detection of HBsAg and anti-HBs. Several monoclonal HBs antibodies directed against the *a* antigen, common to all HBV subtypes, have been produced and used in sensitive screening assays. However, mutations in the *S* region of HBV have led to *a*-deficient 'escape' mutants, which could not be detected by assays based solely on monoclonal anti-*a* (Carman *et al.* 1990). These mutants are not neutralized by anti-HBs *in vivo* or *in vitro*. In addition, if polyclonal assays based on anti-*ad* are used and the mutating virus was originally *ay*, infectious donors will be missed.

The British Standard Unit (BSU) has now been adopted as the International Standard Unit (ISU, shortened to IU) and is approximately equal to 1 ng of HBsAg/ml. Because of the ready availability of several commercial assays for HBsAg based on monoclonal antibodies, which can detect as little as 0.25 ng/ml, the minimum sensitivity requirement in the UK is 0.5 IU/ml (0.5 ng/ml) (UKBTS/NIBSC Liaison Group 2001).

Transmission of hepatitis B virus

HBV is spread by transfusion of infected blood, plasma or coagulation factor concentrates and by a variety of other percutaneous exposures (accidental needle-stick, shared syringes and needles by drug addicts, contaminated needles used in acupuncture, dentistry or tattooing, and by the sharing of razors). HBV can also be transmitted by sexual contact and by close contact between children leading to crossinfection, presumably by blood (e.g. biting) and other infected body fluids. In endemic areas with a high frequency of HbeAg-positive carriers, transmission from mother to infant in the perinatal period is common and often leads to chronic carriage in the infected infant.

In PTH due to the transmission of HBV by blood or blood components, the mean incubation period was found to be 63 days (range 30–150 days) by Gocke (1972) and 73 days (range 39–107 days) by Prince (1975). Highly sensitive assays now detect the presence of viral DNA 2–6 weeks earlier (Biswas *et al.* 2003). Less than 5% of those infected develop chronic hepatitis (Seeff *et al.* 1987).

Washing of red cells reduces the viral load and can render units seronegative. However, washing does not eliminate the risk of transmission of HBV. Red cells from blood that is only lightly contaminated with HBV and is washed, or frozen with glycerol and washed, although apparently HBsAg negative, can still transmit HBV to chimpanzees (Alter *et al.* 1978a) and humans (Rinker and Galambos 1981).

HBV transmitted by HBsAg-negative blood

Carriers with HBsAg below the detection level can transmit HBV by blood transfusion. Patients who were seronegative for all HBV serological markers, but positive for HBV-DNA by PCR, transmitted hepatitis B to two chimpanzees (Thiers *et al.* 1988). Moreover, subjects infected with HBV may be HBsAg negative owing to point mutations in the pre-core region, which may result in inability to synthesize HBsAg. Fulminant hepatitis developed in recipients of HBsAg-negative blood from donors infected with this mutated virus. In all of these donors, high levels of anti-HBc were present (Kojima *et al.* 1991). Extremely sensitive assays for HBV-DNA are defining a disparate group of subjects with occult HBV infection (Allain 2004). The frequency of such occult infections depends on the sensitivity of the assays for HBsAg and HBV as well as the prevalence of HBV infection in the population. Small samples of serum and cells containing HBV-DNA, anti-Hbc and anti-HBs (but not HBsAg) from three subjects who had recovered from HBV infection many years earlier failed to infect three chimpanzees followed for 15 months (Prince *et al.* 2001). However, the infectivity of larger volumes of blood and the prevalence and clinical importance of occult HBV needs further investigation.

In acute infections there are two periods when HBsAg may be undetectable although the subject can transmit HBV: (1) during the early stages of the incubation period when neither HBsAg nor anti-HBc may be detectable (see below) and (2) after clearance of HBsAg but before anti-HBs has become detectable ('diagnostic window'); in this phase anti-HBc, and often anti-HBe, can be detected (Tedder *et al.* 1980). Testing all blood donations for anti-HBc as well as anti-HBsAg has decreased the incidence of HBV infection by transfusion in the USA. About 50% of cases of hepatitis B that could be transmitted by blood from HBsAg-negative donors can be prevented by screening for anti-HBc (Mosley *et al.* 1995).

Inadvertent transmission of HBV from an asymptomatic subject in the early stages of the incubation period has been described (Rinker and Galambos 1981). The donor's washed red cells were given to 32 healthy volunteers (to stimulate antibodies) at a time when the donor was HBsAg negative. Between 36 and 76 days later, the donor turned HBsAg positive and subsequently developed hepatitis. Of 32 subjects who received the donor's blood, 19 developed HBsAg and 14 of these contracted hepatitis. A further nine subjects developed anti-HBs.

Serological findings in cases of HBV hepatitis

In persons exposed to HBV, HBsAg appears first in the incubation period, followed by anti-HBc. HBV-DNA, DNA polymerase, HBeAg and pre-S2 antigen also appear during the incubation period. In acute clinical hepatitis B, HBsAg reaches a peak at the onset of symptoms and then declines during the illness and convalescence, disappearing from the blood in most subjects after a period that varies from a week to several months. Clinical hepatitis B can be a serious disease with approximately 1–3% of acute cases presenting with fulminant hepatitis. Early experience suggested that 5–10% of infected subjects developed chronic hepatitis, but the number appears to be much lower

(Seeff *et al.* 1987; Zuckerman 1990). Subjects who recover have anti-HBs, anti-HBc and anti-pre-S2 in their plasma. The carrier state most commonly develops after asymptomatic infections, especially if infection is acquired in infancy. A study of children from Senegal showed that 80% of infants infected in the first 6 months of life became carriers compared with 15% of children infected between the ages of 2 and 3 years (Coursaget *et al.* 1987). In the UK, where acute HBV infections occur mainly in young adults, about 5% of those infected become carriers (Barbara 1983). Approximately 2 billion people have been infected worldwide with HBV and more than 350 million are chronic carriers. Approximately 15–40% of infected patients will develop cirrhosis, liver failure or hepatocellular carcinoma (Lok 2002).

Management of HBsAg-positive subjects

A survey carried out by Alter (1975) indicated that carriers of HBsAg are not commonly a danger to those with whom they come into ordinary social contact (excluding sexual contact). However, a few instances have been reported in which infected health-care workers have transmitted HBV to their patients while carrying out invasive surgical or dental procedures. Twelve such outbreaks involving 91 HBV-infected surgical patients who acquired the infection from 11 surgeons and one perfusion technician were reported in England, Wales and Northern Ireland between 1975 and 1990 (Heptonstall 1991). Staff of transfusion laboratories should be tested for HBsAg and those who are found to be positive should not assist in the preparation by an open process of blood or blood components intended for clinical use. In carriers of HBsAg, viral replication as revealed by the presence of HBeAg and HBV-DNA in serum is a useful index of infectivity. However, there are patients with severe liver disease who have HBV-DNA but no detectable HBeAg. These HBeAg-negative variants are due to point mutations in the pre-core region, which prevent the synthesis of HBeAg (Carman *et al.* 1989; Harrison and Zuckerman 1992).

A study of HBsAg-positive blood donors in the UK between 1971 and 1981 identified 2880 men and 1054 women who were traced until 1986. Male carriers had a significantly higher risk of dying from hepatocellular carcinoma or of acquiring chronic liver disease than did the general population (Hall 1988).

Protection against HBV by antibody

Subjects whose serum contains anti-HBs are protected from HBV infection (Grady and Lee 1975; Seeff *et al.* 1977). The administration of immunoglobulin prepared from the small proportion of donors with relatively potent anti-HBs was found to reduce the risk of hepatitis in subjects accidentally exposed to HBV infection compared with a control group treated with standard immunoglobulin (Grady and Lee 1975). Standard immunoglobulin, prepared from large pools of unselected donor plasma, contains a titre of anti-HBs too low to be of value in the prophylaxis of hepatitis B (Seeff *et al.* 1977).

The major indication for hepatitis B immunoglobulin (HBIg) is following a single acute exposure to HBV, as when blood known or strongly suspected to contain HBsAg is accidentally inoculated, ingested orally or splashed on to open wounds or mucous membranes of non-immune subjects. In such cases HBIg should be given in a dose of approximately 600 IU (for adults) as soon as possible after exposure; the subject should also be vaccinated. When appropriate, a further dose should be given 1 month later (Deinhardt and Zuckerman 1985). Newborn infants in endemic areas should also be given HBIg (see below).

HBV vaccine

Two types of HBV vaccine are available and have proven to be safe, immunogenic and efficacious; the first was derived from plasma of carriers as a source of surface antigen and the other is a recombinant DNA product synthesized in yeast (Szmuness *et al.* 1982; Eddleston 1990). Protective antibodies develop in 80–97% of subjects receiving the full immunization course. Protection conferred by either type of vaccine may not be permanent and, in a proportion of subjects, lasts no longer than 2–5 years or even less. However, most subjects appear to be protected for 15 years or more (McMahon *et al.* 2005). Reinforcing doses may be needed to prevent HBV infection.

Individuals with levels of anti-HBs below 10 IU/l are susceptible to infection, but it is not clear whether previous immunization helps to prevent the development of the carrier state (Eddleston 1990; Zuckerman 1990).

Universal immunization of infants against HBV has been recommended in the USA since 1991.

Immunization of patients requiring multiple transfusions of blood or blood products, such as patients with haemophilia or thalassaemia and those in need of renal dialysis, as well as health-care workers and medical or dental students exposed to blood, has long been advised by the Advisory Committee on Immunization Practice of the Centers for Disease Control and Prevention (CDC) (http://www.cdc.gov/nip/publications/acip-list.htm). In areas where HBV is endemic and access to vaccine is limited, subjects at risk should be immunized; infants born to HBeAg-positive mothers should be treated with HBIg, as well as with vaccine (Ip *et al.* 1989).

HBV variants

Occasional cases of hepatitis may be caused by variants of HBV that fail to react in conventional screening tests for HBsAg. Sera found negative for HbsAg on routine screening with polyclonal antibodies, but positive with monoclonal antibody as well as positive for HBV-DNA, were shown to transmit hepatitis to HBV-immune chimpanzees (Wands *et al.* 1986). Other HBV mutants have arisen by point mutations in the pre-core region of the genome; some have caused fulminant hepatitis (Kosaka *et al.* 1991; Liang *et al.* 1991) and others have been found in survivors of fulminant hepatitis or in asymptomatic contacts (Carman *et al.* 1991). The majority of these pre-core mutants do not synthesize HBeAg, which requires intact pre-core and core regions. Hence, there are patients with severe liver disease who have HBV-DNA but no HBeAg in their serum. In such patients there may be continuous viral replication despite the presence of anti-HBe (Tong *et al.* 1990).

In subjects immunized with HBV vaccine, the neutralizing antibody is directed against the *a* determinant of HBsAg. Point mutations have given rise to 'escape mutants' of HBV with *a* epitopes that are not neutralized by anti-HBs. If immunized subjects are infected with these mutants, they will have a variant HBsAg in addition to anti-HBs in their plasma (Carman *et al.* 1990; Harrison and Zuckerman 1992).

Hepatitis D (delta virus, HDV)

Delta virus, a 35-nm defective RNA virus found originally in northern Italians, occurs only in HBsAg-positive subjects because it requires HBV as a 'helper' virus (Tiollais 1988). The structure and replication of HDV are well described at the molecular level (Taylor 2003). Fewer than 10% of carriers of HBV are co-infected with HDV and the agent appears to be disappearing (Gaeta *et al.* 2003). Immunization to HBV should hasten its demise. HDV multiplies in the liver and is transmitted by blood and body fluids. The commonest mode of transmission in Europe and the USA is by parenteral inoculation, which explains its association with intravenous drug use (Smedile *et al.* 1982; Rizzetto 1983; Shattock *et al.* 1985). Anti-HDV has been found in the plasma of infected subjects in Europe, Australia, Asia and America; in the USA it is found in 3.8% of blood donations positive for HBsAg (CDC 1984), but it is found only very rarely in British blood donors (Tedder *et al.* 1982). Sexual transmission is particularly common in endemic areas of the Far East.

Superinfection of a carrier of HBsAg with HDV is associated with a chronic course of the delta infection in 70–90% of cases and with an increase in severity of the underlying chronic hepatitis (Smedile *et al.* 1982; Monjardino and Saldanha 1990). Simultaneous infection with HBV and HDV in a previously healthy subject tends to be followed by clearance of both HDV and HBV, although in some instances fulminant hepatitis or a more severe acute course has been reported (Shattock *et al.* 1985; Reynes *et al.* 1989; Fagan and Williams 1990). In HDV infection the delta antigen is present in liver and serum; viral RNA and anti-HDV can also be found in serum. As HDV depends upon the host HBV for its viral coat, chronic HDV infection depends on the persistence of HBV.

Screening for HBsAg in blood donors minimizes but does not abolish the risk of PTH delta in HBsAg-positive recipients (Rosina *et al.* 1985). The simultaneous presence of HDV and HBeAg in the absence of detectable HBsAg has been reported (Shattock *et al.* 1985). HDV has been transmitted not only by blood and blood components but also by coagulation factor concentrates (Purcell *et al.* 1985). Prior to universal use of pathogen-inactivated or recombinant clotting factor in the USA, 75% of patients with haemophilia A had serological evidence of exposure to HBV, and 13% to HDV (Kumar *et al.* 1993). Such exposure from clotting factor should be all but eliminated in the future.

Hepatitis C virus (HCV) and non-A, non-B hepatitis

Non-A, non-B hepatitis

By 1988, three distinct hepatitis viruses had been well characterized: hepatitis A virus (HAV), HBV and HDV. In 1977, the term 'NANBH' was coined for those cases of hepatitis not associated with the above three viruses, or to CMV, Epstein–Barr virus or toxic substances (Dienstag *et al.* 1977). A year later, NANBH was demonstrated to be transmitted by blood (Alter *et al.* 1978b; Tabor *et al.* 1978). Subsequent studies have determined, however, that transfusion accounts for only a small fraction of community-acquired cases of NANBH (Alter *et al.* 1990).

Several NANBH viruses have now been recognized. One of them, hepatitis E virus (HBE), is endemic and transmitted primarily by the faecal–oral route. The others are parenteral (see below). After the introduction of routine screening of blood donations for HBsAg, the great majority of cases of PTH were due to NANBH. Hepatitis C virus (HCV), a flavivirus, has been found to be the cause of most of these cases (Alter *et al.* 1989a; Kuo *et al.* 1989) (see below).

Indirect ('surrogate') markers to detect non-A, non-B hepatitis

Because the search for the specific agent or agents that cause NANBH was unsuccessful for so long, blood collectors looked for 'surrogate' markers to detect infectious donors. Two such markers, the presence of anti-HBc and elevated ALT levels, were proposed as the result of two independent prospective studies conducted in the USA. Both the multicentre Transfusion Transmitted Virus Study (TTVS) and the intramural investigators at the National Institutes of Health (NIH) Clinical Center showed that the incidence of NANB PTH was almost three times greater in recipients of anti-HBc-positive blood than in recipients of anti-HBc-negative blood (Stevens *et al.* 1984; Koziol *et al.* 1986). Although the significance of testing for anti-HBc in the prevention of PTH has been much reduced since the introduction of testing for anti-HCV (see below), its significance for preventing hepatitis B remains. In both of the above studies, elevated ALT levels in blood donors were associated with a significantly increased incidence of NANB PTH in the recipients. However, since testing for anti-HCV has become mandatory, the benefit of testing for ALT levels has declined to such an extent that its value in ensuring blood safety is minimal (Busch *et al.* 1995).

Identification of hepatitis C virus

The early efforts to characterize the agent responsible for NANBH indicated that it had a diameter of 30–60 nm, was chloroform sensitive and could be transmitted to chimpanzees, suggesting a small lipid-coated virus. In general, the concentration of the agent in plasma of infected chimpanzees was not high (Bradley *et al.* 1985). Collaboration between scientists at the CDC in Atlanta, with access to a source of confirmed infectious NANBH material and a group at Chiron Corporation with experience in molecular genetics led to the cloning and identification of the agent responsible for most cases of NANB PTH (Choo *et al.* 1989).

Structure of hepatitis C virus

HCV is a positive, single-stranded, enveloped RNA virus. The size of its RNA varies in different isolates but is about 10 kilobases long. Its genomic organization is similar to that of Flaviviridae and Pestiviruses (Miller and Purcell 1990). The genome is approximately 10 000 nucleotides and encodes a single polyprotein of 3010–3011 amino acids which is subsequently processed by host cell and viral proteases into three major structural proteins and several non-structural proteins necessary for viral replication (see Plate 16.3). The structural proteins include the core and the envelope proteins E1 (glycoprotein 33/35) and E2/NS1 (gp72). The non-structural proteins comprise the N2–N5 proteins, the function of which is not entirely clear; however, the region does code critical enzymes such as an NS3 helicase and an NS5 polymerase (Takeuchi *et al.* 1990; Choo *et al.* 1991; Weiner *et al.* 1991).

At present, six major types (types I–VI) and several subtypes have been described (Simmonds *et al.* 1994; Robertson *et al.* 1998). The distribution of the subtypes varies in different geographical areas. The genotypes are of clinical importance. HCV type II (subtype 1b), for example, is associated with a low response to therapy with alpha-interferon and with relapse after treatment (Yoshioka *et al.* 1992; Brouwer *et al.* 1993).

Evidence that hepatitis C virus is the main agent of non-A, non-B post-transfusion hepatitis

Using the first available test for anti-HCV, all of 15 well-characterized patients with NANBH had detectable antibody, but only three out of five patients with acute resolving NANBH gave positive results. HCV antibodies were detected in six out of seven NANBH sera infectious for chimpanzees (Alter *et al.* 1989b). Similar results were obtained in Japan and Italy (Kuo *et al.* 1989). With the first commercial assay for anti-HCV, an antiglobulin ELISA based on the c100/3 (or c100) antigen, a positive correlation was found between the presence of HCV antibodies and NANB PTH (Alter *et al.* 1989b). Furthermore, anti-HCV was present in all of 27 haemophiliacs who had been transfused at some stage with untreated clotting factor concentrates, but in none of 28 patients who had received only products subjected to viral inactivation procedures (Skidmore *et al.* 1990). Subsequent generations of the anti-HCV assay, with improved sensitivity and specificity, have confirmed the primacy of HCV as the NANB agent; however, evidence from multiple episodes in single patients and chimpanzee crosschallenge studies suggests the presence of additional agents (Mosley *et al.* 1977; Yoshizawa *et al.* 1981).

The incidence of PTH has significantly decreased since screening for anti-HCV was introduced. Whereas 38 (12.4%) of 226 patients who underwent cardiovascular surgery and received blood transfusions developed PTH before screening was begun, none of 87 patients developed PTH after receiving anti-HCV-negative blood (Wang *et al.* 1994). In a study of a Spanish population, HCV screening seemed to be far less effective, although false-negative test results may have played a role in these findings (Esteban *et al.* 1989). In the 40-year prospective studies at the NIH, PTH rates fell from more than 30% in the 1960s to < 1% in 1995 and close to zero by 1997 (Alter and Houghton 2000).

Clinical course of hepatitis C

Most cases of hepatitis C are mild and non-icteric, but 50–70% of the cases become chronic and present as chronic persistent hepatitis or chronic active hepatitis. About 20% of patients infected with HCV develop cirrhosis, although the rate is variable and progression to cirrhosis may take 50 years (Ghany *et al.* 2003). Patients infected with HCV are particularly susceptible to the hepatotoxic effects of alcohol (Corrao and Arico 1998; Harris *et al.* 2001). A strong association between HCV infection and carcinoma of the liver has been found. Differences in the clinical course of HCV infection in different parts of the world may be due to different genetic types of the virus or, given the chronicity of the infection, to the time of origin of the HCV epidemic in each country (Tanaka *et al.* 2002).

Prior to viral inactivation of fractionated plasma, some 80% of severe haemophilia A patients, who received numerous infusions of factor VIII derived from pooled plasma donations, developed chronic hepatitis, almost certainly related to HCV exposure (Aledort *et al.* 1985; Hay *et al.* 1985). Long-term studies of patients with PTH, most of whom were middle-aged when infected, show no increase in mortality, but a distinct increase in liver-related mortality (Seeff *et al.* 2001). Cohorts of women of child-bearing age infected with Rh immunoglobulin exhibit low percentages of inflammation and cirrhosis when followed for 17–20 years (Kenny-Walsh 1999). Although HCV infection clearly progresses over time and is exacerbated by alcohol and co-infection with HIV (Goedert *et al.* 2002), as many as 20% of adults and 45% of children appear to clear the infection spontaneously (Vogt *et al.* 1999; Seeff *et al.* 2001).

Screening and confirmatory assays for HCV antibodies

When populations at low risk were screened with the first ELISAs ('first-generation' assays) 60% of the reactive samples proved to be falsely positive (van der Poel *et al.* 1989). The sensitivity of these assays was poor in the early stage of infection (Esteban *et al.* 1990; Contreras *et al.* 1991). The anti-HCV window ranged from 3–6 months and some patients with PTH never seroconverted with this assay. The limited sensitivity of the 'first-generation' assay was attributed to the use of the c100/3 non-structural antigen alone, which represents only 12% of the viral genome (van der Poel *et al.* 1990) (see Plate 16.3 shown in colour between pages 528 and 529).

Second-generation assays, in which additional viral antigens are used, derived from both the structural and the non-structural part of the HCV genome (the c22, c33c and 5.1.1 antigens; Plate 16.3), proved more sensitive than first-generation assays (Aach *et al.* 1991; McHutchinson *et al.* 1992; Lai *et al.* 1993). In the third-generation assays, an additional non-structural antigen (NS5) is included. These assays are slightly more sensitive than second-generation assays and the percentage of false positives is lower than in second-generation assays (Uyttendaele *et al.* 1994; Lee *et al.* 1995).

To address the problem of false-positive reactions, screening strategies confirm reactive samples with a supplemental assay. For confirmation, recombinant immunoblot assays (RIBAs) are used in which reactions with individual antigens can be visualized. Because of poor sensitivity and specificity, the first-generation RIBAs were rapidly replaced by second-generation assays (RIBA-2) in which four recombinant proteins are used (c22-3, c100-3, c33c and 5.1.1) (Leon *et al.* 1991; Alter 1992).

The RIBA is considered to be positive if a reaction occurs with at least two antigens. A reaction with only one antigen is considered to be an indeterminate result. Evaluation of indeterminate results in RIBA-2 showed that these may be specific (HCV RNA positive) or non-specific (HCV RNA negative). In the third-generation RIBA (RIBA-3), in addition to the initial c33c antigen, a mixture of the recombinant proteins c100-3 and 5.1.1. is used together with a conformationally modified recombinant c22-3 antigen. The recombinant c22-3 protein is replaced by a four-epitope synthetic c22 protein and a second NS5 protein is added. The RIBA-3 has been found to be more sensitive and specific than the RIBA-2 (Pawlotsky 1994; Damen *et al.* 1995). Nevertheless, indeterminate results are still obtained, in which case HCV RNA detection by PCR is mandatory. Recent studies of a cohort of women infected with hepatitis C anti-Rh immune globulin during pregnancy suggests that many 'false-positive' RIBA assays do in fact represent exposure to HCV in the distant past when assays of cellular immunity are performed (Takaki *et al.* 2000). Similar results have been confirmed with a cohort of otherwise healthy blood donors (Semmo *et al.* 2005). Long-term prospective studies will determine whether these findings indicate that spontaneous recovery from HCV infection is higher than conventionally taught.

An alternative approach to using a RIBA for confirmation relies on two sequential, different screening assays, a strategy found to be reliable for screening blood donors (Allain *et al.* 1996). Most laboratories still rely on some form of immunoblotting assay for confirmation of positive results before counselling. Others perform PCR for HCV if two ELISAs are positive.

Polymerase chain reaction for the detection of hepatitis C virus RNA

The most sensitive method for screening for HCV relies on detection of RNA by some gene amplification technique, NAT. NATs turn positive within 3 weeks of infection. HCV NAT using the minipool technique is now used to screen all blood and plasma donors. Although NAT is extremely sensitive and has reduced the HCV window significantly, HCV RNA levels fluctuate during the window period and during the course of chronic infection. High rates of HCV transmission have been found at all levels of viraemia, and donor blood may be infectious even when RNA is undetectable in the TMA assay (Fang *et al.* 2003; Operskalski *et al.* 2003). Current HCV RNA testing will not interdict all infectious units, even with single-donation testing, and serological testing remains essential for screening blood donors.

Transmission of hepatitis C virus

HCV is transmitted by blood components and blood products including IVIG, anti-D Ig for i.v. use and factor VIII concentrate submitted to some of the virus inactivation procedures (Yap *et al.* 1993; Bjoro *et al.* 1994; Bergman 1995; Meisel *et al.* 1995; Power *et al.* 1995). HCV has never been transmitted by albumin concentrates or by anti-D for i.m. use. The risk of transmission from mother to infant is small, although increased when co-infection with HIV exists. The risk is directly related to the amount of virus in the maternal blood, approaching 36% if the viral titre exceeds 10^6 and almost non-existent at lower titres. The HCV genotype in mothers and infants was identical in nearly all cases (Ohto *et al.* 1994; Ferrero *et al.* 2003). The importance of sexual transmission of HCV is controversial. In most studies the techniques used were insensitive and other (mainly shared) risk factors in the sexual partners were not always taken into account. In a study of 50 heterosexual partners of infected subjects over a mean of 13 years, no partner was found positive (Bresters *et al.* 1993). Among 895 monogamous heterosexual partners of HCV chronically infected individuals in a long-term prospective study, 776 (86.7%) spouses were followed for 10 years, corresponding to 7760 person-years of observation. Three HCV infections were observed during follow-up corresponding to an incidence rate of 0.37 per 1000 person-years. However, the infecting HCV genotype in one spouse (2a) was different from that of the partner (1b), clearly excluding sexual transmission. The remaining two couples had concordant genotypes, but sequence analysis of the NS5b region of the HCV genome showed that the corresponding partners carried different viral isolates (Vandelli *et al.* 2004). Sexual transmission of HCV within heterosexual monogamous couples must be extremely low. Different results were obtained in China and Japan where 7 out of 38 and 14 out of 195 spouses of infected subjects were found positive (Anahane *et al.* 1992; Kao *et al.* 1992). However, the prevalence of HCV in these countries is very high and the results may have been confounded by infection of both partners by an external source. The prevalence of HCV in homosexual men is much lower than that of anti-HBc or anti-HIV (Esteban *et al.* 1989).

An episode of HCV infection does not necessarily confer protective immunity (Farci *et al.* 1993). An important feature of HCV is its high degree of genetic variability, which is due to the inherent low fidelity of the viral replication machinery. HCV circulates *in vivo* as a population of genetic variants that have been called 'quasispecies' (Farci 2001). Quasispecies develop in response to immune pressure and represent an escape mechanism for the virus to evade neutralization and clearance. The clinical significance of quasispecies development in transmission, infectivity and in the natural history of the disease is unclear.

Residual risk of post-transfusion hepatitis: beyond the hepatitis alphabet

Since the introduction of testing for HBsAg, anti-HBc, anti-HCV and HCV NAT, the risk of PTH has been reduced dramatically. Nevertheless, cases of PTH due to HBV and HCV still occur, generally caused by transfusion of blood from donors in the early stages of HBV or HCV infection. In the USA, where screening for anti-HBc is done routinely in addition to screening for HBsAg, anti-HCV and HCV NAT, the residual risk of the transmission of HBV or HCV has been calculated as one in 205 000 donations and one in 1 935 000 donations respectively (Dodd *et al.* 2002). Cases of non-A, non-B, non-C PTH also occur but accurate estimates of frequency are not available.

Hepatitis E virus

Hepatitis E virus (HEV) is a non-enveloped RNA virus responsible for epidemic hepatitis in Asia, Africa, Latin America and the Middle East and sporadic hepatitis in developed countries. The agent has been cloned (Reyes *et al.* 1990; Worm *et al.* 2000), which led to the development of molecular tests and a sensitive ELISA assay for detecting anti-HEV (Dawson *et al.* 1992). HEV is nearly always transmitted by the faecal–oral route. However, like HAV, transient viraemia develops after infection, and transmission by blood transfusion does occur (Matsubayashi *et al.* 2004). In Germany, the prevalence of anti-HEV in patients with coagulation disorders has been found to be low (Klarmann *et al.* 1995). HEV is of negligible importance in blood transfusion.

GB viruses (GBV/HGV)

Blind molecular cloning, similar to the strategy used to discover HCV, has resulted in the detection of several other transfusion-transmitted viruses. The first agents associated with acute icteric hepatitis that were passaged serially in marmosets came from the blood of a 34-year-old surgeon (GB) (Deinhardt *et al.* 1967). Later, these agents were characterized extensively and appeared to be distinct from the other hepatitis viruses (Schlauder *et al.* 1995). Using amplification techniques, cloning and sequencing, at first two viruses, GBV-A and GBV-B, found only in tamarins, and later a third virus, GBV-C, from a human serum, were identified (Simons *et al.* 1995; Yoshiba *et al.* 1995). Of the three 'GB' viruses, GBV-C seems to be the only human virus. GBV-C has been recovered from the blood of several patients with hepatitis, from multitransfused patients, haemophiliacs and i.v. drug users. The GB viruses are flavivirus-like agents similar to HCV, with a similar genomic organization. However, there is only 26% homology between the GB viruses and HCV. Homology between GBV-A and GBV-C is fairly strong (48%), but between GBV-A and GBV-B and between GBV-C and GBV-B only about 27% (Zuckerman 1996). In relatively small studies, the prevalence of GBV-C has been found to be quite high: 2% in blood donors in the USA and the UK and 12–14% in drug addicts and multiply transfused patients. Viral RNA has been detected in 20% of seropositives and viraemia can persist for months or years (Denis *et al.* 1996). GBV-C has been detected in three out of six patients with fulminant non-A, -B, -C or -E hepatitis but the real significance of the virus as a cause of hepatitis, PTH and chronic liver disease has still to be established (Yoshiba *et al.* 1995). Lack of a temporal relationship between peak viraemia and raised ALT levels has cast doubt as to whether GBV-C can cause liver disease (Alter *et al.* 1997). Indeed, GBV-C may not even be a hepatotropic agent.

A virus, provisionally designated HGV, was isolated from the blood of a patient with chronic hepatitis (Linnen *et al.* 1995). The virus has been cloned and found to have 95% homology with GBV-C but to be only distantly related to GBV-A, GBV-B and HCV. GBV-C and HGV are almost certainly independent isolates of the same virus that can be transmitted by transfusion but do not result in hepatitis.

TT virus

Using representational difference analysis to compare pre- and post-hepatitis specimens, investigators in Japan discovered a novel non-enveloped, single-stranded DNA virus that correlated with patient elevations of ALT (Nishizawa *et al.* 1997). TT virus (TTV), named after the initials of the index case, is readily transmitted by transfusion and appears to replicate in the liver (Rodriguez-Inigo *et al.* 2000). Although 7.5% of the USA blood donor population carries this virus, an almost identical percentage of transfusion recipients (> 20%) are infected whether or not they develop hepatitis (Matsumoto *et al.* 1999). Although TT virus does not appear to be a cause of PTH, a broad range of isolates have now been identified in this family of circoviridae and it is possible that one of the variants may turn out to be hepatotoxic.

SEN virus

Another transfusion-transmitted member of the family of circoviridae was isolated from, and named after, an Italian patient with the initials 'SEN' (Tanaka *et al.*

2001). The prevalence of SEN virus (SEN-V) in 436 volunteer donors was 1.8%. Two SEN-V variants (SENV-D and SENV-H) were unequivocally transmitted by transfusion and associated statistically with transfusion-transmitted non-A to -E hepatitis (Umemura *et al.* 2001). Even if this association is confirmed, the clinical importance of this agent still remains to be established (Sagir *et al.* 2004).

Hepatitis A virus

Hepatitis A virus (HAV), a 27-nm, non-enveloped picornavirus and the infectious agent of epidemic hepatitis transmitted by the faecal–oral route, causes only transient viraemia and does not induce a carrier state. Although the incubation period following infection lasts for several weeks, viraemia lasts only a day or two during acute illness. HAV rarely causes PTH. In 14 published series, relating to transfusions given to about 9000 subjects, not a single case of PTH due to HAV was observed (Blum and Vyas 1982). Transmission of HAV, leading to the development of PTH, can occur in special circumstances (Seeberg *et al.* 1981; Hollinger *et al.* 1983; Sherertz *et al.* 1984). In London, 21% of donors are immune to HAV, whereas almost all subjects in the developing world have been infected by the age of 10 years (Purcell 1988).

In cases where hepatitis A has followed the transfusion of blood, red cells or fresh-frozen plasma, the donor has been in the early stages of incubating the disease, and then only when the recipient is susceptible to HAV, and when any other units transfused are devoid of anti-HAV that would otherwise neutralize the virus. A single unit of blood transmitted HAV to 11 infants in a neonatal intensive care unit (Noble *et al.* 1984). Acute infection with HAV is most readily recognized by the finding of specific IgM antibodies to the virus.

An unusual outbreak of transfusion-transmitted HAV occurred in 41 Italian haemophiliacs. The source of infection seems to have been factor VIII concentrate from a local plasma fractionation plant. HAV, with a non-lipid envelope, would be resistant to the solvent–detergent method used for viral inactivation (Mannucci 1992). Further outbreaks of HAV transmission due to solvent–detergent-treated factor VIII and factor IX concentrates have been reported by commercial fractionators.

In general, normal Ig for i.m. use contains enough anti-HAV to protect travellers to areas endemic for

HAV. Now that a hepatitis A vaccine is available, haemophiliacs and frequent travellers have an alternative to receiving repeated injections of normal Ig (Craig and Schaffner 2004).

Human immunodeficiency viruses

Retroviruses and blood transfusion

Although retroviruses were among the first known viruses, for almost a century they were only found in animals, usually in association with neoplastic diseases. Until 1980, retroviruses had not been linked to human disease, let alone to transfusion-transmitted infection. However, the sensitive immunological, biochemical and molecular approaches that became available in the 1970s led to the discovery of the first human retroviruses, isolated from lymphocytes of a patient with T-cell leukaemia and appropriately named human T-lymphotropic virus type I (Poiesz et al. 1980). Knowledge of the existence of prototype retroviruses encouraged a search for a human retrovirus as the aetiological agent of AIDS. The causative agent, originally referred to as LAV, or HTLV III and now called human immunodeficiency virus (HIV) was discovered in 1983 (Barre-Sinoussi et al. 1983). Numerous isolates of the different human retroviruses have been reported.

Retroviruses owe their name to their ability to reverse the normal sequence of events in macromolecular synthesis; they are RNA viruses, which, after entering host cells and losing their envelope, use 'reverse transcriptase' (RNA-dependent DNA polymerase) together with cell-derived RNA as a primer to transcribe a double-stranded DNA copy of the single-stranded viral RNA genome. The DNA copy enters the nucleus and is permanently integrated as a DNA provirus into the DNA of the host cells, mainly lymphocytes, but also monocytes, macrophages and other cells. The provirus remains latent and replicates as an integral part of the host genome. The synthesis of new viral proteins and viral messenger RNA is programmed by proviral DNA and mediated by host enzymes. The virus consists of two identical molecules of single-stranded RNA, in a protein core containing several molecules of reverse transcriptase and cell-derived molecules. The core is surrounded by an envelope consisting of virally encoded glycoproteins (gps) and host-derived lipids that are acquired when the

newly assembled viruses bud out through the cell membrane. The progeny viruses will then infect other cells within the same host (Greene and Peterlin 2002).

All retroviruses contain three main structural genes: the gag gene codes for different molecular weight proteins that are integral to the nuclear core; the pol gene codes for reverse transcriptase; and the env gene specifies the envelope glycoproteins. The primary products of these three genes are larger parent polypeptides that can be enzymatically split into smaller peptides. Human retroviruses, especially HTLV-I and -II, have regions of homology between them (Wong-Staal and Gallo 1985; Gallo 2003). Retroviruses are composed of 60–70% protein, 30–40% lipid (confined to the envelope), 2–4% carbohydrate and 1% RNA. The proteins are immunogenic. The integrity of the envelope is essential for infectivity. The high lipid content of the retroviral envelope renders these agents very susceptible to disruption by detergents and organic solvents.

Human retroviruses all share a tropism for lymphocytes inducing fusion and giant cell formation in vitro and impairing function in vivo. To enter the cell they bind to cell receptors for the retroviral glycoproteins. The high-affinity receptor for HIV has been identified as CD4 on helper T lymphocytes, macrophages and other cells. Accessory cell surface molecules called coreceptors, shown to be chemokine receptors (either CCR5 or CXCR4), are required for fusion with the cell membrane (Berger et al. 1999; Weiss 2002). The HTLV-I and -II virus receptor is the transporter of glucose GLUT1 (Manel et al. 2003). All human retroviruses code for a small crossreactive major core protein, p24, and have similar modes of transmission, i.e. sexual, congenital and by blood or body fluid (Wong-Staal and Gallo 1985).

HIV-1 and HIV-2

The causative agent of AIDS was originally described as LAV (lymphadenopathy-associated virus) (Barre-Sinoussi et al. 1983; Vilmer et al. 1984). Gallo and his colleagues succeeded in culturing the same virus, which they called HTLV-III, in large quantities in continuously replicating T cells (Popovic et al. 1984). This virus, together with visna virus, belongs to the lentivirus subfamily of retroviruses. HIV was found to induce premature death of its host cells and to replicate rapidly (Gallo et al. 1984). HIV has a great propensity for genetic variability, especially within the env gene coding for the major external glycoprotein (Wain-Hobson *et al.* 1985; Wong-Staal *et al.* 1985), which carries the epitopes that react with the scarce viral neutralizing antibodies. Extreme genetic diversity, with variants classified as group M (main) with subtypes (clades) A–K, group O and group N, has implications for screening, diagnosis and treatment (Stebbing and Moyle 2003).

A second distinct retrovirus named HIV-2 (LAV-2) causes a somewhat milder disease. Although this virus is also lymphotropic, cytotoxic and neurotropic, and shares epitopes of the core and *pol* proteins with HIV-1, HIV-2 nucleotide sequence identity with HIV-1 isolates is only 40–50%. The main differences between HIV-1 and -2 lie within the envelope nucleotides and proteins. HIV-2 has closer sequence identity with the simian retrovirus SIV (Clavel *et al.* 1986; Brucker *et al.* 1987; Brun-Vezinet *et al.* 1987). The different subtypes of HIV-2 are analogous to the different groups of HIV-1 (Damond *et al.* 2004).

The *env* gene of HIV-1 codes for a major precursor polyprotein p85. This protein becomes heavily glycosylated to form the exterior glycoprotein gp160, which is processed into gp120 and gp41 by a viral protease (Wong-Staal and Gallo 1985). Gp41 is a transmembrane protein that anchors gp120 in the membrane and has specific amino acid domains for binding to the CD4 molecule on target cells, allowing the entry of the virus into the cell (Plate 16.3; Weiss 2002). The gp41 protein is also important for syncytial fusion of cells (Brun-Vezinet *et al.* 1987). There is no crossreactivity between the envelope glycoproteins of HIV-1 and -2. The *gag* gene of HIV-1 codes for the large precursor protein of 55 kDa, p55, which is enzymatically cleaved into the smaller fragments p24, p17 and p15 (Veronese *et al.* 1988). The p24 protein encloses the two strands of RNA and the reverse transcriptase. The antigen p17 encircles the viral core and is attached to the fatty acid myristate. Myristoylation appears to be required for infectivity (Bryant and Ratner 1990). The *gag* proteins p9 and p7, derived from p15, surround the two strands of RNA and form part of the core; p24 and p17 share epitopes with the less well-defined HIV-2 core proteins, p26 and p16 (Brun-Vezinet *et al.* 1987). The *pol* gene products of HIV-1 are derived from the large precursor molecule Pr 180 *gag-pol* and comprise reverse transcriptase, viral integrase and viral protease, the last named being responsible for cleaving both the large Pr 180 *gag-pol* and the p55 *gag* precursor into the core proteins (Schochetman 1992; Weiss 2002).

The cell membrane protein CD4 is the main receptor for HIV (Dalgleish *et al.* 1984). The HIV envelope glycoprotein gp120 binds specifically to CD4-bearing cells and interacts with gp41 for virus–cell and cell–cell fusion events, with the formation of syncytia between infected and uninfected cells. Two molecules act as secondary receptors for HIV-1: one is a G-protein 'receptor-associated' molecule CCR-4 (Feng *et al.* 1996); the other is the β-chemokine receptor CCR-5 (Deng *et al.* 1996; Dragic *et al.* 1996). Most viral isolates use CCR-5. Penetration of HIV into the cell occurs by fusion of the viral and cellular membranes. Once the virus enters the cytoplasm, its partial uncoating activates its reverse transcriptase, which converts RNA into double-stranded DNA. Viral DNA is then integrated as provirus into the host DNA. There are other less efficient routes for entry of HIV into cells; antibody-coated HIV can adhere to monocytes and macrophages via Fc receptors and possibly via complement receptors (Markovic and Clouse 2004).

Once the virus enters susceptible cells, it either remains latent or establishes 'factories' of progeny virus in the infected host, so that all subjects who are shown to be infected with HIV should be assumed to have persistent infection and hence to be infectious to others (Schochetman 1992). The cells most susceptible to HIV infection, carrying significant amounts of CD4 receptors, are T-helper lymphocytes, macrophages, monocytes, megakaryocytes and some bone marrow stem cells. Cells carrying low levels of CD4, such as the epidermal Langerhans cells, dendritic cells and certain cells of the central nervous system, are also susceptible. Some cells such as glial cells, colorectal and fetal brain cells are susceptible to HIV infection despite their lack of CD4 receptors (Takeda *et al.* 1988; Levy 1989).

Course of HIV infection (Fig. 16.2)

For the first few days after infection, no markers of HIV can be detected in blood, an interval known as the 'eclipse' phase. Viraemia follows for a period of several weeks, first with intermittent 'blips' of virus interrupting periods of undetectable markers in blood. This stage is followed by a 'ramp up' phase at about day 10 when HIV viral copy number rises rapidly (Fiebig *et al.* 2003). At about day 17, p24 antigen becomes detectable in serum and at about day 22,

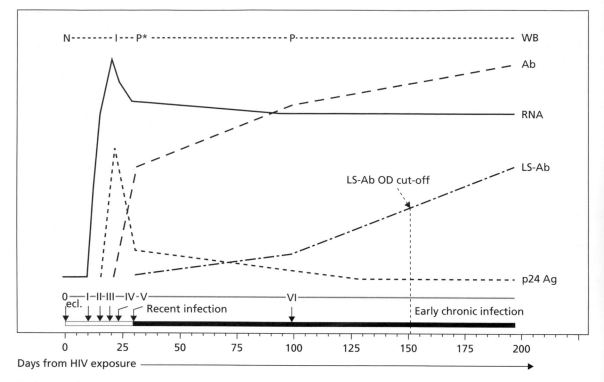

Fig 16.2 A schematic, semi-quantitative display of the progression of HIV markers. From top to bottom: WB, Western blot; Ab, HIV antibody; RNA, HIV RNA; LS-Ab, HIV antibody determined by sensitive/less sensitive enzyme immunoassay testing strategy; p24 Ag, HIV p24 antigen, from time of exposure (day 0) through the first 200 days of infection. As each of the markers appears in the bloodstream, the infection is assigned a new stage from 0 (eclipse period, ecl.), characterized by undetectable viral markers in blood samples; reported to last on average up to 11 days from viral exposure through stage I (definitive HIV RNA viraemia), stage II (p24 antigenaemia), stage III (HIV EIA antibody reactive), stage IV (Western blot indeterminate, 'I'), stage V (Western blot positive without p31 band, 'P*') and stage VI (Western blot positive, 'P' with p31 band). Stages I–VI were derived from an analysis of the 'A' set of plasma donor seroconversion panels as described here. The standardized optical density (OD) cut-off for the sensitive/less sensitive EIA may be varied with recommended cutoffs from 0.5 to 1.0. Cutoffs of 0.5 and 1.0 would result in average demarcations of recent from early chronic infection at 124 and 186 days respectively. Adapted from Fiebig *et al.* (2003).

anti-HIV seroconversion occurs. During this period, more than 40% of patients develop an acute, flu-like or mononucleosis-like syndrome (Kahn and Walker 1998). Two to four months after sexually transmitted infection, and 1–2 months after transfusion-transmitted infection, more than 95% of HIV-infected subjects exhibit a wide range of antibodies to the structural *env, gag* and *pol* viral proteins, mostly IgG with some IgA and transient IgM at the start of the immune response (Horsburgh *et al.* 1989; Seligmann 1990). The period between infection and the detection of HIV, the 'window' period, has not been as clearly defined after sexual exposure as it has after blood

transfusion because the precise date of infection is usually unknown (Seligmann 1990).

As soon as anti-p24 develops, p24 antigenaemia disappears. A long asymptomatic period follows primary infection; however, disease progression is relentless during this interval (Pantaleo *et al.* 1993). Antigenaemia may reappear in the late stages of AIDS and intermittently during the asymptomatic phase of infection, which may last for more than 10 years. Levels of all HIV antibody specificities are usually very high during the asymptomatic period but which antibodies combat infection and which if any enhance disease progression is unknown. Although some correlation has been found between high levels of neutralizing antibodies (mainly anti-gp120) and better clinical outcome (Robert-Guroff *et al.* 1988), protective humoral and cellular immune responses to HIV are either poor or short-lived (Seligmann 1990). The cellular response appears to put selective pressure on viral mutation (Soudeyns *et al.* 1999). Disease develops when the CD4 helper cells have almost completely disappeared, leading to impairment of the immune system and spread of HIV with signs of disease in multiple organs; anti-p24 declines or disappears and p24 antigen reappears at this stage. Other antibodies also decline, with the exception of anti-gp41. CD4 T-cell depletion leads to progressive immunological unresponsiveness to foreign stimuli with increased susceptibility to opportunistic infections (*Pneumocystis carinii*, CMV, atypical mycobacteria) and malignancies such as Kaposi's sarcoma and lymphomas (Mawle 1992). In the absence of treatment, disease progression is usually relentless and almost invariably fatal.

A correlation has been found between the biological phenotype of HIV-I and the clinical course of AIDS. Fast-replicating, syncytium-inducing (SI) variants of the virus are found in 50% of HIV-1-seropositive subjects, preceding progression to AIDS, whereas slowly replicating, non-syncytium-inducing (NSI) variants are predominant in the asymptomatic stage of HIV infection (Tersmette *et al.* 1989). The third variable domain (V3) of the envelope gene has been found to be responsible for differences in phenotype (York-Higgins *et al.* 1990; Shioda *et al.* 1991).

Epidemiology of HIV infection and spread of AIDS

Since AIDS was first described in the USA in 1981 in young, previously healthy, homosexual men, the disease has spread worldwide. As of the end of 2003, an estimated 37.8 million people, 35.7 million adults and 2.1 million children younger than 15 years, were living with HIV/AIDS (UNAIDS 2004). Approximately two-thirds of these people (25.0 million) live in sub-Saharan Africa; another 20% (7.4 million) live in Asia and the Pacific. Between 2002 and 2004, an estimated 10 million people were infected with HIV and just under 6 million people died from AIDS (Piot *et al.* 2004).

The disease is transmitted by sexual intercourse, sharing of needles, transfusion of blood and blood products and vertical transmission from mother to child. In the USA and Europe, sexual transmission by homosexual and bisexual men is still much more important than is heterosexual transmission, but the latter is increasing and appears to be the most important route of spread in Africa, Thailand, India and countries in South America and the Caribbean.

HIV-2 is more restricted in its geographical distribution and is concentrated mainly in West Africa, from the Cape Verde Islands to Benin (e.g. Gambia, Guinea Bissau) with limited spread to those countries in western Europe historically associated with West Africa (Fleming 1990). Cases of HIV-2 infection have also been reported in East Africa, Asia, Latin America and North America. In several West African countries, the frequency of HIV-1 and HIV-2 infections is very similar. In children, AIDS caused by HIV-2 is more likely to be due to transmission by blood transfusion than perinatal transmission (Poulsen *et al.* 1989). Nevertheless, both serotypes have the same modes of transmission and AIDS caused by either is indistinguishable. Both HIV-1 and HIV-2 must be excluded from blood donations.

Transmission of HIV by blood transfusion

Recognition of a possible relationship between blood transfusions and the acquired immune deficiency syndrome (AIDS) provided early clues that AIDS might have an infectious cause. In July 1982, three patients with severe classic haemophilia who developed *Pneumocystis carinii* pneumonia were reported by the Centers for Disease Control in the Morbidity and Mortality Weekly Report (MMWR) (CDC 1982). Two of these patients had also developed oral candidiasis, and one was infected with *Mycobacterium avium-intracellulare*. All had been treated with large doses of commercially prepared factor VIII concentrate. Laboratory and clinical studies of these patients revealed evidence of impaired cell-mediated immunity. In quick succession, several additional reports linked haemophilia and AIDS, two relatively uncommon disorders (Ragni *et al.* 1983; White and Lesesne 1983). The association seemed unlikely to have happened by chance alone. In subsequent studies, some apparently healthy patients with haemophilia, including those treated only with cryoprecipitate obtained from volunteer blood donors, demonstrated abnormalities in cell-mediated immunity (Lederman *et al.* 1983).

The first reported case of transfusion-associated AIDS (TAA) turned out to be an 18-month-old infant with severe combined immunodeficiency who had been transfused repeatedly at birth and had received a unit of platelets from a donor who subsequently developed AIDS (Amman *et al.* 1983). By 1984, 38 cases of AIDS had been reported in patients with no risk factors other than a history of transfusion. Nineteen of the patients were adults who, during the previous 5 years, had received blood components derived from unpooled donations. In those cases in which all the donors could be followed up, an individual in a 'high-risk' group could always be identified (Curran *et al.* 1984). An expanded study of 194 patients showed that in most cases the high-risk donor was anti-HIV positive, and in those few cases in which the high-risk donor lacked anti-HIV, another donor tested positive (Peterman *et al.* 1985). A total of 157 525 cases of AIDS was reported in the USA by the end of 1990, and 5371 (3.4%) of these were attributed to the transfusion of blood or blood components. The median incubation period, estimated as the time from exposure by transfusion to diagnosis of AIDS, has been estimated to be 34 months in adults and 22 months in children (Peterman 1987), although later estimates indicated a longer period with a median of 7–8 years for adults and 3–5 years for children (Rogers 1992). In total, 50% of untreated subjects infected with HIV by transfusion will develop AIDS within 7 years compared with 33% of subjects infected by other routes (Ward *et al.* 1989).

Following the first reports, the number of cases of TAA in the USA increased rapidly. By the end of 1991, out of a total of 206 392 cases of AIDS, there were 6060 adults and 472 infants or children who had acquired the disease by transfusion of blood or blood products, representing 3% and 13.6% of the total cases in adults and children respectively (CDC 1992). The risk of transmission of HIV by blood transfusion is now trivial in countries without major heterosexual spread and in which donor education, encouragement of self-exclusion and screening for HIV antibodies have been established since 1985. In these countries, the risk of transmission of HIV is almost solely attributable to donations given during the window period (see below).

In western Europe, HIV prevalence among blood donors has declined progressively since the onset of systematic testing and, according to the European Centre for Epidemiologic Monitoring of AIDS, approximated 1.3 positives per 100 000 donations in 2002 (www.eurohiv.org). Since 1995, the prevalence has remained relatively constant in Belgium, Scandinavia, Ireland, the Netherlands and the UK, has decreased regularly in France and Spain, but has remained above 2 per 100 000 in Italy, Greece and Portugal (Hamers and Downs 2004). In Eastern Europe, prevalence has increased markedly since 1995, now exceeding 30 per 100 000 in 2002. The highest levels are reported in the Ukraine (93), Estonia (54) followed by Azerbaijan, Georgia and the Russian Federation.

Because HIV is both cell associated and present in plasma, all blood components are potentially infectious (Curran 1985). The viral load has been estimated at between 1.5×10^4 tissue culture infective doses in a 250-ml unit of blood from an asymptomatic donor, to 1.75×10^6 from a unit drawn from a symptomatic person (Ho *et al.* 1989). The relative importance of the viral strain, concurrent infection by other blood-borne agents, cellular receptors for HIV and other genetic and acquired host factors, both for infection and for clinical course of HIV in transfusion recipients, has received a great deal of attention, but is still an area of intense research (Vicenzi *et al.* 1997; Keoshkerian *et al.* 2003; Zaunders *et al.* 2004).

Follow-up studies have shown that 90–95% of patients receiving blood or blood components from anti-HIV-positive donors have become infected (Ward *et al.* 1987; Donegan *et al.* 1990b). The virus is well preserved in refrigerated and frozen blood; however, components that are washed, leucoreduced or cold stored for several weeks, procedures that diminish the number of viable leucocytes or the amount of virus, reduce the likelihood of transfusion transmission (Donegan *et al.* 1990a). Neither donor status nor recipient characteristics affect the likelihood of HIV transmission (Busch *et al.* 1990a). However, when AIDS developed in the donor shortly after donation, the period of asymptomatic infection in the recipient was also shortened (Ward *et al.* 1989). Albumin preparations, immunoglobulins, antithrombin III and hepatitis B vaccine have not been associated with HIV infection (Desmyter 1986; Melbye 1986; Morgenthaler 1989; Cuthbertson 1991). Furthermore, when HIV is added to plasma and the plasma is then fractionated by the cold-ethanol process, HIV does not appear in the Ig fraction (Morgenthaler 1989).

TAA in infants, and AIDS in infants and children in general, has a shorter incubation period than in adults and many of the clinical manifestations of the disease are different (Rogers 1992). Infants born to anti-HIV-positive mothers who become infected perinatally and infants transfused during the first years of life have the shortest median incubation period (less than 5 years), and usually develop AIDS in the first year of life. The increased susceptibility of infants to AIDS may be related to their immature immune system and to the larger viral load relative to body size. Children likely to develop TAA are those who are likely to be transfused: premature infants and children with haemophilia, thalassaemia and sickle cell anaemia. In the USA, of 2734 children with AIDS, 250 (9.1%) were transfusion associated and 138 (5.0% of the total) occurred in children with coagulation factor deficiencies (CDC 1991).

In much of Asia and Africa, the transmission of HIV by blood transfusion is still an important source of infection. Reasons for an alarmingly high rate of transmission, reported to be up to 10% of all cases, include: (1) the high demands for blood for inpatients with severe anaemia and haemorrhage, mainly in obstetrics, gynaecology and paediatrics; (2) the prevalence of HIV infection amongst the donor population, which can be as high as 20%; (3) the fact that HIV infection is not confined to a minority of the population who can be requested to refrain from blood donation; and (4) the inability of many laboratories to test for HIV or to perform and control the tests properly. The patient groups at greatest risk of acquiring HIV-1 or -2 by blood transfusion in tropical Africa are children with malaria and anaemia, patients with sickle cell anaemia (120 000 infants with sickle cell disease are born each year in Africa), anaemic antenatal patients, women with severe obstetric haemorrhage and trauma victims (Fleming 1990).

Transfusion-associated AIDS and haemophilia

To December 1996, 4674 cases of AIDS were reported in patients with haemophilia, accounting for less than 1% of the 581 429 AIDS cases reported in adults and children. Of the 7629 cases of AIDS reported in children under the age of 13 years, 373 (5%) were recipients of blood or tissue and 231 (3%) were haemophiliacs (Centers for Disease Control and Prevention 1997). All but 39 of these infections occurred prior to testing blood and plasma donors for HIV.

Studies of patient cohorts and specimens in serum repositories revealed that more than 90% of severe haemophiliacs (subjects with less than 1% factor VIII activity) treated with factor VIII concentrate had been infected prior to 1984 (Evatt *et al.* 1985). In a study of a 16-centre cohort of haemophiliacs in the USA and Europe, infections first appeared in 1978, peaked in October 1982 and declined to an estimated four infections per 100 person-years by July 1984 (Kroner *et al.* 1994). For patients who were high-dose recipients, peak risk appeared even earlier, indicating that the majority of patients with haemophilia were infected before the disease was widely recognized and long before it was attributed to transfusion. The risk was related to each patient's mean annual dose of clotting factor concentrate. As clotting factor concentrates are prescribed on the basis of patient weight or plasma volume, older patients with severe disease generally received more concentrate, had more 'donor exposures' and seroconverted sooner than did children and patients with milder disease. When corrected for dose and severity of disease, the association between age and early seroconversion disappears. The cumulative incidence of infection was 96% for high-dose recipients, 92% for moderate-dose recipients and 56% for low-dose recipients. Subjects who received only single-donor products (plasma and/or cryoprecipitate) had the lowest cumulative incidence of infection, 16% (Kroner *et al.* 1994). This experience is consistent with other reports (Andes *et al.* 1988; Gjerset *et al.* 1991). These startling numbers underscore the potential public health risks of using transfusion products manufactured from pools of plasma drawn from 20 000 donors or more.

Although AIDS was first reported in three haemophiliacs in 1982, studies of serum samples stored from as far back as 1968 have shown that the first cases of the development of anti-HIV in haemophiliacs occurred in 1978 in the USA and in 1981 in the UK (Evatt *et al.* 1983; Machin *et al.* 1985; Ragni *et al.* 1986). Plasma for preparing the implicated clotting factor concentrates may have been collected a year prior to that. The prevalence of HIV seropositivity and of AIDS varies from one haemophilia centre to another depending on the source, volume and type of concentrate used. In a study of 13 haemophilia centres in western Europe, Canada and Australia involving

2370 patients with haemophilia A and 434 patients with haemophilia B, the overall incidence of anti-HIV was 53.6% (CDC 1987a). The percentage of haemophiliacs infected with HIV in different countries has varied from 4% to more than 60%, with the higher rates in those countries using mainly concentrates from plasma imported from the USA. Some batches of factor VIII concentrate from European plasma have also transmitted HIV (Madhok and Forbes 1990). A clear correlation was also found between the severity of haemophilia and HIV seropositivity (Melbye 1986; UK Haemophilia Centre 1986). Haemophiliacs treated before 1985 with cryoprecipitate alone have shown a low risk of HIV infection (Ragni et al. 1986; UK Haemophilia Centre 1986).

Patients with haemophilia B fared somewhat better (Evatt et al. 1984; Mannucci et al. 1985; Ragni et al. 1986; UK Haemophilia Centre 1986). The difference may be due partly to the uneven partitioning of HIV in infected plasma during fractionation, with HIV separating preferentially in the cryoprecipitate fraction (Aronson 1979; Morgenthaler 1989; Madhok and Forbes 1990). The source of plasma used for fractionation is also partly responsible for this difference. In many countries all the factor IX is prepared locally, whereas at least part of the factor VIII is imported from the USA. Approximately 70% of patients in the USA with haemophilia A and 35% with haemophilia B developed HIV antibodies before the introduction of methods for viral inactivation in blood products (CDC 1987b). In a multicentre study of haemophiliacs treated in the UK between 1980 and 1984, 896 (44%) of 2025 patients with haemophilia A were positive for anti-HIV; 20 (6%) of 324 patients with haemophilia B and 11 (5%) of 215 patients with von Willebrand's disease were seropositive.

Although a large number of severe haemophiliacs in the UK were treated up to 1983 with unheated factor VIII concentrate imported from the USA, the incidence of anti-HIV in haemophiliacs in the UK is much lower than in countries such as Germany, Spain and the USA, where the frequency of anti-HIV ranges between 68% and 94% (Kitchen et al. 1984; 1985). On the other hand, in Groningen, in the Netherlands, only 1 out of 18 severe haemophiliacs treated with commercial factor VIII concentrates between 1978 and 1983 developed HIV antibodies (van der Meer et al. 1986).

There has been no transmission of HBV, HCV or HIV by US-licensed plasma derivatives since the introduction of effective virus inactivation procedures (Tabor 1999).

Prevention of transfusion-transmitted HIV infection

Reducing the residual risk

The reduction in risk of transfusion-transmitted HIV over the past 15 years has been dramatic and reassuring. Nevertheless, enormous public concern persists. As in almost no other area, blood safety, and specifically the possibility of HIV transmission, provokes emotions and measures to further reduce risks that defy the conventional cost–benefit calculus. Actions to reduced residual risk fall into three general categories: (1) measures that can be introduced by blood collection facilities, such as improved donor screening, testing, education and exclusion techniques; (2) enlightened transfusion practice, such as judicious use of allogeneic blood components, appropriate use of autologous blood, and alternatives to transfusion (see Chapter 17); and (3) measures that depend on the development of new technologies, such as viral inactivation of cellular components and safe substitutes for blood.

Donor demographics have proved effective at identifying and excluding donors at high risk for infection and transmission of HIV (Busch et al. 1991a). Donors with high-risk profiles include men who have had sexual contact with other men since 1977, intravenous drug users, residents of high prevalence regions, prisoners, prostitutes, haemophiliacs who have received 'unsafe' clotting factor concentrates and the sexual partners of people in all of these groups. The year 1977 was chosen as the point of reference, because the first clinical cases of AIDS in the USA were diagnosed retrospectively as far back as 1978 (Jaffe et al. 1985). The rate of seropositivity has been higher in paid plasma donors than in volunteers. Seven HIV positives were found out of 35 000 plasma donors attending centres located outside high prevalence areas (Stramer et al. 1989).

Measures to exclude such subjects from blood donor rolls are among the most important means of preventing the spread of AIDS by transfusion. Nevertheless, predonation medical screening and donor education are not infallible (Leitman et al. 1989). Between 1% and 2% of donors do not report risks that would disqualify them from blood donation, and donation incentives such as complimentary laboratory testing increases this rate (Glynn *et al.* 2001). In a study of blood donors found positive for hepatitis C antibody, 42% admitted to intravenous drug use on subsequent questioning, despite denying such use on predonation screening (Conry-Cantilena *et al.* 1996). In an anonymous mail survey of 50 162 volunteer allogeneic blood donors, 1.9% of the 34 726 respondents reported one or more risk factors that should have led to their deferral at the time of their last donation (Williams *et al.* 1997). Refinements in blood donor screening techniques, such as the use of illustrated risk-related activities, expansion of the screening questionnaire and interactive computer-based screening, have been proposed, but data supporting the effectiveness of such measures are lacking (Mayo *et al.* 1991). However, the reasons why some volunteer blood donors appear to disregard certain screening criteria are unknown and may have more to do with donor psychology than with inadequate screening and education.

Donors who are confirmed positive for HIV should be counselled and referred to specialized centres for follow-up. Counselling should be performed by specially trained staff. Appropriate interventions will not only help the donor to obtain long-term supportive care and to prevent further spread, but will also aid transfusion services to understand which groups of the population are HIV seropositive and still come forward to donate (Lefrere *et al.* 1992). Donor education and selection methods can then be modified accordingly.

Self-exclusion ('self-deferral') of donors

Retrospective analysis indicates that the risk of contracting AIDS from the transfusion of blood and blood components (other than products of plasma fractionation) prior to focused screening and testing was far higher than the one infection per million units transfused that had been estimated during the 1983–1985 interval. The risk of HIV transmission from transfusion in San Francisco has been calculated from its first appearance in 1978 to rise exponentially to a peak risk of approximately 1.1% per unit transfused in 1983 (Busch *et al.* 1991a). A retrospective study of heavily transfused patients with leukaemia in New York City revealed an overall risk between 0.02% and 0.11% per component transfused (Minamoto *et al.* 1988). The major blood collectors published a Joint

Statement of Recommendations in January 1983 (American Association of Blood Banks *et al.* 1983), and the Public Health Service published recommendations in March 1983 (CDC 1983) that proposed such measures as public education, self-deferral for donors engaging in high-risk activity and confidential unit exclusion procedures (Pindyck *et al.* 1984, 1985). These measures proved unusually effective. An estimated 90% of men in high-risk cat-egories self deferred. By 1984, the risk in San Francisco had dropped to less than 0.2% per unit. Screening with anti-HIV-1 in 1985 reduced the risk to about 1 in 40 000 units (Busch *et al.* 1991a).

Routine screening tests for HIV in blood donors

In most countries, screening tests for anti-HIV by the enzyme immunoassay (EIA) format are now compulsory for all blood donations. If reactive ('repeat reactive'), additional tests for HIV using independent methods are used to confirm the diagnosis of HIV infection (Stramer *et al.* 2004). The current algorithm in the USA requires that anti-HIV-1/2 repeat reactive specimens be further tested with the HIV-1 Western blot (see below) and a specific anti-HIV-2 EIA. Early ELISA assays using disrupted purified virus were plagued by false-positive reactions. Current generation screening assays, using recombinant and synthetic antigens, have reduced false reactives dramatically while increasing test sensitivity for both the predominant and the variant viral strains (Busch and Alter 1995). Less than 10% of reactive assays confirm positive using this strategy. Western blot is notoriously subjective and complicated by non-viral bands (Kleinman *et al.* 1998). Alternative strategies use a second EIA or a NAT assay of HIV RNA.

Approximately 25.6 million donations were screened by the American National Red Cross from September 1999 to 30 June 2003, resulting in 17 090 HIV repeat reactive blood donations (Stramer *et al.* 2004). Only 4.8% of these donors (818) were Western blot positive and approximately 90% (759) of those also tested positive by NAT. Follow-up testing of the remaining 10% demonstrated that almost all of these donors represent Western blot false-positive results.

Although some antibodies to core and other antigens of HIV-1 and HIV-2 crossreact (Sazama *et al.* 1992), currently available tests are designed to detect both anti-HIV-1 and anti-HIV-2. Such combined assays are available as antiglobulin ELISAs and as sandwich ELISAs and are routinely used in several countries. Seroconversion in infection with HIV-1 is detected earlier in these combined assays than by anti-HIV-1 assays (Gallarda *et al.* 1994; Fiebig *et al.* 2003). Most of the combined assays have been found to be less sensitive for the detection of anti-HIV-2 than most anti-HIV-2 specific tests (Christiansen *et al.* 1996).

Some samples with anti-HIV are repeatedly positive in some, but negative in other screening assays. If only one screening test is used, such samples may give false-negative results (Hancock *et al.* 1993). One cause of such false negatives is that antibodies against subtype O, a variant found predominantly in West Africa, are not recognized in all screening assays (Loussert-Ajaka *et al.* 1994; Schable *et al.* 1994). At present group O prevalence is low in the USA and in western Europe (Sullivan *et al.* 2000). False-negative reactions have also been found to be due to contamination with glove powder, inhibition by serum proteins, haemoglobin and certain anticoagulants (Sazama 1995).

Currently available ELISAs for HIV-1 antibodies detect HIV-1 subtype group 0. Soon after the discovery of an assay for HIV-Ab, transmission of HIV by blood from seronegative donors had been recognized (Esteban *et al.* 1985; Raevsky *et al.* 1986; Ward *et al.* 1988; Cohen and Munoz 1989). Studies reported detection of HIV-1 p24 antigen in analyses of stored blood specimens from plasma donors as early as 1986, and confirmed cases of HIV-Ag-positive, Ab-negative blood in primary HIV infection were reported by 1988 (Allain *et al.* 1986; Clark *et al.* 1991; Irani *et al.* 1991). The utility of this test as a screening assay was not so obvious. Antigen tests are positive for only part of the initial antibody-negative viraemic phase. In some subjects antigen can be detected as early as 2 weeks after infection, persisting for between 3 weeks and 3 months, and is no longer detectable when anti-p24 appears in the serum, although it may reappear intermittently during the asymptomatic phase (Allain *et al.* 1986; Fiebig *et al.* 2003). Later, antigen may reappear with a loss of anti-p24. A prospective study of 515 494 units donated at 13 blood centres in the USA failed to detect a single instance of Ag-positive/Ab-negative donated blood. A retrospective analysis of 200 000 repository specimens and prospective studies of blood donors in Europe confirmed these findings (Backer *et al.* 1987; Busch *et al.* 1990a). However, after three

anti-HIV seroconversions followed transfusion of p24 antigen-positive units, testing of donated blood for p24 antigen was mandated in the USA in 1996 (Busch and Alter 1995). Mathematical models predicted that universal antigen screening would detect eight additional potentially infectious units per year. In fact it took 5 years before eight antigen-positive/antibody-negative units were interdicted (Kleinman *et al.* 1997; Kleinman and Busch 2000). Because of this limited usefulness and troubling frequency of false positives, HIV p24 antigen screening was not adopted widely outside of the USA. With the adoption of universal NAT for HIV in the USA in 1999 and its licensure in 2002, HIV-Ag screening was rendered unnecessary (Busch *et al.* 2000).

Confirmatory tests: they do not always confirm

The Western blot is the most widely used additional or 'confirmatory' test for HIV. The criteria for the interpretation of Western blot results have been re-evaluated several times because of greater sensitivity and specificity of screening assays and Western blot reagents, better insight into the serological patterns of HIV infection, experience with patterns of non-specific reactivity in low- and high-risk populations and knowledge of the serological basis of non-specificity (Sayre *et al.* 1996). Samples are now considered to be WB positive demonstrate reaction with the gp41 and gp120/160 *env* bands or with either of these bands and the p24 *gag* band. The earlier requirement for a reaction with a third gene product (e.g. p31 or p66 *pol* bands) has been abandoned and reactivity with more than one *env* antigen alone is enough for confirmation (O'Gorman *et al.* 1991). If there is reactivity with only one band, the result of the Western blot is considered to be indeterminate. The absence of reactivity in the Western blot indicates that the donor has not developed anti-HIV (Dodd 1991).

In the original Western blot assay, viral lysate was used as a source of antigen. In the newer assays, recombinant or synthetic viral antigens are applied. These assays have been found to be both more sensitive and specific than the original WB (Soriano *et al.* 1994). Nevertheless, the assay is still relatively subjective and beset by indeterminate and false-positive results when compared with NAT as the 'gold standard' or when investigated with sequential sampling follow-up (Kleinman *et al.* 1998; Mahe *et al.* 2002; Stramer 2004).

Detection of HIV DNA and HIV RNA

Donations during the window period constitute the predominant risk for HIV transmission through transfusion (Busch *et al.* 2000). A more sensitive and specific alternative to testing for p24 antigen is NAT for HIV DNA in PBMC (Ou *et al.* 1988) or HIV-1 RNA in plasma by reverse transcription PCR or a similar amplification assay (Henrard *et al.* 1992). All blood in the USA, Japan and most European countries is tested by NAT in pools of 16–90 specimens. Ultrasensitive assays can detect fewer than 10 genomic copies/ml (Busch *et al.* 2000). However, tests have been optimized for HIV subtype B and may lack sensitivity when applied to non-B subtypes (Triques *et al.* 1999). Single-donor assays are inevitable, but await the development of fully automated combination (HIV/ HCV/HBV) assays.

Current risk of transmission of HIV by blood transfusion

Although the various measures outlined above have dramatically reduced the risk of TAA-AIDS, a small residual risk remains (Delwart *et al.* 2004; Phelps *et al.* 2004). Most of this risk results from 'window period' donations. Before the introduction of HIV-Ag and NAT, prospective studies estimated this risk at about one infection in 60 000 units (Busch *et al.* 1991b; Nelson *et al.* 1992). Subsequent estimates rely on models based on calculations of HIV incidence and window period. In the USA, residual risk has been calculated as 1 per 2 135 000 repeat donors (Dodd *et al.* 2002). The incidence rate is approximately two times greater among first-time donors. In most European countries where the prevalence of HIV in blood donors is lower than in the USA, the residual risk is probably lower still. However, in countries with a high percentage of infected subjects and where HIV is spread mainly by heterosexual intercourse, the risk of transmission of HIV by blood transfusion is still considerable.

Human T-cell leukaemia viruses types I and II

The human T-cell leukaemia virus type I (HTLV-I), the first human retrovirus to be described, was isolated from cultured cells from a patient with an aggressive variant of *Mycosis fungoides* and from a patient with Sézary syndrome (Poiesz *et al.* 1980; Gallo *et al.* 1981). The virus has subsequently been shown to be identical to the adult T-cell leukaemia virus (Yoshida *et al.* 1982; Watanabe *et al.* 1984). HTLV-I is the causative agent of adult T-cell leukaemia (ATL) and is associated with a chronic demyelinating neurological disease called tropical spastic paraperesis (TSP), known in Japan as HTLV-associated myelopathy (HAM) (Vernant *et al.* 1987; Roman and Osame 1988). HTLV-seropositive individuals appear to have a 0.25% lifetime risk of developing TSP, compared with a 2–5% risk of developing ATL (Kaplan *et al.* 1990). The virus is also associated with lung infections, cancer of other organs, monoclonal gammopathy, renal failure, infection with *Strongyloides stercoralis*, intractable non-specific dermatomycosis, lymphadenitis and uveitis. These effects may be due to the immunodeficiency induced by HTLV-I infection (Takatsuki 1996). The association of HTLV-I with *Mycosis fungoides* is controversial, as no HTLV-related DNA sequences could be detected in patients with this disease (Bazarbachi *et al.* 1993; Vallejo *et al.* 1995). In Japan, only 2.5% of HTLV-I carriers develop ATL (Takatsuki 1996).

HTLV-I and -II belong to the oncovirus subtype of the retrovirus family and are able to induce polyclonal proliferation of T lymphocytes *in vitro* and *in vivo*. Like the lentiviruses HIV-1 and -2, these viruses are lymphotropic and neurotropic, and have the essential structural genes *gag* (group antigen), *pol* (reverse transcriptase) and *env* (envelope) in addition to regulatory genes. In HTLV-I, the *gag* gene codes for the structural proteins p55/24/19; *pol* codes for a protein of approximately 100 kDa, and *env* codes for glycoproteins gp61/46/21. In HTLV-II the structural proteins are similar to those in HTLV-I with a high degree of cross-reactivity; *gag* encodes the polypeptides p53/24/19; *pol* a protein of approximately 100 kDa; and *env* codes for the glycoproteins gp61/46/21.

Areas endemic for HTLV have been found, particularly in south-west Japan, with prevalence as high as 15% (Maeda *et al.* 1984), in the Caribbean with a 1–8% prevalence (Clark *et al.* 1985), in regions of Central and South America and in parts of sub-Saharan Africa (Gessain *et al.* 1986; Vrielink and Reesink 2004). Populations in these areas show different prevalence rates for anti-HTLV-I, as do emigrants from these regions (Sandler *et al.* 1991; Vrielink and

Reesink 2004). It has been estimated that more than 1 million Japanese people are healthy carriers of HTLV-I. Carriers of HTLV have also been found in the USA, especially in Florida and states on the Pacific, and in France, UK, the Netherlands and many other countries. The prevalence in blood donors has been reported to be one in 6250 in the USA (CDC 1990), about one in 30 000 in France (Pillonel *et al.* 1996), one in 45 000 in the Netherlands (Zaaijer *et al.* 1994) and one in 20 000 in London (Brennan 1992).

HTLV-II, the second human retrovirus to be discovered, has a 65% nucleotide sequence identity with HTLV-I and a significant serological crossreactivity (Hjelle 1991). However, HTLV-II antibodies are not detected by all HTLV-I assays. The distinction between HTLV-I and -II can be made by DNA PCR (Reesink *et al.* 1994), and in the recently developed WB assays in which specific HTLV-I and -II recombinant antigens are used. The relative prevalence of the two viruses in blood donors in the USA was found to be about equal (Glynn *et al.* 2000), but in many other countries HTLV-I predominates in blood donors. There is a high prevalence of HTLV-II among i.v. drug users and their sexual contacts in the USA and other countries (Vrielink and Reesink 2004). A large proportion of HTLV-II-positive subjects in the USA were Hispanics and American Indians (Hjelle *et al.* 1990a; Sandler *et al.* 1991). HTLV-II has been found to be associated with a HAM-like neurological disease (Hjelle *et al.* 1992; Murphy *et al.* 1997). Although the virus was first found in a patient with hairy cell leukaemia (Kalyanaraman *et al.* 1982) and subsequently in other T-cell malignancies, no viral RNA could be detected in the malignant cells (Manns and Blattner 1991).

Transmission of human T-cell leukaemia virus

HTLV is mainly transmitted by sexual contact, by the sharing of infected needles and from mother to child, particularly by breast-feeding (Kajiyama *et al.* 1986). If infected mothers refrain from breast-feeding, transmission of HTLV to their infants is prevented in 80% of cases (Hino *et al.* 1996). Infection of infants is also prevented when the milk is freeze-thawed or heated at 56°C for 30 min (Ando *et al.* 1986; Hino *et al.* 1987). Transmission from mother to fetus has been demonstrated by culture studies of cord blood lymphocytes in

2 out of 40 cord blood samples from HTLV-I-positive mothers (Satow *et al.* 1991).

Human T-cell leukaemia virus and blood transfusion

HTLV-I has been transmitted by cellular components, but not by cell-free plasma or plasma derivatives (Okochi 1985). However, HTLV-RNA is detectable in plasma from infected subjects. The lack of infectivity of HTLV-positive plasma may be explained by the presence of neutralizing antibodies, the fact that it is integrated in viral DNA and the requirement of cell–cell interactions for infectivity (Rios *et al.* 1996).

Antibodies are usually first detectable 14–30 days after transfusion, although the interval may be as long as 98 days (Inaba *et al.* 1989; Gout *et al.* 1990). Of 85 recipients of anti-HTLV-I-positive cell concentrates in Japan, 53 (62%) developed antibodies 3–6 weeks after transfusion: IgM antibodies were present only in the early stages, whereas IgG antibodies persisted at high titre throughout the period of follow-up (Sato and Okochi 1986). Storage of blood appears to decrease the risk of transmission of HTLV. This may explain the lower rate of transmission reported in USA transfusion recipients, whose blood may have been stored for a longer period than the units in Japan and the Caribbean (Donegan *et al.* 1994). Antibodies became detectable in 79.2% of recipients of blood stored for 1–5 days, but in only 55% of recipients of blood stored 11–16 days (Okochi 1989).

Recipients of HTLV-I-infected concentrates may develop HAM (Gout *et al.* 1990; Araujo and Hall 2004). It has been estimated that 2–8% of subjects infected with HTLV-I by blood transfusion will eventually develop HAM (Murphy *et al.* 1997; Araujo and Hall 2004). ATL developed in two immunosuppressed patients who had received multiple transfusions 6 and 11 years earlier (Chen *et al.* 1989). HTLV-II has also been transmitted by blood transfusion (Hjelle *et al.* 1990b).

Screening tests for human T-cell leukaemia virus antibodies

For the detection of HTLV antibodies, ELISAs are used as well as gelatin particle assays. In the ELISAs for the detection of anti-HTLV-I, viral lysate has been used. Although there is considerable (65%) crossreactivity between HTLV-I and -II, the sensitivity of anti-HTLV-I assays for detecting anti-HTLV-II was found to be only 55–91% (Wiktor *et al.* 1991; Cossen *et al.* 1992). As infection with HTLV-II is probably associated with HAM and as many HTLV-positive donors (more than 50% in the USA) are HTLV-II positive, tests designed to detect both antibodies are now used (US Food and Drug Administration 1998). In these ELISAs, recombinant proteins, including HTLV-I and -II-specific ones, have been added to lysate or are used exclusively (Hartley *et al.* 1991). The sensitivity of such assays has been claimed to be 100% (Vrielink *et al.* 1996a).

In Japan, an agglutination test in which gelatin particles are coated with HTLV-I-antigens has been developed and used extensively. The sensitivity of the commercially available agglutination test Serodia HTLV-I has been claimed to be 100% for detecting anti-HTLV-I; all of 12 anti-HTLV-II-containing sera gave positive reactions (Vrielink *et al.* 1996a). An ELISA for the combined detection of anti-HIV-1 and -2 and anti-HTLV-I and -II in which synthetic peptides of all four viruses are used, has been developed (McAlpine *et al.* 1992). In a study 242 samples from anti-HIV-1/-2 or HTLV-I/-II panels, two HTLV-II-positive samples and two very weak anti-HIV-1-positive samples were negative. The specificity of the test was slightly less than that of specific assays (Flanagan *et al.* 1995).

Despite the improved specificity of anti-HTLV-I/-II screening tests, many repeatedly positive reactions that cannot be confirmed are still found and all repeatedly reactive samples must therefore be tested in confirmatory assays.

Human T-cell leukaemia virus confirmatory assays

Confirmatory testing for HTLV-I/-II continues to be challenging, primarily because of a dearth of licensed reagents. Western blot and radioimmunoprecipitation assays (RIPAs) are used (Anderson *et al.* 1989; Hartley *et al.* 1990). For a positive reaction, antibody reactivity with both a *gag* (p19 and/or p24) and an *env* protein (gp46 and/or gp68) are required (WHO 1990). All other reaction patterns were considered to be indeterminate. As the sensitivity of the Western blot in detecting antibodies against *env* proteins was low, many indeterminate results had to be checked in RIPA, a much more elaborate assay (Lillehoj *et al.* 1990; Lal

et al. 1992). A report on the transmission of HTLV-I by blood from a donor with an indeterminate pattern in the WB and RIPA (p19 and gp68 reactivity) to four out of six recipients, confirmed by PCR, demonstrated the insufficient sensitivity of these original confirmation assays (Donegan *et al.* 1992). A modified WB has been developed in which both shared (r21e) and specific (rgp46[I] and rgp46[II]) HTLV-I and -II recombinant *env* proteins are used (Lillehoj *et al.* 1990; Lal *et al.* 1992). For a positive reaction in this modified Western blot, a reaction with at least one *gag* protein (p19 and/or p24) and with *env* r21e as well as rgp46[I] or rgp46[II] is required. All other patterns are indeterminate. This Western blot, in which a reaction with HTLV-I or -II can be distinguished, has been found to be more sensitive and specific than the original Western blot. Instead of 66, only two positive samples required confirmation by RIPA and none of 158 indeterminate samples (original Western blot) reacted (Brodine *et al.* 1993). A recombinant immunoblot assay (RIBA) in which the same antigens are applied gave similar results (Vrielink *et al.* 1996b). NAT has not been licensed for confirmatory testing.

Cytomegalovirus

Characteristics of the virus and of cytomegalovirus infection

Cytomegalovirus (CMV) is a large, enveloped, double-stranded DNA, beta herpes virus that is cell associated, but may also be found free in plasma and other body fluids (Drew *et al.* 2003). CMV has a direct cytopathic effect on infected cells. The result may lead to neutropenia, some depression of cellular immunity and inversion of T-cell subset ratios, with a consequent increase in susceptibility to bacterial, fungal and protozoa infections in immunosuppressed patients (Grumet 1984; Landolfo *et al.* 2003). CMV infection causes parenchymal damage, such as retinitis, pneumonitis, gastroenteritis and encephalitis, and can result in substantial morbidity and mortality.

CMV can cause primary acute clinical and subclinical infections. Chronic subclinical infections may occur in which the virus is shed in saliva and urine. CMV remains latent in a large proportion of infected subjects. The presence of anti-CMV does not guarantee immunity. As with HIV and HCV infection, specific antibody is a marker of potential infectivity although only in the case of CMV, a relatively small proportion of seropositive subjects seem to be infectious (Drew *et al.* 2003). CMV antibody-positive subjects may infect others through sexual contact, breast-feeding, transplacental transmission or transfusion (Tegtmeier 1986). In subjects with antibody, CMV infection may be reactivated, or the subject may become re-infected with exogenous strains of CMV.

Primary CMV infection is generally more severe than is re-infection (co-infection with a different strain) or reactivation. In view of the difficulty of distinguishing between reactivation and re-infection, the term *recurrent infection* has been coined to embrace both. However, when necessary to distinguish between the two, donor viral DNA can be distinguished from recipient viral DNA by restriction enzyme analysis (Glazer *et al.* 1979; Chou 1990). In practice, the diagnosis of recurrent infection is limited to demonstrating a fourfold increase in antibody titre or the presence of IgM anti-CMV. In immunosuppressed patients, serological tests cannot be relied upon for a diagnosis of CMV partly because the patients may not make antibody and partly because any anti-CMV detected may have been derived from transfused blood. Viral culture is impractical because the virus grows slowly *in vitro*. On the other hand, immunofluorescence techniques to detect viral antigen using monoclonal antibodies on biopsies or bronchial washings provide results within hours (Griffiths 1984).

Prevalence of anti-CMV

The frequency of subjects with anti-CMV varies widely in different populations. Seroprevalence is lower (30–80%) in developed than in developing countries, where the figure may reach 100% (Krech 1973; Preiksaitis 1991). The prevalence of anti-CMV correlates with age and socioeconomic status (Lamberson 1985; Tegtmeier 1986). The frequency of anti-CMV-positive donors may vary widely within a given country, for example 25% in southern California and 70% in Nashville, Tennessee (Grumet 1984; Tegtmeier 1986).

Transmission of cytomegalovirus by transfusion

The transmission of CMV by blood transfusion was first reported in the 1960s (Kaariainen *et al.* 1966; Paloheimo *et al.* 1968; Klemola *et al.* 1969). CMV is now known as one of the infectious agents most frequently transmitted by transfusion. The pathogenesis of transfusion-transmitted CMV infection is not clearly understood. In most cases CMV appears to be transmitted in a latent, particulate state only by cellular blood components, and the virus reactivates from donor leucocytes after transfusion. Host as well as donor factors are involved in CMV infection (Tegtmeier 1989; Preiksaitis 1991). CMV has been isolated from the mononuclear and polymorphonuclear cells of patients with acute infections. The specific cell type responsible for carrying the virus has not been identified, although mononuclear cells are the favourite candidates as hosts of CMV in latent infection. Fresh blood appears more likely than stored blood to transmit CMV infection, although no controlled studies document this impression (Tegtmeier 1986).

Some 3–12% of units have the potential to transmit CMV (Adler 1984), although most authors have reported a carrier rate of 1% or less (Tegtmeier 1986; Drew *et al.* 2003). The discrepancy may be related to the frequency of donor testing and the sensitivity and specificity of the assay used. Primary infection rates depend on the number of transfusions, age of blood, time of year and immunocompetence of the recipient (Tegtmeier 1989; Preiksaitis *et al.* 1988; Preiksaitis 2000). Donors with IgM anti-CMV appear to be more likely than others to transmit CMV (Lamberson *et al.* 1984). One large study found that only 0.5% of antibody-positive donors have detectable CMV DNA in their leucocytes (Roback *et al.* 2003).

At present, no rapid, easy way to identify infectious subjects exists. Viral excretion in urine is a good index of infectivity, but blood donors would probably rebel at this screening strategy. Virus can also be cultured from saliva, and PCR-based assays are available for the detection of viral genome in peripheral blood. Detection of pp65 antigen in leucocytes (pp65 antigenaemia) is considered the 'gold standard' among diagnostic tools for diagnosing CMV infection and initiating antiviral therapy. Both CMV DNA and immediate early-messenger RNA detection have been compared with pp65 antigenaemia, but none of them showed advantages in terms of earlier diagnosis and better prognosis. PCR's major advantage is its semi-automation compared with the immunofluorescence employed for pp65 antigenaemia. Isolation of CMV by culture is reliable for the diagnosis of active infection, but is less sensitive and requires more time for viral detection.

Transfusion-transmitted cytomegalovirus infection in immunocompetent subjects

Before the era of universal (or near universal) leuco-reduction, some 30% of anti-CMV-negative recipients undergoing cardiac surgery involving transfusion developed infection, as confirmed by virus isolation or the development of anti-CMV. In addition, some anti-CMV-positive patients developed recurrent infection. In almost all cases, the infection is asymptomatic. Of patients who develop a primary or recurrent CMV infection following transfusion, fewer than 10% develop a mononucleosis-like syndrome. This syndrome, originally termed the post-perfusion syndrome, but now referred to as the post-transfusion syndrome, appears 3–6 weeks after transfusion. Common features include fever, exanthema, hepatosplenomegaly, enlargement of lymph nodes and the presence in peripheral blood of atypical lymphocytes resembling those found in infectious mononucleosis (Foster 1966). Recovery is usually complete. The development of atypical lymphocytes due to post-transfusion CMV infection should be distinguished from the development of atypical lymphocytes 1 week after transfusion as a response to allogeneic lymphocytes.

Consequences of transfusion in patients with impaired immunity

During the past decade, major advances have been achieved regarding the management of CMV infection through the development of new diagnostic techniques for the detection of the virus and through the performance of prospective clinical trials of antiviral agents (Meijer et al. 2003). Nevertheless, in immunosuppressed patients, or in fetuses and premature infants with an immature immune system, CMV infections, particularly primary infections, still cause severe disease that can be fatal.

1 *The fetus in utero.* Following maternal primary CMV infection, the fetus becomes infected in 30–40% of cases. Approximately 5–10% of infected infants develop sequelae such as mental retardation, hearing loss or chorioretinitis (Stagno et al. 1986).

2 *Premature infants.* The risk of serious CMV infection is high when the infant's birthweight is less than about 1300 g and when the mother is anti-CMV negative. In two large prospective studies, 25–30% of infants with these risk factors, transfused with a total of 50 ml or more of blood, some of which was anti-CMV positive, acquired CMV infection, and 25% of these infants died. Infants transfused with anti-CMV-negative blood did not develop CMV infection (0 out of 90) (Yeager et al. 1981; Adler et al. 1983). A lower incidence of CMV infection (7–9%) has been reported from two other centres: in infants weighing less than 1500 g born to anti-CMV-negative mothers and transfused with blood, some of which was anti-CMV positive (Smith et al. 1984; Tegtmeier 1984). All reports agree that clinically significant CMV infection in newborn infants develops only when the infant is premature and of low birthweight, when the mother lacks anti-CMV and when anti-CMV-positive blood is transfused (Tegtmeier 1986).

3 *Bone marrow transplant recipients* frequently develop primary or recurrent CMV infections that may prove fatal (Tegtmeier 1986). Blood transfusion represents the main risk factor for CMV acquisition in CMV-negative patients receiving bone marrow from a CMV-negative donor. In a prospective randomized trial of 97 anti-CMV-negative patients, 57 received anti-CMV-negative marrow: 32 out of the 57 received anti-CMV-negative blood components and only one of these developed a CMV infection; of the 25 who received blood components unscreened for anti-CMV, eight developed CMV infection. Among the 40 recipients of anti-CMV-positive bone marrow, the rate of CMV infection was no lower in those who received only anti-CMV-negative blood components (Bowden et al. 1986). Granulocyte concentrates, which contain large numbers of leucocytes that can harbour CMV, reportedly carry the greatest risk of transmitting CMV infection (Winston et al. 1980; Hersman et al. 1982). However, when only two prophylactic transfusions were given, the risk appeared to be no higher in those who received granulocytes than in those who did not (Vij et al. 2003).

4 *Renal transplant recipients* are at high risk of primary or recurrent CMV infection; the main source of infection lies in the transplanted kidney (Tegtmeier 1986). In anti-CMV-negative recipients of a kidney from an anti-CMV-negative donor, blood transfusion plays a significant role in CMV transmission (Rubin et al. 1985).

5 *Heart and heart–lung transplant recipients* may

develop severe primary CMV infection, which can lead to opportunistic infections with fungi or bacteria. In anti-CMV-negative recipients the main sources of infection are anti-CMV-positive transplanted organs or organ blood donor units (Preiksaitis *et al.* 1983). If both donor and recipient are anti-CMV negative, blood transfusion is a major source of CMV disease; infection can be minimized by the use of anti-CMV-negative red cells and platelets (Freeman *et al.* 1990). If a heart or heart–lung from a donor with CMV antibodies is transplanted to an anti-CMV-negative recipient, prophylactic administration of specific CMV hyperimmune IVIG seems to lessen the severity of CMV disease (Freeman *et al.* 1990), although data in support of this practice are unimpressive.

6 *Following splenectomy due to trauma*, patients receiving massive transfusion may develop serious CMV infections (Baumgartner *et al.* 1982; Drew and Miner 1982).

7 *Subjects infected with HIV* and especially those with AIDS, if anti-CMV negative, may acquire primary CMV infection by transfusion (Jackson *et al.* 1988; Sayers *et al.* 1992). In these patients CMV may cause sight-threatening infection that may lead to blindness in up to 25% of patients not receiving antiviral therapy. Because the rate of reactivation of CMV in already infected patients is high, it is difficult to determine the contribution of transfusion-transmitted virus (Bowden 1995).

8 *Liver transplant recipients* should also be considered at risk, especially children or pregnant women. Now that smaller amounts of blood and blood components are needed in liver transplantation, it has been possible to give only anti-CMV-negative blood and platelets to anti-CMV-negative recipients of anti-CMV-negative grafts.

Prevention of transfusion-transmitted cytomegalovirus infection

Subjects who are at highest risk of severe primary CMV infection are anti-CMV-negative patients with impaired immunity. For such patients, preventive measures are available to reduce transmission of CMV by transfusion. The selection of CMV-seronegative donors has proven to be effective, but not infallible (Tegtmeier 1989; Miller *et al.* 1991). Seropositivity, especially the presence of IgM, is a marker of previous infection and latent, but potentially infectious virus.

However, antibody assays vary in sensitivity and a small risk of transmission even from seronegative units remains (Kraat *et al.* 1993; Bowden *et al.* 1995). Window period infections are the most likely source of antibody screening failures. Although the window periods for HIV-1, HCV and HBV have been reasonably well defined, the length of the CMV-seronegative window, estimated at 6–8 weeks, is less well characterized. Several recent studies using PCR technology documented CMV DNA in both plasma and cellular blood components from several weeks before seroconversion to several months after seroconversion, although culture positivity was found for a much shorter period in white blood cells (WBCs) and not observed in plasma (Zanghellini *et al.* 1999).

When only red cells are required, frozen deglycerolysed red cells can be used and have not been shown not to transmit CMV (Brady *et al.* 1984; Taylor *et al.* 1986; Sayers *et al.* 1992).

As CMV is a white cell-associated virus, an alternative approach to preventing CMV transmission involves filtration removal of leucocytes from red cell and platelet concentrates (Graan-Hentzen *et al.* 1989). Leucoreduction by filtration may fail to prevent CMV transmission, as 10^5 to 10^6 WBCs may still be transfused and an estimated 1 in 1000 to 1 in 10 000 WBCs are infected by CMV during latency (Drew *et al.* 2003). In 10 patients whose WBCs were CMV antigen and culture positive before filtration and culture negative afterwards, 2 out of the 10 did, however, have CMV DNA detected in leucocytes after filtration (Lipson *et al.* 2001). Plasma viraemia, if present, would not be diminished by leucoreduction and might also account for CMV transmission following leucoreduced components. Although the exact number of residual leucocytes that is sufficiently small to pose no risk of CMV transmission is unknown and may not exist, a large prospective study has shown that leucocyte removal is as safe as selection of anti-CMV-negative donors. In this study, 502 patients were randomized prior to bone marrow transplantation to receive filtered, three-log leucocyte-depleted cellular components or components from anti-CMV-negative donors. There was no significant difference in the probability of CMV infection between the recipients of anti-CMV-negative or filtered concentrates, although more CMV-associated disease was observed in the filtration group (Bowden 1995). The same investigators have subsequently questioned their finding that filtered red cells are equivalent to CMV-seronegative cells (Nichols *et al.* 2003). When granulocyte transfusions are needed, selection of anti-CMV-negative donors is the only solution.

The success of leucocyte removal in the prevention of CMV transmission has raised the question of the importance of infection with a second strain of CMV in anti-CMV-positive recipients and the value of transfusing such recipients with leucocyte-depleted concentrates. Although co-infection with a second strain of CMV does occur (Boppana *et al.* 2001), the clinical consequences of such infection resulting from transfusion are less clear.

Tests for anti-CMV

Several tests for anti-CMV are available. Complement fixation used to be the diagnostic reference test, but it proved too complicated for routine donor screening. Indirect immunofluorescence, solid-phase fluorescence, ELISA and particle agglutination assays are also available. Competitive ELISAs seem to be the most reliable of the currently available screening tests (Bowden *et al.* 1987). CMV PCR technology has been used in clinical diagnostics since the 1980s (Bowen *et al.* 1997; Lipson *et al.* 1998). Conventional PCR requires detection and confirmatory testing of the amplicon by gel electrophoresis, incorporating an isotopically labelled or non-radioactive hybridization assay or a nested PCR to detect targets present in very low copy numbers (Lipson *et al.* 1995). A simplified, more rapid PCR-solid-phase enzyme immunoassay (EIA) plate technology system has been developed (Davoli *et al.* 1999). The quantitative real-time CMV PCR assay using TaqMan chemistry and an automated sample preparation system has also been applied to CMV detection (Piiparinen *et al.* 2004).

An inexpensive, uncomplicated CMV-Ag (pp65 antigen) assay is available and well suited for most diagnostic microbiology laboratories (Lipson *et al.* 1998). Assay for the early antigen pp65 is considered the 'gold standard' for the initiation of antiviral therapy.

Other viruses

Epstein–Barr virus

Infection with Epstein–Barr virus (EBV), a herpes virus-like CMV, is endemic throughout the world.

EBV can cause primary symptomatic infection (infectious mononucleosis), but most commonly causes asymptomatic infection followed by latent infection (Henle 1985). In most countries more than 90% of blood donors have neutralizing anti-EBV, which coexists with latent virus in B lymphocytes of peripheral blood and lymph nodes. At least one in 10^7 circulating lymphocytes of carriers harbour EBV genomes, but post-transfusion EBV infection is a rare occurrence, and symptomatic infection is even rarer (Rocchi *et al.* 1977). The virus is found in three of every 10^4 peripheral lymphocytes during acute infection. The majority of susceptible recipients are young children. Even in children, the chance of acquiring EBV infection following the transfusion of anti-EBV-positive blood is minimal, because the donor's neutralizing antibodies persist in the recipient's circulation long after the EBV-infected lymphocytes disappear. In a study of 25 EBV antibody-negative patients aged 3 months to 15 years and transfused with 1–11 units of blood stored for not more than 4 days, only one developed EBV antibodies and this patient had no symptoms (Henle 1985).

Of five patients transfused during cardiac bypass, four who were initially anti-EBV negative produced antibody that persisted at high titre for many months postoperatively. Two out of the four patients had concomitant CMV infection and no heterophile antibodies; one developed transient fever, and the other hepatitis. Only one of the four patients developed an infectious mononucleosis-like syndrome with heterophile antibodies (Gerber *et al.* 1969).

Although most cases of 'post-transfusion syndrome' are caused by CMV, two adult patients who were anti-EBV negative before transfusion developed post-transfusion syndrome due to EBV (McMonigal *et al.* 1983). In a survey of some 800 patients, fewer than 8% lacked EBV antibody before transfusion, and only 5% of these developed antibodies following transfusion. These patients suffered no clinical illness or disturbance of liver function (MRC 1974). Possibly, the discrepancy between these observations and those of others may have been related to the use of fresh blood in the last-named series (Gerber *et al.* 1969).

Post-transfusion infectious mononucleosis is seen only rarely in anti-EBV-negative immunocompetent patients and usually occurs when only a single unit of blood or blood component, obtained from the donor during the incubation phase is given within 4 days of collection. When more than 1 unit is transfused, one of the units is almost certain to contain anti-EBV. In the reported cases, the donors developed symptoms of mononucleosis 2–17 days after blood donation. The incubation period in recipients has been 21–30 days (Solem and Jorgensen 1969; Turner *et al.* 1972). Transfusion-transmitted EBV infection with symptomatic mononucleosis has occasionally been reported in patients transfused for splenectomy (Henle 1985).

Post-transfusion EBV infections may contribute to the development of lymphomas in severely immuno-suppressed patients such as haematopoietic graft recipients. T-lymphocyte suppression allows EBV-infected B lymphocytes to outlive the passively trans-fused antibodies and to proliferate (Marker *et al.* 1979; Hanto *et al.* 1983).

Other herpes viruses

Herpes simplex and *Herpes varicella zoster* have never been shown to be transmitted by blood transfusion; viraemia occurs only during primary infections, which usually occur in childhood (Henle 1985).

HHV-6 is a recently characterized human herpes virus, originally named HBLV (human B lymphotropic virus) for its ability to infect freshly isolated B cells. The virus was found in patients with various lympho-proliferative disorders. HHV-6 can infect monocytes, macrophages, T cells and megakaryocytes (Ablashi 1987). The virus is cytopathic for selected T-cell lines. Infection is acquired usually within the first year of life and the virus was found to be ubiquitous in blood donors when tested in London and the USA (Briggs *et al.* 1988; Saxinger *et al.* 1988). No transfusion-associated disease has been reported.

HHV-8, Kaposi's sarcoma-herpes virus is white cell associated and may be present in up to 30% of normal donors. Despite a relatively high HHV-8 seropre-valence in a Texas blood donor cohort (23%), HHV-8 DNA was not detected in any sample of donor whole blood using a highly sensitive PCR assay (Hudnall *et al.* 2003). Blood components from HHV 8-infected donors apparently carry little transfusion risk (Engels *et al.* 1999).

Human parvovirus B19

HPV B19 infection has long been known to cause erythema infectiosum (Fifth disease), a common febrile exanthem of childhood (Anderson *et al.* 1983). HPV is also associated with polyarthritis and rash in adults as a result of antigen–antibody immune complex deposi-tion in skin and joints (Reid *et al.* 1985; White *et al.* 1985). Because of its specific cytotoxic effect on erythroblasts, HPV B19 can precipitate aplastic crises in children who have haematological disorders with shortened red cell survival, such as those with sickle cell anaemia and other chronic haemolytic anaemias, particularly hereditary spherocytosis (Pattison *et al.* 1981; Young and Mortimer 1984). The virus may also cause thrombocytopenic purpura (Pattison 1987). Intrauterine infection may cause hydrops fetalis and spontaneous abortion in early pregnancy (Brown *et al.* 1984; Anand *et al.* 1987).

HPV B19 was discovered by an Australian virologist who noted viral particles in an antigen–antibody line of detection (plate B, well 19) in an assay for hepatitis B (Cossart *et al.* 1975). HPV B19 is a small single-stranded, non-enveloped, thermostable DNA member of the Parvoviridae family (Shade *et al.* 1986; Young and Brown 2004). The parvoviruses are dependent on help from host cells or other viruses to replicate. Parvovirus B19 is the type member of the erythrovirus genus, which propagates best in erythroid progenitor cells. The red cell P antigen, a globoside present on a variety of cells in addition to erythrocytes, has been documented as the specific receptor for HPV (Brown *et al.* 1994). This may account for reports of poly-arthritis nephropathy, myocarditis and cardiomyo-pathy (Young and Brown 2004). Persistent infection with anaemia occurs in immunosuppressed subjects (Kurtzman *et al.* 1987). PCR assays have revealed the presence of viral DNA along with the simultaneous presence of specific IgG in 0.55–1.3% of normal blood donors (Candotti *et al.* 2004), but the long-term persistence, infectivity and clinical importance of the virus in these subjects has not been well studied. Current methods of viral inactivation may not be able to eliminate HPV B19 completely (Williams *et al.* 1990a).

Infection with the virus normally occurs via respir-atory droplets. HPV B19 has been transmitted by plasma fractionation products derived from large pools of plasma, particularly by factor VIII and factor IX concentrates (Santagostino *et al.* 1997; Blumel *et al.* 2002). One episode of fulminant hepatitis has been attributed to the intravenous route of infection (Hayakawa *et al.* 2002). Use of recombinant products should eliminate this risk (Soucie *et al.* 2004). Transmission of the virus by single-donor components is unusual, but a red cell unit has been associated with HPV B19 transmission and possible cardiac involvement in a 22-year-old woman with thalassaemia major (Zanella *et al.* 1995).

The classic diagnosis of infection with HPV B19 is based on the detection of IgM or IgG antibodies with an EIA (Cohen *et al.* 1983). Alternatively viral DNA can be detected by PCR (Salimans *et al.* 1989; McOmish *et al.* 1993). HPV B19 has been detected by PCR in solvent–detergent-treated clotting factor concentrates (Lefrere *et al.* 1994), in heat-treated factor VIII and IX concentrates and in IVIG (McOmish *et al.* 1993; Santagostino *et al.* 1994) and in clotting factor concentrates prepared by different purification and inactivation procedures (Zakrzewska *et al.* 1992; Blumel *et al.* 2002). The virus has also been detected in plasma pools designed for fractionation (in 64 out of 75 pools), in 3 out of 12 albumin preparations, in 3 out of 15 IVIG and in three out of four IMIG preparations, as well as in seven out of seven factor VIII preparations. There is some indication that treatment of IVIG preparations at low pH may result in removal of detectable HPV B19 DNA (Saldanha and Minor 1996). Since 2002, major plasma fractionators have screened plasma units with quantitative measurements of B19 DNA to reduce the risk of transmission. The prevalence of HPV B19 in blood donors has been estimated at 0.03% in the UK (McOmish *et al.* 1993). A similar prevalence was found in Japan (1 in 35 000) but, during an epidemic of erythema infectiosum, the prevalence was much higher (1 in 4000) (Tsujimura *et al.* 1995). B19 prevalence varies according to season and from year to year (Young and Brown 2004).

A rapid test for HPV B19, suitable for large-scale screening of donors has been developed (Sato *et al.* 1996). The test is based on agglutination of blood group P-positive gluteraldehyde-treated red cells by the virus for which the P antigen is the receptor (see Chapter 4). Although only intact viruses can bind to P, the test has been found to be sensitive and it could be used to select donors for patients at risk. Whether routine screening of donors is necessary is an unanswered question. Although 81.6% of 136 haemophiliacs studied had anti-HPV B19, B19 DNA was detectable in none and there were no signs of lasting clinical or haematological sequelae (Ragni *et al.* 1996).

Commercial immune globulins are a good source of antibodies against parvovirus; a persistent B19 infection responds to a 5- or 10-day course of immunoglobulin at a dose of 0.4 g per kilogram of body weight, with a prompt decline in serum viral DNA, as measured by hybridization methods, accompanied by reticulocytosis and increased haemoglobin levels (Kurtzman *et al.* 1987; Frickhofen *et al.* 1990).

West Nile Virus

Since its importation into the USA in 1999, West Nile virus (WNV) has become a significant transfusion-transmitted infection with a calculated mean risk of transfusion transmission of 3.02 per 10 000 donations in high-risk metropolitan areas during epidemic conditions (Biggerstaff and Petersen 2003). Transfusion transmission was first documented when four organs harvested from a common multi-transfused cadaver donor transmitted virus to all four recipients; the donor's pretransfusion sample tested negative for WNV, while one of 63 blood donors tested positive with a nucleic acid assay and developed IgM antibody to WNV over the subsequent 2 months (Iwamoto *et al.* 2003). Using strict case definition criteria, epidemiologists document 23 transmissions and another 19 inconclusive investigations of 61 case investigations during a 12-month period (Pealer *et al.* 2003). The true number of transmissions was probably higher by at least an order of magnitude.

As was the case with HIV and the hepatitis viruses, blood transfusion of WNV represents a small, but highly visible portion of a large epidemic. WNV is a mosquito-borne flavivirus transmitted primarily to birds and some small mammals. Humans serve as an incidental host. Approximately 80% of human infections are asymptomatic; 20% result in a febrile illness known as West Nile fever. About 1 in 150 patients develop meningoencephalitis and residual neurological deficits have been reported. Although there is no particular susceptibility to mosquito-borne infection, elderly and immunosuppressed subjects appear particularly vulnerable to severe, progressive disease. The virus is present for a week or more during initial infection. Most symptomatic subjects describe fever, headache and malaise, although these are not sufficiently specific for effective donor screening. Viral shedding may persist for 7–8 weeks after infection, usually in the presence of specific antibody. The period of infectivity has not been well defined.

Of the 23 well-studied patients with transfusion-transmitted infection, 14 were identified because West Nile virus-associated illness came to the clinician's attention following transfusion. Overall, 15 patients had recognized illness (13 meningoencephalitis, two fever). The illness began between 2 and 21 days after the implicated transfusion. The highly immunosuppressed transplant recipients appeared to have the longest incubation periods (median 13.5 days). Red cells, platelets and fresh-frozen plasma (FFP) have all been implicated in transmissions. Sixteen blood donors were implicated in transmission, with no predilection for age or gender. Nine out of the sixteen recalled symptoms compatible with a viral illness around the time of donation, although all donors passed the donor screening procedures. Three donors developed symptoms prior to donation, one on the day of donation and five post donation. Fever, headache and weakness were the most common symptoms. Samples obtained at the time of donation had virus levels less than 80 pfu per millilitre and all were negative for West Nile virus IgM antibody.

Since screening of blood was undertaken in the USA, approximately 6 million units were tested during the June–December 2003 interval, resulting in the removal of at least 818 viraemic blood donations from the blood supply. Nevertheless, six cases of WNV transmitted by transfusion occurred because of transfusion of components containing low levels of virus not detected by the testing of pooled specimens (Macedo et al. 2004). All blood donations in the USA are currently screened by rtPCR, and it is likely that testing of individual donations will begin in areas of epidemic transmission and eventually be practised universally (Custer et al. 2004).

Other flaviviruses such as St Louis encephalitis virus, Japanese encephalitis virus and dengue virus are likely to be blood transmissible as well, although documentation is lacking.

Simian foamy virus

Simian foamy virus (SFV) (spumaretrovirus) is a highly prevalent primate retrovirus that has been shown to infect human cells, replicate and produce cell-free infectious virus. Tropism is broad and includes B and T lymphocytes, macrophages, fibroblasts, endothelial cells and kidney cells. Simian retroviruses are spread in areas of the world such as Central Africa, where non-human primates are hunted for food and among people who handle non-human primates as pets or laboratory animals. In total, 1% of people living in southern Cameroon were found to harbour antibodies to SFV; all had reported exposure to fresh primate blood or body fluids (Wolfe et al. 2004).

Studies from the USA CDC report a prevalence of infection of 2–5% with simian foamy viruses among laboratory and zoo workers occupationally exposed to non-human primates (Heneine et al. 1998; Switzer et al. 2004). Persistent viraemia has been detected in peripheral blood lymphocytes (PBLs) and 11 SFV-infected workers are known to have donated blood. Six donors were confirmed positive at the time of donation. SFV transmission through transfusion was not identified among four recipients of cellular blood components (two RBC, one filtered RBC, one platelet concentrate) from one SFV-infected donor (Boneva et al. 2002). Derivatives containing plasma from that donor tested negative for SFV.

Evidence of SFV infection included seropositivity, proviral DNA detection and isolation of foamy virus. There is no evidence as yet that SFV causes human disease but, recombination within the host, especially in immunocompromised hosts that may allow persistent infection, remains a concern.

Prion proteins

A fundamental feature of prion diseases involves a normal protein constituent of human tissue, prion protein (PrP) (Bendheim et al. 1992). PrP can exist in either a natural cellular form (PrP^C) or as variant pathological forms known collectively as 'scrapie isoforms' or PrP^{Sc}. Different prion strains result in distinct clinical and pathological diseases (Prusiner 1998). Both forms of prion protein have an identical amino acid sequence, but differ in the secondary structure, beta-pleated structures in the variant forms instead of the alpha-helical structure of the native protein (Pan et al. 1993). The structural difference has two major consequences. First, the beta-pleated conformation allows PrP^{Sc} molecules to form protease-resistant aggregates. Second, the abnormal protein seems to be capable of suborning normal protein to the abnormal form. The molecules with beta-pleated regions cause key alpha-helical regions of the native protein to assume the pleated conformation, thus converting normal protein to abnormal aggregates that cause the spongiform degeneration of the brain that is characteristic of these diseases.

Prion proteins are linked to the cell plasma membrane by the lipid glycophosphatidyl inositol (GPI). GPI-linked proteins are released from cells by several different mechanisms and may be taken up by other cells, thus facilitating dissemination (Devetten *et al.* 1997). Prion proteins are taken up selectively by motile follicular dendritic cells, suggesting that infective proteins may be present in circulating blood (Klein *et al.* 2001).

Creutzfeldt–Jakob disease

Creutzfeldt–Jakob disease (CJD) is a rare, but invariably fatal neurodegenerative disease, with an incidence of about one per million of the UK and USA population (Collinge and Rossor 1996). CJD may be 'sporadic,' arising from a random change in a normal individual, 'familial,' arising from a point mutation in the DNA coding for the protein, which leads to an increased susceptibility to production of the abnormal form, or 'acquired,' by the transfer of infectious material, as in individuals injected with pituitary-derived hormones or treated with dura mater transplants (Brown *et al.* 1992). A single case of transmission from a corneal transplant has also been reported. The proportion of recipients acquiring CJD from growth hormone varies from 0.3% to 4.4% in different countries, and acquisition from dura mater varies between 0.02% and 0.05% in Japan, where most cases occurred (Brown *et al.* 2000). Patient follow-up after point exposures to contaminated materials indicate that clinical latency for iatrogenic CJD may exceed 30 years (Fradkin *et al.* 1991; Brown *et al.* 2000).

Classic CJD typically affects older subjects with a median age of 60 years. Memory loss is an early manifestation, but the disease progresses rapidly after the first symptoms through confusion, motor and cerebellar symptoms and dementia. Death often occurs within a year of the first symptom.

Because of the possibility of transfer of infectious prions by transfusion, donors have been questioned to discover (1) whether there is any family history of CJD; (2) whether they have received pituitary-derived hormones; or (3) in some countries, whether they have received corneal grafts or grafts of dura mater. However, a systematic review of five case–control studies from the UK, Europe, Japan and Australia, involving 2479 patients, failed to find an association between CJD and blood recipients. No evidence of transmission of CJD by blood transfusion exists, despite the identification of individuals who were exposed to blood donated by people who later developed this disease (Wilson *et al.* 2000). A study of preserved brain samples of 25 haemophilic patients who have high exposure to blood transfusions and potentially higher exposure to blood infected with the agent responsible for Creutzfeldt–Jakob disease found no evidence of the disease (Evatt *et al.* 1998). 'Look-back' studies have not identified any cases of Creutzfeldt–Jakob disease developing in recipients who received blood from a donor in whom the disease was later diagnosed. The risk of CJD transmission through transfusion is now considered negligible, and plasma pools are no longer discarded if a contributing donor develops CJD. Deferrals designed to eliminate 'high-risk' donor categories, such as growth hormone and dura mater recipients, remain in force.

Variant Creutzfeldt–Jakob disease

A neurodegenerative disease affecting cattle was first identified in England in 1984 and subsequently branded 'mad cow disease'. Bovine spongiform encephalopathy (BSE) is now recognized as a prion-related disorder with more than 179 000 confirmed clinical cases of BSE, driven by the recycling of infection through the inclusion of bovine protein in cattle feed. A ban on feeding tissues from one ruminant animal to other ruminant animals, introduced in 1988, brought the British BSE epidemic under control. However, because of the long delay between infection and the onset of clinical signs of disease (5 years on average), the annual incidence of clinical cases did not peak until 1992. BSE has been found in several other European countries and in Canada. More rapid and accurate description of the epidemiology of BSE has been hampered by the absence of a diagnostic test that can be applied to live animals to detect those that are incubating the infection.

The human disease equivalent, new variant Creutzfeldt–Jakob disease (vCJD), was not identified until 1996, 7 years after the ban was introduced. A disease-related isoform of prion resembling that of BSE is consistent with the conclusion that BSE has crossed the species barrier, probably from ingestion of infected beef (Collinge and Rossor 1996; Bruce *et al.*

1997). Unlike classic CJD, vCJD usually affects younger subjects (age 18–53 years) and is characterized by early psychiatric and sensory symptoms. The disease progresses over 8 months to 3 years, with progressive dementia, ataxia and myoclonus. Brain biopsy has a characteristic pattern and Western blot analysis shows a diagnostic migration pattern of proteinase-treated PrP^{Sc}. Pathological PrP^{Sc} can be found in tonsils, spleen lymph nodes and appendix (Collinge et al. 1996). Prion protein gene analysis has shown that all cases were homozygous for methionine at codon 129 (Ironside and Head 2004). More than 150 cases have been found in the UK and cases have been described in France and Italy. Although the number of vCJD 'carriers' remains unknown, early estimates of as many as 100 000 cases have in recent years dwindled to a maximum of just a few hundred cases, assuming an estimate of 15 to 20 years as the average incubation period (Valleron et al. 2001). One model indicates that the primary epidemic in the susceptible genotype (methionine-methionine (MM)-homozygous at codon 129 of the prion protein gene) has now peaked, with an estimate of 40 future deaths (Ghani et al. 2003). However, the prevalence of vCJD infection in the UK population, estimated to be as high as 1 per 4000 based on a study of routinely acquired tonsils and appendices, raises the possibility of a second and third 'wave' of clinical cases in subjects heterozygous (methionine-valine) and homozygous for valine at codon 129.

Prion protein has been identified on a wide range of circulating cells including platelets, myeloid cells, lymphocytes and red cells (Dodelet and Cashman 1998; Holada and Vostal 2000; Bessos et al. 2001; Li et al. 2001). Findings in experimental models show that blood not only contains infective agents of prion diseases, but that no barrier to transmission exists with intraspecies transmission, and that the intravenous route of exposure to prions is fairly efficient (Casaccia et al. 1989; Cervenakova et al. 2003). The seminal experiments in sheep have shown transmission of BSE and scrapie by blood transfusion, and blood for transfusion in these experiments was obtained from sheep midway through the incubation period (Houston et al. 2000; Hunter et al. 2002). Infectivity has also been noted in the incubation period and symptomatic phase in a rodent model of vCJD (Cervenakova et al. 2003).

In 1997, the UK set up a surveillance system between the national CJD surveillance unit and the UK national blood services. In 2004, the first probable transfusion-associated case of vCJD was described (Llewelyn et al. 2004):

A 62-year-old man received 5 units of red cells for a surgical procedure. Six and a half years later, the patient developed irritability and depression, followed by a shuffling gait, blurred vision, motor dysfunction and cognitive impairment. Thirteen months after the onset of symptoms, he died of autopsy-confirmed vCJD. One of the red cell units had been donated by a 24-year-old subject who developed symptoms of vCJD 3 years and 4 months later, and subsequently died of vCJD confirmed at autopsy. Red cells from a second donation were traced to a patient who died of cancer 5 months later. Platelets from the donation could not be traced to a recipient.

The clinical presentation of the transfusion recipient was typical of vCJD, and diagnosis was confirmed by neuropathological examination. Transfusion took place before universal leucoreduction. Of particular note in this case is the age of the recipient, the second oldest patient with vCJD, making it even less likely that this case was caused by ingestion of tainted beef.

Statistical analysis, taking account reported vCJD mortality to date and details of the recipients of vCJD donations indicate that the probability of recording a case of vCJD in this population in the absence of transfusion-transmitted infection ranges between about 1 in 15 000 and 1 in 30 000 (Llewelyn et al. 2004).

A case of preclinical vCJD has been reported in a patient who died from a non-neurological disorder 5 years after receiving a blood transfusion from a donor who subsequently developed vCJD:

In 1999, an elderly patient received a unit of non-leucodepleted red blood cells from a donor who developed symptoms of vCJD 18 months after donation. The donor died in 2001 and vCJD was confirmed at autopsy. The recipient, who had no evidence of a neurological disorder, died 5 years after receiving the transfusion. Western blot analysis of splenic tissue showed the presence of PrP^{res} with the mobility and glycoform ratio of the signals similar to those seen in spleen from patients with clinical vCJD and distinct from those of sporadic CJD cases.

Protease-resistant prion protein (PrP^{res}) was detected by Western blot, paraffin-embedded tissue blot and immunohistochemistry in splenic tissue, but not in the brain. However, animal studies suggest that migration is inevitable given sufficient time. Prion protein was also present in a cervical lymph node. Perhaps the most disturbing observation is that this patient was a heterozygote at codon 129 of prion protein gene (PRNP), suggesting that susceptibility to vCJD infection is not confined to the methionine homozygous genotype. This finding suggests that a second, later wave of vCJD cases in heterozygotes and even a third may appear long after the initial peak of the epidemic (Peden *et al.* 2004). The chance of observing vCJD transmission in the absence of a transfusion infection in this second recipient of blood from a donor with vCJD is far less than the 1 in 15 000 to 1 in 30 000 chance for the first reported case.

Transmissable spongiform encephalopathy (TSE) agents are resistant to the range of physical and chemical means that have been used to inactivate viruses in plasma products. However, a range of studies using animal TSE models have demonstrated that the processes used to purify proteins, including factor concentrates, over the course of plasma fractionation can also contribute significantly to removing both abnormal prions and infectivity (Lee *et al.* 2001). Extensive washing of cellular components may also deplete the prion content; however, the risk of infection has not been determined. A prototype prion removal filter has been designed to remove about four logs of PrP, below the level of detection in the Western blot assay, and has prevented infection in a hamster scrapie model (SO Sowemino-Coker, personal communication).

Bacteria

Transmission of bacteria represents the most frequent infectious complication of blood transfusion in the developed world and a major cause of transfusion-associated mortality (Andreu *et al.* 2002). The reported frequency of contamination varies depending upon the nature of the blood component and the method of study technique.

Treponema pallidum

Treponema pallidum is a motile spirochaete that spreads by sexual contact, transfusion, percutaneous exposure and transmission from mother to infant. The incubation period from transfusion to clinical presentation varies from 4 weeks to 4.5 months, averaging 9–10 weeks, and the infected recipient usually exhibits a typical secondary eruption. Donors at any stage of disease, including late, latent syphilis, can transmit the infection (Hartmann and Schone 1942).

Transfusion-transmitted syphilis was once considered a serious problem. Kilduffe and DeBakey (1942) identified more than 100 cases that had been published after 1915, all from direct transfusion. Some 138 cases had been reported by 1941 (De Schryver and Meheus 1990). Since then, few cases have been reported in the developed world. The last case published in the USA was reported from the Clinical Center at the National Institutes of Health (Chambers *et al.* 1969).

In 1966, a patient was admitted to the Clinical Center with a diagnosis of lymphoma. His serological test for syphilis (STS) was negative on admission. He received 5 units of RBCs and 25 units of fresh platelets, none of which reacted in the VDRL test. Two months later, he developed a maculopapular rash consistent with secondary syphilis. Serological tests and confirmatory assays for syphilis turned positive. The patient was treated with penicillin and the rash cleared.

Of the 30 donors, 27 tested negative repeatedly, but two could not be traced and one refused to be retested. The investigators presumed that one out of those three donors, a platelet donor, was infectious for syphilis.

The chief reasons for the decline of transfusion-transmitted syphilis seem to be the almost universal practice of storing blood at 4°C before transfusion, universal donor testing and the decline in the prevalence of syphilis in many countries since the advent of penicillin. Other factors that have probably contributed to the decline include the administration of antibiotics to a large proportion of patients requiring transfusion and the exclusion of donors with high-risk sexual practices.

Spirochaetes are unlikely to survive in citrated blood stored for more than 72 h at 4–6°C (Bloch 1941; Turner and Diseker 1941). However, organisms can be detected for as long as 6 days (Selbie 1943). There is a close relationship between the number of treponemes added to donor blood and the survival times of *T. pallidum* determined by a sensitive assay in rabbits; in blood heavily contaminated with spirochaetes (1.3×10^6 and 2.5×10^7/ml blood), surviving treponema were found at 120 h (Garretta *et al.* 1977; van der Sluis *et al.* 1985).

Several tests are available for screening blood donations for syphilis, including the automated reagin test (ART), the rapid plasma reagin test (PRP) and the Venereal Disease Research Laboratory (VDRL) slide technique in which non-specific reagins (antibodies) are detected and the *T. pallidum* haemagglutination assay (TPHA), the fluorescent treponemal antibodies absorbed with Reiter's treponeme assay (FTA-Abs) and ELISAs for the detection of specific antibodies. Non-specific reagin tests detect antibody to lipoidal antigen and are often considered to be insufficiently sensitive as screening tests (Barbara *et al*. 1982; Young *et al*. 1992). Positive screening tests should be tested for FTA-Abs or some other specific assay in a reference laboratory. A lack of demonstrable *T. pallidum* DNA or RNA suggests that blood donors with confirmed positive results in STS are unlikely to have circulating *T. pallidum* in their blood, and that that their blood is unlikely to be infectious for syphilis (Orton *et al*. 2002).

Serological tests cannot prevent all cases of transfusion syphilis because most remain negative in early primary syphilis, when spirochaetaemia is most prominent (Spangler *et al*. 1964).

The rationale for continued syphilis testing relies upon the increasing demands for fresh blood components, especially platelets and fresh blood for exchange transfusion in newborn infants, the very occasional reported case (Chambers *et al*. 1969; Soendjojo *et al*. 1982; Risseeuw-Appel and Kothe 1983) and its questionable value as a surrogate test to exclude donors who are in high-risk groups for HIV and HBV infection. A positive test in a transfusion recipient may result from antibody acquired passively from the donor (Rossi *et al*. 2002). However, passively acquired antibody rarely remains detectable for more than a few months after transfusion (Ravitch *et al*. 1949; Rossi *et al*. 2002).

In countries with a high incidence of syphilis, some consultants recommend that recipients of fresh blood receive 2 megaunits of penicillin G or its equivalent (Bruce-Chwatt 1985). In endemic areas, subjects who have had non-venereal trepanomatosis, such as yaws or pima caused by *T. pallidum pertenue* or *T. pallidum carateum*, may also have a positive screening test for syphilis.

Brucella abortus

This organism can survive for months in stored blood and there are several reports of blood transfusion-transmitted symptomatic infection, mainly in children and splenectomized patients (Wood 1955; Tabor 1982). Antibody-positive donors are common in Mexico, Greece, Spain and in some rural areas of the USA, although transfusion-transmitted brucellosis has not been reported in the USA. Infected donor blood has very low concentrations of brucella and poses little risk except for immunosuppressed patients (Fernandez *et al*. 1981).

After an incubation period ranging from 6 days to 4 months, recipients of infected blood may develop undulant fever, headache, chills, excessive sweating, muscle pains and fatigue. Hepatosplenomegaly, lymphadenopathy, leucopenia and arthritis occur and, very rarely, complications such as purpura, encephalitis or endocarditis develop (Tabor 1982).

In view of the chronic nature of the disease, persons with a history of brucellosis should not be used as donors. However, 80% of infections are asymptomatic. Even in endemic areas screening tests are not practical; most subjects with high-titre brucella antibodies do not transmit infection by transfusion (Fernandez *et al*. 1981).

Miscellaneous

Lyme disease

The organism responsible for this disease is *Borrelia burgdorferi*, a tick-borne spirochaete whose primary reservoir is the white-footed mouse. Humans are infected in the nymphal stage of the cycle and white-tailed deer are infected during the second year of life of the tick. Most cases of Lyme disease have been reported in the USA, but thousands of cases have also been reported in Europe.

The disease has three stages: in the acute stage of erythema migrans, a skin rash starting at the site of the tick bite spreads locally and is often accompanied by 'flu-like symptoms'. If this stage is not treated promptly with antibiotics, the second stage progresses to disseminated infection with cardiovascular and neurological manifestations. In the third stage, arthritis develops.

Although no cases of transmission of *B. burgdorferi* by blood transfusion have been reported so far, transmission is theoretically possible. Subjects in the primary stage of infection pose the most risk. However, as these patients are generally ill and as spirochaetaemia is of low intensity and of short duration, infectious donors probably do not present often for blood donation (Popovsky 1990; Westphal 1991a). The spirochaete has been isolated and cultured from blood as old as 14 days.

Four transfusion recipients of blood components from a donor who gave blood between the disappearance of erythema migrans and the second stage of the disease have been studied; none of the recipients showed signs of disease or developed antibodies against *B. burgdorferi* (Halkier *et al.* 1990).

Mycobacterium leprae

Mycobacterium leprae is known to have been transfused inadvertently from a donor incubating leprosy to the two recipients without apparent harm. *M. leprae* has also been injected intravenously into human volunteers without the recipients becoming infected, although the period of follow-up is not known (Tabor 1982).

Tick-borne rickettsial disease

Tick-borne rickettsial diseases are caused by two groups of intracellular bacteria belonging to the order *Rickettsiales*: (1) bacteria belonging to the spotted fever group of the genus *Rickettsia* within the family Rickettsiaceae; and (2) bacteria within the family Anaplasmataceae, including several genera, such as *Anaplasma* and *Ehrlichia*. Rickettsiosis (Rocky Mountain spotted fever) has been reported to have been transmitted by blood from a donor incubating the disease who subsequently died (Wells *et al.* 1978). The rarity of the transmission of rickettsiosis by blood transfusion probably reflects the clinical illness suffered during most of the period of rickettsial infection that makes blood donation unlikely (Tabor 1982).

In addition to the spotted fever group rickettsioses, human anaplasmosis (formerly human granulocytic ehrlichiosis) has also emerged in Europe (Parola 2004). This disease was first described in the USA in 1994 and presents most commonly as a febrile illness occurring in summer or spring. The causative organism is *Anaplasma phagocytophilum*, formerly known as *Ehrlichia equi*, *Ehrlichia phagocytophila* and human granulocytic ehrlichia. The vector in Europe is *I. ricinus*, which is also the vector of Lyme borreliosis. Anaplasma are well preserved in refrigerated blood components (McKechnie *et al.* 2000). Transfusion-transmitted ehrlichiosis has been reported (Eastlund *et al.* 1999).

Exogenous and various endogenous bacteria and bacterial products contaminating stored blood or blood components

Bacteria may affect blood or blood components in one of the following ways:

1 Bacteria may contaminate solutions or equipment that are to be used for transfusions but which have not yet been sterilized. After sterilization the solutions or equipment may remain contaminated with heat-stable bacterial products (pyrogens) capable of producing febrile reactions when they are introduced into the circulation (see Chapter 15). In contaminated equipment or solutions such as hydroxyethyl starch used in leucapheresis, bacteria may survive 'sterilization' or may contaminate solutions that have previously been sterilized, for example when a glass container is cracked during shipment (Wang *et al.* 2000). This kind of contamination has become rare.

2 Bacteria originating from skin flora, such as *Staphylococcus epidermidis*, *Micrococcus* species, *Sarcina* species and diphtheroids, may gain entrance to the blood pack during venesection, especially if the site of venepuncture is scarred. It is virtually impossible to disinfect the deeper layers of the skin and a skin plug often enters the blood pack upon collection (Anderson *et al.* 1986; Puckett 1986a).

3 Bacteria in the environment (*Pseudomonas* species, *Flavobacterium* species, *Bacillus* species) may gain entrance to blood components through minute lesions in the packs, during collection or processing in open systems (Szewzyk *et al.* 1993).

4 The ports of packs of cryoprecipitate or FFP may become contaminated, if not protected by a secondary plastic bag, during thawing in waterbaths contaminated with pseudomonas (e.g. *Pseudomonas cepacia*, *P. aeruginosa*) (Casewell *et al.* 1981).

5 Bacteria circulating in the blood of an apparently healthy donor suffering from asymptomatic bacteraemia may proliferate in red cell components stored at 4°C or in platelet concentrates stored at room temperature. Bacteraemia in donors may be chronic and low grade, as in the case of the incubation or convalescence periods of salmonella, *Yersinia enterocolitica* or *Campylobacter jejuni* infections, or acute and transient as occurs within the first few hours after dental extractions when the organisms involved are usually *Streptococcus viridans*, *Bacteroides* species and, less often, *Staphylococcus aureus*. A particularly notorious case reported from the

Clinical Center at NIH involved a repeat platelet donor with asymptomatic *Salmonella cholerasuis* osteomyelitis, whose donations resulted in sepsis in seven patients and death in one of these before platelets were identified as the source of infection (Rhame *et al.* 1973).

Frequency of bacterial contamination of blood components

Bacteria are usually prevented from growing by the antibacterial properties of blood. Complement, even in the absence of specific antibodies may kill bacteria, which may then be phagocytosed by leucocytes (Högman *et al.* 1991; Gong *et al.* 1994). Nevertheless positive cultures in samples from blood or blood components are found fairly frequently. In an extensive survey in which approximately 2500 units of red cells and an equal number of platelet concentrates were sampled annually, over a period of 10 years the mean rates of positive cultures were 0.3% and 0.4% respectively (Goldman and Blajchman 1991). Bacterial contamination of whole blood cultured after 2–20 h of storage at room temperature ranges from 0.34% to 2.2% (Bruneau *et al.* 2001; de Korte *et al.* 2001). Survival of most organisms is reduced by storage at refrigerated temperatures. However, platelet concentrates are stored at room temperature so that bacterial contamination and continued growth present an urgent clinical problem. In one early study, 6 out of 3141 (0.19%) pooled concentrates from random donors were found to contain bacteria just prior to transfusion (Yomtovian *et al.* 1993). In another prospective study, 7 out of 15 838 (0.04%) concentrates were confirmed positive (Blajchman *et al.* 1994). A higher percentage (0.79%) was found in samples taken from freshly prepared concentrates: of 11 positive cultures only one was confirmed on repeated culture from the same concentrate (Högman and Engstrand 1996). Only 5 out of 17 928 (0.03%) single-donor concentrates obtained by apheresis contained bacteria (Barrett *et al.* 1993). A 6-year experience using a semi-automated system for routine platelet cultures in Denmark reported an initial positive reaction in 84 samples (0.38%) from 22 057 platelet units. Growth was confirmed in 70 of these (Munksgaard *et al.* 2004). The risk of collecting a contaminated unit of platelets is estimated at 1 in 2000 (Chiu *et al.* 1994).

A prospective study using a conservative case definition found the rate of transfusion-transmitted bacteraemia (in events/million units) to be 9.98 for single-donor platelets, 10.64 for pooled platelets and 0.21 for RBC units (1/500 000); for fatal reactions, the rates were 1.94, 2.22 and 0.13 respectively (Kuehnert *et al.* 2001). From a 12-year retrospective analysis of transfusion data from a single institution, symptomatic sepsis from transfused platelets was estimated to occur at between 1 in 5000 (pooled whole-blood-derived platelets) and one in 15 000 single-donor apheresis platelet transfusions (Ness *et al.* 2001).

The incidence of clinical reactions due to contaminated blood is much lower than that expected from the reported rates of positive bacterial cultures. Although some contaminated components, especially those containing large numbers of organisms or endotoxin, result in immediate, catastrophic reactions including shock and death, others may be quite mild with little more than low-grade fever or chills (Yomtovian *et al.* 1993). As many patients who receive platelet transfusions already have an infection, febrile reactions or symptoms of septicaemia may not be ascribed to the transfusion (Chiu *et al.* 1994). Furthermore many of these patients are being treated with antibiotics that blunt detection and diagnosis of septic reactions.

Autologous blood

As might be anticipated, autologous donations are also susceptible to bacterial contamination. At least five such cases have been reported. The majority of the infected units contained *Y. enterocolitica*, and the donors recalled in retrospect gastrointestinal episodes in the weeks prior to donation (Haditsch *et al.* 1994).

Some properties of organisms that grow in stored blood

Organisms isolated from refrigerated blood are usually Gram-negative rods capable of metabolizing citrate (Pittman 1953). Many strains of organisms isolated from contaminated stored blood cause clot formation by consuming citrate, yet another reason to examine all units carefully at the time of issue (Braude *et al.* 1952; Pittman 1953). Blood that is heavily contaminated with organisms is not necessarily haemolysed. Among bacteria isolated from stored blood, 25% produce no haemolysis (Braude *et al.* 1952). Many organisms that grow in stored blood are psychrophilic – organisms that grow preferentially in the cold.

Unless blood is heavily contaminated with organisms, microscopic examination is an unreliable method of detecting infection. After serial dilutions of an inoculum of a coliform organism to blood, 24×10^5 organisms/ml could be detected readily but 24×10^4/ml (one organism in every 100 fields) could be detected only with difficulty (Walter et al. 1957). On the other hand, when an aliquot of 0.3 ml was cultured for 24 h, contamination could be detected when the number of organisms added was as low as 24/ml.

The effect of antibiotics on bacteria in stored blood has been investigated. Chlortetracycline, oxytetracycline and polymyxin B in concentrations as low as 10 mg in 500 ml of blood (i.e. 20 µg/ml) would all prevent the inocula of either cold- or warm-growing bacteria from multiplying in human blood either in the cold or at room temperature. Nevertheless, routine addition of antibiotics to stored blood cannot be recommended. First, antibiotics cannot be autoclaved and would therefore have to be added later, and this addition might itself contaminate the collection. Second, no antibiotics are effective against all organisms. Third, there is the risk of immunizing patients to particular antibiotics or of inducing a hypersensitivity reaction in a patient already immunized.

Importance of maintaining refrigeration

After the first 24 h or so of storage, strict maintenance of refrigeration at a temperature of 4°C becomes essential. When blood has to be transported for any considerable distance the use of refrigerated containers can maintain blood below 10°C for as long as 48 h. Some transfusion centres routinely keep blood at approximately 20°C for up to 24 h after collection before it is processed. The storage at room temperature does not seem to affect the yields of factor VIII in plasma subsequently frozen and fractionated or the shelf-life of platelets or red cells (Pietersz et al. 1989). Leucocytes in fresh blood have a bactericidal effect for a few hours after collection and before processing into blood components with removal of the buffy coats. From experiments in which defined numbers of colony-forming units of different bacteria were added to fresh blood, leucocytes were shown to effect clearing of bacteria, the efficiency varying according to the bacterial species: *Staphylococcus epidermidis* and *Escherichia coli* were cleared more readily than *S. aureus*, which was engulfed by the leucocytes and then released after

causing cell death (Högman et al. 1991). The clearing effect of leucocytes sometimes requires as long as 24 h. Some Gram-negative bacteria are killed by plasma factors, presumably antibodies and complement. Certain anaerobic bacteria such as *Propionibacterium* species do not grow in stored blood, regardless of the presence or absence of white cells. *Yersinia enterocolitica* was cleared temporarily, but reappeared within a few hours; if leucocytes were removed from the blood after 5 h, the units remained sterile. Although some bacteria are killed intracellularly, others kill the cells, which then disintegrate releasing the bacteria (Högman et al. 1991).

Bacteria contaminating different blood components

The type of bacterial contamination largely depends on the type of blood component:

1 *Red cells involved in cases of bacterial infection* have been contaminated mainly with *Pseudomonas fluorescens*, *P. putida* and *Y. enterocolitica*. Yersinia is normally sensitive to complement and is phagocytosed by leucocytes in fresh blood. However, it is capable of producing a virulence plasmid that expresses a surface protein rendering the organism resistant to complement and intracellular killing after phagocytosis (Lian et al. 1987). Yersinia grows well at 4°C, uses citrate as a source of energy and, owing to its lack of siderophores, requires iron for optimum growth. Red cell concentrates provide an ideal culture medium. The organism produces a potent endotoxin during storage. Transfusion of contaminated red cells can cause fatal septicaemia. In almost all serious reactions due to *Y. eneterocolitica*, the red cell concentrates had been stored for more than 3 weeks. Phagocytes containing live bacteria may persist after a donor has otherwise contained a yersinia infection. During storage of red cell concentrates the leucocytes may disintegrate, releasing live bacteria, which can then multiply (Högman et al. 1992). Leucocyte-depleted red cell concentrates, previously inoculated with *Y. eneterocolitica* remain sterile, whereas growth develops after 2–3 weeks in leucocyte-containing concentrates (Gong et al. 1994). Between April 1987 and the end of February 1991, eight fatalities associated with the transfusion of red cells contaminated with bacteria were reported to the FDA; seven of these were due to *Y. enterocolitica*. During the same period, 10 cases of *Y. enterocolitica* caused by contaminated red cell

transfusions were reported in the USA, three cases in France, one in Belgium and one in Australia. The patients developed fever and hypotension within 50 min of the start of transfusion. In the 10 cases that occurred in the USA, the blood had been stored in the cold for a mean of 33 days (range 25–42 days). Although reports of septicaemia due to yersinia are rare, the numbers have increased in the past 10 years. If patients are taking antibiotics, infection by blood contaminated with yersinia can be asymptomatic (Jacobs *et al.* 1989).

2 *Platelet concentrates* stored at 20–24°C have caused fatal bacterial sepsis when contaminated with any of several Gram-negative or -positive organisms such as staphylococci, streptococci, *Serratia* species, flavobacteria and salmonellae (Goldman and Blajchman 1991). One plateletpheresis donor with subclinical *Salmonella cholerae suis* osteomyelitis caused sepsis in seven platelet recipients (Rhame *et al.* 1973).

3 *Cryoprecipitates and FFP* can become contaminated with P. cepacia and P. aeruginosa during thawing in contaminated waterbaths (Goldman and Blajchman 1991).

4 *Any of the above* (1–3) can become infected if the exterior of blood packs is massively contaminated during manufacture by bacteria such as *Serratia marcescens*. Septicaemia has been reported in recipients of such contaminated units (Heltberg *et al.* 1992).

Effect of transfusing bacterially contaminated blood

Shock following the injection of bacteria is presumably due to bacterial toxins, although an immune reaction between naturally occurring antibodies and bacteria may also produce ill effects. The transfusion of contaminated blood may produce immediate collapse, followed by profound shock and hyperpyrexia; haemorrhagic phenomena due to disseminated intravascular coagulation are common; in a series of 25 cases, mortality was 58% (Habibi *et al.* 1973).

A review of more than 30 reports of post-transfusion sepsis due to contaminated red cells, platelets or a few other blood components showed that septic shock developed in many cases and that the overall mortality rate was 26%. Common signs and symptoms reported were fever, chills, vomiting, tachycardia and hypotension, often during the transfusion, but sometimes developing a few hours later. In the case of *Pseudomonas cepacia*, septicaemia or wound infection developed several days or weeks after transfusion (Goldman and Blajchman 1991). However, atypical presentations have been well documented in prospective studies and suggest that clinical syndromes are under-reported (Yomtovian *et al.* 1993).

Investigations following the suspected transfusion of injected blood

Any blood remaining in the container should be cultured at various temperatures, including 4°C and 20°C, in appropriate culture media. A negative culture excludes the possibility that the blood was heavily infected at the time of transfusion. A positive culture does not enable one to say with certainty whether the blood was contaminated before the transfusion or became contaminated during or after transfusion, or upon sampling. Techniques to exclude contamination upon sampling have been described (Puckett 1986b). It is still useful to culture implicated containers that have been left at room temperature for 24 h. Most sterile units remain sterile or at worst lightly contaminated. In fatal cases, blood for culture should be collected from the body (e.g. by cardiac puncture) as soon as possible after death. Blood contaminated with a coliaerogenes bacterium cultured positive, although when pseudomonads were involved, blood collected at autopsy was sterile (Pittman 1953).

Specific identification of the contaminating organism can be important for determining the extent of donor follow-up and the donor counselling message (Haimowitz 2005).

Inspection of red cells: the dark side of transfusion

Colour change in stored red cell concentrates may indicate that the unit has been contaminated with bacteria. In 13 units of red cells that supported the growth of Y. enterocolitica, a darkening related to haemolysis and a decrease in PO_2 was observed in the primary container (Kim *et al.* 1992). The attached sample segments, which were sealed from the main unit, remained sterile and did not darken. The colour change was apparent in all the contaminated units by day 35, or 1.5 to 2 weeks after the bacteria were first detected in cultures of the blood. A keen observer can identify units grossly contaminated with Y. enterocolitica by comparison of the colour of the segment tubing with that of the unit (Kim *et al.* 1992). Review of photographs on file at the Centers for Disease Control revealed this colour change in 2 units of blood that caused transfusion-transmitted sepsis (*Enterobacter agglomerans* and an unidentified Gram-negative bacillus), which demonstrates that the colour change is not limited to contamination by *Y. enterocolitica*.

Screening for bacterial contamination

Avoidance of bacterial contamination is preferable to detecting organisms downstream. Examination of the donor's arms and rigorous skin preparation reduce quantitative bacterial growth by as much as 50% (Goldman *et al.* 1997) (see Chapter 1). Diversion of an aliquot of the initial blood collection removes some of the organisms that populate the phlebotomy site (de Korte *et al.* 2002). Screening collected blood for bacterial contamination is complicated by the small initial inoculum (sampling error), differential growth rates of various species, and the potential for introduction of organisms at the time of the screening procedure. Despite the absence of convenient and inexpensive detection methods, routine surveillance of platelet preparations for bacterial contamination has been instituted in several countries. The two most commonly used methods are culture based. A sensitive and specific automated, continuous monitoring culture system measures carbon dioxide production as a marker of bacterial growth (Brecher *et al.* 2001, 2004). Both aerobic and anaerobic cultures are possible. The procedure increases the storage interval before platelets can be released and cultures may turn positive after platelets have been issued or transfused. A second system monitors consumption of oxygen after 24 h at room temperature in aliquots of platelet concentrates as a marker of microbial growth (Rock *et al.* 2004). The disadvantages include inability to detect anaerobic organisms, reliance on analysis at a single time point and limited ability to detect slow-growing bacteria. However only one example of a fatality associated with an anaerobic organism has been reported (McDonald *et al.* 1998). Both methods have interdicted contaminated transfusions.

Malaria

Transmission of malaria by blood transfusion

Malaria can be transmitted by the transfusion of any blood component likely to contain even small numbers of red cells; platelet and granulocyte concentrates, fresh plasma and cryoprecipitate have all been incriminated. An inoculum containing as few as 10 parasites can cause *Plasmodium vivax* malaria (Bruce-Chwatt 1972).

Despite intensive eradication programmes, the prevalence of malaria in tropical and subtropical countries is extremely high, with about 300 million cases reported each year, and more than 1 million annual fatalities attributed to malaria in tropical Africa (Wyler 1983). The increasing resistance of the mosquitoes to insecticides and the increasing appearance of drug-resistant strains, particularly of *P. falciparum* and the recurrence of malaria in areas where the disease had previously been eradicated, have greatly increased the incidence of malaria in recent years.

Malaria parasites of all species can remain viable in stored blood for at least 1 week (Hutton and Shute 1939). Cases of *P. falciparum* malaria have been transmitted by blood stored for 14 days (Grant *et al.* 1960) and for 19 days (De Silva *et al.* 1988). Malaria parasites may survive longer in blood stored in adenine-containing solutions (WHO 1986). In a review of nearly 2000 cases of transfusion malaria due to *P. malariae*, in the great majority of cases the blood had been stored for less than 5 days and cases following the transfusion of blood stored for 2 weeks were rare (Bruce-Chwatt 1974). The parasites survive well in frozen blood (Kark 1982). Plasma that has been frozen or fractionated has never been known to transmit malaria.

In non-malarious countries, mainly because of delay in diagnosis, post-transfusion malaria has a relatively high fatality rate. Malaria is particularly serious in pregnant women and in splenectomized or immunosuppressed patients (Kark 1982; Bruce-Chwatt 1985).

Transfusion-transmitted malaria usually responds to conventional drug therapy. In severe cases in which the diagnosis has been delayed and in fulminant cases, the patient may benefit from exchange transfusion in the period before antimalarial drugs have had time to become effective (Yarrish *et al.* 1982; Kramer *et al.* 1983; Files *et al.* 1984). However, no controlled trials have been performed and antimalarial medical therapy is effective in most cases (Mordmuller and Kremsner 1998).

The red cells in a renal allograft and in a bone marrow graft have been known to transmit *P. falciparum* malaria (Kark 1982; Dharmasena and Gordon-Smith 1986). The plasmodia can also be transmitted by transplacental passage.

Frequency of post-transfusion malaria

Estimates of the frequency of post-transfusion malaria vary from less than 0.2 cases per million units of blood transfused in non-endemic countries to 50 or more cases per million in some endemic countries (Bruce-Chwatt 1985). In countries where malaria is non-endemic the frequency of reported transfusion malaria is relatively low. The UK has reported eight cases in 50 years, the USA 26 cases in 10 years from 1972 to 1981, and France 110 cases in 20 years (Bruce-Chwatt 1985), although between 1980 and 1986 only 14 cases were observed. On the other hand, nine cases of transfusion-transmitted malaria were reported to the Centers for Disease Control (CDC) in the USA in 1982, although only 11 cases in the following 4 years (Westphal 1991b). In Canada, only three cases of transfusion-transmitted malaria were reported between 1994 and 1999, a rate of 0.67 cases per million donations (Slinger *et al.* 2001). The rate of transfusion-transmitted malaria in the USA since 1992 has fluctuated from 0.18 to 0.6 per million units transfused (Mungai *et al.* 2001). In many malarious areas where reporting is inefficient, the frequency of post-transfusion malaria is unknown.

Frequency with which the different parasites are involved

In the period 1950–72, *P. malariae* was responsible for about 50% of cases of transfusion malaria and *P. vivax* for 20% (Bruce-Chwatt 1974). In the period 1973–80 a global survey showed a large relative increase of cases due to *P. vivax*, which, with a few cases of *P. ovale*, accounted for 42% of all cases; cases due to *P. malariae* fell to 38% whereas those due to *P. falciparum* increased four-fold (Bruce-Chwatt 1982). In more than one-half of the cases reported, the species involved was not identified. The relative increase in cases due to two of the parasites has been attributed to the failure of donors from highly endemic areas to comply with rules laid down by transfusion services (Guerrero *et al.* 1983; Shulman *et al.* 1984). The simultaneous transmission of two different strains of malaria (*P. falciparum* and *P. malariae*) by trans-

fusion has been described (Aymard *et al.* 1980). Of 93 cases of transfusion-transmitted malaria reported to the CDC from 1963 to 1999, 33 (35%) were due to *P. falciparum*, 25 (27%) were due to *P. vivax*, 25 (27%) were due to *P. malariae*, 5 (5%) were due to *P. ovale*, 3 (3%) were mixed infections and 2 (%) were due to unidentified species; 10 out of the 93 patients (11%) died.

Incubation period

The incubation period of transfusion malaria depends on the numbers and strain of plasmodia transfused, on the host and on the use of antimalarial prophylaxis; with *P. falciparum* and *P. vivax* it is between 1 week and 1 month, but with *P. malariae* it may be many months (Bruce-Chwatt 1974).

Period for which donors remain infectious

P. falciparum infections, prevalent in West Africa, are usually eliminated within 1 year but have been known to persist for as long as 5 years after the last exposure to infected mosquitoes (Guerrero *et al.* 1983). *P. falciparum* transmitted from asymptomatic blood donors can cause fulminant infection and death in an already ill, non-immune recipient in whom the diagnosis, being unexpected, is usually delayed. *P. vivax* infections, prevalent on the Indian subcontinent, may relapse for up to 2.5 years after infection but only rarely after more than 3 years. With *P. ovale* a clinical attack may occur up to 4 years after returning from an endemic area. In immune carriers who have lived in endemic areas for most of their lives, *P. falciparum* or *P. vivax* may reappear long after the limits given above. *P. malariae* infections persist for longer than those of any of the other malaria parasites. Transmission of malaria has been known to occur up to 46 years after the last exposure to infection (Miller 1975).

Rules to prevent transmission of malaria in non-endemic areas

In non-endemic areas, eligibility of potential blood donors who have visited endemic areas is restricted. Regulations and standards are not harmonized and not always consistent. Two different approaches have been adopted: the USA relies solely on the deferral of subjects who have been in endemic areas, whereas in

Europe deferral and testing for malaria parasites can be combined.

All donor clinics should have an up-to-date WHO map showing the areas endemic for malaria together with an alphabetical list of the countries.

In the USA, those who normally live in a non-endemic area but have travelled in an area considered to be endemic for malaria may be accepted as regular blood donors 1 year after returning to a non-malarious area, provided that they have had no symptoms. Prospective donors who have had malaria are deferred for 3 years after the cessation of therapy or after leaving the malarial area if they have been asymptomatic meanwhile. In the USA, of 64 implicated donors whose country of origin was reported, 38 (59%) were foreign born. Among those for whom complete information was available, 37 out of 60 donors (6%) would have been excluded from donating according to guidelines in place since 1994, and 30 out of 48 donors (62%) should have been excluded under the guidelines in place at the time of donation (Mungai *et al.* 2001).

The Council of Europe in 1995 adopted the recommendation that individuals born or brought up in endemic areas may be accepted as donors of whole blood 6 months after their arrival in a non-endemic area, provided that an approved immunological test has given a negative result (Council of Europe 2003). Others from non-endemic areas, for example travellers, can be accepted as blood donors 6 months after their return if they have been afebrile and have not taken antimalarial prophylaxis; those who have had febrile illnesses may be accepted if an antibody test is negative at 6 months. Although a proportion of antibody-positive subjects are non-infectious and are thus unnecessarily rejected, application of these procedures makes it possible to use 75–90% of units of blood from donors returning from malarious areas to France, the UK and Belgium (Soulier 1984; Wells and Ala 1985).

The foregoing rules will not prevent the occasional transmission of *P. malariae* and, especially, of *P. vivax*.

Donations to be used for the preparation of plasma for fractionation may be accepted from donors who do not meet the above criteria.

Tests to detect carriers

When blood films are examined by simple microscopy, a density of less than 100 parasites per microlitre of blood cannot be detected, although a unit from a donor whose blood contained even one parasite per microlitre would contain about half a million parasites (Bruce-Chwatt 1985).

The indirect fluorescent antibody test or ELISA offers a good chance of detecting latent malarial infection (Deroff *et al.* 1982; Voller and Draper 1982). ELISA is more suitable for large-scale screening in the blood transfusion service and its specificity is improving with the use of chromogenic substrates. A commercial ELISA for malarial antibodies has undergone a successful trial in the UK. Ideally, potential carriers who volunteer as blood donors in non-malarious areas should be screened for malaria antibodies using a test covering three homologous antigens. However, only *P. falciparum* is readily available for *in vitro* tests: although there is some degree of crossreactivity between the different strains of malaria parasites it is not known how valuable a test based on the use of *P. falciparum* would be in a country such as Mexico, where none of the 44 cases of transfusion malaria reported in 5 years was due to this strain (Olivares-Lopez *et al.* 1985).

Sensitive tests, using monoclonal antibodies, are being developed for use in endemic areas for detection of parasites in red cells, and soluble antigens and antibodies in plasma (Soulier 1984; Prou 1985). In a study in blood donors in Chandigarh, India, a comparison of different screening techniques for malaria carriers showed that a test for malaria antigen, using monoclonal antibodies, had good sensitivity and specificity. The test was considerably more sensitive than the direct examination of blood films (Choudhury *et al.* 1991). Serological tests for malarial antibodies and tests for malarial antigens are useful in the identification of donors implicated in cases of transfusion-transmitted malaria in non-endemic countries when blood films are negative. PCR has been used to determine the prevalence of malaria in potential blood donors identified as being at high risk of having malaria. Only 4% of blood donors tested positive for malaria by PCR. Furthermore, 42% of blood donors who were negative on PCR testing returned to donate, and no cases of transfusion-transmissible malaria were reported (Shehata *et al.* 2004).

Prevention of transfusion malaria in malarious countries

In countries such as Nigeria, Zambia and Papua New Guinea, where up to 10% of donors have plasmodia detectable by simple microscopy, the contribution of blood transfusion to the overall problem of the transmission of malaria is negligible. In such countries, the transmission of malaria to the recipient can be prevented by giving antimalarial treatment to donor or recipient. Officer (1945) injected blood containing some 300 million malaria parasites into each of five healthy volunteers. All volunteers were given antimalarial treatment after transfusion and none developed malaria.

Trypanosoma cruzi Chagas' disease – American trypanosomiasis

In Latin America 24 million people are infected with *Trypanosoma cruzi*. Infection is most commonly transmitted to humans, usually in childhood, by triatomid bugs. Until recently, Chagas' disease was limited to rural areas with mud huts and thatched roofs but, due to migration of the rural population, infected people are also found in urban areas (Wendel 1995). The next most common mode of transmission is by blood transfusion.

Treatment of acute infection cures 50–90% of patients, but most acute infections are subclinical and untreated individuals remain infected throughout life. Depending on the country, between 5% and 40% of untreated patients may develop serious chronic complications such as cardiomyopathy, megaoesophagus and megacolon, 10 or more years after infection (Marsden 1984; Schmunis 1991).

In chronic infection, antibodies can be detected by complement fixation, direct or indirect haemagglutination, immunofluorescence or ELISA (Schmunis 1991). ELISA appears to be more sensitive than indirect immunofluorescence and haemagglutination (Magnaval *et al.* 1985). Although tests for antibody are positive in about 95% of chronic cases and in 50% of acute cases, they are often negative during the first few months of infection (Wolfe 1975). At least 50% of those infected have parasitaemia and are thus likely to be able to transmit infection by blood transfusion (Cerisola *et al.* 1972). Parasitaemia is diagnosed by allowing triatomid bugs to feed on the patient's blood and then examining the insects for infestation ('xenodiagnosis'). Most Latin American countries test part, but not all, of their blood donations for *T. cruzi* antibodies; the frequency of a positive test amongst donors varies from about 0.3% to 28% and is as high

as 62% in parts of Bolivia (Schmunis 1991). Owing to migration to urban areas and to the existence of paid donors, antibody-positive donors are often found in cities that lack the triatomid vector. When blood from an antibody-positive donor is transfused, the incidence of infection in recipients is between 12% and 18% and can be as high as 50% (Schmunis 1991). The parasites of Chagas' disease survive well in stored blood, and blood stored for more than 10 days can still be infectious (Cerisola *et al.* 1972). *T. cruzi* can be transmitted by plasma as well as by whole blood: the parasite survives in plasma which has been frozen at –20°C for 24 h but it does not resist lyophilization (Wendel and Gonzaga 1992). The addition of 125 mg of crystal (gentian) violet to a unit of stored blood kills the parasites after storage at 4°C for 24 h without damaging the red cells. Blood treated with gentian violet causes no obvious toxic reaction in the recipient, but can cause minor side-effects and rouleaux formation of the red cells. Artificial light and sodium ascorbate accelerate the effect and reduce the dose of gentian violet required to kill the parasites. Gentian violet has been reported to have mutagenic effects *in vitro* (Wendel and Gonzaga 1992).

Latin Americans who migrate do so mainly to North America where more than 5 million now live. More than 100 000 may be infected with Chagas' disease (Wendel 1993). Chagas' disease acquired by blood transfusion has been reported in the USA, Canada and Spain (Villalba *et al.* 1992). Six cases of transfusion-transmitted *T. cruzi* have been reported in the USA and Canada (four and two cases respectively), with the implicated donor in at least five of these cases from a *T. cruzi* endemic country (Leiby *et al.* 2002a). Platelets may be the blood component that is most often implicated in transfusion-transmitted Chagas' disease, possibly because of their relatively short storage period at temperatures favouring parasite survival (22–24°C) or because platelet recipients are more likely to be immunocompromised and therefore are more likely to manifest clinical infection than recipients of other components (Leiby *et al.* 1997).

Other protozoa

Toxoplasma gondii

Toxoplasma gondii is an obligate intracellular protozoan that replicates in the intestine of members of the cat family, its definitive host. Humans may be infected by eating undercooked lamb or pork or by exposure to the faeces of infected cats. Seroprevalence of *T. gondii* rises with age and the incidence of infection varies with the population group and geography. In the USA, almost one-quarter of the population has been infected (Jones *et al.* 2001). *T. gondii* has been isolated from donors' blood up to 4 years after the onset of infection; entry of parasites into the blood occurs for only a few weeks, but as *T. gondii* is an obligate intracellular parasite it persists in the white cells and can survive storage at 4°C for 4–7 weeks (Tabor 1982). Congenital transmission occurs, particularly in women infected shortly before or during pregnancy.

Most infections with toxoplasma are asymptomatic or result in mild fever and lymphadenopathy. However, infection in immunocompromised patients is potentially life threatening. Transmission of *T. gondii* from seropositive solid organ donor to seronegative recipient is well documented, but for recipients of haematopoietic stem cell transplants, reactivation of latent infection appears to be more important. Leucocyte transfusions from donors with high levels of toxoplasma antibodies have resulted in severe acute toxoplasmosis in immunosuppressed patients (Siegel *et al.* 1971; Tabor 1982). As the risk of severe transfusion-acquired toxoplasmosis is confined almost entirely to immunosuppressed patients transfused with leucocyte concentrates, some centres have elected to maintain a panel of donors negative for toxoplasma antibodies for leucapheresis and for the provision of granulocyte concentrates for premature babies (M Contreras, personal communication).

Babesia

In North America, the parasite causing babesiosis in humans is *Babesia microti*, which occurs most often in the north-east and in Wisconsin and Minnesota. However, the geographic range of *B. microti* is expanding. Other babesia species have been implicated in transfusion transmission in the western USA, and the mobility of blood donors and blood components may result in the appearance of transfusion-transmitted babesiosis in areas less familiar with these parasites (Cable and Leiby 2003). In Europe, the responsible parasite is *Babesia bovis*. Transfusion-transmitted cases have been reported only in the USA (Popovsky 1990; Mintz *et al.* 1991). *Babesia microti*,

like *Anaplasma phagocytophila* and *B. burgdorferi*, is transmitted to humans from animal reservoirs (primarily deer and mice) by black-legged ticks of the genus *Ixodes* (Cable and Leiby 2003). For donor screening purposes, self-reported tick bites are neither sensitive nor specific indicators of serological status (Leiby *et al.* 2002b).

B. microti reproduce only in red cells, and on blood smear the organisms appear similar to *Plasmodium falciparum*. The clinical symptoms also resemble those of malaria. The diagnosis must be confirmed by testing for *Babesia* antibodies and by inoculating hamsters with the patient's blood. Parasites can survive for up to 35 days in blood stored at 4°C, and persist in frozen red cells for years.

Although normally mild and frequently asymptomatic, the disease can be fulminant and rapidly fatal for immunosuppressed and splenectomized patients. Since 1980, more than 40 USA cases of post-transfusion babesiosis, including at least two cases of WA-1, the western US variant, have been reported, most of them in immunocompromised or splenectomized patients. In two splenectomized patients infected by transfusion (one by a platelet concentrate), exchange transfusion using whole blood helped bring about control of the disease (Jacoby *et al.* 1980; Cahill *et al.* 1981). As in the case of malaria, the role of exchange transfusion is not well documented, but the combination of clindamycin and quinine seems to eradicate the parasite from most immunosuppressed patients (Smith *et al.* 1986).

Microfilariae

Microfilariae of five common species have been shown to persist in the circulation of infected subjects for years and to survive in stored blood. *Wuchereria bancrofti* can be detected in refrigerated blood for 3 weeks. Microfilariae can be transmitted to transfusion recipients. Three varieties of filariae can cause disease in humans: *Brugia malayi* in South-East Asia, *Loa loa* in Africa and *W. bancrofti* in southern Asia, tropical Africa and some tropical areas of Latin America. However, blood transfusion-transmitted microfilariae never reach the adult stage in non-endemic areas because of the absence of the vector necessary for the second passage to humans. Recipients of infected blood usually have no symptoms, although they may occasionally experience acute inflammation of the spleen, lymph nodes or lungs, sometimes with tropical pulmonary eosinophilia. Recipients may develop fever, headache and rash as a hypersensitivity response to the dead microfilariae (Choudhury *et al.* 2003). Signs and symptoms are self-limited and so is the survival of microfilariae in transfusion recipients (Tabor 1982; Westphal 1991a).

Leishmaniasis

In 1903, Leishman and Donovan independently described the protozoan now called *Leishmania donovani* in patients from India with the life-threatening disease now called *visceral leishmaniasis* or *kala-azar*. Leishmaniasis and its major syndromes (visceral, cutaneous and mucosal) have changed little over the past century, but information regarding the endemic areas, the vectors and the transfusion risks have evolved considerably (Herwaldt 1999). More than 20 different species of Leishmania have been recognized, some anthroponotic but most zoonotic. The organism is transmitted by the female phlebotomine sand fly, of which some 30 species are vectors. Visceral leishmaniasis or kala-azar caused primarily by *Leishmania donovani* is found most often in China, India and the eastern Mediterranean. *L. major*, *L. tropica* and *L. infantum* are found in the Middle East. However, the organisms are found in jungles, deserts, rural areas and cities of some 88 countries. Leishmaniasis is endemic in much of Latin America between northern Argentina (*L. braziliensis*, *L. panamensis*) and southern-central Texas (*L. mexicana*), and in south-western Europe (France, Spain, Portugal, Italy, Greece) and, because the sand fly has a limited range, microfoci of activity are found within countries where the disease is considered endemic. The cutaneous form of the disease goes by many names, including Baghdad Aleppo boil, Oriental sore and bush yaws. These characteristics make screening questions difficult to formulate. There is no screening test and no licensed drug therapy. No vaccine has been developed, although paediatric inoculation using preparations from active sores is widely practised in endemic areas.

Leishmania multiply in mononuclear phagocytes and clinical disease transmitted by blood transfusion has been reported in transplant recipients, in haemodialysis patients and in newborn infants. When present in blood, the parasite has been found in large mononuclear cells and granulocytes (Shulman 1990). The incubation period can vary from 10 days to 2 years, but is generally 2–6 months and results in chronic infection. Leishmania species are clearly blood transmitted, although fewer than 15 transfusion cases have been reported, one of which was fatal. Canine transmission is well recognized (Owens *et al.* 2001). Studies of asymptomatic blood donors in southern France indicated that *L. infantum* circulates intermittently at low levels and mononuclear cells from these donors can infect Syrian hamsters (le Fichoux *et al.* 1999). Although the conventional teaching holds that visceral leishmaniasis poses the greatest risk of blood transmission, 'dermatotropic' organisms such as *L. tropica*, *L. braziliensis* and *L. panamensis* have been found in blood decades after the patient's exposure. Human transfusion transmission results in viscerocutaneous disease.

L. tropica has been demonstrated to survive in stored blood under blood bank conditions for 25 days (Grogl *et al.* 1993). A 1-year deferral was instituted by the USA Department of Defense in 1991 and again in 2003 for service personnel stationed in endemic areas in Iraq. Deferral for diagnosed infection is indefinite. Cases of possible transmission of kala-azar by transfusion in India, China, Brazil and four European countries have been reported (Chung *et al.* 1948; Cummins *et al.* 1995; Singh *et al.* 1996). Subjects with a history of visceral leishmaniasis must not be accepted as donors (Council of Europe 1992).

African trypanosomiasis (sleeping sickness) has rarely been transmitted by transfusion (Wolfe 1975; Tabor 1982).

Methods of inactivating pathogens in blood and blood products

Despite careful donor selection and sensitive laboratory testing, a small risk of transmission of infectious agents by transfusion remains, particularly with products obtained from large pools of plasma. The fractions obtained at an early stage of the cold-ethanol fractionation, for example fibrinogen, factor VIII, factor IX and prothrombin complex concentrate, contain intact virus. Plasma fractions obtained later in the fractionation process, such as the immunoglobulins and albumin, are safer, although HCV can be detected in the fraction from which IVIG is prepared (Yei and Yu 1992). HCV has been transmitted by IVIG preparations (Weiland *et al.* 1986; Bjoro *et al.* 1994; Meisel *et al.* 1995; Power *et al.* 1995).

Inactivation of viruses in blood products or their removal, or both, should further increase the safety of transfusion and might protect against unknown pathogens or those for which no screening tests are available. The ideal inactivation technology should reduce the risk of infection from the blood component, result in minimal damage to the component cell or protein content and function, and pose minimal toxicological risk to the recipient, particularly to susceptible patients such as gravid women and neonates. The risk–benefit estimates have clearly favoured inactivation technologies for protein concentrates derived from large plasma pools. The calculus differs for cellular components derived from single donors.

Plasma and plasma products

Heat treatment

Pasteurization and vapour treatment of liquid clotting factor concentrates and heat treatment of lyophilized concentrates ('dry heat') have been used for decades (Kingdon and Lundblad 2002). The efficacy of these methods differs. Hepatitis viruses have been transmitted by lyophilized concentrates heated between 60°C and 68°C for periods of between 24 and 72 h (Colombo *et al.* 1985; Blanchette *et al.* 1991). Even the more heat-labile HIV has been transmitted by such concentrates (Mariani *et al.* 1987; Williams *et al.* 1990b). Dry heating at 80° for 72 h, however, effectively inactivates HIV and hepatitis viruses. No evidence of infection with these viruses was detected in 38 previously untreated haemophiliacs treated with dry-heated concentrates (Skidmore *et al.* 1990; Williams *et al.* 1990b). Pasteurized concentrates are also free from the risk of transmitting HIV (Schimpf *et al.* 1987) and in prospective studies have been found not to transmit hepatitis viruses (Mannucci *et al.* 1990; Azzi *et al.* 1992; Kreuz *et al.* 1995). On the other hand, several cases of hepatitis B or C have been ascribed to the use of pasteurized concentrates in patients not enrolled in controlled studies (Kernoff *et al.* 1987; Brackmann and Egli 1988; Shulman *et al.* 1992).

A major disadvantage of the heat treatment methods is that they may not inactivate non-enveloped viruses such as HAV and parvovirus B19. Some recipients have developed signs of parvovirus B19 infection (Azzi *et al.* 1992). However, dry heat treatment at 100°C for 1 h more effectively inactivates both lipid-enveloped and non-enveloped viruses and, when applied to IVIG preparations, leads to only a very small loss of IgG (Rubinstein *et al.* 1994).

Solvent–detergent treatment

The combination of a solvent and a detergent disrupts lipid-enveloped viruses such as HIV and hepatitis viruses. A non-volatile solvent, tri-(*n*-butyl) phosphate (TNBP) is used in combination with a detergent such as sodium cholate (Prince *et al.* 1986). The solvent–detergent (S–D) mixture is removed at the end of the procedure by precipitation of the product or by chromatography. The viral safety of S–D treatment has been shown by clinical trials in over 100 haemophiliacs and in hundreds of thousands of transfusions (Mannucci 1993; Klein *et al.* 1998).

The S–D method has been adapted for whole plasma and involves incubation of pooled thawed plasma with the organic solvent TNBP and the detergent Triton X-100 for 4 h at 30°C (Horowitz *et al.* 1992; Klein *et al.* 1998). A drawback of the S–D method is that non-enveloped viruses are not inactivated. Several reports of transmission of HAV and parvovirus B-19 by S–D-treated concentrates have been documented (Mannucci 1992; Temperley *et al.* 1992; Peerlinck and Vermylen 1993). Factor VIII or IX concentrates contain diminished levels of anti-HAV which in other fractions, such as IVIg, neutralizes the virus.

S–D treatment has a few other flaws. The reduced level of alpha(2)-antiplasmin in S–D plasma has caused concern when the product is used in patients with liver disease; however, controlled studies have not confirmed a clinical problem (Williamson *et al.* 1999). S–D plasma also has reduced levels of protein S, a plasma factor with anticoagulant properties. Reduced protein S may contribute to reports of venous thrombosis during massive plasma infusion. In 68 consecutive patients with thrombotic thrombocytopenic purpura (TTP) (25 men, 43 women), eight documented thromboembolic events (six deep venous thromboses, three pulmonary emboli) were identified in seven patients during therapeutic plasma exchange. All six were associated with central venous lines at the site of thrombosis (Yarranton *et al.* 2003).

One little appreciated benefit of S–D plasma is the absence of association with TRALI, almost certainly as a result of the pooling of 12 000 units per batch. However, for a variety of reasons, including safety and commercial failure, S–D plasma is no longer available in the USA.

Heating in supension with n-heptane

Heating with n-heptane at 60°C for 20 h has been used for factor VIII and IX concentrates but, as hepatitis viruses have been transmitted by concentrates treated in this way, S–D treatment is preferred.

Methylene blue treatment

Methylene blue was first used clinically by Paul Ehrlich in the nineteenth century and has been used as a virucidal agent for more than half a century. As with other photoactive chemicals, methylene blue and similar phenothiazine dyes have a high affinity for both nucleic acids and the surface structures of viruses. On exposure to red (visible) light at 620–670 nm, excitation of the dye causes chemical modification of adjacent molecules, a process which involves oxygen radicals (Lambrecht et al. 1991). Methylene blue treatment is currently the only method that can be applied to individual units of plasma. Residual dye is minimal (1 μM) and can be further reduced 10-fold from the final product by filtration.

Methylene blue treatment does not inactivate intracellular viruses efficiently but, as the plasma is frozen and thawed, leucocytes are disrupted with release of viral particles. Neither does it effectively reduce transmission of bacteria or protozoa. For reasons that remain unexplained, non-enveloped viruses, especially HAV, are relatively resistant to methylene blue (Wagner 2002). An unfortunate consequence of methylene blue treatment of plasma is the loss of 10% or more of some clotting factors, particularly factor VIII and fibrinogen (Cardigan et al. 2002; Williamson et al. 2003). Cryoprecipitate prepared from this plasma has not been extensively studied and is not in current use.

Commercial manufacturing systems have been developed and millions of single units of plasma treated with methylene blue have now been transfused in Europe without unexpected side-effects (Williamson et al. 2003). Concern remains in some quarters about the potential mutagenic effects of methylene blue and its derivatives, even in low concentration. To date, no immediate problems have been encountered in transfusion recipients, although the number of neonates, children and parous women treated remains small.

Other methods of inactivation: at the bench but not yet at the bedside

Other methods include the use of the virucidal agent hypericin (Lavie et al. 1995) and photochemical treatment with virucidal short-wavelength ultraviolet light with the addition of rutin or psoralen (Chin et al. 1995; Hambleton et al. 2002).

Cellular components

Some viruses such as CMV and HTLV are transmitted exclusively by leucocytes, whereas others, such as HIV, HBV and HCV are transmitted both by cellular components and by plasma. HIV can be internalized by platelets, which may contain large amounts of the virus (Zucker-Franklin et al. 1990; Lee et al. 1993). HIV associates with red cells, probably as antibody–complement adherent complexes, but it is not clear whether this 'pool' of virus is associated with transmission (Hess et al. 2002). HPV B19 is known to adhere to red cells. To be effective, inactivation methods should deal with free virus, virus attached to cells and intracellular virus.

Physical methods

As mentioned above, the removal of leucocytes from red cell and platelet concentrates reduces transmission of CMV and HTLV-I and -II (Kobayashi 1993). Extensive washing and the process of freezing and deglycerolization are also effective in reducing transmission (Brady et al. 1984; Taylor et al. 1986; Sayers et al. 1992).

Chemical and photochemical techniques

Several chemical and photochemical processes target nucleic acid to inactivate residual contaminating viruses, bacteria and protozoa in blood components (Klein 2005). As an added benefit, nucleic acid-targeted processes have the potential to inactivate residual lymphocytes and prevent transfusion-associated graft-versus-host disease (Fast et al. 2002, 2003, 2004).

Whole blood and red cells: the hurdles remain

For red cell concentrates, agents must be selected that are photoactivated with a wavelength above that of haemoglobin that would otherwise absorb the agent. Optimal properties of sensitizing dyes for use in red cell suspensions include selection of dyes that traverse cell and viral membranes, bind to nucleic acids, absorb light in the red region of the spectrum, inactivate a wide range of pathogens, produce little red cell photo-damage from dye not bound to nucleic acid and do not haemolyse red cells in the dark. Some agents inactivate both free and cell-associated virus, but subtle changes in the red cell membrane may affect storage, survival or immunogenicity (Sieber *et al.* 1992; Wagner *et al.* 1993).

A red cell additive, S-303 or frangible anchor linker effector, is an alkylating agent that inactivates nucleated pathogens by crosslinking DNA and RNA in a rapid, light-independent reaction (Klein 2005). The initial enthusiasm for this agent has been tempered by the report of red cell antibody formation in two subjects enrolled in clinical trials (L Corash, personal communication). Antibody formation has also been reported during a trial of chronic transfusion of patients with sickle cell disease using red cells treated with PEN110 (J. Chapman, personal communication). PEN110, a binary ethyleneimine that binds covalently to nucleic acid is also light independent and interferes with polymerase-mediated replication (Lazo *et al.* 2002; Ohagen *et al.* 2002).

A 50-µM riboflavin solution added to diluted red cells that are exposed to visible light of 450 nm, a wavelength with minimal absorbance by haemoglobin, effects a two- to four-log reduction of a number of pathogens (Klein 2005). Clinical data for riboflavin treatment of red cells are not yet available. No method has been licensed for inactivating pathogens in whole blood or red cells.

Methods for treating platelets

PEN110 treatment, which involves covalent binding of drug to nucleic acids (see above), requires an extensive washing procedure to remove residual additive, so the process has not been applied to plasma or platelet components. Riboflavin, an essential nutrient (vitamin B2) that absorbs both visible and UVA light, has been investigated with both components (Li *et al.* 2004). Riboflavin's three-ringed planar structure intercalates between bases of DNA and RNA, and upon light exposure, oxidizes guanosine through electron transfer reactions, resulting in single-strand breaks of nucleic acids and formation of covalent adducts (Dardare and Platz 2002). The process has proved effective against a wide range of human and animal pathogens, including bacteria, intracellular HIV-1, West Nile virus and porcine parvovirus in preclinical studies of platelets and plasma (Goodrich 2000; Ruane *et al.* 2004). Initial toxicology assessment of the photoproducts of riboflavin generated under proposed treatment conditions have been encouraging.

By far the greatest experience with pathogen reduction of platelet components involves the use of psoralen additives and UVA light activation. Psoralens pass through the cell membrane and the capsids of viruses and intercalate reversibly into helical regions of nucleic acids. Upon illumination with UVA (300–400 nm) covalent crosslinks to pyrimidines in RNA and DNA form and block the replication and transcription of nucleic acids (Hanson 1992). 8-Methoxypsoralen (8-MOP) inactivates free virus and even HIV incorporated in the genome (Corash *et al.* 1992). This very high-energy dose of UV damages platelets, but when aminomethyl-trimethyl psoralen (amotosalen, AMT, S-59) is used, lower doses of UV can be applied for shorter periods without loss of virucidal activity (Corash *et al.* 1992; Benade *et al.* 1994). When psoralens are used, the platelets must be suspended in plasma-reduced medium, as plasma inhibits the inactivation of virus (Moroff *et al.* 1992). The addition of agents that neutralize oxygen radicals further protects the platelet membrane (Margolis-Nunno *et al.* 1994). Some psoralen derivatives also limit platelet damage (Goodrich 1994). Moreover, the derivatives do not appear to be mutagenic in the absence of UVA (Wollowitz *et al.* 1994; Yerram *et al.* 1994). The potential mutagenicity of psoralen is also avoided by absorbing excess agent on a ligand, C18, fixed on silicon as used for S–D-treated plasma (Margolis-Nunno *et al.* 1995). Extensive preclinical toxicology studies for S-59-treated platelets showed no CNS, cardiac or reproductive toxicity, and no evidence of genotoxicity or phototoxicity. In a heterozygote p53 knockout mouse model, exposure to S-59-treated plasma over 6 months or 26 weeks did not produce excess carcinogenicity. This system (INTERCEPT) is licensed in Europe as a medical device.

Three clinical trials in 166 thrombocytopenic patients were conducted in Europe, two with buffy coat platelets and one with apheresis platelets. These studies demonstrated that, for equal platelet doses, INTERCEPT platelets provided similar platelet count increments to conventional platelets; the adverse reaction profile appeared comparable (van Rhenen *et al.* 2003). A USA phase III study evaluating haemostatic efficacy and safety of transfusions of apheresis platelet concentrates randomized 645 patients to receive either S-59 photochemically treated or conventional platelets for up to 28 days. Although the mean 1-h post-transfusion platelet corrected count increment (CCI) (11.1×10^3 treatment vs. 16.0×10^3 control), average number of days to next platelet transfusion (1.9 treatment vs. 2.4 control) and number of platelet transfusions (8.4 treatment vs. 6.2 control) differed, the trial demonstrated equivalence in prevention and treatment of grade 2 and higher grade bleeding according to WHO criteria (McCullough *et al.* 2004).

References

Aach RD, Stevens CE, Hollinger FB *et al.* (1991) Hepatitis C virus infection in post-transfusion hepatitis. An analysis with first- and second-generation assays. N Engl J Med 325: 1325–1329

Ablashi DV, Salahuddin SZ, Josephs SF *et al.* (1987) HBLV (or HHV-6) in human cell lines (Letter). Nature (Lond) 329: 207.

Adler SP (1984) International forum: Transfusion transmitted CMV infections. Vox Sang 46: 387–414

Adler SP, Chandrika T, Lawrence L *et al.* (1983) Cytomegalovirus infections in neonates acquired by blood transfusions. Pediatr Infect Dis 2: 114–118

Aledort LM, Levine PH, Hilgartner M *et al.* (1985) A study of liver biopsies and liver disease among hemophiliacs. Blood 66: 367–372

Allain JP (2000) Genomic screening for blood-borne viruses in transfusion settings. Clin Lab Haematol 22: 1–10

Allain JP (2004) Occult hepatitis B virus infection: implications in transfusion. Vox Sang 86: 83–91

Allain JP, Laurian Y, Paul DA *et al.* (1986) Serological markers in early stages of human immunodeficiency virus infection in haemophiliacs. Lancet ii: 1233–1236

Allain, J-P, Coghlan PJ, Kenrick KG *et al.* (1996) Safety and efficacy of anti-hepatitis C virus screening of blood donors with two sequential screening assays. Transfusion 36: 401–406

Alter HJ (1975) Hepatitis B surface antigen and the health care professions. In: Transmissable Disease and Blood Transfusion. TJ Greenwalt, GA Jamieson (eds). New York, NY: Grune & Stratton

Alter HJ (1992) New kit on the block: evaluation of second generation assays for detection of antibody to hepatitis C virus. Hepatology 15: 350–353

Alter HJ, Houghton M (2000) Clinical Medical Research Award. Hepatitis C virus and eliminating post-transfusion hepatitis. Nature Med 6: 1082–1086

Alter HJ, Tabor E, Meryman HT *et al.* (1978a) Transmission of hepatitis B virus infection by transfusion of frozen-deglycerolized red blood cells. N Engl J Med 298: 637

Alter HJ, Purcell RH, Holland PV *et al.* (1978b) Transmissible agent in non-A, non-B hepatitis. Lancet 1: 459–463

Alter HJ, Purcell RG, Shih JW *et al.* (1989a) Detection of antibody to hepatitis C virus in prospectively followed transfusion recipients with acute and chronic non-A, non-B hepatitis. N Engl J Med 321: 1495–1500

Alter MJ, Hadler SC, Judson FN *et al.* (1990) Risk factors for acute non-A, non-B hepatitis in the United States and association with hepatitis C virus infection. JAMA 264: 2231–2235

Alter HJ, Nakatsuji Y, Melpolder J *et al.* (1997) The incidence of transfusion-associated hepatitis G virus infection and its relation to liver disease. N Engl J Med 336: 747–754

American Association of Blood Banks, American Red Cross, Council of Community Blood Centers (1983) Joint statement on acquired immune deficiency syndrome (AIDS) related to transfusion (1983a). Transfusion 23: 87–88

Amman AJ, Cowan MJ, Wara DM *et al.* (1983) Acquired immunodeficiency in an infant: possible transmission by means of blood products. Lancet i: 956–957

Anahane Y, Aikawa T, Sugai Y *et al.* (1992) Transmission of HCV between spouses. Lancet 339: 1059–1060

Anand A, Gray ES, Brown T *et al.* (1987) Human parvovirus infection in pregnancy and hydrops fetalis. N Engl J Med 316: 183–186

Anderson MJ, Jones SE, Fisher-Hoch SP *et al.* (1983) Human parvovirus. The cause of erythema infectiosum (Fifth disease). Lancet i: 1378

Anderson KC, Lew MA, Gorgone BC *et al.* (1986) Transfusion-related sepsis after prolonged platelet storage. Am J Med 81: 405–411

Anderson DW, Epstein JS, Lee TH *et al.* (1989) Serological confirmation of human T-lymphocytotropic virus type I infection in healthy blood and plasma donors. Blood 74: 2585–2591

Andes WA, Daul CB, deShazo RD *et al.* (1988) Seroconversion to human immunodeficiency virus (HIV) in hemophiliacs. Relation to lymphadenopathy. Transfusion 28: 98–102

Ando Y, Nakano S, Saito K *et al.* (1986) Prevention of HTLV-I transmission through the breast milk by a freeze-drying process. Jap J Cancer Res (Gann) 77: 974–977

Andreu G, Morel P, Forestier F *et al.* (2002) Hemovigilance network in France: organization and analysis of immediate transfusion incident reports from 1994 to 1998. Transfusion 42: 1356–1364

Araujo A, Hall WW (2004) Human T-lymphotropic virus type II and neurological disease. Ann Neurol 56: 10–19

Aronson DL (1979) Factor IX complex. Semin Thromb Hemost 6: 28–43

Aymard JP, Vinet E, Lederlin P et al. (1980) Paludisme post-transfusionnel: un cas de double infestation a *Plasmodium falciparum* et *Plasmodium* malariae. Rev Fr Transfusion Immunohematol 23: 491–493

Azzi A, Ciappi S, Zakvrezeska K (1992) Human parvovirus B 19 infection in hemophiliacs first infused with two high-purity virally attenuated factor VIII concentrates. Am J Hematol 39: 228–230

Backer U, Weinauer F, Gathof G et al. (1987) HIV antigen screening in blood donors (Letter). Lancet ii: 177–180

Barbara JAJ (1983) Microbiology. In: Blood Transfusion. Bristol: John Wright

Barbara JAJ, Briggs M (1981) Follow-up of HBsAg-positive donors to determine the proportion undergoing acute infections (Abstract). Transfusion 21: 605–606

Barbara JAJ, Mijovic V, Cleghorn et al. (1978) Liver enzyme concentrations as a measure of possible infectivity in chronic asymptomatic carriers of hepatitis B. BMJ 12: 1600–1602

Barbara JAJ, Salker R, Lalji F et al. (1982) TPHA compared with cardiolipin tests for serological detection of early primary syphilis. J Clin Pathol 35: 1394–1395

Barre-Sinoussi F, Chermann JC, Rey F et al. (1983) Isolation of a T-lymphotropic retrovirus from a patient at risk for acquired immune deficiency syndrome (AIDS). Science 220: 868–871

Barrett BB, Andersen JW, Anderson KC (1993) Strategies for the avoidance of bacterial contamination of blood components. Transfusion 33: 228–233

Baumgartner JD, Glauser MP, Burgo-Black AL et al. (1982) Severe cytomegalovirus infection in multiply transfused, splenectomised, trauma patients. Lancet ii: 63–66

Bazarbachi A, Soal F, Laroche L et al. (1993) HTLV-I provirus and mycosis fungoides. Science 259: 1470

Benade LE, Shumaker J, Xu Y et al. (1994) Inactivation of free and cell-associated human immunodeficiency virus in platelet suspensions by aminomethyltrimethylpsoralen and ultraviolet light. Transfusion 34: 680–684

Bendheim PE, Brown HR, Rudelli RD et al. (1992) Nearly ubiquitous tissue distribution of the scrapie agent precursor protein. Neurology 42: 149–156

Berger EA, Murphy PM, Farber JM (1999) Chemokine receptors as HIV-1 coreceptors: roles in viral entry, tropism, and disease. Annu Rev Immunol 17: 657–700

Bergman GE (1995) Transmission of hepatitic C virus by monoclonal-purified viral-attenuated factor VII concentrate. Lancet 346: 1296–1297

Bessos H, Drummond O, Prowse C et al. (2001) The release of prion protein from platelets during storage of apheresis platelets. Transfusion 41: 61–66

Biggerstaff BJ, Petersen LR (2003) Estimated risk of transmission of the West Nile virus through blood transfusion in the US, 2002. Transfusion 43: 1007–1017

Biswas R, Tabor E, Hsia CC et al. (2003) Comparative sensitivity of HBV NATs and HBsAg assays for detection of acute HBV infection. Transfusion 43: 788–798

Bjoro K, Froland SS, Yun Z et al. (1994) Hepatitis C infection in patients with primary hypogammaglobulinemia after treatment with contaminated immunoglobulin. N Engl J Med 331: 1607–1611

Blajchman MA, Ali AM, Richardson HL (1994) Bacterial contamination of blood components. Vox Sang 67, S3: 25–33

Blanchette VS, Vorstman E, Shore A et al. (1991) Hepatitis C infection in children with hemophilia A and B. Blood 78: 285–289

Bloch O (1941) Loss of *Treponema pallidum* in citrated blood at 5 °C. Bull Johns Hopkins Hosp 68: 412

Blum HE, Vyas GN (1982) Non-A, non-B hepatitis: a contemporary assessment. Haematologia 15: 162–183

Blumberg BS, Sutnick AI, London WT (1968) Hepatitis and leukaemia: their relation to Australia antigen. Bull NY Acad Med 44: 1566

Blumel J, Schmidt I, Effenberger W et al. (2002) Parvovirus B19 transmission by heat-treated clotting factor concentrates. Transfusion 42: 1473–1481

Boneva RS, Grindon AJ, Orton SL et al. (2002) Simian foamy virus infection in a blood donor. Transfusion 42: 886–891

Boppana SB, Rivera LB, Fowler KB et al. (2001) Intrauterine transmission of cytomegalovirus to infants of women with preconceptional immunity. N Engl J Med 344: 1366–1371

Bowden RA (1995) Transfusion-transmitted cytomegalovirus infection. Immunol Invest 24: 117–128

Bowden RA, Sayers M, Flournoy N et al. (1986) Cytomegalovirus immune globulin and seronegative blood products to prevent primary cytomegalovirus infection after marrow transplantation. N Engl J Med 314: 1006–1010

Bowden RA, Sayers M, Gleaves et al. (1987) Cytomegalovirus-seronegative blood components for the prevention of primary cytomegalovirus infection after marrow transplantation. Considerations for blood banks. Transfusion 27: 478–481

Bowden RA, Slichter SJ, Sayers M et al. (1995) A comparison of filtered leukocyte-reduced and cytomegalovirus (CMV) seronegative blood products for the prevention of transfusion-associated CMV infection after marrow transplant. Blood 86: 3598–3603

Bowen EF, Sabin CA, Wilson P et al. (1997) Cytomegalovirus (CMV) viraemia detected by polymerase chain reaction identifies a group of HIV-positive patients at high risk of CMV disease. AIDS 11: 889–893

Brackmann HH, Egli H (1988) Acute hepatitis B infection after treatment with heat-inactivated Factor VIII concentrate. Lancet ii: 967

Bradley DW, McCaustland, Karen A *et al*. (1985) Post-transfusion non-A, non-B hepatitis in chimpanzees. Physicochemical evidence that the tubule-forming agent is a small, enveloped virus. Gastroenterology 88: 773–779

Brady MT, Milam JD, Anderson DC *et al*. (1984) Use of deglycerolized red blood cells to prevent posttransfusion infection with cytomegalovirus in neonates. J Infect Dis 150: 334–339

Braude AJ, Sandford JP, Bartlett JE *et al*. (1952) Effects and clinical significance of bacterial contaminants in transfused blood. J Lab Clin Med 39: 902

Brecher ME, Means N, Jere CS *et al*. (2001) Evaluation of an automated culture system for detecting bacterial contamination of platelets: an analysis with 15 contaminating organisms. Transfusion 41: 477–482

Brecher ME, Hay SN, Rothenberg SJ (2004) Validation of BacT/ALERT plastic culture bottles for use in testing of whole-blood-derived leukoreduced platelet-rich-plasma-derived platelets. Transfusion 44: 1174–1178

Brennan MT, Runganga J, Barbara JAJ *et al*. (1992). The prevalence of anti-HTLV in North London blood donors. HTLV Symposium (Abstract), Montpellier, France

Bresters D, Mauser-Bunschoten EP, Reesink HW *et al*. (1993) Sexual transmission of hepatitis C virus. Lancet 342: 210–211

Briggs M, Fox J, Tedder RS (1988) Age prevalence of antibody to human herpes virus 6 (Letter). Lancet i: 1058–1059

Brodine SK, Kaime EM, Roberts C *et al*. (1993) Simultaneous confirmation and differentiation of human T-lymphotropic virus types I and II infection by modified Western blot containing recombinant envelope proteins. Transfusion 33: 925–929

Brouwer J, Nevens F, Kleter G *et al*. (1993) Which hepatitis patient will benefit from interferon? Multivariate analysis of 350 patients treated in a Benelux multicentre study. J Hepatol 18 (Suppl. 1): S10

Brown KE, Hibbs JR, Gallinella G *et al*. (1994) Resistance to parvovirus B19 infection due to lack of virus receptor (erythrocyte P antigen). N Engl J Med 330: 1192–1196

Brown P, Preece MA, Will RG (1992) Friendly fire in medicine: hormones, homografts and Creutzfeld-Jacob disease. Lancet 340: 24–27

Brown P, Preece M, Brandel JP *et al*. (2000) Iatrogenic Creutzfeldt-Jakob disease at the millennium. Neurology 55: 1075–1081

Brown T, Anaud A, Ritchie JP *et al*. (1984) Intrauterine parvovirus infection in pregnancy and hydrops fetalis. Lancet ii: 1033–1034

Bruce-Chwatt LJ (1972) Blood transfusion and tropical disease. Trop Dis Bull 69: 825

Bruce-Chwatt LJ (1974) Transfusion malaria. Bull WHO 50: 337

Bruce-Chwatt LJ (1982) Transfusion malaria revisited. Trop Dis Bull 79: 827–840

Bruce-Chwatt LJ (1985) Transfusion associated parasitic infections. In: Infection, Immunity and Blood Transfusion. RY Dodd, LF Barker (ed.). New York: Alan R Liss, pp. 101–125

Bruce ME, Will RG, Ironside JW *et al*. (1997) Transmissions to mice indicate that 'new variant' CJD is caused by the BSE agent. Nature 389: 498–501

Brucker G, Brun-Vezinet F, Rosenheim M *et al*. (1987) HIV-2 infection in two homosexual men in France. Lancet i: 223

Brun-Vezinet F, Rey MA, Katlama C (1987) Lymphadenopathy-associated virus type 2 in AIDS and AIDS related complex. Clinical and virological features in four patients. Lancet i: 128–132

Bruneau C, Perez P, Chassaigne M *et al*. (2001) Efficacy of a new collection procedure for preventing bacterial contamination of whole-blood donations. Transfusion 41: 74–81

Bryant ML, Ratner L (1990) Myristoylation-dependent replication and assembly of human immunodeficiency virus 1. Proc Natl Acad Sci USA 87: 523–527

Busch MP, Alter HJ (1995) Will human immunodeficiency virus p24 antigen screening increase the safety of the blood supply and, if so, at what cost? Transfusion 35: 536–539

Busch MP, Donegan E, Stuart M *et al*. (1990a) Donor HIV-1 p24 antigenaemia and course of infection in recipients. Transfusion Safety Study Group. Lancet 335: 1342

Busch MP, Taylor PE, Lenes BA *et al*. (1990b) Screening of selected male blood donors for p24 antigen of human immunodeficiency virus type 1. N Engl J Med 323: 1308–1312

Busch MP, Young MJ, Samson SM *et al*. (1991a) Risk of human immunodeficiency virus (HIV) transmission by blood transfusions before the implementation of HIV-1 antibody screening. The Transfusion Safety Study Group. Transfusion 31: 4–11

Busch MP, Eble BE, Khayam-Bashi H *et al*. (1991b) Evaluation of screened blood donations for human immunodeficiency virus type 1 infection by culture and DNA amplification of pooled cells. N Engl J Med 325: 1–5

Busch MP, Korelitz SH, Kleinman SR *et al*. (1995) Declining value of alanine aminotransferase in screening of blood donors to prevent posttransfusion hepatitis B and C virus infection. Transfusion 35: 903–910

Busch MP, Kleinman SH, Jackson B *et al*. (2000) Committee report. Nucleic acid amplification testing of blood donors for transfusion-transmitted infectious diseases: Report of the Interorganizational Task Force on Nucleic Acid Amplification Testing of Blood Donors. Transfusion 40: 143–159

Cable RG, Leiby DA (2003) Risk and prevention of transfusion-transmitted babesiosis and other tick-borne diseases. Curr Opin Hematol 10: 405–411

Cahill KM, Benach JL, Reich LM et al. (1981) Red cell exchange: treatment of babesiosis in a splenectomized patient. Transfusion 21: 193–198

Candotti D, Etiz N, Parsyan A et al. (2004) Identification and characterization of persistent human erythrovirus infection in blood donor samples. J Virol 78: 12169–12178

Cardigan R, Allford S, Williamson L (2002) Levels of von Willebrand factor-cleaving protease are normal in methylene blue-treated fresh-frozen plasma. Br J Haematol 117: 253–254

Carman WF, Jacyna MR, Hadziyannis S et al. (1989) Mutation preventing formation of hepatitis e antigen in patients with chronic hepatitis B virus infection. Lancet ii: 588–591

Carman WF, Zanetti AR, Karayiannis P et al. (1990) Vaccine induced escape mutant of hepatitis B virus. Lancet ii: 325–329

Carman WF, Fagan EA, Hadziyannis S et al. (1991) Association of a precore variant of hepatitis B virus with fulminant hepatitis. Hepatology 14: 219–222

Casaccia P, Ladogana A, Xi YG et al. (1989) Levels of infectivity in the blood throughout the incubation period of hamsters peripherally injected with scrapie. Arch Virol 108: 145–149

Casewell MW, Slater NG, Cooper JE (1981) Operating theatre water-baths as a cause of pseudomonas septicaemia. J Hosp Infect 2: 237–247

CDC (1982) Pneumocystis carinii pneumonia among persons with haemophilia A. MMWR 31: 365–367

CDC (1983) Prevention of acquired immune deficiency syndrome (AIDS): Report of interagency recommendations. MMWR 32: 101–103

CDC (1984) Delta hepatitis – Massachusetts. MMWR 33: 493–494

CDC (1987a) Survey of non-US haemophilia treatment centers for HIV seroconversion following therapy with heat treated factor concentrates. MMWR 36: 121–124

CDC (1987b) Human immunodeficiency virus infection in the United States. MMWR 36: 801–804

CDC (1990) Human T-lymphotropic virus type I screening in volunteer blood donors – United States, 1989. MMWR 39: 915–924

CDC (1991) HIV/AIDS Surveillance Report. Atlanta:

CDC (1992) HIV/AIDS. Surveillance report. MMWR 9:

CDC (1997) HIV/AIDS. Surveillance Report 8(2): 10

Cerisola JA, Rabinovich A, Alvarez M (1972) Enfermedad de Chagas y la transfusión de sangre. Bol Of Sanit Panam 73: 203–206

Cervenakova L, Yakovleva O, McKenzie C et al. (2003) Similar levels of infectivity in the blood of mice infected with human-derived vCJD and GSS strains of transmissible spongiform encephalopathy. Transfusion 43: 1687–1694

Chambers RW, Foley HT, Schmidt PJ (1969) Transmission of syphilis by fresh blood components. Transfusion 9: 32–34

Chen Y-C, Wang C-H, Su I-J et al. (1989) Infection of human T-cell leukemia virus type I and. Development of human T-cell leukemia/lymphoma in patients with hematologic neoplasms: a possible linkage to blood transfusion. Blood 74: 388–394

Cherubin CE, Prince AM (1971) Serum hepatitis specific antigen (SH) in commercial and volunteer sources of blood. Transfusion 11: 25

Chin S, Williams B, Cottlieb P et al. (1995) Virucidal short wavelength ultraviolet light treatment of plasma and Factor VIII concentrate: protection of proteins by antioxidants. Blood 86: 4331–4336

Chiu EKW, Yuen KY, Lie AKW et al. (1994) A prospective study of symptomatic bacteremia following platelet transfusion and its management. Transfusion 34: 950–954

Choo Q-L, Kuo G, Weiner AJ et al. (1989) Isolation of a cDNA clone derived from a blood-borne non-A, non-B viral hepatitis genome. Science 244: 359–361

Choo Q-L, Richmond KH, Han JH (1991) Genetic organization and diversity of the hepatitis C virus. Proc Natl Acad Sci USA 88: 2451–2455

Chou SW (1990) Differentiation of cytomegalovirus strains by restriction analysis of DNA sequences amplified from clinical specimens. J Infect Dis 162: 738–742

Choudhury N, Jolly JG, Mahajan RC et al. (1991) Malaria screening to prevent transmission by transfusion: an evaluation of techniques. Med Lab Sci 48: 206–211

Choudhury N, Murthy PK, Chatterjee RK et al. (2003) Transmission of filarial infection through blood transfusion. Indian J Pathol Microbiol 46: 367–370

Christiansen CB, Jessen TE, Nielsen C et al. (1996) False negative anti-HIV-1/HIV-2 ELISAs in acute HIV-2 infection. Vox Sang 70: 144–147

Chung H-L, Chow H-K, Lu J-P (1948) The first two cases of transfusion kala-azar. Chinese Med J 66: 325–326

Clark J, Saxinger C, Gibbs WN (1985) Seroepidemiologic studies of human T-cell leukemia/lymphoma virus type I in Jamaica. Int J Cancer 36: 37–41

Clark SJ, Saag MS, Decker WD et al. (1991) High titers of cytopathic virus in plasma of patients with symptomatic primary HIV-1 infection. N Engl J Med 324: 954–960

Clavel F, Guetard D, Brun-Vezinet F et al. (1986) Isolation of a new human retrovirus from West African patients with AIDS. Science 233: 343–346

Cohen BJ, Mortimer PP, Pereira MS (1983) Diagnostic assays with monoclonal antibodies for the human serum parvovirus-like virus (SPLV). J Hyg 91: 113–130

Cohen ND, Munoz AR (1989) Transmission of retroviruses by transfusion of screened blood in patients undergoing cardiac surgery. N Engl J Med 320: 1172–1176

Collinge J, Rossor M (1996) A new variant of Prion disease. Lancet 347: 1996–1997

Collinge J, Sidle KCL, Meads J et al. (1996) Molecular analysis of prion strain variation and the aetiology of 'new variant' CJD. Nature (Lond) 383: 685–690

Colombo M, Mannucci PM, Carnelli V et al. (1985) Transmission of non-A, non-B hepatitis by heat-treated Factor VIII concentrate. Lancet ii: 1–4

Conry-Cantilena C, VanRaden M, Gibble J et al. (1996) Routes of infection, viremia, and liver disease in blood donors found to have hepatitis C virus infection. N Engl J Med 334: 1691–1696

Contreras M, Barbara JAJ, Anderson CC et al. (1991) Low incidence of non-A, non-B post-transfusion hepatitis in London confirmed by hepatitis C virus serology. Lancet i: 753–757

Corash L, Lin L, Wiesehahn G (1992) Use of 8-methoxypsoralen and longwavelength ultraviolet irradiation for decontamination of platelet concentrates. Blood Cells 18: 57–74

Corrao G, Arico S (1998) Independent and combined action of hepatitis C virus infection and alcohol consumption on the risk of symptomatic liver cirrhosis. Hepatology 27: 914–919

Cossart YE, Field AM, Cant B et al. (1975) Parvovirus-like particles in human sera. Lancet 1: 72–73

Cossen C, Hagens D, Fukuchi R et al. (1992) Comparison of six commercial human T-cell lymphotropic virus type I (HTLV-I) enzyme immunoassay kits for detection of antibody to HTLV-I and -II. J Clin Microbiol 30: 724–725

Council of Europe (1995) Guide to the Preparation, Use and Quality Assurance of Blood Components, 9th edn. Strasbourg: Council of Europe Press, p. 45

Coursaget P, Yvonnet B, Chotard J et al. (1987) Age- and sex-related study of hepatitis B virus chronic carrier state in infants from an endemic area (Senegal). J Med Virol 22: 1–5

Craig AS, Schaffner W (2004) Clinical practice. Prevention of hepatitis A with the hepatitis A vaccine. N Engl J Med 350: 476–481

Cummins D, Amin S, Halil O et al. (1995) Visceral leishmaniasis after cardiac surgery. Arch Dis Child 72: 235–236

Curran JW, Lawrence DN, Jaffe H et al. (1984) Acquired immunodeficiency syndrome (AIDS) associated with transfusions. N Engl J Med 310: 69–75

Curran JW, Jaffe HW, Peterman TA et al. (1985) Epidemiologic aspects of acquired immunodeficiency syndrome (AIDS) in the United States: cases associated with transfusions. In: Infection, Immunity and Blood Transfusion. RY Dodd, LF Barker (eds). New York: Alan R Liss, pp. 259–269

Custer B, Tomasulo PA, Murphy EL et al. (2004) Triggers for switching from minipool testing by nucleic acid technology to individual-donation nucleic acid testing for West Nile virus: analysis of 2003 data to inform 2004 decision making. Transfusion 44: 1547–1554

Cuthbertson B (1991) Viral contamination of human plasma and procedures for preventing virus transmission by plasma products. In: Blood Separation and Plasma Fractionation. JR Harris (ed.). New York: Wiley-Liss, pp. 385–435

Dalgleish AG, Beverley PCL, Clapham PR et al. (1984) The CD4 (T4) antigen is an essential component of the receptor for the AIDS retrovirus. Nature (Lond) 312: 763–767

Damen M, Zaaijer HL, Cuypers HTM et al. (1995) Reliability of the third-generation recombinant immunoblot assay for hepatitis C virus. Transfusion 35: 745–749

Damond F, Worobey M, Campa P et al. (2004) Identification of a highly divergent HIV type 2 and proposal for a change in HIV type 2 classification. AIDS Res Hum Retroviruses 20: 666–672

Dane DS, Cameron CH, Briggs M (1970) Virus-like particles in serum of patients with Australia-antigen associated hepatitis. Lancet i: 695–698

Dardare N, Platz MS (2002) Binding affinities of commonly employed sensitizers of viral inactivation. Photochem Photobiol 75: 561–564

Davoli EH, Lipson SM, Match ME et al. (1999) Evaluation of the PrimeCapture CMV DNA detection plate system for detection of cytomegalovirus in clinical specimens. J Clin Microbiol 37: 2587–2591

Dawson GJ, Chan KH, Cabal CM et al. (1992) Solid-phase enzyme-linked immunosorbent assay for hepatitis E virus IgG and IgM antibodies utilising recombinant antigens and synthetic peptides. J Virol Methods 38: 174–186

Deinhardt F, Zuckerman AJ (1985) Immunization against hepatitis B: report on a WHO meeting on viral hepatitis in Europe. J Med Virol 17: 209–217

Deinhardt F, Holmes AW, Capps RB et al. (1967) Studies on the transmission of human viral hepatitis to marmoset monkeys: transmission of disease: serial passages and description of liver lesions. J Exp Med 125: 673–687

Delwart EL, Kalmin ND, Jones TS et al. (2004) First report of human immunodeficiency virus transmission via an RNA-screened blood donation. Vox Sang 86: 171–177

Deng HK, Lin R, Ellmeyer W et al. (1996) Identification of a major co-receptor for primary isolates of HIV-1. Nature (Lond) 381: 661–666

Denis F, Ranger-Rogez S, Nicot T (1996) Les nouveaux virus des hepatites. Transfusion Clin Biol 1: 19–25

Deroff P, Regner M, Simitzis AM et al. (1982) Screening of blood donors likely to transmit falciparum malaria. Rev Fr Transfusion Immunohematol 25: 3–10

Desmyter J (1986) AIDS and blood transfusion. Vox Sang 51 (Suppl.): 1, 21

De Schryver A, Meheus A (1990) Syphilis and blood transfusion: a global perspective. Transfusion 30: 844–847

De Silva M, Contreras M, Barbara J (1988) Two cases of transfusion-transmitted malaria (TTM) in the UK (letter). Transfusion 28: 86

Devetten MP, Liu JM, Ling V et al. (1997) Paroxysmal nocturnal hemoglobinuria: new insights from murine Pig-a-deficient hematopoiesis. Proc Assoc Am Phys 109: 99–110

Dharmasena F, Gordon-Smith EC (1986) Transmission of malaria by bone marrow transplantation. Transplantation 42: 228

Dienstag JL, Purcell HR, Alter HJ et al. (1977) Non-A, non-B post-transfusion hepatitis. Lancet 1: 560–562

Dodd RY (1991) Donor testing and its impact on transfusion-transmitted infection. In: Transfusion Transmitted Infections. DM Smith, RY Dodd (eds). Chicago: ASCP, pp. 243–269

Dodd RY, Notari EP, Stramer SL (2002) Current prevalence and incidence of infectious disease markers and estimated window-period risk in the American Red Cross blood donor population. Transfusion 42: 975–979

Dodelet VC, Cashman NR (1998) Prion protein expression in human leukocyte differentiation. Blood 91: 1556–1561

Donegan E, Lenes BA, Tomasulo PA et al. (1990a) Transmission of HIV-1 by component type and duration of shelf storage before transfusion. Transfusion 30: 851–852

Donegan E, Stuart M, Niland JC et al. (1990b) Infection with human immunodeficiency virus type 1 (HIV-1) among recipients of antibody-positive blood donations. Ann Intern Med 113: 733–739

Donegan E, Pell P, Lee H (1992) Transmission of human T-lymphotropic virus type I by blood components from a donor lacking anti-p24: a case report. Transfusion 32: 68–71

Donegan E, Lee H, Operskalski EA et al. (1994) Transfusion transmission of retroviruses: human T-lymphotropic virus types I and II compared with human immunodeficiency virus type 1. Transfusion 34: 478–483

Dow BC, MacVarish I, Barr A et al. (1980) Significance of tests for HBeAg and anti-HBe in HBsAg positive blood donors. J Clin Pathol 33: 1106–1109

Dragic T, Litwin V, Allaway GP et al. (1996) HIV entry into CD4+ cells is mediated by the chemokine receptor for CC-CKR-5. Nature (Lond) 381: 667–673

Drew WL, Miner RC (1982) Transfusion-related cytomegalovirus infection following noncardiac surgery. JAMA 247: 2389–2391

Drew WL, Tegtmeier G, Alter HJ et al. (2003) Frequency and duration of plasma CMV viremia in seroconverting blood donors and recipients. Transfusion 43: 309–313

Eastlund T, Persing D, Mathiesen D et al. (1999) Human granulocytic ehrlichiosis after red cell transfusion. Transfusion 39 (Suppl.): 117S

Eddleston A (1990) Modern vaccines. Hepatitis. Lancet i: 1142–1145

Engels EA, Eastman H, Ablashi DV et al. (1999) Risk of transfusion-associated transmission of human herpesvirus 8. J Natl Cancer Inst 91: 1773–1775

Esteban JI, Shih JW, Tai CC et al. (1985) Importance of western blot analysis in predicting infectivity of anti-HTLV-III/LAV positive blood. Lancet 2: 1083–1086

Esteban JI, Estban R, Viladomiu L et al. (1989) Hepatitis C virus antibodies among risk groups in Spain. Lancet ii: 294–297

Esteban JI, Gonzalez A, Hernandez M et al. (1990) Evaluation of antibodies to hepatitis C virus in a study of transfusion associated hepatitis. N Engl J Med 323: 1107–1112

Evatt B, Austin H, Barnhart E et al. (1998) Surveillance for Creutzfeldt-Jakob disease among persons with hemophilia. Transfusion 38: 817–820

Evatt BL, Stein SF, Francis DP et al. (1983) Antibodies to human T-cell leukemia virus-associated membrane antigens in hemophiliacs: evidence for infection before 1980. Lancet ii: 698

Evatt BL, Ramsey RB, Lawrence DN et al. (1984) The acquired immunodeficiency syndrome in patients with hemophilia. Ann Intern Med 100: 499

Evatt BL, Gomperts ED, McDougal JS et al. (1985) Coincidental appearance of LAV/HTLV-III antibodies in hemophiliacs and the onset of the AIDS epidemic. N Engl J Med 312: 483–486

Fagan EA, Williams R (1990) Fulminant viral hepatitis. Br Med Bull 46: 462–480

Fang CT, Tobler LH, Haesche C et al. (2003) Fluctuation of HCV viral load before seroconversion in a healthy volunteer blood donor. Transfusion 43: 541–544

Farci P (2001) Hepatitis C virus. The importance of viral heterogeneity. Clin Liver Dis 5: 895–916

Farci P, Alter HJ, Govindaragan S et al. (1993) Lack of protective immunity against reinfection with hepatitis C virus. Science 258: 135–140

Fast LD (2003) The effect of exposing murine splenocytes to UVB light, psoralen plus UVA light, or gamma-irradiation on in vitro and in vivo immune responses. Transfusion 43: 576–583

Fast LD, DiLeone G, Edson CM et al. (2002) PEN110 treatment functionally inactivates the PBMNCs present in RBC units: comparison to the effects of exposure to gamma irradiation. Transfusion 42: 1318–1325

Fast LD, Semple JW, DiLeone G et al. (2004) Inhibition of xenogeneic GVHD by PEN110 treatment of donor human PBMNCs. Transfusion 44: 282–285

Feng Y, Broder CC, Kennedy PE et al. (1996) HIV entry cofactor; functional cDNA cloning of a seven-transmembrane G protein-coupled receptor. Science 272: 872–877

Fernandez MN, Daza RM, Orden B *et al.* (1981) Anticuerpos a Brucela en donantes de sangre. Sangre 26: 360–366

Ferrero S, Lungaro P, Bruzzone BM *et al.* (2003) Prospective study of mother-to-infant transmission of hepatitis C virus: a 10-year survey (1990–2000). Acta Obstet Gynecol Scand 82: 229–234

le Fichoux Y, Quaranta JF, Aufeuvre JP *et al.* (1999) Occurrence of Leishmania infantum parasitemia in asymptomatic blood donors living in an area of endemicity in southern France. J Clin Microbiol 37: 1953–1957

Fiebig EW, Wright DJ, Rawal BD *et al.* (2003) Dynamics of HIV viremia and antibody seroconversion in plasma donors: implications for diagnosis and staging of primary HIV infection. AIDS 17: 1871–1879

Files JC, Case CJ, Morrison FS (1984) Automated erythrocyte exchange in fulminant falciparum malaria. Ann Intern Med 100: 396–397

Flanagan P, McAlpine L, Ramskill SJ *et al.* (1995) Evaluation of a combined HIV-1/2 and HTLV-I/II assay for screening blood donors. Vox Sang 68: 220–224

Fleming AF (1990) AIDS in Africa. In: Haematology in HIV Disease. C Costello (ed.). Baillières Clinical Haematology 3: 177–206

Foster KM (1966) Post-transfusion mononucleosis. Aust Ann Med 15: 305

Fradkin JE, Schonberger LB, Mills JL *et al.* (1991) Creutzfeldt-Jakob disease in pituitary growth hormone recipients in the United States. JAMA 265: 880–884

Freeman R, Gould FK, McMaster A (1990) Management of cytomegalovirus antibody negative patients undergoing heart transplantation. J Clin Pathol 43: 373–376

Frickhofen N, Abkowitz JL, Safford M *et al.* (1990) Persistent B19 parvovirus infection in patients infected with human immunodeficiency virus type 1 (HIV-1): a treatable cause of anemia in AIDS. Ann Intern Med 113: 926–933

Gaeta GB, Stornaiuolo G, Precone DF *et al.* (2003) Epidemiological and clinical burden of chronic hepatitis B virus/hepatitis C virus infection. A multicenter Italian study. J Hepatol 39: 1036–1041

Gallarda JL, Henrard DR, Liu D *et al.* (1994) Early detection of antibody to human immuno-deficiency virus type 1 by using an antigen conjugate immunoassay correlated with the presence of IgM antibody. J Clin Microbiol 30: 2379–2384

Gallo RC (2003) A journey with T cells, primate/human retroviruses and other persisting human T-cell tropic viruses. Rev Clin Exp Hematol 7: 329–335

Gallo RC, De-The GB, Ito Y (1981) Kyoto workshop on some specific recent advances in human tumor virology. Cancer Res 41: 4738–4739

Gallo RC, Salahuddin SZ, Popovic M *et al.* (1984) Frequent detection and isolation of cytopathic retroviruses (HTLV-III) from patients with AIDS and at risk for AIDS. Science 224: 500–503

Ganem D, Prince AM (2004) Hepatitis B virus infection – natural history and clinical consequences. N Engl J Med 350: 1118–1129

Garretta M, Paris-Hamelin A, Vaismam A (1977) Syphilis et transfusion. Rév Fr Transfusion Immunohematol 2: 287–308

Gerber P, Walsh JH, Rosenblum EN *et al.* (1969) Association of EB-virus infection with the post-perfusion syndrome. Lancet i: 593

Gessain A, Francis H, Sonan T *et al.* (1986) HTLV-1 and tropical spastic paraparesis in Africa. Lancet ii: 698

Ghani AC, Donnelly CA, Ferguson NM *et al.* (2003) Updated projections of future vCJD deaths in the UK. BMC Infect Dis 3: 4

Ghany MG, Kleiner DE, Alter H *et al.* (2003) Progression of fibrosis in chronic hepatitis C. Gastroenterology 124: 97–104

Gjerset GF, Clements MJ, Counts RB *et al.* (1991) Treatment type and amount influenced human immunodeficiency virus seroprevalence of patients with congenital bleeding disorders. Blood 78: 1623–1627

Glazer JP, Friedman HM, Grossman RA *et al.* (1979) Live cytomegalovirus vaccination of renal transplant candidates: a preliminary trial. Ann Intern Med 91: 676–683

Glynn SA, Kleinman SH, Schreiber GB *et al.* (2000) Trends in incidence and prevalence of major transfusion-transmissible viral infections in US blood donors, 1991 to 1996. Retrovirus Epidemiology Donor Study (REDS). JAMA 284: 229–235

Glynn SA, Smith JW, Schreiber GB *et al.* (2001) Repeat whole-blood and plateletpheresis donors: unreported deferrable risks, reactive screening tests, and response to incentive programs. Transfusion 41: 736–743

Gocke DJ (1972) A prospective study of post-transfusion hepatitis. The role of Australia antigen. JAMA 219: 1165

Goedert JJ, Eyster ME, Lederman MM *et al.* (2002) End-stage liver disease in persons with hemophilia and transfusion-associated infections. Blood 100: 1584–1589

Goldman MB, Blajchman MA (1991) Blood product-associated bacterial sepsis. Transfusion Med Rev 5: 73–83

Goldman M, Roy G, Frechette N *et al.* (1997) Evaluation of donor skin disinfection methods. Transfusion 37: 309–312

Gong J, Rawal BD, Högman CF *et al.* (1994) Complement killing of *Yersinia enterocolitica* and retention of the bacteria by leucocyte removal filters. Vox Sang 66: 166–170

Goodrich RP (2000) The use of riboflavin for the inactivation of pathogens in blood products. Vox Sang 78 (Suppl. 2): 211–215

Goodrich RP, Yerram NR, Tay-Goodrich BH *et al.* (1994) Selective inactivation of viruses in the presence of human platelets: UV sensitization with psoralen derivatives. Proc Natl Acad Sci USA 91: 5552–5556

Gout O, Baulac M, Gessain A et al. (1990) Rapid development of myelopathy after HTLV-1 infection acquired by transfusion during cardiac transplantation. N Engl J Med 322: 383–388

Graan-Hentzen YC, Gratama JW, Mudde GC et al. (1989) Prevention of primary cytomegalovirus infection in patients with hematologic malignancies by intensive white cell depletion of blood products. Transfusion 29: 757–760

Grady GF, Lee VA (1975) Prevention of hepatitis from accidental exposure among medical workers. N Engl J Med 293: 1067

Grant DB, Perinpanayagam MS, Shute PG et al. (1960) A case of malignant tertian (Plasmodium falciparum) malaria after blood-transfusion. Lancet ii: 469

Greene WC, Peterlin BM (2002) Charting HIV's remarkable voyage through the cell: Basic science as a passport to future therapy. Nature Med 8: 673–680

Griffiths PD (1984) Diagnostic techniques for cytomegalovirus infection. Clin Haematol 13: 631–644

Grogl M, Daugirda JL, Hoover DL et al. (1993) Survivability and infectivity of viscerotropic Leishmania tropica from Operation Desert Storm participants in human blood products maintained under blood bank conditions. Am J Trop Med Hyg 49: 308–315

Grumet FC (1984) In International Forum: Transfusion-transmitted CMV infections. Vox Sang 46: 387–414

Guerrero IC, Weniger BC, Schultz MG (1983) Transfusion malaria in the United States 1972–1981. Ann Intern Med 99: 221–226

Högman CF, Gong J, Erikkson L et al. (1991) Transfusion transmitted bacterial infection (TTBI). (Abstracts) 2nd Congr W. Hong Kong: Pacific Region Int Soc Blood Transf

Högman CF, Gong J, Hamkraens A et al. (1992) The role of leucocytes in the transmission of Yersinia enterocolitica with blood components. Transfusion 32: 654–657

Habibi B, Kleinknecht D, Vachon F et al. (1973) Le choc transfusionnel par contamination bacté, rienne du sang conservé. Analyse de 25 observations. Rev Fr Transfusion 16: 41

Haditsch M, Binder L, Gabriel C et al. (1994) Yersinia enterocolitica septicemia in autologous blood transfusion. Transfusion 34: 907–909

Haimowitz MD, Hernandez LA, Herron RM Jr (2005) A blood donor with bacteremia. Lancet 365: 1596

Halkier-Sørensen, L, Kragballe K, Nedergaard ST et al. (1990) Lack of transmission of Borrelia burgdorferi by blood transfusion. Lancet i: 550

Hall AJ, Alveyn CG, Winter PD et al. (1988) Mortality of hepatitis B-positive blood donors in England and Wales. In: Viral Hepatitis and Liver Disease. AJ Zuckerman (ed.). New York: Alan R Liss, pp. 192–194

Hambleton J, Wages D, Radu-Radulescu L et al. (2002) Pharmacokinetic study of FFP photochemically treated with amotosalen (S-59) and UV light compared to FFP in healthy volunteers anticoagulated with warfarin. Transfusion 42: 1302–1307

Hamers FF, Downs AM (2004) The changing face of the HIV epidemic in western Europe: what are the implications for public health policies? Lancet 364: 83–94

Hancock JS, Taylor RN, Johnson CE et al. (1993) Quality of laboratory performance in testing for human immunodeficiency virus type I antibodies: identification of variables associated with laboratory performance. Arch Pathol Lab Med 117: 1148–1155

Hanson CV (1992) Photochemical inactivation of viruses with psoralenes: an overview. Blood Cells 18: 7–25

Hanto DW, Gajl-Peczalska KJ, Frizzera G et al. (1983) Epstein-Barr virus (EBV)-induced polyclonal and monoclonal B-cell lymphoproliferative diseases occurring after renal transplantation. Ann Surg 198: 356–369

Harris DR, Gonin R, Alter HJ et al. (2001) The relationship of acute transfusion-associated hepatitis to the development of cirrhosis in the presence of alcohol abuse. Ann Intern Med 134: 120–124

Harrison TJ, Zuckerman AJ (1992) Variants of hepatitis B virus. Vox Sang 63: 161–167

Harrison TJ, Bal V, Wheeler EG et al. (1985) Hepatitis B virus DNA and e antigen in serum from blood donors in the United Kingdom positive for hepatitis B surface antigen. BMJ 290: 663–664

Hartley TM, Khabbaz RF, Cannon RO et al. (1990) Characterization of antibody reactivity to human T-cell lymphotropic virus types I and II using immunoblot and radioimmunoprecipitation assays. J Clin Microbiol 28: 646–650

Hartley TM, Malone GE, Khabbatz RF et al. (1991) Evaluation of a recombinant T-cell lymphotropic virus type I (HTLV-I) p21e antibody detection enzyme immunoassay as a supplementary test in HTLV-I/II antibody testing algorithms. J Clin Microbiol 29: 1125–1129

Hartmann O, Schone R (1942) Syfilis overfort ved blodtransfusion. Nord T Milit-Med 45: 1

Hawkins A, Davidson F, Simmonds P (1997) Comparison of plasma virus loads among individuals infected with hepatitis C virus (HCV) genotypes 1, 2, and 3 by quantiplex HCV RNA assay versions 1 and 2, Roche Monitor assay, and an in-house limiting dilution method. J Clin Microbiol 35: 187–192

Hay CR, Preston FE, Triger DR et al. (1985) Progressive liver disease in haemophilia: an understated problem? Lancet 1: 1495–1498

Hayakawa F, Imada K, Towatari M et al. (2002) Life-threatening human parvovirus B19 infection transmitted by intravenous immune globulin. Br J Haematol 118: 1187–1189

Heltberg O, Skov F, Gerner-Smidt P *et al.* (1992) Nosocomial epidemic of *Serratia marcescens* septicemia ascribed to contaminated blood transfusion bags. Transfusion 33: 221–227

Heneine W, Switzer WM, Sandstrom P *et al.* (1998) Identification of a human population infected with simian foamy viruses. Nature Med 4: 403–407

Henle W (1985) Epstein-Barr virus and blood transfusion. In: Infection, Immunity and Blood Transfusion. RY Dodd, LF Barker (eds). New York: Alan R Liss, pp. 201–209

Henrard DR, Mehaffey WF, Allain JP (1992) A sensitive viral capture assay for detection of plasma viremia in HIV-infected individuals. AIDS Res Hum Retroviruses 8: 47–52

Heptonstall J (1991) Outbreaks of hepatitis B virus infection associated with infected surgical staff. CDR 1: 81–85

Hersman J, Meyers JD, Thomas ED *et al.* (1982) The effect of granulocyte transfusions on the incidence of cytomegalovirus infection after allogeneic marrow transplantation. Ann Intern Med 96: 149–152

Herwaldt BL (1999) Leishmaniasis. Lancet 354: 1191–1199

Hess C, Klimkait T, Schlapbach L *et al.* (2002) Association of a pool of HIV-1 with erythrocytes *in vivo*: a cohort study. Lancet 359: 2230–2234

Hino S, Sugiyama H, Doi H *et al.* (1987) Breaking the cycle of HTLV-I transmission via carrier mother's milk. Lancet ii: 158–159

Hino S, Katamine S, Miyata H *et al.* (1996) Mother to child transmission of HTLV-I. Vox Sang 70 (Suppl. 2): 1

Hjelle B (1991) Human T-cell leukaemia/lymphoma viruses. Life cycle, pathogenicity, epidemiology and diagnosis. Arch Pathol Lab Med 115: 440–450

Hjelle B, Scalf R, Swenson, S (1990a) High frequency of human T-cell leukemia-lymphoma virus type II infection in New Mexico blood donors: determination by sequence-specific oligonucleotide hybridization. Blood 76: 450–454

Hjelle B, Mills R, Mertz G *et al.* (1990b) Transmission of HTLV-II via blood transfusion. Vox Sang 59: 119–122

Hjelle B, Mills R, Mertz G *et al.* (1992) Chronic neurodegenerative disease associated with HTLV-II infection. Lancet 339: 645–646

Ho DD, Moudgil T, Alam M (1989) Quantitation of human immunodeficiency virus type 1 in the blood of infected persons. N Engl J Med 321: 1621–1625

Högman CF, Engstrand L (1996) Factors affecting growth of *Yersinia enterocolitica* in cellular blood products. Transfus Med Rev 10: 259–275

Högman CF, Gong J, Eriksson L *et al.* (1991) White cells protect donor blood against bacterial contamination. Transfusion 31: 620–626

Holada K, Vostal JG (2000) Different levels of prion protein (PrPc) expression on hamster, mouse and human blood cells. Br J Haematol 110: 472–480

Hollinger FB, Khan NC, Oefinger PE *et al.* (1983) Post transfusion hepatitis type A. JAMA 250: 2313–2317

Hoofnagle JH, Seeff LB, Bales ZB *et al.* (1978) Type B hepatitis after transfusion with blood containing antibody to hepatitis B core antigen. N Engl J Med 298: 1379

Horowitz B, Bonomo R, Prince AM *et al.* (1992) Solvent/detergent treated plasma. A virus-inactivated substitute of fresh frozen plasma. Blood 79: 826–831

Horsburgh C Ou CY, Jason J Jr (1989) Duration of human immunodeficiency virus infection before detection of antibody. Lancet ii: 637–640

Houston F, Foster JD, Chong A *et al.* (2000) Transmission of BSE by blood transfusion in sheep. Lancet 356: 999–1000

Hu KQ (2002) Occult hepatitis B virus infection and its clinical implications. J Viral Hepatol 9: 243–257

Hudnall SD, Chen T, Rady P *et al.* (2003) Human herpesvirus 8 seroprevalence and viral load in healthy adult blood donors. Transfusion 43: 85–90

Hunter N, Foster J, Chong A *et al.* (2002) Transmission of prion diseases by blood transfusion. J Gen Virol 83: 2897–2905

Hutton EL, Shute PG (1939) The risk of transmitting malaria by blood transfusion. J Trop Med Hyg 42: 309

Inaba S, Sato H, Okochi K *et al.* (1989) Prevention of transmission of human T-lymphotrophic virus type 1 (HTLV-1) through transfusion, by donor screening with antibody to the virus. Transfusion 29: 7–11

Ip HM, Wong VC, Lelie PN *et al.* (1989) Hepatitis B infection in infants after neonatal immunization. Acta Paediatr Jpn 31: 654–658

Irani MS, Dudley AW, Lucco LJ (1991) Case of HIV-1 transmission by antigen-positive, antibody-negative blood (Letter). N Engl J Med 325: 1174–1175

Ironside JW, Head MW (2004) Neuropathology and molecular biology of variant Creutzfeldt-Jakob disease. Curr Topics Microbiol Immunol 284: 133–159

Iwamoto M, Jernigan DB, Guasch A *et al.* (2003) Transmission of West Nile virus from an organ donor to four transplant recipients. N Engl J Med 348: 2196–2203

Jackson JB, Englund EA, Edson JR *et al.* (1988) Prevalence of cytomegalovirus antibody in hemophiliacs and homosexuals infected with human immunodeficiency virus type 1. Transfusion 28: 187–189

Jacobs J, Jamaer D, Vandeven J *et al.* (1989) *Yersinia enterocolitica* in donor blood: a case report and review. J Clin Microbiol 27: 1119–1121

Jacoby GA, Hunt JV, Kosinski KS *et al.* (1980) Treatment of transfusion-transmitted babesiosis by exchange transfusion. N Engl J Med 303: 1098–1100

Jaffe, HW, Darrow WW, Echenberg DF *et al.* (1985) The acquired immunodeficiency syndrome in a cohort of homosexual men: a six-year follow-up study. Ann Intern Med 103: 210–214

Jones JL, Kruszon-Moran D, Wilson M *et al.* (2001) *Toxoplasma gondii* infection in the United States: seroprevalence and risk factors. Am J Epidemiol 154: 357–365

Kaariainen L, Klemola E, Paloheimo J *et al.* (1966) Rise of cytomegalovirus antibodies in an infectious-mononucleosis-like syndrome after transfusion. BMJ 5498: 1270–1272

Kahn JO, Walker BD (1998) Acute human immunodeficiency virus type 1 infection. N Engl J Med 339: 33–39

Kajiyama W, Kashiwagi S, Ikematsum H *et al.* (1986) Intrafamilial transmission of adult T cell leukaemia virus. J Infect Dis 154: 851–857

Kalyanaraman VS, Sarngadharan MG, Robert-Guroff M (1982) A new subtype of human T cell leukaemia virus (HTLV-II) associated with a T-cell variant of hairy cell leukaemia. Science 218: 571–573

Kao JH, Chen PJ, Yang PM *et al.* (1992) Intrafamilial transmission of hepatitis C virus: the important role of infections between spouses. J Infect Dis 166: 900–903

Kao JH, Chen PJ, Lai MY *et al.* (2000) Hepatitis B genotypes correlate with clinical outcomes in patients with chronic hepatitis B. Gastroenterology 118: 554–559

Kaplan JE, Osame M, Kubota H *et al.* (1990) The risk of development of HTLV-1 associated myelopathy/tropical spastic paraparesis among persons infected with HTLV-1. J. AIDS 3: 1096–1101

Kark JA (1982) Malaria transmitted by blood transfusion. In: E. Tabor (ed.) New York: Academic Press, pp. 93–126

Kato H, Gish RG, Bzowej N *et al.* (2004) Eight genotypes (A-H) of hepatitis B virus infecting patients from San Francisco and their demographic, clinical, and virological characteristics. J Med Virol 73: 516–521

Kenny-Walsh E (1999) Clinical outcomes after hepatitis C infection from contaminated anti-D immune globulin. Irish Hepatology Research Group. N Engl J Med 340: 1228–1233

Keoshkerian E, Ashton LJ, Smith DG *et al.* (2003) Effector HIV-specific cytotoxic T-lymphocyte activity in long-term nonprogressors: associations with viral replication and progression. J Med Virol 71: 483–491

Kernoff PBA, Miller EJ, Savidge GF *et al.* (1987) Reduced risk of non-A, non-B hepatitis after a first exposure to 'wet heated' Factor VIII concentrate. Br J Haematol 67: 207–211

Kilduffe RA, DeBakey M (1942) The Blood Bank and the Techniques and Therapeutics of Transfusion. St Louis, MO: CV Mosby

Kim DM, Brecher ME, Bland LA *et al.* (1992) Visual identification of bacterially contaminated red cells. Transfusion 32: 221–225

Kingdon HS, Lundblad RL (2002) An adventure in biotechnology: the development of haemophilia A therapeutics – from whole-blood transfusion to recombinant DNA to gene therapy. Biotechnol Appl Biochem 35: 141–148

Kitchen LW, Barin F, Sullivan JL *et al.* (1984) Aetiology of AIDS-antibodies to human T-cell leukaemia virus (type III) in haemophiliacs. Nature (Lond) 312: 367–369

Kitchen LW, Leal M, Wichman F *et al.* (1985) Antibodies to HTLV-III in haemophiliacs from Spain. Blood 66: 1473–1475

Klarmann D, Kreuz W, Kornhuber B (1995) Low prevalence of hepatitis E virus antibodies in hepatitis C virus-positive patients with coagulation disorders. Transfusion 35: 969–970

Klein HG (2005) Pathogen inactivation technology: cleansing the blood supply. J Intern Med 257: 224–237

Klein HG, Dodd RY, Dzik WH *et al.* (1998) Current status of solvent/detergent-treated frozen plasma. Transfusion 38: 102–107

Klein MA, Kaeser PS, Schwarz P *et al.* (2001) Complement facilitates early prion pathogenesis. Nature Med 7: 488–492

Kleinman SH, Busch MP (2000) The risks of transfusion-transmitted infection: direct estimation and mathematical modelling. Baillieres Best Pract Res Clin Haematol 13: 631–649

Kleinman S, Busch MP, Korelitz JJ *et al.* (1997) The incidence/window period model and its use to assess the risk of transfusion-transmitted human immunodeficiency virus and hepatitis C virus infection. Transfus Med Rev 11: 155–172

Kleinman S, Busch MP, Hall L *et al.* (1998) False-positive HIV-1 test results in a low-risk screening setting of voluntary blood donation. Retrovirus Epidemiology Donor Study. JAMA 280: 1080–1085

Klemola E, von Essen R, Paloheimo J *et al.* (1969) Cytomegalovirus antibodies in donors of fresh blood to patients submitted to open-heart surgery. Scand J Infect Dis 1: 137–140

Kobayashi M (1993) Leukocyte depletion of HTLV-1 carrier red cell concentrates by filters. In: Clinical Application of Leukocyte Depletion. S Sekiguchi (ed.). Boston, MA: Blackwell Scientific, pp. 138–148

Kojima M, Shimizu M, Tsuchimochi T *et al.* (1991) Posttransfusion fulminant hepatitis B associated with precore-defective HBV mutants. Vox Sang 60: 34–39

de Korte D, Marcelis JH, Soeterboek AM (2001) Determination of the degree of bacterial contamination of whole-blood collections using an automated microbe-detection system. Transfusion 41: 815–818

de Korte D, Marcelis JH, Verhoeven AJ, Soeterboek AM (2002) Diversion of first blood volume results in a reduction of bacterial contamination for whole-blood collections. Vox Sang 83: 13–16

Kosaka Y, Takase K, Kojima M *et al.* (1991) Fulminant hepatitis B: induction by hepatitis B virus mutants defective in the precore region and incapable of encoding e antigen. Gastroenterol 100: 1087–1094

Koziol DE, Holland PV, Alling DW *et al.* (1986) Antibody to hepatitis B core antigen as a paradoxical marker for non-A, non-B hepatitis agents in donated blood. Ann Intern Med 104: 488–495

Kraat YJ, Stals FS, Landini MP *et al.* (1993) Cytomegalovirus IgM antibody detection: comparison of five assays. New Microbiol 16: 297–307

Kramer SL, Campbell CC, Moncrieff RE (1983) Fulminant *Plasmodium falciparum* infection treated with exchange blood transfusion. JAMA 249: 244–245

Krech U (1973) Complement fixing antibodies against cytomegalovirus in different parts of the world. Bull WHO 49: 103–106

Kreuz W, Auerswald G, Bruckmann C *et al.* (1995) Prevention of hepatitis C virus infection in children with hemophilia A and B and von Willebrand's disease (Letter). Thromb Haemos 67: 184

Kroner BL, Rosenberg PS, Aledort LM *et al.* (1994) HIV-1 infection incidence among persons with hemophilia in the United States and western Europe, 1978–1990. Multicenter Hemophilia Cohort Study. J AIDS 7: 279–286

Kuehnert MJ, Roth VR, Haley NR *et al.* (2001) Transfusion-transmitted bacterial infection in the United States, 1998 through 2000. Transfusion 41: 1493–1499

Kumar A, Kulkarni R, Murray DL *et al.* (1993) Serologic markers of viral hepatitis A, B, C, and D in patients with hemophilia. J Med Virol 41: 205–209

Kuo G, Choo QL, Alter HJ *et al.* (1989) An assay for circulating antibodies to a major etiologic virus of human non-A, non-B hepatitis. Science 244: 362–364

Kurtzman GJ, Ozawa K, Cohen B *et al.* (1987) Chronic bone marrow failure due to persistent B19 parvovirus infection. N Engl J Med 317: 287–294

Lai ME, De Virgilis S, Argiolu F *et al.* (1993) Evaluation of antibodies to hepatitis C virus in a long-term prospective study of posttransfusion hepatis among thalassemic children: comparison between first- and second-generation assays. J Pediatr Gastroenterol Nutr 16: 458–464

Lal RB, Brodine S, Kazura J (1992) Sensistivity and specificity of a recombinant transmembrane glycoprotein (rgp21)-spiked western immunoblot for serological confirmation of human T-cell lymphotropic virus type I and type II. J Clin Microbiol 30: 296–299

Lamberson H, McMillan J, Weiner L *et al.* (1984) Nursery acquired CMV infection in transfused neonates (Abstract). Transfusion 24: 430

Lamberson HV (1985) Cytomegalovirus (CMV): the agent, its pathogenesis and its epidemiology. In: Infection, Immunity and Blood Transfusion. RY Dodd, LF Baker (eds). New York: Alan R Liss, pp. 149–173

Lambrecht B, Mohr H, Knuver-Hopf *et al.* (1991) Photo-inactivation of viruses in human fresh plasma by pheno-thiazine dyes in combination with visible light. Vox Sang 60: 207–213

Landolfo S, Gariglio M, Gribaudo G *et al.* (2003) The human cytomegalovirus. Pharmacol Ther 98: 269–297

Larsen J, Hetland G, Skaug K (1990) Posttransfusion hepatitis B transmitted by blood from a hepatitis B surface antigen-negative hepatitis B virus carrier. Transfusion 30: 431–432

Lavie G, Mazur Y, Lavie D *et al.* (1995) Hypericin as an inactivator of infectious viruses in blood components. Transfusion 35: 392–400

Lazo A, Tassello J, Jayarama V *et al.* (2002) Broad-spectrum virus reduction in red cell concentrates using INACTINE PEN110 chemistry. Vox Sang 83: 313–323

Lederman MM, Ratnoff OD, Scillian JJ (1983) Impaired cell-mediated immunity in patients with classic haemophilia. N Engl J Med 308: 79–83

Lee DC, Stenland CJ, Miller JL *et al.* (2001) A direct relationship between the partitioning of the pathogenic prion protein and transmissible spongiform encephalopathy infectivity during the purification of plasma proteins. Transfusion 41: 449–455

Lee SR, Wood CL, Lane MJ *et al.* (1995) Increased detection of hepatitis C virus infection in commercial plasma donors by a third-generation screening assay. Transfusion 35: 845–849

Lee TH, Stromberg RR, Henrard D (1993) Effect of platelet-associated virus on assays of HIV-1 in plasma. Science 262: 1585

Lefrere J-J, Elghouzzi M-H, Paquez F *et al.* (1992) Interviews with anti-HIV-positive individuals detected through the systematic screening of blood donations: consequences on predonation medical interview. Vox Sang 62: 25–28

Lefrere J-J, Mariotti M, Thauvin M (1994) B19 parvovirus DNA in solvent/detergent-treated anti-haemophilia concentrates. Lancet 343: 211–212

Leiby DA, Read EJ, Lenes BA *et al.* (1997) Seroepidemiology of *Trypanosoma cruzi*, etiologic agent of Chagas' disease, in US blood donors. J Infect Dis 176: 1047–1052

Leiby DA, Herron RM Jr, Read EJ *et al.* (2002a) *Trypanosoma cruzi* in Los Angeles and Miami blood donors: impact of evolving donor demographics on seroprevalence and implications for transfusion transmission. Transfusion 42: 549–555

Leiby DA, Chung AP, Cable RG *et al.* (2002b) Relationship between tick bites and the seroprevalence of *Babesia microti* and *Anaplasma phagocytophila* (previously Ehrlichia sp.) in blood donors. Transfusion 42: 1585–1591

Leitman SF, Klein HG, Melpolder JJ *et al.* (1989) Clinical implications of positive tests for antibodies to human immunodeficiency virus type 1 in asymptomatic blood donors. N Engl J Med 321: 917–924

Leon A, Canton R, Elia M (1991) Second generation RIBA to confirm diagnosis of HCV infection. Lancet 337: 912

Levy JA (1989) Human immunodeficiency viruses and the pathogenesis of AIDS. JAMA 261: 2997–3006

Li J, de Korte D, Woolum MD et al. (2004) Pathogen reduction of buffy coat platelet concentrates using riboflavin and light: comparisons with pathogen-reduction technology-treated apheresis platelet products. Vox Sang 87: 82–90

Li R, Liu D, Zanusso G et al. (2001) The expression and potential function of cellular prion protein in human lymphocytes. Cell Immunol 207: 49–58

Lian CJ, Hwang WS, Pai CH (1987) Plasmid-mediated resistance to phagocytosis in Yersinia enterocolitica. Infect Immunol 55: 1176–1183

Liang TJ, Hasegawa K, Rimon N (1991) A hepatitis-B virus mutant associated with an epidemic of fulminant hepatitis. N Engl J Med 324: 1705–1709

Lieberman HM, La Brecque DR, Kew MC (1983) Detection of hepatitis B virus DNA directly in human serum by a simplified molecular hybridisation test: comparison to HBeAg/anti-HBe status in HBsAg carriers. Hepatology 3: 285–291

Lillehoj EP, Alexander SS, Dubrule CJ (1990) Development and evaluation of a human T-cell leukaemia virus type 1 serologic confirmatory assay incorporating a recombinant envelope polypeptide. J Clin Microbiol 28: 2653–2658

Linnen J, Wages JJ, Zhen-Yong Z-K (1995) Molecular cloning and disease association of hepatitis G virus: a transfusion-transmittable agent. Science 271: 505–508

Lipson SM, Ashraf AB, Lee SH et al. (1995) Cell culture-PCR technique for detection of infectious cytomegalovirus in peripheral blood. J Clin Microbiol 33: 1411–1413

Lipson SM, Match ME, Toro AI et al. (1998) Application of a standardized cytomegalovirus antigenemia assay in the management of patients with AIDS. Diagn Microbiol Infect Dis 32: 75–79

Lipson SM, Shepp DH, Match ME et al. (2001) Cytomegalovirus infectivity in whole blood following leukocyte reduction by filtration. Am J Clin Pathol 116: 52–55

Llewelyn CA, Hewitt PE, Knight RS et al. (2004) Possible transmission of variant Creutzfeldt-Jakob disease by blood transfusion. Lancet 363: 417–421

Lok AS (2002) Chronic hepatitis B. N Engl J Med 346: 1682–1683

Loussert-Ajaka I, Ly TD, Chaix ML (1994) HIV-1/HIV-2 seronegativity in HIV-1 subtype O infected patients. Lancet 343: 1393–1394

Macedo dOA, Beecham BD, Montgomery SP et al. (2004) West Nile virus blood transfusion-related infection despite nucleic acid testing. Transfusion 44: 1695–1699

McAlpine L, Parry JV, Tosswill JHC (1992) An evaluation of an enzyme immunoassay for the combined detection of antibodies to HIV-1, HIV-2, HTLV-I and HTLV-II. AIDS 6: 387–391

McCullough J, Vesole DH, Benjamin RJ et al. (2004) Therapeutic efficacy and safety of platelets treated with a photochemical process for pathogen inactivation: The SPRINT Trial. Blood 104:1534–41

McDonald CP, Hartley S, Orchard K et al. (1998) Fatal Clostridium perfringens sepsis from a pooled platelet transfusion. Transfusion Med 8: 19–22

Machin SJ, McVerry BA, Cheingsong-Popov R (1985) Seroconversion for HTLV-III since 1980 in British haemophiliacs. Lancet i: 336

McHutchinson JG, Person JL, Govindarajan S (1992) Improved detection of hepatitis C virus antibodies in high risk population. Hepatology 15: 19–25

McKechnie DB, Slater KS, Childs JE et al. (2000) Survival of Ehrlichia chaffeensis in refrigerated, ADSOL-treated RBCs. Transfusion 40: 1041–1047

McMahon BJ, Bruden DL, Petersen KM et al. (2005) Antibody levels and protection after hepatitis B vaccination: results of a 15-year follow-up. Ann Intern Med 142: 333–341

McMonigal K, Horwitz CA, Henle W (1983) Postperfusion syndrome due to Epstein-Barr virus. Report of two cases and review of the literature. Transfusion 23: 331–335

McOmish F, Yap PL, Jordan A (1993) Detection of parvovirus B19 in donated blood: a model system for screening by polymerase chain reaction. J Clin Microbiol 31: 323–328

Madhok R, Forbes CD (1990) HIV-1 infection in haemophilia. The treatment of haemophilia: a double-edged sword. In: Haematology in HIV Disease. C Costello (ed.). Baillière's Clinical Haematology 3: 79–101

Maeda Y, Furukawa M, Takehara Y (1984) Prevalence of possible adult T-cell leukemia virus-carriers among volunteer blood donors in Japan: a nation-wide study. Int J Cancer 33: 717–720

Magnaval JF, Brochier B, Charlet JP et al. (1985) Dépistage de la maladie de Chagas par immunoenzymologie. Comparaison de l'ELISA avec l'immunofluoresence et l'hémagglutination indirecte chez 976 donneurs de sang. Rev Fr Transfus Immunohematol 28: 201–212

Mahe C, Kaleebu P, Ojwiya A et al. (2002) Human immunodeficiency virus type 1 Western blot: revised diagnostic criteria with fewer indeterminate results for epidemiological studies in Africa. Int J Epidemiol 31: 985–990

Manel N, Kim FJ, Kinet S et al. (2003) The ubiquitous glucose transporter GLUT-1 is a receptor for HTLV. Cell 115: 449–459

Manns A, Blattner WA (1991) The epidemiology of the human T-cell lymphotrophic virus type I and type II: etiologic role in human disease. Transfusion 31: 67–75

Mannucci PM (1992) Outbreak of hepatitis A among Italian patients with haemophilia. Lancet 339: 819

Mannucci PM (1993) Clinical evaluation of viral safety of coagulation factor VIII and IX concentrates. Vox Sang 64: 197–203

Mannucci PM, Amnassari M, Gringeri A et al. (1985) Anti-LAV and concentrate consumption in Italian haemophiliacs. Thromb Haemost 54: 556

Mannucci PM, Schimpf K, Brettler DB et al. (1990) Low risk for hepatitis in hemophiliacs given high-purity, pasteurized factor VIII concentrate. Ann Intern Med 113: 27–32

Margolis-Nunno H, Robinson R, Ben Hur E (1994) Quencher-enhanced specificity of psoralen-photosensitized virus inactivation in platelet concentrates. Transfusion 34: 802–810

Margolis-Nunno H, Robinson R, Ben Hur E (1995) Elimination of potential mutagenicity in platelet concentrates that are virally inactivated with psoralens and ultraviolet A light. Transfusion 35: 855–862

Mariani G, Ghirardini A, Mandelli F et al. (1987) Heated clotting factor and seroconversion for human immunodeficiency virus in three hemophilic patients (Letter). Ann Intern Med 107: 113

Marker SC, Asher NL, Kalis JM et al. (1979) Epstein-Barr virus antibody responses and clinical illness in renal transplant recipients. Surgery 85: 433–440

Markovic I, Clouse KA (2004) Recent advances in understanding the molecular mechanisms of HIV-1 entry and fusion: revisiting current targets and considering new options for therapeutic intervention. Curr HIV Res 2: 223–234

Marsden PD (1984) Chagas' disease: clinical aspects. In: Recent Advances in Tropical Medicine. HM Gilles (ed.). Edinburgh: Churchill Livingstone, pp. 63–87

Matsubayashi K, Nagaoka Y, Sakata H et al. (2004) Transfusion-transmitted hepatitis E caused by apparently indigenous hepatitis E virus strain in Hokkaido, Japan. Transfusion 44: 934–940

Matsumoto A, Yeo AE, Shih JW et al. (1999) Transfusion-associated TT virus infection and its relationship to liver disease. Hepatology 30: 283–288

Mawle AC, McDougall JS (1992) Immunologic aspects of human immunodeficiency virus infection. In: AIDS Testing. Methodology and Management Issues. G Schochetman, JR George (eds). New York: Springer Verlag, pp. 30–47

Mayo DJ, Rose AM, Matchett SE et al. (1991) Screening potential blood donors at risk for human immunodeficiency virus. Transfusion 31: 466–474

Meijer E, Boland GJ, Verdonck LF (2003) Prevention of cytomegalovirus disease in recipients of allogeneic stem cell transplants. Clin Microbiol Rev 16: 647–657

Meisel H, Reip A, Faltus B (1995) Transmission of hepatitis C virus to children and husbands by women infected with contaminated anti-D immunoglobulin. Lancet 345: 1209–1211

Melbye M (1986) The natural history of human T-lymphotropic virus-III infection: the cause of AIDS. BMJ 292: 5–12

Miller LH (1975) Transfusion malaria. In: Transmissible Disease and Blood Transfusion. TJ Greenwalt, GA Jamieson (eds). New York: Grune & Stratton

Miller RH, Purcell RH (1990) Hepatitis C virus shares amino acid sequence similarity with pestiviruses and flaviviruses as well as members of two plant virus supergroups. Proc Natl Acad Sci USA 87: 2057–2061

Miller WJ, McCullough J, Balfour HH Jr et al. (1991) Prevention of cytomegalovirus infection following bone marrow transplantation: a randomized trial of blood product screening. Bone Marrow Transplant 7: 227–234

Minamoto GY, Scheinberg DA, Dietz K et al. (1988) Human immunodeficiency virus infection in patients with leukemia. Blood 71: 1147–1149

Mintz ED, Anderson JF, Cable RG (1991) Transfusion-transmitted babiosis: a case report from a new endemic area. Transfusion 31: 365–368

Monjardino JP, Saldanha JA (1990) Delta hepatitis. The disease and the virus. Br Med Bull 46: 399–407

Mordmuller B, Kremsner PG (1998) Hyperparasitemia and blood exchange transfusion for treatment of children with falciparum malaria. Clin Infect Dis 26: 850–852

Morgenthaler J-J (1989) Effect of ethanol on viruses. In: Virus Inactivation in Plasma Products. JJ Morgenthaler (ed.). Basel: S Karger, pp. 109–121

Moroff G, Wagner S, Benade L et al. (1992) Factors influencing virus inactivation and retention of platelet properties following treatment with aminomethyltrimethylpsoralen and ultraviolet A light. Blood Cells 18: 43–56

Mosley JW, Redeker AG, Feinstone SM et al. (1977) Mutliple hepatitis viruses in multiple attacks of acute viral hepatitis. N Engl J Med 296: 75–78

Mosley JW, Stevens CE, Aach RD et al. (1995) Donor screening for antibody to hepatitis B core antigen and hepatitis B virus infection in transfusion recipients. Transfusion 35: 5–12

Medical Research Council (1974) Post-transfusion hepatitis in a London hospital: results of a two-year prospective study. J Hyg (Lond) 73: 173–188

Mullis KB, Faloona FA (1987) Specific synthesis of DNA in vitro via a polymerase-catalyzed chain reaction. Methods Enzymol 155: 335–350

Mungai M, Tegtmeier G, Chamberland M et al. (2001) Transfusion-transmitted malaria in the United States from 1963 through 1999. N Engl J Med 344: 1973–1978

Munksgaard L, Albjerg L, Lillevang ST et al. (2004) Detection of bacterial contamination of platelet components:

six years' experience with the BacT/ALERT system. Transfusion 44: 1166–1173

Murphy EL, Fridey J, Smith JW, Engstrom J et al. (1997) HTLV-associated myelopathy in a cohort of HTLV-I and HTLV-II-infected blood donors. The REDS investigators. Neurology 48: 315–320

Nagington J, Cossart YE, Cohen BJ (1977) Reactivation of hepatitis B after transplantation operations. Lancet i: 558–560

Nelson KE, Donahue JG, Munoz A et al. (1992) Transmission of retroviruses from seronegative donors by transfusion during cardiac surgery. A multicenter study of HIV-1 and HTLV-I/II infections. Ann Intern Med 117: 554–559

Ness P, Braine H, King K et al. (2001) Single-donor platelets reduce the risk of septic platelet transfusion reactions. Transfusion 41: 857–861

Nichols WG, Price TH, Gooley T et al. (2003) Transfusion-transmitted cytomegalovirus infection after receipt of leukoreduced blood products. Blood 101: 4195–4200

Nishizawa T, Okamoto H, Konishi K et al. (1997) A novel DNA virus (TTV) associated with elevated transaminase levels in posttransfusion hepatitis of unknown etiology. Biochem Biophys Res Commun 241: 92–97

Noble RC, Kane MA, Reeves SA (1984) Post-transfusion hepatitis A in a neonatal intensive care unit. JAMA 252: 2711–2715

Nolte FS, Fried MW, Shiffman ML et al. (2001) Prospective multicenter clinical evaluation of AMPLICOR and COBAS AMPLICOR hepatitis C virus tests. J Clin Microbiol 39: 4005–4012

O'Gorman MR, Weber D, Landis SE (1991) Interpretive criteria of the Western blot assay for serodiagnosis of human immunodeficiency virus type I infection. Arch Pathol Lab Med 115: 26–30

Officer R (1945) Experimental transfusion with malaria infected blood. Med J Aust i: 271

Ohagen A, Gibaja V, Aytay S et al. (2002) Inactivation of HIV in blood. Transfusion 42: 1308–1317

Ohto H, Terazawa S, Sasaki N (1994) Transmission of hepatitis C virus from mothers to infants. N Engl J Med 330: 744–750

Okochi K (1985) Adult T-cell leukemia virus, blood donors and transfusion: experience in Japan. In: Infection, Immunity and Blood Transfusion. RY Dodd, LF Barker (eds). New York: Alan R Liss, pp. 245–256

Okochi K (1989) Blood transfusion and HTLV-I in Japan. In: HTLV-I and the Nervous System. CG Roman, JC Vernant, M Osame (eds). New York: Alan R Liss, pp. 527–532

Olivares-Lopez F, Cruz-Carranza G, Peterz-Rodriguez GE (1985) Malaria inducida por transfusión de sangre. Analisis de 44 casos. Rev Med Inst Mex Seg Soc 23: 153–157

Operskalski EA, Mosley JW, Tobler LH et al. (2003) HCV viral load in anti-HCV-reactive donors and infectivity for their recipients. Transfusion 43: 1433–1441

Orton SL, Liu H, Dodd RY et al. (2002) Prevalence of circulating Treponema pallidum DNA and RNA in blood donors with confirmed-positive syphilis tests. Transfusion 42: 94–99

Ou CY, Kwok S, Mitchell SW (1988) DNA amplification for direct detection of HIV-1 in DNA of peripheral blood mononuclear cells. Science 239: 295–297

Owens SD, Oakley DA, Marryott K et al. (2001) Transmission of visceral leishmaniasis through blood transfusions from infected English foxhounds to anemic dogs. J Am Vet Med Assoc 219: 1076–1083

Paloheimo JA, von Essen R, Klemola E et al. (1968) Subclinical cytomegalovirus infections and cytomegalovirus mononucleosis after open heart surgery. Am J Cardiol 22: 624–630

Pan KM, Baldwin M, Nguyen J et al. (1993) Conversion of alpha-helices into beta-sheets features in the formation of the scrapie prion proteins. Proc Natl Acad Sci USA 90: 10962–10966

Pantaleo G, Graziosi C, Demarest JF et al. (1993) HIV infection is active and progressive in lymphoid tissue during the clinically latent stage of disease. Nature 362: 355–358

Pao CC, Yao D-S, Lin C-Y et al. (1991) Serum hepatitis B virus DNA in hepatitis B virus seropositive and seronegative patients with normal liver function. Am J Clin Pathol 95: 591–596

Parola P (2004) Tick-borne rickettsial diseases: emerging risks in Europe. Comp Immunol Microbiol Infect Dis 27: 297–304

Pattison JR (1987) B19 virus – a pathogenic human parvovirus. Blood Rev 1: 58–64

Pattison JR, Jones SE, Hogdson J et al. (1981) Parvovirus infections and hypoplastic crisis in sickle-cell anaemia. Lancet i: 664

Pawlotsky JM (1994) Significance of indeterminate second generation RIBA and resolution by third generation RIBA. In: Hepatitis C Virus: New Diagnostic Tools. Paris: John Libbey Eurotext, pp. 17–29

Pealer LN, Marfin AA, Petersen LR et al. (2003) Transmission of West Nile virus through blood transfusion in the United States in 2002. N Engl J Med 349: 1236–1245

Peden AH, Head MW, Ritchie DL et al. (2004) Preclinical vCJD after blood transfusion in a PRNP codon 129 heterozygous patient. Lancet 364: 527–529

Peerlinck K, Vermylen J (1993) Acute hepatitis A in patients with haemophilia A. Lancet 341: 179

Peterman TA (1987) Transfusion-associated acquired immunodeficiency syndrome. World J Surg 11: 36–40

Peterman TA, Jaffe HW, Feorino PM *et al.* (1985) Transfusion-associated acquired immunodeficiency syndrome in the United States. JAMA 254: 2913–2917

Phelps R, Robbins K, Liberti T *et al.* (2004) Window-period human immunodeficiency virus transmission to two recipients by an adolescent blood donor. Transfusion 44: 929–933

Pietersz RNI, de Korte D, Reesink HW (1989) Storage of whole blood for up to 24 hours at ambient temperature prior to component preparation. Vox Sang 56: 145–150

Piiparinen H, Hockerstedt K, Gronhagen-Riska C *et al.* (2004) Comparison of two quantitative CMV PCR tests, Cobas Amplicor CMV Monitor and TaqMan assay, and pp65-antigenemia assay in the determination of viral loads from peripheral blood of organ transplant patients. J Clin Virol 30: 258–266

Pillonel J, Courouc, AM, Elghouzzi MH (1996) Seroconversion to HTLV in blood donors. Vox Sang 70: 47

Pindyck J, Waldman A, Oleszkow W *et al.* (1984) Prevalence of viral antibodies and leukocyte abnormalities among blood donors considering themselves at risk of exposure to AIDS. Ann NY Acad Sci 437: 472–484

Pindyck J, Waldman A, Zang E (1985) Measures to decrease the risk of acquired immune deficiency transmission by blood transfusion. Transfusion 25: 3–9

Piot P, Feachem RG, Lee JW *et al.* (2004) Public health. A global response to AIDS: lessons learned, next steps. Science 304: 1909–1910

Pittman M (1953) A study of bacteria implicated in transfusion reactions and of bacteria isolated from blood products. J Lab Clin Med 42: 273

van der Poel CL, Reesink HW, Lelie PN (1989) Anti-hepatitis C antibodies and non-A, non-B post-transfusion hepatitis in The Netherlands. Lancet ii: 297–298

van der Poel CL, Reesink HW, Lelie PN (1990) Anti-HCV and transaminase testing of blood donors. Lancet ii: 187–188

Poiesz BJ, Ruscetti FW, Gazdar AF *et al.* (1980) Detection and isolation of type C retrovirus particles from fresh and cultured lymphocytes of a patient with cutaneous T-cell lymphoma. Proc Natl Acad Sci USA 77: 7415–7419

Popovic M, Sarngadharan MG, Read I *et al.* (1984) Detection, isolation and continuous production of cytopathic retrovirus HTLV-III from patients with AIDS and pre-AIDS. Science 224: 497–500

Popovsky MA (1990) Babesiosis and lyme disease: a transfusion medicine perspective. In: Emerging Global Patterns in Transfusion Transmitted infections. RG Westphal, KB Carlson, JM Ture (eds). Arlington, VA: Am Assoc Blood Banks, pp. 45–64

Poulsen A-G, Kvinesdal B, Aaby P (1989) Prevalence of and mortality from human immunodeficiency virus type 2 in Bissau, West Africa. Lancet i: 827–831

Power JP, Lawlor E, Davidson F (1995) Molecular epidemiology of an outbreak of infection with hepatitis C virus in recipients of anti-D immunoglobulin. Lancet 345: 1211–1213

Preiksaitis J (1991) Indications for the use of cytomegalovirus-seronegative blood products. Transfusion Med Rev 5 1: 1–17

Preiksaitis JK (2000) The cytomegalovirus-'safe' blood product: is leukoreduction equivalent to antibody screening? Transfusion Med Rev 14: 112–136

Preiksaitis JK, Rosno S, Grumet C *et al.* (1983) Infections due to herpes viruses in cardiac transplant recipients: role of the donor heart and immunosuppressive therapy. J Infect Dis 147: 974–981

Preiksaitis JK, Brown L, McKenzie M (1988) The risk of cytomegalovirus infection in seronegative transfusion recipients not receiving exogenous immunosuppression. J Infect Dis 157: 523–529

Prince AM (1968) An antigen detected in the blood during the incubation period of serum hepatitis. Proc Natl Acad Sci USA 60: 814

Prince AM (1975) Post-transfusion hepatitis: etiology and prevention. In: Transfusion and Immunology. 14th Congr Int Soc Blood Transfus, Helsinki

Prince AM, Horowitz B, Brotman B (1986) Sterilization of hepatitis and HTLV-III viruses by exposure to tri(n-butyl) phosphate and sodium cholate. Lancet 1: 706

Prince AM, Lee DH, Brotman B (2001) Infectivity of blood from PCR-positive, HBsAg-negative, anti-HBs-positive cases of resolved hepatitis B infection. Transfusion 41: 329–332

Prou O (1985) Mise en evidence de *Plasmodium falciparum* par immunofluorescence indirecte a l'aide d'anticorps monoclonaux murins specifiques. Rev Fr Transfus Immunohématol 28: 659–670

Prusiner SB (1998) Prions. Proc Natl Acad Sci USA 95: 13363–13383

Puckett A (1986a) Bacterial contamination of blood for transfusion: a study of the growth characteristics of four implicated organisms. Med Lab Sci 43: 252–257

Puckett A (1986b) A sterility testing method for blood products. Med Lab Sci 43: 249–251

Purcell RH, Ticehurst JR (1988) Enterically transmitted non-A, non-B hepatitis: epidemiology and clinical characteristics. In: Viral Hepatitis and Liver Disease. AJ Zuckerman (ed.) New York: Alan R Liss, pp. 131–137

Purcell RH, London WT, Newman J (1985) Hepatitis B virus, hepatitis non-A, non-B virus and hepatitis delta virus in lyophilized anti-hemophilic factor; relative sensitivity to heat. Hepatology 5: 1091–1099

Raevsky CA, Cohn DL, Wolf FC (1986) Transfusion-associated human T-lymphotropic virus type III/ lymphadenopathy-associated virus infection from a seronegative donor – Colorado. MMWR 35: 389–391

Ragni MV, Lewis JH, Spero JA et al. (1983) Acquired-immunodeficiency-like syndrome in two haemophiliacs. Lancet 1: 213–214

Ragni MV, Tegtmeier GE, Levy JA (1986) AIDS retrovirus antibodies in hemophiliacs treated with factor VIII or factor IX concentrates, cryoprecipitate, or fresh frozen plasma: prevalence, seroconversion rate, and clinical correlations. Blood 67: 592–595

Ragni MV, Koch WC, Jordan JA (1996) Parvovirus B19 infection in patients with hemophilia. Transfusion 36: 238–241

Ravitch MM, Farmer TW, Davis B (1949) Use of blood donors with positive serologic tests for syphilis-with a note on the disappearance of passively transferred reagin. J Clin Invest 28: 18

Reesink HW, Vrielink H, Zaaijer HL (1994) Evaluation of a new HTLV-I/II PCR: Amplicor HTLVI/II test (Abstract). Transfusion 34 (Suppl.): 48S

Reesink HW, Wesdorp ICE, Grijm R (1980) Follow-up of blood donors positive for hepatitis B surface antigen. Vox Sang 38: 138

Rehermann B, Nascimbeni M (2005) Immunology of hepatitis B virus and hepatitis C virus infection. Nature Rev Immunol 5: 215–229

Reid PM, Brown T, Reid TSM (1985) Human parvovirus associated arthritis: a clinical and laboratory description. Lancet ii: 422–425

Reyes GR, Purdy MA, Kim JP (1990) Isolation of a cDNA from the virus responsible for enterically transmitted non-A, non-B hepatitis. Science 247: 1335–1339

Reynes M, Zignego L, Samuel D (1989) Graft hepatitis delta virus infection after orthotopic liver transplantation in HDV cirrhosis. Transplant Proc 21: 2424–2425

Rhame FS, Root RK, MacLowry JD (1973) Salmonella septicemia from platelet transfusions: study of an outbreak traced to a hematogenous carrier of Salmonella cholera suis. Ann Intern Med 78: 633–641

van Rhenen D, Gulliksson H, Cazenave JP et al. (2003) Transfusion of pooled buffy coat platelet components prepared with photochemical pathogen inactivation treatment: the euroSPRITE trial. Blood 101: 2426–2433

Rinker J, Galambos JT (1981) Prospective study of hepatitis B in thirty-two inadvertently infected people. Gastroenterology 81: 686–691

Rios M, Duran E, Wong-Schneider S (1996) RNA sequence of HTLV-I and HTLV-II can be detected in the plasma of infected individuals. Vox Sang 70 (Suppl.) 2: 2

Risseeuw-Appel IM, Kothe FC (1983) Transfusion syphilis: a case report. Sex Transmitted Dis 10: 200–201

Rizzetto M (1983) The delta agent. Hepatology 3: 729–737

Roback JD, Drew WL, Laycock ME et al. (2003) CMV DNA is rarely detected in healthy blood donors using validated PCR assays. Transfusion 43: 314–321

Robert-Guroff M, Goedert JJ, Naugle CJ (1988) Spectrum of HIV-1 neutralizing antibodies in a cohort of homosexual men: results of a 6 year prospective study. AIDS Res Hum Retroviruses 4: 343–350

Robertson B, Myers G, Howard C et al. (1998) Classification, nomenclature, and database development for hepatitis C virus (HCV) and related viruses: proposals for standardization. International Committee on Virus Taxonomy. Arch Virol 143: 2493–2503

Rocchi G, deFelici A, Ragona G (1977) Quantitative evaluation of Epstein-Barr virus-infected mononuclear peripheral blood leukocytes in infectious mononucleosis. N Engl J Med 296: 131–134

Rock G, Neurath D, Toye B et al. (2004) The use of a bacteria detection system to evaluate bacterial contamination in PLT concentrates. Transfusion 44: 337–342

Rodriguez-Inigo E, Casqueiro M, Bartolome J et al. (2000) Detection of TT virus DNA in liver biopsies by in situ hybridization. Am J Pathol 156: 1227–1234

Rogers MF, Schochetman G (1992) Human immunodeficiency virus infection in children. In: AIDS Testing. Methodology and Management Issues. G Schochetman, JR George (eds). New York: Springer Verlag, pp. 152–167

Roman GC, Osame M (1988) Identity of HTLV-I associated tropical spastic paraparesis and HTLV-I-associated myelopathy (Letter). Lancet i: 651

Romano JW, van Gemen B, Kievits T (1996) NASBA: a novel, isothermal detection technology for qualitative and quantitative HIV-1 RNA measurements. Clin Lab Med 16: 89–103

Rosina F, Saracco G, Rizzetto M (1985) Risk of posttransfusion infection with the hepatitis delta virus. A Multicenter Study. N Engl J Med 312: 1488–1491

Rossi KQ, Nickel JR, Wissel ME et al. (2002) Passively acquired treponemal antibody from intravenous immunoglobulin therapy in a pregnant patient. Arch Pathol Lab Med 126: 1237–1238

Ruane PH, Edrich R, Gampp D et al. (2004) Photochemical inactivation of selected viruses and bacteria in platelet concentrates using riboflavin and light. Transfusion 44: 877–885

Rubin RH, Tolkoff-Rubin NE, Oliver D (1985) Multicenter seroepidemiologic study of the impact of cytomegalovirus infection on renal transplantation. Transplantation 40: 243–249

Rubinstein AJ, Rubinstein DB, Tom W (1994) Terminal 100°C dry heat treatment of intravenous immunoglobulin preparations to assure sterility. Vox Sang 66: 295–296

Sagir A, Kirschberg O, Heintges T et al. (2004) SEN virus infection. Rev Med Virol 14: 141–148

Saldanha J, Minor P (1996) Detection of human parvovirus B19 DNA in plasma pools and blood products derived from these pools: implications for efficiency and consistency of removal of B19 DNA during manufacture. Br J Haematol 93: 714–719

Salimans MMM, Holsappel S, van de Rijke FM (1989) Rapid detection of parvovirus B19 DNA by dot-hybridisation and the polymerase chain reaction. J Virol Methods 23: 19–23

Sampliner RE, Hamilton FA, Iseri OA (1979) The liver histology and frequency of clearance of the hepatitis B surface antigen (HBsAg) in chronic carriers. Am J Med Sci 277: 17–22

Sandler SG, Fang CT, Williams AE (1991) Human T-cell lymphotropic virus type I and II in transfusion medicine. Transfus Med Rev 5: 93–107

Santagostino E, Mannucci PM, Gringeri A (1994) Eliminating parvovirus B19 from blood products. Lancet 343: 798–799

Santagostino E, Mannucci PM, Gringeri A et al. (1997) Transmission of parvovirus B19 by coagulation factor concentrates exposed to 100 degrees C heat after lyophilization. Transfusion 37: 517–522

Sarkodie F, Adarkwa M, Adu-Sarkodie Y et al. (2001) Screening for viral markers in volunteer and replacement blood donors in West Africa. Vox Sang 80: 142–147

Sarrazin C, Teuber G, Kokka R et al. (2000) Detection of residual hepatitis C virus RNA by transcription-mediated amplification in patients with complete virologic response according to polymerase chain reaction-based assays. Hepatology 32: 818–823

Sato H, Okochi K (1986) Transmission of human T cell leukaemia virus (HTLV-I) by blood transfusion: demonstration of proviral DNA in recipients' blood lymphocytes. Int J Cancer 37: 397–400

Sato H, Takakura F, Kojima E (1996) Human parvovirus B19. Vox Sang 70 (Suppl. 2): 17

Satow Y-I, Hashido M, Ishikawa K-I (1991) Detection of HTLV-I antigen in peripheral and cord blood lymphocytes from carrier mothers. Lancet ii: 915–916

Saxinger C, Polesky H, Eby N (1988) Antibody reactivity with HBLV (HHV-6) in US populations. J Virol Methods 21: 199–208

Sayers MH, Anderson KC, Goodnough LT (1992) Reducing the risk for transfusion-transmitted cytomegalovirus infection. Ann Intern Med 116: 55–62

Sayre KR, Dodd RY, Tegtmeier G (1996) Falsepositive human immunodeficiency virus type 1 Western blot tests in noninfected blood donors. Transfusion 36: 45–52

Sazama K (1995) Existing problems in the testing for infectious diseases. Immunol Invest 24: 131–146

Sazama K, Kuramoto IK, Holland PV et al. (1992) Detection of antibodies to human immunodeficiency virus type 2 (HIV-2) in blood donor sera using United States assay methods for anti-HIV type 1. Transfusion 32: 398–401

Schable C, Zekeng L, Pau CP et al. (1994) Sensitivity of United States HIV antibody tests for detection of HIV-1 group O infections. Lancet 244: 1333–1334

Schimpf K, Mannucci PM, Krentz W et al. (1987) Absence of hepatitis after treatment with a pasteurised Factor VIII concentrate in patients with haemophilia and no previous transfusion. N Engl J Med 316: 918–922

Schlauder GS, Dawson GJ, Simons JJ et al. (1995) Molecular and serologic analysis in the transmission of the GB hepatitis agents. J Med Virol 46: 81–90

Schmunis GA (1991) Trypanosoma cruzi, the etiologic agent of Chagas' disease: status in the blood supply in endemic and nonendemic countries. Transfusion 31: 547–557

Schochetman G (1992) AIDS Testing. Methodology and Management Issues. New York: Springer-Verlag

Seeberg S, Brandberg, Hermodsson S (1981) Hospital outbreak of hepatitis A secondary to blood exchange in a baby (Letter). Lancet i: 1155–1156

Seeff LB, Zimmerman HJ, Wright EC et al. (1977) A randomized, double blind controlled trial of the efficacy of immune serum globulin for the prevention of posttransfusion hepatitis. Gastroenterology 72: 111

Seeff LB, Beebe GW, Hoofnagle JH et al. (1987) A serologic follow-up of the 1942 epidemic of post-vaccination hepatitis in the United States Army. N Engl J Med 316: 965–970

Seeff LB, Hollinger FB, Alter HJ et al. (2001) Long-term mortality and morbidity of transfusion-associated non-A, non-B, and type C hepatitis: A National Heart, Lung, and Blood Institute collaborative study. Hepatology 33: 455–463

Selbie FR (1943) Viability of Treponema pallidum in stored plasma. Br J Exp Pathol 24: 150

Seligmann M (1990) Immunological features of human immunodeficiency virus disease. In: Haematology in HIV Disease. C Christine (ed.). London: Baillière Tindall, pp. 37–63

Semmo N, Barnes E, Taylor C et al. (2005) T-cell responses and previous exposure to hepatitis C virus in indeterminate blood donors. Lancet 365: 327–329

Shade RO, Blundell MC, Cotmer SS et al. (1986) Nucleotide sequence and genome organization of human parvovirus B19 isolated from the serum of a child during aplastic crisis. J Virol 58: 921–926

Shattock AG, Irwin FM, Morgan BM et al. (1985) Increased severity and morbidity of acute hepatitis in drug abusers with simultaneously acquired hepatitis B and hepatitis D virus infections. BMJ 290: 1377–1380

Shehata N, Kohli M, Detsky A (2004) The cost-effectiveness of screening blood donors for malaria by PCR. Transfusion 44: 217–228

Sherertz RJ, Russell BA, Reuman PD (1984) Transmission of hepatitis A by transfusion of blood products. Arch Intern Med 144: 1579–1580

Shioda T, Levy JA, Cheng-Mayer C (1991) Macrophage and T-cell-line tropisms of HIV-1 are determined by specific regions of the envelope gp 120 gene. Nature (Lond) 349: 167–169

Shulman IA, Appleman MD (1990) An overview of unusual diseases transmitted by blood transfusion within the United States. In: Emerging Global Patterns in Transfusion Transmitted Infections. RG Westphal, KB Carlson, JM Turc (eds). Arlington, VA: Am Assoc Blood Banks

Shulman IA, Saxena S, Nelson JM et al. (1984) Neonatal exchange transfusions complicated by transfusion-induced malaria. Pediatrics 73: 330–332

Shulman S, Lindgren AM, Petrini P et al. (1992) Transmission of hepatitis C with pasteurized factor VIII (Letter). Lancet ii: 305–306

Sieber F, O'Brien JM, Gaffney DK (1992) Merocyaninesensitized photoinactivation of enveloped viruses. Blood Cells 18: 117–128

Siegel SE, Lunde MN, Gelderman AH et al. (1971) Transmission of toxoplasmosis by leukocyte transfusion. Blood 37: 388

Simmonds P, Alberti A, Bonnio F et al. (1994) The proposed system for the nomenclature of Hepatitis C virus genotypes. Hepatology 19: 1321–1324

Simons JN, Pilot-Matias TJ, Leary TP et al. (1995) Identification of two flavivirus-like genomes in the GB hepatitis agent. Proc Natl Acad Sci USA 93: 3401–3405

Singh S, Chaudhry VP, Wall JP (1996) Transfusion-transmitted kala-azar in India (Letter). Transfusion 36: 848–849

Skidmore SJ, Pasi KJ, Mawson SJ et al. (1990) Serological evidence that dry heating of clotting factor concentrates prevents transmission of non-A, non-B hepatitis. J Med Virol 30: 50–52

Slinger R, Giulivi A, Bodie-Collins M et al. (2001) Transfusion-transmitted malaria in Canada. CMAJ 164: 377–379

van der Sluis JJ, Ten KFJW, Vuzevski VD (1985) Transfusion syphilis, survival of Treponema pallidum in stored donor blood. II-Dose dependence of experimentally determined survival times. Vox Sang 49: 390–399

Smedile A, Farci P, Verme G et al. (1982) Influence of delta infection on severity of hepatitis B. Lancet ii: 945–947

Smith D, Wright P, Estes W (1984) Posttransfusion cytomegalovirus infection in neonates weighing less than 1,250 grams (Abstract). Transfusion 24: 430

Smith RP, Evans AT, Popovsky M (1986) Transfusion-acquired babesiosis and failure of antibiotic treatment. JAMA 256: 2726–2727

Soendjojo A, Boedisantoso M, Ilias MI et al. (1982) Syphilis d'emblee due to blood transfusion. Case report. Br J Vener Dis 58: 149–150

Solem JH, Jorgensen W (1969) Accidentally transmitted infectious mononucleosis. Acta Med Scand 186: 433

Soriano V, Gutiérrez M, Hereda A et al. (1994) Evaluation of different supplementary assays for the confirmation of HIV-1 and HIV-2 infections. Vox Sang 66: 82–83

Soucie JM, Siwak EB, Hooper WC et al. (2004) Human parvovirus B19 in young male patients with hemophilia A: associations with treatment product exposure and joint range-of-motion limitation. Transfusion 44: 1179–1185

Soudeyns H, Paolucci S, Chappey C et al. (1999) Selective pressure exerted by immunodominant HIV-1-specific cytotoxic T lymphocyte responses during primary infection drives genetic variation restricted to the cognate epitope. Eur J Immunol 29: 3629–3635

Soulier JP (1984) Diseases transmissible by blood transfusion. Vox Sang 47: 1–6

Spangler AS, Jackson JH, Fiumara NJ et al. (1964) Syphilis with a negative blood test reaction. JAMA 189: 87–90

Stagno S, Pass RF, Cloud G (1986) Primary cytomegalovirus infection in pregnancy. Incidence, transmission to fetus and clinical outcome. JAMA 256: 1904–1908

Stebbing J, Moyle G (2003) The clades of HIV: their origins and clinical significance. AIDS Rev 5: 205–213

Stevens CE, Aach RD, Hollinger FB et al. (1984) Hepatitis B virus antibody in blood donors and the occurrence of non-A, non-B hepatitis in transfusion recipients. An analysis of the transfusion-transmitted viruses study. Ann Intern Med 101: 733–737

Stramer SL (2004) Viral diagnostics in the arena of blood donor screening. Vox Sang 87 (Suppl.) 2: 180–183

Stramer SL, Heller IS, Coombs RW et al. (1989) Markers of HIV infection prior to IgG antibody seropositivity. JAMA 262: 64–69

Stramer SL, Glynn SA, Kleinman SH et al. (2004) Detection of HIV-1 and HCV infections among antibody-negative blood donors by nucleic acid-amplification testing. N Engl J Med 351: 760–768

Sullivan PS, Do AN, Ellenberger D et al. (2000) Human immunodeficiency virus (HIV) subtype surveillance of African-born persons at risk for group O and group N HIV infections in the United States. J Infect Dis 181: 463–469

Switzer WM, Bhullar V, Shanmugam V et al. (2004) Frequent simian foamy virus infection in persons occupationally exposed to nonhuman primates. J Virol 78: 2780–2789

Szewzyk U, Szewzyk R, Stenstrom TA (1993) Growth and survival of Serratia marcescens under aerobic and anaerobic conditions in the presence of materials from blood bags. J Clin Microbiol 31: 1826–1830

Szmuness W, Stevens CE, Harley EJ et al. (1982) Hepatitis B vaccine in medical staff of hemodialysis units: efficacy and subtype cross-protection. N Engl J Med 307: 1481–1486

Tabor E (1982) Infectious Complications of Blood Transfusion. New York: Academic Press

Tabor E (1999) The epidemiology of virus transmission by plasma derivatives: clinical studies verifying the lack of transmission of hepatitis B and C viruses and HIV type 1. Transfusion 39: 1160–1168

Tabor E, Gerety RJ, Drucker JA et al. (1978) Transmission of non-A, non-B hepatitis from man to chimpanzee. Lancet 1: 463–466

Takahashi K, Imai M, Nomura M et al. (1981) Demonstration of the immunogenicity of hepatitis B core antigen in a hepatitis B e antigen polypeptide (P19). J Gen Virol 57: 325–330

Takaki A, Weise M, Maertens G, et al. (2000) Cellular immune responses persist and humoral responses decrease two decades after recovery from a single source outbreak of hepatitis C. Nature Med 6: 578–582

Takatsuki K (1996) HTLV-I associated diseases. Vox Sang 70 (Suppl.) 3: 123–126

Takeda A, Tuazon CU, Ennis FA (1988) Antibody-enhanced infection by HIV-1 via Fc receptor-mediated entry. Science 242: 580–583

Takeuchi K, Kubo Y, Boonmar S et al. (1990) The putative nucleocapsid and envelope protein genes of hepatitis C virus determined by comparison of the nucleotide sequences of two isolates derived from an experimentally infected chimpanzee and healthy human carriers. J Gen Virol 71: 3027–3033

Tanaka Y, Primi D, Wang RY et al. (2001) Genomic and molecular evolutionary analysis of a newly identified infectious agent (SEN virus) and its relationship to the TT virus family. J Infect Dis 183: 359–367

Tanaka Y, Hanada K, Mizokami M et al. (2002) Inaugural Article: A comparison of the molecular clock of hepatitis C virus in the United States and Japan predicts that hepatocellular carcinoma incidence in the United States will increase over the next two decades. Proc Natl Acad Sci USA 99: 15584–15589

Taylor JM (2003) Replication of human hepatitis delta virus: recent developments. Trends Microbiol 11: 185–190

Taylor BJ, Jacobs RF, Baker RL et al. (1986) Frozen deglycerolyzed blood prevents transfusion-acquired cytomegalovirus infections in neonates. Pediatr Infect Dis 5: 188–191

Tedder RS, Cameron CH, Wilson-Croome R et al. (1980) Contrasting patterns and frequency of antibodies to the surface, core, and e antigens of hepatitis B virus in blood donors and in homosexual patients. J Med Virol 6: 323–332

Tedder RS, Briggs M, Howell DR et al. (1982) UK prevalence of delta infection. Lancet ii: 764–765

Tegtmeier GE (1986) Transfusion-transmitted cytomegalovirus infections: significance and control. Vox Sang 51 (Suppl.) 1: 22–30

Tegtmeier GE (1989) Posttransfusion cytomegalovirus infections. Arch Pathol Lab Med 113: 236–245

Tegtmeier GE, Buckley SA, Jenkins DC et al. (1984) Acquired cytomegalovirus infections in transfused, premature neonates. 18th Congr Int Soc Blood Transfusion, Munich, 180 (Abstract)

Temperley IJ, Cotter KP, Walsh TJ et al. (1992) Clotting factors and hepatitis A. Lancet 340: 1466

Tersmette M, Gruters HA, de Wolf F et al. (1989) Evidence for a role of virulent human immuno-deficiency virus (HIV) variants in the pathogenesis of acquired immunodeficiency syndrome: studies on sequential HIV isolates. J Virol 63: 2118–2125

Thiers V, Nakajima E, Kermsdorf D et al. (1988) Transmission of hepatitis B from hepatitis-B-seronegative subjects. Lancet ii: 1273–1276

Tiollais P (1988) Structure, genetic organization, and transcription of Hepadna viruses. In: Viral Hepatitis and Liver Disease. AJ Zuckerman (ed.). New York: Alan R Liss, pp. 295–300

Tong S, Li J, Vitvitski L et al. (1990) Active hepatitis B virus replication in the presence of anti-HBe is associated with viral variants containing an inactive pre-C region. Virology 176: 596–603

Triques K, Coste J, Perret JL et al. (1999) Efficiencies of four versions of the AMPLICOR HIV-1 MONITOR test for quantification of different subtypes of human immunodeficiency virus type 1. J Clin Microbiol 37: 110–116

Tsujimura M, Matsushita K, Shiraki H (1995) Human parvovirus B19 infection in blood donors. Vox Sang 69: 206–212

Turner AR, MacDonald RN, Cooper BA (1972) Transmission of infectious mononucleosis by transfusion of pre-illness plasma. Ann Intern Med 77: 751

Turner BG, Summers MF (1999) Structural biology of HIV. J Mol Biol 285: 1–32

Turner TB, Diseker TK (1941) Duration of infectivity of Treponema pallidum in citrated blood stored under conditions obtaining in blood banks. Bull Johns Hopkins Hosp 68: 269

US Food and Drug Administration (1998) Guidance for Industry: donor screening for antibodies to HTLV-2. Rockville, MD

UK Haemophilia Centre (1986) Prevalence of antibody to HTLV-III in haemophiliacs in the United Kingdom. BMJ 293: 175–176

UKBTS/NIBSC Liaison Group (2001) Guidelines for the Blood Transfusion Services. London: HMSO

Umemura T, Yeo AE, Sottini A et al. (2001) SEN virus infection and its relationship to transfusion-associated hepatitis. Hepatology 33: 1303–1311

UNAIDS (2004) Report on the Global AIDS Epidemic, July, 2004. Joint United Nations program on HIV/AIDS

Uyttendaele S, Claeys H, Mertens HW (1994) Evaluation of third-generation screening and confirmatory assays for HCV antibodies. Vox Sang 66: 122–129

Vallejo A, Lopez-Estebaranz JL, Ortiz-Romero P (1995) Is *Mycosis fungoides* associated with HTLV-I? Vox Sang 69: 84

Valleron AJ, Boelle PY, Will R *et al.* (2001) Estimation of epidemic size and incubation time based on age characteristics of vCJD in the United Kingdom. Science 294: 1726–1728

van der Meer J, Daenen S, van Imhoff GW *et al.* (1986) Absence of seroconversion for HTLV-III in haemophiliacs intensively treated with heat treated factor VIII concentrate. BMJ 1292: 1049

Vandelli C, Renzo F, Romano L *et al.* (2004) Lack of evidence of sexual transmission of hepatitis C among monogamous couples: results of a 10-year prospective follow-up study. Am J Gastroenterol 99: 855–859

Vernant JC, Maurs L, Gessain A *et al.* (1987) Endemic tropical spastic paraparesis associated with T-lymphotropic virus type I: a clinical and seroepidemiological study of 25 cases. Ann Neurol 21: 123–130

Veronese FD, Copeland TD, Oroszlan S *et al.* (1988) Biochemical and immunological analysis of human immunodeficiency virus gag gene products p17 and p24. J Virol 62: 795–801

Vicenzi E, Bagnarelli P, Santagostino E *et al.* (1997) Hemophilia and nonprogressing human immunodeficiency virus type 1 infection. Blood 89: 191–200

Vij R, DiPersio JF, Venkatraman P *et al.* (2003) Donor CMV serostatus has no impact on CMV viremia or disease when prophylactic granulocyte transfusions are given following allogeneic peripheral blood stem cell transplantation. Blood 101: 2067–2069

Villalba R, Fornés C, Alvarez MA *et al.* (1992) Acute Chagas' disease in a recipient of a bone marrow transplant in Spain: case report. Clin Infect Dis 14: 594–595

Vilmer E, Montagnier L, Chermann JC *et al.* (1984) Isolation of a new lymphotropic retrovirus from two siblings with haemophilia B, one with AIDS. Lancet i: 753–757

Vogt M, Lang T, Frosner G *et al.* (1999) Prevalence and clinical outcome of hepatitis C infection in children who underwent cardiac surgery before the implementation of blood-donor screening. N Engl J Med 341: 866–870

Voller A, Draper CC (1982) Immunodiagnosis and seroepidemiology of malaria. Br Med Bull 38: 173–177

Vrielink H, Reesink HW (2004) HTLV-I/II prevalence in different geographic locations. Transfusion Med Rev 18: 46–57

Vrielink H, Zaaijer HL, van der Poel CL *et al.* (1996a) New strip immunoblot for the confirmation of HTLVI/II infection. Vox Sang 70: 114–116

Vrielink H, Reesink HW, Zaaijer HL *et al.* (1996b) Sensitivity and specificity of four assays to detect human T-lymphotropic virus type I/II antibodies. Transfusion 36: 344–346

Wagner SJ (2002) Virus inactivation in blood components by photoactive phenothiazine dyes. Transfusion Med Rev 16: 61–66

Wagner SJ, Storry JR, Mallory DA *et al.* (1993) Red cell alterations associated with virucidal methylene blue phototreatment. Transfusion 33: 30–36

Wain-Hobson S, Sonigo P, Danos O *et al.* (1985) Nucleotide sequence of the AIDS virus, LAV. Cell 40: 9–17

Wallace J, Milne GR, Barr A (1972) Total screening of blood donations for Australia (hepatitis associated) antigen and its antibody. BMJ i: 663

Walsh JH, Purcell RH, Morrow AG *et al.* (1970) Posttransfusion hepatitis after open-heart operations. JAMA 211: 261

Walter CW, Kundsin RB, Button LN (1957) New technique for detection of bacterial contamination in a blood bank using plastic equipment. N Engl J Med 257: 364

Wands JR, Fujita YK, Isselbacher KJ *et al.* (1986) Identification and transmission of hepatitis B virus-related variants. Proc Natl Acad Sci USA 83: 6608–6612

Wang SA, Tokars JI, Bianchine PJ *et al.* (2000) *Enterobacter cloacae* bloodstream infections traced to contaminated human albumin. Clin Infect Dis 30: 35–40

Wang YJ, Lee SO, Hwang SJ *et al.* (1994) Incidence of posttransfusion hepatitis before and after screening for hepatitis C virus antibody. Vox Sang 67: 187–190

Ward JW, Deppe DA, Samson S *et al.* (1987) Risk of human immunodeficiency virus infection from blood donors who later developed the acquired immunodeficiency syndrome. Ann Intern Med 106: 61–62

Ward JW, Holmberg SD, Allen JR *et al.* (1988) Transmission of human immunodeficiency virus (HIV) by blood transfusions screened as negative for HIV antibody. N Engl J Med 318: 473–478

Ward JW, Bush TJ, Perkins HA *et al.* (1989) The natural history of transfusion-associated infection with human immunodeficiency virus. N Engl J Med 321: 947–952

Watanabe T, Seiki M, Yoshida M (1984) HTLV type I (US isolate) and ATLV (Japanese isolate) are the same species of human retrovirus. Virology 133: 238–241

Weiland D, Mattsson L, Glaumann H (1986) Non-A, non-B hepatitis after intravenous gammaglobulin. Lancet i: 976–977

Weiner AJ, Brauer MJ, Rosenblatt J *et al.* (1991) Variable and hypervariable domains are found in the regions of HCV corresponding to the flavivirus envelope and NS1 proteins and the pestivirus envelope glycoproteins. Virology 180: 842–848

Weiss RA (2002) HIV receptors and cellular tropism. IUBMB Life 53: 201–205

Wells GM, Woodward TE, Fiset P *et al.* (1978) Rocky mountain spotted fever caused by blood transfusion. JAMA 239: 2763–2765

Wells L, Ala FA (1985) Malaria and blood transfusion. Lancet i: 1317–1319

Wendel S (1993) Chagas' disease: an old entity in new places. Int J Artif Organs 16: 117–119

Wendel S (1995) Current concepts on transmission of bacteria and parasites by blood transfusion. Vox Sang 67, Suppl. 3: 161–175

Wendel S, Gonzaga AL (1993) Chagas' disease and blood transfusion: a new world problem? Vox Sang 64: 1–12:

Westphal R (1991a) Other parasitic organisms transmitted by transfusion. In: Transfusion-transmitted Infections. DM Smith, RY Dodd (eds). Chicago, IL: ASCP Press, pp. 181–193

Westphal R (1991b) Transfusion-transmitted malarial infections. In: Transfusion-transmitted Infections. DM Smith, RY Dodd (eds). Chicago, IL ASCP Press, pp. 167–180

White DG, Mortimer PP, Blake AD et al. (1985) Human parvovirus arthropathy. Lancet ii: 419–421

White GC, Lesesne HR (1983) Hemophilia, hepatitis, and the acquired immunodeficiency syndrome. Ann Intern Med 98: 403–404

WHO (1986) Severe and complicated malaria. Trans R Soc Trop Med Hyg 80: 1–50

WHO (1990) Acquired immunodeficiency syndrome (AIDS). Proposed criteria for interpreting results from Western blot assays for HIV-1, HIV-2 and HTLV-I/HTLV-II. Weekly Epidemiol Record 65: 281–288

Wiktor SZ, Pate EJ, Weiss SH (1991) Sensitivity of HTLV-I antibody assays for HTLV-II (Letter). Lancet ii: 512–513

Williams AE, Thomson RA, Schreiber GB et al. (1997) Estimates of infectious disease risk factors in US blood donors. Retrovirus Epidemiology Donor Study. JAMA 277: 967–972

Williams MD, Cohen BJ, Bedall AC (1990a) Transmission of human parvovirus B19 by coagulation factor concentrates. Vox Sang 58: 177–181

Williams MD, Skidmore SJ, Hill FGH (1990b) HIV seroconversion in hemophilic boys receiving heat-treated factor VIII concentrate. Vox Sang 58: 135–136

Williamson LM, Llewelyn CA, Fisher NC et al. (1999) A randomized trial of solvent/detergent-treated and standard fresh-frozen plasma in the coagulopathy of liver disease and liver transplantation. Transfusion 39: 1227–1234

Williamson LM, Cardigan R, Prowse CV (2003) Methylene blue-treated fresh-frozen plasma: what is its contribution to blood safety? Transfusion 43: 1322–1329

Wilson K, Code C, Ricketts MN (2000) Risk of acquiring Creutzfeldt-Jakob disease from blood transfusions: systematic review of case-control studies. BMJ 321: 17–19

Winston DJ, Ho WG, Howell CL (1980) Cytomegalovirus infections associated with leukocyte transfusions. Ann Intern Med 93: 671–675

Wolfe MS (1975) Parasites, other than malaria, transmissible by blood transfusion. In: Transmissible Disease and Blood Transfusion. TJ Greenwalt, GA Jamieson (eds). New York: Grune & Stratton

Wolfe ND, Switzer WM, Carr JK et al. (2004) Naturally acquired simian retrovirus infections in central African hunters. Lancet 363: 932–937

Wollowitz S, Fano Y, Jiatao P (1994) Novel psoralens with enhanced UVA dependent inactivation of human immunodeficiency virus and reduced mutagenicity in the absence of UVA light. Transfusion (Suppl.): 715

Wong-Staal F, Gallo RC (1985) Human T-lymphotropic retroviruses. Nature (Lond) 317: 395–403

Wong-Staal F, Shaw GM, Hahn BH (1985) Genomic diversity of human T-lymphotrophic virus type III (HTLV-III). Science 229: 759–762

Wood EE (1955) Brucellosis as a hazard of blood transfusion. BMJ i: 27

Worm HC, Schlauder GG, Wurzer H et al. (2000) Identification of a novel variant of hepatitis E virus in Austria: sequence, phylogenetic and serological analysis. J Gen Virol 81: 2885–2890

Wyler DJ (1983) Resurgence, resistance and research. N Engl J Med 308: 875–940

Yap PL, McOmish F, Webster ADB (1993) Hepatitis C virus transmission by intravenous immunoglobulin. Hepatology 21: 455–468

Yarranton H, Cohen H, Pavord SR et al. (2003) Venous thromboembolism associated with the management of acute thrombotic thrombocytopenic purpura. Br J Haematol 121: 778–785

Yarrish RL, Janas JAS, Nosanchuk JS (1982) Transfusion malaria. Treatment with exchange transfusion after delayed diagnosis. Arch Intern Med 142: 187–188

Yeager AS, Grumet FC, Hafleigh EB (1981) Prevention of transfusion-acquired cytomegalovirus infections in newborn infants. J Pediatr 98: 281–287

Yei S, Yu MW (1992) Partitioning of hepatitis C virus during Cohn-Oncley fractionation of plasma. Transfusion 32: 824–828

Yerram N, Forster P, Goodrich T (1994) Comparison of virucidal properties of brominated psoralen with 8-methoxy psoralen (8-MOP) and aminomethyltrimethylpsoralen (AMT) in platelet concentrates. Transfusion 34 (Suppl.): 402a

Yomtovian R, Lazarus HM, Goodnough LT (1993) A prospective microbiologic surveillance program to detect and prevent the transfusion of bacterially contaminated platelets. Transfusion 33: 902–909

York-Higgins D, Cheng-Mayer C, Bauer D (1990) Human immunodeficiency virus type 1 cellular host range, replication and cytopathy are linked to the envelope region of the viral genome. J Virol 64: 4016–4020

Yoshiba M, Okamoto H, Mishiro S (1995) Detection of the GBV-C hepatitis virus genome in serum from patients with fulminant unknown aetiology. Lancet 346: 1131–1132

Yoshida M, Miyoshi I, Hinuma Y (1982) Isolation and characterization of retrovirus from cell lines of human adult T-cell leukemia and its implications in the disease. Proc Natl Acad Sci USA 79: 2031–2035

Yoshioka K, Kakuma S, Wakita T (1992) Detection of hepatitis C virus by polymerase chain reaction and response to interferon-alpha therapy: relationship to genotypes of hepatitis C virus. Hepatology 16: 293–299

Yoshizawa H, Itoh Y, Iwakiri S et al. (1981) Demonstration of two different types of non-A, non-B hepatitis by reinjection and cross-challenge studies in chimpanzees. Gastroenterology 81: 107–113

Young H, Moyes A, McMillan A (1992) Enzyme immunoassay for anti-treponemal IgG: screening or confirmatory test? J Clin Pathol 45: 37–41

Young N, Mortimer P (1984) Viruses and bone marrow failure. Blood 63: 729–737

Young NS, Brown KE (2004) Parvovirus B19. N Engl J Med 350: 586–597

Zaaijer HL, Cuijpers HTM, Dudok DW (1994) Results of 1-year screening of donors in the Netherlands for human T-lymphotropic virus (HTLV) type I: significance of Western blot patterns for confirmation of HTLV infection. Transfusion 34: 877–880

Zakrzewska K, Azzi A, Patou G (1992) Human parvovirus B19 in clotting concentrates: B19 DNA detection by the nested polymerase chain reaction. Br J Haematol 81: 407–412

Zanella A, Rossi F, Cesana C (1995) Transfusion-transmitted human parvovirus B19 infection in a thalassemic patient. Transfusion 35: 769–772

Zanghellini F, Boppana SB, Emery VC et al. (1999) Asymptomatic primary cytomegalovirus infection: virologic and immunologic features. J Infect Dis 180: 702–707

Zaunders JJ, Dyer WB, Wang B et al. (2004) Identification of circulating antigen-specific CD4+ T lymphocytes with a CCR5+, cytotoxic phenotype in an HIV-1 long-term nonprogressor and in CMV infection. Blood 103: 2238–2247

Zucker-Franklin D, Seremetis S, Zheng ZY (1990) Internalization of human immunodeficiency virus type 1 and other retrovirus by megakaryocytes and platelets. Blood 75: 1920–1923

Zuckerman AJ (1990) Viral hepatitis. Br Med Bull 46: 1–564

Zuckerman AJ, Taylor PE (1969) Persistence of the serum hepatitis (SH-Australia) antigen for many years. Nature (Lond) 223: 81

Zuckerman AR (1996) Alphabet of hepatitis viruses. Lancet 347: 558–559

17 Exchange transfusion and haemapheresis

Exchange transfusion

An impressive exchange transfusion was carried out in dogs by Dr Richard Lower of Oxford in February 1666. The donors were two very large mastiffs and the recipient was a smaller dog. After drawing a large quantity of blood from the jugular vein of the smaller dog, blood from one of the donors was taken from its cervical artery and allowed to flow through a silver tube into the vein of the smaller dog. Blood was drawn from the recipient at intervals. After the first donor had been exsanguinated, the second was used in a similar fashion. Lower calculated that by the end of the experiment the recipient had received (and lost) an amount of blood equal to the weight of the whole body. 'Yet, once its jugular vein was sewn up and its binding shackles tossed off it promptly jumped down from the table and apparently oblivious of its hurts soon began to fondle its master and to roll on the grass to clean himself of the blood, exactly as it would have done if it had merely been thrown into a stream and with no more sign of discomfort or displeasure' [Lower, 1669, translated from the Latin (Keynes 1949)].

Another account of Lower's experiments was communicated through the Royal Society by Robert Boyle (Boyle 1666a). Some practical notes of the method are followed by some reflections, the final one of which reads: 'The most probable use of this Experiment may be conjectured to be that one Animal may live with the bloud of another: and consequently that those Animals, that want bloud, or have corrupt bloud, may be supplied from other with a sufficient quantity, and of such as is good, provided the Transfusion be often repeated, by reason of the quick expence that is made of the bloud'.

Following the account of the operation, mention was made of planned blood exchanges of old and young, sick and healthy, hot and cold, fierce and fearful, tame and wild animals, etc. although it was predicted 'that the exchange of bloud will not alter the nature or disposition of the animals on which it shall be practised'.

In a later volume of the *Philosophical Transactions* (Boyle 1666b), Boyle proposed to Dr Lower various questions that might be answered by transfusion experiments, for example: 'Whether a Dog that is sick of some disease chiefly imputable to the mass of bloud, may be cured by exchanging it with that of a sound Dog? And whether a sound Dog may receive such diseases from the bloud of a sick one, as are not otherwise of an infectious nature?'.

Exsanguination–transfusion seems to have been first used in man to treat severe toxaemias. Initial experiments were carried out in rabbits; blood was withdrawn from one vein and donor blood simultaneously transfused into another. The method was then applied to humans with various toxaemias (including a case of resorcin poisoning) and appeared to have reduced mortality substantially (Robertson 1924). Although exchange transfusion continued to be used up to about 1975 for removing toxic substances from plasma, plasma exchange has now replaced the procedure for this purpose. On the other hand, a few conditions still require removal of the subject's red cells, for example haemolytic disease of the newborn (see Chapter 12) and sickle cell anaemia (see Chapter 9), and in these conditions exchange transfusion using whole blood or red cells is indicated.

Exchange transfusion of whole blood is more practicable than plasma exchange for removing toxic substances from the plasma of infants, as blood cell separators suitable for use in small children have not been developed.

Principles of haemapheresis exchange transfusion

The objective of haemapheresis is efficient removal of some circulating blood component, either cells (cytapheresis) or some plasma solute (plasmapheresis). For therapeutic applications, the treatment goal is to deplete the circulating cell or substance directly responsible for the disease process. For collection of blood components for transfusion, the aim is efficient removal of the most specific element(s) without causing sufficient depletion to harm the donor (see below).

Calculation of volume replaced

Formulae that predict the percentage of blood exchanged in replacement transfusion were designed by Wallerstein and Brodie (1948). When replacement is being carried out continuously and one homogeneous fluid is being replaced by another, for example plasma by 5% albumin, the percentage of original plasma remaining at time $t = 100e^{(v/V)t}$. The exchange of a volume equivalent to the subject's blood volume leaves 37% of the original fluid and an exchange equivalent to twice the blood volume leaves 13.5%.

When exchange is carried out by an intermittent method, as for example in exchange transfusion in newborn infants, and again assuming that one homogeneous fluid is being replaced by another, the percentage of the original blood remaining after n operations, where V = the original blood volume and v the volume of blood removed at each operation = $[(V - v)/V]^n$. Even when the packed cell volumes (PCVs) of the transfused blood and of the patient's blood happen to be the same, the formula is not applicable because the red cells are not uniformly distributed throughout the vascular system; a more elaborate formula is needed to predict the rate of red cell exchange. If the blood volume of the infant (assumed to be constant during exchange transfusion) is V ml, v ml is removed and replaced at each operation, H_o is the initial venous haematocrit of the infant's blood, H_d is the haematocrit of the donor's blood and k is the ratio of the whole body haematocrit to the venous haematocrit (see Appendix 4), the fraction of the infant's original

cells remaining after n operations is calculated by the formula:

$$\frac{H_n}{H_o} = \left(1 - \frac{v}{kV}\right)^n \qquad (17.1)$$

where H_n is the venous haematocrit of the recipient's own red cells after n operations. The total PCV after n operations is calculated by:

$$H_n = H_o\left(1 - \frac{v}{kV}\right)^n + H_d\left(1 - \left(1 - \frac{v}{kV}\right)^n\right) \qquad (17.2)$$

The first term represents the patient's residual red cells and the second term the donor's red cells (Veall and Mollison 1950).

When the method of intermittent substitution is used for plasma exchange, a similar formula can be derived for calculating the rate of exchange (Veall and Mollison 1950; Mollison et al. 1950) (see also 'Therapeutic plasma exchange', below).

Sophisticated equations are not necessary in practice. Removal of most blood components follows a logarithmic curve (Fig. 17.1) (McCullough and Chopek 1981). This model assumes that the component removed is neither synthesized nor degraded substantially during the procedure, remains within the intravascular compartment and mixes instantaneously and completely with any replacement solution. When

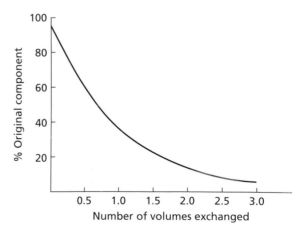

Fig 17.1 Relation between volumes removed by apheresis and percentage of the target component remaining. The relation is valid for blood volumes during red cell exchange or for plasma volumes during plasmapheresis if the target solute remains primarily within the intravascular space. Adapted from Chopek and McCullough (1981) Lab Med 12: 745.

the goal of plasmapheresis is to supply a deficient substance, for example plasma factors in the treatment of thrombotic thrombocytopenic purpura, replacement follows logarithmic kinetics similar to those developed for solute removal. From Fig. 17.1, it should be evident that removal of 1.5–2 volumes will reduce an intravascular substance by about 60% and that processing larger volumes results in little additional gain.

Indications for red cell exchange (erythrocytapheresis)

Sickle cell disease

Red cell exchange (erythrocytapheresis) is used most often to manage or prevent the acute vaso-occlusive complications of sickle cell disease. Automated blood cell separators are faster and easier than manual exchange transfusion (Klein *et al.* 1980; Klein 1982). Most new instruments calculate the exchange conditions after the patient's laboratory and clinical data are entered into a pre-programmed exchange protocol.

Sickle cell anaemia occurs in individuals who are homozygous for a single mutation in codon 6 of the beta globin gene, resulting in substitution of a single amino acid. Although the defect appears simple, the genetics may be further complicated by other polymorphisms in the haemoglobin molecule or mutations in control of chain synthesis. The pathophysiology of the vaso-occlusive crises is even more complex, involving haemoglobin polymerization, change in cell shape, adhesion to endothelial cells, release of inflammatory cytokines and nitric oxide binding by free haemoglobin (Kaul *et al.* 1996, 1998, 2000; Reiter and Gladwin 2003). Clinical manifestations vary from patient to patient and there may be distinct clinical phenotypes (Alexander *et al.* 2004). The rationale behind exchange transfusion involves improving tissue oxygenation and preventing microvascular sickling by diluting the patient's abnormal red cells, and simultaneously correcting anaemia and favourably altering whole blood viscosity and rheology. No clinical data support a single optimal level of haemoglobin A (HbA); however, as few as 30% of transfused cells markedly decrease blood viscosity; at mixtures of > 50%, resistance to membrane filterability approaches normal (Anderson *et al.* 1963; Lessin *et al.* 1978; Kurantsin-Mills *et al.* 1988). In non-emergency situations, such levels can often be achieved with a simple transfusion regimen. For simple and exchange transfusions, raising the level of HbA to 60–70% while lowering the level of HbS to 30% is generally efficacious, although even higher levels of HbA may be required to treat an ongoing crisis. The percentage of HbA in a sample of patient's blood may continue to rise after transfusion as the short survival of the sickle cells results in a survival advantage for the transfused cells.

Clinical indications for exchange transfusion in patients with sickle cell anaemia remain controversial. Limited controlled study data are available. Simple transfusion has been shown to improve renal concentrating ability and splenic function in young sickle cell patients; exchange transfusion improves exercise tolerance and reverses the periodic oscillations in cutaneous blood flow associated with this disease (Keitel *et al.* 1956; Pearson *et al.* 1970; Miller *et al.* 1980; Rodgers *et al.* 1984). Such observations have encouraged the use of exchange transfusion for acute complications of sickle cell disease such as chest syndrome, priapism, cerebrovascular accident, and hepatic and retinal infarction. Exchange transfusion for sickle cell patients has also been used for prophylaxis during pregnancy and before surgery, although prophylactic transfusion in these settings is controversial. The only randomized trial of transfusion during pregnancy has shown that prophylactic transfusion sufficient to reduce the incidence of painful crises did not reduce other maternal morbidity or perinatal mortality (Koshy *et al.* 1988). In a randomized study of sickle cell disease patients undergoing surgery, a conservative simple transfusion regimen to increase the haemoglobin level to 10 g/dl was as effective as an aggressive regimen (to lower the HbS level to < 30%) with respect to perioperative non-transfusion-related complications (Vichinsky *et al.* 1995). The patients in the aggressive regimen group received twice as many units of blood, had a proportionally increased red blood cell alloimmunization rate and suffered more haemolytic transfusion reactions. The results of this and other studies suggest that if prophylactic preoperative exchange transfusion is used, it should be limited to patients undergoing high-risk procedures in whom simple transfusion could not effectively raise the HbA level to > 70%.

Transfusion prophylaxis is now clearly indicated for children at high risk for stroke. A randomized controlled study demonstrated a risk reduction of 90%

in the patients who were maintained at levels of HbS < 30% by simple or exchange transfusion (Adams *et al.* 1998). This result confirms earlier experience (Russell *et al.* 1984) and indicates that in this group of children with sickle cell anaemia, transfusion therapy should begin before the first event and continue indefinitely. Long-term erythrocytapheresis may be preferable for patients at high risk for stroke who have developed iron overload to levels associated with organ damage (Kim *et al.* 1994). However, patients remain in positive iron balance, although iron accumulation is slow and chelation is rarely required to prevent transfusional haemosiderosis. Use of exchange transfusion for adults is extrapolated from the paediatric experience, as no equivalent systematic data have been collected.

Exchange transfusion, although relatively safe, carries all the complications of red cell transfusion. Patients are exposed to a large number of donors and are at a small but significant risk of contracting hepatitis and other blood-borne infections (see Chapter 16). As many as 33% of all patients develop alloantibodies, and life-threatening delayed haemolytic transfusion reactions have been reported (Diamond *et al.* 1980; Coles *et al.* 1981). In addition, a study of multiply transfused sickle cell patients found that 85% of heavily transfused patients had been alloimmunized to HLA and/or platelet-specific antigens (Friedman *et al.* 1996). Extended red blood cell phenotyping at diagnosis and provision of phenotypically matched blood can reduce the risk of red cell alloimmunization and associated haemolytic transfusion reactions (Rosse *et al.* 1990; Vichinsky *et al.* 1990; Castro *et al.* 2002). However, providing extended matching may be difficult for chronic transfusion programmes, and a reasonable compromise concentrates on matching for the most immunogenic, clinically important antigens, D, E, K and C.

Haemolytic disease of the newborn

See Chapter 12 and Appendix 13.

Exchange transfusion in other conditions

Other indications for red cell exchange are rare. The procedure has been used for patients with overwhelming red cell parasitic infections, such as severe and complicated malaria and babesiosis (Miller *et al.*

1989). In these situations, red cell exchange decreases the concentration of circulating parasites and may help sustain life until conventional therapy and natural immunity take effect. Although the efficacy of this therapy has not been evaluated by controlled trials, prospective studies and review of published cases consider erythrocytapheresis prudent when parasitaemia exceeds 10–15%, and even at lower levels in selected patients (Powell and Grima 2002). Automated red cell removal with volume replacement (isovolaemic haemodilution) can be performed rapidly and safely in polycythaemic subjects. This manoeuvre should be reserved for polycythaemic patients with an urgent clinical indication to lower the haematocrit (e.g. evolving thrombotic stroke) for which standard single-unit manual phlebotomy might be inadvisably slow. Automated double red cell apheresis technology has been used more recently to treat individuals with hereditary haemochromatosis (Leitman *et al.* 2003a) (see Chapter 1). This procedure removes excess iron more rapidly than manual phlebotomy, and may be more tolerable to patients due to the lower frequency of maintenance procedures required. Red cell exchange is occasionally indicated when a patient is found to have been recently transfused with incompatible red cells or as an adjunct to RH-Ig therapy when a D-negative woman of child-bearing age who is not already immunized to D has been inadvertently transfused with a large volume of D-positive cells.

Plasmapheresis

A short history of plasmapheresis

Plasmapheresis is a distant relative of ancient bloodletting but, unlike phlebotomy, apheresis has its origins in the research laboratory and relies heavily on science and technology. John Jacob Abel in 1914 coined the term *plasmapheresis*, from a Greek verb meaning 'to take away or withdraw', to describe removal of plasma and return of the remaining blood components to the donor. Abel and colleagues (1914) described the technique of plasma removal as an investigational treatment for toxaemia in nephrectomized dogs, but foresaw a variety of additional potential applications. Their studies, like those of contemporaries in Germany and Russia, relied upon cumbersome phlebotomy, centrifugation and resuspension techniques, as well as anticoagulation with the leech-derived protein, hirudin. The results of Abel and colleagues were clouded by technique-related deaths of several experimental animals.

The first manual plasmapheresis procedures in humans were likewise conducted for experimental purposes to determine the normal rate of protein regeneration in six volunteer donors (Tui *et al.* 1944). The procedure proved safe, although one volunteer experienced a pyrogenic reaction, most likely related to contamination of the reusable glass bottle system that was employed for blood donation in the 1940s. A similar manual technique was put into practice by Grifols-Lucas (1952), the first use of an apheresis procedure to provide components for transfusion. Whole blood was removed from the donor, and red cells were either allowed to sediment by gravity or packed by centrifugation, removed and returned to the donor, often as long as a week after the initial phlebotomy. In the same report, Grifols-Lucas described the use of manual plasmapheresis to treat a few patients with hypertension and recorded what is arguably the first placebo effect with therapeutic apheresis, 'striking subjective improvement, which, however, is not matched by a corresponding betterment of the objective symptoms'. A further refinement of manual plasmapheresis relied upon a closed-system vacuum bottle technique to remove plasma from a patient with macroglobulinaemia (Adams *et al.* 1952).

Although the early manual methods demonstrated the feasibility of plasmapheresis for collecting components and for therapy, glass bottles proved awkward, and reusable equipment raised concern about contamination with bacteria and pyrogens. With the introduction of sterile, disposable, interconnected plastic blood bags, plasmapheresis became relatively safe and easy (Skoog and Adams 1959). The integral-bag procedure required only minor modifications in centrifuge technique for single-donor platelet collections (Kliman *et al.* 1961). However, manual apheresis proved too slow, inefficient and labour intensive for large component volumes and engendered concerns that the separated units of red cells might be returned accidentally to the wrong donor or patient, with potentially fatal consequences (Cumberland *et al.* 1991). The introduction of automated on-line blood cell separators solved these problems.

Automated on-line blood processing arose from the seminal studies of Edwin J Cohn and collaborators, who developed an *ex vivo* refrigerated, sealed-bowl system for centrifugal separation of blood components (Tullis *et al.* 1956). This system evolved into a single-arm instrument capable of separating plasma or cellular blood elements in a plastic, disposable bowl and returning the unwanted components to the donor in a batch-processing fashion (Latham 1986). Almost concurrently, a scientific team from the IBM Corporation and the National Cancer Institute was developing a continuous-flow instrument, modelled after the first mechanical heart–lung oxygenator, for collecting granulocytes and platelets from blood donors (Freireich *et al.* 1965; Jones 1988). These early instruments had reusable parts, rotating seals on the centrifuge bowls and numerous rings and external connections. A system that eliminates seals for continuous-flow centrifuges has been designed and is now used by several manufacturers (Ito *et al.* 1975).

Although centrifugal cell separation was the earliest and most widely used apheresis technique, automated equipment was also designed to collect granulocytes by filtration or, more accurately, by granulocyte adhesion to nylon filters (Djerassi and Kim 1977). Problems with haemocompatibility and donor reactions led to the abandonment of this technique. However, the success of haemodialysis and the desire to effect more selective separation of plasma proteins spurred further development of filtration and column technology.

Plasmapheresis vs. plasma exchange

When relatively small amounts of plasma, for example 500–650 ml, are removed, without infusing any fluid as a replacement, or infusing only saline, plasmapheresis is the appropriate term for the whole operation. When more than this amount of plasma is removed it becomes advisable to infuse a crystalloid or colloid such as albumin or, occasionally, plasma to replace part or all of the lost plasma protein. This operation constitutes plasma exchange.

The need for plasma for fractionation is still greater than the need for red cells. As a consequence, plasmapheresis is used in some countries, such as the USA, as a method of collecting fresh plasma from normal donors for fractionation into plasma derivatives. Plasma from particular donors, for example donors hyperimmunized to Rh D, tetanus or HBsAg, needed to obtain specific immunoglobulins, is also collected by apheresis. As described in a later section, plasma exchange is carried out for therapeutic purposes with the object of removing some particular constituent from a patient's plasma.

Plasmapheresis: from plastic packs to blood cell separators

In early practice, whole blood was drawn into a primary pack with anticoagulant and a series of attached satellite packs. The blood was centrifuged while the intravenous line was maintained with a saline drip. The plasma or platelet-rich plasma (PRP) was extracted and retained, and the red cells were returned to the donor. The whole procedure was repeated ('double plasmapheresis'), yielding a total of approximately 500 ml of citrated plasma. With modern blood bank refrigerated centrifuges, double plasmapheresis can be completed in less than 1 h.

Because manual plasmapheresis is cumbersome and time consuming and carries some additional hazards, automated equipment is now used routinely (see below). The most serious hazard is that red cell units may be interchanged so that a donor suffers a haemolytic transfusion reaction (Cumberland *et al.* 1991).

The advantages of automated apheresis are that (1) donors are never disconnected from their own blood, thus eliminating the risk of introducing the red cells or other blood components from another donor, (2) the speed of collection is considerably faster than in manual apheresis, (3) the procedure is preferred to manual apheresis by donors and (4) the total extracorporeal volume at any one time is less than in double (manual) plasmapheresis. A major advantage is the use of totally disposable harnesses, the majority of which are available prepacked as sterile, closed systems.

Several machines have been designed exclusively for plasma removal based on the principle of either separation of blood components by centrifugation or filtration through a spinning cylindrical membrane. Cell separators use special sterile tubing preconnected to the centrifugation receptacle, containers with fluids (anticoagulant, saline) and collection bags, all known as the harness or 'kit'. With modern instruments, the anticoagulant is metered in an automated way, often controlled by a microprocessor.

Centrifugal separation involves either continuous or discontinuous flow. Both systems allow centrifugation of the blood without twisting or kinking of the external tubing connected to the moving centrifuge parts either by the use of a rotary seal with one face stationary and the other moving, or by using a flexible jump-rope type of seal-less connector based on the Adams principle (Ito *et al.* 1975; Stong 1975; Suaudeau *et al.* 1978). In the discontinuous system, following the separation and removal of the plasma, centrifugation stops while the cells are returned to the donor (Fig. 17.2). Depending on the size of the bowl, approximately 250–500 ml of blood is processed with each cycle. The cycles are repeated as often as necessary to obtain the required volume of platelet-poor

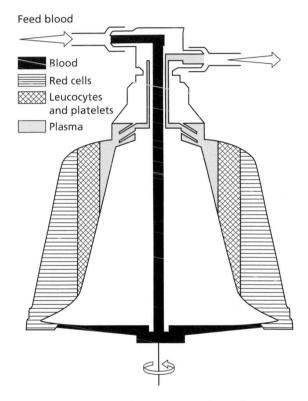

Fig 17.2 Cross-section of an intermittent-flow cell separator bowl (Haemonetics Model A-30 Latham bowl), redrawn from a diagram supplied by the Haemonetics Corporation. Blood is fed into the bottom of a disposable, polycarbonate, rotating bowl and, after separation of the components of blood into layers, different fractions may be harvested sequentially into separate plastic bags. The required fraction, for example that containing the platelets, is retained for transfusion to a patient and the remaining components are returned to the donor. The whole operation may then be repeated.

plasma (PPP). The disadvantages of the discontinuous system are slower performance and greater extra-corporeal volume; the main advantages, which make the system ideal for plasmapheresis, are simplicity and the need for a single venous access.

The advantages of apheresis plasma for fractionation are: (1) in general it can be frozen more rapidly after collection than plasma derived from whole blood donation ('recovered plasma'), yielding 5% higher recovery of factor VIII; (2) donors with blood groups (A, B and AB) with higher factor VIII yields can be selected; and (3) small volume, metered anticoagulants designed for maximum recovery of plasma (such as 4% citrate) can be used rather than larger proportions of anticoagulant-preservative solutions needed for red cell storage. A further advantage of plasma collected by apheresis is that the size of the donor panel is limited. Small pools prepared from such plasma, and subjected to pasteurization or solvent–detergent treatment to inactivate viruses, are used at present in several European countries. In addition, single units of apheresis plasma can be treated with methylene blue. Plasma collected by apheresis may differ from plasma collected by simple centrifugation, and apheresis plasma itself is not a uniform product. The platelet content in plasma for fractionation varies from $8 \pm 2.4 \times 10^9/l$, obtained with some cell separators to $60 \pm 30 \times 10^9/l$ in some plasma from routine donations.

Effects of intensive or long-continued plasmapheresis

Plasmapheresis of donors may be performed at three levels (WHO 1989b): (1) The donor gives plasma at the same frequency as that allowed for whole blood; (2) the volume of plasma taken and the frequency of donations are two or three times that allowed for routine donations; and (3) 1000–1200 ml of plasma are collected weekly, reaching an annual volume of 50–60 l of plasma per donor, depending on whether the weight of the donor is below or above 80 kg. With this programme, protein levels do not return to initial values although, in most healthy well-nourished donors, levels remain within the normal range.

Intensive plasmapheresis equivalent to levels 2 and 3, and long-term plasmapheresis, appear to be well tolerated in healthy subjects (Cohen and Oberman 1970; Friedman *et al.* 1975). However, when 1000 ml of plasma is removed weekly for long periods, if

equilibrium is to be maintained, an extra 6 g of albumin and 2 g of immunoglobulin G (IgG) must be synthesized daily. These amounts are considerable in relation to the normal production of these proteins, estimated at approximately 12 g of albumin and 2 g of IgG per day (Schultze 1966).

The maximum amount of plasma that may be donated is 50–60 l a year according to regulations in the USA, but only 15 l per year in Europe. As discussed above, when 1 l is donated each week, albumin synthesis must increase by 50% if equilibrium is to be maintained. This figure seems uncomfortably close to the maximum possible increase in albumin synthesis which, in both humans and experimental animals, seldom exceeds 100%. Subjects who donate 1 l of plasma per week lose as much albumin as does a patient with nephrotic syndrome and severe proteinuria (Lundsgaard-Hansen 1977a). Other theoretical risks of intensive plasmapheresis are atherosclerosis due to increased synthesis of low-density and very low-density lipoproteins stimulated by enhanced protein synthesis and platelet aggregation (Lundsgaard-Hansen 1977b). No evidence of increased atherosclerosis in frequent plasma donors has been reported. There is also a reduction in the level of immunoglobulins, especially IgM, although the capacity to mount a normal immune response is maintained (Friedman *et al.* 1975). In donors undergoing long-term third-level plasmapheresis, the plasma concentrations of antithrombin, plasminogen and factor VIII are not significantly affected (Cohen and Oberman 1970; Jaffe and Mosher 1981). In view of the relatively sparse scientific information about the long-term effects of the considerable extra load on protein synthesis and of a depleted total albumin pool, continued careful monitoring of donors is warranted. Several hundreds of donors in London underwent level 2 plasmapheresis (15 l of plasma per year and 600 ml per session with an interval not shorter than 2 weeks between donations) for more than 10 years with no adverse effects; reduced total protein and albumin concentrations have been found only in donors on 'slimming' diets (Brozovic 1984).

During plasmapheresis, most of the platelets are returned to the donor. When PRP is harvested, the donor's platelet count is well maintained until about 5 l of plasma is collected per week; even then, platelet counts return to normal within 3 days of the last donation (Kliman *et al.* 1964).

Care of plasmapheresis donors

The criteria for the acceptability of plasmapheresis donors are slightly stricter than those for routine blood donors. In the UK, plasma donors are accepted for the first time only if they have given blood previously on at least two occasions, if they are under 50 years of age and if their complete blood count and total serum protein are within the normal range. In the USA, annual examination of frequent plasmapheresis donors is required (Solomon 1985). Laboratory tests are carried out periodically and include a full blood count, determination of total serum proteins, of serum albumin and of immunoglobulins as well as screening for urinary protein and glucose.

No donor should be subjected to plasmapheresis without detailed informed consent about the possible hazards (WHO 1989b). If donors are to undergo immunization with vaccines, red cells or blood group substances for the provision of specific immunoglobulins, guidelines to safeguard the donor should be followed (WHO 1975, 1989b).

If plasma donors give whole blood or do not have their red cells returned during apheresis, a period of 8 weeks should elapse before the next plasma donation, unless the physician in charge and the donor agree on the need for and safety of the procedure (WHO 1989a; American Association of Blood Banks 2003).

Harvesting of platelets, leucocytes, red cells and progenitor cells

For the collection of platelets, leucocytes or peripheral blood stem cells (PBSCs), automated blood cell separators use microprocessor technology to draw and anticoagulate blood, separate components either by centrifugation or by filtration, collect the desired component and recombine the remaining components for return to the donor (Hester et al. 1979; Burgstaler 2003).The equipment contains disposable plastic software in the blood path and uses anticoagulants containing citrate or combinations of citrate and heparin that do not result in clinical anticoagulation of the patient or donor. Most instruments function well at blood flow rates of 30–80 ml/min and can operate from peripheral venous access or from a variety of multilumen central venous catheters. Centrifugal separation involves either a discontinuous or a continuous flow.

Intermittent (discontinuous)-flow cell separators

There are several varieties of instruments, all of which have in common a stationary tube, a rotating bowl and a rotating seal (Burgstaler 2003). These seals are now designed to maintain sterility, so that the system is considered 'closed' and the components can be stored for more than 24 h.

PRP can be collected in 30 min. From the PRP, 450 ml of plasma for fractionation and 150 ml of platelet concentrate, containing $2–3 \times 10^{11}$ platelets, can be obtained depending on the donor's platelet count. Platelet concentrates in a volume of approximately 300 ml and containing $3–6 \times 10^{11}$ platelets require twice this time. In-line filters can effect acceptable levels of leucoreduction of the platelet concentrate (Seghatchian et al. 2001). An intermittent-flow cell separator has been designed with the flexibility to collect red cells, platelets or plasma (for clinical use or for fractionation), or any combination of these options depending on the programme chosen (Bandarenko et al. 2001).

Continuous-flow cell separators

Continuous-flow devices were developed initially for the collection of granulocytes (Freireich et al. 1965). Anticoagulated blood is fed continuously into a rapidly rotating chamber or channel in which red cells, leucocytes, platelets and plasma separate into layers (see Figs 17.3 and 17.4). Any layer or layers can be removed through special ports, depending on the harness and programme, and the remainder, together with a replacement fluid, if plasma or red cells are being removed, returned to the patient.

The CS-3000 has two chambers within one centrifugation bowl; citrated blood enters into the first chamber, where red cells are separated from PRP. The chambers are plastic bags fitted into moulds. The PRP is pumped into the second chamber, where the platelets or white cells are removed from plasma depending on the computerized programme and the collection chamber selected. The red cells are returned to the donor and most of the processing is carried out through computer-assisted devices. The donor's extracorporeal volume is much lower, about 300 ml, than with intermittent-flow machines. The absence of a seal in the CS-3000 permits collection of platelets in a closed system, making it safe to store them for more

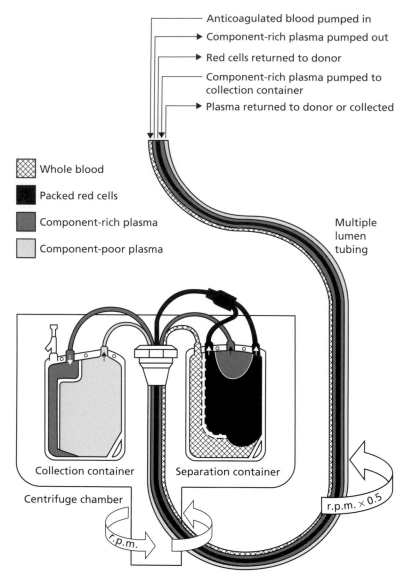

Anticoagulated blood pumped in
Component-rich plasma pumped out
Red cells returned to donor
Component-rich plasma pumped to collection container
Plasma returned to donor or collected

Whole blood
Packed red cells
Component-rich plasma
Component-poor plasma

Multiple lumen tubing

Collection container
Separation container
Centrifuge chamber

r.p.m.
r.p.m. × 0.5

Fig 17.3 Diagram of continuous-flow blood cell separator (Baxter Transfusion Technologies CS-3000). Blood is pumped through one of the five channels of the multiple lumen tube into the separation container. As the centrifuge chamber revolves, the multiple lumen tube revolves round the outside of the chamber at half the speed so that twisting of the tube is avoided and there is no need for a rotating seal. Component-rich, (platelet-rich) plasma is pumped out of the separation container and back into the collection chamber, which can be used directly for transfusion. For further details, see text (diagram supplied by Fenwal Laboratories).

than 24 h. High platelet yields ($3–5 \times 10^{11}$ per 90–110 min procedure) are obtained with the standard platelet separation chamber. Even higher yields (more than 6×10^{11} in 70–90 min) seem possible with a high-efficiency separation chamber insert, although with considerably greater white cell contamination. For this reason, the manufacturer has developed the CS-3000 Plus TNX-6 machine that supersedes the CS-3000 in all aspects of platelet collection: yields of platelets are higher (sufficient for two therapeutic doses), there is

less white cell contamination, and the platelets have a 5-day shelf-life.

The Amicus is smaller than the CS-3000, uses the same basic seal-less harness technology, but has a novel disposable series of cassettes and drive mechanism (Burgstaler 2003). The instrument is fully automated and has a relatively short processing time that yields a predictable, leucoreduced platelet concentrate. This instrument has single- and dual-needle capability, although the dual-needle procedure is used almost exclusively.

Fig 17.4 Diagram of the Spectra LRS Continuous flow separation channel: whole blood entering the channel is separated in the first stage into PRP flowing clockwise and red cells flowing anticlockwise, leaving the channel through the 'RBC out' line. Transfer of all fluids to and from the pumps and the donor is through a closed loop system. The PRP enters the second stage by passing over a dam and is separated into a platelet concentrate and plasma, which is further processed in the LeukoReduction System (LRS) chamber into a leucocyte-poor platelet concentrate. The plasma leaves the channel partly through the 'plasma out' line and partly through the control tube, where it sustains the interface at the desired level in the second stage. Advanced fluid dynamics and fluidized particle bed technology separate out virtually all of the few remaining passenger leucocytes from the platelet concentrate, resulting in a final product with very few leucocytes (diagram supplied by Gambro BCT, Lakewood, CO, USA).

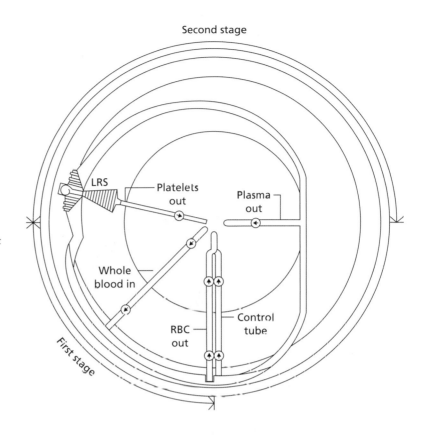

The Spectra models (Gambro BCT, Lakewood, CO, USA) separate the different components of anticoagulated blood on the basis of density; they have a hollow, loop-like, rotating channel in which the blood travels circumferentially and in which centrifugal forces act radially. The centrifugal force and flow rate can be varied by the operator to adjust the composition of the buffy coat, which is then extracted via a tubing manifold into a collection chamber. The outlet port of each component is controlled by a separate pump. There are two types of channel designs, with different positionings and sizes of the exit ports, which are used to collect white cells or perform plasma and white cell exchange by one channel, or plasma exchange alone by another. A third type is configured for red cell exchange. A two-stage channel is available to collect a purer preparation of platelets; in the first stage PRP is separated from the red cells, and in the second stage the PRP enters a spiral and narrow channel in which

the concentrated platelets and PPP are separated (Fig. 17.4). The Spectra cell separator can use any of the three channel designs; the platelets collected with the dual-stage separation channel have little white cell contamination (less than 0.5×10^7 per concentrate) with a yield, after 90-min collection, often above 6×10^{11}, sufficient to enable partitioning of the concentrate into two full adult therapeutic doses. The use of a sterile disposable harness and micropore filters for the anticoagulant and saline makes extended platelet storage safe. A leucoreduction enhancement to the software and harness (LRS in Fig. 17.4) has reduced white cell contamination to less than 1×10^6 in more than 99% of uneventful platelet procedures. The instrument has a small extracorporeal volume and, depending on the programme chosen, is adaptable to different processes, such as platelet collection, plasma exchange, PBSC collection, etc. A programme is available with the Spectra model for single venous access

783

procedures, which is only slightly slower than when two arms are used. Continuous-flow cell separators such as the Spectra tend to use more citrate per procedure giving rise to a greater frequency of hypocalcaemic symptoms.

Several continuous-flow blood cell separators have been designed as on-site component processing systems capable of collecting red cells and other blood components on-line so that donor collections can be matched to blood inventory needs (Leitner *et al.* 2003). These instruments are intended for blood donation only. The intermittent-flow MCS plus has been described above. The Gambro BCT Trima and Trima Accel are continuous-flow devices that use single-needle access and either single-stage or dual-stage chambers similar to those of the Spectra (Rock *et al.* 2003). The Baxter ALYX system is a single-needle, continuous-flow instrument that uses a reservoir system to achieve this match. All of these systems emphasize ease of use, programmed protocols, standardized component collection and flexible programming.

Continuous-flow cell separators have the advantages of speed and, because of the small extracorporeal volume involved, minimal blood volume fluctuations. The disadvantages of these separators are that, in general they are relatively immobile and require two sites of vascular access, although the Spectra is an exception in that it is lighter and more mobile and can be used with one vascular site of access. Detailed technical descriptions of centrifugal systems of cell separation have been compiled by Burgstaler (2003).

Collection of platelets by cell separators

If platelet concentrates are to be stored, gas exchange through an appropriate plastic container is vital to avoid hypoxic conditions that lead to accelerated production of lactic acid and fall in pH. The availability of more permeable or thinner plastics has prolonged the shelf-life of platelet concentrates from 3 to 5 days, and containers suitable for 7-day storage have been produced (see Chapter 14).

Large quantities – at least 3×10^{11} platelets (a 'full dose') – can be collected from single donors using intermittent-flow centrifugation or by continuous-flow centrifugation, which not infrequently yields $6–10 \times 10^{11}$ platelets (a double dose) per collection. The number, 3×10^{11}, is an arbitrary one arrived at by consensus, rather than by some scientific or medical

principle, at a time when instrumentation could not reliably collect greater numbers. The procedure normally requires 1–2 h and a relatively large volume of citrate anticoagulant is returned to the donor. Regardless of the system used, the platelet yield will depend mainly on the donor's platelet count and blood volume before thrombapheresis and on the volume of blood processed. On the other hand, the volume of the platelet concentrate and the degree of white cell contamination will depend on the instrument used. Several studies have shown that platelets collected by apheresis have *in vitro* and *in vivo* functions similar or superior to platelets obtained from units of whole blood, although different collection protocols, containers, preservatives and processing complicate comparisons (Seghatchian and Krailadsiri 2000). Platelets for extended storage should be kept in the appropriate large plastic containers at a concentration suitable to maintain pH between 6.4 and 7.4. In the case of high platelet yields, with double adult doses, i.e. $> 6 \times 10^{11}$ platelets, the concentrate may be split into two storage containers.

The percentage of platelets collected by apheresis in different countries varies and is influenced by historical practice, cost, regulatory hurdles and perhaps by litigation as clinicians strive to limit the number of exposures to allogeneic donors. Some North American centres supply 100% of the platelets as apheresis donations. In the USA approximately 70% of platelet units derive from apheresis collections and more than 40% of collections are split into multiple doses, thus making more efficient use of the platelet donor (National Blood Data Resource Center 2002). When platelets from only one or two donors are needed, as when transfusing infants or using HLA-matched platelets collected by apheresis, donors should avoid aspirin-containing medication within the previous week, as aspirin impairs platelet function. On the other hand, when transfusing pooled concentrates obtained from many different donors, it is unnecessary to reject platelets from donors taking aspirin, as it is unlikely that all donors contributing to a pool will be taking the drug (Slichter 1985).

Yields of platelets with different modern cell separators are similar. Most continuous-flow systems meet the criteria of the Council of Europe for leucodepletion, 75% of products tested have white cell counts below 5×10^6 per 3×10^{11} platelets (equivalent to 1×10^6 per 0.6×10^{11} platelets). However, to achieve a white cell count below 1×10^6 per adult dose of platelets consistently, the platelets in the concentrate need to be counted and, if needed, platelet leucodepletion filters designed for this purpose can be used. Filtration adds an additional processing step, involving a loss of 4–18% of the platelets collected, depending on the filter used (Heaton 1993; Kao et al. 1995).

Donor reactions

Thrombapheresis is generally safe and well tolerated (see also Chapter 15). However, rapid infusion of citrate anticoagulant solutions induces a fall in total and ionized calcium (30% decrease at 90 min) and a sharp rise in parathormone levels, both of which are blunted by oral calcium taken 30 min before the procedure (Bolan et al. 2001). A rise in osteocalcin levels as well as a striking increase in urinary calcium and magnesium excretion occur and persist for at least 24 h. Whether repeated procedures over years will result in long-term loss of total body calcium and bone density remains to be determined. Clinical impressions notwithstanding, the common practice of administering oral calcium prior to the procedure, at least in a commercially available tablet preparation, has at best a minimal affect on relieving citrate-related symptoms in thrombapheresis donors (Bolan et al. 2003c) (see below). Reducing flow rate is more effective.

Transient but significant decreases in platelet counts have been documented to occur in donors undergoing single and serial short-term plateletpheresis collections (Glowitz and Slichter 1980; Rock et al. 1992). Regular plateletpheresis donors develop sustained decreases in platelet count of up to 50 000 per μl, which correlate directly with donation frequency in all but the most frequent donors. However, clinically significant thrombocytopenia is unusual (Lazarus et al. 2001).

Vasovagal reactions are common at the first donation, but appear to occur less frequently in apheresis donors than in whole blood donors (McLeod et al. 1998). Venepuncture pain, haematoma, nausea and vomiting occur in only about 1% of donors, and no life-threatening adverse events were encountered in a survey of 19 611 procedures at seven centres (McLeod et al. 1998).

Collection of granulocytes by leucapheresis

A unit of fresh blood contains $1.5–2 \times 10^9$ leucocytes. As only one-half can be retrieved by centrifugation, at least 10–12 and preferably double this number of units of blood would be required to provide a sufficient daily dose for an adult (2 units for a newborn infant) (see Chapter 14). The provision of leucocyte concentrates from routine donations entails exposing the recipients to large numbers of donors as well as sacrificing the red cells from those units because of the additives and manipulation needed in the processing. Granulocytes for adult transfusions are therefore not prepared routinely from whole blood units, but rather collected by leucapheresis from a single donor.

Three methods have been widely used, separately or more often in combination, to increase the yield of granulocytes: the administration of steroids to the donor to increase the peripheral granulocyte count, the introduction into the cell separator of a red cell sedimenting agent such as hydroxyethyl starch (HES) and stimulation of the donor with a haematopoietic cytokine such as granulocyte colony-stimulating factor (filgrastim, G-CSF). Stimulating donors with G-CSF or G-CSF with dexamethasone increases the yield of granulocytes compared to the yield from the traditional collection regimen of dexamethasone alone (Dale et al. 1998; Liles et al. 2000; Stroncek et al. 2001). The need for agents that cause rouleaux formation and thus help to separate red cells from granulocytes arises from the fact that the specific gravity of red cells and granulocytes is very similar (1.093–1.096 for red cells; 1.087–1.092 for granulocytes), so that centrifugation alone is a very inefficient means of separation (Mishler 1975).

Use of donor bone marrow stimulation

The yield of granulocytes correlates directly with the donor's circulating granulocyte count. Granulocyte collection from normal volunteer donors by continuous-flow centrifugal separation yields insufficient numbers of cells unless the donor can be stimulated or 'mobilized' prior to the collection. The original stimulant was etiocholanalone, which releases marginating granulocytes from the peripheral pool (McCredie et al. 1974). The effect was transient and donor side-effects unacceptable.

The administration of corticosteroids increases the granulocyte count by stimulating the release of neutrophils from bone marrow reserves and by inhibiting the escape of granulocytes from the circulation. A single dose of oral steroids may be given at least 2 h and preferably > 4 h before collection. For practical purposes, dexamethasone (6–12 mg) or prednisone (40–60 mg) is routinely administered the evening (8–12 h) before donation. For optimal results, 2–3 oral doses of dexamethasone can be given 12–18 h before leucapheresis. The pretreatment of donors within a 10- to 12-h period prior to leucapheresis with a double dose of dexamethasone significantly increased the total quantity and efficiency of granulocyte collected compared with a donor group receiving a single dose of dexamethasone (Winton and Vogler 1978). A mean of 25.5×10^9 total granulocytes were collected in addition to an efficiency of 2.11×10^9 granulocytes harvested per litre of blood processed in the double dose-treated donors, in contrast with 19.6×10^9 total granulocytes collected and an efficiency of 1.82×10^9 granulocytes harvested per litre of blood processed in the single-dose donor group (Higby et al. 1975).

Donor mobilization with G-CSF results in a 10-fold increase in the circulating granulocyte count and a six-fold increase in the number of cells collected compared with historical collections (Bensinger et al. 1993). A single subcutaneous dose of G-CSF administered 12–16 h before collection resulted in a five-fold increase in granulocyte yields and normal function of the collected cells (Caspar et al. 1993). Dexamethasone administration potentiates this effect and results in no immediate increased donor toxicity (Liles et al. 2000; Stroncek et al. 2001). Granulocyte mobilization response to subcutaneous G-CSF plus dexamethasone is sustained at peak levels for 8–24 h after co-administration of the two drugs, and even although the cytokine can be administered intravenously, no advantage accrues from doing so (Stroncek et al. 2002).

Use of erythrocyte sedimenting agents

The yield of granulocytes can be increased by adding an erythrocyte sedimenting (rouleaux-forming) agent with the citrate anticoagulant to the input line of the cell separator. HES has been used extensively in the USA. The increased granulocyte yield with HES administration may not be due solely to its sedimenting properties, but may have a specific effect independent of an increase in erythrocyte sedimentation rate (ESR) (Mishler 1982). Both ESR and granulocyte collection efficiency (GCE) vary widely among donors, yet may remain relatively constant for a given donor. Baseline ESR correlates with hydroxyethyl starch-modified

ESR and with GCE (Lee and Klein 1995). The HES commonly used is pentastarch, which has a lower molecular weight and is more rapidly excreted than hetastarch; it is used as a 10% solution in a 500-ml dose (Strauss et al. 1986). However, HES results in superior granulocyte collection and almost double the efficiency and has become the standard agent despite the longer in vivo retention time (Lee et al. 1995).

Plasmagel (a modified fluid gelatin) has been used widely in France as a red cell sedimenting agent. Plasmagel is eliminated more rapidly from the body than is HES, although allergic reactions are more frequent (Huestis et al. 1985), and plasma volume is also expanded (Rock et al. 1984).

Donor complications

Donors who receive a single 5-μg/kg dose of G-CSF experience headache, bone pain, myalgia, arthralgia, insomnia, dizziness, nausea and fatigue (Dale et al. 1998; Liles et al. 2000). When donors were given dexamethasone, 58% reported one or more symptoms on at least 1 day, compared with 85% when they were given G-CSF alone and 75% when they were given G-CSF plus dexamethasone (Stroncek et al. 2001). The largest proportion of donors reported symptoms on day 2. When donors were given G-CSF, they were more likely to report two or more symptoms on day 2 than when they were given dexamethasone. Some donors continued to experience symptoms 3 and 4 days later. Donors given G-CSF or G-CSF plus dexamethasone are more likely to experience arthralgias than when they are given dexamethasone alone, and donors given G-CSF are more likely to report headaches than when they receive dexamethasone alone (Stroncek et al. 2001).

Because corticosteroids are known to induce posterior subcapsular cataracts, concern has been expressed that repeated leucapheresis might increase the risk of cataract formation (Ghodsi and Strauss 2001). Confirmatory data are lacking. However, donors who have undergone repeated collections of granulocytes may benefit from an annual ocular examination and indication of cataract formation should preclude further donation. No other long-term risks of mobilization regimens have been reported, but few studies have been performed.

Solutions of hetastarch used for volume expansion produce significant abnormalities in some laboratory measurements of haemostasis (Strauss *et al.* 2002). It is unlikely that the modest haemostatic abnormalities produced at these doses would contribute to a risk of bleeding in volunteer granulocyte donors, even when infused on consecutive days. Hetastarch causes more haemostatic abnormalities than pentastarch.

Collection of red cells by apheresis

An estimated 273 000 red cell units were collected by apheresis in the USA in 2001, an increase of 135% compared with collections in 1999 (National Blood Data Research Center 2001). The growth in the number of instruments capable of performing red cell collection and increasing acceptance by collectors and donors indicates that the trend is likely to continue worldwide. A procedure for 2-unit ('double red cell') collection has been licensed. The several advantages include fewer donor visits per year, decreased testing costs and decreased donor exposures when both units are given to one recipient (Shi and Ness 1999). The procedure is particularly applicable to donors with haemochromatosis, as depletion of iron stores develops rapidly with repeated procedures (Leitman *et al.* 2003b). Other donors may benefit from iron supplementation (1994). At present donor suitability is limited to larger (by weight) donors and the donation interval is extended to 112 days. The incidence of immediate adverse effects related to 2-unit RBC apheresis is about 3%, similar to that of other apheresis procedures. The majority of reactions involve discomfort from venepuncture, citrate intolerance and vasovagal reactions. Donor tolerance of 2-unit red cell donations (400 ml), a volume of red cells twice that in a standard 450-ml blood donation, does not seem to differ substantially from donor tolerance of standard or sham donations (Smith *et al.* 1996).

Collection of progenitor (stem) cells from peripheral blood

Collection of peripheral blood haematopoietic stem (progenitor) cells

It has not proved possible to identify pluripotent progenitor (stem) cells by microscopy, cell surface markers or cell culture techniques. However, good correlation exists between the dose of mononuclear cells expressing the CD34 surface marker, the presence

of long-term culture initiating cells (LT-CIC) and haematopoietic engraftment in animal models and in human haematopoietic reconstitution. Most centres rely on CD34$^+$ cells because they are readily quantified and the kinetics of CD34$^+$ cell mobilization have been well studied. Individual centres have defined a minimum graft dose, for example 2.5×10^6 CD34$^+$ cells/kg of patient's body weight (Haynes *et al.* 1995). The cells seem to be qualitatively similar to those found in bone marrow (Korbling *et al.* 1995; Prosper *et al.* 1997). Most available centrifugal instruments can achieve adequate doses for transplantation, although the efficiency of each collection varies with donor characteristics, operator experience and the particular instrument and protocol used; 10–20 l are routinely processed per procedure, and two to three procedures may be required to reach the target dose. Intravenous electrolyte (primarily calcium) supplementation has permitted longer, more efficient collection procedures (Bolan *et al.* 2003b, 2004).

PBSC mobilization requires multiple daily injections of cytokine (G-CSF or GM-CSF) and the increase in circulating cells is temporary (Stroncek *et al.* 1996a). After the first 48 h of daily injections, no increase in circulating CD34$^+$ cells can be detected. By the third day, cell counts begin to increase and reach a peak on the fifth or sixth day. The peak number varies among individuals (Stroncek *et al.* 1997). When 5- to 10-μg/kg per day G-CSF is administered, circulating CD3$^+$ cells on day 6 range from 8×10^6 cells/l to 155×10^6 cells/l (Stroncek *et al.* 1997). After the sixth day, CD34$^+$ cell counts fall even if injections are continued, achieve only one-third of peak by day 10 and one-quarter by day 11. Doses of up to 16 μg/kg per day have been administered and some centres have found that doses injected twice a day appear more effective than a single dose (Waller *et al.* 1996). Other centres have not confirmed this split dose effect (Anderlini *et al.* 2000). Cytokine mobilization also increases the colony-forming units in peripheral blood, and LTC-IC in particular appear to mobilize well (Prosper *et al.* 1996). No increase in these progenitors or in CD34$^+$ cells is found in the marrow, suggesting that mobilization does not result from expansion of cells in the marrow cavity, but from release from the marrow or expansion from peripheral blood. The marrow itself may be depleted at least transiently of progenitors responsible for long-term engraftment, as late graft failures have been reported when patients receive marrow grafts from donors stimulated with G-CSF (Mavroudis *et al.* 1998). The cytokine GM-CSF has also been studied as a mobilizing agent but does not appear to have any advantage over G-CSF and may result in more severe side-effects (Fritsch *et al.* 1994; Lane TA *et al.* 1995).

The mechanism(s) involved in the process of mobilization are incompletely understood (Kessinger and Sharp 2003). The G-CSF effect appears to be mediated by cytokine release and enzymatic action on $CD34^+$ cell ligands. As noted, multiple doses over several days are necessary for maximum mobilization effect. Dividing the daily dose may increase yields, at least in healthy volunteers (Kroger *et al.* 2004). AMD3100 (160 µg/kg × 1 on day 5), a selective antagonist of the CXCR4 molecule that also appears to attach progenitors to their marrow niche, rapidly mobilizes $CD34^+$ haematopoietic progenitor cells from marrow to peripheral blood after a single dose. AMD3100-mobilized leucapheresis products contained significantly greater numbers of T and B cells compared with G-CSF-stimulated leucapheresis products (Liles *et al.* 2005). Combined administration of AMD 3100 and G-CSF produces more rapid and effective mobilization of $CD34^+$ cells than does G-CSF alone (Flomenberg 2005).

Collections of PBSC contain large numbers of platelets, leucocytes and red cells. The mean number of T lymphocytes, $CD3^+$ cells, is about 10 times that of a bone marrow collection. Red cell volume ranges up to 22 ml, but ordinarily does not exceed 1.5 ml/l (Leitman and Read 1996).

Stimulation of donors with G-CSF is not without discomfort, risk and adverse events. Bone pain, insomnia and malaise occur in 40–80% of mobilized donors. These symptoms respond to paracetamol or ibuprofen. Cutaneous reactions including folliculitis, urticaria, pyoderma gangrenosum and exacerbations of psoriasis have been reported (Brumit *et al.* 2003). Transient laboratory abnormalities include increases in sodium, lactate dehydrogenase (LDH), alkaline phosphatase, serum glutamate pyruvate transaminase and uric acid levels and decreases in potassium, bilirubin, blood urea nitrogen and magnesium levels. Platelet counts drop in PBPC concentrate donors during the administration of G-CSF and following collection of PBPC. WBC counts rise during the administration of G-CSF, but then fall below baseline levels 2–3 weeks after PBSC collection (Stroncek *et al.* 1996b, 1997). Daily

G-CSF administration results in splenic enlargement and, rarely, spontaneous rupture of the spleen (Falzetti *et al.* 1999). Enlargement is transient, but may be marked in some donors and may place them at risk for splenic rupture, especially if the abdomen is subjected to blunt force trauma in the several weeks following mobilization (Stroncek *et al.* 2003). Side-effects with administration of single doses of AMD3100 appear to be minimal, but experience with this drug is far more limited than with the other mobilizing agents.

Effects of repeated cytapheresis

Volunteer subjects undergoing repeated apheresis should be monitored to prevent levels of red cells, platelets and lymphocytes from falling below normal limits. Neutrophils are so rapidly produced and released that their number in the circulation remains unchanged.

Platelet loss: inadequate components but no donor purpura

When platelets or granulocytes are collected with blood cell separators, the donor's platelet count may not return to pre-donation levels for 6–7 days. Low platelet count limits the frequency of platelet donations by relatives of patients requiring HLA-compatible platelets. On occasion the platelet count can fall below $100 \times 10^9/l$ and, although this poses no risk to the donor, thrombocytopenia to this degree makes further platelet collection inefficient (Strauss *et al.* 1983). Platelet donation is ordinarily deferred if the pre-apheresis platelet count falls below $150 \times 10^9/l$. Regular plateletpheresis donors develop sustained decreases in platelet count that correlate directly with donation frequency (see above) (Lazarus *et al.* 2001).

Lymphocyte losses: does immune compromise result?

Large losses of lymphocytes may occur during intensive thrombapheresis owing to the similar density of lymphocytes and platelets. Broadly similar losses of lymphocytes were found in three different studies: 3.5×10^9 in donors from whom platelets or granulocytes were harvested by intermittent-flow cytapheresis, using a six-cycle procedure (Koepke *et al.* 1981); 6×10^9 per plateletpheresis donation (Fratantoni and French 1980) and 3×10^9 (T lymphocytes) in donors given prednisone and a sedimenting agent (Dwyer *et al.* 1981). The long-term effects of this loss of lymphocytes might seem potentially serious, however no adverse health problems have been reported. After 10 weekly donations, a fall in the lymphocyte count of 20%, with a decrease in B cells in one-half of the donors, has been observed (Koepke *et al.* 1981).

In a study of 21 healthy blood donors subjected to 9–17 cytaphereses over a period of 12 months, absolute lymphocyte count decreased 23%, T cells decreased 25% and B cells fell by 46%, with a reduction of 14% in serum IgG concentration (Senhauser *et al.* 1982). Similar results were obtained in 21 out of 113 donors who gave platelets regularly by apheresis with the Haemonetics H-30 model, with a mean number of 13.1 procedures a year over a mean period of 162.7 weeks (Robbins *et al.* 1985). The lymphocyte count was inversely related to the total number of thrombaphereses and the CD4$^+$ and CD8$^+$ lymphocyte subsets were reduced in all 13 lymphocytopenic donors tested. However, CD4/CD8 ratios were found to be normal and no adverse effects were noted in any of the donors. Lymphocytes are also lost in large numbers when the CS-3000 instrument is used to collect platelets, particularly with the isoradial chamber. Donors who develop lymphocytopenia (lymphocyte count $< 1 \times 10^9$/l) are ordinarily excluded from donation until the lymphocyte count is $> 1.5 \times 10^9$/l. Donors who fail to revert to normal within 8 weeks are often referred for further investigations (Strauss *et al.* 1983). On the other hand, short-term removal of lymphocytes has little measurable effect. Following a total of six lymphapheresis procedures over a 12-day period in 12 blood donors with a mean removal of 41.6×10^9 lymphocytes, no significant changes in absolute lymphocyte counts, immunoglobulin levels or *in vitro* tests of the immune response were measured (Blanchette *et al.* 1985).

Depletion of haematopoietic progenitors. Few donors have been mobilized repeatedly for PBSC collection. As yet there is no evidence that depletion of the stem cell compartment poses a risk to donors.

Symptoms and signs in donors giving blood via cell separators

Apheresis donation is a safe undertaking, suitable for voluntary blood donors, with a very low risk of serious adverse effects. Many of the symptoms and signs such as vasovagal reactions are similar to those experienced by donors giving a routine blood donation or by patients during plasma exchange. Factors that may cause symptoms or signs include changes in the donor's blood volume, chilling of returned blood and the administration of pharmaceutical agents such as citrate or HES. Of a total 195 372 donor apheresis procedures, complications were reported in 9.6% of cases, including 5.2% donor-related problems (e.g. fainting, citrate toxicity), 4% machine and harness problems and 0.4% operator errors (Robinson 1990). When transient paraesthesia and mild vasovagal events are excluded, a survey of 17 USA centres reporting on 19 611 apheresis donations recorded 600 adverse events in 428 donations (2.18% of donations and 4.84% of the 2295 first donations). Only 203 donations (1.04%) sustained non-venepuncture adverse effects. No life-threatening adverse effects were reported. Procedure-specific non-venepuncture rates were 1.05% of 17 584 platelet donations, 0.67% of 594 white cell donations and 0.37% of 1354 plasma donations. Centre-specific rates varied from 0.32% to 6.81% of donations for total adverse effects and from 0.11% to 2.92% of donations for non-venepuncture events (McLeod *et al.* 1998). Most of the immediate complications can be dealt with by the operator and apheresis need not be halted. Reactions can usually be controlled by adjusting the return flow of blood or the rate of saline infusion into the receiving arm.

Syncope, seizures and vasovagal effects occur more frequently when using intermittent-flow devices as the extracorporeal blood volume is larger than with continuous-flow blood cell separators especially during the last cycles. Extracorporeal volume should not exceed 15% of the donor's own volume at any time (Huestis 1989). Severe vasovagal episodes were reported in 32 donors undergoing leucapheresis; 10 donors lost consciousness and had seizures (Sandler and Nusbacher 1982). However, if experienced blood donors are used for plasmapheresis and thrombapheresis, syncope occurs in only 0.2% of procedures although fainting and nausea are 10 times more likely when cells rather than plasma components are collected. From the UK apheresis registry, the chance of severe syncope requiring resuscitation has been estimated at 1 in 100 000 procedures (Robinson 1990). In the USA, vasovagal nausea and/or vomiting occurred in 0.87% of first-time and 0.13% of repeat donors, whereas the experience for syncope and/or seizure was 0.39% and 0.04% respectively (McLeod *et al.* 1998).

Chills are relatively common and may be due partly to extracorporeal chilling of blood and partly to undetermined factors. In the USA, chills and/or rigors were noted in 0.31% of first-time and 0.01% of repeat donors (McLeod *et al.* 1998). In most cases, a blanket or a blood warmer will prevent the chills.

Vascular effects such as venous spasm, collapse, infiltration and haematoma formation are more frequent in apheresis than in routine donations because one or two needles have to be in place for 60–90 min and the needles are usually larger because of the pumped red cell return (Robinson 1990; Simon 1994). Pain or haematoma at a venepuncture site was the most common complaint in the USA survey complicating 1.15% of donations (McLeod *et al.* 1998).

Citrate toxicity is related to the concentration of citrate used, the rate of re-infusion, the duration of the procedure, the volumes processed and whether a continuous or discontinuous procedure is used. Citrate 'effect', mild tingling, is common as contrasted with citrate toxicity. The distinction is a matter of degree, but toxicity can be aborted by early recognition of donor or patient discomfort. Common manifestations include circumoral paraesthesia, vibratory sensations, nausea, vomiting and overt tetany that may be exacerbated by the alkalosis that follows hyperventilation.

Citrate-induced nausea and/or vomiting occur in less than 1% of donors and tetany is less frequent by an order of magnitude (McLeod *et al.* 1998). In the collection of plasma components, the return of citrated plasma is small and the incidence of toxicity is 10 times lower than when leucocytes or platelet concentrates are collected (Robinson 1990). Signs of citrate toxicity closely parallel the fall in ionized calcium when standard concentrations of ACD-A (Olson *et al.* 1977; Bolan *et al.* 2001) or sodium citrate (Mishler *et al.* 1977) are used (see above). Signs of toxicity may be avoided by slowing the rate of infusion or by using a lower concentration of citrate, combined if necessary with a small amount of heparin (Huestis 1986a). In the treatment of citrate toxicity during voluntary donation, the administration of intravenous calcium is not recommended routinely as it can cause clotting in the extracorporeal circuit or arrhythmia in the donor (Westphal 1984). However, in the USA, where the recommended citrate load (ACD-A) should not exceed 1 ml/l of the total blood volume, i.v.

calcium has been administered to donors to prevent symptoms of citrate toxicity (Bolan *et al.* 2002). Oral tablets of calcium are not particularly effective in preventing either hypocalcaemia or donor symptoms (Bolan *et al.* 2003a,c). In the UK, there are recommendations for maximum flow rates for the different anticoagulant ratios in different instruments to avoid the need to use calcium supplementation (Robinson 1990).

Adverse effects of hydroxyethyl starch – febrile and allergic reactions due to HES are discussed in Chapter 2. Frequent infusions of HES over a short period are potentially hazardous. Four healthy donors were given infusions of 500 ml of HES (molecular weight 450 000) daily for 4 days. After the fourth infusion, the average increase in plasma volume was 0.85 l; 24 h later, in all but one of the donors, plasma volume was still 0.5 l above the donor's initial value (Rock and Wise 1979). In subjects who donate granulocytes regularly by apheresis and receive repeated infusions of HES, plasma HES levels are still raised 3 months after the last infusion (Ring *et al.* 1980). In such donors, headache, mild hypertension, swollen fingers and peripheral or periorbital oedema may be present (Westphal 1984). Abnormalities of coagulation assays occur, but bleeding does not appear to be a concern (Strauss *et al.* 2002) (see above).

Transitory side-effects due to *steroid administration* such as headache, insomnia, flushing, palpitations and euphoria occur in some donors and are dose related.

Allergic reactions consisting of sneezing, urticaria or even angioedema are seen in occasional donors and are five times more likely to occur in donors giving cells than in donors giving plasma components (Robinson 1990). Severe reactions due to sensitization to ethylene oxide are discussed in Chapter 15.

Mild haemolysis is seen occasionally and is caused by kinks in the plastic tubing (Huestis 1986a, 1989; McLeod *et al.* 1998).

Infections at the site of venesection are more likely to occur in cytapheresis donors who have two needles in their veins for a period of 1–3 h. There is also the more remote, although more serious, danger of infection from contaminated bottles of solutions used in cytapheresis or from leaking harnesses (Kosmin 1980).

Mortality

Fatalities attributed to the donation of plasma or cells by apheresis are rare. Nine deaths were reported to the

FDA for the 10 years between 1976 and 1985; eight of these were attributed to plasma donations and one to leucapheresis (Sazama 1990). No deaths attributed to apheresis have occurred either in 289 385 procedures analysed in the UK registry from mid-1985 to April 1989 or in the USA survey.

Therapeutic plasma exchange

The exchange of large volumes of plasma and their replacement with other colloids such as albumin or allogeneic plasma became possible with the introduction of automated plasmapheresis performed with centrifugal blood cell separators or with hollow fibre or membrane filters. Filtration can occur at a high flow rate through continuous-flow systems, and with a pore diameter between 0.2 and 0.5 μm, immunoglobulins and most immune complexes can be removed while the cells pass through the separator and return to the patient with the replacement fluid. However, large immune complexes and IgM may not be removed effectively and cryoglobulins may gel in the extracorporeal circuit, impairing their clearance. Several variations of filtration using combinations of filters or filters and columns have been devised to remove plasma components of a specific molecular weight or a particular physical characteristic ('cascade filtration, cryofiltration'), but with the exception of columns for removal of low-density lipoproteins (see below), these procedures are not widely used (Pineda 1991; Griffin 1996). Virtually all therapeutic exchanges are performed with centrifugal blood cell separators.

The main criteria for the application of therapeutic plasma exchange and more particularly for immunoadsorption are: (1) the existence of a known pathogenic substance in the plasma; and (2) the possibility of removing this substance more rapidly than it can be renewed in the body. However, clinical improvement does not necessarily follow the removal of a pathogenic substance. On the other hand, some conditions improve after plasma exchange even when the concentration of the substance in the plasma does not fall (Huestis 1986c). Moreover, in uncommon conditions such as thrombotic thrombocytopenic purpura (TTP), there appears to be, in addition to unwanted substances that need to be removed, a missing plasma factor that is supplied in sufficient quantities by replacement with fresh-frozen plasma (FFP) or cryoprecipitate-poor plasma (Levy *et al.* 2005)

(see below). In general, plasma exchange is used to treat severely ill patients not responding to conventional therapy. As plasma exchange has short-lived benefits and because it is a complex and expensive form of therapy which is not without risk, it should be used in only two circumstances: in well-controlled clinical trials, and in treating patients with one of the few conditions in which there is good evidence of its efficacy (Strauss *et al.* 1993; Griffin *et al.* 1996).

Volumes of fluid exchanged

The volume of fluid exchanged at each therapeutic plasma exchange (TPE) is usually equivalent to the patient's plasma volume. The usual practice consists of a course of four or five procedures carried out within 7–10 days, although the volume and frequency of plasma exchanges vary depending on the individual patient, the clinical condition and the protocols of each centre.

In TPE, the amount of a specific pathogenic substance removed depends on the volume of plasma exchanged and on the frequency of the procedure. The concentration X_t of a pathogenic substance X after a time t (in h) of plasma exchange is given by the equation:

$$X_t = X_0 e^{-rt} \qquad (17.3)$$

where X_0 represents the initial concentration of the pathogenic component and r the fractional rate of exchange or volume of plasma exchanged per hour divided by the plasma volume (Calabrese *et al.* 1980). The equation is valid only if the following conditions are met: complete mixing, no change in the patient's blood volume and no influx of the component from the extravascular space. In these circumstances, each plasma exchange equivalent to one plasma volume will remove approximately 60% of a (pathogenic) intravascular component. The removal of 40 ml of plasma per kilogram of body weight gives roughly the same results as predicted by the equation (Huestis 1986c). In practice, the conditions outlined above are rarely met. For molecules that are mainly intravascular, such as immune complexes or IgM, the final concentration is nearer the calculated value than for smaller molecules such as IgG, which diffuse freely to the extravascular space. Other factors that need to be taken into consideration are the catabolism, half-life and rate of renewal of the substance being removed. If resynthesis is very rapid, greater numbers of procedures will be required. Rebound phenomena tend to occur after plasma exchange when antibodies or immune complexes need to be removed. In these cases the concurrent use of immunosuppressive therapy has proved the treatment of choice, as plasma exchange reduces the required dose of immunosuppression with a consequent reduction in hazards (Huestis 1986c).

Vascular access

An antecubital vein is used whenever possible. For children, and when more effective blood flow is needed, a catheter can be passed into a femoral or subclavian vein, or arteriovenous shunts, arteriovenous fistulae or prosthetic grafts can be established. Temporary rigid polyethylene and Teflon catheters and semi-rigid polyurethane ones are used for emergency and short-term access. A semi-permanent catheter, made of soft silicone rubber with a subcutaneous anchoring system inserted through a subcutaneous tunnel is indicated for medium- and long-term use. Although catheter design has benefited greatly from technical advances and material haemocompatability, catheter-related morbidity still remains high and is associated with significant rates of infection and thrombosis that can extend proximally and distally. The morbidity includes gangrene, aneurysm formation, cardiac arrhythmia, pneumothorax, perforation of great vessels and even of the heart (Huestis 1986b; Couriel and Weinstein 1994; Stegmayr and Wikdahl 2003).

Replacement fluid

In general, in TPE, replacement fluids are given in a volume equal to that of plasma removed, although patients with fluid overload may be given smaller volumes of replacement fluids and those with contracted plasma volumes may be given additional fluids to avoid hypotension. Colloid osmotic pressure and electrolyte balance are generally maintained. Except for TTP, for which plasma is the treatment of choice (see below), the composition of the replacement fluid is rarely important. If the patient's protein levels are normal, 1 l of crystalloids may be used at the beginning of the procedure; the replacement fluid given first will be partially removed at the end of the exchange (Urbaniak 1983). A large number of centres routinely use equal volumes of 0.9% saline and 4–5% albumin as a replacement fluid. Much has been made of the removal of coagulation factors, but clinically important bleeding does not often occur. Immediately after exchange, significant prolongation of the prothrombin, partial thromboplastin and thrombin times occurs, with reduction of the fibrinogen and antithrombin III levels. Within 4 h of exchange, almost all factors, including platelets, return to pre-exchange values, and at 24 h all are corrected (Flaum *et al.* 1979). Plasma exchange with solutions devoid of coagulation factors results in a coagulation defect that may be of clinical significance in a haemostatically compromised patient. Partial replacement with FFP may be needed for patients with a risk of bleeding such as those with liver disease or disseminated intravascular coagulation (DIC). Patients with hypoalbuminaemia or contracted plasma volume may require total replacement with 5% albumin. Patients undergoing multiple, intensive exchanges may become hypofibrinogenaemic; this is rarely of clinical significance. The plasma Ig levels may also fall considerably in such patients, but it is not clear that replacement IVIG is needed. The levels of certain complement components such as C3 may drop precipitously and, similarly, cholinesterase levels may become so low as to lead to apnoea in patients injected with suxamethonium prior to surgery (Evans *et al.* 1980).

The disadvantages of the use of plasma as replacement include: increased incidence of citrate toxicity and of urticarial and anaphylactic reactions, transmission of viral infections and passive transfer of antibodies such as leucoagglutinins, thought to be responsible for the severe and even fatal pulmonary complications (TRALI, see Chapter 15) of plasma exchange. If plasma needs to be used in the UK, it is obtained from male volunteers and subjected to viral inactivation. However, the ideal replacement fluid is the patient's own plasma from which the pathogenic component had been removed. Unfortunately, methods for the selective removal of plasma constituents are not without risk and are, at present, applicable only to a small number of diseases (see below).

Indications for plasma exchange

Plasma exchange is indicated for conditions in which well-controlled trials have shown the treatment to be of value and in others in which the pathogenic plasma component can be removed or replaced. Although reports claim benefit for plasma exchange in more than 100 disorders, scientific studies and well-controlled clinical trials are sparse (Strauss *et al.* 1993; Griffin *et al.* 1996; Shehata *et al.* 2002). There are only a few conditions in which plasma exchange has been shown to be of definite benefit, namely the hyperviscosity syndrome, cryoglobulinaemia, myasthenia gravis, Guillain–Barré syndrome, chronic inflammatory demyelinating polyneuropathy, homozygous familial hypercholesterolaemia, Goodpasture syndrome, Refsum disease, post-transfusion purpura and TTP. In many other conditions, suggestive evidence of the value of plasma exchange has been obtained, but the absence of control subjects makes it impossible to reach definite conclusions; plasma exchange in D-immunized pregnant women is one example. Reviews of the effects of plasma exchange in various other conditions abound (Strauss *et al.* 1993; McLeod 2002; Shehata *et al.* 2002; Smith *et al.* 2003). Increasingly, IVIG has become the preferred initial form of therapy for autoantibody-mediated immune disorders such as PTP, refractory immune thrombocytopenia (ITP), acute Guillain–Barré syndrome, myasthenia gravis and systemic vasculitis in patients with Wegener granulomatosis (Jayne 1990; Kasprisin 1991; Knezevic-Maramica and Kruskall 2003).

Several professional societies have published evidence-based consensus guidelines for therapeutic plasmapheresis (Strauss *et al.* 1993; Smith *et al.* 2003). A summary listing of the most common indications can be found in Table 17.1.

Removal of antibodies

Alloantibodies. Plasmapheresis to remove anti-HPA-1a in PTP is standard therapy (see Chapter 15). Removal of anti-D and anti-P during pregnancy reportedly salvages some fetuses and allows some women with recurrent spontaneous abortion to carry the pregnancy to term (Robinson and Tovey 1980; Rock *et al.* 1985) (see Chapter 12). Removal of HLA antibodies has been undertaken before renal transplantation and for hyperacute rejection (Alarabi *et al.* 1995). In the former case, specific and durable elimination was achieved, whereas in the latter case, the data on graft survival are impressive, although uncontrolled (Sonnenday *et al.* 2002; Montgomery and Zachary 2004). The removal of anti-A and anti-B is now seldom necessary in ABO-

Table 17.1 Common indications for therapeutic plasmapheresis.

Haematological diseases (including blood cell-specific autoimmune diseases)
Thrombotic thrombocytopenic purpura
Idiopathic thrombocytopenic purpura
Hyperviscosity
Post-transfusion purpura
Cold agglutinin syndrome
Coagulation factor inhibitors
ABO-mismatched marrow transplant (recipient)

Alloimmune disease
Antibody removal for hyperimmune renal allograft rejection

Autoimmune diseases
Cryoglobulinaemia
Rheumatoid arthritis (immunoadsorption, lymphoplasmapheresis)
Myasthenia gravis
Lambert–Eaton myasthenic syndrome
Goodpasture syndrome
Acute Guillain–Barré syndrome
Chronic inflammatory demyelinating polyneuropathy
HIV-related polyneuropathy

Metabolic diseases
Homozygous familial hypercholesterolaemia (selective adsorption)
Refsum disease

Other
Drug overdose and poisoning

incompatible bone marrow transplants (see Chapter 14), although it has proved useful prior to ABO-incompatible renal grafts (Griffin *et al.* 1996; Gloor *et al.* 2003). An instance of successful renal allografting in the face of both ABO and HLA incompatibility using a preconditioning regimen of TPE and low-dose CMV hyperimmune globulin (CMVIg) delivered every other day has been published (Warren *et al.* 2004).

Autoantibodies. For example, anti-acetylcholine receptor (AChR) in myasthenia gravis; anti-basement membrane in Goodpasture syndrome; factor VIII inhibitor in unresponsive haemophiliacs with severe haemorrhage and in the rare antibody-mediated, pure red cell aplasia; autoantibodies to epidermal cell membrane glycoproteins in pemphigus; platelet autoantibodies in refractory immune thrombocytopenia, although IVIG is now the treatment of choice; and peripheral nerve myelin autoantibodies in Guillain–Barré syndrome, where TPE has been shown to be of benefit in two large clinical trials (McKhann *et al.* 1988). IVIG appears to be equally effective (van der Meche and Schmitz 1992).

In myasthenia gravis, removal of AChR autoantibodies by plasma exchange is associated with clinical improvement, relieving weakness of respiration and swallowing after about 2 days (Dau *et al.* 1977; Richman and Agius 2003). However, there is little role for TPE in the long-term management of this condition. Patients with the Lambert–Eaton myasthenic syndrome, caused by autoantibodies to the calcium channel on the pre-synaptic nerve terminal, also benefit from TPE (Griffin *et al.* 1996; Newsom-Davis 2001). IVIG affords equal benefit in the acute phase and immunosuppressive therapy provides long-term control in both conditions.

In Goodpasture syndrome, a rapidly progressive glomerulonephritis accompanied by pulmonary haemorrhage, autoantibodies to type IV collagen in the glomerular and alveolar basement membranes can be removed by plasma exchange; the procedure is particularly effective in the early stages of the disease. Suppression of further antibody synthesis can be achieved with immunosuppressive medication such as cyclophosphamide, azathioprine and corticosteroids (Lockwood *et al.* 1975). Early treatment is essential, as renal impairment is irreversible (Levy *et al.* 2001). A small controlled trial confirmed that the addition of plasmapheresis not only results in the expected rapid decline in antibody to glomerular basement membrane (anti-GBM), but in improvement in renal function, renal histology and disease outcome (Johnson *et al.* 1985). Combination of TPE and immunosuppression proved similarly successful in a small controlled study of rapidly progressive glomerulonephritis (excluding Goodpasture syndrome), even when patients had become dependent on dialysis (Pusey *et al.* 1983). Experience with dialysis-independent patients in a large multicentre trial failed to confirm these results (Glockner *et al.* 1988). In severe systemic vasculitis (Wegener granulomatosis, Churg–Strauss syndrome) with pulmonary haemorrhage, even in the absence of renal involvement, plasma exchange combined with immunosuppression has a chequered history, but seems to provide reasonable adjunctive therapy in patients with rapidly progressing disease, especially when a patient's organ or life is threatened (Guillevin *et al.* 1995; Gaskin and Pusey 2001). Plasma exchange removes anti-neutrophil cytoplasmic autoantibodies (ANCAs) and immune complexes as well as inflammatory mediators such as cytokines, complement factors and coagulation components, but improvements in clinical outcome have been difficult to document.

Removal of immune complexes and macromolecules (e.g. rapidly progressive glomerulonephritis (see above), systemic lupus erythematosus and cryoglobulinaemia)

Symptomatic treatment of cryoglobulinaemia with plasma exchange has proved successful on a short-term basis. The cold-precipitating properties of cryoglobulins make it possible to deplete them selectively, although cold ultrafiltration has not gained many supporters (Pineda 1991; Siami and Siami 1998, 2004). Removal of the cryoprotein does not always improve the clinical syndrome. Plasma exchange has enjoyed some success in treating patients with recurrent focal segmental glomerulosclerosis (FSGS) after renal transplantation and less commonly in the native kidney. A circulating plasma factor that increases glomerular permeability to albumin has been isolated from these patients, but this may not be the pathogenic agent. TPE is often used, but appears to be less efficacious in adults than in children with this disease (Matalon *et al.* 2000).

Plasma exchange effectively removes antibodies, immune complexes and inflammatory mediators from the blood of patients with systemic lupus erythematosis. Despite a wealth of anecdotal reports that point to efficacy, controlled trials have failed to define a treatment strategy that would benefit patients with lupus nephritis or other manifestations of the disease (Wei *et al.* 1983; Lewis *et al.* 1992; Doria *et al.* 1994; Wallace *et al.* 1998).

Removal of monoclonal proteins (e.g. hyperviscosity syndrome)

The hyperviscosity syndrome is most commonly due to an increase of serum IgM (Waldenström macroglobulinaemia), although it is occasionally due to high-molecular-weight polymers of IgG or IgA (in patients with multiple myeloma). One of the most effective

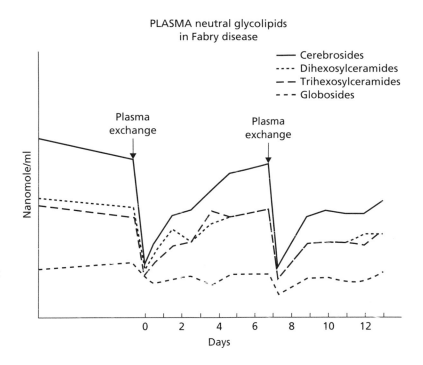

PLASMA neutral glycolipids
in Fabry disease

—— Cerebrosides
---- Dihexosylceramides
— — Trihexosylceramides
- - - Globosides

Fig 17.5 Plasma exchange to remove plasma neutral glycolipids in a patient with Fabry disease. The plasma lipid recovery kinetics appear biphasic, reflecting initial re-equilibration from tissue stores and subsequent new synthesis of that glycolipid.

applications of plasma exchange is the treatment of the acute cardiovascular, neurological and haemorrhagic complications of this disease before there has been time for chemotherapy to become effective (Solomon and Fahey 1963). In most cases, only two or three plasma exchanges are needed; the replacement fluid should be plasma free and, if the volume replaced is moderate, protein free as well. Patients who are refractory to, or intolerant of, chemotherapy can be maintained on plasma exchange at regular (4- to 6-weekly) intervals. Comprehensive reviews describing the rationale and treatment schedules for plasmapheresis in patients with a variety of paraproteinaemias, including cryoglobulinaemia and Waldenstrom's macroglobulinaemia, and other haematological/oncological indications have been published (Drew 2002).

Removal of excess plasma constituent (e.g. phytanic acid as an adjunct to restrictive diet in Refsum disease)

Simple plasma exchange may be used in patients with other inherited metabolic diseases, such as Refsum disease (Gibberd *et al.* 1979). The frequency of exchange depends primarily on total body burden, rate of synthesis and plasma concentration of the solute to be removed (Fig. 17.5). Less evidence exists to support a role for repeated treatments in these diseases.

Homozygous familial hypercholesterolaemia is characterized by a high level of LDL that is virtually confined to the plasma. TPE has proved effective in reducing the levels of cholesterol and LDL and is now an accepted form of therapy in this condition (see Table 17.1), in conjunction with drugs such as simvastatin or, more recently, atrovastatin. Most signs and symptoms improve, except for aortic stenosis (Thompson *et al.* 1995).

Replacement of a specific plasma component: thrombotic thrombocytopenic purpura

Long before the mechanisms responsible for the majority of TTP cases were described, a missing plasma factor was thought to be responsible for the syndrome (Upshaw 1978). The pathological process was aborted in some cases with the infusion of small volumes of plasma, whereas other cases seemed to require plasma exchange to reverse thrombosis and haemolysis and to prevent thrombosis (Byrnes and

795

Khurana 1977; Bukowski *et al.* 1981). It now appears that, in the majority of cases, the syndrome results from lack of a normal plasma constituent, from immune destruction of this factor and, less commonly, from some platelet-aggregating factor that is inhibited by normal plasma (Tsai 1996; Tsai and Lian 1998; Vesely *et al.* 2003; Levy *et al.* 2005). The effectiveness of plasma exchange now seems to result from removal of antibody to and/or replacement of the von Willebrand factor-cleaving metalloprotease, designated ADAMTS13 (Furlan and Lammle 2002; Furlan 2003; Zheng *et al.* 2004). However, patients with clinical features of TTP and only moderate ADAMTS13 deficiency or even normal activity may respond to plasma exchange (Vesely *et al.* 2003). The infusion about every 3 weeks of normal ADAMTS13 into familial TTP patients who produce defective ADAMTS13 molecules is sufficient to prevent TTP episodes. As the plasma $T_{1/2}$ of infused ADAMTS13 activity is about 2 days, ADAMTS13 molecules may adhere to fixed platelet–von Willebrand factor (VWF) complexes and effect disassociation (Moake 2004; Zheng *et al.* 2004). Treatment of adults and children with acquired idiopathic TTP usually involves episodes associated with ADAMTS13 deficiency, and often requires daily single-volume plasma exchange. Both frequency and duration of treatment are guided by clinical response, increase in platelet count to 100 000/µl or more and evidence of declining haemolysis, as measured by normalization of serum LDH and decline in the number of schistocytes on the peripheral blood smear.

All of the theories of pathogenesis provide a rational basis for the use of plasma as a form of therapy in TTP. Plasma exchange removes circulating ultra-large VWF multimer–platelet complexes that stimulate endothelial cells to secrete VWF multimers, and the autoantibodies against ADAMTS13 whereas the infusion of fresh-frozen plasma or cryosupernatant supplies the protein (see Chapter 14). Solvent–detergent-treated plasma and methylene blue/light-treated plasma both contain active ADAMTS13.

The results of the only large prospective, controlled trial in 102 TTP patients favours plasma exchange over simple transfusion. On 7 of the first 9 days of entry into the trial, patients underwent either a plasma exchange (with FFP) or a simple infusion of FFP. All patients received aspirin and dipyridamole. At the end of 9 days, platelet counts had risen in 24 of 51 patients

in the plasma exchange group but in only 13 out of 51 in the infusion group; after 6 months, 11 patients in the plasma exchange group and 19 patients in the infusion group had died (Rock *et al.* 1991). Whether the superior effect of plasma exchange is due to the more intensive replacement of deficient factors or to removal of antibody or other pathogenic factors remains unclear (Griffin 1996).

The difficulty in evaluating efficacy of plasmapheresis in many disorders, especially when the procedure is combined with other treatments, is epitomized by the controversy concerning its role in the management of multiple sclerosis (MS). The only large double-blind, randomized, controlled trial had a significant effect in improving disability in chronic MS (Khatri *et al.* 1985). However, the statistical management of this study has been questioned. Significant patient improvement was observed at 5 months, but not at 11 months, and patient response has suggested to some that they were in the relapsing–remitting phase of the disease rather than the chronic progressive phase. Studies of chronic progressive disease fail to find a benefit from repeated plasmapheresis (Weiner *et al.* 1989; Bitsch and Bruck 2002). A recent review of published studies of therapeutic plasmapheresis in MS concludes that plasmapheresis may be an effective therapy in acute or chronic progressive MS when conventional corticosteroid or other immunosuppressive drug therapies have failed (Khatri 2000). The long-term benefit for patients with chronic progressive disease remains controversial (McLeod 2003).

Methods for the selective removal of plasma components

The ideal method for treating disorders mediated by abnormal plasma components is to remove the offending substance selectively. A variety of on-line filtration and column adsorption techniques have been introduced or proposed. Several methods for the selective removal of plasma components are based either on separation filtration according to the physical characteristics of the component or on immunoaffinity binding. Ligands bound to a column matrix may be relatively non-specific chemical sorbents, such as charcoal or heparin, or specific ligands, such as monoclonal antibodies and recombinant protein antigens. Two such columns are commercially available; one using staphylococcal protein A and the other using dextran sulphate–cellulose beads (Pineda 1991). Staphylococcal protein A has high affinity for the Fc portion of IgG1, 2 and 4 and for immune complexes containing these IgG subtypes. This column is approved for use in therapeutic apheresis procedures for patients with chronic idiopathic thrombocytopenia and selected adult patients with rheumatoid arthritis. The dextran sulphate–cellulose columns selectively remove low-density lipoproteins and have proved effective in managing patients with homozygous hypercholesterolaemia who have not responded to diet and cholesterol-lowering drug therapy. The combination of apheresis with column or ultrafiltration technology has several advantages: (1) it avoids the need for allogeneic plasma by returning the patient's own treated plasma; (2) only separated plasma is passed through the column, so there is little danger of cellular damage or platelet depletion; (3) there is little risk of depletion of coagulation factors, allowing more intensive plasma exchange; (4) there is a wider choice of type and concentration of anticoagulant; and (5) the possibility of using small bead packings allows fast and efficient adsorption (Pepper 1983; Pineda 1991).

Development of methods for the selective removal of unwanted substances from the patient's plasma to be followed by the return of the remaining plasma to the patient is clearly desirable. Unfortunately, for many diseases, the causative agent or agents that need to be removed by apheresis and their pathogenetic mechanisms are unknown.

Immunoaffinity apheresis

The basic affinity chromatography technology employs a substance (ligand) with a selective binding affinity, firmly coupled to an insoluble carrier, which binds its complementary substance from a mixture of materials in solution or suspension. The ligand can be an antigen, an antibody or an immune reactant able to absorb its reciprocal material, although non-immunological substances can also be removed by immune-mediated processing.

Staphylococcal protein A–agarose columns consist of Cowan I strain *Staphylococcus aureus* protein linked covalently to beaded agarose. The protein binds strongly to Ig 1, 2 and 4 and even more avidly with these IgG subclasses bound to antigen, as with circulating immune complexes. Binding to IgG3, IgM and IgA is variable. This technology, dual columns that

receive separated plasma over one column while a second one is regenerated, has been used primarily in Europe for patients with antibodies to coagulation factors VIII and IX, and for removing HLA and auto-antibodies from patients awaiting renal allografting (Hakim *et al.* 1990; Watt *et al.* 1992). Whereas patient response is variable, column immunoadsorption does reduce alloreactivity in the patient's serum and small, uncontrolled series report improved renal allograft survival (Gjorstrup 1991; Hiesse *et al.* 1992; Ross *et al.* 1993). Immunoadsorption has been used to treat or reduce bleeding in patients with clotting factor inhibitors and as part of tolerance induction regimens (Gjorstrup *et al.* 1991). Treatment clearly reduces inhibitor titre, but often does not eliminate inhibitor activity, so that immunoadsorption is ordinarily combined with other means of eliminating these antibodies. Staphylococcal protein A–silica columns have been licensed in the USA for treating selected patients with ITP and rheumatoid arthritis (Mittelman *et al.* 1992; Snyder *et al.* 1992; Felson *et al.* 1999). In practice, immunoadsorption is usually limited to severely afflicted patients unresponsive to other therapies. Whether the mechanism of action involves removal of antibody and immune complexes or some more obscure immuno-modulatory effect is the source of some speculation (Bertram *et al.* 1985; Snyder *et al.* 1989). Passage of plasma over these columns does activate complement, which may be involved both in the efficacy and in the toxicity of the treatment. About one-third of procedures and 70% of treated patients experience adverse effects of treatment. Common side-effects include fever, headache, nausea, vomiting, pain and severe cardiopulmonary toxicity (Huestis and Morrison 1996).

LDL-apheresis. Patients with homozygous familial hypercholesterolaemia are notoriously difficult to manage with drug therapy and, prior to methods of mechanical removal of lipid, died in early adulthood from accelerated coronary artery disease. Early experience with repeated plasmapheresis demonstrated that the disease could be retarded and even reversed, and that patients survived into middle age (Thompson *et al.* 1975, 1985). One such patient, treated for more than 45 years at NIH, has now reached her late sixties and enjoys travelling and a variety of activities in her retirement.

ApoB-containing lipoproteins with well-defined biochemistry and physical characteristics became ideal targets for selective removal. Methods using filtration, heparin-mediated precipitation, antibody-mediated immunadsorption, and most recently dextran sulphate adsorption have been incorporated into apheresis systems (Stoffel *et al.* 1981; Borberg *et al.* 1990; Lane DM *et al.* 1995). LDL-apheresis is a convenient, effective, life-saving measure for the small number of patients with homozygous familial hypercholesterolaemia. Whereas modern drug therapy is effective for most heterozygotes, a subset of patients with severe disease and relative refractoriness to drugs clearly benefits from LDL-apheresis. Repeated treatments lower LDL cholesterol, induce coronary plaque regression and reduce the number of coronary events (Mabuchi *et al.* 1998; Matsuzaki *et al.* 2002). Few adverse events have been reported with any of the systems.

Side-effects of plasma exchange

The effects of intensive plasmapheresis in which small amounts of plasma are removed on numerous occasions have been considered above. In plasma exchange, large amounts of plasma are removed on any one occasion.

Effects of therapeutic plasma exchange on the circulation

Pronounced tiredness and malaise, presumably due to shifts in fluid balance and extracorporeal circulation, are seen not infrequently in patients undergoing plasma exchange. Hypotension, hypovolaemia and vasovagal attacks are more common after plasma exchange than after routine blood donations. Most of these reactions can be controlled by temporary interruption of the procedure and by the re-infusion of some extra fluid (Huestis 1986a).

Plasma protein levels

The extent of protein depletion will depend on the volume exchange, the number of procedures and the replacement fluid. Several studies have shown that plasma levels of immunoglobulins, C3, cholesterol, alkaline phosphatase and serum glutamic oxaloacetic transaminase (SGOT) are considerably reduced after plasma exchange and that it may take weeks for them to return to normal levels (Keller and Urbaniak 1978; Orlin and Berkman 1980; Stellon and Moorhead 1981; Nilsson *et al.* 1983). Immunoglobulin depletion

combined with immunosuppression may increase the possibility of infection.

Coagulation factors

Intensive or prolonged plasma exchange has the potential to induce haemorrhagic complications, through reduction in antithrombin III (ATIII) levels, but few such complications have been reported, and these may have been due to the patient's underlying state (Huestis 1983). Repeated plasma exchanges of 4–5 l resulted in a fall in fibrinogen levels to 25% after one exchange and to 1% after 10 exchanges; haemorrhagic complications were rare, although platelet transfusion was sometimes given when the platelet count was low (Flaum *et al.* 1979; Keller *et al.* 1979). In another series, 40–50% of patients undergoing repeated plasma exchanges with plasma-free solutions had platelet counts below $30 \times 10^9/l$ but bleeding episodes attributed to thrombocytopenia were observed in only 5 out of 815 (0.6%) procedures (Urbaniak 1983).

ATIII levels fell by about 84% in myasthenic patients undergoing 51 plasma exchanges, prothrombin and thrombin times shortened progressively and two patients showed hypercoagulability (Sultan *et al.* 1979). On the other hand, in seven alloimmunized pregnant women undergoing plasma exchanges equivalent to 60% of their plasma volume five times a week, coagulation factors remained within normal limits (Nilsson *et al.* 1983). The rarity of thrombotic complications in the presence of low levels of ATIII may be due to the concomitant reduction in fibrinogen and other procoagulant factors (Urbaniak 1983).

Citrate toxicity

The manifestations of citrate toxicity have been considered in the section on cell separators. The effects are exacerbated if the plasma is infused without first being warmed or if it is delivered through large-bore catheters situated close to the heart (Sutton *et al.* 1981).

Mortality

Plasma exchange is often used to treat severely ill patients and it is difficult to determine from most of the published reports whether to attribute death directly or indirectly to the exchange procedure or to the patient's underlying condition. The mortality rate attributable to plasma exchange has been estimated as 3 per 10 000 procedures. Of 59 deaths associated with plasma exchange, 30 were attributed to cardiac arrhythmia leading to cardiac arrest or to severe respiratory complications, such as the adult respiratory distress syndrome; plasma was used as a replacement fluid in the majority of these cases (Huestis 1989). In the UK, where albumin is the main replacement fluid and plasma is seldom used, no deaths attributed to plasma exchange have been reported. In France, five deaths attributed to plasma exchange were reported in 9437 procedures carried out in 1130 patients, and in Canada one death was reported in 3840 procedures in 640 patients (Robinson 1990). The most recent survey in the USA reported 89 adverse events in 1140 procedures that used plasma and 42 events in 1255 procedures that used non-plasma replacement solutions. There were no deaths reported (McLeod et al. 1999).

Therapeutic cytapheresis

Red cell exchange (therapeutic erythrocytapheresis)

Red cell exchange has been discussed above.

Therapeutic leucapheresis

Therapeutic leucapheresis has been used most successfully to help manage patients with acute leukaemia and extremely high white blood cell (WBC) numbers, so-called acute hyperleucocytic leukaemias (AHLs). The first instances of fatal cerebrovascular haemorrhage with hyperleucocytosis were reported almost 50 years ago (Fritz et al. 1959; Freireich et al. 1960). Their patients showed a characteristic histological finding at autopsy: circumscribed nodules of leukaemic cells surrounded by haemorrhage. The syndrome came to be called 'white ball disease'. A characteristic microscopic finding showed small vessels packed with leukaemic cells, so-called 'leucostasis'. Whereas changing neurological findings implicated the central nervous system as the most important target organ, leucostasis affects other organs, notably lung and kidney, as well. Increasing dyspnoea, hypoxaemia and pulmonary infiltrates in the setting of a high and rising blast count should signal severe leucostasis and necessitate urgent treatment.

Leucostasis occurs most often during the acute phase of myelocytic (AML) and myelomonocytic leukaemia. However, chronic myelocytic leukaemia (CML) in the accelerated or blast phases can also lead to leucostasis, particularly when the percentage of immature myeloid cells rises precipitously. This is particularly true of childhood CML (Rowe and Lichtman 1984). Neither the leucocyte count nor the blast count reliably predicts the onset of the leucostasis syndrome. However, all patients with AML and CML and a WBC count exceeding 200 000/μl have evidence of intravascular thrombi or aggregates at autopsy and 40% of those whose count ranged from 50 000 to 200 000 did as well (McKee and Collins 1974). The WBC count is generally higher (> 300 000) before aggregates occur in chronic lymphocytic leukaemia (CLL) owing to the smaller size and different rheology of the cells. Clinical evidence of leucostasis is unusual in this disease. One of the authors (HGK) has followed a patient with a WBC count exceeding 1 million/μl without any evidence of symptomatology; virtually all of the cells were mature, small lymphocytes. When the fractional volume of leucocytes (leucocrit) exceeds 20%, blood viscosity increases and leucocytes can interfere with pulmonary and cerebral blood flow and compete with tissue for oxygen in the microcirculation (Lichtman and Rowe 1982). These values, WBC count, percentage of blasts, rate of rise and leucocrit, in the presence of symptoms suggestive of early leucostasis, can guide therapy. Recent investigations of the expression and function of adhesion receptors on leukaemic cells and the role of adhesion molecules in leucocyte-induced acute lung injury in sepsis suggest that the pathophysiology of leucostasis may also be related to leukaemic blast–endothelial cell interactions mediated by locally released adhesion molecules (Porcu et al. 2002).

A single leucapheresis procedure processing one to three blood volumes and using a sedimenting agent such as HES generally reduces the WBC count by 20–50%, depending on the differing sedimentation characteristics of the specific blast cell population. Cells appear to be mobilized from the spleen and other tissue sites (Vallejos et al. 1973; Lowenthal et al. 1975). Ordinarily, leucapheresis is initiated in an AML patient when the blast count is > 100 000/mm³ or when rapidly rising blast counts are > 50 000/mm³, especially when evidence of central nervous system or pulmonary symptoms appears. The threshold for initiation of leucapheresis in patients with ALL is generally higher (WBC count > 200 000/mm^3). Other immediate measures for treatment of patients with AHL include infusion of i.v. fluids, administration of hydroxyurea and allopurinol, and correction of coagulopathy and thrombocytopenia.

Mechanical cytoreduction for managing other leukaemic processes has limited value. Although repeated leucapheresis has adequately reduced the WBC count in a series of patients with chronic myeloid leukaemia, the median patient survival rate was not significantly different from that of similar patients treated with conventional chemotherapy (Hester *et al.* 1982). Leucapheresis reduces early mortality in AML and improves the rate of initial remission, but does not improve survival (Cuttner *et al.* 1983; Giles *et al.* 2001). Chronic leucapheresis can provide acceptable control of the peripheral WBC count in clinical situations such as pregnancy, when cytotoxic agents may best be avoided, but cytoreduction alone does not appear to alter the course of CML. Some studies of patients with CLL suggested short-term clinical benefit, but long-term support of patients when the disease is refractory to chemotherapy does not appear to prolong life (Cooper *et al.* 1979; Goldfinger *et al.* 1980).

Lymphocyte removal by apheresis has also been used to modify immune responsiveness in patients with autoimmune diseases, to enhance solid organ allograft survival and to reverse solid organ graft rejection, but evidence of clinical efficacy in these situations is sparse. Removal of large numbers of lymphocytes over a period of a few weeks can suppress peripheral lymphocyte counts in rheumatoid arthritis patients for up to 1 year and alter skin-test reactivity and lymphocyte mitogen responsiveness to a variety of stimulants (Wright *et al.* 1981). Selected patients experience a modest but significant reduction in disease activity; however, the subset of patients who may derive substantial benefit from this therapy is difficult to identify (Wallace *et al.* 1979; Karsh *et al.* 1981). Most patients with this disorder find the degree of improvement insufficient to justify the time and inconvenience of repeated apheresis.

Therapeutic thrombocytapheresis

Thrombocytosis is generally categorized as 'reactive', as is seen with iron deficiency or post splenectomy, or 'clonal' as is the case with the myeloproliferative disorders (Schafer 2004). Therapeutic plateletpheresis is generally reserved for patients with myeloproliferative disorders and clonal thrombocytosis who suffer haemorrhage or thrombosis associated with an increase in circulating platelets. Thrombosis is more common in polycythaemia vera and essential thrombocythaemia regardless of the absolute platelet count, and haemorrhage is more common in CML. In addition to the common signs and symptoms of impending thrombotic events, paraesthesias, digital pain and erythromelalgia, evidence of microvascular ischaemia, may presage such events in patients with clonal thrombocytosis. Many centres consider using plateletpheresis when the patient's peripheral platelet count is > 10^6/mm^3, although no consistent relation between the level of platelet elevation and the occurrence of symptoms has been found, and no generally accepted assay of platelet dysfunction predicts which patients are at risk (Chievitz and Thiede 1962; Kessler *et al.* 1982; Schafer 2004) A single cytapheresis procedure can lower the platelet count by 30–50%. There is no target platelet count that can avoid additional clinical events. Attempts to maintain thrombocythaemic patients at normal platelet counts by cytapheresis alone have not been successful; more practical long-term chemotherapy should be instituted concurrently. A variety of regimens have been used (Tefferi *et al.* 2000). As most patients with thrombocytosis do not develop symptoms, including patients with myeloproliferative disorders, prophylactic plateletpheresis is unwarranted regardless of the platelet count.

Extracorporeal photopheresis: tanning the white cells to suppress immune response

Photopheresis is a form of automated photochemotherapy in which the patient's own leucocytes collected by apheresis are exposed outside the body (*ex vivo*) to 8-methoxy-psoralen (8-MOP) photoactivated with ultraviolet A (UVA) light and then returned i.v. to the patient. In the classical treatment, a high dose of 8-MOP is given orally followed by leucapheresis and UVA irradiation with an instrument licensed for this purpose. Alternatively, the light-sensitizing agent may be delivered directly to the extracorporeal leucocyte fraction, which may reduce the adverse effects such as nausea and vomiting associated with oral administration. The mechanism of action of photopheresis is unclear, but may involve generating an anti-idiotype cytotoxic T-cell response or inducing apoptosis in pathogenic T lymphocytes and antigen-presenting dendritic cells (Fimiani *et al.* 2004). This therapy has minimal toxicity and is highly effective in the treatment of patients with advanced cutaneous T-cell lymphoma (Lim and Edelson 1995). Other disorders reported to respond to photopheresis therapy include systemic sclerosis and other autoimmune diseases (Mayes 2000; Sapadin and Fleischmajer 2002), solid organ graft rejection (Dall'Amico *et al.* 1998; Lehrer *et al.* 2001) and graft-versus-host disease (GvHD) following haematopoietic stem cell transplantation (Seaton *et al.* 2003; Fimiani *et al.* 2004). Optimum frequency and duration of treatment are unknown, but responders have often required multiple procedures per week for months. Controlled experience with photopheresis in these clinical settings is limited.

References

Abel JJ, Rowntree LG, Turner BB (1914) Plasma removal with return of corpuscles. J Pharmacol Exp Ther 5: 625

Adams WS, Blahd WH, Bassett SH (1952) A method of human plasmapheresis. Proc Soc Exp Biol Med 80: 377–379

Adams RJ, McKie VC, Brambilla D *et al.* (1998) Stroke prevention trial in sickle cell anemia. Control Clin Trials 19: 110–129

Alarabi A, Backman U, Wikstrom B *et al.* (1995) Pretransplantation plasmapheresis in HLA-sensitized patients: five years experience. Transplant Proc 27: 3448

Alexander N, Higgs D, Dover G *et al.* (2004) Are there clinical phenotypes of homozygous sickle cell disease? Br J Haematol 126: 606–611

American Association of Blood Banks (AABB) (1994) Guidelines for Therapeutic Hemapheresis. Bethesda, MD: AABB Press

American Association of Blood Banks (AABB) (2003) Standards for Blood Banks and Transfusion Services. Bethesda, MD: AABB Press

Anderlini P, Donato M, Lauppe MJ *et al.* (2000) A comparative study of once-daily versus twice-daily filgrastim administration for the mobilization and collection of CD34+ peripheral blood progenitor cells in normal donors. Br J Haematol 109: 770–772

Anderson R, Cassell M, Mullinax GL *et al.* (1963) Effect of normal cells on viscosity of sickle-cell blood. *In vitro* studies and report of six years' experience with a prophylactic program of 'partial exchange transfusion'. Arch Intern Med 111: 286–294

Bandarenko N, Rose M, Kowalsky RJ *et al.* (2001) *In vivo* and *in vitro* characteristics of double units of RBCs collected by apheresis with a single in-line WBC-reduction filter. Transfusion 41: 1373–1377

Bensinger WI, Price TH, Dale DC (1993) The effects of daily recombinant human granulocyte colony-stimulating factor administration on normal granulocyte donors undergoing leukapheresis. Blood 81: 1883–1888

Bertram JH, Grunberg SM, Shulman I *et al.* (1985) Staphylococcal Protein A column: correlation of mitogenicity of perfused plasma with clinical response. Cancer Res 45: 4486–4494

Bitsch A, Bruck W (2002) Differentiation of multiple sclerosis subtypes: implications for treatment. CNS Drugs 16: 405–418

Blanchette VS, Dunne J, Steele D (1985) Immune function in blood donors following short-term lymphocytapheresis. Vox Sang 49: 101–109

Bolan CD, Greer SE, Cecco SA *et al.* (2001) Comprehensive analysis of citrate effects during plateletpheresis in normal donors. Transfusion 41: 1165–1171

Bolan CD, Cecco SA, Wesley RA *et al.* (2002) Controlled study of citrate effects and response to i.v. calcium administration during allogeneic peripheral blood progenitor cell donation. Transfusion 42: 935–946

Bolan CD, Wesley RA, Yau YY *et al.* (2003a) Randomized placebo-controlled study of oral calcium carbonate administration in plateletpheresis: I. Associations with donor symptoms. Transfusion 43: 1403–1413

Bolan CD, Carter CS, Wesley RA *et al.* (2003b) Prospective evaluation of cell kinetics, yields and donor experiences during a single large-volume apheresis versus two smaller volume consecutive day collections of allogeneic peripheral blood stem cells. Br J Haematol 120: 801–807

Bolan CD, Cecco SA, Yau YY *et al.* (2003c) Randomized placebo-controlled study of oral calcium carbonate supplementation in plateletpheresis: II. Metabolic effects. Transfusion 43: 1414–1422

Bolan CD, Yau YY, Cullis HC *et al.* (2004) Pediatric large-volume leukapheresis: a single institution experience with heparin versus citrate-based anticoagulant regimens. Transfusion 44: 229–238

Borberg H, Gaczkowski A, Oette K *et al.* (1990) Immunosorptive apheresis of LDL. Prog Clin Biol Res 337: 163–167

Boyle R (1666a) Phil Trans 20: 353

Boyle R (1666b) Phil Trans 22: 385

Brozovic B (1984) International forum: How much plasma, relative to his body weight, can a donor give over a certain period without a continuous deviation of his plasma protein metabolism in the direction of plasma protein deficiency? Vox Sang 47: 435–436

Brumit MC, Shea TC, Brecher ME (2003) G-CSF-associated rash in an allogeneic PBPC donor. Transfusion 43: 1343

Bukowski RM, Hewlett JS, Reimer RR *et al.* (1981) Therapy of thrombotic thrombocytopenic purpura: an overview. Semin Thromb Hemost 7: 1–8

Burgstaler EA (2003) Current apheresis instruments. In: Apheresis: Principles and Practice. BC McLeod, TH Price, R Weinstein (eds). Bethesda, MD: Am Assoc Blood Banks, pp. 95–130.

Byrnes JJ, Khurana M (1977) Treatment of thrombotic thrombocytopenic purpura with plasma. N Engl J Med 297: 1386–1389

Calabrese LH, Clough JD, Krakauer RS (1980) Plasmapheresis therapy of immunologic disease. Cleve Clin Quart 47: 53–72

Caspar CB, Seger RA, Burger J *et al.* (1993) Effective stimulation of donors for granulocyte transfusions with recombinant methionyl granulocyte colony-stimulating factor. Blood 81: 2866–2871

Castro O, Sandler SG, Houston-Yu P *et al.* (2002) Predicting the effect of transfusing only phenotype-matched RBCs to patients with sickle cell disease: theoretical and practical implications. Transfusion 42: 684–690

Chievitz E, Thiede T (1962) Complications and causes of death in polycythaemia vera. Acta Med Scand 172: 513–523

Cohen MA, Oberman HA (1970) Safety and long-term effects of plasmapheresis. Transfusion 10: 58

Coles SM, Klein HG, Holland PV (1981) Alloimmunization in two multitransfused patient populations. Transfusion 21: 462–466

Cooper IA, Ding JC, Adams PB *et al.* (1979) Intensive leukapheresis in the management of cytopenias in patients with chronic lymphocytic leukaemia (CLL) and lymphocytic lymphoma. Am J Hematol 6: 387–398

Couriel D, Weinstein R (1994) Complications of therapeutic plasma exchange: a recent assessment. J Clin Apheresis 9: 1–5

Cumberland GD, Titford M, Riddick L (1991) Demonstration of a fatal hemolytic transfusion reaction using immunoperoxidase techniques. Am J Forensic Med Pathol 12: 250–251

Cuttner J, Holland JF, Norton L *et al.* (1983) Therapeutic leukapheresis for hyperleukocytosis in acute myelocytic leukemia. Med Pediatr Oncol 11: 76–78

Dale DC, Liles WC, Llewellyn C *et al.* (1998) Neutrophil transfusions: kinetics and functions of neutrophils mobilized with granulocyte-colony-stimulating factor and dexamethasone. Transfusion 38: 713–721

Dall'Amico R, Murer L, Montini G *et al.* (1998) Successful treatment of recurrent rejection in renal transplant patients with photopheresis. J Am Soc Nephrol 9: 121–127

Dau PC, Lindstrom JM, Cassel CK *et al.* (1977) Plasmapheresis and immunosuppressive drug therapy in myasthenia gravis. N Engl J Med 297: 1134–1140

Diamond WJ, Brown FL Jr, Bitterman P *et al.* (1980) Delayed hemolytic transfusion reaction presenting as sickle-cell crisis. Ann Intern Med 93: 231–234

Djerassi I, Kim JS (1977) Problems and solutions with filtration leukapheresis. Prog Clin Biol Res 13: 305–313

Doria A, Piccoli A, Vesco P *et al.* (1994) Therapy of lupus nephritis. A two-year prospective study. Ann Med Interne (Paris) 145: 307–311

Drew MJ (2002) Plasmapheresis in the dysproteinemias. Ther Apheresis 6: 45–52

Dwyer JM, Wade MJ, Katz AJ (1981) Removal of thymic-derived lymphocytes during pheresis procedures. Vox Sang 41: 287–294

Evans RT, MacDonald R, Robinson A (1980) Suxamethonium apnoea associated with plasmapheresis. Anaesthesia 35: 198–201

Falzetti F, Aversa F, Minelli O *et al.* (1999) Spontaneous rupture of spleen during peripheral blood stem-cell mobilisation in a healthy donor. Lancet 353: 555

Felson DT, LaValley MP, Baldassare AR *et al.* (1999) The Prosorba column for treatment of refractory rheumatoid arthritis: a randomized, double-blind, sham-controlled trial. Arthritis Rheum 42: 2153–2159

Fimiani M, Di Renzo M, Rubegni P (2004) Mechanism of action of extracorporeal photochemotherapy in chronic graft-versus-host disease. Br J Dermatol 150: 1055–1060

Flaum MA, Cuneo RA, Appelbaum FR *et al.* (1979) The hemostatic imbalance of plasma-exchange transfusion. Blood 54: 694–702

Flomenberg N, Devine SM, Dipersio JF *et al.* (2005) The use of AMD3100 plus G-CSF for autologous hematopoietic progenitor cell mobilization is superior to G-CSF alone. Blood 106: 1867–1874

Fratantoni JC, French JE (1980) International Forum. Which are the principal established or potential risks for donors undergoing cytapheresis procedures and how can they be prevented? Vox Sang 39: 174–176

Freireich EJ, Thomas LB, Frei E III *et al.* (1960) A distinctive type of intracerebral hemorrhage associated with 'blastic crisis' in patients with leukemia. Cancer 13: 146–154

Freireich EJ, Judson G, Levin RH (1965) Separation and collection of leukocytes. Cancer Res 25: 1516–1520

Friedman BA, Schork MA, Mocniak JL (1975) Short-term and long-term effects of plasmapheresis on serum proteins and immunoglobulins. Transfusion 15: 467

Friedman DF, Lukas MB, Jawad A *et al.* (1996) Alloimmunization to platelets in heavily transfused patients with sickle cell disease. Blood 88: 3216–3222

Fritsch G, Fischmeister G, Haas OA *et al.* (1994) Peripheral blood hematopoietic progenitor cells of cytokine-stimulated healthy donors as an alternative for allogeneic transplantation. Blood 83: 3420–3421

Fritz RD, Forkner CE Jr, Freireich EJ et al. (1959) The association of fatal intracranial hemorrhage and blastic crisis in patients with acute leukemia. N Engl J Med 261: 59–64

Furlan M (2003) Deficient activity of von Willebrand factor-cleaving protease in thrombotic thrombocytopenic purpura. Expert Rev Cardiovasc Ther 1: 243–255

Furlan M, Lammle B (2002) Assays of von Willebrand factor-cleaving protease: a test for diagnosis of familial and acquired thrombotic thrombocytopenic purpura. Semin Thromb Hemost 28: 167–172

Gaskin G, Pusey CD (2001) Plasmapheresis in antineutrophil cytoplasmic antibody-associated systemic vasculitis. Ther Apheresis 5: 176–181

Ghodsi Z, Strauss RG (2001) Cataracts in neutrophil donors stimulated with adrenal corticosteroids. Transfusion 41: 1464–1468

Gibberd FB, Billimoria JD, Page NGR (1979) Heredopathia atactica polineuritiformis (Refsum's disease) treated by diet and plasma exchange. Lancet i: 575–578

Giles FJ, Shen Y, Kantarjian HM et al. (2001) Leukapheresis reduces early mortality in patients with acute myeloid leukemia with high white cell counts but does not improve long-term survival. Leuk Lymphoma 42: 67–73

Gjorstrup P (1991) Anti-HLA antibody removal in hyperimmunized ESRF patients to allow transplantation. The Collaborative Study Group on Anti-HLA Antibody Removal. Transplant Proc 23: 392–395

Gjorstrup P, Berntorp E, Larsson L et al. (1991) Kinetic aspects of the removal of IgG and inhibitors in hemophiliacs using protein A immunoadsorption. Vox Sang 61: 244–250

Glockner WM, Sieberth HG, Wichmann HE et al. (1988) Plasma exchange and immunosuppression in rapidly progressive glomerulonephritis: a controlled, multi-center study. Clin Nephrol 29: 1–8

Gloor JM, Lager DJ, Moore SB et al. (2003) ABO-incompatible kidney transplantation using both A2 and non-A2 living donors. Transplantation 75: 971–977

Glowitz RJ, Slichter SJ (1980) Frequent multiunit plateletpheresis from single donors: effects on donors' blood and the platelet yield. Transfusion 20: 199–205

Goldfinger D, Capostagno V, Lowe C et al. (1980) Use of long-term leukapheresis in the treatment of chronic lymphocytic leukemia. Transfusion 20: 450–454

Griffin SV, Lockwood CM, Pusey CD (1996) Plasmapheresis and immunoadsorption. In: Therapeutic Immunology. KF Austen, SJ Burakoff (eds). Cambridge, MA: Blackwell Science, pp. 636–651

Grifols-Lucas J (1952) Use of plasmapheresis in blood donors. BMJ 1: 854

Guillevin L, Lhote F, Cohen P et al. (1995) Corticosteroids plus pulse cyclophosphamide and plasma exchanges versus corticosteroids plus pulse cyclophosphamide alone in the treatment of polyarteritis nodosa and Churg-Strauss syndrome patients with factors predicting poor prognosis. A prospective, randomized trial in sixty-two patients. Arthritis Rheum 38: 1638–1645

Hakim RM, Milford E, Himmelfarb J et al. (1990) Extracorporeal removal of anti-HLA antibodies in transplant candidates. Am J Kidney Dis 16: 423–431

Haynes AP, Hunter A, McQuaker G (1995) Engraftment characteristics of peripheral blood stem cells mobilised with cyclophosphamide and delayed addition of G-CSF. Bone Marrow Transplant 16: 359–363

Heaton WAL, Holme S (1993) Storage of platelet concentrates. In: Quality Assurance in Transfusion Medicine: Vol. II. Methodological Advances and Clinical Aspects. G Rock (ed.). Boca Raton, FL: CRC Press, pp. 121–146

Hester JP, Kellogg RM, Mulzet AP et al. (1979) Principles of blood separation and component extraction in a disposable continuous-flow single-stage channel. Blood 54: 254–268

Hester JP, McCredie KB, Freireich EJ (1982) Response to chronic leukapheresis procedures and survival of chronic myelogenous leukemia patients. Transfusion 22: 305–307

Hiesse C, Kriaa F, Rousseau P et al. (1992) Immunoadsorption of anti-HLA antibodies for highly sensitized patients awaiting renal transplantation. Nephrol Dial Transplant 7: 944–951

Higby DJ, Mishler JM, Rhomberg W et al. (1975) The effect of a single or double dose of dexamethasone on granulocyte collection with the continuous flow centrifuge. Vox Sang 28: 243–248

Huestis DW (1983) Mortality in therapeutic haemapheresis (Letter). Lancet i: 1043

Huestis DW (1986a) Complications of therapeutic apheresis. In: Therapeutic Hemapheresis. M Valbonesi (ed.). Milan: Wichtig Editore, pp. 179–186

Huestis DW (1986b) Therapeutic plasmapheresis. In: Progress in Transfusion Medicine. JD Cash (ed.). Edinburgh: Churchill Livingstone, pp. 78–94

Huestis DW (1989) Risks and safety practices in hemapheresis procedures. Arch Pathol Lab Med 113: 273–278

Huestis DW, Morrison FS (1996) Adverse clinical effects of immune sorption with staphylococcal protein A columns. Transfusion Med Rev 10: 62–70

Huestis DW, Loftus TJ, Gilcher R (1985) Modified fluid gelatin. An alternative macromolecular agent for centrifugal leukapheresis. Transfusion 25: 343–348

Ito Y, Suaudeau J, Bowman RL (1975) New flow-through centrifuge without rotating seals applied to plasmapheresis. Science 189: 999–1000

Jaffe JP, Mosher DF (1981) Plasma antithrombin III and plasminogen levels in chronic plasmapheresis. N Engl J Med 304: 789

Jayne DRW (1990) New strategies for plasma exchange in systemic vasculitis Transfus Sci 11: 263–269

Johnson JP, Moore J Jr, Austin HA III et al. (1985) Therapy of anti-glomerular basement membrane antibody disease: analysis of prognostic significance of clinical, pathologic and treatment factors. Medicine (Baltimore) 64: 219–227

Jones AL (1988) The IBM Blood Cell Separator and Blood Cell Processor: a personal perspective. J Clin Apheresis 4: 171–182

Kao KJ, Mickel M, Braine HG et al. (1995) White cell reduction in platelet concentrates and packed red cells by filtration: a multicenter clinical trial. The Trap Study Group. Transfusion 35: 13–19

Karsh J, Klippel JH, Plotz PH et al. (1981) Lymphapheresis in rheumatoid arthritis. A randomized trial. Arthritis Rheum 24: 867–873

Kasprisin DO, Hoffman KC (1991) Hemapheresis vs intravenous immune globulin. In: Cellular and Humoral Immunotherapy and Apheresis. RA Sacher, DB Brubaker, DD Kasprisin (eds). Arlington, VA: Am Assoc Blood Banks, pp. 17–29

Kaul DK, Fabry ME, Nagel RL (1996) The pathophysiology of vascular obstruction in the sickle syndromes. Blood Rev 10: 29–44

Kaul DK, Liu XD, Nagel RL et al. (1998) Microvascular hemodynamics and in vivo evidence for the role of intercellular adhesion molecule-1 in the sequestration of infected red blood cells in a mouse model of lethal malaria. Am J Trop Med Hyg 58: 240–247

Kaul DK, Tsai HM, Liu XD et al. (2000) Monoclonal antibodies to alphaVbeta3 (7E3 and LM609) inhibit sickle red blood cell-endothelium interactions induced by platelet-activating factor. Blood 95: 368–374

Keitel H, Thompson D, Itano H (1956) Hyposthenuria in sickle cell anemia: a reversible defect. J Clin Invest 35: 998–1001

Keller AJ, Urbaniak SJ (1978) Intensive plasma exchange on the cell separator: effects on serum immunoglobulins and complement components. Br J Haematol 38: 531

Keller AJ, Chirnside A, Urbaniak SJ (1979) Coagulation abnormalities produced by plasma exchange on the cell separator with special reference to fibrinogen and platelet levels. Br J Haematol 42: 593–603

Kessinger A, Sharp JG (2003) The whys and hows of hematopoietic progenitor and stem cell mobilization. Bone Marrow Transplant 31: 319–329

Kessler CM, Klein HG, Havlik RJ (1982) Uncontrolled thrombocytosis in chronic myeloproliferative disorders. Br J Haematol 50: 157–167

Keynes G (1949) Blood transfusion. In: The History of Blood Transfusion. G Keynes (ed.). Bristol: John Wright & Sons

Khatri BO (2000) Therapeutic apheresis in multiple sclerosis and other central nervous system disorders. Ther Apheresis 4: 263–270

Khatri BO, McQuillen MP, Harrington GJ et al. (1985) Plasmapheresis in progressive MS. Neurology 35: 614

Kim HC, Dugan NP, Silber JH et al. (1994) Erythrocytapheresis therapy to reduce iron overload in chronically transfused patients with sickle cell disease. Blood 83: 1136–1142

Klein HG (1982) Cell separators for red cell exchange. In: Advances in the Pathophysiology, Diagnosis, and Treatment of Sickle Cell Disease. RB Scott (ed.). Progress in Clinical and Biological Research 98. New York: Alan R Liss, pp 109–116

Klein HG, Garner RJ, Miller DM et al. (1980) Automated partial exchange transfusion in sickle cell anemia. Transfusion 20: 578–584

Kliman A, Gaydos LA, Schroeder LR et al. (1961) Repeated plasmapheresis of blood donors as a source of platelets. Blood 18: 303–309

Kliman A, Carbone PP, Gaydos LA (1964) Effects of intensive plasmapheresis on normal blood donors. Blood 23: 647

Knezevic-Maramica I, Kruskall MS (2003) Intravenous immune globulins: an update for clinicians. Transfusion 43: 1460–1480

Koepke JA, Parks WM, Gocken JA (1981) The safety of weekly plateletpheresis: effect on the donors' lymphocyte population. Transfusion 21: 59–63

Korbling M, Huh YO, Durett A et al. (1995) Allogeneic blood stem cell transplantation: peripheralization and yield of donor-derived primitive hematopoietic progenitor cells (CD34+ Thy-1dim) and lymphoid subsets, and possible predictors of engraftment and graft-versus-host disease. Blood 86: 2842–2848

Koshy M, Burd L, Wallace D et al. (1988) Prophylactic red-cell transfusions in pregnant patients with sickle cell disease. A randomized cooperative study. N Engl J Med 319: 1447–1452

Kosmin M (1980) Bacteremia during leukapheresis. Transfusion 20: 115

Kroger N, Sonnenberg S, Cortes-Dericks L et al. (2004) Kinetics of G-CSF and CD34+ cell mobilization after once or twice daily stimulation with rHu granulocyte-stimulating factor (lenograstim) in healthy volunteers: an intraindividual crossover study. Transfusion 44: 104–110

Kurantsin-Mills J, Klug PP, Lessin LS (1988) Vaso-occlusion in sickle cell disease: pathophysiology of the microvascular circulation. Am J Pediatr Hematol Oncol 10: 357–372

Lane DM, Alaupovic P, Knight-Gibson C et al. (1995) Changes in plasma lipid and apolipoprotein levels between heparin-induced extracorporeal low-density lipoprotein precipitation (HELP) treatments. Am J Cardiol 75: 1124–1129

Lane TA, Law P, Maruyama M *et al.* (1995) Harvesting and enrichment of hematopoietic progenitor cells mobilized into the peripheral blood of normal donors by granulocyte-macrophage colony-stimulating factor (GM-CSF) or G-CSF: potential role in allogeneic marrow transplantation. Blood 85: 275–282

Latham A Jr (1986) Early developments in blood cell separation technology. Vox Sang 51: 249–252

Lazarus EF, Browning J, Norman J *et al.* (2001) Sustained decreases in platelet count associated with multiple, regular plateletpheresis donations. Transfusion 41: 756–761

Lee JH, Klein HG (1995) The effect of donor red cell sedimentation rate on efficiency of granulocyte collection by centrifugal leukapheresis. Transfusion 35: 384–388

Lee JH, Leitman SF, Klein HG (1995) A controlled comparison of the efficacy of hetastarch and pentastarch in granulocyte collections by centrifugal leukapheresis. Blood 86: 4662–4666

Lehrer MS, Rook AH, Tomaszewski JE *et al.* (2001) Successful reversal of severe refractory cardiac allograft rejection by photopheresis. J Heart Lung Transplant 20: 1233–1236

Leitman SF, Read EJ (1996) Hematopoietic progenitor cells. Semin Hematol 33: 341–358

Leitman SF, Browning JN, Yau YY *et al.* (2003) Hemochromatosis subjects as allogeneic blood donors: a prospective study. Transfusion 43: 1538–1544

Leitner GC, Jilma-Stohlawetz P, Stiegler G *et al.* (2003) Quality of packed red blood cells and platelet concentrates collected by multicomponent collection using the MCS plus device. J Clin Apheresis 18: 21–25

Lessin LS, Kurantsin-Mills J, Klug PP *et al.* (1978) Determination of rheologically optimal mixtures of AA and SS erythrocytes for transfusion. Prog Clin Biol Res 20: 123–137

Levy JB, Turner AN, Rees AJ *et al.* (2001) Long-term outcome of anti-glomerular basement membrane antibody disease treated with plasma exchange and immunosuppression. Ann Intern Med 134: 1033–1042

Levy GG, Motto DG, Ginsburg D (2005) ADAMTS13 Turns 3. Blood 106: 11–17

Lewis EJ, Hunsicker LG, Lan SP *et al.* (1992) A controlled trial of plasmapheresis therapy in severe lupus nephritis. The Lupus Nephritis Collaborative Study Group. N Engl J Med 326: 1373–1379

Lichtman MA, Rowe JM (1982) Hyperleukocytic leukemias: rheological, clinical, and therapeutic considerations. Blood 60: 279–283

Liles WC, Rodger E, Dale DC (2000) Combined administration of G-CSF and dexamethasone for the mobilization of granulocytes in normal donors: optimization of dosing. Transfusion 40: 642–644

Liles WC, Rodger E, Broxmeyer HE *et al.* (2005) Augmented mobilization and collection of CD34+ hematopoietic cells from normal human volunteers stimulated with granulocyte-colony-stimulating factor by single-dose administration of AMD3100, a CXCR4 antagonist. Transfusion 45: 295–300

Lim HW, Edelson RL (1995) Photopheresis for the treatment of cutaneous T-cell lymphoma. Hematol Oncol Clin North Am 9: 1117–1126

Lockwood CM, Boulton-Jones FM, Lowenthal RM *et al.* (1975) Recovery from Goodpasture's syndrome after immunosuppressive treatment and plasmapheresis. BMJ 2: 252–254

Lowenthal RM, Buskard NA, Goldman JM *et al.* (1975) Intensive leukapheresis as initial therapy for chronic granulocytic leukemia. Blood 46: 835–844

Lundsgaard-Hansen P (1977a) Volume limitations of plasmapheresis. Vox Sang 32: 20

Lundsgaard-Hansen P (1977b) Intensive plasmapheresis as a risk factor for arteriosclerotic cardiovascular disease? Vox Sang 33: 1–4

Mabuchi H, Koizumi J, Shimizu M *et al.* (1998) Long-term efficacy of low-density lipoprotein apheresis on coronary heart disease in familial hypercholesterolemia. Hokuriku-FH-LDL-Apheresis Study Group. Am J Cardiol 82: 1489–1495

McCredie KB, Freireich EJ, Hester JP *et al.* C (1974) Increased granulocyte collection with the blood cell separator and the addition of etiocholanolone and hydroxyethyl starch. Transfusion 14: 357–364

McCullough J, Chopek M (1981) Therapeutic plasma exchange. Lab Med 12: 745

McKee LC Jr, Collins RD (1974) Intravascular leukocyte thrombi and aggregates as a cause of morbidity and mortality in leukemia. Medicine (Baltimore) 53: 463–478

McKhann GM, Griffin JW, Cornblath DR *et al.* (1988) Role of therapeutic plasmapheresis in the acute Guillain-Barre syndrome. J Neuroimmunol 20: 297–300

McLeod BC (2002) An approach to evidence-based therapeutic apheresis. J Clin Apheresis 17: 124–132

McLeod BC (2003) Plasmapheresis in multiple sclerosis. J Clin Apheresis 18: 72–74

McLeod BC, Price TH, Owen H *et al.* (1998) Frequency of immediate adverse effects associated with apheresis donation. Transfusion 38: 938–943

McLeod BC, Sniecinski I, Ciavarella D *et al.* (1999) Frequency of immediate adverse effects associated with therapeutic apheresis. Transfusion 39: 282–288

Matalon A, Valeri A, Appel GB (2000) Treatment of focal segmental glomerulosclerosis. Semin Nephrol 20: 309–317

Matsuzaki M, Hiramori K, Imaizumi T *et al.* (2002) Intravascular ultrasound evaluation of coronary plaque regression by low density lipoprotein-apheresis in familial hypercholesterolemia: the Low Density Lipoprotein-Apheresis Coronary Morphology and Reserve Trial (LAC-MART). J Am Coll Cardiol 40: 220–227

Mavroudis DA, Read EJ, Molldrem J et al. (1998) T cell-depleted granulocyte colony-stimulating factor (G-CSF) modified allogenic bone marrow transplantation for hematological malignancy improves graft CD34+ cell content but is associated with delayed pancytopenia. Bone Marrow Transplant 21: 431–440

Mayes MD (2000) Photopheresis and autoimmune diseases. Rheum Dis Clin North Am 26: 75–79

van der Meche FG, Schmitz PI (1992) A randomized trial comparing intravenous immune globulin and plasma exchange in Guillain-Barre syndrome. Dutch Guillain-Barre Study Group. N Engl J Med 326: 1123–1129

Miller DM, Winslow RM, Klein HG et al. (1980) Improved exercise performance after exchange transfusion in subjects with sickle cell anemia. Blood 56: 1127–1131

Miller KD, Greenberg AE, Campbell CC (1989) Treatment of severe malaria in the United States with a continuous infusion of quinidine gluconate and exchange transfusion. N Engl J Med 321: 65–70

Mishler JM (1982) Pharmacology of Hydroxyethyl Starch. Oxford: Oxford University Press

Mishler JM, Higby DJ, Romberg W et al. (1975) Leucapheresis: increased efficiency of collection by the use of hydroxyethyl starch and dexamethasone. In: Leucocytes: Separation, Collection and Transfusion. JM Goldman, RM Lowenthal (eds). New York: Academic Press

Mishler IM, Borberg H, Reuter J (1977) The utilization of a new strength citrate anticoagulant during centrifugal plateletpheresis. II. Assessment of in vitro platelet function. Blut 34: 237

Mittelman A, Puccio C, Ahmed T et al. (1992) Response of refractory thrombotic thrombocytopenic purpura to extracorporeal immunoadsorption. N Engl J Med 326: 711–712

Moake JL (2004) von Willebrand factor, ADAMTS-13, and thrombotic thrombocytopenic purpura. Semin Hematol 41: 4–14

Mollison PL, Veall N, Cutbush N (1950) Red cell volume and plasma volume in newborn infants. Arch Dis Child 25: 242

Montgomery RA, Zachary AA (2004) Transplanting patients with a positive donor-specific crossmatch: a single center's perspective. Pediatr Transplant 8: 535–542

National Blood Data Resource Center (2001). Comprehensive report on blood collection and transfusion in the United States in 1999. National Blood Data Resource Center. Am Assoc Blood Banks, Bethesda, MD

National Blood Data Resource Center (2002) Comprehensive report on blood collection and transfusion in the United States in 2001. National Blood Data Resource Center, Bethesda, MD

Newsom-Davis J (2001) Lambert-Eaton myasthenic syndrome. Curr Treat Options Neurol 3: 127–131

Nilsson T, Rudolphi O, Cedergren B (1983) Effects of intensive plasmapheresis on the haemostatic system. Scand J Haematol 30: 201–206

Olson PR, Cox C, McCullough J (1977) Laboratory and clinical effects of the infusion of ACD solution during plateletpheresis. Vox Sang 33: 79

Orlin JB, Berkman EM (1980) Partial exchange using albumin replacement: removal and recovery of normal plasma constituents. Blood 56: 1055–1059

Pearson HA, Cornelius EA, Schwartz AD et al. (1970) Transfusion-reversible functional asplenia in young children with sickle-cell anemia. N Engl J Med 283: 334–337

Pepper DS (1983) A review of column technology as applied to apheresis. Apheresis Bull 1: 114–124

Pineda AA (1991) Immunoaffinity apheresis columns: clinical applications and therapeutic mechanisms of action. In: Cellular and Humoral Immunotherapy and Apheresis. RA Sacher, DB Brubaker, DO Kasprisin et al. (eds). Arlington, VA: Am Assoc Blood Banks, pp. 31–42

Porcu P, Farag S, Marcucci G et al. (2002) Leukocytoreduction for acute leukemia. Ther Apheresis 6: 15–23

Powell VI, Grima K (2002) Exchange transfusion for malaria and Babesia infection. Transfusion Med Rev 16: 239–250

Prosper F, Stroncek D, Verfaillie CM (1996) Phenotypic and functional characterization of long-term culture-initiating cells present in peripheral blood progenitor collections of normal donors treated with granulocyte colony-stimulating factor. Blood 88: 2033–2042

Prosper F, Vanoverbeke K, Stroncek D et al. (1997) Primitive long-term culture initiating cells (LTC-ICs) in granulocyte colony-stimulating factor mobilized peripheral blood progenitor cells have similar potential for ex vivo expansion as primitive LTC-ICs in steady state bone marrow. Blood 89: 3991–3997

Pusey CD, Lockwood CM, Peters DK (1983) Plasma exchange and immunosuppressive drugs in the treatment of glomerulonephritis due to antibodies on the glomerular basement membrane. Int J Artif Organs 6 Suppl. 1: 15–18

Reiter CD, Gladwin MT (2003) An emerging role for nitric oxide in sickle cell disease vascular homeostasis and therapy. Curr Opin Hematol 10: 99–107

Richman DP, Agius MA (2003) Treatment of autoimmune myasthenia gravis. Neurology 61: 1652–1661

Ring J, Sharkofl D, Richter W (1980) Using HES in man. Vox Sang 39: 181–185

Robbins G, Petersen CV, Brozovic B (1985) Lymphocytopenia in donors undergoing regular platelet apheresis with cell separators. Clin Lab Haematol 7: 225–230

Robertson LB (1924) Exsanguination-transfusion. A new therapeutic measure in the treatment of severe toxemias. Arch Surg 9: 1–15

Robinson EAE (1990) Hazards of apheresis and the UK approach to guidelines. Transfusion Sci 11: 305–308

Robinson EAE, Tovey LAD (1980) Intensive plasma exchange in the management of severe Rh disease. Br J Haematol 45: 621–631

Rock G, Wise P (1979) Plasma expansion during granulocyte procurement: cumulative effects of hydroxyethyl starch. Blood 53: 1156–1163

Rock G, Wise P, Kardish R (1984) Modified fluid gelatin in leukapheresis; accumulation and persistence in the body. Transfusion 24: 68–73

Rock JA, Shirey RS, Braine HG et al. (1985) Plasmapheresis for the treatment of repeated early pregnancy wastage associated with anti-P. Obstet Gynecol 66: 57S–60S

Rock GA, Shumak KH, Buskard NA (1991) Comparison of plasma exchange with plasma infusion in the treatment of thrombotic thrombocytopenic purpura. N Engl J Med 325: 393–397

Rock G, Tittley P, Sternbach M et al. (1992) Repeat plateletpheresis: the effects on the donor and the yield. Vox Sang 63: 102–106

Rock G, Moltzan C, Alharbi A et al. (2003) Automated collection of blood components: their storage and transfusion. Transfusion Med 13: 219–225

Rodgers GP, Schechter AN, Noguchi CT et al. (1984) Periodic microcirculatory flow in patients with sickle-cell disease. N Engl J Med 311: 1534–1538

Ross CN, Gaskin G, Gregor-Macgregor S et al. (1993) Renal transplantation following immunoadsorption in highly sensitized recipients. Transplantation 55: 785–789

Rosse WF, Gallagher D, Kinney TR (1990) Transfusion and alloimmunization in sickle cell disease. Blood 76: 1431–1437

Rowe JM, Lichtman MA (1984) Hyperleukocytosis and leukostasis: common features of childhood chronic myelogenous leukemia. Blood 63: 1230–1234

Russell MO, Goldberg HI, Hodson A et al. (1984) Effect of transfusion therapy on arteriographic abnormalities and on recurrence of stroke in sickle cell disease. Blood 63: 162–169

Sandler SG, Nusbacher J (1982) Health risks of leukapheresis donors. Haematologia 15: 57–69

Sapadin AN, Fleischmajer R (2002) Treatment of scleroderma. Arch Dermatol 138: 99–105

Sazama K (1990) Reports of 355 transfusion-associated deaths: 1976 through 1985. Transfusion 30: 583–590

Schafer AI (2004) Thrombocytosis. N Engl J Med 350: 1211–1219

Schultze HE, Heremans JF (1966) Molecular Biology of Human Proteins with Special Reference to Plasma Proteins, vol. 1. Amsterdam: Elsevier

Seaton ED, Szydlo RM, Kanfer E et al. (2003) Influence of extracorporeal photopheresis on clinical and laboratory parameters in chronic graft-versus-host disease and analysis of predictors of response. Blood 102: 1217–1223

Seghatchian J, Krailadsiri P (2000) Current position on preparation and quality of leucodepleted platelet concentrates for clinical use. Transfusion Sci 22: 85–88

Seghatchian J, Beard MJ, Krailadsiri P (2001) Studies on the improvement of leucodepletion performance of the Haemonetics MCS+ for production of leucodepleted platelet concentrate. Platelets 12: 298–301

Senhauser DA, Westphal RG, Bohman JE (1982) Immune system changes in cytapheresis donors. Transfusion 22: 302–304

Shehata N, Kouroukis C, Kelton JG (2002) A review of randomized controlled trials using therapeutic apheresis. Transfusion Med Rev 16: 200–229

Shi PA, Ness PM (1999) Two-unit red cell apheresis and its potential advantages over traditional whole-blood donation. Transfusion 39: 218–225

Siami FS, Siami GA (2004) A last resort modality using cryofiltration apheresis for the treatment of cold hemagglutinin disease in a Veterans Administration hospital. Ther Apheresis Dial 8: 398–403

Siami GA, Siami FS (1998) Cryofiltration apheresis in the United States. Ther Apheresis 2: 228–235

Simon TL (1994) The collection of platelets by apheresis procedures. Transfusion Med Rev 8: 132–145

Skoog WF, Adams WS (1959) Plasmapheresis in a case of Waldenstrom's macroglobulinemia. Clin Res 7: 96

Slichter SJ (1985) Optimal platelet concentrate preparation and storage. In: Current Concepts in Transfusion Therapy. G Garratty (ed.). Arlington, VA: Am Assoc Blood Banks

Smith JW, Weinstein R for The AABB Hemapheresis Committee KL (2003) Therapeutic apheresis: a summary of current indication categories endorsed by the AABB and the American Society for Apheresis. Transfusion 43: 820–822

Smith KJ, James DS, Hunt WC et al. (1996) A randomized, double-blind comparison of donor tolerance of 400 mL, 200 mL, and sham red cell donation. Transfusion 36: 674–680

Snyder HW Jr, Balint JP Jr, Jones FR (1989) Modulation of immunity in patients with autoimmune disease and cancer treated by extracorporeal immunoadsorption with PROSORBA columns. Semin Hematol 26: 31–41

Snyder HW Jr, Cochran SK, Balint JP Jr et al. (1992) Experience with protein A-immunoadsorption in treatment-resistant adult immune thrombocytopenic purpura. Blood 79: 2237–2245

Solomon JM (1985) Federal regulation of commercial plasmapheresis centers. J Clin Apheresis 2: 368–371

Solomon A, Fahey JL (1963) Plasmapheresis therapy in macroglobulinemia. Ann Intern Med 58: 789–800

Sonnenday CJ, Ratner LE, Zachary AA et al. (2002) Preemptive therapy with plasmapheresis/intravenous immunoglobulin allows successful live donor renal transplantation in patients with a positive cross-match. Transplant Proc 34: 1614–1616

Stegmayr B, Wikdahl AM (2003) Access in therapeutic apheresis. Ther Apheresis Dial 7: 209–214

Stellon AJ, Moorhead PJ (1981) Polygeline compared with plasma protein fraction as the sole replacement fluid in plasma exchange. BMJ i: 696–697

Stoffel W, Borberg H, Greve V (1981) Application of specific extracorporeal removal of low density lipoprotein in familial hypercholesterolaemia. Lancet 2: 1005–1007

Stong CL (1975) The amateur scientist. Sci Am 23: 120–122

Strauss RG, Huestis DW, Wright DG (1983) Cellular depletion by apheresis (Panel V). J Clin Apheresis 1: 158–165

Strauss RG, Hester JP, Vogler WR et al. (1986) A multicenter trial to document the efficacy and safety of a rapidly excreted analog of hydroxyethyl starch for leukapheresis with a note on steroid stimulation of granulocyte donors. Transfusion 26: 258–264

Strauss RG, Ciavarella D, Gilcher RO (1993) Clinical applications of therapeutic hemapheresis. An overview of current management. J Clin Apheresis 8: 189–194

Strauss RG, Pennell BJ, Stump DC (2002) A randomized, blinded trial comparing the hemostatic effects of pentastarch versus hetastarch. Transfusion 42: 27–36

Stroncek DF, Clay ME, Petzoldt ML et al. (1996a) Treatment of normal individuals with granulocyte-colony-stimulating factor: donor experiences and the effects on peripheral blood CD34+ cell counts and on the collection of peripheral blood stem cells. Transfusion 36: 601–610

Stroncek DF, Clay ME, Smith J et al. (1996b) Changes in blood counts after the administration of granulocyte-colony-stimulating factor and the collection of peripheral blood stem cells from healthy donors. Transfusion 36: 596–600

Stroncek DF, Clay ME, Herr G et al. (1997) The kinetics of G-CSF mobilization of CD34+ cells in healthy people. Transfusion Med 7: 19–24

Stroncek DF, Yau YY, Oblitas J et al. (2001) Administration of G-CSF plus dexamethasone produces greater granulocyte concentrate yields while causing no more donor toxicity than G-CSF alone. Transfusion 41: 1037–1044

Stroncek DF, Matthews CL, Follmann D et al. (2002) Kinetics of G-CSF-induced granulocyte mobilization in healthy subjects: effects of route of administration and addition of dexamethasone. Transfusion 42: 597–602

Stroncek D, Shawker T, Follmann D et al. (2003) G-CSF-induced spleen size changes in peripheral blood progenitor cell donors. Transfusion 43: 609–613

Suaudeau J, Kolobow T, Vaillancourt R et al. (1978) The Ito 'Flow-Through' Centrifuge. A new device for long-term (24 hours) plasmapheresis without platelet deterioration. Transfusion 18: 312–319

Sultan Y, Bussel A, Maisonneuve P (1979) Potential danger of thrombosis after plasma exchange in the treatment of patients with immune disease. Transfusion 19: 588–593

Sutton DMC, Cardella CJ, Uldall PR (1981) Complications of intensive plasma exchange. Plasma Ther 2: 19–23

Tefferi A, Solberg LA, Silverstein MN (2000) A clinical update in polycythemia vera and essential thrombocythemia. Am J Med 109: 141–149

Thompson GR, Lowenthal R, Myant NB (1975) Plasma exchange in the management of homozygous familial hypercholesterolaemia. Lancet 1: 1208–1211

Thompson GR, Miller JP, Breslow JL (1985) Improved survival of patients with homozygous familial hypercholesterolaemia treated with plasma exchange. BMJ (Clin Res Ed) 291: 1671–1673

Tsai HM (1996) Physiologic cleavage of von Willebrand factor by a plasma protease is dependent on its conformation and requires calcium ion. Blood 87: 4235–4244

Tsai HM, Lian EC (1998) Antibodies to von Willebrand factor-cleaving protease in acute thrombotic thrombocytopenic purpura. N Engl J Med 339: 1585–1594

Tui B, Barrter FC, Wright AM et al. (1944) Red cell reinfusion and the frequency of plasma donations: preliminary report of multiple donations in eight weeks by each of six donors. JAMA 124: 331–336

Tullis JL, Surgenor DM, Tinch RD et al. (1956) New principle of closed system centrifugation. Science 124: 792–797

Upshaw JD Jr (1978) Congenital deficiency of a factor in normal plasma that reverses microangiopathic hemolysis and thrombocytopenia. N Engl J Med 298: 1350–1352

Urbaniak SJ (1983) Replacement fluids in plasma exchange. Apheresis Bull 1: 104–113

Vallejos CS, McCredie KB, Brittin GM et al. (1973) Biological effects of repeated leukapheresis of patients with chronic myelogenous leukemia. Blood 42: 925–933

Veall N, Mollison PL (1950) The rate of red cell exchange in replacement transfusion. Lancet ii: 792

Vesely SK, George JN, Lammle B et al. (2003) ADAMTS13 activity in thrombotic thrombocytopenic purpura-hemolytic uremic syndrome: relation to presenting features and clinical outcomes in a prospective cohort of 142 patients. Blood 102: 60–68

Vichinsky EP, Earles A, Johnson RA (1990) Alloimmunization in sickle cell anaemia and transfusion of racially unmatched blood. N Engl J Med 322: 1617–1622

Vichinsky EP, Haberkern CM, Neumayr L *et al.* (1995) A comparison of conservative and aggressive transfusion regimens in the perioperative management of sickle cell disease. The Preoperative Transfusion in Sickle Cell Disease Study Group. N Engl J Med 333: 206–213

Wallace DJ, Goldfinger D, Gatti R *et al.* (1979) Plasmapheresis and lymphoplasmapheresis in the management of rheumatoid arthritis. Arthritis Rheum 22: 703–710

Wallace DJ, Goldfinger D, Pepkowitz SH *et al.* (1998) Randomized controlled trial of pulse/synchronization cyclophosphamide/apheresis for proliferative lupus nephritis. J Clin Apher 13: 163–166

Waller CF, Bertz H, Wenger MK *et al.* (1996) Mobilization of peripheral blood progenitor cells for allogeneic transplantation: efficacy and toxicity of a high-dose rhG-CSF regimen. Bone Marrow Transplant 18: 279–283

Wallerstein H, Brodie SS (1948) The efficiency of blood substitution. Am J Clin Pathol 18: 857

Warren DS, Zachary AA, Sonnenday CJ *et al.* (2004) Successful renal transplantation across simultaneous ABO incompatible and positive crossmatch barriers. Am J Transplant 4: 561–568

Watt RM, Bunitsky K, Faulkner EB *et al.* (1992) Treatment of congenital and acquired hemophilia patients by extracorporeal removal of antibodies to coagulation factors: a review of US clinical studies 1987–1990. Hemophilia Study Group. Transfusion Sci 13: 233–253

Wei N, Klippel JH, Huston DP *et al.* (1983) Randomised trial of plasma exchange in mild systemic lupus erythematosus. Lancet 1: 17–22

Weiner HL, Dau PC, Khatri BO *et al.* (1989) Double-blind study of true vs. sham plasma exchange in patients treated with immunosuppression for acute attacks of multiple sclerosis. Neurology 39: 1143–1149

Westphal RG (1984) Health risks to cytapheresis donors in blood transfusion and blood banking. Clin Haematol 13: 289–301

WHO (1975) Meeting on the utilization and supply of human blood and blood products, Bern, Switzerland. In: Resolutions, Recommendations and Decisions on Blood Transfusion. Geneva: League of Red Cross and Red Crescent Societies

WHO (1989a) Expert Committee on Biological Standardization, 39th Report, Annex 4. Geneva: World Health Organization, pp. 94–176

WHO (1989b) Requirements for the Collection, Processing and Quality Control of Blood, Blood Components and Plasma Derivatives. WHO Technical Series Report 786. Geneva: WHO, pp. 94–176

Winton EF, Vogler WR (1978) Development of a practical oral dexamethasone premedication schedule leading to improved granulocyte yields with the continuous-flow centrifugal blood cell separator. Blood 52: 249–253

Wright DG, Karsh J, Fauci AS *et al.* (1981) Lymphocyte depletion and immunosuppression with repeated leukapheresis by continuous flow centrifugation. Blood 58: 451–458

Zheng XL, Kaufman RM, Goodnough LT *et al.* (2004) Effect of plasma exchange on plasma ADAMTS13 metalloprotease activity, inhibitor level, and clinical outcome in patients with idiopathic and nonidiopathic thrombotic thrombocytopenic purpura. Blood 103: 4043–4049

18 Alternatives to allogeneic transfusion

Bloodless surgery has become a mantra. Blood conservation falls into two general categories: re-infusion of the patient's own (autologous) blood, and techniques to limit blood loss. Autologous transfusions, although not truly 'bloodless', contribute to bloodless management. Furthermore, a variety of drugs and biologicals are available to stimulate autologous cell production, replace blood components and help manage haemostasis in patients who might otherwise require transfusion. This chapter will address strategies for autologous transfusion, various blood-derived biologicals, non-blood-derived drugs and strategies to prevent haemorrhage and manage haemostatic disorders.

Autologous transfusion

Preoperative ('pre-deposit') autologous blood collections

The transfusion requirements of a significant number of surgical patients can be met completely with autologous blood (Anderson and Tomasulo 1988; Maffei 1988). The criteria for accepting donors for autologous transfusion need not be as strict as those for allogeneic transfusion. For example, vast experience supports inclusion of patients over the age of 70 or under 17 and patients with haemoglobin of about 110 g/l in pre-deposit programmes (Mann et al. 1983; Ness et al. 1987; Silvergleid 1987; Daneshvar 1988). Patients taking medication, pregnant women with a high risk of bleeding during delivery and patients with a history of cardiac disease or recent surgery are acceptable in specialized centres for the collection of autologous blood (Britton et al. 1989; McVay et al.

1989; Owings et al. 1989). A study conducted by the American Red Cross showed that in 5660 pre-deposit donations given in donor clinics outside hospitals, serious untoward effects occurred in less than 1%. Some patients not meeting the usual criteria for donors had an overall rate of reaction (mostly fainting) of 4.2% compared with 2.7% of those who met the criteria. Patients not meeting criteria for donors, for example those who were less than 17 years old, weighed less than 100 lbs (45.4 kg) or had suffered previous reactions, were more likely to have a reaction. On the other hand, donors over 75 years of age, with a history of cardiac disease, medication or surgery, did not have an increased risk of reacting adversely to donation (Aubuchon et al. 1988).

When planning an autologous donation programme, it is important to select patients who are expected to require transfusion. Patients most likely to benefit are those undergoing orthopaedic procedures (joint replacement, spinal surgery), cardiovascular procedures and radical prostatectomy where significant blood loss is anticipated (Goodnough et al. 1996). Several reports show that a significant number of units of blood collected preoperatively will not be transfused to the patient donor; in fact the number can be as high as 50%, which leads to the question of the cost-effectiveness of the procedure (Birkmeyer et al. 1994; Etchason et al. 1995). A hospital's maximum surgical blood ordering schedule (MSBOS, see Chapter 8) can be helpful in predicting which patients will benefit from a pre-deposit programme (Goodnough et al. 1992a).

The theory behind preoperative autologous donation presumes that the red cell mass removed before elective surgery will regenerate sufficiently before the operation so that less allogeneic blood will be required during the procedure and in the immediate postoperative period. This is not ordinarily the case. Despite the potential for 6-week refrigerated storage, autologous red cells are generally collected just a week or two prior to surgery, too short an interval to expect significant marrow regeneration of red cell mass (Brecher and Goodnough 2002). For patients donating autologous blood in the few weeks immediately before surgery, the procedure achieves no better result than does acute normovolaemic haemodilution at the time of surgery (Ness et al. 1992; Goodnough et al. 2000). Unless patients are selected carefully, preoperative autologous collection can result in discarded units, inappropriately transfused autologous units or a patient with no allogeneic exposure, but a lower red cell mass in the postoperative period than might have obtained had no preoperative procedure been performed. Efforts to use predictors of erythropoiesis to define patients most likely to benefit from preoperative autologous donation are promising, but require validation (Klein 2000; Nuttall et al. 2000). Mathematical models have been developed using the patient's presenting haematocrit and the physician's 'transfusion trigger' to predict the estimated blood loss at which transfusion (or autologous blood) might be needed (Cohen and Brecher 1995).

The ability to donate sufficient numbers of red cell units to prevent allogeneic transfusion depends primarily on the patient's initial haematocrit (Goodnough et al. 1994). For most patients, donation of a unit of blood every 5–7 days does little to stimulate endogenous erythropoietin or a brisk marrow response (Kickler and Spivak 1988). Recombinant erythropoietin supplemented with oral iron therapy has been administered to patients to improve red cell regeneration and augment autologous donations. These strategies are effective, but costly. When recombinant human erythropoietin (600 units per kilogram of body weight intravenously, twice per week, for 21 days, and ferrous sulphate, 325 mg orally, three times daily) was administered to 47 adults scheduled for elective orthopaedic procedures in a randomized controlled trial, the patients who received erythropoietin were able to donate a mean red cell volume that was 41% greater than that donated by the patients who received placebo (Goodnough et al. 1989). Although this result seems impressive and has been confirmed repeatedly, patients who present with a normal haematocrit do

not benefit from this regimen (Goodnough et al. 1992b; Biesma et al. 1994). Erythropoietin administration in a pre-deposit programme may allow patients with mild to moderate anaemia to avoid allogeneic exposures, but patients with poorly responsive anaemia and those with iron deficiency are unlikely to benefit even from aggressive management (Goodnough et al. 1991; Mercuriali et al. 1993; Price et al. 1996).

Not all patients are eligible for autologous donation; the ultimate responsibility for ensuring the patient's safety rests with the physician undertaking the collection. Although the restrictions vary in different countries, with the USA taking a more liberal approach than the UK, contraindications for pre-deposit autologous transfusion exist: (1) bacteraemia; (2) significant cardiovascular problems (e.g. unstable angina, cardiac failure, severe aortic stenosis, cyanotic heart disease, uncontrolled hypertension or respiratory or cerebrovascular diseases); (3) pregnancy with anaemia, hypovolaemia, pre-eclampsia or any condition associated with retardation of fetal growth, or impaired placental blood flow; and (4) epilepsy. Patients who would not qualify as blood donors must be bled in a hospital under the supervision of a clinician. When patients on beta-blockers or angiotensin-converting enzymes are bled, saline is often infused as the blood is drawn to maintain intravascular volume (Lee et al. 1993). Pregnant women likely to need blood transfusion for conditions such as placenta praevia and bleeding in the third trimester are bled in the left lateral position by some, but with no special precautions by others (McVay et al. 1989). Although pregnant women can give blood with no significant adverse effects to themselves, very few data are available on the effect of blood donation in the third trimester on fetal circulation and iron status. For this reason, if specific indications for autologous donation exist, blood should be collected early in pregnancy, whenever possible, and cryopreserved. Although for appropriately selected patients autologous donation is safe (see above), a reported 1 in 16 783 autologous donations results in a severe outcome (an adverse event that leads to hospitalization), a rate that is 11.8 times higher than the risk associated with healthy volunteers (Popovsky et al. 1995).

Only 2% of children between the ages of 8 and 18 years had adverse reactions to autologous donation, provided that they had no cardiac or respiratory problems (Depalma and Luban 1990). However, the collection of blood from children is difficult. Children weighing between 28 and 50 kg can be bled of 250 ml into paedipaks, which contain 35 ml of CPD-A1. If these packs are not available, a standard-sized pack can be used with a satellite pack attached so that excess anticoagulant can be removed while retaining a closed system. The amount of blood to be taken should not exceed 12% of the blood volume and is calculated as: [weight (kg)/50] × 450 ml, and the volume of anticoagulant to be used as: [volume of donation (ml)/450] × 63 ml.

It is prudent to perform the same tests on autologous blood as on blood donated by routine blood donors. The main reasons for this recommendation are: (1) to address the possibility that a mistake in identification may be made, leading to the transfusion of blood of the wrong ABO group or of blood contaminated with an infectious agent and (2) to discover whether the patient is already infected with a virus that he or she fears might be acquired by transfusion with allogeneic blood. UK collection and transfusion centres will not store autologous units found positive for HBsAg or for anti-HIV, -HCV or -HTLV. In any case, autologous donations should be clearly labelled and stored separately from routine blood donations (Lee *et al.* 1993).

Although the use of platelets is rarely indicated in elective surgery, except perhaps in complicated cardiac or vascular surgery, the collection of platelets with cell separators taken either 1–2 days or immediately before surgery has been reported (Giordano *et al.* 1988, 1989).

The practice of collecting blood from healthy subjects for long-term frozen storage in case they should require future transfusion is expensive, wasteful and impractical. On the other hand, long-term storage of autologous blood is indicated for: (1) subjects with rare blood groups or with multiple red cell antibodies, for whom compatible blood may be difficult to find and (2) those rare patients who have had more than one unexplained haemolytic transfusion reaction. Even then, these frozen units often remain unused in storage and even the patient may forget that they exist (Depalma *et al.* 1990).

In the UK, blood taken for autologous transfusion should not, if unused, be put into the general stocks of allogeneic blood ('crossover'). The main reasons for this recommendation are that: (1) as, at the time of withdrawal, the donation was not intended for allogeneic transfusion, the criteria for donor acceptance could have been less stringent (e.g. the patient might have been taking medications or might have been transfused within the last year); (2) the labelling will be inappropriate; (3) most autologous blood is collected in hospitals, using different documentation from that used at transfusion centres; (4) the risk of errors increases as donation details transfer from one database to another; (5) the donor may have an increased chance of being positive for markers of infectious disease (Grossman *et al.* 1988; Starkey *et al.* 1989); and (6) a considerable proportion of the autologous units will be near expiry date before it is determined that they will not be needed for the patient donor. In any case, if programmes of autologous transfusion are properly planned, the volume of blood left unused after surgery should be small. In fact, in well-conducted programmes not less than 3% and at the most 9% of autologous units would be available for allogeneic blood transfusion. The complexities of record keeping in order to transfer such small numbers of units to the voluntary donor pool argue against the practice of 'crossover' (Silvergleid 1991).

Intraoperative haemodilution

Details of the haemodilution procedure are discussed in Chapter 2. Mathematical modelling indicates that deep acute normovolaemic haemodilution must be performed and substantial blood loss must occur before a practical red cell mass of autologous blood is 'saved' (Cohen and Brecher 1995). Put a different way, acute haemodilution appears to be as effective as pre-donation, and the same caveats regarding patient selection apply (Ness *et al.* 1992; Monk *et al.* 1999). Although most patients tolerate the reduced red cell mass that accompanies haemodilution and surgical bleeding without problems, cardiac ischaemia remains a concern and the procedure is best left to experienced practitioners (Carvalho *et al.* 2003).

Red cell salvage: harvesting the operative field

Intraoperative red cell salvage

It was once a fairly common practice to collect blood shed into the peritoneal cavity, particularly when operating on patients with a ruptured ectopic gestation or ruptured spleen, and to re-inject the blood immediately, or after filtration and citration, into the patient's circulation (for details, see eighth edition). Nowadays, when blood is salvaged at operation, special devices are used for the purpose. At least two types are available: (1) The simpler, less expensive, lightweight, canister type in which salvaged blood is anticoagulated and aspirated, using a vacuum supply, into a disposable liner bag contained in a reusable rigid canister. The liner bag has a capacity of 1900 ml and an integral filter. Once the liner is full, the red cells can be concentrated and washed in the blood bank or re-infused directly through the filter. (2) The more automated type, based on centrifuge-assisted, semi-continuous-flow technology and requiring some technical expertise, anticoagulates, washes and concentrates the red cells before re-infusion. Automated, microprocessor-controlled devices use disposable bowls, bags and tubing and can produce processed blood within 3–5 min, depending on the PCV of the aspirated red cells (Leach 1991; Williamson and Taswell 1991). As the simpler system has the potential for the transfusion of activated clotting factors, procoagulants, complement components, haemolysed blood, excess anticoagulant, particulate matter and tissue fluids, as well as for producing air embolism, large volumes of blood salvaged in this way cannot be used unless it is washed (Pineda 1990; Williamson and Taswell 1991). However, there is little risk of systemic complement activation or disseminated intravascular coagulation if less than 500 ml of unwashed salvaged blood is re-infused (Dzik and Sherburne 1990; Tawes *et al.* 1994). Cell salvage instruments of all types induce mechanical injury to the red cells collected, resulting in a fall in the Hb level, although the 2,3-DPG levels and red cell survival are satisfactory (Pineda 1990).

Salvaged red cells are ordinarily not used if the blood is contaminated by microorganisms, tumour cells or substances such as topical disinfectants or bovine collagen (AuBuchon 1989; Williamson and Taswell 1991). However data to support these prohibitions are limited and the contraindications should not be considered absolute. For example, malignant cells can be found in the circulation prior to surgery and many more enter the circulation as soon as the surgeon manipulates the tumour. No randomized, controlled studies have been performed in the setting of malignancy and it is unlikely that any will be contemplated. However, uncontrolled studies do not suggest that intraoperative blood salvage increases the risk of tumour spread or shortens the life of the

cancer patient (Osawa *et al.* 1992; Thomas 1999). For patients who decline transfusion for religious reasons, intraoperative salvage can enable major surgical procedures such as hepatic resection for the cancer patient (Nieder *et al.* 2004). Favourable results associated with the transfusion of significant volumes of salvaged washed red cells during operation have been reported in various type of patients, i.e. those with trauma or ruptured ectopic pregnancy or those receiving liver transplants or undergoing cardiovascular, vascular or orthopaedic surgery. However, despite the apparent value of cell salvage in procedures such as vascular surgery, there are as yet surprisingly few controlled data to support its use (Alvarez *et al.* 2004). When very large volumes of salvaged red cells are transfused, supplementary transfusions of platelets and fresh-frozen plasma (FFP) are likely to be needed.

More than 7000 cases of red cell salvage with no major untoward effects have been reported from the Mayo Clinic over a period of 5 years, using both types of technology, the choice depending on the indications, cost and required speed of return of blood. Automated cell savers are used when blood loss is expected to be rapid and large. Processing blood collected with canisters takes not less than 45 min; hence, the use of this method is suitable only for prolonged collection periods, and then only if the red cells are washed (Williamson and Taswell 1991).

In a multiyear community autologous blood programme, efficacy of blood salvage was measured by both reduction in allogeneic transfusion and the volumes salvaged and re-transfused (Giordano *et al.* 1993). An analysis of 9918 consecutive procedures in various surgical specialties revealed that the average return of autologous blood salvaged was equivalent to 2.61 units of erythrocytes. Cardiac operation had the greatest average number of units recovered (4.65), whereas orthopaedic operation had the least (1.05).

Postoperative red cell salvage

Several devices are available for the collection and re-infusion of blood from thoracic, mediastinal and orthopaedic drainages after surgery. Extensive experience has been reported with postoperative collection of both washed and unwashed wound drainage from patients who have undergone orthopaedic or cardiac surgery. The results are conflicting (Schaff *et al.* 1979; Eng *et al.* 1990; Martin *et al.* 1992; Ward *et al.* 1993;

Ritter *et al.* 1994). As with the other methods of auto-logous collection and transfusion, patient selection is the key to effective use of these procedures (Goodnough *et al.* 1995). Febrile reactions are not uncommon with infusion of unwashed collections. Concerns about transfusion of activated plasma proteins and wound detritus, especially after orthopaedic procedures, has led to the recommendation that the red cells should be washed prior to re-infusion and infused through a microaggregate filter within 6 h of starting the collection (Leach 1991; Tawes *et al.* 1994).

Pharmacological alternatives

Haematopoietic growth factors

Haemopoietic growth factors produced by recombinant technology have enjoyed increasing use in clinical medicine, and in many instances their administration has either complemented or replaced transfusion therapy. The use of G-CSF and GM-CSF for mobilizing marrow progenitor cells and the effectiveness of G-CSF for granulocyte mobilization have been discussed in Chapter 14. Use of recombinant human erythropoietin (rhEPO) as an adjunct to autologous transfusions has been discussed previously in this chapter.

Erythropoietin

Erythropoietin (EPO) is a 36-kDa glycoprotein that is the primary regulator of erythropoiesis. EPO is produced primarily by the peritubular cells in the kidney in response to hypoxia. A small amount is made in the liver in adults. Administration of rhEPO results in egress of immature reticulocytes from the bone marrow and gradual elevation of the haematocrit (Spivak 1993, 2001). The EPO gene was cloned in 1985. Clinical-grade rhEPO became available and became a standard treatment for anaemic patients with end-stage renal disease by 1989 (Fisher 2003). The drug is now administered in a variety of settings in addition to uraemia where it may replace the use of allogeneic blood (Cazzola *et al.* 1997).

Treatment of patients with renal failure. The major cause of anaemia in patients with end-stage renal disease is a lack of production of erythropoietin, and recombinant human erythropoietin (rhEPO) is now used successfully to treat the anaemia in these patients (Winearls *et al.* 1986; Eschbach *et al.* 1989). The approved dose of rhEPO in renal failure is 50–150 U/kg intravenously or subcutaneously three times a week until the haematocrit reaches 0.30–0.34 (Eschbach 2002). The clinical response to rhEPO will probably not improve at doses above 500 U/kg intravenously three times weekly. On average, subcutaneous (s.c.) administration is more effective than i.v., as the drug is released more slowly from the tissues, which results in a longer circulating half-life and lower but more sustained plasma levels (Sisk *et al.* 1991). Pharmacokinetic studies indicate that rhEPO has a half-life of 4–9 h after i.v. administration, but > 24 h after s.c. injection. Treatment with rhEPO leads to functional iron deficiency as red cell production outstrips the mobilization of iron stores, and patients must be monitored appropriately (Brugnara *et al.* 1993). A randomized, open label study comparing intravenous iron with oral iron supplementation and controls in 157 cancer patients with chemotherapy-related anaemia suggested that intravenous iron raises haematocrit more effectively than does ferrous sulphate (Auerbach *et al.* 2004). Although patient randomization was not stratified for a variety of clinical factors, the study supports the notion that iron is necessary for at least a portion of patients treated with rhEPO.

The major side-effects of treatment with rhEPO are hypertension and thrombotic episodes, originally thought to be related primarily to excessive doses and too rapid correction of anaemia (Johnson *et al.* 1990; Spivak 2001). However, rhEPO appears to have haematocrit-independent, vasoconstrictive activity that can result in hypertension (Bode-Boger *et al.* 1996; Banerjee *et al.* 2000). EPO-related pure red cell aplasia has been reported in association with the appearance of circulating EPO-neutralizing antibodies (Casadevall *et al.* 2002; Bennett *et al.* 2004). Incidence is 10-fold higher when the Eprex® formulation is administered (Cournoyer *et al.* 2004). Discontinuation of drug and immunosuppressive therapy are associated with haematological recovery, and a majority (56%) regain responsiveness to rhEPO therapy, 89% of those without evidence of antibody at the time of re-exposure (Bennett *et al.* 2005). A novel erythropoiesis-stimulating recombinant cytokine (darbepoetin) has been synthesized, which has a higher carbohydrate content resulting in a longer plasma half-life and an amino acid sequence different from that of native human EPO. Darbopoietin reportedly is as effective as rhEPO at maintaining haemoglobin level but with less frequent dosing (Locatelli *et al.* 2001).

In the USA, the use of EPO almost immediately decreased consumption of red cells by 0.5 million units per year (Adamson 1991a,b).

Treatment of patients without renal disease. Those patients with AIDS and zidovudine-induced anaemia, whose levels of erythropietin are decreased (< 500 mu/ml), respond to treatment with rHuEPO (100 U/kg three times a week) (Spivak *et al.* 1989). Good results have also been obtained in anaemia related to chemotherapy in patients with cancer whose EPO level is < 200 mu/ml (Abels 1991). The dose advised is 100–150 U/kg three times weekly (Miller *et al.* 1990). In a randomized, double-blind, placebo-controlled study of 375 patients with anaemia receiving nonplatin chemotherapy with solid or non-myeloid haematolog ical malignancies, decreased transfusion requirements and increased haematocrit followed rhEPO treatment of 150 –300 IU/kg three times per week subcutaneously for 12–24 weeks (Littlewood *et al.* 2001). rhuEPO has been used for bone marrow transplantation (Steegmann *et al.* 1992), myelodysplastic syndrome (Di Raimondo *et al.* 1996), rheumatoid arthritis (Pincus *et al.* 1990) and the anaemia of prematurity (Bader *et al.* 1996; Maier *et al.* 2002). All require further study.

Colony-stimulating factors

Myeloid growth factors

For use as mobilizing agents for granulocyte and progenitor cell collection, see Chapter 14.

Febrile neutropenia with cancer chemotherapy. More than a dozen studies have evaluated the benefit of administering myeloid cytokines (granulocyte colony-stimulating factor, G-CSF; granulocyte–macrophage colony-stimulating factor, GM-CSF) to febrile neutropenic patients with malignancies. Although such therapy is more convenient than granulocyte transfusion, the results are no more satisfying. A Cochrane analysis found that overall mortality was not influenced by the use of colony-stimulating factor (CSF) (Clark *et al.* 2003). The benefit in reducing infection-related mortality is marginal, and even this result was highly influenced by one study. The prophylactic use of these cytokines for patients with febrile neutro-

penia due to cancer chemotherapy did not reduce the number of hospital days or the neutrophil recovery period. Although primary prophylaxis with a myeloid growth factor can reduce the incidence of febrile neutropenia by as much as 50%, such use is hard to justify if there is no improvement in response or survival (Ozer *et al.* 2000). The collective results of eight treatment trials provide consistent support for the recommendation that cytokines should not be used routinely as adjunct therapy for the treatment of uncomplicated fever and neutropenia (Ozer *et al.* 2000).

Chronic neutropenia. Severe chronic neutropenia, an absolute neutrophil count of less than $0.5 \times 10^9/l$ lasting from months to years, was one of the original indications for G-CSF treatment. Congenital, cyclic and idiopathic neutropenia fall into this category. A sustained increase of the neutrophil count, a reduction of the number of infections and reduced requirement for antibiotics was obtained in 40 out of 44 children with congenital neutropenia. Treatment for 4–6 years was well tolerated in the majority of patients and resulted in a long-term improvement of the clinical condition (Bonilla *et al.* 1989). More than 850 patients, most treated with daily or alternate-day recombinant human G-CSF (or filgrastim), have been followed on the Chronic Neutropenia Registry (Dale *et al.* 2003). G-CSF treatment increased the ANC 10-fold during the first year of treatment. For most patients, the responses were durable and patients remained on the same dose of G-CSF for years. Most patients remained free of bacterial infection. Thrombocytopenia developed in 4% of patients and myelodysplasia or acute myelocytic leukaemia has occurred in 35 out of 387 patients with congenital neutropenia with a cumulative risk of 13% after 8 years of G-CSF treatment. These events occurred without a predictable relationship to the duration or dose of G-CSF treatment. It is not clear whether the drug had any causative role in these disorders. No patient with cyclic or idiopathic neutropenia developed myelodysplasia or leukaemia. Growth and development and the outcome of pregnancy appeared to be unaffected by G-CSF treatment (Dale *et al.* 2003).

Neonatal neutropenia. In infants of very low birth-weight, GM-CSF has been found to produce a significant increase in the neutrophil and platelet counts and in the bone marrow neutrophil storage pool (Cairo *et al.* 1995).

Thrombopoietin

For almost 50 years scientists have looked for 'thrombopoietin', a humoral factor that regulates platelet production and might be used to treat patients with thrombocytopenia (Kelemen *et al.* 1958). Clinical trials with cytokines such as interleukin 6 (IL-6) and IL-11 showed that these proteins stimulate platelet production, and IL-11 has been given to reduce the need for platelet transfusions in patients with chemotherapy-induced thrombocytopenia (D'Hondt *et al.* 1995; Gordon *et al.* 1996). However, IL-11 is not a true thrombopoietin. Although its administration can reduce the need for platelet transfusions by one-third in selected patients with severe thrombocytopenia, it is accompanied by significant side-effects such as fever, fatigue, chills, dyspnoea, hypotension, peripheral oedema, atrial arrhythmias and syncope (Gordon *et al.* 1996; Vredenburgh *et al.* 1998).

In contrast with IL-11, thrombopoietin (TPO), also called c-Mpl ligand, is a 95-kDa, 332-amino-acid, lineage-specific glycoprotein with considerable homology to erythropoietin, which stimulates megakaryocyte growth and maturation (De Sauvage *et al.* 1994; Foster 1994; Lok *et al.* 1994). TPO is synthesized primarily in the liver (Peck-Radosavljevic *et al.* 2000). Various recombinant preparations of TPO have been developed including recombinant human thrombopoietin (rhTPO) and pegylated recombinant human megakaryocyte growth and development factor (PEG-rHuMGDF). TPO levels usually increase as platelet mass declines, and remain elevated during the course of thrombocytopenia. Platelet transfusions ordinarily decrease the plasma TPO levels, as TPO binds to the c-Mpl receptor on platelets and is removed from the circulation (Scheding *et al.* 2002).

Chemotherapy-induced thrombocytopenia. Of the two recombinant thrombopoietins, PEG-rHuMGDF, the most widely studied, produces dose-dependent increases in platelet counts in patients with advanced malignancies and chemotherapy-induced thrombocytopenia (Basser *et al.* 1997; Fanucchi *et al.* 1997). When administered before chemotherapy as a daily subcutaneous injection, PEG-rHuMGDF produced a dose dependent increase in peripheral blood platelet count. No evidence of platelet activation or altered platelet function has been observed. In a randomized, dose-escalation study, the platelet nadir in 53 patients with lung cancer treated with PEG-rHuMGDF after chemotherapy was higher than that of control subjects, but the need for platelet transfusions was unchanged because few patients developed severe thrombocytopenia (Basser *et al.* 1997). Similar results have been reported in other studies of chemotherapy for non-myeloid malignancies. Some reduction in the need for platelet transfusion may be found, but the effect is usually limited to the early cycles of chemotherapy.

Similar experience has been reported with recombinant human thrombopoietin. When administered as a single intravenous dose before chemotherapy, rhTPO was associated with a dose-dependent increase in platelets that began about day 4 and peaked about day 12 (Vadhan-Raj *et al.* 1997). rhTPO administered subcutaneously to previously treated patients with gynaecological malignancies before and after chemotherapy produced a modest dose-dependent rise in circulating platelet count. The need for platelet transfusions decreased by 75% (Vadhan-Raj *et al.* 1997). PEG-rHuMGDF and rhTPO have not improved thrombocytopenia significantly when administered to patients receiving intensive chemotherapy for acute leukaemia or stem cell transplantation, and failed to reduce the requirement for platelet transfusion (Nash *et al.* 2000; Schiffer *et al.* 2000).

Immune thrombocytopenia. TPO administration may have a role in management of ITP. Six HIV-infected patients with ITP and normal or slightly elevated endogenous TPO levels experienced a 10-fold rise in platelet count within 14 days of the start of PEG-rHuMGDF (Harker *et al.* 1998). A similar response has been reported in patients with non-HIV-related ITP treated with intravenous PEG-rHuMGDF. One patient with ITP has been successfully treated twice weekly with subcutaneous PEG-rHuMGDF for more than 3 years (Kuter and Begley 2002). These patients appear to have a suboptimal endogenous TPO response to thrombocytopenia, possibly as a result of their megakaryocyte mass, and appear to be able to increase the rate of effective platelet production when recombinant drug is administered.

Thrombapheresis. Healthy thrombapheresis donors increase their platelet count at 10–14 days after a single injection of PEG-rHuMGDF (Goodnough *et al.* 2001; Kuter *et al.* 2001). The rise in platelet count is dose

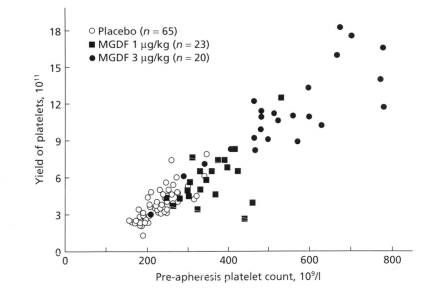

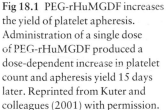

Fig 18.1 PEG-rHuMGDF increases the yield of platelet apheresis. Administration of a single dose of PEG-rHuMGDF produced a dose-dependent increase in platelet count and apheresis yield 15 days later. Reprinted from Kuter and colleagues (2001) with permission.

dependent and effects a significant increase in the apheresis platelet yield (Fig. 18.1). The platelets appear to aggregate normally and retain normal function after transfusion into thrombocytopenic recipients. The corrected count increment was significantly higher in patients transfused with cells mobilized by PEG-rHuMGDF than in those whose platelets came from control donors. No serious adverse events were seen in these donors.

Safety of recombinant thrombopoietin. Administration of multiple doses of PEG-rHuMGDF to some cancer patients and healthy volunteers was associated with the development of neutralizing antibodies and thrombocytopenia (Li *et al.* 2001). Thrombocytopenia occurred in 4 out of 665 cancer/stem cell transplantation/leukaemia patients given multiple doses, in 2 of 210 healthy volunteers who received two doses and in 11 out of 124 healthy volunteers given three doses of PEG-rHuMGDF (Li *et al.* 2001). No subject developed neutralizing antibodies or thrombocytopenia after a single injection. Evaluation of these thrombocytopenic subjects showed that the thrombocytopenia was due to the formation of an IgG antibody to PEG-rHuMGDF that crossreacted with endogenous TPO (Li *et al.* 2001). Neutralizing antibodies have not appeared in patients treated with intravenous rhTPO, although one non-neutralizing antibody was detected after subcutaneous injection of rhTPO (Vadhan-Raj *et al.* 2000).

Naturally occurring antibodies have been discovered in some patients with thrombocytopenia, and one would expect that platelet transfusion, not rhTPO, would be the treatment of choice should such patients require haemostasis support (Aledort *et al.* 2004).

Adjuncts to haemostasis

Pharmaceutical and biological agents occasionally replace transfusion therapy, but are more commonly used as adjuncts in the treatment of patients with haemostatic disorders (Counts *et al.* 1979; Mannucci 1998). A wide range of agents is available. Recombinant factor VIIa has emerged not as a replacement therapy, although it is licensed for this purpose in Europe, but as a treatment for bleeding haemophiliacs with inhibitors (Chapter 14), and as both prophylaxis and therapy for patients with surgically induced massive bleeding. A synthetic analogue of L-vasopressin, DDAVP, has been used to minimize haemorrhage for most mild forms of haemophilia A and VWD, and is increasingly recognized to have multiple less well-defined haemostatic effects when administered empirically in other circumstances. Lysine analogues that inhibit fibrinolysis are used both systemically and locally for acquired and inherited defects in haemostasis and thrombocytopenia. Aprotinin, a bovine-derived serine protease inhibitor with potent antifibrinolytic activity, is widely employed to enhance surgical haemostasis after cardiopulmonary bypass. Vitamin preparations in the naphthoquinone family (vitamin K) are used to prevent neonatal bleeding syndromes as well as to reverse warfarin anticoagulation or to treat ingestion of warfarin-like rodenticides. Still other agents such as oestrogens and protamine sulphate have proved valuable adjuncts to transfusion therapy.

Recombinant factor VIIa

The effectiveness of plasma fractions containing activated clotting factors in treating factor VII-deficient patients as well as other haemophiliacs with coagulation factor inhibitors led to the appreciation of the singular role of factor VII and the development of recombinant factor VIIa (rFVIIa) for human use (see also Chapter 14) (Hedner and Kisiel 1983). Recombinant factor VIIa, a two-chain procoagulant enzyme of approximately 50 000 molecular weight, becomes active when complexed with tissue factor in the extrinsic clotting cascade (Butenas et al. 2003). The circulating half-life is between 2 and 3 h, although it appears to be somewhat shorter in children than in adults (Villar et al. 2004). Dosage remains contentious. Most studies have used a dose of 90 μg/kg repeated every 2 h; however, doses as low as 30 μg/kg and as high as 120 μg/kg have been administered. The mechanism of action remains controversial. Preclinical studies in dogs indicate that functional platelets are critical to achieve normal haemostasis, although FVIIa can induce localized fibrin deposition on the surface of platelets with defective aggregation and induce platelet aggregates (Lisman et al. 2004). At pharmacological doses, rFVIIa binds directly to activated platelets and may generate a burst of thrombin that is localized to the site of bleeding (Lisman et al. 2004). For this reason, administration of rFVIIa has not been recommended for thrombocytopenic patients, although anecdotal reports suggest that even with severe, refractory thrombocytopenia, haemostasis may be improved (Vidarsson and Onundarson 2000; Gerotziafas et al. 2002; Tranholm et al. 2003). Whether the absolute platelet count or the mechanism of thrombocytopenia is important has yet to be determined.

Additional indications. Recombinant VIIa has been administered for a wide range of bleeding problems in addition to replacement therapy and management of haemophiliacs with inhibitors. The drug reduces the prothrombin time and controls bleeding in patients who require rapid reversal of warfarin anticoagulation (Deveras and Kessler 2002; Freeman et al. 2004). Changes in the laboratory test do not correlate with cessation of bleeding. There is no assay suitable for monitoring drug efficacy. rFVIIa infusion may provide one option for reversing treatment with newer anticoagulants such as those that target factor Xa– or tissue factor, but as yet little experience has been reported in this setting (Levi et al. 2004). rVIIa has reportedly controlled bleeding in a variety of inherited and acquired disorders of platelet function, such as Glanzmann thrombasthenia, Hermansky–Pudlak syndrome, Bernard–Soulier syndrome, VWD and uraemia (Monroe et al. 2000; Pozo Pozo et al. 2002; Poon et al. 2004). Patients with liver disease and profuse variceal bleeding have responded promptly to bolus infusions and the drug has been used prophylactically for patients undergoing liver biopsy (Bosch et al. 2004; Caldwell et al. 2004; Romero-Castro et al. 2004). Although bleeding has been well controlled in a subgroup of patients with variceal haemorrhage, reduction in mortality has not yet been seen. rFVIIa is reportedly effective and well tolerated as an option for managing central nervous system bleeding in patients with VII deficiency, anticoagulation, haemophilia with inhibitors and possibly other conditions such as aneurysms and trauma (Schmidt et al. 1994; Freeman et al. 2004; Huang et al. 2004). In a proof-of-concept study, rVIIa (160 μg/kg) administered within 4 h of symptoms reduced haematoma expansion at 24 h in patients who sustained intracerebral haemorrhage (Mayer et al. 2005). Each of three treatment groups realized improvements in functional scores when compared to a placebo control group at 3 months. However, arterial and venous thromboembolic events were more than three times as common in the treatment groups (7% vs. 2%) than in the control group.

Trauma and surgery. The earliest and perhaps most promising applications for rVIIa seemed to be in the settings of trauma and surgery with profuse bleeding. The observation that after a bolus of rVIIa, bleeding may cease virtually instantaneously in patients with desperate wounds or profuse bleeding at operation has produced many advocates but few controlled trials (Kenet et al. 1999; Martinowitz et al. 2001). In the largest series of trauma patients, coagulopathy was reversed in 61 out of 81 cases, with an associated reduction in prothrombin time from 19.6 to 10.8 s,

However, these findings did not translate into improved mortality compared to historical controls (Dutton *et al.* 2004). The same dramatic improvements in haemostasis have been reported with cardiac surgery and surgery for extensive, disfiguring facial haemangiomas (Tanaka *et al.* 2003; Waner 2004). In a controlled trial of rVIIa during retropubic prostatectomy, the patients who received drug sustained less blood loss and required on the average 2 units fewer red cell transfusion. Seven out of twelve placebo-treated patients were transfused, whereas no patients who received 40 μg/kg of rVIIa needed transfusion (Friederich *et al.* 2003).

One surprise has been the apparent lack of side-effects related to the administration of an activated clotting factor even in patients, who may be predisposed to thrombosis. In several hundred thousand administrations to patients with haemophilia, only a 1% incidence of serious adverse reactions has been reported (Abshire and Kenet 2004). Although experience in non-haemophilic patients is much less extensive, the concern about excessive thrombosis with resultant stroke and myocardial infarction has not been realized. It is still too early to conclude that the concern is unwarranted.

DDAVP (1-deamino-8-D-arginine vasopressin or desmopressin)

DDAVP is a synthetic analogue of the antidiuretic hormone L-vasopressin that has been used to control bleeding in patients with mild congenital or acquired bleeding disorders for more than 25 years (Richardson and Robinson 1985; Mannucci 1986; Lee *et al.* 1999). The drug has been used to reduce blood loss in a variety of surgical settings; however, with the possible exceptions of patients who have ingested aspirin or have other disorders of platelet function, benefit appears to be minimal (Dilthey *et al.* 1993; Despotis *et al.* 1999b; Carless *et al.* 2004).

Mechanisms of action and tachyphylaxis. DDAVP administration raises circulating FVIII and VWF levels, which account in part for the drug's haemostatic effect (Edelson *et al.* 1974; Richardson and Robinson 1985). Compared with vasopressin, DDAVP has increased affinity for V-1 receptors, which results in rapid release of FVIII and VWF from preformed cellular stores, and markedly decreased affinity for V-2 receptors that

mediate vasoconstriction (Richardson and Robinson 1985; Mannucci 1986). In normal subjects, DDAVP increases FVIII and VWF levels within 30 min after infusion. Levels peak at 300–400% of baseline in 1–2 h, and persist for 6–12 h (Mannucci *et al.* 1981). Response is faster with intravenous infusion than with intranasal administration.

Both red blood cell (RBC) and platelet adhesion to endothelial cells are increased by DDAVP when studied *in vitro* (Tsai *et al.* 1990; Rosse and Nishimura 2003). These effects might be produced by direct action on the vessel wall (Rosse and Nishimura 2003) or by release of high-molecular-weight VWF at the endothelial cell surface (Barnhart *et al.* 1983; Takeuchi *et al.* 1988). DDAVP also increases procoagulant platelet microparticle formation (Horstman *et al.* 1995), expression of tissue factor on endothelial cells (Galvez *et al.* 1997) and expression of p-selectin and the adhesive glycoprotein Ib on platelet membranes (Sloand *et al.* 1994; Wun *et al.* 1995). One or more of these or other unidentified effects may explain the observation that DDAVP shortens the bleeding time in patients with severe VWD who have already received cryoprecipitate infusions (Cattaneo *et al.* 1989), and in qualitative platelet disorders such as uraemia (Mannucci *et al.* 1983), liver disease (Mannucci *et al.* 1986) or other acquired or congenital conditions (Kentro *et al.* 1987) in which levels of FVIII and VWF are usually normal.

DDAVP infusion for haemophilia A and VWD produces short-term increases of circulating FVIII and VWF as preformed cell stores are released (Mannucci 1997). DDAVP alone has been used to control bleeding associated with minor surgical procedures or dental work, but is inadequate for procedures that require prolonged haemostasis. Repeat administration of DDAVP at intervals shorter than 24 h or repeatedly for several days is associated with decreased laboratory and clinical response (tachyphylaxis) (Mannucci *et al.* 1992; Mannucci 2004). The blunted response apparently results from depletion of intracytoplasmic stores of FVIII and VWF. The pattern of tachyphylaxis is not predictable. Patients with VWD are less likely to respond poorly or fail to respond after repeated doses. Although the haemostatic response to initial administration of DDAVP varies among patients, it is usually reproducible on each occasion for a given patient (Mannucci *et al.* 1992). If management with DDAVP is planned, patients should receive a test infusion to establish response several days prior to any planned invasive procedure.

Dose and administration. DDAVP may be administered by intravenous, subcutaneous and intranasal routes. The intravenous dose is 0.3 µg/kg, administered over 30 min in 50 ml of normal saline for adults (in 10 ml for children weighing less than 10 kg). The maximum response, factor elevations of three to five times baseline levels, occur within 30 to 60 min at intravenous doses of 0.3 µg/kg (Mannucci *et al.* 1981, 1992). The subcutaneous dose is 0.3–0.4 µg/kg, with peak responses approximately 230% above baseline at 60 min after administration, slightly lower and later than the peak dose after intravenous administration. The intranasal dose is an order of magnitude higher than the intravenous or subcutaneous dose, 300 µg for adults. Higher doses do not enhance efficacy, but may be associated with increased toxicity. A concentrated nasal spray formulation is available in both the USA and Europe. However, a concentrated preparation for subcutaneous use is not available in the USA, and the substantial volume (7 ml) required for subcutaneous treatment of a 70-kg individual may be uncomfortable. DDAVP is cleared by the liver and kidneys and has a plasma half-life of 124 min (Mannucci 1997).

Indications. As the bleeding tendency in haemophilia A, and to a lesser degree in VWD, correlates with measured blood levels of the deficient factor, the ability of DDAVP to transiently raise FVIII and VWF has resulted in its approval for use in these disorders. Experience has confirmed its usefulness and DDAVP is now the treatment of choice for minor and even moderately invasive procedures in patients with these disorders who respond to a test infusion (Mannucci 1997; Porte and Leebeek 2002; Mannucci 2004). Response is estimated from prospective studies at about 28% for VWD type I, 18% for type IIA, 14% for type IIM and 75% for type IIN (Federici *et al.* 2004). Genotype predicts response better than does phenotype for type IIA and IIN. The use of DDAVP in type IIB VWD remains controversial, but is generally contraindicated because these patients develop mild thrombocytopenia related to the affinity of the VWF for the platelets. Infusion of DDAVP and release of endogenous VWF stores into circulation may worsen thrombocytopenia (Mannucci 2004). Nevertheless

improved haemostasis in type IIB VWD after infusion of DDAVP associated with little or only mild thrombocytopenia has been reported (McKeown *et al.* 1996). In patients with severe haemophilia A, FVIII levels do not increase after DDAVP infusion; however, DDAVP may still provide potential benefit by increasing VWF levels, with an associated increased response in activity of infused FVIII concentrates (Deitcher *et al.* 1999).

DDAVP has been found to augment haemostasis in a variety of acquired and congenital conditions with impaired haemostasis in which other treatment options are limited. In a double-blind placebo-controlled study of patients with congenital platelet defects, DDAVP lowered the bleeding time most effectively in subjects with normal platelet-dense granule stores (Rao *et al.* 1995). In other studies, DDAVP has been shown to improve the bleeding time or be associated with adequate surgical haemostasis in patients with storage pool defect (Schulman *et al.* 1987; Kobrinsky *et al.* 1991), Bernard Soulier disease (Noris *et al.* 1998), aspirin ingestion (Flordal and Sahlin 1993; Reiter *et al.* 2003) and other defects in platelet hemostasis. DDAVP shortens the bleeding time in some haemorrhagic diseases of multifactorial origin such as cirrhosis and uraemia. Extrapolation of the utility of DDAVP in these conditions should be done with caution. Most studies have determined the efficacy of DDAVP by observing a shortening of the bleeding time, a notoriously poor predictor of haemostasis in most settings, or by assessing surgical haemostasis in uncontrolled studies of small numbers of patients.

Initial reports that DDAVP decreased blood loss and transfusion requirements after cardiac and spinal surgery have not been confirmed in follow-up studies (Mannucci 1997; Porte and Leebeek 2002). One large meta-analysis revealed no reduction in bleeding after the use of DDAVP in cardiac surgery, in contrast with comparative studies with lysine analogue antifibrinolytics and aprotinin (Levi *et al.* 1999). DDAVP had no effect on mortality or need for repeat thoracotomy, but was associated with a two- to four-fold increased risk of coronary thrombosis. A Cochrane analysis arrived at a similar conclusion (Carless *et al.* 2004). The subset of patients with preoperative platelet defects, including those that have ingested aspirin, appears to benefit from administration of DDAVP prior to surgery. Blood loss was markedly reduced in patients with preoperative defects in platelet function (identified by point-of-care testing) who received DDAVP compared with those who received placebo (Despotis *et al.* 1999b). Three randomized double-blind placebo-controlled trials have shown clinically significant reductions in blood loss and transfusion requirements after the use of DDAVP in patients who have ingested aspirin before cardiac surgery (Gratz *et al.* 1992; Dilthey *et al.* 1993; Sheridan *et al.* 1994). DDAVP also reduced bleeding in an unblinded comparison with placebo in patients who ingested aspirin before cholecystectomy (Gratz *et al.* 1992). In addition, DDAVP has been demonstrated to shorten the bleeding time in normal volunteers after aspirin ingestion, perhaps due to direct effects on platelets or increases in VWF (Lethagen *et al.* 2000). Whereas some studies have indicated that DDAVP is not effective in patients with thrombocytopenia or Glanzman disease, other patients with Glanzman disease or thrombocytopenia have been reported to respond (Mannucci *et al.* 1986; DiMichele and Hathaway 1990).

Toxicity. Most side-effects of DDAVP are minor. Facial flushing, often marked, and minimal elevation in pulse rate or blood pressure are observed, more frequently with the intravenous than with the subcutaneous or intranasal routes. The most common, clinically significant adverse event is hyponatraemia, which results from the antidiuretic effect of this vasopressin analogue. Hyponatraemic seizures have been reported in children aged 1 month to 8 years, especially when hypotonic intravenous fluids and multiple doses of DDAVP are administered concurrently in the surgical setting (Sutor 2000). Less severe but significant symptoms of headache, nausea or lethargy have been reported in adults after intranasal or repeated intravenous and subcutaneous administration (Dunn *et al.* 2000). Careful monitoring of i.v. fluids, urine output and electrolytes is therefore important, especially for children who receive DDAVP perioperatively, and in older patients when mild renal insufficiency decreases their ability to excrete free water. Patients should be instructed to restrict fluid intake for 24 h.

Isolated cases of thrombosis such as myocardial infarction, cerebral thrombosis and unstable angina have been reported after use of DDAVP in patients at risk for thrombotic events. In the surgical setting, one randomized, placebo-controlled study specifically designed to detect deep venous thrombosis in 50 patients undergoing hip surgery did not detect an increased incidence of thrombosis following DDAVP therapy (Flordal *et al.* 1992). However, meta-analysis has found a two- to four-fold increased risk of myocardial infarction in cardiac surgery patients who received DDAVP (Levi *et al.* 1999). It therefore seems prudent to evaluate patients receiving DDAVP for possible occult coronary artery disease and to avoid the concurrent use of antifibrinolytic agents in these patients under most circumstances.

Lysine analogue antifibrinolytic agents

Fibrinolysis occurs when plasmin generated from the proenzyme plasminogen by plasminogen activators digests fibrin clots (Collen 1999). Both plasmin and plasminogen bind to fibrin through specific lysine binding sites. The synthetic lysine analogues, tranexamic acid (AMCA) and epsilon-aminocaproic acid (EACA), delay fibrinolysis by reducing the binding of plasminogen to fibrin that is required for activation by plasminogen activators (Mannucci 1998). These agents have been available for more than 30 years to inhibit fibrinolysis and ensure clot stability (Dunn and Goa 1999).

AMCA was developed within a few years of EACA. AMCA is 10-fold more potent on a molar basis, and tends to cause less gastrointestinal discomfort at equivalent antifibrinolytic doses in healthy volunteers (Verstraete 1985). Much of the early use of antifibrinolytics in the USA involved EACA, whereas AMCA was used relatively more frequently in Europe. Although AMCA and EACA have been considered equivalent agents, optimal dosing regimens have not been determined for either agent and reported toxicities vary (Bluemle 1965; Porte and Leebeek 2002).

Lysine analogue antifibrinolytic drugs are effective and clearly indicated in rare inherited conditions associated with excessive fibrinolysis such as congenital $\alpha2$-antiplasmin deficiency (Aoki *et al.* 1979). However, much of the enthusiasm for these drugs has focused on acquired disorders with evidence of excessive systemic fibrinolysis, especially cardiac bypass surgery and, to a lesser degree, orthopaedic surgery performed with the use of tourniquets. Both agents are useful when administered topically in areas with excessive local fibrinolysis such as the oral cavity and uterine cavity. In these instances, efficacy has been well established, and side-effects are minimal compared with systemic administration (Nilsson 1975, 1980; Mannucci 1998; Fung *et al.* 2004). AMCA and EACA are also administered to reduce bleeding in such conditions as amegakaryocytic and peripheral immunemediated thrombocytopenia, where the indication is less obvious, and efficacy is presumably related to stabilization of fibrin clots (Gardner and Helmer 1980; Bartholomew *et al.* 1989; Fricke *et al.* 1991).

Dose and administration. Both agents may be administered orally, intravenously or topically. EACA and AMCA are well absorbed orally, and are cleared virtually unchanged by the kidney (Verstraete 1985). The drugs are distributed widely throughout the body. AMCA crosses into cerebrospinal fluid, semen, synovial fluid and cord blood, but is not secreted in saliva (Dunn and Goa 1999). In the non-operative setting, the half-life for both agents is approximately 1–2 h in patients with normal renal function. The dose should be reduced in renal failure (Dunn and Goa 1999). A typical total daily oral dose for EACA is 10–24 g, administered as 2–4 g every 3–4 h, and for AMCA 3–4 g, administered as 1 g every 6–8 h. Dosage in individual studies varies widely. Recent studies have attempted to optimize dosing for both agents in conditions such as cardiac surgery where the clearance and distribution of these agents is altered (Butterworth *et al.* 1999, 2001; Dowd *et al.* 2002).

Indications. A randomized, double-blind placebo-controlled study of AMCA administered to reduce bleeding in 38 patients with acute myeloid leukaemia found a significant reduction in bleeding episodes and platelet transfusions during consolidation, but not during induction therapy (Shpilberg *et al.* 1995). A smaller study of eight patients with amegakaryocytic thrombocytopenia (seven with severe aplastic anaemia and one with myelodysplasia) treated with AMCA in a placebo-controlled, double-blind, crossover design found no such reduction. Bleeding increased in patients while receiving AMCA (Fricke *et al.* 1991).

Lysine analogues are often used in cardiac bypass surgery, where excessive bleeding and fibrinolysis are associated with extracorporeal devices. Although early studies did not reveal a uniformly beneficial effect,

antifibrinolytic use has increased as repeated analyses have found that EACA prophylaxis significantly reduces postoperative blood loss and re-exploration, without increasing thromboembolic events (Fremes *et al.* 1994; Munoz *et al.* 1999). In contrast with DDAVP, lysine analogues are administered prior to bypass. A meta-analysis of placebo-controlled studies of antifibrinolytic agents in cardiac surgery that did not distinguish between AMCA and EACA demonstrated lower rates of re-exploration, improved mortality and no significant increased risk of myocardial infarction in the treatment group (Levi *et al.* 1999). Antifibrinolytic agents have been shown to reduce bleeding in total knee arthroplasty where use of a tourniquet produces excessive fibrinolysis (Hiippala *et al.* 1997), and to correct laboratory evidence of fibrinolysis in liver transplantation (Kaspar *et al.* 1997; Dalmau *et al.* 2004). Transfusion requirements were not reduced in these settings.

Other uses of lysine analogues include those based on well-designed studies as well as anecdote, with the strength of evidence often unrelated to clinical enthusiasm. Two retrospective uncontrolled studies of 31 patients with thrombocytopenia, including amegakaryocytic and immune-mediated aetiologies, demonstrated benefit with oral EACA (Garewal and Durie 1985; Bartholomew *et al.* 1989). Although not widely used for control of gastrointestinal haemorrhage, in which fibrinolytic enzymes may in fact play a role, AMCA has been associated with a reduced incidence of rebleeding and a 30–40% reduction in mortality in a meta-analysis that included 1200 patients from double-blind placebo-controlled trials (Henry and O'Connell 1989). A similar analysis found significant improvement in women with menorrhagia who received antifibrinolytic agents compared to hormonal methods and other modalities (Lethaby *et al.* 2000). Concern for thromboembolism has tempered the widespread use of these agents for excessive menstrual bleeding; however, studies have not confirmed any increase in this complication. AMCA reduced the incidence of rebleeding in patients with subarachnoid haemorrhage in three double-blind placebo-controlled studies subjected to Cochrane analysis (Roos *et al.* 2003). However, based on 1041 patients in three trials, antifibrinolytic treatment did not evidence improved outcome. Treatment increased the risk of cerebral ischaemia in five trials (Roos *et al.* 2003).

Uncontrolled observations have proposed that shorter courses of high-dose EACA, or lower dose AMCA, might reduce rebleeding and avoid the complications associated with long-term use in patients scheduled for early aneurysmal therapy to control subarachnoid hemorrhage. There is insufficient evidence from randomized controlled trials of antifibrinolytic agents in trauma to either support or refute the use of these drugs (Coats *et al.* 2004).

Topical or local administration of the lysine analogues has been successful in a variety of clinical settings. Topical AMCA dramatically reduced the incidence of rebleeding after traumatic hyphaema, decreased systemic symptoms compared to oral administration and improved long-term outcomes compared with untreated control subjects (Crouch *et al.* 1997). Similarly, topical tranexamic acid (1 g in 100 ml of saline) administered during open heart surgery directly into the pericardial cavity and over the mediastinal tissues before closure reduced chest tube drainage, but not transfusion requirements, without detectable AMCA blood levels (De Bonis *et al.* 2000).

The topical use of antifibrinolytic agents to control bleeding in dental surgery for patients with haemophilia and other conditions predisposing to excessive haemorrhage including oral anticoagulation deserves special mention. In this setting, antifibrinolytic treatment probably counteracts excessive fibrinolysis in the oral cavity, which lacks endogenous fibrinolytic inhibitors (Sindet-Pedersen *et al.* 1989). More than 30 years ago, controlled trials demonstrated reduced bleeding and decreased requirements for clotting factor concentrates in patients with haemophilia A and B who received systemic oral administration of EACA, 6 g four times daily for 7–10 days (Walsh *et al.* 1971, 1975). More recently, AMCA mouthwash (10 ml of a 4.8% aqueous solution applied prior to sutures and as a 2-min rinse four times a day for 7 days) dramatically reduced bleeding episodes after dental procedures (Sindet-Pedersen *et al.* 1989). Topical administration of AMCA, along with the use of DDAVP and fibrin sealant, has become standard treatment in haemophilia dental centres.

Toxicity. The most common side-effects of lysine analogue antifibrinolytic therapy are mild dose-dependent gastrointestinal symptoms, such as nausea, cramping and diarrhoea. These symptoms are less frequently reported with AMCA than with EACA (Verstraete 1985; Dunn and Goa 1999). Rhabdomyolysis, possibly due to inhibition of carnitine synthesis, has been described, although rarely, when oral EACA has been continued beyond 4 weeks (Seymour and Rubinger 1997). Rhabdomyolysis has not been reported after AMCA administration. Some patients who have developed this complication while on EACA have been successfully treated for many months with AMCA (Dunn and Goa 1999).

When administered at usual clinical doses, the antifibrinolytic drugs do not appear to differ in their potential to cause thrombosis. Widespread thrombosis has occurred in the setting of disseminated intravascular coagulation (DIC), where increased fibrinolysis may protect against organ ischaemia. Some studies have attempted to pair antifibrinolytic therapy with heparin anticoagulation in DIC and 'excessive' fibrinolysis characterized by low levels of α_2-antiplasmin. Although bleeding decreased in most cases, some patients still developed generalized organ system failure attributed to thrombosis (Williams 1989). High-grade ureteral obstruction due to inhibition of urokinase and clot formation may occur when antifibrinolytics are used to treat patients with haematuria (Schultz and van der Lelie 1995). Topical therapy, administered by irrigation, has been successful for control of intractable urinary bleeding localized to the bladder (Singh and Laungani 1992).

Aprotinin. Aprotinin is a bovine lung-derived 58-residue polypeptide with broad antiprotease activity directed towards trypsin, kallikrein, thrombin and plasmin (Longstaff 1994). Aprotinin activity is ordinarily expressed in kallikrein inactivator units (KIUs). However, the relationship of this activity to the mechanism(s) of its haemostatic action is not clear. Aprotinin has potent antifibrinolytic activity, at least as regards circulating plasmin, and this is believed to be the primary haemostatic mechanism (Ray and Marsh 1997). Other proposed mechanisms for the haemostatic function involve a long-disputed platelet-protective effect and inhibition of protease-activated receptors found on platelets, leucocytes and vascular endothelium (Shigeta *et al.* 1997; Mannucci 1998). Aprotinin does not induce platelet adhesion or aggregation, but inhibits various platelet agonists produced during surgical procedures and cardiopulmonary bypass. Aprotinin also inhibits complement activation, attenuates the release of tissue necrosis factor-alpha (TNF-α), IL-6 and IL-8 and inhibits endogenous cytokine-induced nitric oxide synthase induction (Mahdy and Webster 2004).

Dosage and clearance. As was the case with the other antifibrinolytic agents, aprotinin has been used in different doses and regimens; the most common regimen involves a loading dose of 2 million KIU followed by continuous infusion of 500 000 KIU/h (Royston *et al.* 1987). In cardiac surgery, an additional 2 million KIU may be added to the bypass pump prime. After i.v. injection, aprotinin distributes into the extracellular space, leading to a rapid decrease in plasma concentration. The drug is eliminated in a biphasic pattern: a rapid-phase half-life of approximately 40 min and a slower phase half-life of 7 h (Porte and Leebeek 2002).

Indications. During trials of aprotinin designed to reduce neutrophil activation in patients undergoing repeat open heart surgery, investigators noted that the operative field was dry and that transfusion requirements decreased eight-fold compared with control patients who received no drug (Royston *et al.* 1987). Subsequent trials have demonstrated the effectiveness of aprotinin in patients undergoing procedures requiring cardiopulmonary bypass (Lemmer *et al.* 1994). Aprotinin has been of particular benefit in operations characterized by large volume blood loss, such as those patients undergoing reoperation or heart transplantation (Prendergast *et al.* 1996; Smith 1998). Meta-analyses have confirmed these findings (Fremes *et al.* 1994; Laupacis and Fergusson 1997; Levi *et al.* 1999; Munoz *et al.* 1999). When tested with other inhibitors of fibrinolysis, aprotinin was the only agent associated with reduced mortality, whereas both aprotinin and lysine analogue antifibrinolytic agents reduced overall transfusion requirements and the need for re-exploration (Levi *et al.* 1999). Aprotinin is significantly more expensive than lysine analogue antifibrinolytics, and the cost-effectiveness and other merits of aprotinin compared with these agents continues to be debated (Reddy and Song 2003).

Adverse events. Anaphylaxis is the greatest concern with administration of a foreign protein such as aprotinin and is reported in approximately 0.5% of

initial exposures and up to 9% of repeat exposures (Diefenbach *et al.* 1995; Scheule *et al.* 1997). Mild hypersensitivity reactions are more common. Quantitative detection of anti-aprotinin IgE and IgG have limited predictive value for identifying patients at risk for anaphylaxis following re-exposure to aprotinin, and repeat treatment within 6 months is discouraged (Dietrich *et al.* 1997, 2001).

The possibility of unintended thrombosis, particularly myocardial infarction, bypass graft occlusion and deep vein thrombosis, has raised concerns about using antifibrinolytic therapy during operative procedures (Bohrer *et al.* 1990). However, neither the incidence of myocardial infarction nor the frequency of graft patency appear to be influenced by aprotinin administration in the controlled trials of this drug (Lavee *et al.* 1993; Havel *et al.* 1994; Lemmer *et al.* 1994). Imaging studies have not identified an increased risk of deep vein thrombosis in the setting of orthopaedic surgery (Murkin *et al.* 2000; Samama *et al.* 2002).

As aprotinin is derived from bovine lung, the possibility of prion transmission and variant Creutzfeldt–Jakob disease has been raised. No patients with the disorder have received aprotinin.

Reversal of anticoagulation

Vitamin K and its antagonists (warfarin, bishydroxycoumarin, Dicumoral®)

Henrik Dam (Dam and Glavind 1938) discovered that chicks fed an ether-extracted diet developed a haemorrhagic diathesis that responded to a fat-soluble factor that became known as Koagulationvitamin or vitamin K. Vitamin K was subsequently found to correct the acquired bleeding tendency during the first week of life that has come to be known as haemorrhagic disease of the newborn (Brinkhous and Smith 1937; Dam and Dyggve 1952). With recognition that the bleeding in 'sweet clover disease of cattle' was caused by a compound identified later as bishydroxycoumarin, or Dicumoral®, which interfered with vitamin K-dependent synthesis of active prothrombin, vitamin K acquired a prominent role in the management of excessive anticoagulation due to warfarin, superwarfarin rodenticides and other orally active anticoagulants with similar mechanisms of action. Vitamin K is also indicated in acquired vitamin K deficiency that results from the combination of poor diet and antibiotic therapy that occurs commonly in intensive care settings (Alperin 1987; Cohen *et al.* 1988).

Vitamin K1 is synthesized by plants, possessing the same phytyl side-chain as chlorophyll, and is the major dietary source of vitamin K. The vitamin K1 content varies widely between foods, yet diet is a trivial source of variation in patient response to oral anticoagulants (Schurgers *et al.* 2004). Absorption of dietary vitamin K occurs in the ileum and requires the formation of mixed micelles composed of bile salts and the products of pancreatic lipolysis. Oral absorption is impaired in conditions of either biliary obstruction or pancreatic insufficiency. Vitamin K2 (menadione) is synthesized by bacterial flora of the large intestine and appears to have a reserve function to protect against dietary vitamin K deficiency, a rare occurrence in healthy adults (Vermeer and Schurgers 2000).

Mechanism of action. Vitamin K functions as an essential cofactor for the post-translational gamma carboxylation of glutamic acid moieties in the N-terminal region of a series of proteins (Furie *et al.* 1999). Synthesis of functional prothrombin, as well as of coagulation factors VII, IX, X and naturally occurring anticoagulant proteins C and S, requires vitamin K (Vermeer and Schurgers 2000). The decarboxylated, functionally inactive forms of vitamin K-dependent proteins (also called *proteins induced by vitamin K absence* or *PIVKA*) may be detected in the circulation of patients on oral anticoagulants or in those with vitamin K deficiency due to malabsorption. The enzyme(s) that reduce and recycle vitamin K and vitamin K epoxide have different sensitivities to oral anticoagulant-induced inhibition, which explains why vitamin K functions as an antidote to excessive oral anticoagulation and why patients on warfarin therapy who receive high doses of vitamin K may appear resistant to re-institution of therapy (Furie *et al.* 1999). The primary site of inhibition by warfarin is vitamin K epoxide reductase, which under physiological conditions is also the enzyme that reduces vitamin K to the active hydroquinone required for carboxylation. However, a second, warfarin-insensitive reductase can reduce vitamin K to the active hydroquinone in the presence of high tissue concentrations of vitamin K. Thus, exogenous vitamin K can produce additional active vitamin K hydroquinone via this warfarin-insensitive step, bypassing the warfarin-induced inhibition of vitamin K epoxide reductase and

reversing excessive anticoagulation (Furie *et al.* 1999). If vitamin K levels accumulate, this same process may also lead to warfarin resistance upon resumption of anticoagulation.

Lowered levels of vitamin K-dependent clotting factors of patients taking oral anticoagulants recover at the same rate during the initial 8 h following vitamin K administration, but subsequent recovery depends on the rate of synthesis of new gamma carboxylated factors by the liver. Levels of factor VII reconstitute most rapidly, followed by factors IX and X, and lastly by prothrombin (van der Meer *et al.* 1968). The differential rate of circulating factor levels after vitamin K administration has practical importance. Oral anticoagulation is most frequently monitored using the prothrombin time, which is most sensitive to decreases in factor VII levels. During stable anticoagulant therapy, the several vitamin K-dependent coagulant and anticoagulant proteins are decreased in relatively constant ratios to one another. However, administration of vitamin K for excessive anticoagulation may result in a prothrombin time correction related largely to a rapid increase in the factor VII level and underestimating the bleeding risk from the lower levels of factors IX, II and X.

Dose and administration. Both vitamin K1 and K2 are active when administered orally or intravenously. Liquid preparations are prepared as a colloid solution, each millilitre containing 2 or 10 mg of phytonadione in a polyoxyethylated fatty acid derivative, which functions as a cremaphor to solubilize the vitamin K. Intramuscular administration may cause haemorrhage in anticoagulated patients and should be reserved for prophylaxis against haemorrhagic disease of the newborn (1 μg). The side-effects reported with intravenous administration (see below) have limited its use, even though intravenous administration is more rapid and reliable than the subcutaneous or oral routes (van der Meer *et al.* 1968; Nee *et al.* 1999). Scored tablets are available, containing 5 mg of phytonadione, permitting a dose range as low as 2.5 mg. Although injectable and oral preparations have been available for nearly half a century, the appropriate dose and route of administration remain controversial (Taylor *et al.* 1999).

The response to vitamin K administration depends on the direction, rate of change and degree of prolongation of clotting times, the dose and type of anticoagulant administered and the presence of concurrent liver disease, antibiotics or dietary factors (Cosgriff 1956; Schulman 2003) Anticoagulant reversal is more prompt and more reliable with intravenous than with subcutaneous administration of vitamin K (Nee *et al.* 1999; Raj *et al.* 1999). In a prospective, randomized, single-blind study of 22 patients, the INR decreased from a mean initial value of 8.0 to 4.6 and 3.1 after 8 and 24 h respectively in patients who received 1 mg intravenously, compared with a mean initial value of 8.5, which decreased to 8.0 and 5.0 at the same intervals in patients who received 1 mg subcutaneously (Raj *et al.* 1999). The response after oral ingestion of vitamin K is slower and less predictable than either subcutaneous or intravenous administration, but is more rapid than that observed after simple discontinuation of warfarin, which can be prolonged in elderly patients. Oral vitamin K doses as low as 0.5–2.5 mg (Crowther *et al.* 2000; Gunther *et al.* 2004) have been recommended for patients at risk with mild to moderate prolongation of the INR, but who are not bleeding.

Vitamin K deficiency occurs commonly in malnourished patients in intensive care units, either with or without concomitant antibiotic use, accounting for four or five cases yearly in one tertiary care referral centre (Alperin 1987; Cohen *et al.* 1988; Goldman *et al.* 1997). Administration over 30 min of 5–25 mg of intravenous vitamin K corrected the coagulopathy within 12 h (Alperin 1987). A much smaller dose of vitamin K, 1 mg intravenously, is effective within 24 h when vitamin K deficiency is due to malabsorption in patients who are not critically ill, and the effect lasts 1–2 weeks (van der Meer *et al.* 1968).

When excessive oral anticoagulation occurs in the absence of bleeding, omission of a dose or two of anticoagulant may suffice until the therapeutic range is reached. Correction of the prothrombin time or International Normalized Ratio (INR) may be achieved more rapidly if a small dose of vitamin K1 is administered, most conveniently as a 1-mg oral dose. This approach also reduces the risk of minor haemorrhage for patients with INR values of between 4.5 and 10 (Crowther *et al.* 2000; Wilson *et al.* 2004). Alternatively, 0.5 mg of vitamin K1 may be injected intravenously. Higher doses should be avoided as they may lead to overcorrection and resistance to anticoagulation with vitamin K antagonists for several days. Subcutaneous injection is not recommended, as

absorption is variable, although correction via this route invariably occurs within 72 h.

For excessive anticoagulation associated with bleeding, especially with an INR dangerously outside of the therapeutic range, and with intracranial haemorrhage, administration of vitamin K1 is not sufficient, as full reversal will not occur for 12 to 24 h. FFP is ordinarily the drug of choice in this circumstance. The volume of plasma required for reversal may be large, and if volume overload is a problem, prothrombin complex concentrate is effective (Makris *et al.* 1997) as is administration of factor VIIa, a more expensive alternative (see above) (Deveras and Kessler 2002). When plasma or prothrombin complex is used, the volume (or units) may be calculated as below (Schulman 2003):

1 Determine the target INR – full correction (1.0) is desirable for patients with serious bleeding and a small risk of thrombosis. Low-level anticoagulation may be desirable for patients with mild bleeding and a high risk of thrombosis.

2 Convert the INR to percentage of normal plasma haemostatic activity (Table 18.1):

Table 18.1 Conversion of INR to percentage of normal plasma haemostatic activity.

	INR	Approximate percentage
Excess anticoagulation	> 5	5
	4.0–4.9	10
Therapeutic range	2.6–3.9	15
	2.2–2.5	20
	1.9–2.1	25
Subtherapeutic range	1.7–1.8	30
	1.4–1.6	40
Complete reversal	1.0	100

3 Calculate the dose: [target INR (%) – observed INR (%)] × body weight (kg) = plasma (ml) or prothrombin complex concentrate (IU).

Too often, insufficient plasma is given for correction and, even when plasma infusion is used for reversal, the correction may be temporary, especially as factor VII has a half-life of only 6 h, and may have to be repeated.

A 59-year-old man with atrial fibrillation was placed on chronic oral anticoagulation with coumadin 2 mg a day. Because of a prescription error, he ingested a 5-mg daily dose for 30 days until he developed haematuria. His physician discontinued the medication and drew a prothrombin time. When the laboratory reported an INR of 12.3, he was referred to the emergency room. A repeat INR of 11.9 led to treatment with 2 units of fresh-frozen plasma. INR immediately thereafter was 3.5. The patient was discharged home. Twelve hours later he felt dizzy, developed a headache and was noted to be confused. He developed hemiparesis and radiological studies revealed an extensive intracranial haemorrhage. The INR was recorded at 9.7.

Patients with the severe haemorrhagic diathesis due to ingestion of powerful rodenticides may require initial daily oral administration of 100 mg of vitamin K for 2 months, and then a slow taper over 300 days due to the extreme *in vivo* half-life of the fat-soluble poison (Weitzel *et al.* 1990). In contrast, prolonged INR values associated with the relatively weaker anticoagulant activity of antibiotics with the N-methylthiotetrazole (NMTT, moxalactam, cefoperazone, cefamandole, cefotetan and cefmetazole) side-chain respond rapidly to small doses in many cases (Breen and St Peter 1997).

Toxicity. Anaphylaxis, the major toxicity associated with vitamin K, is rare, but dramatic. It has resulted in fatalities, but is described only after intravenous administration (Rich and Drage 1982). Symptoms of flushing and chest pain after intravenous administration of phytonadione were described as early as 1952, and cardiac irregularities in the 1960s were attributed to injections given more rapidly than 10 mg/min or to the propylene glycol content of an older preparation that has since been withdrawn from the market. However, severe anaphylaxis also occurred in a patient who received an intravenous injection of a mixed micelles vitamin K1 preparation composed of glycolic acid and lecithin designed to reduce anaphylaxis (Havel *et al.* 1987). It is not clear whether the vitamin, the excipient, formation of a hapten between the vitamin K and emulsifying agents or non-immunological mechanisms led to these reactions.

What is known about reactions following vitamin K administration may be summarized as follows:

1 Anaphylactic reactions occur and are unpredictable.
2 Repeated administrations to the same patient do not necessarily carry the same risks.

3 Slow injection does not prevent these reactions, but permits interruption of the injection as soon as the onset of symptoms occurs. Fatalities have occurred even when intravenous administration does not exceed the 1 mg/min guideline (Rich and Drage 1982).
4 Severe reactions have been reported most frequently in elderly patients who have received doses greater than 5 mg, and after repeat dosing. However, anaphylaxis has occurred in young patients, even after the first administration.
5 There is no obvious dose dependency in the frequency of reactions. However, reactions are rare when doses of 1 mg or less are used and no fatalities have been reported at these doses (Soedirman *et al.* 1996; van der Meer *et al.* 1999; Nee *et al.* 1999).
6 The cremaphor excipients in various preparations used in the USA and overseas are not identical but may have the same risks.
7 Shock occurs as a result of severe peripheral vasodilatation, and treatment should be directed to counteract this effect. Caution should be exercised with intravenous vitamin K administration. However, when other routes are not feasible or when rapid, reliable dosing is required, it seems prudent to dissolve the preparation in 125 ml of isotonic solution and administer it carefully over at least 20 min. Small doses usually suffice, and the infusion should be halted if flushing or hypotension occurs.

Protamine sulphate

Protamine sulphate, the specific inhibitor of unfractionated heparin (UFH), is a polycationic, highly positively charged protein of approximately 4500 Da in molecular weight, derived from salmon sperm (Carr and Silverman 1999). Protamine binds to the negatively charged heparin molecules, forms a stable complex and displaces antithrombin III (ATIII) from the heparin–ATIII complex. Protamine is the only effective specific antidote to excessive anticoagulation produced by UFH. Low-molecular-weight heparin contains a protamine-resistant ultra-low-molecular-weight fraction with low sulphate charge density (Crowther *et al.* 2002). Protamine sulphate reverses only about 60% of the anti-factor Xa activity of low-molecular-weight heparin, has negligible effects on danaparoid, a mixture of anticoagulant glycosaminoglycans used to treat heparin-induced thrombocytopenia, and fondaparinux, a synthetic antithrombin-binding pentasaccharide with exclusive anti-factor Xa activity used for anti-thrombotic prophylaxis following orthopaedic surgery (Warkentin and Crowther 2002).

Protamine possesses additional intrinsic anticoagulant activities, including platelet clumping, thrombocytopenia and interference with the formation of fibrin by thrombin so that doses in excess of those calculated to neutralize UFH should be avoided (Warkentin and Crowther 2002). Protamine sulphate is administered by intravenous infusion. Its onset of action is immediate and its duration of action about 2 h. Plasma protamine concentrations decrease rapidly, and become undetectable within about 20 min, with a half-life of 7.4 min. Elimination differs significantly between men and women. The rapid disappearance of protamine from the circulation may contribute to cases of 'heparin rebound' after initial adequate reversal of heparin (Butterworth *et al.* 2002). Dosing strategies to neutralize excessive anticoagulation induced by UFH are often based on the use of 1 mg of protamine to neutralize 80–100 USP units of heparin (Warkentin and Crowther 2002). Ordinarily, the dosage should not exceed 100 mg over 2 h unless blood coagulation tests indicate a need for larger doses.

Protamine is administered at the completion of bypass surgery using dosing algorithms and measurement of the activated clotting time (ACT) to estimate circulating heparin concentration (Despotis *et al.* 1999a). Monitoring protocols can markedly influence protamine doses used to neutralize UFH. Newer point-of-care haemostasis testing systems developed to replace traditional ACT-based empiric regimens have reduced both protamine dosage and postoperative bleeding in some, but not all, prospective studies (Despotis *et al.* 1999a).

Adverse events. Protamine administration may also be associated with hypotension, increased pulmonary artery pressure, pulmonary neutrophil sequestration and anaphylaxis, side-effects that are mediated by complement activation, histamine release, thromboxane and nitric oxide production and antibody production (Carr and Silverman 1999; Viaro *et al.* 2002). Severe acute lung injury has been reported (Urdaneta *et al.* 1999). The frequency of allergic reactions may be increased after rapid administration and in patients with a history of prior insulin allergy, but probably not in those with a history of fish allergy or vasectomy

(Wakefield *et al.* 1996; Carr and Silverman 1999). Methylene blue, another positively charged molecule, has been used to neutralize UFH in patients with a history of severe protamine reactions (Sloand *et al.* 1989). The plasma levels necessary for neutralization of heparin levels of 1 unit/ml are easily achieved using doses routinely used in treatment of methaemoglobinaemia. The toxicity of higher doses has not been extensively studied.

Other agents

Oestrogens

Conjugated oestrogens have been used since the 1960s to augment haemostasis for a wide variety of conditions from surgical procedures to VWD and uraemia (Verstraete *et al.* 1968; Alperin 1982; Livio *et al.* 1986; Ambrus *et al.* 1971). Conjugated oestrogens at a dose of 0.6 mg/kg daily administered intravenously shortened the bleeding time in patients with uraemia; the effect was first observed within 6 h of the initial dose, achieved maximum effect between 5 and 7 days, and lasted 2 weeks (Livio *et al.* 1986). Additional studies in patients with uraemia have confirmed effectiveness in shortening the bleeding time with either single or repeated intravenous doses of 0.6 mg/kg, whereas administration of 0.3 mg/kg was ineffective (Vigano *et al.* 1988). The effect of 4–5 daily doses lasted as long as 2 weeks. Oral oestrogens (50 mg daily of Premarin®) also shorten the bleeding time and may control bleeding symptoms in uraemic patients after 7 days of therapy (Shemin *et al.* 1990). Similarly, transdermal oestradiol administration of 50 or 100 μg/24 h every 3.5 days has been reported to shorten the bleeding time in uraemia and reduce transfusion requirements (Sloand and Schiff 1995).

Oestrogens have also been used for patients with VWD. Three women who previously required blood product therapy for control of bleeding due to VWD were able to undergo successful surgical procedures after being treated with oral oestrogens that had been prescribed as hormone replacement therapy or for contraception for 2 years prior to surgery and supplemented by 5 mg of conjugated oestrogens daily during postoperative recovery. Each patient had previously exhibited a decrease in VWD-related bleeding during pregnancies and subsequent normalization of coagulation tests during oral oestrogen treatment. These same tests were abnormal when measured 8 weeks after discontinuation of treatment (Alperin 1982).

The mechanism of action for oestrogen therapy is not well characterized, and may involve effects on the mucopolysaccharide content of the vessel wall, increased synthesis of VWF by endothelial cells or other less clearly defined effects on haemostasis (Verstraete et al. 1968; Harrison and McKee 1984; Nichols et al. 2003). These actions may explain the efficacy of oral oestrogens in patients with gastrointestinal bleeding due to vascular malformations (van Cutsem et al. 1990). Significant haemostatic toxicity has not been reported. Mild gynaecomastia, weight gain and dyspepsia have been reported in men.

Fibrin sealant

Fibrin sealants, sometimes referred to as fibrin glue (see Chapter 14), are topical haemostatic agents composed of highly concentrated fibrinogen, thrombin and occasionally additional agents such as EACA, aprotinin and factor XIII included to stabilize the fibrin clot and inhibit clot lysis (Jackson 2001; Mankad and Codispoti 2001). Sealants were derived initially from units of cryoprecipitate and subsequently by methods for preparing autologous fibrinogen of somewhat higher concentration. Several commercial sealants are now available that have been treated to inactivate infectious agents. The sealants are used primarily as surgical tissue adhesives in which the fibrinogen and thrombin components are either combined at the surgical site or sprayed along suture lines (Radosevich et al. 1997). The agents must be applied to relatively dry surfaces and do not replace the need for sutures.

Indications. Fibrin sealant has been used extensively in cardiovascular, orthopaedic, urological, gastrointestinal, neurological and vascular surgery (Spotnitz et al. 1987). The most widespread use remains in cardiovascular surgery where sealant has been used for everything from vascular anastamoses to haemostasis for median sternotomy, synthetic grafts and muscle flaps. Sealant use reportedly reduces bleeding and time to achieve haemostasis (von Segesser et al. 1995; Milne et al. 1996). Collagen sealant combinations have been used to treat pulmonary resection, air leakage during

thoracic surgery and to close small bronchopulmonary fistulae (Nomori et al. 2000; Fabian et al. 2003). Topical haemostatics have reduced blood loss and accelerated coagulation when used to secure skin grafts in burn victims (Nervi et al. 2001). In addition to its use as an adhesive, fibrin sealant has been used to introduce antibiotics and to deliver growth factors in a variety of surgical settings (Schlag and Redl 1988; Marone et al. 1999).

Adverse events. Early concerns with the use of commercial fibrin sealant produced from pooled human plasma involved viral transmission. Although pasteurization, ultrafiltration and chemical pathogen inactivation methods have reduced this risk dramatically, agents such as parvovirus B19 can still be transmitted and may infect up to 20% of susceptible patients (Radosevich et al. 1997). Hypersensitivity reactions, including anaphylaxis, have been reported and may be more common in the sealants that contain bovine thrombin, aprotinin or lysine analogues (Scheule et al. 1998; Oswald et al. 2003). Development of antibodies to bovine thrombin that crossreact to factor V have been detected and have caused a severe haemorrhagic disorder in some patients (Rapaport et al. 1992; Kajitani et al. 2000). Fibrin sealant preparations that use only human-derived proteins appear to avoid this complication (Streiff and Ness 2002).

Red cell substitutes

The popular term 'blood substitute' is a misnomer. Most candidate substitutes replace only one or two functions of transfused blood. By this definition, several blood substitutes are already in common use: dextran and starch solutions that act as volume expanders, recombinant proteins and even anticoagulants such as warfarin and heparin that are used on occasion to substitute for naturally occurring anticoagulant proteins. For other functions of blood, those of the platelet and leucocytes, no substitute is likely to emerge in the near future. The 'holy grail' of blood substitute research has been the development of a red cells substitute (RCS), a small molecule that delivers oxygen efficiently, requires no compatibility testing, can be sterilized, has a long shelf-life at room temperature, reconstitutes easily, persists in the circulation for days or weeks and can be provided at a price

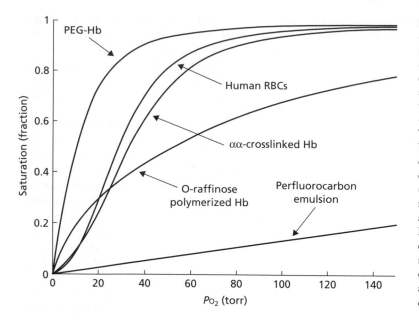

Fig 18.2 Oxyhaemoglobin equilibrium curves (fractional saturation vs. P_{O_2}) for representatives of the main classes of oxygen carriers. The PEG-Hb curve is for surface-modified human Hb, and the polymerized Hb curve is for o-raffinose-modified human Hb. The crosslinked Hb curve is for the US Army's $\alpha\alpha$-Hb. Small changes in oxygen partial pressure in the ranges of low-tissue P_{O_2}, mixed venous P_{O_2} (40 mmHg) and arterial P_{O_2} (100 mmHg) result in large changes in the amount of oxygen bound or released. In contrast, perfluorochemicals dissolve oxygen in a linear fashion and require high P_{O_2} (supplemental oxygen) to carry clinically relevant amounts of oxygen. From Stowell et al. (2001) with permission.

competitive with that of human blood. Although no such substance is licensed, candidate agents with several of these qualities are in clinical trials.

Potential RCS fall into three general classes: perfluorochemicals (PFCs), haemoglobin-based oxygen carriers (HBOCs) and liposome-encapsulated haemoglobin. Although it is convenient to review these drugs as 'classes', each formulation should be considered a unique drug with its own physical characteristics, biological activities and adverse reaction profile.

Perfluorochemical emulsions

Perfluorochemicals are synthetic, inert, hydrophobic molecules with an almost unlimited ability to dissolve gases including oxygen. They are excreted unchanged through the lungs. Because these molecules are structurally similar to hydrocarbons, they are not water soluble and therefore must be emulsified with surfactants before they are suitable for intravenous use. This property has complicated their preparation and storage and the nature of the emulsifier turns out to be as important as the PFC itself. The classic early experiments in which a mouse was submerged in a beaker of pre-oxygenated PFC emulsion and shown to breathe liquid continues to fascinate medical journalists as do the exchange-transfused 'bloodless rat' experiments (Clark and Gollan 1966; Geyer 1975).

However, early PFC formulations were impure, persisted for long periods in the reticuloendothelial system, appeared to inhibit macrophage function and proved unsuitable for clinical trials (Ohnishi and Kitazawa 1980; Vercellotti et al. 1982).

Broad application of PFC as RCS may be limited by their oxygen-loading and off-loading properties (Fig. 18.2). Unlike blood and haemoglobin constructs, PFC dissolve oxygen in a linear fashion related directly to the partial pressure of oxygen. What this means in practice is that these emulsions can carry a great deal of oxygen, but only if the patient inspires high concentrations of supplemental oxygen. Furthermore, the compounds may release much of the oxygen as blood passes through less well-oxygenated environments and long before it reaches the most ischaemic tissues. The latter property, the need for refrigerated storage and the relatively short-circulating half-life have led some investigators to postulate that these chemicals will prove most suitable for in-hospital use.

During a 10-year period, thousands of patients with a wide variety of illnesses received an early PFC formulation, Fluosol DA. However, in controlled clinical trials, patients receiving Fluosol failed to show substantial physiological benefit and were plagued with adverse reactions attributed by some to complement activation (Gould et al. 1986). Production of this drug ceased in 1994.

Newer PFC formulations containing more perfluorocarbon and carrying up to five times more dissolved oxygen have undergone clinical trials. The troubling side-effects associated with Fluosol DA, complement activation and cytokine release, seem to have been attenuated by newer formulations containing smaller emulsion particles. However, a flu-like syndrome attributed to macrophage-mediated clearance of the emulsion and a curious sequestration of 15–20% of circulating platelets are commonly observed. A European multicentre, randomized trial of orthopaedic surgery patients reported reduced need for allogeneic blood during profound intraoperative haemodilution (Spahn et al. 1999). A study of general surgery patients indicated that acute normovolaemic haemodilution with PFC reduced transfusion needs in patients, but whereas the number of adverse events in the treatment and control groups were similar, more serious adverse events were reported in the PFC group (Spahn et al. 2002). Further trials using PFC to augment profound perisurgical haemodilution have been suspended while an increased frequency of stroke in the treatment arm is investigated. It is not clear whether stroke was related to the PFC or to trial design, which included rapid, deep haemodilution at the onset of surgery (Keipert 2003).

Haemoglobin-based oxygen carriers

In total, 98% of blood oxygen is carried by encapsulated haemoglobin, nature's oxygen transport protein. The well-known sigmoid shape of the oxygen equilibrium curve describes how haemoglobin in human red cells binds oxygen rapidly in the lung and releases it efficiently in the low-oxygen environment of the tissues (see Fig. 18.2) (Stowell et al. 2001). For this reason, cell-free haemoglobin with similar characteristics seemed the logical candidate for a RCS. However, inside the red cell membrane, the haemoglobin tetramer is stabilized, provided with organic phosphates that modify oxygen delivery and protected from harmful oxidants, while outside the red cell, haemoglobin is vulnerable to oxidative inactivation and its chains dissociate into dimers. The oxygen affinity of human haemoglobin in solution is much higher than that of intracellular haemoglobin, in part because of the absence of 2,3-diphosphoglycerate within the red cell stroma, and in part because of the relatively alkaline pH of plasma in comparison with

the interior of the red cell (Bohr effect). Haemoglobin solutions have a high colloid osmotic pressure that might limit preparations to a concentration less than 7 g/dl (Moss et al. 1984). Unless stored in an oxygen-free environment, haemoglobin in solution gradually oxidizes to methaemoglobin (Vandegriff 1992).

Early clinical studies of purified haemoglobin solutions were notable primarily for a pattern of hypertension and bradycardia in the recipients as well as evidence of renal toxicity, in part related to dissociation of the haemoglobin tetramer subunits into alpha-beta dimers (Amberson et al. 1949; Savitsky et al. 1978). A variety of chemical modifications have been pursued to prevent subunit dissociation and to achieve different characteristics of the haemoglobin solution. Dissociation curves of a crosslinked, cell-free haemoglobin, haemoglobin molecules that have been polymerized to increase extravascular persistence and decrease colloidal osmotic pressure, and haemoglobin coupled to polyethylene glycol (PEG) are compared with red cells and perfluorocarbon solution in Fig. 18.2.

Most HBOCs are derived from human or bovine blood washed to remove cellular debris, pasteurized, filtered and passed over chromatographic columns to ensure purity. The tetramer is then chemically modified by any of a bewildering variety of methods to provide molecules of different size, molecular weight, oxygen affinity, viscosity and oncotic activity (Stowell et al. 2001). The most widely used method involves treatment with pyridoxal phosphate to lower oxygen affinity, followed by internal crosslinking and linkage of haemoglobin with glutaraldehyde to polymerize the molecules (Payne 1973). Recombinant haemoglobin molecules with features not found in nature have also been prepared (Looker et al. 1992). RCS can thus be customized for their intended use, provided that the characteristics necessary for that use are well defined. Most candidate HBOCs have been engineered to copy the characteristics of the whole blood oxygen dissociation curve, and the solutions have frequently been prepared to mimic many of the characteristics of blood, albeit at a lower haemoglobin concentration. However, as with PFC emulsions, the physiology of oxygen delivery by small molecules that extravasate beyond the microcirculation is incompletely understood and it is possible that different affinity, viscosity and oncotic pressure may eventually prove superior

(Winslow 2003). Finally, in an ironic recapitulation of red cell evolution, haemoglobin has been encapsulated in liposomes to prolong its intravascular circulation. However, liposomal haemoglobin has yet to realize the success of other liposome-encapsulated pharmaceuticals (MacGregor and Hunt 1990).

Clinical studies. It has been surprisingly difficult to demonstrate efficacy with the candidate HBOC. In a detailed report of a single patient, Mullon and colleagues (2000) described a 21-year-old woman with life-threatening autoimmune haemolytic anaemia, treated with a polymerized bovine haemoglobin preparation after severe reactions to repeated incompatible transfusions, and her rapidly falling haematocrit left few options other than oxygen carriers devoid of red cell membrane antigens. In this situation, proof of drug efficacy is still indirect, as the lower limits of haemoglobin that humans tolerate have not been defined (Weiskopf *et al.* 1998). However, the reversal of signs, symptoms and electrocardiographic evidence of ischaemia in this symptomatic anaemic patient are compelling, as is the laboratory evidence of reduced end-organ ischaemia. In this instance, it seems reasonable to conclude that the 11 HBOC infusions over a 7-day period helped to sustain this patient until her autoimmune process remitted.

Refractory autoimmune haemolytic anaemia illustrates an extremely limited indication for RCS. Most clinical trials use 'blood sparing' or 'blood avoidance' during surgery as primary study endpoints. However, the short 12- to 48-h half-life of these small molecules limits their blood-sparing utility. Mathematical modelling suggests that benefits will be confined primarily to non-anaemic patients who undergo extreme haemodilution and sustain large perioperative blood losses (Brecher *et al.* 1999). A randomized trial of polymerized haemoglobin solution for acute blood loss in trauma patients has reported that infusion of a polymerized HBOC was able to maintain total Hb concentration despite the marked fall in red cell Hb, and to reduce the use of allogeneic blood (Gould *et al.* 1998). Up to 20 units (each unit 50 g of Hb) of this product have been infused without evidence of toxicity. In a randomized, double-blind efficacy trial of a bovine polymerized HBOC, a total of 98 patients undergoing cardiac surgery and requiring transfusion was randomly assigned to receive either red blood cell units or the HBOC for the first three postoperative transfusions. In 34% of cases, the HBOC eliminated the need for red blood cell transfusion, although substantial doses were needed to produce a modest degree of blood conservation (Levy *et al.* 2002). In a previous study of 72 patients prospectively randomized two-to-one to HBOC or allogeneic RBC at the time of the first transfusion decision, this HBOC eliminated the need for allogeneic RBC transfusion in 27% of patients undergoing infrarenal aortic reconstruction, but did not reduce the median allogeneic RBC requirement. The preparation was well tolerated and did not influence morbidity or mortality rates (LaMuraglia *et al.* 2000). However the infusion of up to 1000 ml of a diaspirin crosslinked human haemoglobin in a multicentre, randomized, controlled single-blinded trial in 112 patients with traumatic haemorrhagic shock resulted in excessive unpredicted deaths in the treatment group (Sloan *et al.* 1999). When the same product was administered to 85 patients with acute ischaemic stroke in a randomized, single-blind, controlled trial, more serious adverse events and deaths occurred in the treated patients than in control patients (Saxena *et al.* 1999). Trials of this solution have been discontinued.

There has been limited experience with HBOC in patients with sickle cell disease, where small-molecule oxygen delivery might in theory benefit areas of the microcirculation occluded by sickled cells. In an uncontrolled series, polymerized bovine haemoglobin was administered to treat aplastic and vaso-occlusive crises in nine African children with sickle cell disease. All patients reportedly improved and no adverse effects were noted (Feola *et al.* 1992). In a single case report, a patient who refused transfusion on religious grounds received 12 units of human polymerized Hb solution over 13 days to treat acute chest syndrome in the setting of sepsis. The authors considered the treatment life saving as the patient's respiratory status improved and she was discharged without receiving RBC transfusions (Lanzkron *et al.* 2002).

Adverse effects of haemoglobin solutions

A large number of pre-clinical abnormalities have been described with different HBOC formulations (Buehler and Alayash 2004). The clinical importance of these observations is unclear but, given the unfortunate experience of several clinical trials, careful investigation is warranted.

Vasoactivity. Acute normovolaemic haemodilution with crystalloid or colloid solutions is accompanied by increased cardiac output. Blood replacement with several of the HBOCs has caused systemic and pulmonary hypertension in animal models and in human subjects (Amberson *et al.* 1934; Savitsky *et al.* 1978; Hess 1995). This pressor effect is related in part to scavenging of the vasodilator nitric oxide, but a direct action on the microvasculature involving oxygen autoregulation of capillary blood flow has been proposed as well (Murad *et al.* 1978; Schultz *et al.* 1993; Winslow 2003). The pressor effect has been implicated in symptoms related to smooth muscle contractility such as gastroenteric motility abnormalities, cardiovascular abnormalities and changes in vascular tone. When blood is removed from experimental animals and replaced with polymerized haemoglobin or haemoglobin modified by polyethylene glycol, the pressor effect appears to be attenuated or eliminated (Gould *et al.* 1990; Vlahakes *et al.* 1990; Winslow 2004). The ability of haemoglobin to pass through the vascular endothelium depends on the size of the haemoglobin molecule. Polymerized haemoglobin (such as PolyHeme) should penetrate the endothelium less readily than stabilized single tetramers (such as DCLHb and rHbl.l), and so might be expected to have fewer cardiovascular effects.

Nephrotoxicity. Elements of red cell stroma damage the kidneys (Rabiner *et al.* 1970). Infusions of tetrameric, stroma-free haemoglobin have been shown to cause renal damage in human volunteers (Savitsky *et al.* 1978). Obvious evidence of renal impairment seems to have been eliminated from the HBOCs currently in clinical trials.

Applications

The current generation of RCS has an intravascular survival time suitable for a resuscitation solution or as an oxygen-carrying adjuvant in haemodiluted patients undergoing surgery. They are not suitable substitutes for red cells in the treatment of chronic anaemia. Furthermore, chronic binding of nitric oxide to some of the candidate molecules might lead to unanticipated toxicities, such as pulmonary hypertension (Rother *et al.* 2005). Avoidance of allogeneic blood transfusion would benefit the individual patient only if the toxicity of the solution proves to be lower than that of the current red cell components. Blood transfusion has a long history and its adverse effects and toxicity have been studied for centuries. In the developed world, blood components are relatively safe and available. For the developing world, where blood is in short supply and fully tested blood often unavailable, an inexpensive RCS might save hundreds of thousands of lives (Blank *et al.* 1984).

References

Abels RJ, Larholt KM, Krantz KD (1991) Blood cell growth factors: their present and future use. In: Hematology and Oncology. J Murphy Jr (ed.). Dayton, OH: Alpha Med Press, p. 121

Abshire T, Kenet G (2004) Recombinant factor VIIa: review of efficacy, dosing regimens and safety in patients with congenital and acquired factor VIII or IX inhibitors. J Thromb Haemost 2: 899–909

Adamson JW (1991a) Cytokine biology: implications for transfusion medicine. Cancer 67: 2708–2711

Adamson JW (1991b) Erythropoietin: its role in the regulation of erythropoiesis and as a therapeutic in humans. Biotechnology 19: 351–363

Aledort LM, Hayward CP, Chen MG et al. (2004) Prospective screening of 205 patients with ITP, including diagnosis, serological markers, and the relationship between platelet counts, endogenous thrombopoietin, and circulating antithrombopoietin antibodies. Am J Hematol 76: 205–213

Alperin JB (1982) Estrogens and surgery in women with von Willebrand's disease. Am J Med 73: 367–371

Alperin JB (1987) Coagulopathy caused by vitamin K deficiency in critically ill, hospitalized patients. JAMA 258: 1916–1919

Alvarez GG, Fergusson DA, Neilipovitz DT et al. (2004) Cell salvage does not minimize perioperative allogeneic blood transfusion in abdominal vascular surgery: a systematic review. Can J Anaesth 51: 425–431

Amberson WR, Flexner J, Steggarda FR (1934) On the use of Ringer-Locke solutions containing hemoglobin as a substitute for normal blood in animals. J Cell Comp Physiol 5: 359

Amberson WR, Jennings JJ, Rhode CM (1949) Clinical experience with hemoglobin-saline solutions. J Appl Physiol I: 469

Ambrus JL, Schimert G, Lajos TZ et al. (1971) Effect of antifibrinolytic agents and estrogens on blood loss and blood coagulation factors during open heart surgery. J Med 2: 65–81

Anderson BV, Tomasulo PA (1988) Current autologous transfusion practices. Implication for the future. Transfusion 28: 394–396

Aoki N, Saito H, Kamiya T *et al.* (1979) Congenital deficiency of alpha 2-plasmin inhibitor associated with severe hemorrhagic tendency. J Clin Invest 63: 877–884

AuBuchon JP (1989) Autologous transfusion and directed donations: current controversies and future directions. Transfusion Med Rev 3: 290–306

AuBuchon JP, Popovsky MA (1988) Autologous donor safety in non-hospital programs (Abstract). Transfusion 28: 345

Auerbach M, Ballard H, Trout JR *et al.* (2004) Intravenous iron optimizes the response to recombinant human erythropoietin in cancer patients with chemotherapy-related anemia: a multicenter, open-label, randomized trial. J Clin Oncol 22: 1301–1307

Babcock RB, Dumper CW, Scharfman WB (1976) Heparin-induced immune thrombocytopenia. N Engl J Med 295: 237–241

Bader D, Blondheim O, Jonas R *et al.* (1996) Decreased ferritin levels, despite iron supplementation, during erythropoietin therapy in anaemia of prematurity. Acta Paediatr 85: 496–501

Banerjee D, Rodriguez M, Nag M *et al.* (2000) Exposure of endothelial cells to recombinant human erythropoietin induces nitric oxide synthase activity. Kidney Int 57: 1895–1904

Barnhart MI, Chen S, Lusher JM (1983) DDAVP: does the drug have a direct effect on the vessel wall? Thromb Res 31: 239–253

Bartholomew JR, Salgia R, Bell WR (1989) Control of bleeding in patients with immune and nonimmune thrombocytopenia with aminocaproic acid. Arch Intern Med 149: 1959–1961

Basser RL, Rasko JE, Clarke K *et al.* (1997) Randomized, blinded, placebo-controlled phase I trial of pegylated recombinant human megakaryocyte growth and development factor with filgrastim after dose-intensive chemotherapy in patients with advanced cancer. Blood 89: 3118–3128

Bennett CL, Luminari S, Nissenson AR *et al.* (2004) Pure red cell aplasia and epoetin therapy. N Engl J Med 351: 1403–1408

Bennett CL, Cournoyer D, Carson KR *et al.* (2005) Long-term outcome of individuals with pure red cell aplasia and anti-erythropoietin antibodies in patients treated with recombinant epoetin: A follow-up report from the Research on Adverse Drug Events and Reports (RADAR) Project. Blood: Epub, 11 August 2005

Biesma DH, Marx JJ, van de Wiel A (1994) Collection of autologous blood before elective hip replacement. A comparison of the results with the collection of two and four units. J Bone Joint Surg Am 76: 1471–1475

Birkmeyer JD, AuBuchon JP, Littenberg B *et al.* (1994) Cost-effectiveness of preoperative autologous donation in coronary artery bypass grafting. Ann Thorac Surg 57: 161–168

Blank JP, Sheagren TG, Vajaria J (1984) The role of rbc transfusion in the premature neonate. Am J Dis Child 138: 831–833

Bode-Boger SM, Boger RH, Kuhn M *et al.* (1996) Recombinant human erythropoietin enhances vasoconstrictor tone via endothelin-1 and constrictor prostanoids. Kidney Int 50: 1255–1261

Bohrer H, Fleischer F, Lang J *et al.* (1990) Early formation of thrombi on pulmonary artery catheters in cardiac surgical patients receiving high-dose aprotinin. J Cardiothorac Anesth 4: 222–225

Bonilla MA, Gillio AP, Ruggiero M (1989) Effects of recombinant human granulocyte colony-stimulating factor on neutropenia in patients with congenital agranulocytosis. N Engl J Med 320: 1574–1580

Bosch J, Thabut D, Bendtsen F *et al.* (2004) Recombinant factor VIIa for upper gastrointestinal bleeding in patients with cirrhosis: a randomized, double-blind trial. Gastroenterology 127: 1123–1130

Brecher ME, Goodnough LT (2002) The rise and fall of preoperative autologous blood donation (Editorial). Transfusion 41: 1459–1462

Brecher ME, Goodnough LT, Monk T (1999) The value of oxygen-carrying solutions in the operative setting, as determined by mathematical modeling. Transfusion 39: 396–402

Breen GA, St Peter WL (1997) Hypoprothrombinemia associated with cefmetazole. Ann Pharmacother 31: 180–184

Brinkhous KM, Smith H (1937) Plasma prothrombin level in normal infancy and in hemorrhagic disease of the newborn. Am J Med Sci 193: 475

Britton LW, Eastland DT, Dziuban SW (1989) Predonated autologous blood use in elective cardiac surgery. Ann Thorac Surg 47: 529–532

Brugnara C, Chambers LA, Malynn E *et al.* (1993) Red blood cell regeneration induced by subcutaneous recombinant erythropoietin: iron-deficient erythropoiesis in iron-replete subjects. Blood 81: 956–964

Buehler PW, Alayash AI (2004) Toxicities of hemoglobin solutions: in search of in-vitro and in-vivo model systems. Transfusion 44: 1516–1530

Butenas S, Brummel KE, Bouchard BA *et al.* (2003) How factor VIIa works in hemophilia. J Thromb Haemost 1: 1158–1160

Butterworth J, James RL, Lin Y *et al.* (1999) Pharmacokinetics of epsilon-aminocaproic acid in patients undergoing aortocoronary bypass surgery. Anesthesiology 90: 1624–1635

Butterworth J, James RL, Lin YA *et al.* (2001) Gender does not influence epsilon-aminocaproic acid concentrations in adults undergoing cardiopulmonary bypass. Anesth Analg 92: 1384–1390

Butterworth J, Lin YA, Prielipp R et al. (2002) The pharmacokinetics and cardiovascular effects of a single intravenous dose of protamine in normal volunteers. Anesth Analg 94: 514–522

Cairo MS, Christensen R, Sender LS et al. (1995) Results of a phase I/II trial of recombinant human granulocyte–macrophage colony-stimulating factor in very low birthweight neonates: significant induction of circulatory neutrophils, monocytes, platelets and bone marrow neutrophils. Blood 86: 2509–2515

Caldwell SH, Chang C, Macik BG (2004) Recombinant activated factor VII (rFVIIa) as a hemostatic agent in liver disease: a break from convention in need of controlled trials. Hepatology 39: 592–598

Carless PA, Henry DA, Moxey AJ et al. (2004) Desmopressin for minimising perioperative allogeneic blood transfusion. Cochrane Database Syst Rev CD001884

Carr JA, Silverman N (1999) The heparin-protamine interaction. A review. J Cardiovasc Surg (Torino) 40: 659–666

Carvalho B, Ridler BM, Thompson JF et al. (2003) Myocardial ischaemia precipitated by acute normovolaemic haemodilution. Transfusion Med 13: 165–168

Casadevall N, Nataf J, Viron B et al. (2001) Pure red cell aplasia and antierythropoietin antibodies in patients treated with recombinant erythropoietin. N Engl J Med 346: 469–475

Castle V, Andrew M, Kelton J et al. (1986) Frequency and mechanism of neonatal thrombocytopenia. J Pediatr 108: 749–755

Cattaneo M, Moia M, Delle VP et al. (1989) DDAVP shortens the prolonged bleeding times of patients with severe von Willebrand disease treated with cryoprecipitate. Evidence for a mechanism of action independent of released von Willebrand factor. Blood 74: 1972–1975

Cazzola M, Mercuriali F, Brugnara C (1997) Use of recombinant human erythropoietin outside the setting of uremia. Blood 89: 4248–4267

Clark LC Jr, Gollan F (1966) Survival of mammals breathing organic liquids equilibrated with oxygen at atmospheric pressure. Science 152: 1755–1756

Clark OA, Lyman G, Castro AA et al. (2003) Colony stimulating factors for chemotherapy induced febrile neutropenia. Cochrane Database Syst Rev CD003039

Coats T, Roberts I, Shakur H (2004) Antifibrinolytic drugs for acute traumatic injury. Cochrane Database Syst Rev CD004896

Cohen JA, Brecher ME (1995) Preoperative autologous blood donation: benefit or detriment? A mathematical analysis. Transfusion 35: 640–644

Cohen H, Scott SD, Mackie IJ et al. (1988) The development of hypoprothrombinaemia following antibiotic therapy in malnourished patients with low serum vitamin K1 levels. Br J Haematol 68: 63–66

Collen D (1999) The plasminogen (fibrinolytic) system. Thromb Haemost 82: 259–270

Cosgriff SW (1956) The effectiveness of an oral vitamin K1 in controlling excessive hypoprothrombinemia during anticoagulant therapy. Ann Intern Med 45: 14–22

Cournoyer D, Toffelmire E, Wells G et al. (2004) Anti-erythropoietin antibody-mediated pure red cell aplasia after treatment with recombinant erythropoietin products: recommendations for minimization of risks. J Am Soc Nephrol 15: 2728–2734

Cregan P, Donegan E, Gotelli G (1991) Hemolytic transfusion reaction following autologous frozen and washed red cells. Transfusion 31: 172–175

Crouch ER Jr, Williams PB, Gray MK et al. (1997) Topical aminocaproic acid in the treatment of traumatic hyphema. Arch Ophthalmol 115: 1106–1112

Crowther MA, Julian J, McCarty J et al. (2000) Treatment of warfarin-induced coagulopathy with oral vitamin K: a randomized controlled trial. Lancet 356: 1551–1553

Crowther MA, Berry LR, Monagle PT et al. (2002) Mechanisms responsible for the failure of protamine to inactivate low-molecular weight heparin. Br J Haematol 116: 178–186

van Cutsem E, Rutgeerts P, Vantrappen G (1990) Treatment of bleeding gastrointestinal vascular malformations with oestrogen-progesterone. Lancet 335: 953–955

Dale DC, Cottle TE, Fier CJ et al. (2003) Severe chronic neutropenia: treatment and follow-up of patients in the Severe Chronic Neutropenia International Registry. Am J Hematol 72: 82–93

Dalmau A, Sabate A, Koo M et al. (2004) The prophylactic use of tranexamic acid and aprotinin in orthotopic liver transplantation: a comparative study. Liver Transpl 10: 279–284

Dam H, Dyggve H (1952) Relation of Vitamin K deficiency to hemorrhagic disease of the newborn. Adv Pediatr 5: 129

Dam H, Glavind J (1938) Vitamin K in human pathology. Lancet 1: 720–721

Daneshvar A (1988) Fluid replacement after blood donation: implications for elderly and autologous blood donors. Maryland Med J 37: 787–791

De Bonis M, Cavaliere F, Alessandrini F et al. (2000) Topical use of tranexamic acid in coronary artery bypass operations: a double-blind, prospective, randomized, placebo-controlled study. J Thorac Cardiovasc Surg 119: 575–580

Deitcher SR, Tuller J, Johnson JA (1999) Intranasal DDAVP induced increases in plasma von Willebrand factor alter the pharmacokinetics of high-purity factor VIII concentrates in severe haemophilia A patients. Haemophilia 5: 88–95

Depalma L, Luban NLC (1990) Autologous blood transfusion in pediatrics. Pediatrics 85: 125–128

Depalma L, Palmer R, Leitman SF *et al.* (1990) Utilization patterns of frozen autologous red blood cells. Experience in a referral center and a community hospital. Arch Pathol Lab Med 114: 516–518

De Sauvage FJ, Hass PE, Spencer SD (1994) Stimulation of megakaryocytopoiesis and thrombopoiesis by the c-Mpl ligand. Nature (Lond) 369: 533–538

Despotis GJ, Gravlee G, Filos K *et al.* (1999a) Anti-coagulation monitoring during cardiac surgery: a review of current and emerging techniques. Anesthesiology 91: 1122–1151

Despotis GJ, Levine V, Saleem R *et al.* (1999b) Use of point-of-care test in identification of patients who can benefit from desmopressin during cardiac surgery: a randomised controlled trial. Lancet 354: 106–110

Deveras RA, Kessler CM (2002) Reversal of warfarin-induced excessive anticoagulation with recombinant human factor VIIa concentrate. Ann Intern Med 137: 884–888

D'Hondt V, Humblet Y, Guillaume T *et al.* (1995) Thrombopoietic effects and toxicity of interleukin-6 in patients with ovarian cancer before and after chemotherapy: a multicentric placebo-controlled, randomized phase Ib study. Blood 85: 2347–2353

Diefenbach C, Abel M, Limpers B *et al.* (1995) Fatal anaphylactic shock after aprotinin reexposure in cardiac surgery. Anesth Analg 80: 830–831

Dietrich W, Spath P, Ebell A *et al.* (1997) Prevalence of anaphylactic reactions to aprotinin: analysis of two hundred forty-eight re-exposures to aprotinin in heart operations. J Thorac Cardiovasc Surg 113: 194–201

Dietrich W, Spath P, Zuhlsdorf M *et al.* (2001) Anaphylactic reactions to aprotinin reexposure in cardiac surgery: relation to antiaprotinin immunoglobulin G and E antibodies. Anesthesiology 95: 64–71

Dilthey G, Dietrich W, Spannagl M *et al.* (1993) Influence of desmopressin acetate on homologous blood requirements in cardiac surgical patients pretreated with aspirin. J Cardiothorac Vasc Anesth 7: 425–430

DiMichele DM, Hathaway WE (1990) Use of DDAVP in inherited and acquired platelet dysfunction. Am J Hematol 33: 39–45

Di Raimondo F, Longo G, Cacciola E Jr *et al.* (1996) A good response rate to recombinant erythropoietin alone may be expected in selected myelodysplastic patients. A preliminary clinical study. Eur J Haematol 56: 7–11

Dowd NP, Karski JM, Cheng DC *et al.* (2002) Pharmacokinetics of tranexamic acid during cardiopulmonary bypass. Anesthesiology 97: 390–399

Dunn CJ, Goa KL (1999) Tranexamic acid: a review of its use in surgery and other indications. Drugs 57: 1005–1032

Dunn AL, Powers JR, Ribeiro MJ *et al.* (2000) Adverse events during use of intranasal desmopressin acetate for haemophilia A and von Willebrand disease: a case report and review of 40 patients. Haemophilia 6: 11–14

Dutton RP, McCunn M, Hyder M *et al.* (2004) Factor VIIa for correction of traumatic coagulopathy. J Trauma 57: 709–719

Dzik WH, Sherburne B (1990) Intraoperative blood salvage: medical controversies. Transfusion Med Rev 4: 208–235

Edelson RN, Chernik NL, Posner JB (1974) Spinal subdural hematomas complicating lumbar puncture. Arch Neurol 31: 134–137

Eng J, Kay PH, Murday AJ *et al.* (1990) Postoperative autologous transfusion in cardiac surgery. A prospective, randomised study. Eur J Cardiothorac Surg 4: 595–600

Eschbach JW (2002) Anemia management in chronic kidney disease: role of factors affecting epoetin responsiveness. J Am Soc Nephrol 13: 1412–1414

Eschbach JW, Kelly MR, Haley NR *et al.* (1989) Treatment of the anemia of progressive renal failure with recombinant human erythropoietin. N Engl J Med 321: 158–163

Etchason J, Petz L, Keeler E *et al.* (1995) The cost effectiveness of preoperative autologous blood donations. N Engl J Med 332: 719–724

Fabian T, Federico JA, Ponn RB (2003) Fibrin glue in pulmonary resection: a prospective, randomized, blinded study. Ann Thorac Surg 75: 1587–1592

Fanucchi M, Glaspy J, Crawford J *et al.* (1997) Effects of polyethylene glycol-conjugated recombinant human megakaryocyte growth and development factor on platelet counts after chemotherapy for lung cancer. N Engl J Med 336: 404–409

Federici AB, Mazurier C, Berntorp E *et al.* (2004) Biologic response to desmopressin in patients with severe type 1 and type 2 von Willebrand disease: results of a multicenter European study. Blood 103: 2032–2038

Feola M, Simoni J, Angelillo R *et al.* (1992) Clinical trial of a hemoglobin based blood substitute in patients with sickle cell anemia. Surg Gynecol Obstet 174: 379–386

Fisher JW (2003) Erythropoietin: physiology and pharmacology update. Exp Biol Med (Maywood) 228: 1–14

Flordal PA, Sahlin S (1993) Use of desmopressin to prevent bleeding complications in patients treated with aspirin. Br J Surg 80: 723–724

Flordal PA, Ljungstrom KG, Fehrm A (1992) Desmopressin and postoperative thromboembolism. Thromb Res 68: 429–433

Foster DC, Sprecker CA, Grant FJ *et al.* (1994) Human thrombopoietin: gene structure, cDNA sequence, expression and chromosomal localization. Proc Natl Acad Sci USA 91: 13023–13027

Freeman WD, Brott TG, Barrett KM *et al.* (2004) Recombinant factor VIIa for rapid reversal of warfarin anticoagulation in acute intracranial hemorrhage. Mayo Clin Proc 79: 1495–1500

Fremes SE, Wong BI, Lee E *et al.* (1994) Metaanalysis of prophylactic drug treatment in the prevention of postoperative bleeding. Ann Thorac Surg 58: 1580–1588

Fricke W, Alling D, Kimball J *et al.* (1991) Lack of efficacy of tranexamic acid in thrombocytopenic bleeding. Transfusion 31: 345–348

Friederich PW, Henny CP, Messelink EJ *et al.* (2003) Effect of recombinant activated factor VII on perioperative blood loss in patients undergoing retropubic prostatectomy: a double blind placebo-controlled randomised trial. Lancet 361: 201–205

Furie B, Bouchard BA, Furie BC (1999) Vitamin K-dependent biosynthesis of gamma-carboxyglutamic acid. Blood 93: 1798–1808

Galvez A, Gomez-Ortiz G, Diaz-Ricart M *et al.* (1997) Desmopressin (DDAVP) enhances platelet adhesion to the extracellular matrix of cultured human endothelial cells through increased expression of tissue factor. Thromb Haemost 77: 975–980

Gardner FH, Helmer RE III (1980) Aminocaproic acid. Use in control of hemorrhage in patients with amegakaryocytic thrombocytopenia. JAMA 243: 35–37

Garewal HS, Durie BG (1985) Antifibrinolytic therapy with aminocaproic acid for the control of bleeding in thrombocytopenic patients. J Scand Haematol 35: 497–500

Gerotziafas GT, Zervas K, Arzoglou P *et al.* (2002) On the mechanism of action of recombinant activated factor VII administered to patients with severe thrombocytopenia and life-threatening haemorrhage: focus on prothrombin activation. Br J Haematol 117: 705–708

Geyer RP (1975) 'Bloodless' rats through the use of artificial blood substitutes. Fed Proc 34: 1499–1505

Giordano GF, Rivers SL, Chung GK *et al.* (1988) Autologous platelet-rich plasma in cardiac surgery: effect on intraoperative and postoperative transfusion requirements. Ann Thorac Surg 46: 416–419

Giordano GF Sr, Giordano GF Jr, Rivers SL *et al.* (1989) Determinants of homologous blood usage utilizing autologous platelet-rich plasma in cardiac operations. Ann Thorac Surg 47: 897–902

Giordano GF, Giordano DM, Wallace BA *et al.* (1993) An analysis of 9918 consecutive perioperative autotransfusions. Surg Gynecol Obstet 176: 103–110

Goodnough LT, Rudnick S, Price TH *et al.* (1989) Increased preoperative collection of autologous blood with recombinant human erythropoietin therapy. N Engl J Med 321: 1163–1168

Goodnough LT, Price TH, Rudnick S (1991) Iron-restricted erythropoiesis as a limitation to autologous blood donation in the erythropoietin-stimulated bone marrow. J Lab Clin Med 118: 289–296

Goodnough LT, Saha P, Hirschler NV *et al.* (1992a) Autologous blood donation in nonorthopaedic surgical procedures as a blood conservation strategy. Vox Sang 63: 96–101

Goodnough LT, Price TH, Rudnick S *et al.* (1992b) Preoperative red cell production in patients undergoing aggressive autologous blood phlebotomy with and without erythropoietin therapy. Transfusion 32: 441–445

Goodnough LT, Vizmeg K, Verbrugge D (1994) The impact of autologous blood ordering and blood procurement practices on allogeneic blood exposure in elective orthopedic surgery patients. Am J Clin Pathol 101: 354–357

Goodnough LT, Verbrugge D, Marcus RE (1995) The relationship between hematocrit, blood lost, and blood transfused in total knee replacement. Implications for postoperative blood salvage and reinfusion. Am J Knee Surg 8: 83–87

Goodnough LT, Monk TG, Brecher ME (1996) Autologous blood procurement in the surgical setting: lessons learned in the last 10 years. Vox Sang 71: 133–141

Goodnough LT, Despotis GJ, Merkel K *et al.* (2000) A randomized trial comparing acute normovolemic hemodilution and preoperative autologous blood donation in total hip arthroplasty. Transfusion 40: 1054–1057

Goodnough LT, Kuter DJ, McCullough J *et al.* (2001) Prophylactic platelet transfusions from healthy apheresis platelet donors undergoing treatment with thrombopoietin. Blood 98: 1346–1351

Gordon MS, McCaskill-Stevens WJ, Battiato LA *et al.* (1996) A phase I trial of recombinant human interleukin-11 (neumega rhIL-11 growth factor) in women with breast cancer receiving chemotherapy. Blood 87: 3615–3624

Gould SA, Rosen AL, Sehgal LR *et al.* (1986) Fluosol-DA as a red-cell substitute in acute anemia. N Engl J Med 314: 1653–1656

Gould SA, Sehgal LR, Rosen AL *et al.* (1990) The efficacy of polymerized pyridoxylated hemoglobin solution as an O2 carrier. Ann Surg 211: 394–398

Gould SA, Moore EE, Hoyt DB *et al.* (1998) The first randomized trial of human polymerized hemoglobin as a blood substitute in acute trauma and emergent surgery. J Am Coll Surg 187: 113–120

Gratz I, Koehler J, Olsen D *et al.* (1992) The effect of desmopressin acetate on postoperative hemorrhage in patients receiving aspirin therapy before coronary artery bypass operations. J Thorac Cardiovasc Surg 104: 1417–1422

Grossman BJ, Stewart NC, Grindon AJ (1988) Increased risk of a positive test for antibody to hepatitis B core antigen (anti-HBc) in autologous blood donors. Transfusion 28: 283–285

Gunther KE, Conway G, Leibach J *et al.* (2004) Low-dose oral vitamin K is safe and effective for outpatient management of patients with an INR > 10. Thromb Res 113: 205–209

Harker LA, Carter RA, Marzek UM *et al.* (1998) Correction of thrombocytopenia and ineffective platelet production in patients infected with human immunodeficiency virus (HIV) by PEG-rHuMGDF therapy. Blood 92 (Suppl. 1): 707a

Harrison RL, McKee PA (1984) Estrogen stimulates von Willebrand factor production by cultured endothelial cells. Blood 63: 657–664

Havel M, Muller M, Graninger W *et al.* (1987) Tolerability of a new vitamin K1 preparation for parenteral administration to adults: one case of anaphylactoid reaction. Clin Ther 9: 373–379

Havel M, Grabenwoger F, Schneider J *et al.* (1994) Aprotinin does not decrease early graft patency after coronary artery bypass grafting despite reducing postoperative bleeding and use of donated blood. J Thorac Cardiovasc Surg 107: 807–810

Hedner U, Kisiel W (1983) Use of human Factor VIIa in the treatment of two haemophilia A patients with high titre inhibitors. J Clin Invest 71: 1836–1841

Henry DA, O'Connell DL (1989) Effects of fibrinolytic inhibitors on mortality from upper gastrointestinal haemorrhage. BMJ 298: 1142–1146

Hess JR (1995) Review of modified hemoglobin research at Letterman: attempts to delineate the toxicity of cell-free tetrameric hemoglobin. Artif Cells Blood Substit Immobil Biotechnol 23: 277–289

Hiippala ST, Strid LJ, Wennerstrand MI *et al.* (1997) Tranexamic acid radically decreases blood loss and transfusions associated with total knee arthroplasty. Anesth Analg 84: 839–844

Horstman LL, Valle-Riestra BJ, Jy W *et al.* (1995) Desmopressin (DDAVP) acts on platelets to generate platelet microparticles and enhanced procoagulant activity. Thromb Res 79: 163–174

Huang WY, Kruskall MS, Bauer KA *et al.* (2004) The use of recombinant activated factor VII in three patients with central nervous system hemorrhages associated with factor VII deficiency. Transfusion 44: 1562–1566

Jackson MR (2001) New and potential uses of fibrin sealants as an adjunct to surgical hemostasis. Am J Surg 182: 36S–39S

Johnson WJ, McCarthy JT, Yamagihara TEA (1990) Effects of recombinant human erythropoietin on cerebral and cutaneous blood flow and on blood coagulability. Kidney Int 38: 919–924

Kajitani M, Ozdemir A, Aguinaga M *et al.* (2000) Severe hemorrhagic complication due to acquired factor V inhibitor after single exposure to bovine thrombin product. J Card Surg 15: 378–382

Kaspar M, Ramsay MA, Nguyen AT *et al.* (1997) Continuous small-dose tranexamic acid reduces fibrinolysis but not transfusion requirements during orthotopic liver transplantation. Anesth Analg 85: 281–285

Keipert PE (2003) Oxygen therapeutics ('blood substitutes') where are they, and what can we expect? Adv Exp Med Biol 540: 207–213

Kelemen E, Cserhati I, Tanos B (1958) Demonstration and some properties of human thrombopoietin in thrombocythaemic sera. Acta Haematol 20: 350–355

Kenet G, Walden R, Eldad A *et al.* (1999) Treatment of traumatic bleeding with recombinant factor VIIa. Lancet 354: 1879

Kentro TB, Lottenberg R, Kitchens CS (1987) Clinical efficacy of desmopressin acetate for hemostatic control in patients with primary platelet disorders undergoing surgery. Am J Hematol 24: 215–219

Kickler TS, Spivak JL (1988) Effect of repeated whole blood donations on serum immunoreactive erythropoietin levels in autologous donors. JAMA 260: 65–67

Klein HG (2000) Transfusion safety: avoiding unnecessary bloodshed. Mayo Clin Proc 75: 5–7

Kobrinsky NL, Israels ED, Bickis MG (1991) Synergistic shortening of the bleeding time by desmopressin and ethamsylate in patients with various constitutional bleeding disorders. Am J Pediatr Hematol Oncol 13: 437–441

Kuter DJ, Begley CG (2002) Recombinant human thrombopoietin: basic biology and evaluation of clinical studies. Blood 100: 3457–3469

Kuter DJ, Goodnough LT, Romo J *et al.* (2001) Thrombopoietin therapy increases platelet yields in healthy platelet donors. Blood 98: 1339–1345

LaMuraglia GM, O'Hara PJ, Baker WH *et al.* (2000) The reduction of the allogenic transfusion requirement in aortic surgery with a hemoglobin-based solution. J Vasc Surg 31: 299–308

Lanzkron S, Moliterno AR, Norris EJ *et al.* (2002) Polymerized human Hb use in acute chest syndrome: a case report. Transfusion 42: 1422–1427

Laupacis A, Fergusson D (1997) Drugs to minimize perioperative blood loss in cardiac surgery: meta-analyses using perioperative blood transfusion as the outcome. The International Study of Peri-operative Transfusion (ISPOT) Investigators. Anesth Analg 85: 1258–1267

Lavee J, Raviv Z, Smolinsky A *et al.* (1993) Platelet protection by low-dose aprotinin in cardiopulmonary bypass: electron microscopic study. Ann Thorac Surg 55: 114–119

Leach PZ, Friedman LI, Stromberg RR (1991) Blood cell salvage equipment. In: Autologous Transfusion and Hemotherapy. HF Taswell, AA Pineda (eds), pp. 164–193. Cambridge, MA: Blackwell Scientific Publications

Lee D, Chapman C, Contreras M (1993) Guidelines for autologous transfusion. I. Pre-operative autologous donation. Transfusion Med 3: 307–316

Lemmer JH Jr, Stanford W, Bonney SL *et al.* (1994) Aprotinin for coronary bypass operations: efficacy, safety, and influence on early saphenous vein graft patency. A multi-center, randomized, double-blind, placebo-controlled study. J Thorac Cardiovasc Surg 107: 543–551

Lethaby A, Farquhar C, Cooke I (2000) Antifibrinolytics for heavy menstrual bleeding. Cochrane Database Syst Rev CD000249

Lethagen S, Olofsson L, Frick K et al. (2000) Effect kinetics of desmopressin-induced platelet retention in healthy volunteers treated with aspirin or placebo. Haemophilia 6: 15–20

Levi M, Cromheecke ME, de Jonge E et al. (1999) Pharmacological strategies to decrease excessive blood loss in cardiac surgery: a meta-analysis of clinically relevant endpoints. Lancet 354: 1940–1947

Levi M, Bijsterveld NR, Keller TT (2004) Recombinant factor VIIa as an antidote for anticoagulant treatment. Semin Hematol 41: 65–69

Levy JH, Goodnough LT, Greilich PE et al. (2002) Polymerized bovine hemoglobin solution as a replacement for allogeneic red blood cell transfusion after cardiac surgery: results of a randomized, double-blind trial. J Thorac Cardiovasc Surg 124: 35–42

Li J, Yang C, Xia Y et al. (2001) Thrombocytopenia caused by the development of antibodies to thrombopoietin. Blood 98: 3241–3248

Linden JV, Kruskall MS (1997) Autologous blood: always safer? Transfusion 37: 455–456

Lisman T, Adelmeijer J, Heijnen HF et al. (2004) Recombinant factor VIIa restores aggregation of alphaIIb-beta3-deficient platelets via tissue factor-independent fibrin generation. Blood 103: 1720–1727

Littlewood TJ, Bajetta E, Nortier JW et al. (2001) Effects of epoetin alfa on hematologic parameters and quality of life in cancer patients receiving nonplatinum chemotherapy: results of a randomized, double-blind, placebo-controlled trial. J Clin Oncol 19: 2865–2874

Livio M, Mannucci PM, Vigano G et al. (1986) Conjugated estrogens for the management of bleeding associated with renal failure. N Engl J Med 315: 731–735

Locatelli F, Olivares J, Walker R et al. (2001) Novel erythropoiesis stimulating protein for treatment of anemia in chronic renal insufficiency. Kidney Int 60: 741–747

Lok S, Kaushanski K, Holly RD (1994) Cloning and expression of murine thrombopoietin cDNA and stimulation of platelet production in vivo. Nature (Lond) 369: 565–568

Longstaff C (1994) Studies on the mechanisms of action of aprotinin and tranexamic acid as plasmin inhibitors and antifibrinolytic agents. Blood Coagul Fibrinolysis 5: 537–542

Looker D, Abbott-Brown D, Cozart P et al. (1992) A human recombinant haemoglobin designed for use as a blood substitute. Nature 356: 258–260

MacGregor RD, Hunt CA (1990) Artificial red cells. A link between the membrane skeleton and RES detectability?. Biomater Artif Cells Artif Organs 18: 329–343

McKeown LP, Connaghan G, Wilson O et al. (1996) 1-Desamino-8-arginine-vasopressin corrects the hemostatic defects in type 2B von Willebrand's disease. Am J Hematol 51: 158–163

McVay PA, Hoag RW, Hoag MS (1989) Safety and use of autologous blood donation during the third trimester of pregnancy. Am J Obstet Gynecol 160: 1479–1488

Maffei LM, Thurer RL (1988) Foreword. In: Autologous Blood Transfusion. Current Issues. LM Maffei, RL Thurer (eds), pp. xi–xii. Arlington, VA; Am Assoc Blood Banks

Mahdy AM, Webster NR (2004) Perioperative systemic haemostatic agents. Br J Anaesth 93: 842–858

Maier RF, Obladen M, Muller-Hansen I et al. (2002) Early treatment with erythropoietin beta ameliorates anemia and reduces transfusion requirements in infants with birth weights below 1000 g. J Pediatr 141: 8–15

Makris M, Greaves M, Phillips WS et al. (1997) Emergency oral anticoagulant reversal: the relative efficacy of infusions of fresh frozen plasma and clotting factor concentrate on correction of the coagulopathy. Thromb Haemost 77: 477–480

Mankad PS, Codispoti M (2001) The role of fibrin sealants in hemostasis. Am J Surg 182: 21S–28S

Mann M, Sacks HJ, Goldfinger D (1983) Safety of autologous blood donation prior to elective surgery for a variety of potentially 'high-risk' patients. Transfusion 23: 229–232

Mannucci PM (1986) Desmopressin (DDAVP) for treatment of disorders of hemostasis. Prog Hemost Thromb 8: 19–45

Mannucci PM (1997) Desmopressin (DDAVP) in the treatment of bleeding disorders: the first 20 years. Blood 90: 2515–2521

Mannucci PM (1998) Hemostatic drugs. N Engl J Med 339: 245–253

Mannucci PM (2004) Treatment of von Willebrand's disease. N Engl J Med 351: 683–694

Mannucci PM, Canciani MT, Rota L et al. (1981) Response of factor VIII/von Willebrand factor to DDAVP in healthy subjects and patients with haemophilia A and von Willebrand's disease. Br J Haematol 47: 283–293

Mannucci PM, Remuzzi G, Pusineri F et al. (1983) Deamino-8-D-arginine vasopressin shortens the bleeding time in uremia. N Engl J Med 308: 8–12

Mannucci PM, Vicente V, Vianello L et al. (1986) Controlled trial of desmopressin in liver cirrhosis and other conditions associated with a prolonged bleeding time. Blood 67: 1148–1153

Mannucci PM, Bettega D, Cattaneo M (1992) Patterns of development of tachyphylaxis in patients with haemophilia and von Willebrand disease after repeated doses of desmopressin (DDAVP). Br J Haematol 82: 87–93

Margulies DH (1997) Interactions of TCRs with MHC-peptide complexes: a quantitative basis for mechanistic models. Curr Opin Immunol 9: 390–395

Marone P, Monzillo V, Segu C et al. (1999) Antibiotic-impregnated fibrin glue in ocular surgery: in vitro antibacterial activity. Ophthalmologica 213: 12–15

Martin JW, Whiteside LA, Milliano MT et al. (1992) Postoperative blood retrieval and transfusion in cementless total knee arthroplasty. J Arthroplasty 7: 205–210

Martinowitz U, Kenet G, Segal E et al. (2001) Recombinant activated factor VII for adjunctive hemorrhage control in trauma. J Trauma 51: 431–438

Mayer SA, Brun NC, Begtrup K et al. (2005) Recombinant activated factor VII for acute intracerebral hemorrhage. N Engl J Med 352: 777–785

Mercuriali F, Zanella A, Barosi G et al. (1993) Use of erythropoietin to increase the volume of autologous blood donated by orthopedic patients. Transfusion 33: 55–60

Miller CB, Jones RJ, Piantadosi S (1990) Decreased erythropoietin response in patients with the anemia of cancer. N Engl J Med 322: 1689–1692

Milne AA, Murphy WG, Reading SJ et al. (1996) A randomised trial of fibrin sealant in peripheral vascular surgery. Vox Sang 70: 210–212

Mollison PL, Engelfriet CP, Contreras M (1987) Blood Transfusion in Clinical Medicine, 8th edn. Oxford: Blackwell Scientific Publications

Monk TG, Goodnough LT, Brecher ME et al. (1999) A prospective randomized comparison of three blood conservation strategies for radical prostatectomy. Anesthesiology 91: 24–33

Monroe DM, Hoffman M, Allen GA et al. (2000) The factor VII-platelet interplay: effectiveness of recombinant factor VIIa in the treatment of bleeding in severe thrombocytopathia. Semin Thromb Hemost 26: 373–377

Moss GS, Gould SA, Sehgal LR et al. (1984) Hemoglobin solution – from tetramer to polymer. Surgery 95: 249–255

Mullon J, Giacoppe G, Clagett C et al. (2000) Transfusions of polymerized bovine hemoglobin in a patient with severe autoimmune hemolytic anemia. N Engl J Med 342: 1638–1643

Munoz JJ, Birkmeyer NJ, Birkmeyer JD et al. (1999) Is epsilon-aminocaproic acid as effective as aprotinin in reducing bleeding with cardiac surgery?: a meta-analysis. Circulation 99: 81–89

Murad F, Mittal CK, Arnold WP et al. (1978) Guanylate cyclase: activation by azide, nitro compounds, nitric oxide, and hydroxyl radical and inhibition by hemoglobin and myoglobin. Adv Cyclic Nucleotide Res 9: 145–158

Murkin JM, Haig GM, Beer KJ et al. (2000) Aprotinin decreases exposure to allogeneic blood during primary unilateral total hip replacement. J Bone Joint Surg Am 82: 675–684

Nash RA, Kurzrock R, DiPersio J et al. (2000) A phase I trial of recombinant human thrombopoietin in patients with delayed platelet recovery after hematopoietic stem cell transplantation. Biol Blood Marrow Transplant 6: 25–34

National Blood Data Resource Center (2003) Nationwide Blood Collection and Utilization Survey. Bethesda, MD; Am Assoc Blood Banks

Nee R, Doppenschmidt D, Donovan DJ et al. (1999) Intravenous versus subcutaneous vitamin K1 in reversing excessive oral anticoagulation. Am J Cardiol 83: 286–287

Nervi C, Gamelli RL, Greenhalgh DG et al. (2001) A multicenter clinical trial to evaluate the topical hemostatic efficacy of fibrin sealant in burn patients. J Burn Care Rehabil 22: 99–103

Ness PM, Baldwin ML, Walsh PC (1987) Pre-deposit autologous transfusion in radical retropubic prostatectomy (Abstract). Transfusion 27: 518

Ness PM, Bourke DL, Walsh PC (1992) A randomized trial of perioperative hemodilution versus transfusion of preoperatively deposited autologous blood in elective surgery. Transfusion 32: 226–230

Nieder AM, Simon MA, Kim SS et al. (2004) Intraoperative cell salvage during radical prostatectomy: a safe technique for Jehovah's Witnesses. Int Braz J Urol 30: 377–379

Nilsson IM (1975) Local fibrinolysis as a mechanism for haemorrhage. Thromb Diathesis Haemorrh 34: 623–633

Nilsson IM (1980) Clinical pharmacology of aminocaproic and tranexamic acids. J Clin Pathol Suppl (R Coll Pathol) 14: 41–47

Nomori H, Horio H, Suemasu K (2000) Mixing collagen with fibrin glue to strengthen the sealing effect for pulmonary air leakage. Ann Thorac Surg 70: 1666–1670

Noris P, Arbustini E, Spedini P et al. (1998) A new variant of Bernard-Soulier syndrome characterized by dysfunctional glycoprotein (GP) Ib and severely reduced amounts of GPIX and GPV. Br J Haematol 103: 1004–1013

Nuttall GA, Santrach PJ, Oliver WC Jr et al. (2000) Possible guidelines for autologous red blood cell donations before total hip arthroplasty based on the surgical blood order equation. Mayo Clin Proc 75: 10–17

Ohnishi Y, Kitazawa M (1980) Application of perfluorochemicals in human beings – a morphological report of a human autopsy case with some experimental studies using rabbit. Acta Pathol Jpn 30: 489–504

Osawa T, Nakamura S, Imai T (1992) [Intraoperative blood recovery in transurethral resection of prostate (TURP)]. Nippon Hinyokika Gakkai Zasshi 83: 1276–1283

Oswald AM, Joly LM, Gury C et al. (2003) Fatal intraoperative anaphylaxis related to aprotinin after local application of fibrin glue. Anesthesiology 99: 762–763

Owings DV, Kruskall MS, Thurer RL (1989) Autologous blood donations prior to elective cardiac surgery: safety and effect on subsequent blood use. JAMA 262: 1963–1968

Ozer H, Armitage JO, Bennett CL et al. (2000) 2000 update of recommendations for the use of hematopoietic colony-stimulating factors: evidence-based, clinical practice guidelines. American Society of Clinical Oncology Growth Factors Expert Panel. J Clin Oncol 18: 3558–3585

Payne JW (1973) Polymerization of proteins with glutaraldehyde. Soluble molecular-weight markers. Biochem J 135: 867–873

Peck-Radosavljevic M, Wichlas M, Zacherl J et al. (2000) Thrombopoietin induces rapid resolution of thrombocytopenia after orthotopic liver transplantation through increased platelet production. Blood 95: 795–801

Pincus T, Olsen NJ, Russell IJ et al. (1990) Multicenter study of recombinant human erythropoietin in correction of anemia in rheumatoid arthritis. Am J Med 89: 161–168

Pineda AA, Valbonesi M (1990) Intraoperative blood salvage. In: Blood Transfusion: the Impact of New Technologies. M Contreras (ed.). Baillière's Clincial Haematology 3: 385–403

Poon MC, D'Oiron R, Von Depka M et al. (2004) Prophylactic and therapeutic recombinant factor VIIa administration to patients with Glanzmann's thrombasthenia: results of an international survey. J Thromb Haemost 2: 1096–1103

Popovsky MA, Whitaker B, Arnold NL (1995) Severe outcomes of allogeneic and autologous blood donation: frequency and characterization. Transfusion 35: 734–737

Porte RJ, Leebeek FW (2002) Pharmacological strategies to decrease transfusion requirements in patients undergoing surgery. Drugs 62: 2193–2211

Pozo AI, Jimenez-Yuste V, Villar A et al. (2002) Successful thyroidectomy in a patient with Hermansky-Pudlak syndrome treated with recombinant activated factor VII and platelet concentrates. Blood Coagul Fibrinolysis 13: 551–553

Prendergast TW, Furukawa S, Beyer AJ III et al. (1996) Defining the role of aprotinin in heart transplantation. Ann Thorac Surg 62: 670–674

Price TH, Goodnough LT, Vogler WR et al. (1996) Improving the efficacy of preoperative autologous blood donation in patients with low hematocrit: a randomized, double-blind, controlled trial of recombinant human erythropoietin. Am J Med 101: 22S–27S

Rabiner SF, O'Brien K, Peskin GW (1970) Further studies with stroma-free hemoglobin solution. Ann Surg 171: 615

Radosevich M, Goubran HI, Burnouf T (1997) Fibrin sealant: scientific rationale, production methods, properties, and current clinical use. Vox Sang 72: 133–143

Raj G, Kumar R, McKinney WP (1999) Time course of reversal of anticoagulant effect of warfarin by intravenous and subcutaneous phytonadione. Arch Intern Med 159: 2721–2724

Rao AK, Ghosh S, Sun L et al. (1995) Mechanisms of platelet dysfunction and response to DDAVP in patients with congenital platelet function defects. A double-blind placebo-controlled trial. J Thromb Haemost 74: 1071–1078

Rapaport SI, Zivelin A, Minow RA et al. (1992) Clinical significance of antibodies to bovine and human thrombin and factor V after surgical use of bovine thrombin. Am J Clin Pathol 97: 84–91

Ray MJ, Marsh NA (1997) Aprotinin reduces blood loss after cardiopulmonary bypass by direct inhibition of plasmin. J Thromb Haemost 78: 1021–1026

Reddy P, Song J (2003) Cost comparisons in open-heart surgery. Pharmacoeconomics 21: 249–262

Reiter RA, Mayr F, Blazicek H et al. (2003) Desmopressin antagonizes the in vitro platelet dysfunction induced by GPIIb/IIIa inhibitors and aspirin. Blood 102: 4594–4599

Rich EC, Drage CW (1982) Severe complications of intravenous phytonadione therapy. Two cases, with one fatality. Postgrad Med 72: 303–306

Richardson DW, Robinson AG (1985) Desmopressin. Ann Intern Med 103: 228–239

Ritter MA, Keating EM, Faris PM (1994) Closed wound drainage in total hip or total knee replacement. A prospective, randomized study. J Bone Joint Surg Am 76: 35–38

Romero-Castro R, Jimenez-Saenz M, Pellicer-Bautista F et al. (2004) Recombinant-activated factor VII as hemostatic therapy in eight cases of severe hemorrhage from esophageal varices. Clin Gastroenterol Hepatol 2: 78–84

Roos YB, Rinkel GJ, Vermeulen M et al. (2003) Antifibrinolytic therapy for aneurysmal subarachnoid haemorrhage. Cochrane Database Syst Rev CD001245

Rosse WF, Nishimura J (2003) Clinical manifestations of paroxysmal nocturnal hemoglobinuria: present state and future problems. Int J Hematol 77: 113–120

Rother RP, Bell L, Hillmen P et al. (2005) The clinical sequelae of intravascular hemolysis and extracellular plasma hemoglobin: a novel mechanism of human disease. JAMA 293: 1653–1662

Royston D, Bidstrup BP, Taylor KM et al. (1987) Effect of aprotinin on need for blood transfusion after repeat open-heart surgery. Lancet 2: 1289–1291

Sachs UJ, Bux J (2003) TRALI after the transfusion of cross-match-positive granulocytes. Transfusion 43: 1683–1686

Samama CM, Langeron O, Rosencher N et al. (2002) Aprotinin versus placebo in major orthopedic surgery: a randomized, double-blinded, dose-ranging study. Anesth Analg 95: 287–293

Savitsky JP, Doczi J, Black J (1978) A clinical safety trial of stroma-free hemoglobin. Clin Pharmacol Ther 23: 73–80

Saxena R, Wijnhoud AD, Carton H et al. (1999) Controlled safety study of a hemoglobin-based oxygen carrier, DCLHb, in acute ischemic stroke. Stroke 30: 993–996

Schaff HV, Hauer J, Gardner TJ *et al.* (1979) Routine use of autotransfusion following cardiac surgery: experience in 700 patients. Ann Thorac Surg 27: 493–499

Scheding S, Bergmann M, Shimosaka A *et al.* (2002) Human plasma thrombopoietin levels are regulated by binding to platelet thrombopoietin receptors *in vivo*. Transfusion 42: 321–327

Scheule AM, Jurmann MJ, Wendel HP *et al.* (1997) Anaphylactic shock after aprotinin reexposure: time course of aprotinin-specific antibodies. Ann Thorac Surg 63: 242–244

Scheule AM, Beierlein W, Lorenz H *et al.* (1998) Repeated anaphylactic reactions to aprotinin in fibrin sealant. Gastrointest Endosc 48: 83–85

Schiffer CA, Miller K, Larson RA *et al.* (2000) A double-blind, placebo-controlled trial of pegylated recombinant human megakaryocyte growth and development factor as an adjunct to induction and consolidation therapy for patients with acute myeloid leukemia. Blood 95: 2530–2535

Schlag G, Redl H (1988) Fibrin sealant in orthopedic surgery. Clin Orthop 227: 269–285

Schmidt ML, Gamerman S, Smith HE *et al.* (1994) Recombinant activated factor VII (rFVIIa) therapy for intracranial hemorrhage in hemophilia A patients with inhibitors. Am J Hematol 47: 36–40

Schulman S (2003) Clinical practice. Care of patients receiving long-term anticoagulant therapy. N Engl J Med 349: 675–683

Schulman S, Johnsson H, Egberg N *et al.* (1987) DDAVP-induced correction of prolonged bleeding time in patients with congenital platelet function defects. Thromb Res 45: 165–174

Schultz M, van der Lelie H (1995) Microscopic haematuria as a relative contraindication for tranexamic acid. Br J Haematol 89: 663–664

Schultz SC, Grady B, Cole F (1993) A role for endothelin and nitric oxide in the pressor response to diaspirin cross-linked hemoglobin. J Lab Clin Med 122: 301–308

Schurgers LJ, Shearer MJ, Hamulyak K *et al.* (2004) Effect of vitamin K intake on the stability of oral anticoagulant treatment: dose-response relationships in healthy subjects. Blood 104: 2682–2689

von Segesser LK, Fasnacht MS, Vogt PR *et al.* (1995) Prevention of residual ventricular septal defects with fibrin sealant. Ann Thorac Surg 60: 511–515

Seymour BD, Rubinger M (1997) Rhabdomyolysis induced by epsilon-aminocaproic acid. Ann Pharmacother 31: 56–58

Shemin D, Elnour M, Amarantes B *et al.* (1990) Oral estrogens decrease bleeding time and improve clinical bleeding in patients with renal failure. Am J Med 89: 436–440

Sheridan DP, Card RT, Pinilla JC *et al.* (1994) Use of desmopressin acetate to reduce blood transfusion requirements during cardiac surgery in patients with acetylsalicylic-acid-induced platelet dysfunction. Can J Surg 37: 33–36

Shigeta O, Kojima H, Jikuya T *et al.* (1997) Aprotinin inhibits plasmin-induced platelet activation during cardiopulmonary bypass. Circulation 96: 569–574

Shpilberg O, Blumenthal R, Sofer O *et al.* (1995) A controlled trial of tranexamic acid therapy for the reduction of bleeding during treatment of acute myeloid leukemia. Leuk Lymphoma 19: 141–144

Silvergleid AJ (1987) Safety and effectiveness of predeposit autologous transfusion in preteen and adolescent children. JAMA 257: 3403–3404

Silvergleid AJ (1991) Preoperative autologous donation: what have we learned? (Editorial). Transfusion 31: 99–101

Sindet-Pedersen S, Ramstrom G, Bernvil S *et al.* (1989) Hemostatic effect of tranexamic acid mouthwash in anticoagulant-treated patients undergoing oral surgery. N Engl J Med 320: 840–843

Singh I, Laungani GB (1992) Intravesical epsilon aminocaproic acid in management of intractable bladder hemorrhage. Urology 40: 227–229

Sisk JE, Gianfrancesco FD, Coster JM (1991) Recombinant erythropoietin and medicare payment. JAMA 266: 247–249

Sloan EP, Koenigsberg M, Gens D *et al.* (1999) Diaspirin cross-linked hemoglobin (DCLHb) in the treatment of severe traumatic hemorrhagic shock: a randomized controlled efficacy trial. JAMA 282: 1857–1864

Sloand JA, Schiff MJ (1995) Beneficial effect of low-dose transdermal estrogen on bleeding time and clinical bleeding in uremia. Am J Kidney Dis 26: 22–26

Sloand EM, Kessler CM, McIntosh CL *et al.* (1989) Methylene blue for neutralization of heparin. Thromb Res 54: 677–686

Sloand EM, Alyono D, Klein HG *et al.* (1994) 1-Deamino-8-D-arginine vasopressin (DDAVP) increases platelet membrane expression of glycoprotein Ib in patients with disorders of platelet function and after cardiopulmonary bypass. Am J Hematol 46: 199–207

Smith CR (1998) Management of bleeding complications in redo cardiac operations. Ann Thorac Surg 65: S2–S8

Soedirman JR, De Bruijn EA, Maes RA *et al.* (1996) Pharmacokinetics and tolerance of intravenous and intramuscular phylloquinone (vitamin K1) mixed micelles formulation. Br J Clin Pharmacol 41: 517–523

Spahn DR, van Brempt R, Theilmeier G *et al.* (1999) Perflubron emulsion delays blood transfusions in orthopedic surgery. European Perflubron Emulsion Study Group. Anesthesiology 91: 1195–1208

Spahn DR, Waschke KF, Standl T *et al.* (2002) Use of perflubron emulsion to decrease allogeneic blood transfusion in high-blood-loss non-cardiac surgery: results of a European phase 3 study. Anesthesiology 97: 1338–1349

Spivak JL (1993) The clinical physiology of erythropoietin. Semin Hematol 30: 2–11

Spivak JL (2001) Erythropoietin use and abuse: When physiology and pharmacology collide. Adv Exp Med Biol 502: 207–224

Spivak JL, Barnes PC, Fuchs E (1989) Serum immunoreactive erythropoietin in HIV-infected patients. JAMA 261: 3104–3107

Spotnitz WD, Dalton MS, Baker JW et al. (1987) Reduction of perioperative hemorrhage by anterior mediastinal spray application of fibrin glue during cardiac operations. Ann Thorac Surg 44: 529–531

Starkey JM, MacPherson JL, Bolgiano DC (1989) Markers for transfusion-transmitted disease in different groups of blood donors. JAMA 262: 3452–3454

Steegmann JL, Lopez J, Otero MJ et al. (1992) Erythropoietin treatment in allogeneic BMT accelerates erythroid reconstitution: results of a prospective controlled randomized trial. Bone Marrow Transplant 10: 541–546

Stowell CP, Levin J, Spiess BD et al. (2001) Progress in the development of RBC substitutes. Transfusion 41: 287–299

Streiff MB, Ness PM (2002) Acquired FV inhibitors: a needless iatrogenic complication of bovine thrombin exposure. Transfusion 42: 18–26

Sutor AH (2000) DDAVP is not a panacea for children with bleeding disorders. Br J Haematol 108: 217–227

Takeuchi M, Nagura H, Kaneda T (1988) DDAVP and epinephrine-induced changes in the localization of von Willebrand factor antigen in endothelial cells of human oral mucosa. Blood 72: 850–854

Tanaka KA, Waly AA, Cooper WA et al. (2003) Treatment of excessive bleeding in Jehovah's Witness patients after cardiac surgery with recombinant factor VIIa (NovoSeven). Anesthesiology 98: 1513–1515

Tawes RL, Sydorak GR, DuVall TB (1994) Postoperative salvage: A technological advance in the 'washed' versus 'unwashed' blood controversy. Semin Vasc Surg 7: 98–103

Taylor CT, Chester EA, Byrd DC et al. (1999) Vitamin K to reverse excessive anticoagulation: a review of the literature. Pharmacotherapy 19: 1415–1425

Thomas MJ (1999) Infected and malignant fields are an absolute contraindication to intraoperative cell salvage: fact or fiction? Transfusion Med 9: 269–278

Thomas MJ, Gillon J, Desmond MJ (1996) Consensus conference on autologous transfusion. Preoperative autologous donation. Transfusion 36: 633–639

Toy PT, Strauss RG, Stehling LC et al. (1987) Predeposited autologous blood for elective surgery. A national multicenter study. N Engl J Med 316: 517–520

Tranholm M, Rojkjaer R, Pyke C et al. (2003) Recombinant factor VIIa reduces bleeding in severely thrombocytopenic rabbits. Thromb Res 109: 217–223

Tsai HM, Sussman II, Nagel RL et al. (1990) Desmopressin induces adhesion of normal human erythrocytes to the endothelial surface of a perfused microvascular preparation. Blood 75: 261–265

Urdaneta F, Lobato EB, Kirby RR et al. (1999) Non-cardiogenic pulmonary edema associated with protamine administration during coronary artery bypass graft surgery. J Clin Anesth 11: 675–681

Vadhan-Raj S, Murray LJ, Bueso-Ramos C et al. (1997) Stimulation of megakaryocyte and platelet production by a single dose of recombinant human thrombopoietin in patients with cancer. Ann Intern Med 126: 673–681

Vadhan-Raj S, Verschraegen CF, Bueso-Ramos C et al. (2000) Recombinant human thrombopoietin attenuates carboplatin-induced severe thrombocytopenia and the need for platelet transfusions in patients with gynecologic cancer. Ann Intern Med 132: 364–368

van der Meer J, Hemker HC, Loeliger EA (1968) Pharmacological aspects of vitamin K1. A clinical and experimental study in man. Thromb Diath Haemorrh 29 (Suppl.): 1–96

Vandegriff KD (1992) Blood substitutes: engineering the haemoglobin molecule. Biotechnol Genet Eng Rev 10: 403–453

Vercellotti GM, Hammerschmidt DE, Craddock PR et al. (1982) Activation of plasma complement by perfluorocarbon artificial blood: probable mechanism of adverse pulmonary reactions in treated patients and rationale for corticosteroids prophylaxis. Blood 59: 1299–1304

Vermeer C, Schurgers LJ (2000) A comprehensive review of vitamin K and vitamin K antagonists. Hematol Oncol Clin North Am 14: 339–353

Verstraete M (1985) Clinical application of inhibitors of fibrinolysis. Drugs 29: 236–261

Verstraete M, Vermylen J, Tyberghein J (1968) Double blind evaluation of the haemostatic effect of adrenochrome monosemicarbazone, conjugated oestrogens and epsilon-aminocaproic acid after adenotonsillectomy. Acta Haematol 40: 154–161

Viaro F, Dalio MB, Evora PR (2002) Catastrophic cardiovascular adverse reactions to protamine are nitric oxide/cyclic guanosine monophosphate dependent and endothelium mediated: should methylene blue be the treatment of choice? Chest 122: 1061–1066

Vidarsson B, Onundarson PT (2000) Recombinant factor VIIa for bleeding in refractory thrombocytopenia. J Thromb Haemost 83: 634–635

Vigano G, Gaspari F, Locatelli M et al. (1988) Dose-effect and pharmacokinetics of estrogens given to correct bleeding time in uremia. Kidney Int 34: 853–858

Villar A, Aronis S, Morfini M et al. (2004) Pharmacokinetics of activated recombinant coagulation factor VII (NovoSeven) in children vs. adults with haemophilia A. Haemophilia 10: 352–359

Vlahakes GJ, Lee R, Jacobs EE Jr *et al.* (1990) Hemodynamic effects and oxygen transport properties of a new blood substitute in a model of massive blood replacement. J Thorac Cardiovasc Surg 100: 379–388

Vredenburgh JJ, Hussein A, Fisher D *et al.* (1998) A randomized trial of recombinant human interleukin-11 following autologous bone marrow transplantation with peripheral blood progenitor cell support in patients with breast cancer. Biol Blood Marrow Transplant 4: 134–141

Wakefield TW, Hantler CB, Wrobleski SK *et al.* (1996) Effects of differing rates of protamine reversal of heparin anticoagulation. Surgery 119: 123–128

Walsh PN, Rizza CR, Matthews JM *et al.* (1971) Epsilon-Aminocaproic acid therapy for dental extractions in haemophilia and Christmas disease: a double blind controlled trial. Br J Haematol 20: 463–475

Walsh PN, Rizza CR, Evans BE *et al.* (1975) The therapeutic role of epsilon-aminocaproic acid (EACA) for dental extractions in hemophiliacs. Ann NY Acad Sci 240: 267–276

Waner M (2004) Novel hemostatic alternatives in reconstructive surgery. Semin Hematol 41: 163–167

Ward HB, Smith RR, Landis KP *et al.* (1993) Prospective, randomized trial of autotransfusion after routine cardiac operations. Ann Thorac Surg 56: 137–141

Warkentin TE, Crowther MA (2002) Reversing anticoagulants both old and new. Can J Anaesth 49: S11–S25

Weiskopf RB, Viele MK, Feiner J *et al.* (1998) Human cardiovascular and metabolic response to acute, severe isovolemic anemia. JAMA 279: 217–221

Weitzel JN, Sadowski JA, Furie BC *et al.* (1990) Surreptitious ingestion of a long-acting vitamin K antagonist/rodenticide, brodifacoum: clinical and metabolic studies of three cases. Blood 76: 2555–2559

Williams EC (1989) Plasma alpha 2-antiplasmin activity. Role in the evaluation and management of fibrinolytic states and other bleeding disorders. Arch Intern Med 149: 1769–1772

Williamson KR, Taswell HF (1991) Intraoperative blood salvage. In: Autologous Transfusion and Hemotherapy. HF Taswell (ed.), pp. 122–154. Cambridge, MA; AA Pineda Blackwell Scientific Publications

Wilson SE, Watson HG, Crowther MA (2004) Low-dose oral vitamin K therapy for the management of asymptomatic patients with elevated international normalized ratios: a brief review. Can Med Assoc J 170: 821–824

Winearls CG, Oliver DO, Pippard MM (1986) Effect of human erythropoietin derived from recombinant DNA on the anaemia of patients maintained by chronic haemodialysis. Lancet ii: 1175–1178

Winslow RM (2003) Current status of blood substitute research: towards a new paradigm. J Intern Med 253: 508–517

Winslow RM (2004) MP4, a new nonvasoactive polyethylene glycol-hemoglobin conjugate. Artif Organs 28: 800–806

Wun T, Paglieroni TG, Lachant NA (1995) Desmopressin stimulates the expression of P-selectin on human platelets *in vitro*. J Lab Clin Med 126: 401–409

Appendices

Appendix 1
Preparation of platelet concentrates

From platelet-rich plasma

The following method yields $0.72 \pm 0.3 \times 10^{11}$ platelets per concentrate with minimal lymphocyte and granulocyte contamination ($0.032 \pm 0.02 \times 10^9$ and $0.009 \pm 0.004 \times 10^9$ cells respectively): blood is collected into standard multi-unit (triple) bags containing the volume of CPD-A. The bags are centrifuged at $1600\,g$ for 3 min; the platelet-rich plasma (PRP) is transferred into a plastic satellite bag (PL-146 for 3 days' storage or PL-732 for 5–7 days' storage) and is centrifuged at $1850\,g$ for 7 min; the platelet-poor plasma is transferred to the third satellite bag and frozen for issue as fresh-frozen plasma (FFP), leaving 50 ml of residual plasma with the platelets. The platelet concentrate is left undisturbed for 1 h to allow the platelets to disaggregate spontaneously. The platelet pellet is then resuspended in the 50 ml of residual plasma by gentle manual agitation. The unit of blood is kept at room temperature from the time of collection onwards and all procedures are carried out at room temperature. Constant gentle mixing is essential to maintain viability of platelets stored at 22°C (Slichter and Harker 1976).

From buffy coat

The following method yields $79 \pm 8\%$ of the platelets, with a leucocyte count in the concentrate of $13 \pm 7 \times 10^6$; blood is taken into the collecting bag of a quadruple blood bag system (e.g. Terumo, Baxter,

NPBI) with CPD as an anticoagulant. The bag is then stored in such a way in a 'cooling unit' containing butane-1,4-diol that the collecting bag is in contact with the unit. The temperature of the blood is reduced to 22°C in 2 h. After a variable period of storage at 22°C, the blood is centrifuged for 10 min at 3600 r.p.m. in a Beckman JFM centrifuge with the shielded six-place JS 4.2 rotor. The plasma is pressed into an empty satellite bag and the buffy coat into the 300-ml bag, which is the second in the row of four. The saline–adenine–glucose mannitol (SAG-M) solution in the fourth bag is then added to the red cells and 30 ml of plasma is returned to the bag containing the buffy coat. The bags with the red cells and the plasma are then detached. The buffy coat is mixed gently with the plasma and once more centrifuged at 22°C for 6 min at 1250 r.p.m. The PRP is then slowly transferred to the bag that originally contained the SAG-M solution. Inserts can be made in the oval cups of the Beckman JGM centrifuge so that four sets of bags can be centrifuged per cup (Pietersz et al. 1987).

In a modification of this method, part of the plasma in which the platelets are stored is replaced by a platelet additive solution (PAS), containing 70.0 mmol/l, KCl 10.0 mmol, $Na_2HPO_4 . 2H_2O$ 5.0 mmol/l, Na_3 citrate. $2H_2O$ 30.0 mmol/l, D-mannitol 30.0 mmol/l; for further details, see the work of Eriksson and co-workers (1993).

Sterile connecting devices make it possible to pool four buffy coats with the plasma from only one of the donations, yielding a product with a better yield of platelets ($3–4 \times 10^{11}$) and significantly fewer white cells.

Using automated instrumentation

The following method yields buffy coat platelets containing 91.7×10^9 platelets and 2.8×10^9 leucocytes in 55 ml (van Rhenen *et al.* 1998). Then, 500 ± 50 ml of blood is collected into a primary 'bottom-and-top' container filled with 70 ml of CPD anticoagulant–preservative solution, a secondary conventional container filled with 110 ml of SAG-M solution and an empty transfer bag (Optipac®, Baxter, La Châtre, France). Blood units are cooled (see above) to 20 ± 2 °C and stored overnight at room temperature (20 ± 2 °C) before being centrifuged at high speed (4657 g) for 10 min. The automated blood cell processing device (Optipress, Baxter) is set for the primary separation for buffy coat volume: 55 ml, buffy coat level: 6.7, pressplate force: 25 kg. The instrument may be set for the secondary separation of platelets from pooled buffy coats using the following parameters: time: 5 min, sensitivity: 40, red cell level (RCL): 40, pressplate force: 8 kg. A volume of 300 ml of acetate containing additive solution (PAS II) is added to the pool containing the equivalent of five buffy coats.

Buffy coat platelets containing 90% of the platelets of whole blood in 40 ml can be prepared as follows (Li *et al.* 2004): whole blood units are collected into bottom-and-top bags (Compoflex; Fresenius Hemocare, Emmer-Compascuum, the Netherlands) and stored at 22°C between collection and processing using butane-diol cooling plates (see above). After centrifugation (3000 g, 9 min), the buffy coat is separated from the plasma and red cells using the automatic Compomat G4 separator (Fresenius Hemocare). The instrument may be set for the secondary separation of platelets from five pooled buffy coats (each with a volume of 40 ml) and dilution with 300 ml of autologous plasma, by a further centrifugation (900 g, 5 min), followed by PC extraction using the Compomat separation. The final BCPC component can be leucoreduced by gravity filtration (Imuguard III-PL filters, Terumo, Somerset, NJ, USA) and transferred to a 1-L ELP™ bag (Extended Life Platelet; Gambro BCT, Lakewood, CO, USA).

References

Eriksson L. (1995) Platelet concentrates in an addictive solution prepared from pooled buffy coats. Vox Sang 64: 133–138

Li J, de Korte D, Woolum MD *et al.* (2004) Pathogen reduction of buffy coat platelet concentrates using riboflavin and light. Vox Sang 87: 82–90

Pietersz RNI, Reesink HW, Dekker WJA (1987) Preparation of leucocyte poor platelet concentrates from buffy coats. Vox Sang 53: 203–208

van Rhenen DJ, Vermeij J, de Voogt J *et al.* (1998) Quality and standardization in blood component preparation with an automated blood processing technique. Transfus Med 8: 319–324

Slichter SJ, Harker LA (1976) Preparation and storage of platelet concentrates. Transfusion 16: 8–12

Appendix 2
Estimation of red cell volume, using ^{99m}Tc, ^{111}In and ^{51}Cr

Although ^{51}Cr has by far the lowest rate of elution from red cells, ^{99m}Tc and ^{111}In should be used in preference for estimating red cell volume: first, because of their far lower radiotoxicity and, second, because the rate of elution is not of great importance when samples are being taken over a period of less than 1 h after injecting labelled red cells.

Labelling with ^{99m}Tc

^{99m}Tc-pertechnetate is obtained from a molybdenum generator; ^{99m}Tc has a $T_{1/2}$ of 6.0 h but ^{99}Mo (the generator) has a $T_{1/2}$ of 72 h. Pertechnetate will not bind firmly to red cells (actually, to Hb) unless it is first reduced; labelling is accomplished by first treating the cells with a very small amount of a stannous compound and then incubating the cells with ^{99m}Tc-pertechnetate. In 5 min at room temperature, red cells take up approximately 95% of the added ^{99m}Tc (Smith and Richards 1976). The optimal amount of Sn (as $SnCl_2$) to use with heparinized red cells is 0.02 µg per millilitre of red cells (Jones and Mollison 1978). This amount can conveniently be added using commercially available vials (Technescan PYP, supplied by Amersham International). These vials contain 3.4 mg of $SnCl_2$ (with pyrophosphate) in 5 ml of saline; 1 ml of the solution is added to 500 ml of saline; addition of 0.1 ml of the diluted solution to red cells from 10 ml of heparinized blood gives the required ratio of tin to red cells. The red cells should be washed once in saline before being incubated for 5 min with the tin.

Red cells that have been treated with tin are incubated at room temperature with 25 µCi (0.9 mBq) of ^{99m}Tc, then washed once in saline before being made up to a convenient volume (e.g. 20 ml) for injection. They should be kept on ice until injected (for further details, see Jones and Mollison 1978; ICSH 1980).

The loss of ^{99m}Tc from the red cells during the 60 min after re-injection into the circulation has been found to be about 4% (Smith and Richards 1976; Jones and Mollison 1978); variable loss rates have been reported in the first 24 h, for example about 50% (Atkins et al. 1985), 33% (Holt et al. 1983) and about 23% as judged by the ratio of ^{99m}Tc to ^{51}Cr in surviving red cells (Marcus et al. 1987).

Labelling with ^{111}In

^{111}In has a $T_{1/2}$ of 2.8 days. For red cell labelling a chelating agent must be used: oxine, acetylacetone and tropolone have been found to be equally suitable (AuBuchon and Brightman 1989). In 11 subjects in whom red cells were labelled using oxine on one occasion and tropolone on another, with both methods uptake exceeded 96%; during the first 15 min after injection of the labelled cells, there was a loss of 3–4% of the label but there was no further loss at 60 min; loss in the first 24 h was 10–13%.

Labelling with ^{51}Cr

Radioactive chromium is obtained as sodium chromate (Na$_2$^{51}CrO$_4$) with a specific activity that may be as high as 200 μCi (7.4 mBq)/μg Cr. It is convenient to dilute the stock in 9 g/l sodium chloride solution and then to put suitable amounts into ampoules that are sealed and autoclaved. ^{51}Cr has a half-life of 27.7 days and if the ampoules are to be used over a period of several weeks the amounts placed in them must be increased to take account of this. For the estimation of red cell volume, the amount of ^{51}Cr added should be such that the patient receives no more than 0.2 μCi (7.4 kBq)/kg. The amount of ^{51}Cr actually added to the red cells must be greater than this by about 25%, as only about 90–95% of the ^{51}Cr will be taken up by the red cells and part of the final suspension must be retained as a standard.

The added Na$_2$^{51}CrO$_4$ should be in a volume of at least 0.2 ml. The amount of red cells labelled should be such that the dose of chromium does not exceed 2 μg/ml of red cells.

When Na$_2$^{51}CrO$_4$ is added to blood, the rate of uptake by the red cells is more rapid at pH 6.8–7.0 than at physiological pH, is approximately three times more rapid at 37°C than at 22°C and is more rapid when the ^{51}Cr is added to packed red cells than when it is added to the same red cells suspended in their own plasma (Mollison and Veall 1955). In practice, if the ^{51}Cr is added to packed red cells from ACD blood, uptake will exceed 90% after 15 min at room temperature.

Obtain blood by venepuncture and add 10 ml to 1.5 ml of ACD A (see Appendix 10). Centrifuge the citrated blood at 1000–1500 g for 5–10 min. Remove and discard the supernatant plasma, taking care not to remove any red cells. However, if the leucocyte count is greater than 25×10^9/l, also remove and discard the buffy coat. Add the ^{51}Cr sodium chromate solution slowly and with continuous gentle mixing to the packed red cells. Allow the mixture to stand at room temperature for 15 min or place it in a waterbath at 37°C for 10 min. Wash the labelled cells twice in four to five volumes of isotonic saline.

Standards

A volume (e.g. 3 ml) of the washed, labelled red cell suspension should be set aside for the preparation of standards, one in 100 dilutions are suitable and should be prepared in duplicate.

Injection of labelled red cells

Several methods of injecting a known amount of cells can be used. For example, a precalibrated syringe, known to deliver a certain volume, can be used. Alternatively, the syringe can be weighed before and after injection and the exact volume injected can be calculated as:

weight of suspension/specific gravity of suspension

Assuming that packed red cells have an Hb concentration of 34 g/dl and a specific gravity of 1.097, the specific gravity of the suspension can be deduced from the Hb concentration of the suspension as:

$$1.0 + \frac{\left[\begin{array}{c}\text{(Hb concentration of}\\ \text{suspension in g/dl)}\end{array} \times (1.097 - 1.000)\right]}{34 \text{ g/dl}}$$

(A2.1)

Blood samples

Normally, a blood sample should be taken about 10 min after injection, but when it is suspected that mixing will not be complete in 10 min, as, for example, in a patient with gross splenomegaly, the sample should be taken at 60 min instead. Corrections to apply for elution of ^{99m}Tc and ^{111}In can be deduced from data given above; with ^{51}Cr, no correction is necessary, as the loss in the first 60 min is not more than 0.5% (Mollison 1961).

The packed cell volume (PCV) of the 10- or 60-min sample is determined in duplicate and duplicate volumes (e.g. 2 ml) are pipetted into vials, together with duplicate volumes of each of two dilutions of the standard. Saponin is added to each vial and the samples are counted in a gamma counter; when possible, 10 000 counts are recorded for each sample.

In determining the PCV, the spun haematocrit, applying appropriate corrections for trapped plasma (Chaplin and Mollison 1952), remains the most accurate method (ICSH Expert Panel on Blood Cell Sizing 1980).

For further details of estimating red cell volume (RCV), see ICSH (1980).

Formula for estimating red cell volume

$$\text{RCV (ml)} = \frac{\text{total counts injected}}{\text{counts per millilitre of red cells at time zero}} \quad \text{(A2.2)}$$

For example, suppose a 1 in 100 dilution of the injection suspension has a counting rate of 1100 per min and 20 ml of suspension have been injected, so that the total counts injected = $20 \times 100 \times 1100$, or 2.2×10^6/min, and that a blood sample taken 10 min after injection has a PCV of 0.45 (after correction for trapped plasma) and a counting rate of 460/min, so that counts/min/ml at zero time are:

$$\left(460 \times \frac{100}{45}\right) \times \frac{100}{98.5}, \quad \text{or } 1.04 \times 10^3 \quad \text{(A2.3)}$$

then

$$\text{RCV} = \frac{2.2 \times 10^6}{1.04 \times 10^3} = 2100 \text{ ml} \quad \text{(A2.4)}$$

References

Atkins AL, Srivastava HC, Meinken GE (1985) Biological behaviour of erythrocytes labelled in vivo and in vitro with technetium-99m. J Nucl Med Technol 13: 136–139

AuBuchon JP, Brightman A (1989) Use of Indium-III as a red cell label. Transfusion 29: 143–147

Chaplin H Jr, Mollison PL (1952) Correction for plasma trapped in the red cell column of the hematocrit, Blood 7: 1227

Holt JT, Spitealnik SL, McMican AE (1983) A technetium-99m red cell survival technique for in vivo compatibility testing. Transfusion 23: 148–151

ICSH (1980) Recommended methods for measurement of red-cell and plasma volume. J Nucl Med 21: 793–800

ICSH Expert Panel on Blood Cell Sizing (1980) Recommendation for reference method for determination by centrifugation of packed cell volume of blood. J Clin Pathol 33: 1–2

Jones J, Mollison PL (1978) A simple and efficient method of labelling red cells with 99mTc for determination of red cell volume. Br J Haematol 38: 141

Marcus CS, Mythre BA, Angulo MC (1987) Radiolabelled red cell viability I, Comparison of 51Cr, 99mTc, and 111In for measuring the viability of autologue stored red cells. Transfusion 27: 415–419

Mollison PL (1961) Further observations on the normal survival curve of ^{51}Cr-labelled red cells. Clin Sci 21: 21

Mollison PL, Veal N (1955) The use of isotope ^{51}Cr as a label for red cells. Br J Haematol 1: 62

Smith TD, Richards P (1976) A simple kit for the preparation of 99mTc-labelled red blood cells. J Nucl Med 17: 126

Appendix 3
Estimation of plasma volume

Use of ^{125}I-labelled albumin

In preparing a dilution of 'stock' ^{125}I-albumin for injection it is best to add the labelled albumin to a few millilitres (e.g. 7 ml) of heparinized plasma obtained from the subject whose plasma volume is to be estimated. Dilution of labelled albumin in a large volume of saline should be avoided, as there would then be a risk of loss of protein by adsorption on to glass surfaces. However, the mixture of labelled albumin and plasma can be diluted with saline to a convenient volume such as 25 ml, of which 20 ml can be injected into an arm vein.

In diluting an aliquot of the injection solution for counting as a standard, the injection solution may either be diluted in saline to which bovine albumin has been added to give a final concentration of at least 0.05% or alternatively may be diluted in saline containing 1% detergent to prevent the adsorption of protein on to glass.

Following injection of the labelled albumin, blood samples should be taken at 10, 20 and 30 min; the concentration of the label at zero time is determined by extrapolating a line fitted to the points (ICSH 1980). Plasma volume is given by the expression: total c.p.m. injected (i.e. c.p.m./ml of standard × dilution of standard × volume of labelled albumin injected) divided by c.p.m./ml of recipient's plasma at zero time. There is evidence that in a wide variety of disease states, measurements with labelled albumin overestimate blood volume, presumably due to extra loss of albumin from the circulation (Strumia *et al.* 1968; Valeri *et al.* 1973).

References

ICSH (1980) Recommended methods for radioisotope red-cell survival studies. Br J Haemat 45: 659–666

Strumia MM, Strumia PV, Dugan A (1968) Significance of measurement of plasma volume and of indirect estimation of red cell volume. Transfusion 8: 197

Valeri CR, Cooper AG, Pivacek LE (1973) Limitations of measuring blood volume with iodinated I^{125} serum albumin. Arch Intern Med 132: 534

Appendix 4
Derivation of blood volume from red cell volume or plasma volume

If the haematocrit (PCV) of blood in peripheral veins (H_v) were representative of the blood in the whole circulation, blood volume could be derived from RCV as $RCV \times 1/H_v$ and from plasma volume (PV) as $PV \times 1/(1 - H_v)$. In fact, the haematocrit of blood in the whole body, H_B, is lower than H_v, the ratio H_B/H_v being about 0.91 (Chaplin *et al.* 1953). Accordingly, $BV = RCV \times 1/(H_v \times 0.91)$ or $PV \times 1/(1 - [H_v \times 0.91])$.

In subjects with splenomegaly, the ratio H_B/H_v is increased and may exceed 1.1 (Fudenberg *et al.* 1961). For other references, see eighth edition.

References

Chaplin H Jr, Mollison PL, Vetter H (1953) The body/venous hematocrit ratio: its constancy over a wide hematocrit range. J Clin Invest 32: 1309

Fudenberg HH, Kunkel HG, Franklin EC (1961) The body hematocrit/venous hematocrit ratio and the splenic 'reservoir'. Blood 16: 71

Appendix 5
Prediction of normal blood volume from height and weight

Prediction of blood volume (BV) from height (H) and weight (W) cannot be highly accurate, partly because no allowance is made for variation in the ratio of fat, with a blood content of 11–22 ml/kg, to lean body mass, with a blood content of 92 ml/kg. The effect of this variation can be reduced by using formulae in which the subject's height is cubed (Allen *et al.* 1956). Slight improvements on predictions from these formulae were obtained by 'computer correction' (Nadler *et al.* 1962). The standard error of estimates was found to be about 0.4 l. Similarly, in a series in which the BV of 38 men was deduced from RCV (estimated with ^{51}Cr) and compared with the values obtained by Nadler and colleagues, the standard deviation of the estimates was 0.5 l (see fifth edition, p. 86). In one obese subject, measured BV was more than 1 l less than the predicted value and in one muscular subject was 1 l more than the predicted value.

Nadler and colleagues measured only plasma volume and in predicting RCV (as BV − PV) they used values for normal PCV, which were probably too high. In any case, their predictions of RCV were found to be consistently higher than those based on formulae derived from direct measurements of RCV and PV taken from selected published papers (Pearson *et al.* 1995). Mean normal values were given by the following formulae:

For males:

$$RCV\ (ml) = (1486 \times S) - 825 \qquad (A5.1)$$

$$PV\ (ml) = 1578 \times S \qquad (A5.2)$$

For females:

$$RCV\ (ml) = (1.06 \times age) + (822 \times S) \qquad (A5.3)$$

$$PV\ (ml) = 1395 \times S \qquad (A5.4)$$

where S = surface area (m²) = $W^{0.425} \times H^{0.725} \times 0.007184$; age = age (years); H = height (cm); W = weight (kg).

In total, 98–99% of measured values were within ± 25% of the mean normal values predicted from the above formulae.

References

Allen TH, Peng MT, Chen KP (1956) Prediction of blood volume and adiposity in man from body weight and cube of height. Metabolism 5: 328, 346, 353

Nadler SB, Hidalgo JU, Bloch T (1962) Prediction of blood volume in normal human adults. Surgery 51: 224

Pearson ES, Hartley HO (eds) (1954) Biometrika Tables for Statisticians, 2nd edn, vol. I, p. 203. Cambridge University Press (for the Biometrika Trustees)

Appendix 6
Estimation of red cell survival using ^{51}Cr

Autologous or presumed compatible allogeneic red cells

Red cells are labelled exactly as described in Appendix 2 except that the amount of ^{51}Cr must be increased, for example when survival is to be followed for as long as a month, about 0.8 μCi (30 kBq)/kg will be needed.

Blood samples should be taken at 10 min and 24 h, and three further samples should be taken between days 2 and 7; thereafter, at least two further samples should be taken each week for the duration of the study.

Interpretation of results

Uncorrected Cr results, as counts/g Hb or counts/ml red cells, should first be plotted on semi-logarithmic paper and a straight line fitted to them by eye so as to determine the T_{50}Cr. [Strictly speaking, the points cannot be fitted by a straight line, as the disappearance curve is not an exponential (see Chapter 9), but for the present purpose the error is not serious.] If the T_{50}Cr is within normal limits, i.e. about 25–37 days, the interpretation is that red cell survival has not been shown to be abnormal and nothing further should be done. If the T_{50}Cr is less than 25 days the estimates are corrected for Cr elution using the correction values given in Table 9.1. The values are now plotted on semi-logarithmic and linear graph paper, and the best straight-line fits determined by a least-squares fitting procedure. When the best fit is obtained with a semi-logarithmic plot, mean red cell lifespan is given by the time taken for survival to fall to 37%. When the best fit is obtained with a linear plot, mean lifespan is given

by the point at which the line cuts the time axis (Dornhorst 1951). If it is not obvious by simple inspection which plot gives the best fit, a statistical fitting criterion can be applied to decide which one to use. If the data are not fitted well on either a semi-logarithmic or a linear plot, one can use only the first few points, plotted on linear paper, to obtain the initial slope (ICSH 1971).

Estimation of survival of red cells known to be, or suspected of being, incompatible

As described in Chapter 10, when an estimate of the survival of incompatible red cells is being made, and red cell volume is not determined using a second red cell label, the first sample should be taken at 3 min and further samples should be taken at suitable intervals (see pages 408 and 435).

References

Dornhorst AC (1951) The interpretation of red cell survival curves. Blood 6: 1284

ICSH (1971) Recommended methods for radioisotope red cell survival studies. Br J Haematol 21: 241

Appendix 7
Red cell survival methods based on antigenic differences between donor and recipient

Differential agglutination or haemolysis

When transfused red cells are present in the circulation of a recipient it may be possible to recognize them serologically either: (1) indirectly, i.e. by their failure to be agglutinated by a serum that agglutinates the recipient's red cells (e.g. when group O red cells have been transfused to a group A recipient they may be recognized by their failure to be agglutinated by anti-A) or (2) directly, i.e. by their being agglutinated by a serum that fails to agglutinate the recipient's red cells (e.g. when group M red cells have been transfused to a group N recipient they may be recognized by their reaction with anti-M serum).

Indirect differential agglutination. If quantitative estimates are required, agglutination of the recipient's red cells must be virtually complete; the number of cells remaining unagglutinated should not exceed $10 \times 10^9/l$. The importance of using potent antisera cannot be over-stated. Either a manual technique (Dacie and Mollison 1943) or flow cytometry (Garratty and Arndt 1999) can be used. In the manual technique, one volume (approximately 0.2 ml) of a 1:50 dilution of blood is mixed with one volume of antiserum in a small test tube. The mixture is incubated at room temperature for 1 h, centrifuged at 150 g for 1 min and tapped to break up the agglutinated mass into fragments. After repeating the process to ensure agglutination, a drop of supernatant suspension is transferred to a haemocytometer for counting and comparison with the pre-transfusion count (see third edition, p. 140).

Indirect differential haemolysis. Potent haemolytic anti-A or anti-B sera can be used to produce virtually complete lysis of A or B red cells and the unhaemolysed cells can then be counted as in differential agglutination. Alternatively, the red cells can be labelled with ^{51}Cr and then either the unhaemolysed or the haemolysed cells counted (for details see ninth edition, p. 795).

Combined indirect and direct method using ^{51}Cr. Red cells from 0.1 ml of blood are labelled with 20 μCi (0.7 mBq) of ^{51}Cr. Saline is added to washed, labelled cells to provide a 2% suspension. The following mixtures are prepared in vials suitable for analysis in a gamma counter:

1 *Test*: 0.5 ml of cell suspension and 0.5 ml of antibody + 0.1 ml of complement source (guinea pig serum).
2 *100% lysis*: 0.5 ml of cell suspension + 0.6 ml of distilled water + 'pinch' of dry saponin.
3 *Blank*: 0.5 ml of cell suspension + 0.5 ml of EDTA-treated antibody + 0.1 ml of EDTA-treated complement.
4 *Control of antibody potency*: 0.5 ml of 2% labelled cells + 0.5 ml of antibody + 0.1 ml of complement.

The tubes are incubated at 37 °C for 30 min, mixed and centrifuged. The supernatants are removed, transferred to counting vials and counted together with all cell residues. The percentage of transfused cells (as Hb) in (1) is given by [the counts in supernatant of (1) – counts in supernatant of (3) divided by counts in (2)]. In (4), virtually all counts (> 99%) should be in the supernatant.

The method works best with potent antibodies such as anti-A or anti-A,B.

References

Dacie JV, Mollison PL (1943) Survival of normal erythrocytes after transfusion to patients with familial haemolytic anaemia (acholuric jaundice). Lancet i: 550

Garratty G, Arndt PA (1999) Applications of flow cytometry to red blood cell immunology. Cytometry 38: 259–267

Appendix 8
Platelet recovery and survival: radioisotopic labelling and infusion of fresh or stored platelets with ^{111}indium oxine and $Na_2^{51}CrO_4$ (^{51}chromium)

Elements of this method derive from several protocols (Snyder *et al.* 1986; Holme *et al.* 1993).

Equipment/supplies/reagents

The equipment/supplies/reagents required are as follows:
- calibrated, temperature-controlled, variable speed, swinging bucket centrifuge;
- calibrated electronic balance, accurate to ± 0.0002;
- 19- to 21-G butterfly or straight needles;
- sterile transfer pipettes (3.2-ml draw);
- 15- and 50-ml sterile conical polypropylene plastic tubes;
- evacuated sample tubes with EDTA;
- ACD-A: anticoagulant citrate dextrose solution – formula A;
- ACD-A/saline solution: 1 part ACD-A to seven parts of sterile 0.9% saline, adjusted to pH 6.5 to 6.8 with 1 N NaOH; sterilize by filtration;
- 0.22-μm sterilizing filter unit;
- ^{111}indium oxine;
- ^{111}indium oxine labelling solution: aseptically add 4.0 ml of sterile ACD-A/saline solution to the vial of ^{111}indium oxine to make 5.0 ml of sterile ^{111}indium oxine solution for labelling, mix well;
- $NA_2^{51}CRO_4$, chromium-51;
- 18-G spinal needles sterile;
- assorted sterile syringes;
- positive displacement pipettes for whole blood aliquots;
- assorted sizes of pipettes and tips;
- SDS (sodium dodecyl sulphate) 20%: dissolve 20 g of sodium dodecyl sulphate in 100 ml of distilled water.

Preparation of platelets for labelling with [111]indium oxine

Using a 19-G needle, collect 51 ml of venous blood into a 60-ml sterile plastic syringe containing 9 ml of ACD-A. A clean 'non-traumatic' venepuncture is important. Avoid excessive negative pressure in the syringe during draw to prevent activation of the platelets. Simultaneously, collect one 5- or 7-ml blood sample from the subject into an EDTA tube and mix well. This specimen is reserved for determination of radiolabel elution (see below).

Using sterile technique, in a laminar flow hood, remove the needle and express the contents of the syringe into two sterile 50-ml screw-cap conical centrifuge tubes. Centrifuge (soft spin) the conical tubes at 180–200 g for 15 min at 20 to 24°C with the brake off to produce red cell-poor platelet–rich plasma (PRP). Remove the PRP from both tubes with a sterile transfer pipette or spinal needle and syringe and place into a single 50-ml sterile conical plastic centrifuge tube. Avoid aspirating any contaminating red cells. Add a volume of sterile ACD-A equal to 15% of the volume of PRP to the PRP. Cap the tube and mix gently by inversion.

Preparation of aliquot from stored platelet unit

Mix unit thoroughly and resuspend platelets completely. Using sterile technique, in a laminar flow hood, gently remove 10 ml from the stored platelet unit using a 20-ml syringe and 16-G needle. Remove the needle and express the contents of the syringe into a 15-ml screw-cap conical labelled centrifuge tube containing 1.5 ml of sterile ACD-A. Cap and mix gently by inversion. Centrifuge (soft spin) the conical tubes at 180–200 g for 5 min at 20–24°C with the brake off to produce red cell-poor platelet-rich plasma (PRP). Remove the PRP with a sterile transfer pipette or spinal needle and syringe and place into a new 15-ml sterile conical plastic centrifuge tube. Avoid aspirating any contaminating red cells. Centrifuge (hard spin) the ACD-PRP at 1500–2000 g for 15 min with brake off. Remove the platelet-poor plasma (PPP) produced as completely as possible and transfer to a new 50-ml sterile conical tube. Spin PPP for a second time (1500–2000 g for 15 min with brake off), discard pellet and reserve supernatant PPP in a sterile tube for later use. Resuspend the harvested platelet pellet with 2 ml of ACD-A/saline solution. Resuspend completely (no visible aggregates or clumps) before initiating radiolabelling.

Platelet labelling with [111]indium oxine

Add 50–60 µCi of [111]indium oxine labelling solution to the washed platelet suspension. Incubate at 20–24°C for 20 min to achieve labelling. At the end of incubation, add 3.5 ml of ACD-A/saline and 0.5 ml of the reserved PPP directly to the incubation tube containing the platelets in ACD-A/saline and [111]indium oxine. Centrifuge the tube at 1250 g at 20–24°C for 10 min. Remove the supernatant and retain in a separate test tube. Determine the activity of this supernatant and the labelled pellet in a dose calibrator. Calculate and note the efficiency of labelling by dividing the activity of the pellet by the combined activities of the pellet and supernate.

Hard spin the platelet pellet in 2 ml of PPP reserved previously, then gently resuspend. After complete resuspension, add an additional 4 ml of PPP.

Injectate and standard preparation

Label five 100-ml volumetric flasks and five 12 × 75 mm polystyrene tubes with the isotope used, subject name and/or unit identification, date prepared and In STD, Cr STD and STD I, II or III. Add 1.8 ml of 0.9% saline to each 12 × 75-mm standard capped tube. Weigh each tube and record the weights. Take care to avoid touching saline to the cap. Add 10 ml of 2% SDS/saline solution (one part saturated (20%) SDS + 99 parts 0.9% saline) to each flask. Mix each single labelled platelet aliquot. Draw 0.3 cc of each suspension into its own 1-cc syringe through a 16-G needle. Weigh the filled syringe, needle and needle cover accurately. Record the weight.

Carefully add 0.2 ml of each injectate directly into each flask, 'Cr STD' or 'In STD', as appropriate. Add 0.9% saline to the flask to bring to volume. Mix carefully. Weigh the syringe, needle and needle cover accurately and determine the mass of labelled injectate placed in each standards flask. Draw the appropriate radioactive dose of ^{51}Cr-labelled platelets into a labelled syringe. Weigh the syringe and record the radioactive dose. The activity needed to be injected is dependent on a number of variables, such as the gamma counter's crystal size. In general, 10–20 µCi is required to be injected for accurate determinations. The injectates of the fresh and stored platelets should have approximately the same activities.

Remove enough ^{111}In-labelled platelets from the centrifuge tube to leave the tube containing the radioactive dose of ^{111}In that is intended to be injected. Measure and record the radioactive dose. Record the weight of the tube. Verify subject identification on the chromium syringe and indium tube. Inject the ^{51}Cr-labelled platelets into the centrifuge tube containing the ^{111}In-labelled platelets. Mix the labelled injectate in the tube. Prepare final mixed injectate for infusion by using an 18-G spinal needle and a syringe labelled with subject information to aspirate all but at least 1 ml of labelled solution in conical tube. (This remaining amount will be used for preparation of standards and determination of cell-bound activity.)

Remove the spinal needle and replace with a sterile syringe cap. Record the weight of the final injectate syringe and cap. Draw approximately 0.8 ml of the remaining labelled solution from the tube containing the ^{51}Cr- and ^{111}In-labelled platelets into a 1-cc syringe through a 16-G needle to be used for standard preparation. Record the weight of the filled syringe, needle and needle cover. Carefully add 0.2 ml of the injectate directly into the flask labelled 'STD I'. Add 0.9% saline to the flask to bring to volume. Mix carefully.

Reweigh the 1-cc syringe, needle and needle cover and record this weight and the difference between the two weights (this being the net weight of the mixed injectate added to the standards flask). Repeat these steps for the remaining two flasks.

Pipette 0.2 ml of each standard into the appropriate preweighed capped tube containing 1.8 ml of saline, one sample tube per standard. Weigh the capped tubes and record the weight. Avoid allowing the sample touch the cap.

Infusion procedure

Record recipient's pre-infusion vital signs and verify that recipient's identifiers match the information on the infusion syringe. Perform venepuncture with a 19- to 21-G butterfly infusion needle. Draw one 10-ml EDTA tube for the pre-infusion sample. Flush the line with saline to ensure patency of the vein. Inject labelled platelet suspension slowly. Record exact time (starting from the time when one-half of injectate has been infused). Flush butterfly line and needle with 10 ml of sterile 0.9% sodium chloride. Remove butterfly needle and apply pressure to injection site; bandage when bleeding has stopped.

Weigh empty infusion syringe, needle and needle cover. Record weight on the data sheet. Record the net weight of injectate. Dispose of used supplies in receptacle labelled for radioactive waste. Measure and record post-infusion vital signs.

Sampling procedure and sample preparation

One 5–10 ml EDTA tube sample is to be drawn by direct venepuncture at the following times:
1 pre-infusion;
2 5 min post infusion (optional, to be used for investigation of discrepant observation at next sampling time);
3 2 h after infusion – collect from the contralateral arm to that used for infusion;
4 one sample daily between days 1 and 7 and one final sample on day 10, 11 or 12. (The last sample is called the 'baseline' sample and is used to correct for inadvertent labelling of other blood components.)

Sample processing. Processing should be completed as soon as possible after sampling. Prior to the infusion, label and weigh capped 12×75-mm polystyrene tubes: one for each sampling time (including presample) for whole blood, packed cells and plasma and three for standards. Tubes for daily samples may be labelled and weighed on the day of use or beforehand. Immediately prior to aliquoting sample, thoroughly mix each timed sample from the subject manually or for a maximum of 2 min on a rocker. Pipette 2.0 ml of the mixed whole blood into the appropriate preweighed tube, using a positive displacement pipettor and replace cap. Weigh the capped tube and record the weight. Take care that the sample *does not* touch the cap.

Pipette 2.0 ml of blood into the appropriate tube labelled for packed cells. Centrifuge this second set of tubes at 2000 g for 15 min at room temperature. Pipette the plasma from the packed cell tubes to the appropriate tube labelled for plasma. Count the 'splits' (packed cell and plasma tubes, including the injectate) (see Calculations). (When possible, count the 'splits' on the day of sampling.)

Elution of radioactivity from labelled platelets in whole blood

Add 10 μl of the labelled platelets sample into a 5- or 7-ml EDTA tube of blood collected from the subject as soon as possible after the infusion of the labelled cells procedure. This timing is anticipating infusion of the radiolabelled platelets at the earliest possible time. If delay in infusion is anticipated, the elution steps described in this section should be begun so that the separation of the supernatant after the next step occurs approximately coincidently with the infusion.

Mix and incubate the tube for 2 h at 37°C in a wet incubator (waterbath) or a dry incubator in a cylinder of water. Pipette approximately 2 ml into a 12×75-mm capped tube. Spin at 2000 g for 15 min. Transfer the supernatant plasma to a capped 12×75-mm tube. Count the splits. The activity found in the cells and plasma will be used to evaluate the *in vivo* cell-bound activity of the labelled platelets for each of the two radiolabels.

$$\text{Elution} = (\text{CPM}_{\text{supernate}})/[(\text{CPM}_{\text{cells}}) + (\text{CPM}_{\text{supernate}})] \quad \text{(A8.1)}$$

Counting the samples

Load racks into gamma counter and initiate counting. Count whole blood samples once all samples from the subject have been collected and processed. (One can also count standards and splits daily.) Load the gamma counter in a standard order, such as: blank/background, standards, elutions, pre-infusion and post-infusion timed specimens in order collected. Select appropriate counting programme. Set count time to achieve a 2% accuracy, including background. When the tubes have finished counting, label the instrument printout. Verify that the background has not drifted significantly. Verify that all samples counted for expected times. Place the gamma counter printouts in the appropriate file. Transfer all data to appropriate spreadsheets for calculations. Verify accurate transcription.

Calculations

Determine corrected CPM/g for each sample.

Most gamma counters correct automatically for background activity and decay. Using these corrected CPM values reported by the gamma counter ($\text{CPM}_{\text{corrected}}$), determine CPM/g for standards and timed subject samples as follows:

Standards:

$$\text{STD} = \text{CPM}_{\text{corrected}} \times \text{dilution factor/mass counted} \quad \text{(A8.2)}$$

Timed sample activity:

$$\text{Sample} = \text{CPM}_{\text{corrected}}/\text{mass counted} \quad \text{(A8.3)}$$

The volume of each sample counted is based on the gravimetric determination of the weight of the sample.

Determine cell-bound proportion. Using timed split samples, determine the proportion of the activity in each timed sample that can be associated with the cellular fraction: cell-bound fraction ($\text{CbF}_{\text{time } t}$) = (activity of cells)/(activity of cells + activity of plasma) = $(\text{CPM}_{\text{cell bound}})/[(\text{CPM}_{\text{cell bound}}) + (\text{CPM}_{\text{plasma}})]$.

Adjustment for injectate elution. Determine the mean CPM of the standards. Multiply the mean CPM of the standard samples by the elution correction.

$$\text{STD}_{\text{corrected}} = \text{STD}^*\text{elution} \quad \text{(A8.4)}$$

Adjustment for cell-bound proportion and baseline:

The following two adjustments should be made to the timed sample CPM/g counts. These adjustments result in 'fully adjusted counts' used for curve fitting.

Adjustment of timed sample for plasma radioactivity.

$\text{Sample}_{\text{time } t} = \text{timed sample (sample, CPM/g)} \times (\text{CPF}_{\text{time } t})$

Adjust for baseline, according to the day on which the 'baseline' sample was taken. (This results in fully adjusted timed sample counts.)
Day 10:

Fully adjusted count = $\text{sample}_{\text{time } t} - [\text{sample}_{\text{day 10}} \times$
$(1.20-0.20 \text{ (time } t/\text{time of day 10 sample)}] \quad \text{(A8.5)}$

or day 11:

Fully adjusted count = $\text{sample}_{\text{time } t} - [\text{sample}_{\text{day 10}} \times$
$(1.22-0.22 \text{ (time } t/\text{time of day 11 sample)}] \quad \text{(A8.6)}$

or day 12:

Fully adjusted count = $\text{sample}_{\text{time } t} - [\text{sample}_{\text{day 10}} \times$
$(1.24-0.24 \text{ (time } t/\text{time of day 12 sample)}] \quad \text{(A8.7)}$

Note: 'time t' is the elapsed time in hours from the time of infusion; 'time of day 10 sample' is the elapsed time in hours from time of infusion for a timed sample obtained on day 10 following infusion.

Determination of expected time 0 count following infusion. Calculate blood volume:

Male: BV (ml) = $[0.3669^*\text{height (cm)}]^3 +$
$0.03219^*\text{weight (kg)} + 0.6041 \quad \text{(A8.8)}$

Female: BV (ml) = [0.3561*height (cm)]³ +
[0.3308*weight (kg)] + 0.1833   (A8.9)

Convert the blood volume to blood mass by multiplying the volume by the specific gravity of whole blood, 1.05 g/ml. Determine expected time 0 ($t = 0$) count

$STD_{corrected}$*infusate mass (g)/blood mass   (A8.10)

The recovery is determined using the $time_0$ extrapolation of the curve fitting program.

Kinetic curve fitting

The fully adjusted timed sample counts for when times greater than 20 h are used for kinetic curve fitting and estimation of recovery and survival. That is, the 5-min and 2-h time samples are not used for kinetic curve fitting. These parameters may be estimated using a validated non-linear curve fitting routine found in various statistical and pharmacokinetic computer program packages (Lotter et al. 1988). The use of COST software, one of these software packages, is described below.

Recovery is determined as the extrapolated y-axis intercept ($t = 0$) of the survival curve, expressed as the blood cell-bound activity in proportion to the expected activity as projected from the blood volume-based dilution.

The fully adjusted count data (CPM/g) for each timed sample point are entered into the COST program as y values, the time after infusion (in hours) as x values, and the expected $time_0$ count.

Activate the COST program. Select the appropriate group in COST into which the subject's data will be entered. Enter the number of data points to be entered. Enter the x (time in hours) and y fully adjusted timed sample count for each timed sample. Double check entry accuracy. Perform data analyses using the multiple hit model. If outliers are found, determine potential source of error and flag for review by medical director. Remove point from curve only if clearly a spurious result. Save and print results. Append to unit records.

Determination of acceptable recovery and survival

The mean recovery of the platelets under evaluation should be at least two-thirds of that of the fresh platelets, and the mean survival should be at least one-half of that of the fresh platelets. Achievement of these requirements should be determined in a manner to document non-inferiority of the results. The upper limit of the 95% (one-sided) confidence interval of the mean difference between fresh and 'test' platelets' recovery for each subject must be smaller than the difference between the mean recovery of fresh platelets and 0.667 times that value. The upper limit of the 95% (one-sided) confidence interval of the mean difference between fresh and 'test' platelets' survival for each subject must be smaller than the difference between the mean survival of fresh platelets and 0.50 times that value.

Activity is measured in Ci or Bq (Becquerels), Bq being the official SI unit: 1 Bq = 1 decay per second, thus $1 Ci = 3.7 \times 10^{10}$ Bq.

References

Holme S, Heaton A, Roodt J. Concurrent label method with ^{111}In and ^{51}Cr allows accurate evaluation of platelet viability of stored platelet concentrates. Br J Haematol 1993; 84: 717–723.

Lotter MG, Rabe WL, Van Zyl JM et al. A computer program in compiled BASIC for the IBM personal computer to calculate the mean platelet survival time with the multiple-hit and weighted mean methods. Comput Biol Med 1988; 18: 305–315.

Snyder EL, Moroff G, Simon T et al. and Members of the Ad Hoc Platelet Radiolabeling Study Group. Recommended methods for conducting radiolabeled platelet survival studies. Transfusion 1986; 26: 37–42.

Appendix 9
Citrate solutions for storage of whole blood

Citrate–phosphate–dextrose–adenine (CPDA-1)

- trisodium citrate (dihydrate)   26.30 g;
- citric acid (monohydrate)   3.27 g;
- sodium dihydrogen phosphate (monohydrate) 2.22 g;
- dextrose (monohydrate)   31.8 g;
- adenine   0.275 g;
- water to 1 l.

Note: 14 ml to be added to each 100 ml of blood. In CPDA-2, the amount of dextrose is increased to 44.6 g and that of adenine to 0.55 g.

Half-strength CPD (0.5 CPD)

- citric acid (monohydrate)   1.64 g;
- sodium citrate (dihydrate)   13.2 g;
- glucose (anhydrous)   23.2 g;
- sodium dihydrogen phosphate   2.51 g;
- water to 1 l.

Note: 63 ml of solution (pH 5.7) is mixed with 450 ml of blood.

Appendix 10
Red cell additive solutions

Saline–adenine–glucose mannitol (SAG-M)

- sodium chloride   8.77 g;
- dextrose (anhydrous)   8.2 g;
- adenine   0.169 g;
- mannitol   5.25 g;
- water to 1 l.

Note: 100 ml of this solution (pH 5.7) is added to packed red cells (approximately 200 ml) from 450 ml of blood.

Adenine–dextrose solution (Adsol)

- sodium chloride   9.0 g;
- dextrose (monohydrate)   22.0 g;
- adenine   0.27 g;
- mannitol   7.5 g;
- water to 1 l.

Note: 100 ml of this solution (pH 5.6) is added to packed red cells (approximately 200 ml) from 450 ml of blood.

Nutricell (AS-3)

- sodium chloride   4.1 g;
- dextrose (anhydrous)   10.0 g of sodium dihydrogen phosphate (monohydrate)   2.76 g;
- trisodium citrate (dihydrate)   5.88 g;
- citric acid (monohydrate)   0.456 g;
- adenine   0.3 g;
- water to 1 l.

Note: Blood is taken into CP2D (containing twice as much dextrose as CPD) and packed red cells from 450 ml of blood are stored with 100 ml of AS-3 pH 5.8.

Red cell additive solution (RAS2)

- sodium citrate (dihydrate)   7.82 g;
- sodium dihydrogen phosphate (dihydrate)   0.73 g;
- sodium phosphate (dihydrate)   3.03 g;
- adenine   0.215 g;
- mannitol   7.74 g;
- water to 1 l.

Note: 94 ml of this solution (pH 7.3) is mixed with the following solution (sterilized separately in a length of plastic tubing):
- glucose   13.64 g;
- water   6 ml.

Note: Red cells from 450 ml of blood, taken into 63 ml of 0.5 CPD (pH 7.3) is mixed with 100 ml of additive solution.

Appendix 11
Citrate solutions used in apheresis or plasma exchange

Citrate–phosphate–dextrose (CPD)

- trisodium citrate (dihydrate)   26.30 g;
- citric acid (monohydrate)   3.27 g;
- Sodium dihydrogen phosphate (monohydrate) 2.22 g;
- dextrose (monohydrate)   25.50 g;
- water to 1 l.

Note: This solution is almost identical to 'CPD 5' of Gibson and co-workers (1957).

Acid–citrate–dextrose A (ACD-A, NIH–A)
trisodium citrate (dihydrate)   22.0 g

- citric acid (monohydrate)   8.0 g;
- dextrose (monohydrate)   24.6 g;
- water to 1 l.

Note: this solution is also used for labelling red cells with ^{51}Cr: 1.5 ml of the solution (pH 5.0–5.1) is mixed with 10 ml of blood.

Acid–citrate–dextrose B (ACD-B, NIH–B)
trisodium citrate (dihydrate)   13.2 g

- citric acid (monohydrate)   4.8 g;
- dextrose   14.7 g;
- water to 1 l.

Citrate-phosphate-dextrose 50 (CPD-50)

- trisodium citrate (dihydrate)   39.5 g;
- citric acid (monohydrate)   4.9 g;
- sodium dihydrogen phosphate   3.76 g;
- dextrose (monohydrate)   50.0 g;
- water to 1 l.

Acid citrate–phosphate–dextrose (acid CPD)

- trisodium citrate   22.0 g;
- citric acid (monohydrate)   12.0 g;
- dextrose (monohydrate)   50.0 g;
- sodium dihydrogen phosphate   3.76 g;
- water to 1 l.

Reference

Gibson JG, Rees SB, McManus TJ (1957) A citrate-phosphate-dextrose solution for the preservation of human blood. Am J Clin Pathol 28: 569

Appendix 12
Glycerol solutions for storage of red cells

Slow freezing

Storage for later transfusion. A standard CPD unit of blood, stored at 4°C for not more than 5 days, is centrifuged at 3630 *g* for 10 min; plasma is squeezed out of the bag, the bag is weighed and the net weight of red cells deduced. With continuous mixing an appropriate volume of a solution containing 6.2 mmol/l glycerol is added in stages (e.g. 300 ml when the weight of packed red cells is 151–230 g). The bag is centrifuged, the supernatant is expressed and the red cells then stored at −80°C. When needed, the unit is thawed in a water-bath at 37°C and the red cells washed free of glycerol, preferably with an automated cell washer (slightly modified from Valeri *et al.* 1981).

Red cells collected in various anticoagulant preservative solutions may also be cryopreserved for up to 6 days (or longer in AS-1 or AS-3) in polyvinyl chloride or polyolefin containers kept at −65°C or colder in cardboard or metal canisters (Meryman and Hornblower 1972). An aliquot of serum or plasma should be frozen to permit future diagnostic tests.

Storage for blood grouping tests. A convenient solution is 'glycigel', which is made up as follows: 62.9 ml of glycerol is placed in a graduated cylinder and distilled water is added to 100 ml. After adding 0.9 g of NaCl, the solution is warmed; 2.5 g of gelatin is then added and warming continued until the gelatin has liquefied. After adding 0.3 g of EDTA, 0.25- to 1.0-ml quantities are placed in 2 ml of evacuated blood sample tubes and the tubes stored at 1–6°C. For storage, an equal volume of washed red cells is added to a volume of glycigel. For other details see Chapter 8.

Removal of glycerol by washing in hypertonic solutions. Red cells that have been equilibrated with about 3.0 mol/l glycerol (approximately 30% w/v) are first centrifuged and the supernatant discarded. The red cells are then washed first in 12% v/v glycerol in 5% trisodium citrate then in 5% v/v glycerol in 5% trisodium citrate, and finally in saline (MacDonald and Marsh 1958). This method gives too much lysis if the red cells have been stored with glycerol concentrations of the order of 4.5 mol/l (40% w/v). For such cells the red cells are first thawed at 37°C, equilibrated in 12% (v/v) NaCl and washed with at least 2 l of 1.6% (v/v) NaCl until deglycerolization is complete (Meryman and Hornblower 1972).

Removal of glycerol by dialysis. A convenient method is to place a few millilitres of the thawed glycerolized red cells in a length of dialysis tubing and then place the tubing in saline for 30–60 min (Weiner 1961). Lysis can be minimized by dialysis against a citrate–phosphate solution (e.g. the one described by Mollison *et al.* 1958), rather than saline and, after dialysis, giving the cells one wash in citrate–phosphate before washing them in saline. Provided that dialysis is allowed to continue for 60 min and the concentration of glycerol in the original red cell mixture does not exceed 30% (w/v), there should be very little lysis.

References

MacDonald KA, Marsh WL (1958) Frozen red cells. A modified recovery technique. J Med Lab Technol 15: 22

Meryman HT, Hornblower M (1972) A method for freezing and washing red blood cells using a high glycerol concentration. Transfusion 12: 145

Mollison PL, Robinson MA, Hunter DA (1958) Improved method of labelling red cells with radioactive phosphorus. Lancet i: 766

Valeri CR, Valeri DA, Anastasi J *et al*. (1981) Freezing in the primary polyvinylchloride plastic collection bag: a new system for preparing and freezing non-rejuvenated and rejuvenated red blood cells. Transfusion 21: 138–149

Weiner W (1961) Reconstitution of frozen red cells. Lancet i: 1264

Appendix 13
Acid-elution method for the detection of fetal red cells (Betke and Kleihauer 1958)

Technique

From whole fresh blood, mixed with anticoagulant, spread ordinary films on glass slides and allow them to dry in air for not longer than 60 min. Fix the films in 80% ethanol for 5 min. Rinse with tap water and dry. (The films can be left at this stage for up to 2 days in a refrigerator.)

The films are now placed in the following buffer:

- 26.6 ml of 0.2 mol/l Na_2HPO_4;
- 73.4 ml of 0.1 mol/l citric acid.

In making up the buffer, anhydrous Na_2HPO_4 should be used; the final pH should be 3.3.

The buffer must be warmed to 37°C before the slides are put (vertically) into it; the slides should be moved up and down from time to time; 15 min should be allowed for elution. The slides are now washed in tap water, stained with acid haematoxylin for 3 min and finally with erythrosine (0.3% solution in water) for 30 s.

For variations of the original method, see Sebring (1984).

Quantification

Apart from research purposes, quantitative estimates of transplacental haemorrhage (TPH) are required in two circumstances: first, in screening the blood of D-negative women to detect a TPH that is believed to be too large to be covered by the prophylactic dose of anti-D that is being administered and, second, in cases in which a relatively large TPH is detected, to provide an estimate of the size of the TPH and thus determine the dose of anti-D which may be expected to suppress Rh D immunization.

In making quantitative estimates of the size of TPH by the acid-elution method, the density of red cells on the film that is being scanned must be known, i.e. the average number of red cells in a given area. Each laboratory can determine this for itself by counting the average number of adult red cells per high-power field and determining the area of the high-power field from the expression πr^2, r being determined by means of a micrometre scale placed on the stage of a microscope. In one survey (Mollison 1972) the density was found to vary from 1.2 to 13.4×10^3 cells per square millimetre; it is suggested that a density of $5.0 \times 10^3/mm^2$ should be the aim.

In order to draw quantitative conclusions from the average number of red cells seen per low-power field, the area of the low-power field must be determined. Again, this is done by reading a micrometre scale under the low power of the microscope to determine 'r'. Most observers have found that a low-power field with an area of approximately $0.8\ mm^2$ is convenient. When the density of adult red cells is 5000 per mm^2, the number or red cells per low-power field will be 4000.

The size of TPH (as millilitres of fetal red cells) in the mother's circulation can be deduced approximately from the formula:

2400/number ratio of adult to fetal red cells

The indicator rosette test, in which D-positive red cells circulating in a D-negative woman are detected by adding reagent anti-D to a blood specimen followed by D-coated reagent cells and counting the resulting 'rosettes', is a relatively simple and accurate semi-quantitative assay (Sebring 1984).

When the purpose of examining a film for fetal red cells is simply to ensure that not more than a certain number is present, it is evidently unnecessary, when very few cells are seen, to determine the number precisely. As an example, suppose the object is to ensure that the size of TPH does not exceed 4 ml, corresponding to one fetal red cell for every 600 adult cells (see above). Assume that the low-power field usually contains 4000 adult red cells (based on experience of actual counts in the laboratory concerned) but that as a safety factor it is supposed the average number might fall as low as 2400. The average number of fetal red cells expected per low-power field with a TPH of 4 ml is then four. Using tables giving the confidence limits for a Poisson variable (Pearson 2001), the maximum number of cells that can be seen in a given number of low-power fields without arousing the suspicion that the actual number present exceeds an average of four can be determined. For example, if five fields are scanned, the maximum number of cells that can be seen without arousing the suspicion that the average number present is 20 or more is nine at the $P = 0.01$ level and 12 at the $P = 0.05$ level (Mollison 1972).

References

Betke K, Kleihauer E (1958) Fetaler und bleibender Blutfarbstoff in Erythrozyten und Erythroblasten von menschlichen Feten und Neugeborenen. Blut 4: 241

Mollison PL (1972) Quantitation of transplacental haemorrhage. Br Med J iii: 31, 35

Sebring ES (1984) Fetomaternal haemorrhage – incidence and methods of detection and quantitation. In: Haemolytic Disease of the Newborn. G Garratty (ed.), pp. 87–117. Arlington, VA: Am Assoc Blood Banks

Appendix 14
Cryopreservation and storage of human cells and tissue-based products

Human cells and tissue-based products (HCT/Ps) are cryopreserved with a freeze mix containing 5% dimethyl sulphoxide (DMSO), an intracellular cryoprotectant, 6% pentastarch, an extracellular cryoprotectant, and human serum albumin (HSA). Heparin and dornase alpha (rhDNAse) are added to minimize post-thaw clumping. HCT/Ps are frozen in a controlled rate freezer to minimize cell damage. Frozen HCT/Ps are stored in a liquid nitrogen (LN2) freezer at –120 to –196°C until needed. The following procedure applies to peripheral blood progenitor cells, and can be applied to umbilical cord blood and other mononuclear cell preparations (Stiff *et al.* 1987; Areman *et al.* 1992; Kang *et al.* 2002). Preparations are routinely carried out in a biological cabinet. Cryogloves and safety goggles must be used when handling products stored in LN2 to avoid chemical burns.

- HCT/Ps cryopreserved for clinical use are stored temporarily in the vapour phase of liquid nitrogen until transmissible infectious disease test results on the product or pre-collection screening sample are completed and negative. Research HCT/Ps may be stored in the vapour phase of a designated LN2 freezer until distribution.
- Plasma-Lyte A with 4% human serum albumin (HSA) is used to supplement clinical and research products when autologous plasma is removed or not available.

- Freeze mix solution and Plasma-Lyte A with 4% human serum albumin expire 24 h after the time of preparation.
- DMSO is stored at room temperature and may be used to prepare freeze mix for clinical products for a total of 7 days.

Procedure

Prepare freeze mix

Estimate the amount of freeze mix based on type of product, total number of cells and number of components to be cryopreserved. See Calculations, below. Add 5 ml of DMSO and 16 ml of 25% HAS to 31 ml of pentastarch (in plastic bag). For small volume (< 25 ml) freeze mix, use pentastarch in vial. See Calculations, below, to prepare smaller volume of freeze mix. The freeze mix is stored at 2–8°C.

Prepare Plasma-Lyte A with 4% human serum albumin (if required)

Estimate volume of Plasma-Lyte A with 4% HSA required. See Calculations, below. Choose a container based on volume: for volume < 50 ml, use sterile screw-capped conical tube. Use syringe or pipette to transfer Plasma-Lyte A or 25% HSA. For volume > 50 ml, use transfer pack of appropriate size. Use sterile connecting device to transfer Plasma-Lyte A and syringe to transfer 25% HSA. Store at 2–8°C.

Containers for samples and cryopreservation

See Table A14.1.

Concentrate and volume reduce product

See Table A14.2.

1 Remove as much plasma as possible. Add plasma back until volume of concentrated cells is equal to one-half of total volume to be placed in bag (i.e. 12.5 ml for 25-ml total or 25 ml for 50-ml total).

2 Add 20 mg/ml of DNAse and 30 U/ml preservative-free heparin to concentrated cells. See Calculations, below, to determine volumes of DNAse and heparin.

3 Place cell container(s) and freeze mix bags in wet ice to chill for at least 20 min.

Table A14.1 Containers for samples and cryopreservation

Container type	Maximum volume	Minimum cell concentration	Maximum cell concentration	Maximum TNC per container
1.8 ml of cryovial	1 ml	1×10^6/ml	1×10^8/ml	1×10^8
5 ml of cryovial	4.5 ml	2.5×10^6/ml	1×10^8/ml	4.5×10^8
Bag	25 ml or 50 ml	2×10^7/ml	3×10^8/ml	1.5×10^{10}

Table A14.2 Concentrate and volume reduce product

Volume	Container	Centrifuge type	Speed	Time (min)
< 100 ml	50-ml conical tube	Table top	1800	10
> 100 ml	250-ml conical tube	Floor	2500	10
> 200 ml	Transfer pack	Floor	4000	6.5

Add freeze mix and transfer into freezing container(s)

1 Multiple bags

(a) Sterile connect chilled freeze mix to concentrated cells.

(b) Slowly add freeze mix while mixing gently.

(c) Sterile connect product with freeze mix to common end of multilead harness for multiple bags (maximum of four bags per harness). If there are more than four bags or > 200 ml total volume, transfer excess volume into a labelled transfer pack. Sterile connect bag containing excess product to a freeze bag or a second multilead harness if multiple additional freeze bags are required.

(d) Clamp bag with cells and freeze mix and hang bag.

(e) Verify that all clamps leading to freeze bags are open.

(f) Open clamp from cell bag and let cells transfer to freeze bags by gravity. Verify that bags fill to equal volumes ($\pm 10\%$).

(g) If there is a big difference of volume between bags (< 45 ml or > 55 ml) return all cells to original container and repeat steps c to e.

(h) After cells have emptied into freeze bags remove air from each bag and heat seal fill tubing twice at a point that allows fill tubing to be cut and contained within the upper pocket of bag. Seal upper pocket of bag containing fill port with remainder of attached fill tubing using Accu-Seal sealer.

2 Vials

(a) Add chilled freeze mix slowly using a sterile pipette or syringe into concentrated cells while mixing gently.

(b) Transfer cells with freeze mix using sterile pipette into labelled vial(s).

(c) Cryopreservation in controlled rate freezer should occur at a rate of 1–3°C per minute until temperature reaches 45–48°C. The rate is then increased to –10°C per minute until temperature reaches –90°C.

Calculations

1 Calculations for small volume freeze mix with 12% pentastarch, 8% HSA and 10% DMSO

(a) Stock concentrations: pentastarch 20%

HAS 25%

DMSO 100%

Example: For 10 ml of freeze mix (using formula $C_1V_1 = C_2V_2$):

$$\text{Volume of pentastarch} = \frac{12\% \times 10 \text{ ml}}{20\%} = 6 \text{ ml}$$
(A14.1)

$$\text{Volume of 25\% HSA} = \frac{8\% \times 10 \text{ ml}}{25\%} = 3.2 \text{ ml}$$
(A14.2)

$$\text{Volume of DMSO} = \frac{10\% \times 10 \text{ ml}}{100\%} = 1 \text{ ml}$$
(A14.3)

2 Calculations for 4% HSA in Plasma-Lyte A
(a) Stock concentration: HSA   25%
  Example: 100 ml of 4% HSA in Plasma-Lyte A needed, using formula $C_1V_1 = C_2V_2$:

$$\text{Volume of stock HSA} = \frac{100\ \text{ml} \times 4\%}{25\%} = 16\ \text{ml} \tag{A14.4}$$

$$100\ \text{ml} - 16\ \text{ml stock HSA} = 84\ \text{ml of Plasma-Lyte A} \tag{A14.5}$$

3 Estimating number of bags for cryopreservation
(a) Total nucleated cell count $(\times 10^9)$ divided by 15×10^9 (maximum no. of cells in 50-ml bag)
  Example: TNC of a PBSC is 105×10^9

$$\frac{105 \times 10^9}{15 \times 10^9} = \text{seven bags} \tag{A14.6}$$

4 Calculations for volume of DNAse and heparin
(a) Stock concentration: DNAse   1000 µg/ml
                            Heparin   1000 U/ml
  Example: 20 µg/ml of DNAse and 30 U/ml of heparin required to supplement 100 ml of concentrated PBSC using formula $C_1V_1 = C_2V_2$

$$\text{Volume of DNAse} = \frac{20\ \text{µg/ml} \times 100\ \text{ml}}{1000\ \text{µg/ml}} = 2\ \text{ml} \tag{A14.7}$$

$$\text{Volume of heparin} = \frac{30\ \text{U/ml} \times 100\ \text{ml}}{1000\ \text{U/ml}} = 3\ \text{ml} \tag{A14.8}$$

5 Calculation for determining RBC content of product or aliquot: (% haematocrit /100) × volume (ml)
  Example: RBC content of 350 ml of PBSC with haematocrit (hct) of 5% cryopreserved in four bags (aliquots)

$$\text{RBC content} = 0.05 \times 350\ \text{ml} = 17.5\ \text{ml}/4$$
$$= 4.38\ \text{ml per bag} \tag{A14.9}$$

Umbilical cord blood stem cells (CBs) are prepared for cryopreservation using Hespan for red cell sedimentation and hydroxyethl starch (HES) for cryopreservation. The product must have suitable cellular content based on enumeration assays. Umbilical cord blood is collected in CPD anticoagulant-preservative with a maximum volume at the time of collection of 150 ml. CBs should be stored no longer than 48 h between collection and processing..

The container should be checked for bag integrity and clots and excess tubing sealed and removed.

Weight (volume) is recorded. One millilitre is withdrawn for WBC count, smear and flow cytometry. Hetastarch is added to the collection bag in a 1:5 ratio and mixed well. The bag is centrifuged at 650 r.p.m. (floor centrifuge) and the leucocyte-rich plasma *plus* 15–20 ml of the red cells are extracted into a 150–300 ml transfer pack. A 2-ml sample is removed (1 ml for the cell count, smear, flow and 1 ml for CFU). The plasma is removed until the volume is equal to one-half of the volume to be cryopreserved and the plasma saved for TTV testing. Freezing is performed as above. Assays may include colony-forming units, sterility testing, TTV, ABO/ RH, RPR and CMV.

References

Areman EM, Deeg HJ, Sacher RA (1992) Bone Marrow and Stem Cell Processing: A Manual of Current Techniques. Philadelphia, PA: FA Davis Company

Kang EM, Areman EM, David-Ocampo V *et al.* (2002) Mobilization, collection, and processing of peripheral blood stem cells in individuals with sickle trait. Blood 99: 850–855

Stiff PJ, Koestner R, Weidner MK *et al.* (1987) Autologous bone marrow transplantation using unfractionated cells cryopreserved in dimethylsulfoxide and hydroxethyl starch without controlled-rate freezing. Blood 70: 974–978

Appendix 15
Thawing human cells and tissue-based products cryopreserved in 6% pentastarch and 5% DMSO

Each product (PBSC and mononuclear cells cryopreserved in bags or vials) is thawed rapidly in a 37°C waterbath to minimize loss of cell viability and function (Kang *et al.* 2002). After thawing, the product is slowly diluted with thawing media. Product expiration date and time is defined as 2 h after product is removed from freezer unless otherwise specified. The thaw mix expires 24 h after the time of preparation. Cryogloves and safety goggles must be used when handling products stored in LN2 to avoid chemical burns.

Procedure

Preparation for thaw

Cryopreserved product in vial for infusion. Prepare 30-ml thaw mix as follows:

- Obtain a bag of cold Plasma-Lyte A from refrigerator and place in biological safety cabinet (BSC).
- Label one 50-ml sterile conical tube 'Thaw mix' and a second 50-ml sterile conical tube with product type and recipient information.
- Calculate volume of Plasma-Lyte A and preservative-free heparin to prepare 30 ml of 'Thaw mix' for each vial to be thawed (see Calculation, below).
- Using a syringe, aliquot appropriate volume of cold Plasma-Lyte A into labelled conical tube.
- Add 10 U/mL of preservative-free heparin into Plasma-Lyte A.
- Place thaw mix and labelled tube in refrigerator (2–8°C) until needed.

Cryopreserved product in bag for infusion. Prepare Plasma-Lyte A as follows:
- Obtain bag of cold Plasma-Lyte A from refrigerator and place in BSC.
- Aliquot 12 ml of Plasma-Lyte A into a 20-ml syringe for each 50-ml bag to be thawed or 6 ml of Plasma-Lyte A into a 10-ml syringe for each 25-ml bag to be thawed.
- Replace needle with sterile female luer cap and place syringe(s) in a labelled plastic bag at 2–8°C until needed.

Thawing product cryopreserved in bag

1 Place Sepacell adapter in BSC.
2 Inspect over wrap bag and freeze container for breaks. Replace over wrap bag if broken.
3 Immediately immerse product and over wrap bag in 37°C waterbath, gently massage and remove as soon as product has consistency of slush. *If a leak is observed*, isolate leak using a haemostat and position container in waterbath to prevent further leakage.
4 Wipe over wrap to dry and remove product from bag to BSC.
5 Spike bag port with Sepacell.
6 Spike one of the Sepacell ports with a sampling site coupler.
7 Sterilize coupler with iodine swab.
8 Obtain chilled syringe with Plasma-Lyte A and attach a needle.
9 Inject appropriate volume of Plasma-Lyte A into port slowly while gently mixing.
10 Remove sample for post-thaw QC if required and remove product label from pouch to document expiration date and time and correct product volume.
11 Attach product label on cardboard tag and place product in plastic zip lock bag.

Thawing product cryopreserved in vial

1 Inspect over wrap bag and freeze vial for breaks or loose cap: replace over wrap bag if broken.
2 Immediately immerse product and over wrap bag in 37°C waterbath and remove as soon as product is almost completely thawed.
3 Wipe over wrap bag to dry and remove vial from bag to BSC.
4 Place pre-chilled 'Thaw mix' and labelled conical tube in BSC.
5 Remove and discard appropriate volume of thaw mix 4.5 ml or 1 ml (volume of frozen product) to keep final diluted product at 30 ml.
6 Remove vial cap and carefully transfer contents of vial into labelled conical tube using a sterile serological pipette.
7 Using the same pipette, aspirate thaw mix and rinse vial.
8 Aspirate thaw mix used for rinsing vial into pipette and add dropwise to thawed product while gently mixing tube.
9 Add 'Thaw mix' slowly to a volume of about 15 ml and then add remaining 'Thaw mix' more rapidly.
10 Remove sample for post-thaw QC if required.

Product rescue from damaged bag

1 Prepare 15-ml sterile screw-capped tube for sterility sample.
2 Prepare freeze bag with appropriate product label.
3 Locate break or leak on bag (usually on fill port of Teflon bag).
4 Remove over wrap and clamp port with haemostat to isolate and prevent further leakage.
5 Place product into large thawing bag.
6 Immerse product into 37°C waterbath, gently massage and remove as soon as product has consistency of slush.
7 Transfer product carefully into labelled freeze bag, rinse broken bag with pre-chilled Plasma-Lyte A and transfer rinse into new bag.
8 Remove sterility sample, transfer into labelled 15-ml conical tube and perform sterility testing.

Calculation

Calculation for preparation of 30 ml of thaw mix: stock concentration of heparin: 1000 U/ml.

Example: 10 U/ml of heparin to supplement 30 ml of Plasma-Lyte A (using formula $C_1V_1 = C_2V_2$)

$$\text{Volume of heparin} = \frac{10 \text{ U/ml} \times 30 \text{ ml}}{1000 \text{ U/ml}} = 0.3 \text{ ml} \tag{A15.1}$$

$$\text{Volume of Plasma-Lyte A} = 30 \text{ ml} - 0.3 \text{ ml} = 29.7 \text{ ml} \tag{A15.2}$$

Reference

Kang EM, Areman EM, David-Ocampo V et al. (2002) Mobilization, collection, and processing of peripheral blood stem cells in individuals with sickle cell trait. Blood 99: 850–855

Appendix 16
Collection of umbilical cord/placental blood (modified from Fraser et al. 1998)

Materials, equipment and reagents

A list of the materials, equipment and reagents is given below:
- collection stand;
- chux pads (three to four);
- collection kit (contains gauze, alcohol, iodine prep. and scrub sticks, cord clamp, 10-cc syringe, 19-G/1.5-inch needle, personal protective garb, collection basin, biohazard disposal bag);
- collection bag label;
- CPD placental/umbilical cord blood container;
- maternal donor file folder;
- rocker/scale;
- heat sealer;
- scissors;
- haemostat;
- biohazard blood specimen bags (two);
- transporter;
- collection strainer (optional).

Procedure

Upon arrival in the labour and delivery suite, confirm the maternal donor's enrolment and review procedure to obtain placenta with obstetric staff. Plan must identify the person who will hand off the placenta to the collector immediately after it is delivered and the spot where the hand-off is to occur. Ideally the collector will assume responsibility for the collection of hospital-required cord blood specimens.

Position the stand over or near utility sink on a counter top in a clean workplace. Check integrity of collection bag and position tubes for serum and cells, labels and biohazard disposal bag in an easily accessible location. Create a clean area for the collection by spreading a drape or chux pad beneath collection stand. Place the rocker/scale in close proximity to the collection stand and position the collection bag on the scale's bed so that the needles will reach the cord when it is on the rocker/scale. Cut a 1-inch-diameter hole in the centre of a 19×23 biohazard bag and slip the bag into the plastic basin (or strainer) lining up the bag's and the basin's holes. Open up the bag and cover the inside walls of the basin. Pull the remaining portion down over the outside walls of the basin and set the covered basin in clean area at base of stand. Place a drape or chux pad over it until time of collection. When delivery is imminent, unwrap personal protective garb packet and don gown and face mask. Open the remaining wrapped portion of the collection tray, triple-glove and proceed to collection area to receive the container with placenta from the designated person.

Collection

Place placenta, fetal side down, into the covered basin. Replace haemostat on the infant end of the cord with a gomco clamp, gently pull the clamped cord through the hole in the covered basin. Place the basin into the collection stand allowing the cord to hang freely beneath the placenta. Remove and discard outermost soiled gloves. Turn on rocker/scale. Hold cord taut (using gomco clamp) and, with free hand, clean cord from placental to fetal end with alcohol-saturated gauze until it is free of maternal blood. Remove and discard second set of (soiled) gloves. Grasp the cord by the clamp at the base and vigorously scrub the 3- to 5-inch segment of cord directly above the clamp with an iodine soap stick for 30 s. Then, starting at the placental end of the scrubbed segment, moving towards the fetal end, wipe cord clean being careful not to touch the cord after it is fully cleansed. Hold the cord tight using gomco clamp, identify area for venepuncture and perform phlebotomy. With the bevel of the needle facing away, enter the vein at approximately a 10° angle and advance needle no more than 1–4 inches past the bottom of the bevel. Holding needle in place with one hand, open tubing clamp and allow blood to flow into the collection bag. When blood flow ceases (the umbilical vein is collapsed and cord appears whitish), place a haemostat on the cord immediately above the inserted needle, remove needle and clamp. Re-evaluate specimen for additional blood and, if necessary, position the placenta by lifting and/or rotating it. Milk the cord by squeezing gently with alcohol-saturated gauze and simultaneously moving the gauze down the cord in the placenta to fetal direction. Do not contaminate the previously cleansed segment of the cord.

Remove the cover from the bag's other needle and make a second puncture into the umbilical cord, selecting a site above the haemostat. Open the white clamp on the tubing below the unused needle, allowing any blood to flow into bag. When the collection is completed and the cord/placenta appears to have no blood remaining, remove the needle from the cord. Clamp tubing on top of the collection bag in the rocker/scale. Maintain rocking while obtaining cord blood samples for testing (hospital-required cord blood samples, haemoglobin genotyping and HLA samples).

Cord blood specimens for hospital and laboratory analysis

Turn the placenta over, exposing the fetal side, locate a large full vein, wipe area with the remaining alcohol-saturated gauze and insert needle attached to syringe. Needle should be inserted bevel side down into the vein in the direction of blood flow or towards the cord.

Completing collection

Remove the collection bag and tubing from the rocker/scale and strip any blood remaining in the tubing down towards the collection bag. Heat seal the tubing with a set of three to four seals below the junction of the tubing leading to the needles. Break tubing at the seal closest to needles and dispose of the needle section of tubing into sharps container. Record weight of the unit onto the 'Collection and Receipt' form and complete labelling.

Reference

Fraser JK, Cairo MS, Wagner EL *et al.* Cord Blood Transplantation Study (COBLT): cord blood bank standard operating procedures. J Hematother 1998; 7: 521–561

Index

Page numbers in *italics* represent figures, those in **bold** represent tables.